Principles and Practice of NURSE ANESTHESIA

third edition

Principles and Practice of NURSE ANESTHESIA

third edition

Wynne R. Waugaman, CRNA, PhD
Associate Professor and Director
Department of Nursing/Program of Nurse Anesthesia
University of Southern California
Los Angeles, California

Scot D. Foster, CRNA, PhD
Professor and Director
Program of Nurse Anesthesia
School of Nursing
Samuel Merritt College
Oakland, California

Benjamin M. Rigor, Sr., MD
Professor and Chairman
Department of Anesthesiology
School of Medicine
University of Louisville
Louisville, Kentucky

APPLETON & LANGE
Stamford, Connecticut

98 99 00 01 02/ 10 9 8 7 6 5 4 3 2 1

Prentice Hall International (UK) Limited, *London*
Prentice Hall of Australia Pty. Limited, *Sydney*
Prentice Hall Canada, Inc., *Toronto*
Prentice Hall Hispanoamericana, S.A., *Mexico*
Prentice Hall of India Private Limited, *New Delhi*
Prentice Hall of Japan, Inc., *Tokyo*
Simon & Schuster Asia Pte. Ltd. *Singapore*
Editora Prentice Hall do Brasil Ltda, *Rio de Janeiro*
Prentice Hall, *Upper Saddle River, New Jersey*

Library of Congress Cataloging-in-Publication Data

Principles and practice of nurse anesthesia / [edited by] Wynne R.
    Waugaman, Scot D. Foster, Benjamin M. Rigor, Sr.—3rd ed.
        p.   cm.
    Includes bibliographical references and index.
    ISBN 0-8385-8118-8 (case : alk. paper)
    1.   Anesthesiology.   2.   Nurse anesthetists.   I.   Waugaman, Wynne R.
II.   Foster, Scot Douglas.   III.   Rigor, Benjamin M.
    [DNLM: 1.   Nurse Anesthetists.   WY 151 P957 1998]
    RD82.P755   1998
    617.9'6—dc21
    DNLM/DLC
    for Library of Congress   97-46159
                                                                CIP

ISBN-0-8385-8118-8

90000

9 780838 1186

Acquisitions Editor: Patricia Casey
Editorial Assistant: Elisabeth Church Garofalo
Production Service: Spectrum Publisher Services
Designer: Mary Skudlarek

PRINTED IN THE UNITED STATES OF AMERICA

This book is dedicated to all clinical CRNA faculty and preceptors,
the heart of every nurse anesthesia program, who give their time, energy, and wisdom
to teach the next generation of nurse anesthetists.

Contents

Part IV. Applied Pharmacology   343

Part V. Perioperative Management, Techniques, and Applications   497

Part VI. Outcomes and Evaluation   765

Contributors

John G. Aker, CRNA, MS
Chief Nurse Anesthetist
Department of Anesthesia
University of Iowa Hospitals & Clinics
Iowa City, Iowa

Steve L. Alves, CRNA, MSNA
Curriculum Coordinator
Staff Nurse Anesthetist
St. Joseph Hospital School of Anesthesia for Nurses
North Providence, Rhode Island

Debra A. Barber, CRNA, MS
Medical Center Anesthesiologist
Department of Anesthesiology
Jewish Hospital
Louisville, Kentucky

Gene A. Blumenreich, Esq.
Notter, McClennan & Fish
Boston, Massachusetts

Leon F. Deisering, CRNA, MSN
Associate Professor and CRNA Program Director
University of New England
Biddeford, Maine

Cecil B. Drain, CRNA, PhD, FAAN
Dean
School of Allied Health Professions
Medical College of Virginia
Virginia Commonwealth University
Richmond, Virginia

Ilze Ducis, PhD
Assistant Professor
School of Natural & Health Sciences
Barry University
Miami Shores, Florida

Margaret Faut-Callahan, CRNA, DNSc, FAAN
Professor and Program Director
Nurse Anesthesia Program
College of Nursing
Rush University
Chicago, Illinois

Linda S. Finander, CRNA, MS
Senior Nurse Anesthetist
VA Medical Center of West Los Angeles
Los Angeles, California

Lee C. Fosburgh, MLIS, MA
Archivist
American Association of Nurse Anesthetists
Park Ridge, Illinois

Scot D. Foster, CRNA, PhD
Professor and Director
Program of Nurse Anesthesia
School of Nursing
Samuel Merritt College
Oakland, California

Regina Y. Fragneto, MD
Assistant Professor and Director, Obstetric Anesthesia
Department of Anesthesiology
Medical College of Virginia
Virginia Commonwealth University
Richmond, Virginia

Donna Jean Funke, CRNA, MS
Instructor
Kaiser Permanente School of Anesthesia
California State University
Long Beach, California

Francis R. Gerbasi, CRNA, PhD
Director
Anesthesiology Department/Program of Nurse Anesthesia
Hurley Medical Center
Flint, Michigan

Michele E. Gold, CRNA, PhD
Assistant Professor of Clinical Nursing
Department of Nursing/Program of Nurse Anesthesia
University of Southern California
Los Angeles, California

Laurie Hanna, CRNA, MS
Staff Nurse Anesthetist
Kaiser Foundation Hospitals
Lecturer, Department of Nursing
University of Southern California at Los Angeles
Los Angeles, California

Louis Heindel, CRNA, ND
Commander and Clinical Coordinator
Navy Nurse Corps Anesthesia Program
San Diego, California

Evan Koch, CRNA, MSN
Archives Liaison
American Association of Nurse Anesthetists
Park Ridge, Illinois

Michael Kremer, CRNA, DNSc
Assistant Professor, Medical Surgical Nursing
Nurse Anesthesia Program
College of Nursing
Rush University
Chicago, Illinois

Leo A. Le Bel, CRNA, ARNP, MEd, JD
Director
Program of Nurse Anesthesia
Southern Connecticut State University/Bridgeport Hospital
Bridgeport, Connecticut

Susanna K. Cook Lindsey, CRNA, MS, ND
Chief Nurse Anesthetist
Trinity Hospital
Chicago, Illinois

Alfred E. Lupien, CRNA, PhD
Coordinator and Assistant Professor
Nursing Anesthesia Program
Medical College of Georgia
Augusta, Georgia

Denise Martin-Sheridan, CRNA, EdD
Associate Professor and Associate Graduate Director
Department of Anesthesiology/Nurse Anesthesiology Program
Albany Medical College
Albany, New York

Cathy Mastropietro, CRNA, PhD
Staff Nurse Anesthetist
Cleveland Clinic Foundation
Cleveland, Ohio

Dolores A. Maxey, CRNA, MS
Assistant Professor of Anesthesiology
Department of Anesthesiology
University of Southern California
Los Angeles, California

W. Gray McCall, CRNA, MHDL
Program Coordinator
Program of Anesthesia
Trover Foundation/Murray State University
Murray, Kentucky

Charles H. Moore, CRNA, PhD
Clinical Associate Professor
Department of Nurse Anesthesia
Medical College of Virginia
Virginia Commonwealth University
Richmond, Virginia

Lucille Y. Osaki, CRNA, MSN, MS
Staff Nurse Anesthetist
Department of Anesthesiology
VA Medical Center of Long Beach
Long Beach, California

J. L. Reeves-Viets, MD
Associate Professor
Department of Anesthesiology
Baylor College of Medicine
Houston, Texas

Benjamin M. Rigor, Sr., MD
Professor and Chairman
Department of Anesthesiology
School of Medicine
University of Louisville
Louisville, Kentucky

Jane A. Scanlan, CRNA, MS
Staff Nurse Anesthetist
VA Medical Center of West Los Angeles
Los Angeles, California

K. Patman Smith, CRNA, MS
Staff Nurse Anesthetist
Department of Anesthesiology
VA Medical Center of Dallas
Dallas, Texas

Elizabeth Sodbinow, CRNA, MSN
Private Practice
Santa Rosa, California

Brent Sommer, CRNA, MPHA
Assistant Professor and Clinical Coordinator
Program of Nurse Anesthesia
School of Nursing
Samuel Merritt College
Oakland, California

Ceil E. Vercellino, CRNA, MS
Private Practice
Lecturer
Department of Nursing/Program of Nurse Anesthesia
Los Angeles, California

Celeste G. Villanueva, CRNA, MS
Assistant Professor and Associate Director
Program of Nurse Anesthesia
School of Nursing
Samuel Merritt College
Oakland, California

Wynne R. Waugaman, CRNA, PhD
Associate Professor and Director
Department of Nursing/Program of Nurse Anesthesia
University of Southern California
Los Angeles, California

Stephen J. Yermal, CRNA, MSN
Staff Nurse Anesthetist
Department of Anesthesiology
Northwestern University Medical School
Chicago, Illinois

Christine S. Zambricki, CRNA, MS
Director of Anesthesia Services/PACU
William Beaumont Hospital
Royal Oak, Michigan
Director, Nurse Anesthesia Track
School of Nursing
Oakland University
Rochester, Michigan

Lieutenant Colonel Gary D. Zarr, CRNA, MS
US Army Nurse Corps (RET), Former Adjunct Assistant
    Professor of Health Science
US Army Program in Anesthesia Nursing, Phase I
Army Medical Department Center and School
Fort Sam Houston, Texas
Private Practice
Corpus Christi Obstetric Anesthesia Associates
Corpus Christi, Tex

▶ CONTRIBUTORS TO SECOND EDITION

A special thank you and recognition go to those who contributed to the second edition of this book.

John Aker, CRNA, MS
Gerald David Allen, MB, FFARCS
Marianne Bankert
Hollis E. Bivens, BA, MD
Norman H. Blass, MD
Nancy Bruton-Maree, CRNA, MS
Eddie Bowie
Lida Inge Swafford Dahm, MD, FAAP
Michael P. Dosch, CRNA, MS
Colonel Cecil B. Drain, CRNA, PhD, FAAN
Margaret Faut-Callahan, CRNA, DNSc, FAAN
Linda S. Finander, CRNA, MS
Scot D. Foster, CRNA, PhD
Francis R. Gerbasi, CRNA, PhD
Michele E. Gold, CRNA, PhD
Dana Lynn Grogan, CRNA, MS
Thomas J. Grogan, MD
Ira P. Gunn, MLN, CRNA, FAAN
Everard R. Hicks, CRNA, MEd
Don R. Hirschman, CRNA, BA
Lesa J. Hirschman, CRNA, MS
Linda M. Huffman, CRNA, BA
Lorraine M. Jordan, CRNA, MS
Kathleen C. Koerbacher, CRNA, MA
Leo A. Le Bel, CRNA, MEd, JD
Carol Boetger Mann, CRNA, MS

Cathy Mastropietro, CRNA, MEd
Charles H. Moore, CRNA, MS, PhD
Jeanette F. Peter, CRNA, MAEd
M. Regina B. Puno, MD
Joseph T. Rando, CRNA, MN
J. L. Reeves-Viets, MD
Leslie Rendell-Baker
Benjamin M. Rigor, MD
Timothy D. Saye, MD
Barbara Shwiry, CRNA, BA
Janet S. Simpson, CRNA, JD
Jonathan H. Skerman, BDSc, MScD, DSc
Bruce Skolnick, MD, PhD
Jeanne F. Slack, CRNA, DNSc
Michael D. Stanton-Hicks, MB, BS, Drmed, FCAnaesth
D. E. Supkis, Jr, MD
Doris J. Tanaka, CRNA, MS
Ceil E. Vercellino, CRNA, MS
Susan A. Ward, DPhil
Wynne R. Waugaman, CRNA, PhD
Marian Waterhouse, CRNA, MEd
Joel M. Weaver, DDS, PhD
Laura Wong, CRNA, MS
Karen L. Zaglaniczny, CRNA, PhD
Christine S. Zambricki, CRNA, MS
Lieutenant Colonel Gary D. Zarr, CRNA, MS

Reviewers

Sharon A. Horsfall, CRNA, MSN
Clinical Coordinator
Case Western Reserve University
Francis Payne Bolton School of Nursing
Cleveland Clinic Foundation
School of Nurse Anesthesia
Cleveland, Ohio

Alfred E. Lupien, CRNA, PhD
Coordinator and Assistant Professor
Nursing Anesthesia Program
Medical College of Georgia
Augusta, Georgia

Kenneth M. Kirsner, CRNA, MS, JD
Staff Nurse Anesthetist
University of Texas
M. D. Anderson Cancer Center
Houston, Texas

Margaret R. Myers, CRNA, MAE
Program Director
Sacred Heart Medical Center
Gonzaga University
Master of Anesthesiology Education Program
Spokane, Washington

Bernadette T. Roche, CRNA, MS
Administrative Director, Anesthesia Services
Program Director
Ravenswood Hospital Medical Center
School of Anesthesia
Chicago, Illinois

Preface

The editors and contributors are pleased to introduce the third edition of *Principles and Practice of Nurse Anesthesia*. The textbook has been modified from the previous editions to emphasize assessment and a return to health and wellness following anesthesia, to stimulate critical thinking, to incorporate recent changes in the health care environment, and to apply theory to clinical practice situations.

This text is designed primarily for the first-year nurse anesthesia student who seeks a comprehensive and germane discussion of the basic principles of anesthesia practice. The editors also feel that the text will serve as a meaningful tool for learners in other disciplines who may be seeking basic information about anesthesia practice. Above all, this third edition continues the tradition begun with the first edition, of serving as an example of how CRNAs can and should assume the responsibilities for the education of future nurse anesthetists through production of our own educational materials.

The format of this book has undergone substantial updating and rewriting with a focus on comprehensiveness and application of theoretical principles to clinical practice. This third edition incorporates a new organizational structure that more closely approximates the anesthesia process and planning for case management to facilitate students' competence in learning the art and science of nurse anesthesia. Major sections of the book now include From Nurse to Nurse Anesthetist, Environment, Assessment Across the Life Span, Applied Pharmacology, Perioperative Management, Techniques and Applications, and Outcomes and Evaluation.

All specialty anesthesia chapters except those on geriatrics, pediatrics, and obstetrics have been eliminated from this edition to focus content for the entry-level graduate student in the first year of the nurse anesthesia program. Key references in the chapters refer the reader to specialized articles or texts that provide more depth in specific content areas. Each chapter follows a similar format and includes study questions, key references, and key concepts summarizing the important points. Most chapters also have a case study to illustrate the content presented. The section on Assessment Across the Life Span is a systems approach to advanced health assessment and includes pertinent anatomy, physiology, and pathophysiology as well as a thorough discussion of all aspects of the perianesthesia process by body system. Systemic assessment and evaluation and perianesthetic management that differs from that for the adult patient is detailed in the chapters on assessment of the geriatric, pediatric and neonatal, and obstetrical patients.

The editors suggest that the student may wish to begin study of the text by reading Surgical Environments for the Twenty-First Century (Chapter 5). This chapter provides an overview of anesthetic practice and the different environments where the student will receive clinical experience. Strategies for Learning in Graduate Education (Chapter 4) will also assist the student in focusing on critical thinking and managing the graduate educational experience in nurse anesthesia. CRNA Role Evolution (Chapter 2) describes the CRNA role and how the student will be socialized into all aspects of the professional role. From there the student is directed to the section on Assessment Across the Life Span to provide a broad base of clinical knowledge. The student should study the remainder of the text, as it complemen___ first year of graduate education in the spe___

In addition to a new structure and ___ case applications are used throughout ___ tate application of theory to practice ___ Chapter 32, which is devoted entire___ of cases presented through tho___ tions that call on the student to ___ problem-solving anesthetic situations. Another new feature of this edition is the computer diskette with reference information and clinical tips inside the back cover. The diskette includes guidelines for preoperative assessment, care plan templates that can be personalized by

each student, laboratory values, commonly used drugs and dosages, and many other clinical references. The student can either print out the information for reference or personalize the data to meet changing clinical situations.

► ACKNOWLEDGMENTS

In developing the third edition of *Principles and Practice of Nurse Anesthesia,* we were fortunate to retain a number of authors who participated in the first and/or second edition and recruited 23 new authors to provide their subject expertise. The identification of subject experts by the editors and the expertise and dedication of these contributors continue to be the heart of this text. Without the interest, support, and participation of these individuals, the third edition would not have come to fruition.

We would like to give special thanks to Elisabeth Church Garofalo, our Nursing Editorial Assistant from Ap-

pleton & Lange, whose stylistic contribution to this edition has improved it immeasurably. Her patience, guidance, encouragement, and professionalism provided the critical ingredients necessary to help us achieve our goals. We wish to also express our heartfelt gratitude to Pat Bensinger for her outstanding assistance in editing many of the chapters. Finally, we wish to thank our families, friends, and colleagues for their patience and support.

Wynne R. Waugaman
Scot D. Foster
Benjamin M. Rigor, Sr.

Foreword

While there is evidence that nurses were involved in administering anesthesia dating back to the American Civil War and the Franco-Prussian War in Europe, this clinical nursing specialty became formalized during the first two decades of the twentieth century. The history of this specialty demonstrates the dedication of nurse anesthetists to the advancement of the art and science of anesthesia through their involvement in pioneering new anesthetic techniques and working with physicians and engineers to develop new and better equipment. One of the major purposes for these nursing pioneers to come together and found the American Association of Nurse Anesthetists in 1931 was to share their knowledge and develop standards for high quality education for nurses entering this specialty. Their commitment and dedication to this purpose has served as an inspiration throughout the years to succeeding generations of nurse anesthetists.

This book represents no less of a milestone in the history of nurse anesthesia than did many of the individual accomplishments of persons such as Alice Magaw, Agatha Hodgins, Helen Lamb, Hilda Salomon, Olive Berger, and others too numerous to mention. It is the first, multiauthored, comprehensive anesthesia textbook written principally by CRNAs for nurse anesthesia students and their CRNA colleagues. These CRNA authors have been joined by some basic scientists and physicians who have been directly involved in nurse anesthesia education and/or their practice. The contributors to this book have distilled the essence of the basic sciences and meshed them with concepts from the clinical and behavioral sciences in a manner which allows the learner to unify diverse knowledge components into a specific anesthesia care plan to meet the needs of an individual patient. As such, this book primarily deals with anesthesia practice, its concepts and its reality. In addition, the book addresses the environment within which anesthesia is practiced and the necessary management styles, programs, and resources to assess and assure the quality of anesthesia services.

While anesthesia practice is a dynamic, constantly changing field, this textbook provides those basic fundamentals that serve as a sound foundation for future growth and development in this field. It also may serve as a reference book for nurses in other specialties who care for the anesthetized patient. And finally, it will also be of interest to those nurses who have yet to decide upon a nursing specialty, allowing them to become more knowledgeable about this field, its educational requirements, and the clinical demands placed upon CRNAs.

The authors have kept faith with nurse anesthetist pioneers in accepting responsibility for putting something back into the specialty, rather than merely taking from those who were our predecessors. This book should serve as an incentive for other CRNA authors to undertake the writing of other needed texts or reference books from which we all can benefit.

John F. Garde, CRNA, MS

From Nurse to Nurse Anesthetist

Justifiably Proud: A Brief History of Nurse Anesthetists

Evan Koch and Lee C. Fosburgh

Without a knowledge of our professional history, we are deprived of the justifiable pride we can take in the outstanding contributions of past nurse anesthetists: the remarkable quality of the anesthesia services they provided under primitive conditions; significant contributions to the development of the art, science and early technology of anesthesia and their capability for meeting almost insurmountable challenges in the practice environment. History can teach us what it takes of individuals and of the collective body to make the system work for Certified Registered Nurse Anesthetists (CRNAs) even when the opposition is formidable and, most notably, to make needed changes. And, it affords us examples to emulate and infuses us with confidence, for we, too, with the same commitment to the profession and to the quality of our services, have no reason to fear the future or its challenges. (Gunn, 1990, p. 20)

Nurse anesthesia history, as distinct from anesthesia history in general, exists in order to draw attention to the accomplishments of nurse anesthetists. Unfortunately, many of the major published works recounting the history of anesthesiology have either minimized or ignored completely the contributions of CRNAs. That unfortunate situation, however, has not prevented the story from being recorded. Virginia S. Thatcher (1953) wrote *History of Anesthesia with Emphasis on the Nurse Specialist,* shortly after (and because) nurses were excluded

from the centennial celebration of the discovery of modern anesthesia in 1946. In 1989, Marianne Bankert extended the public's understanding about nurse anesthetists in *Watchful Care: A History of America's Nurse Anesthetists*. Both are considered seminal works in the historical literature of the discipline.

This chapter chronicles only the essentials of nurse anesthesia history, relying heavily on the work of Thatcher and Bankert to describe the key individuals and institutions that emerged from and guided the profession in its early years. Unfortunately, only a handful of unpublished research papers, derived largely from interviews and archival data that were dutifully prepared by a few nurse anesthesia students in graduate schools throughout the United States, are still available for historical reference. When more has been written, we may then compile a comprehensive history of anesthesia, one that encompasses a philosophy and anthropology of this great discipline.

▶ ANESTHESIA PRIOR TO 1846

The journey begins with the assumptions that pain and efforts to control pain have been around forever. Examples of traditional efforts to control pain included applying pressure to or elevating an injured limb, invoking voodoo, hypnotism, or acupuncture. Alkaloids of opium, coca, and mandragora were also employed. A universal characteristic of all these methods, and particularly those that relied on magic, was cultural specificity. For people who believed in them, these methods of pain control worked (Knight, 1983, p. 11). What the world lacked before 1846 was a reliable, reversible, and reproducible way to simultaneously produce analgesia and amnesia. A sequence of scientific and experimental revelations between 1800 and 1846 would alter our view of this problem forever.

In the early 19th century, the physical sciences were more advanced than the life sciences. Although Isaac Newton's discoveries had made possible an understanding of the motion of the planets; asepsis, evolution, and cell theory were not yet conceived. Consequently, it was from the physical science of pneumatics that the discipline of anesthesiology was born. Eighteenth-century European scientists led the way. Joseph Black (1728–1799) discovered that when elements were heated, they emitted a large amount of air. Known today as carbon dioxide, he named his discovery "fixed air" and identified it with the "gas sylvestre" that Jean Baptiste van Helmont (1577–1691) had produced earlier from burning charcoal, fermenting beer, and observing the action of vinegar on shells. Robert Boyle (1627–1691) first produced hydrogen from iron filings treated with mineral acid, and Henry Cavendish (1731–1810) compared "fixed air," or carbon dioxide, and "inflammable air," or hydrogen, establishing the existence of two gases different from air (Thatcher, 1953). Karl Wilhelm Scheele (1742–1786) of Sweden probably discovered oxygen independently in 1771 and published his findings in his *Chemical Essay on Air and Fire.* In 1771, Joseph Priestley (1733–1804), a nonconformist minister in England, also discovered oxygen, and 1 year later he produced nitrous oxide from metals heated with nitric acid. These men inhaled the substances they were procuring, so it is not surprising that in 1798, Humphry Davy (1778–1829) discovered the exhilarating effect of breathing nitrous oxide.

In a logical next step, Davy realized that inhalation of nitrous oxide could produce stupefaction. In 1799, Davy introduced nitrous oxide at Beddoes' Pneumatic Institute in Clifton, Bristol. Both Davy and Thomas Beddoes (1760–1808) encouraged visitors to the institute, notably the poets Robert Southey and Samuel Taylor Coleridge, to breath nitrous oxide and relate how it affected them. It later became fashionable for people to indulge in nitrous oxide or "laughing gas" parties. Davy went on to write, in the most famous near miss of anesthesia history, that "as nitrous oxide in its extensive operation appears capable of destroying physical pain, it may probably be used during surgical operations in which no great effusion of blood takes place" (Davy, 1800, p. 533). Why Davy never followed through on his own supposition is un-

known. The discovery of modern anesthesia was still more than 40 years away.

From stupefaction, inhaling gases was taken one step closer to anesthesia by the English surgeon, Henry Hill Hickman (1800–1830). In 1824, Hickman successfully performed small operations on animals made unconscious by rebreathing carbon dioxide and thus discovered for himself how anesthesia might work. However, Hickman was rebuffed by the Royal Society when he attempted to share his work. Ironically, the Royal Society at the time was under the direction of Humphrey Davy, whose denial of any further investigation of carbon dioxide was inexplicable, but fortunate, because carbon dioxide was not the right agent. Nevertheless, it seemed as though European scientists willfully refused to discover anesthesia.

The final steps in the process took place in America, where society was less structured and, therefore, perhaps more receptive to new ideas. Inhaling ether was a preferred form of recreation among medical students at the time. This experience lead the Georgia physician Crawford Williamson Long (1815–1878) to the notion that ether might render surgery painless. On March 30, 1842, in Jefferson, Georgia, Long successfully removed a small tumor from the neck of James Venable under the influence of ether. Venable felt neither the pain nor Long's surgical knife, making Long the first man to use ether for the purpose of producing surgical anesthesia. Unfortunately for him and for every other surgical patient between 1842 and 1846, Long decided not to publish his finding. He claimed that his rural practice, deep in the Antebellum South, kept him too busy and too isolated to verify or publicize his discovery (Hammonds & Steinhaus, 1993). Whatever the cause, Long's delay cost him the recognition he most certainly would have otherwise received. In the December 1849 issue of the *Southern Medical and Surgical Journal,* Long's work finally appeared, three years after ether anesthesia had already been introduced to the world by another investigator.

In the interim, the idea of eliminating pain by inhalation occurred in December, 1844, to a New England dentist named Horace Wells (1815–1848). Wells attended a staged public demonstration on the effects of nitrous oxide in Hartford, Connecticut, where a man, under the influence of nitrous oxide, fell from the stage and cut his leg. He reported no recollection of pain or even of the event taking place. Seeing this, Wells wondered if a man could have a tooth extracted without pain while under nitrous oxide. In a subsequent experiment on himself, Wells underwent a pain-free dental extraction. Realizing the importance of his discovery, Wells exclaimed, "It is the greatest discovery ever made! I didn't feel it so much as the prick of a pin" (Keys, 1978, p. 24). Wells then performed a series of successful painless tooth extractions on patients under nitrous oxide. Taking his discovery to Boston where he hoped to bring it to the attention of the surgeons at Massachusetts General Hospital, Wells gained permission from John Collins Warren (1778–1856), Chief of Surgical Service, to demonstrate nitrous oxide before his class in surgery. This time, the patient screamed because the anesthesia was not complete. Medical students called the discovery a hoax, and Wells left Boston in total disgrace. If Wells had done the procedure correctly, nitrous oxide probably would have been adopted for surgical anesthesia as early as 1844. Although the demonstration ended in failure, Wells was credited with having been the first to use nitrous oxide as an anesthetic (Small, 1994).

Another New England dentist, William T.G. Morton (1819–1868), who learned dentistry from Wells and for a time shared his practice, grew interested in ether as an anesthetic for monetary reasons. Pain-free dentistry would induce his patients to return for follow-up visits. Morton, who had not had the benefit of higher education, went to Charles Jackson, a well-known physician and geologist in Boston, for tutoring. Morton plied Jackson for advice about ether, learning from him that ether applied to the gums would provide analgesia for dental work. Jackson would later claim that the idea of using ether as an inhaled anesthetic was his own.

In the summer of 1846, Morton secretly experimented with ether vapor on himself in his office, and on small animals at his estate in West Needham. On September 30, 1846, Morton painlessly removed the tooth of Eben Frost, a Boston merchant. Henry Jacob Bigelow (1818–1890), a surgeon at Massachusetts General Hospital, observed the effects of ether applied by Morton. Based on Bigelow's advice, John Collins Warren invited Morton to demonstrate ether anesthesia in the surgical amphitheater of the Bulfinch Building at Massachusetts General Hospital. On October 16, 1846, Morton gave ether to Edward Gilbert Abbot during a 10-minute operation performed by Warren. Abbot felt no pain, making Morton's procedure a success. Warren, who had witnessed more than one failed attempt to produce anesthesia by inhalation, told the audience gathered in the amphitheater: "Gentlemen, *this* is no humbug" (Keys, 1978, p. 11). Oliver Wendell Holmes named Morton's procedure "anesthesia." Morton's success marked the beginning of modern anesthesia and is the event celebrated annually.

No sooner had Morton's discovery been made public than desire for the credit as discoverer grew in the minds of Crawford Long, Horace Wells, and Charles Jackson. Each man recognized its phenomenal importance, as well as the fame and wealth that would come to the discoverer. Each man's claim had some justification, and each had his own group of supporters. The dispute quickly escalated into a battle, complete with character assassination, lies, and endless recrimination, waged before the press, the government, and medical societies of the United States, Britain, and France. The disagreements became so bitter that Horace Wells committed suicide. William Morton died in poverty of apoplectic seizures, and Charles Jackson spent the last 12 years of his life in an insane asylum. To this day, followers of each of these men continue to assert credit to their respective "discoverer."

▶ NINETEENTH-CENTURY DEVELOPMENTS

The discovery of anesthesia came at a time when scientific thought was first being applied to the natural world and man could reasonably contemplate pain control (Caton, 1985). The prevailing belief was that pain was providential and surgery was a therapy of last resort. Operations had been limited to superficial procedures and quick surgeons who could finish before the onset of cardiovascular shock. With anesthesia, the scope and developmental growth of surgical technique expanded rapidly. Surgeons were eager to develop new operations once anesthesia made them possible.

It was fortunate that ether anesthesia was discovered before chloroform because ether was safe. Ether and chloroform administered through inhalation remained the only anesthetics in common use until nitrous oxide was reintroduced as a dental anesthetic in the early 1860s. Ether was the more important agent because it was easy to formulate, transport, and administer. Ether was potent and volatile, and could be administered in small doses in room air without causing hypoxia. Unlike other inhaled anesthetics, ether did not cause respiratory or cardiovascular depression (Greene, 1971). Consequently, patients were able to tolerate the often-times rough and inattentive ministrations of the early anesthetists.

At first, there was no recognition of the need for care when administering anesthesia. Ether was usually administered by a disinterested medical student or by some other untrained individual. Induction was compared to asphyxiation, and patients struggled so much they had to be held down. Morbidity and mortality were encountered as a result of poor anesthetic technique. It became clear that in order for surgery to advance there would have to be dedicated professional anesthetists. But doctors were not interested in making anesthesia a full-time practice because anesthesia was totally subordinate to surgery and had a much lower professional status and income potential. For these reasons surgeons drafted nurses into anesthetic practice.

▶ THE FIRST NURSE ANESTHETISTS

Nurses were the obvious and ideal candidates to be anesthetists. Surgeons needed anesthetists who would attend solely to the care of patients under anesthesia and who would present no competitive obstacle to an eager surgeon. This important point was made by, among others, Virginia S. Thatcher. Surgeons turned to nurses because "they wanted a person who would: (1) be satisfied with the subordinate role that the work required; (2) make anesthesia their one absorbing interest; (3) not look on the situation of anesthetist as one that put them in a position to watch and learn from the surgeon's technique; (4) accept relatively low pay; and (5) have natural aptitude and intelligence to develop a high level of skill in providing the smooth anesthesia and relaxation that the surgeon demanded" (Thatcher, 1953, p. 53). As we shall see, nurses excelled in their new role.

It is not known when the first nurse gave anesthesia, but it is likely to have been earlier than we assume. Between 1855 and 1865, nursing changed from a church-run occupation involving menial work and custodial care into a secularized profession based on attendance, cleanliness, and nourishment. Nursing, like teaching, eventually became an accepted path for a bourgeois woman to pursue. History does record a Mrs. John Harris of Baltimore taking chloroform to the battle of Gettysburg, although there is no evidence that she, other women or nurses, actually administered anesthetics during the Civil War (Thatcher, 1953, p. 33). As far as we know, Catholic Church records document the earliest nurse anesthetists, dating to 1877.

The specialty of nurse anesthesia emerged from the midwest in Catholic hospitals that had sprung up along the developing railroad lines. The earliest recorded nurse anesthetist was Sister Mary Bernard, who administered anesthesia at St. Vincent's Hospital in Erie, Pennsylvania in 1877. Sister Secundina Mindrup (1868–1951) a Hospital Sister of the Third Order of St. Francis, was recruited by surgeons in the late 1870s to administer anesthetics. In 1880, the administration of ether and chloroform was taught to Sister Aldoza Eltrich at St. John's Hospital in Springfield, Illinois. By 1889, sisters in Michgan, Iowa, and Minnesota had become nurse anesthetists. Before the end of the century, nurse anesthesia had been extended to both coasts and Hawaii (Thatcher, 1953).

St. Mary's Hospital of Rochester, Minnesota, was established by the Sisters of St. Francis in 1889, and was renamed the Mayo Clinic. The hospital soon became a gathering place for people interested in learning techniques from its surgeons and nurse anesthetists. The

anesthesia was administered at first by sisters Edith (1871–1943) and Dinah Graham (1860–1947), who graduated from the School of Nursing at the Women's Hospital in Chicago, Illinois. "In the first place . . . they had no interns. And when the interns came, the brothers [William and Charles Mayo] decided that a nurse was better suited to the task [of delivering anesthesia] because she was more likely to keep her mind strictly on it" (Clapesattle, 1941, p. 256). Dinah's tenure as a nurse anesthetist was brief; Edith, however, continued giving anesthesia until her marriage to Charles Mayo in 1893.

In 1893, the Grahams were succeeded by the most famous nurse anesthetist of the nineteenth century, Alice Magaw (1860–1928) (Fig. 1-1). Magaw, a graduate of Women's Hospital in Chicago, was said to have "won more widespread notice than that of any other member of the Rochester group apart from the brothers" (Clapesattle, 1941, p. 255). At the time, anesthetic inductions were still accomplished by saturating a towel with ether

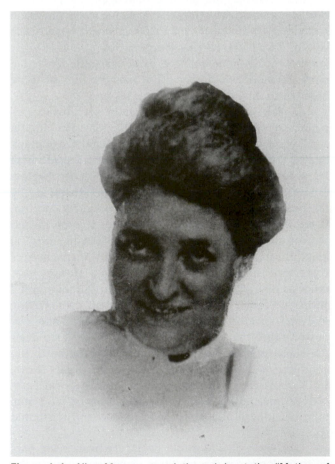

Figure 1–1. Alice Magaw earned the sobriquet the "Mother of Anesthesia" for perfecting the open drop method of ether administration in the nineteenth century. Her published records of superior anesthesia practice became instrumental in the 1930s in a court case establishing the legality of nurse anesthesia practice. (*Photo: AANA Archives.*)

or chloroform and nearly suffocating patients, causing an immense struggle. A visiting German surgeon introduced Magaw to the open drop technique. Dropping ether was merely a means of gradually introducing the irritating ether vapor to the sensitive respiratory tract and titrating a surgical level of anesthesia. Magaw perfected a smooth anesthetic induction by combining the gradual dripping of ether and chloroform with her nursing skills. She earned international respect and the sobriquet "the mother of anesthesia" for her mastery of this technique (Clapesattle, 1941). In a talk given to the Missouri State Medical Society in 1906, Magaw described her approach:

> Suggestion is a great aid in producing a comfortable narcosis. The anesthetist must be able to inspire confidence in the patient, and a great deal depends on the manner of approach. One must be quick to notice the temperament, and decide which mode of suggestion will be the most effective in the particular case: the abrupt, crude, and very firm, or the reasonable, sensible, and natural. The latter mode is far the best in the majority of cases. The subconscious or secondary self is particularly susceptible to suggestive influence; therefore, during the administration, the anaesthetist should make those suggestions that will be most pleasing to this particular subject. Patients should be prepared for each stage of the anaesthesia with an explanation of just how the anaesthetic is expected to affect him; 'talk him to sleep,' with the addition of as little ether as possible. We have one rule; patients are not allowed to talk, as by talking or counting patients are more apt to become noisy and boisterous. Never bid a patient to 'breath deep,' for in so doing a feeling of suffocation is sure to follow, and the patient is also apt to struggle. (Pougiales, 1970, p. 237)

Recognizing that her accomplishments would have value in the education of other anesthetists, Magaw published articles on the practice of anesthesia. Her first paper, "Observations on 1092 cases of anesthesia from January 1, 1899, to January 1, 1900," was published in the *St. Paul Medical Journal.* In December 1906, she published "A review of over 14,000 surgical anesthetics" in *Surgery, Gynecology, and Obstetrics.* These articles reported the use of the open drop method of administering anesthesia without a fatality. What Magaw did not realize was that her excellent record, as documented by her articles, would earn her a measure of immortality. In the 1930s her publications were cited as evidence in a California civil suit that supported the contention that when administering anesthetics nurses do not illegally practice medicine.

Another nurse anesthetist of importance from the Mayo Clinic was Florence Henderson (Fig. 1–2), who from 1903 until 1917 was Dr. Charles Mayo's anesthetist. An innate educator, Henderson had been superintendent

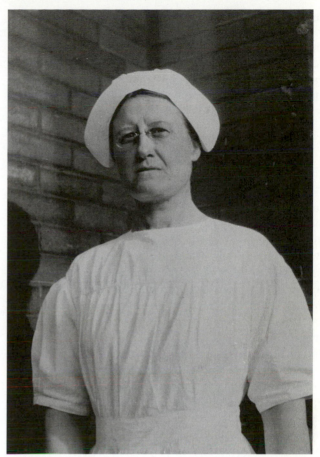

Figure 1–2. Florence Henderson worked with Alice Magaw at the Mayo Clinic, and was among the first to call publicly for formalized anesthesia training for nurses. *(Photo: AANA Archives.)*

at Bishop Clarkson Memorial Hospital School of Nursing in Omaha after graduating there in 1900. In the customary manner of the time, Henderson trained visiting doctors and nurses in anesthesia at the Mayo Clinic. She published her first article on the practice of anesthesia in the September 1909 issue of the *American Journal of Nursing.* Her article discussed the drawbacks of administration of anesthetics by interns, the reasons surgeons were turning to nurse anesthetists, and some factors the nurse anesthetist must bear in mind while administering anesthesia (Harris & Hunziker-Dean, 1997).

Henderson's chief interest was improving anesthesia education. At the time, the training of anesthetists was haphazard, and fell into one of three categories: (1) on the job training of nurses; (2) observation and supervision of visiting clinicians as a courtesy; or (3) through demonstrations given by itinerant manufacturer's representatives to buyers. Anesthesia training was not a part of medical or nursing school curricula. A paper presented by Henderson at the Nurse's Associated Alumni of the United States, also in 1909, lamented the lack of formal training for nurses in anesthesia, and provoked from the audience a call for anesthesia education in schools of nursing. Eventually, Henderson's call was echoed by officers of the American Hospital Association, and by 1912 the first organized programs of anesthesia education in the United States came into being.

► EARLY NURSE ANESTHESIA EDUCATION PROGRAMS

The first formal training programs in anesthesia were begun by nurses. They varied considerably and no doubt the classes and curricula reflected the work and personality of the pioneering nurse anesthetist–educator in charge. Some programs were established solely to meet an immediate local need for anesthetists, but most were begun in response to the growing sentiment that anesthesia training should be formalized. In 1909 nurses at the Massachusetts General Hospital anesthesia training program received some didactic instruction along with practical instruction. At the University of Pennsylvania Hospital, Anna Marie S. Rose, CRNA, was appointed anesthetist in 1909 to the General Surgical Clinic where she also taught anesthesia to both medical students and nurses. A program was begun at St. Vincent's Hospital in Portland, Oregon, in 1909. The six-week course included instruction in anatomy and physiology of the respiratory system, and pharmacology and techniques of administration of the commonly used anesthetic drugs. In 1913, students at the New York Post Graduate Hospital attended heart clinics and lectures by physicians. Two textbooks were used: *Anesthetics and Their Administration* (1901), by Fredrick W. Hewett, and *Anesthetics: Their Uses and Administration* (1907), by Dudley W. Buxton. Experimental work, such as passing of laryngeal tubes, was practiced on cadavers. By graduation, each student had administered ether anesthesia 400 times.

The University Hospitals of Cleveland, Lakeside, was a vitally important center of activity for early nurse anesthetists. The renowned surgeon at Lakeside, George Washington Crile (1864-1943), asked Agatha Cobourg Hodgins, CRNA (1877-1945), to become his anesthetist in 1908. In 1909, Hodgins and Crile developed anoci-association, an anesthetic technique combining nerve blocks with nitrous oxide, to attenuate the cardiovascular shock associated with ether and chloroform. With great success, Hodgins administered nitrous oxide–oxygen anesthesia in a series of 575 operations. Visiting surgeons were so impressed by this method of anesthesia that they sent nurses from their own clinics to be trained by Hodgins. By 1911, Hodgins inaugurated a school of anesthesia at Lakeside that would become as famous for its anesthetic techniques as for its subsequent closure amid much political controversy.

Other nurse anesthesia educators, most trained at the Mayo Clinic, organized programs within academic medical centers along the Eastern Seaboard. Margaret Boise, CRNA (1883-?), at Johns Hopkins Hospital in Baltimore, Maryland, opened a 6-month course where nurses received a certificate at the completion of the program. Boise, in collaboration with surgeon Hugh H. Young, invented a gas–ether machine later known as the Boise–Young apparatus. In 1922, Yale Medical School appointed Alice Hunt, CRNA, to the position of instructor of anesthesia with university rank, where she taught anesthesia to nurses and medical students for 26-years. Hunt authored a textbook entitled *Anesthesia: Principles and Practice* in 1948. Grady Memorial Hospital in Atlanta, Georgia, organized the first school for nurse anesthetists in the southeastern United States. The students were taught how to administer chloroform, ether, nitrous oxide, and oxygen anesthesia. Theoretical instruction consisted of 10 hours of lectures in pharmacology.

By the early twentieth century, nurse anesthesia educators were at the vanguard of nursing and anesthesia practice. They had spread from the Mayo Clinic and the midwest because of their reputations and practice records as superior clinical anesthetists. They were the first to recognize the need to formalize anesthesia training, and convinced their colleagues in surgery and administration to let them undertake this important task. By being the first to establish formal anesthesia training programs, nurse anesthetists moved anesthesia into the world of academe and became the founding pioneers of advanced practice in nursing. As the word of their success spread, it would not take long for physicians to surmise a potentially competitive role as anesthetists in a burgeoning field.

► ANTI-NURSE ANESTHETIST ACTIVITIES

The movement by physician anesthetists to abolish nurse anesthesia began in the twentieth century when competition for work grew more intense (the term *anesthesiologist* was coined by physician anesthetists in the 1930s to differentiate themselves from nurse anesthetists). Once the legality of nurse anesthesia practice had been established in law, physician anesthetists pursued their goal in other ways. Consequently, the courts, state legislatures, and state regulatory bureaucracies all became involved in anti-nurse anesthetist activities in subsequent years.

The first public conflict between nurse and physician anesthetists occurred in 1917 when the well known physician anesthetist, Frank McMechan, moved to close the Lakeside School for nurse anesthetists. Lakeside had sponsored a six-month course open to qualified graduate nurses, physicians, and dentists. Under Agatha Hodgin's leadership, Lakeside was poised to expand when it suddenly faced a resolution passed by the Ohio State Medical Board, that McMechan had sponsored, proclaiming that anesthesia was strictly the practice of medicine. The resolution withheld recognition of Lakeside's nursing graduates until and unless it ceased to train nurses to be anesthetists. At a Medical Board hearing later that same year, Dr. Crile and two other surgeons defended the training of nurses as anesthetists, and prevailed upon the Board to reverse itself. The Lakeside School reopened, increased its class size, and incorporated new didactic instruction, with Hodgins delivering the lectures.

In the clash between the Ohio Medical Board and the Lakeside School, there were themes that would recur in subsequent attempts to eliminate nurse anesthetists. First was the central question: are nurses who deliver anesthesia engaging in the practice of medicine without a license? During the next two decades, physician anesthetists would pose this question to the courts of Kentucky in *Frank v. South* (1917) and California in *Chalmers-Francis v. Nelson* (1936). Second, subsequent to the Ohio conflict, an allegiance formed between surgeons, hospital administrators, and nurse anesthetists that would persist throughout the court cases, doing much to support the nursing cause.

Both *Frank v. South* and *Chalmers-Francis v. Nelson* were decided in favor of nurse anesthetists. Important points cited by the courts in *Frank v. South* were: (1) medical practice laws are designed to protect consumers, and not to benefit the members of one profession at the expense of members of another profession; (2) there can be overlap between the scopes of practice of different professions; and (3) nurses have the right to administer anesthetic medications when directed to do so by a physician, and to use independent judgement in the process. The verdicts rested on the fact that nurses had a documented history of giving safe and effective anesthesia, and that nurse anesthesia had become the customary practice in many communities. The evidence included Alice Magaw's 35-year-old publication. In addition, the court asserted that the knowledge of administering anesthetics was not exclusively within the province of medicine; that when a nurse administered anesthesia, she was practicing nursing (Hanchett, 1995, p. 88).

The Kentucky and California successes not withstanding, the challenge to nurse anesthesia has persisted over the decades. Its focus would shift away from the legality of practice to other legislative, regulatory, and economic areas. To this day however, the American Society of Anesthesiologists insists that anesthesia is the practice of medicine. Antitrust violations, governmental and nongovernmental regulation of health care facilities, control over accreditation of education programs, and clinical privileging are but a few examples of other areas where nurse anesthetist's autonomy has been challenged.

Two positive outcomes of these activities should be noted. Significantly, most nurse anesthetists and anesthesiologists continue to work well together, considering the fact that much of what they each do connotes direct competition between two very distinct provider groups. In fact, today nearly 80% of all nurses and physicians work within some definition of an anesthesia care team where both the nurse and physician provide substantial efforts toward the care of patients. Second, these threats helped galvanize CRNAs as a professional group, motivating them to establish a formidable national organization, the American Association of Nurse Anesthetists, which now represents over ninety percent of America's nurse anesthetists.

▶ ORGANIZING NURSE ANESTHETISTS

Threats to the well-being of CRNAs caused groups of nurse anesthetists to join forces in the late 1920s. The most well-known example occurred in 1928 in California where Adeline Curtis, a feisty and articulate nurse anesthetist in Anaheim, was led to believe by the California Board of Medical Examiners that State law prohibited her from giving anesthesia. Through an attorney, Curtis obtained an opinion from the California Attorney General dispelling this information. Consequently, Curtis resumed practicing anesthesia, and set out to inform other nurse anesthetists of her experiences and urge them to form a state professional organization that would protect their collective interests. For many months, Curtis visited hospitals and clinics and lectured throughout the state. As a result of her efforts, the first meeting of the California Association of Nurse Anesthetists was held in Los Angeles in 1930. A charter was signed, and Sophie Gran Winton was elected president. A national organization of nurse anesthetists (National Association of Nurse Anesthetists) followed in 1931. Before 1940, there would be nurse anesthesia associations in 23 states, and by 1950, professional associations would exist in 33 states.

The National Association of Nurse Anesthetists grew out of the Lakeside School Alumni Association in Cleveland, and strongly reflected the foresight, work, and priorities of its founder, Agatha Hodgins. In 1930, Hodgins presented a paper suggesting that nurse anesthetists organize into a "coherent and acting body" at the biennial convention of the American Nurses Association (ANA). However, philosophical differences with mainstream nursing, as represented by the ANA, eventually prompted nurse anesthetists to remain independent of that group. Through Hodgins' efforts, and with considerable support from surgeons and hospital administrators, the dream of a national professional organization for nurse anes-

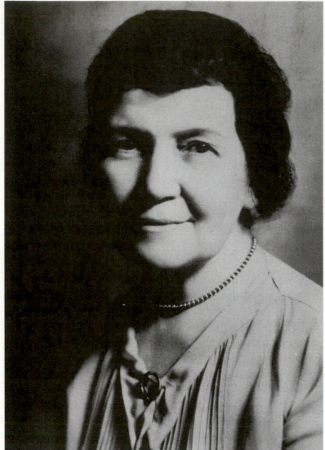

Figure 1–3. Agatha Hodgins, who between 1931 and 1933 organized the National Association of Nurse Anesthetists. Hodgins became the Association's first President. *(Photo: AANA Archives.)*

thetists became reality on June 17, 1931 (Fig. 1–3). A group of 48 anesthetists, representing 12 states, met in a classroom in the Anesthesia Department of University Hospitals of Cleveland, Lakeside, and formed the National Association of Nurse Anesthetists (NANA). The date is now commemorated by a plaque, placed in 1995 at the University Hospital of Cleveland, by the (renamed in 1939) American Association of Nurse Anesthetists (AANA).

The mission of the national association was to improve anesthesia education and advance the clinical discipline. Founders intended to accomplish the mission by placing better qualified people in the field, keeping practitioners abreast of new, more modern developments, and providing protection and recognition for nurse anesthetists as a group of professional providers. Through the 1930s, the new association initiated a campaign to standardize education, accredit schools of anesthesia, and implement a certification examination for entry into practice. These goals would take years to reach fruition, largely due to World War II, which necessarily slowed further efforts at professionalization. In fact, the military's

decision to rely heavily on nurse anesthetists would ultimately help the AANA to carry out its plans to improve the profession.

▶ NURSE ANESTHETISTS IN THE ARMED FORCES

Military utilization of nurses as anesthetists on a large scale began in World War I, and has continued since. Although the United States did not enter World War I until 1917, medical units were formed in the United States and sent overseas at the outbreak of war in Europe. The first unit was organized by the University Hospitals of Cleveland, Lakeside. On December 13, 1914, Agatha Hodgins, the chief anesthetist who would later spearhead the drive to establish NANA, and George Crile as surgeon-in-chief, traveled to France with three other surgeons and a number of nurses and assistants (Fig. 1–4). Hodgins and Crile introduced anoci-association into wartime surgery in England and France. Crile returned to the United States within 2 months and presented a plan to the Surgeon General to create hospital units for service abroad composed of doctors, nurses, and anesthetists. Hodgins stayed in France after Crile's departure to educate others, notably Berkeley George Moynihan's anesthetist, and two groups of English and French nurses in nitrous oxide–oxygen anesthesia (Bankert, 1989).

Sophie Gran Winton (1887-1989) was one of the most distinguished nurse anesthetists to serve in World War I (Fig. 1–5). She was a graduate of Swedish Hospital of Minneapolis, Minnesota, with 5 years of experience and a record of more than 10 000 cases without a fatality. Winton joined the Army Nurse Corps (through the Red Cross) because she felt that it was the patriotic thing to do. Winton and nine other nurses from Minneapolis Hospital were assigned to Mobile Hospital No. 1 in Chateau-Thierry, France with physician anesthetist James T. Gwathmey (1863–1944). All nurses in Winton's unit were awarded the Croix de Guerre. Winton was also awarded six overseas bars as well as honors from the Overseas Nurses Association, the American Legion, and the Veterans of Foreign Wars.

Anne Penland was the first nurse anesthetist on the British front. Penland was with the New York Presbyterian Hospital Unit. Her anesthetics were so well performed that the British, who never permitted nurses to give anesthetics during peacetime, elected to train nurse anesthetists for wartime service.

In World War II, as with World War I, medical preparations were already underway before U.S. involvement and again they had major impact on the profession of nurse anesthesia. The number of schools of anesthesia and applicants rose quickly to fill an expanded civilian and military need. By September 1940, nurse anesthetists

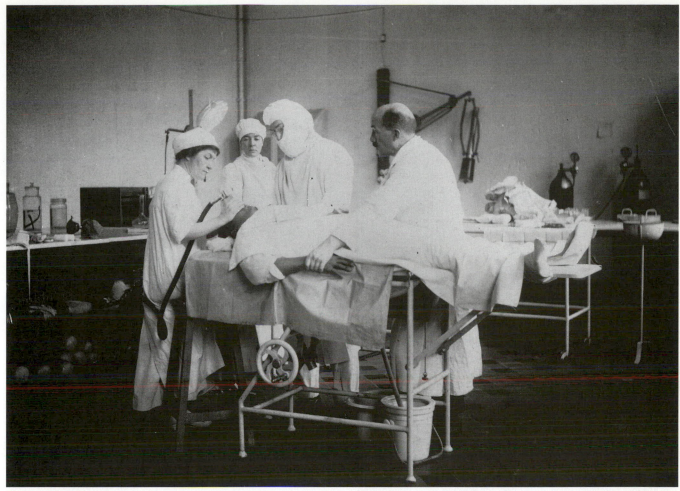

Figure 1–4. Agatha Hodgins administering anesthesia for surgeon George Washington Crile (far right) in France during World War I. *(Photo: AANA Archives.)*

were being recruited into the Army with special incentives. By August 1941, AANA headquarters was inundated with letters from members requesting information about the status of nurse anesthetists in the U.S. Defense Program. These letters expressed a strong desire among members to volunteer their services coupled with concerns that they be allowed to practice as anesthetists, rather than regular duty nurses. Advertisements addressing shortages appeared in the November 1941 issue of *The Bulletin of the American Association of Nurse Anesthetists.* Miriam Shupp, CRNA published in August 1941, the following details:

United States Army, Major Julia O. Flikke, Superintendent Army Nurse Corps: "Nurse anesthetists are appointed to the Army Nurse Corps in the grade of nurse, with the relative rank of 2nd Lieutenant. They are subject to all the regulations governing regular army nurses. Since there is a need for anesthetists in the Nurse Corps at present, they are usually assigned to that duty. However, in some of the smaller Army hospitals, where more than one Nurse Anesthetist is

on duty, they may be assigned to duties other than those of anesthetist." The rate of pay is $70.00 per month, with maintenance.

United States Navy Rear Admiral Ross T. McIntire, Surgeon General, USN: "Under existing Navy Regulations there is no provision whereby nurses may be appointed in the Nurse Corps of the Navy or Naval Reserve for duty limited to the administration of anesthetics. However, if a member of the Navy Nurse Corps is qualified in the administration of anesthetics, she may be assigned to that duty by the Commanding Officer for the Naval Hospital or Station to which she is attached.

"Modification of the present arrangements is not contemplated. It is considered to be in the best interests of the Medical Department not to designate nurses for the administration of anesthetics only, but to appoint applicants who hold this qualification as nurses for general nursing duties." (*AANA Bulletin,* 1941, p. 232)

With the shortage of nurse anesthetists in civilian hospitals, the AANA was reluctant to urge trained nurse

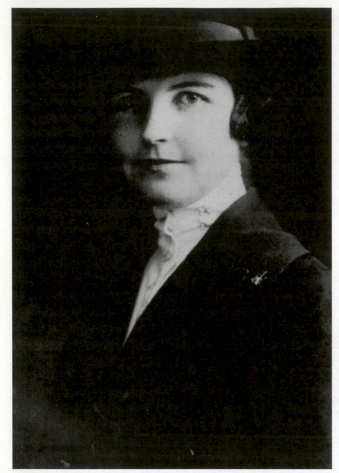

Figure 1–5. Sophie Gran Winton was a nurse anesthetist trained at the Mayo Clinic who was decorated for service in France during World War I. She later became the founding president of the California Association of Nurse Anesthetists. *(Photo: AANA Archives.)*

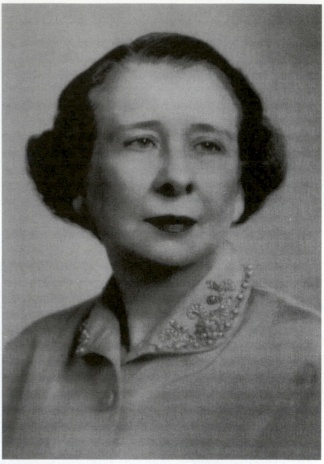

Figure 1–6. Helen Lamb, who led the American Association of Nurse Anesthetists during the turbulent years of World War II. *(Photo: AANA Archives.)*

anesthetists to abandon anesthesia jobs in the civilian sector for possible general nursing service in the military forces under the regulations stated by Shupp. The AANA did recommend that nurse anesthetists volunteer for university hospital units that were subject to be called in an emergency. This approach was similar to the one taken by the Lakeside Hospital Unit in World War I. The issue for the AANA was not whether nurse anesthetists should volunteer for military service, but whether the military would recognize a new clinical specialty within nursing.

An increased demand for students in anesthesia schools in response to the increased need in the military also led the AANA to fear improper training and dilution of standards. Hospitals were opening schools of anesthesia to meet local needs, often with little regard for the quality of education. AANA Education Committee Chair, Helen Lamb, reluctantly supported the increase, but voiced her concern for the hard-won progress made by

the AANA (Fig. 1–6). Lamb stated: "During this critical period, your Committee on Education feels that its greatest contribution may lie in defending the important gains that have been heretofore achieved in the standards of our education. Encouraging in fullest manner the utilization of our already well-organized and effectively functioning Schools of Anesthesia rather than countenance the draining [effect] of inadequately planned new teaching enterprises, whose chief justification only too often lies merely in that particular institution's desire for additional individual staff service" (Bankert, 1989, p. 67). As it would happen, the military utilization of nurse anesthetists actually helped advance the educational interests of the AANA.

The exigencies of war and the proven value of nurse anesthetists in wartime led the Army to formally recognize the specialty of nurse anesthesia by initiating its own educational programs for nurse anesthetists. Fifteen million battle-related hospital admissions and hun-

AANA TIMELINE OF EVENTS

1931	AANA Executive Office established in Cleveland, OH
1933	First AANA Annual Meeting held in Milwaukee, WI
1933	Publication of the *Bulletin of the National Association of Nurse Anesthetists*
1934	*Chalmers-Francis, et al. v. Dagmar Nelson, et al. (Calif.),* 57 P (2d) 1312
1937	AANA Headquarters moved from Cleveland to Chicago, IL
1940	*Bulletin of the National Association of Nurse Anesthetists* was renamed *Bulletin of the American Association of Nurse Anesthetists*
1941	United States enters World War II
1945	First qualifying examination was administered
1944	Inclusion of African Americans into AANA membership
1945	The *Bulletin of the American Association of Nurse Anesthetists* was renamed *The Journal of the American Association of Nurse Anesthetists*
1946	Creation of the AANA Assembly of School Faculty
1947	Inclusion of male nurse anesthetists into AANA membership
1947	Publication of a separate journal, *The Journal of the American Association of Nurse Anesthetists* and *AANA NewsBulletin*
1947	Professional liability insurance is made available to AANA members
1950	Nurse anesthetists serve in Korea
1952	Accreditation program for schools approved with the first one site visit made to Ravenswood Hospital School of Anesthesia in Chicago
1953	Nurse anesthetists were historically recognized in the publication of *History of Anesthesia with Emphasis on the Nurse Specialist*
1955	U.S. Department of Health Education and Welfare recognized the AANA as the accrediting agency for schools of nurse anesthesia
1965	Nurse anesthetists serve in Vietnam
1968	AANA–ASA recognition statements published
1969	Creation of a voluntary continuing education program
1972	AANA–ASA joint statement on qualifications published
1973	AANA became a charter member of the National Federation for Specialty Nursing Organizations
1974	The *Journal of the American Association of Nurse Anesthetists* publication was renamed the *AANA Journal*
1975	Creation of the AANA Councils on Accreditation, Certification, and Practice
1976	First independent AANA annual meeting; past annual meetings were held in conjunction with the American Hospital Association
1977	Mandatory continuing education was approved by AANA members
1978	Formation of the AANA Council on Recertification
1978	Purchase of AANA office building at 216 Higgins, Park Ridge, IL
1979	Nurse Training Act was signed into federal law that specifically includes Nurse Anesthetist Traineeships
1981	Creation of the AANA Education and Research Foundation
1985	*Bhan v. NME Hospitals, Inc.,* 84-2256, D.C. No. CV-S-83-295 LKK (Oct. 2, 1985)
1985	First International Symposium for Nurse Anesthetists was held in Lucerne, Switzerland
1986	Passage of Medicare direct reimbursement legislation for CRNAs was signed by U.S. President Ronald Reagan, making nurse anesthesia the first nursing specialty/nonphysician group to be accorded direct reimbursement rights under the Medicare program
1986	*Oltz v. St. Peters Hospital,* 656, F.Supp. 760
1988	Formation of AANA subsidiary Anesthesia Professional Liability Services
1989	Implementation of direct reimbursement
1989	Formation of the International Federation of Nurse Anesthetists (IFNA) in St. Gallen, Switzerland
1989	Publication of a history of American nurse anesthetists entitled *Watchful Care: A History of America's Nurse Anesthetists*
1991	Nurse anesthetists serve in the Persian Gulf
1992	Purchase of office building at 222 South Prospect, Park Ridge, IL
1993	Formation of AANA subsidiary, Prospect Travel, Inc.
1994	AANA Archives opened for research
1995	Creation of the AANA Managed Care and Direct Reimbursement Department
1995	Establishment of the IFNA Office at the AANA headquarters in Park Ridge, IL

dreds of thousands of surgeries had overwhelmed the number of available trained anesthetists. During the war, 600 nurses were trained in anesthesia by the Army, and in several instances, floor nurses were tapped and quickly prepared for anesthesia duties. Their training period, as the AANA had feared, was necessarily shortened and accelerated, in some places to as little as ninety days. However, the outstanding performance of military nurse anesthetists resulted in 96% of battle wounded being saved, an improvement of 4% over World War I figures, and gave the Army reason to keep training nurse anesthetists for peacetime.

The fact that the Army continued to use nurses as its chief anesthesia provider after World War II impacted civilian anesthesia in positive ways. Prior to the war, the AANA struggled to impose uniform standards on education programs and to implement a certification exam for entry into practice. At that time, education was relatively haphazard, and there was little or no regulation of practice. When the Army established its first post-war training program in 1947, it looked to the AANA for academic guidelines, and designed the curriculum to prepare graduates for the AANA qualifying exam (Balz, 1947). By imposing these standards on its many graduates and programs, the Army helped hasten the acceptance of uniformity among civilian training programs, and gave legitimacy to the AANA as an accrediting agency. The first qualifying exam was given by the AANA in 1945, and accreditation of civilian nurse anesthesia schools began in 1952.

▶ NURSE ANESTHESIA AND INEQUALITY

A professional group is a microcosm of the society in which it exists. It was therefore no surprise that racial and gender-based discrimination played a role in the history of nurse anesthesia. Until 1944, the AANA had no African American members and until 1947, it had no male members. The increasing number of men in the military nurse corps probably accounted for the start of male membership following World War II. AANA leaders have asserted (J. Garde, personal communication, 1995) that integrating the Association along racial lines did not meet with resistance from the membership, but that there were many members who felt men should not be admitted.

Inspired by their predecessors, nurse anesthetists have continued working together to advance the profession. In areas of reimbursement for services, control of educational programing, and entry into practice, equitable regulatory treatment, maintenance of antitrust protections, and promotion of professional autonomy, nurse anesthetists have made significant advances. In the 1970s, the AANA formed independent councils to protect the integrity of the accreditation, certification, and recertification functions. In the 1980s, the organization was instrumental in forming an international association of nurse anesthetists, known today as the International Federation of Nurse Anesthetists. In the 1990s, the AANA initiated a formal archival program.

▶ SUMMARY

Approximately 30 years after the discovery of modern anesthesia in 1846, nurses were introduced to anesthesia practice by surgeons who sought to improve the quality of anesthesia care for their patients. Since then, nurse anesthetists have advanced the discipline of anesthesiology in numerous ways. Nursing's contributions to the discipline have been historically related to patient care and education. However, in recent years, with the preparation of all CRNAs at the master's level and increasingly more at the doctoral level, they have contributed much to research, administration, and formulation of health policy for their states and nation. CRNAs have become a powerful agent for change as health care moves into new and emerging paradigms of delivery. The numbers and demand for CRNA providers has continued unabated for the last century—a clear message that success has only two requirements, vigilance and the expert care of patients.

▶ KEY CONCEPTS

- Modern anesthesia was discovered in 1846, by a Boston dentist named William Morton whose demonstration of ether culminated the thoughts and work of many individuals who preceded him.
- Nurses were drafted into anesthesia in the 1880s and retained as anesthetists because they were reliable and cost-effective clinicians solely devoted to the care of patients under anesthesia.
- As nursing's first specialty group, nurse anesthetists made important strides in the young discipline through organizing the first education programs and standards of clinical practice.

- During World War I, nurse anesthetists created such an impressive record that nurses were again used as anesthetists during World War II; in 1947, the Army decided to use nurse anesthetists exclusively, which effectively strengthened and codified civilian nurse anesthesia training.
- The challenge of whether nurse anesthesia was the practice of medicine or nursing was litigated in two landmark cases, *Frank v. South* (1971) in Kentucky and *Chalmers-Francis v. Nelson* (1936) in California.
- The National Association of Nurse Anesthetists (NANA) was founded in 1931 by Agatha Hodgins. In 1939, the organization was renamed the American Association of Nurse Anesthetists (AANA), whose purpose it was to improve anesthesia education and advance the clinical discipline.
- The first qualifying examination was given in 1945. Accreditation of civilian nurse anesthesia programs began in 1952.

▶ STUDY QUESTIONS

1. Why were nurses given the opportunity to practice anesthesia?

2. Once opposition arose, why and how were nurses able to retain their role as anesthetists?

3. What impact did wartime have on nurse anesthesia?

4. How have nurses advanced the field of anesthesia?

5. Name five pioneer nurse anesthetists and their role in history.

KEY REFERENCES

Bankert, M. (1989). *Watchful care: A history of America's nurse anesthetists.* New York: Continuum.

Thatcher, V. S. (1953). *History of Anesthesia: With emphasis on the nurse specialist.* Philadelphia: J. B. Lippincott.

REFERENCES

Balz, K. E. (1947). The value of special training in anesthesia for the Army nurse. *JAANA. 1,* 138.

Bankert, M. (1989). *Watchful care: A history of America's nurse anesthetists.* New York: Continuum Publishing Co.

Calverly, R. K., (1989). Anesthesia as a specialty: Past, present, and future. In P. G. Barash, B. F. Cullen, & R. K. Stoelting, (Eds.), *Clinical anesthesia* (pp. 3–33). Philadelphia: J. B. Lippincott.

Caton, D. (1985). The secularization of pain. *Anesthesiology, 62, 4.*

Clapesattle, H. (1941). *The doctors Mayo.* Minneapolis: University of Minnesota Press.

Davy, H. (1800). *Researches chemical and physical chiefly concerning nitrous oxide.* London: J. Johnson.

Flikke, J. O. (1941). Present status of nurse anesthetists in the United States Army and Navy [letter in unsigned editorial.] *Bulletin of the American Association of Nurse Anesthetists,* 9(3), 232–233.

Greene, N. M. (1971). A consideration of factors in the discovery of anesthesia and their effects on its development. *Anesthesiology. 33,* 515.

Gunn, I. P. (1990). Notes from the Editor. *CRNA Forum, 6, 20.*

Hammonds, W. D., Steinhaus, J. E. (1993). Pioneer physician in anesthesia. *Journal of Anesthesia, 5,* 553

Hanchett, S. (1995). *Nurse anesthesia is nursing: A historic review of the Chalmers-Francis case.* Unpublished master's degree thesis. Los Angeles, CA: University of California.

Harris, N., & Hunziker-Dean, J. (1997). *The art of Florence Henderson: Pioneer Nurse and Anesthetist.* Unpublished master's degree thesis. Rochester, MN: Mayo School of Health and Related Sciences.

Hunt, A. M. (1948). *Anesthesia: Principles and practice.* New York: Putnam.

Keys, T. E. (1978). *The history of surgical anesthesia.* Huntington, NY: Robert E. Krieger.

Knight, N. (1983). *Pain & its relief.* Washington, DC: The Smithsonian Institute.

Pougiales, J. (1970). The first anesthetizers at the Mayo Clinic. *Journal of the American Association of Nurse Anesthetists, 2,* 237.

Small, S. D. (1994). Implications of the personal library of Horace Wells: Refocusing on the discovery of anesthesia. *Anesthesia History Association Newsletter, 12,* 3.

Thatcher, V. S. (1953). *History of anesthesia with emphasis on the nurse specialist.* Philadelphia: J. B. Lippincott.

The Evolution of the Role of the Certified Registered Nurse Anesthetist

Scot D. Foster

For over a century, Certified Registered Nurse Anesthetists (CRNAs) have proudly and successfully practiced the art and science of anesthesiology. Our successes have been predicted largely on a clearly defined professional identification, that is, who we are and what we do. Additionally our ancestors described the values on which our practice would be based. These values provided a strong and reliable foundation for the profession during the times it was forced to weather a variety of challenges from external sources. Those values bear repeating in this text if for no other reason than our continued growth and influence will in part depend on our collective understanding of them. However, as we move into a new century of providing anesthesia services, we must develop additional values and skills that will help us to remain professionally viable. It is the purpose of this chapter to describe the evolutionary growth of the role of the CRNA within the context of both our historical values and those which we will need in the next century to ensure that our second century of service will be as successful as our first. The challenges are substantial and our commitment must remain firm.

▶ WHAT HAVE WE LEARNED FROM HISTORY?

It has often been said of and by CRNAs that the success we enjoy today stems directly from two sources. First, an uncompromised commitment to patient care, or in today's lexicon, quality management services and second, our cost effectiveness. Although the second point may be argued by some, the first clearly cannot be disputed. Our history is replete with examples of early CRNAs who were recognized nationally and internationally for their commitment to patient care and developing the pioneering techniques of anesthesia delivery.

For instance, Alice Magaw, known to us as the mother of anesthesia, was the first nurse anesthetist to publish articles on her clinical practice, reviewing 14 000 chloroform and ether cases without a death. With Magaw, Florence Henderson perfected the technique of using combinations of chloroform and ether by open drop methods. Agatha Hodgins perfected the administration of nitrous oxide–oxygen anesthesia and became responsible for training literally hundreds of nurse and physicians anesthetists both in the United States and France during World War I (Garde, 1996).

Today, clinical excellence is still the mantra of CRNAs as evidenced by a steadily decreasing professional liability insurance rate, decreasing nationwide between 6% and 13% from 1988 to 1993 and remaining stable thereafter. In addition, CRNAs administer 65% of all anesthetics given in this country annually; further evidence of the acceptance of CRNAs within the health care community as professionals committed to quality care (AANA, 1997).

Quality of patient care was also driven by our second value, and that was a commitment to service: a recognition on the part of the profession that it must uphold its social contract to the public who requires a staunch commitment to quality of care in return for social sanction of the specialty as one worthy of autonomy, competitive pay, and internal professional control. History provides many examples of how these social sanctions have been aggressively challenged by organized medicine including *Frank et al. v. South et al.* (1917), and the most noted, *Chalmers-Francis et al. v. Nelson* (1934), both of which reaffirmed that nurse anesthetists in administering anesthesia were not practicing medicine. CRNAs have learned the worth of their social contract to the public and the professional strength derived from it from history. We have come to know that anesthesia, when administered by a nurse, constitutes the practice of nursing, not medicine. CRNAs must remain most vigilant about this tenet.

History has also taught us to value professional organizations of providers that must assume the responsibilities of leadership for the sake of patients as well as for members. The lesson is simple: you either lead or you are led. Our forebearers realized the necessity of this step in actualizing our profession. In 1930, Agatha Hodgins suggested organizing nurse anesthetists into "a coherent and acting body" and those efforts came to fruition on June 17, 1931, when a group of 48 nurse anesthetists representing 12 states met in a classroom of the anesthesia department of University Hospitals of Cleveland, Lakeside, to form the National Association of Nurse Anesthetists (NANA) (Garde, 1996).

The American Association of Nurse Anesthetists (AANA; renamed in 1939) has since become a strong and progressive organization. The role and function of the national organization includes crafting federal legislative efforts to restructure the current health care delivery system, gaining rightful reimbursement from payers, eliminating barriers to practice, strengthening antitrust law, promoting antidiscrimination legislation, as well as engaging in a variety of patient safety/quality service activities through national accreditation activities (eg, the Joint Commission on the Accreditation of Hospitals and Organizations and the AANA Foundation). These efforts, among hundreds of others, have been aided by the development of highly effective state professional organizations of CRNAs to manage the increasingly complex job of monitoring and influencing local politics. They remain on the cutting edge of change, and are invaluable in sustaining a presence for CRNAs. For decades now, the AANA and its state affiliate organizations have been at the forefront of health care policy development both at the state and federal levels, promoting clinical standards in education and practice, ensuring that CRNAs have an active voice and role in health affairs.

Our more recent history has taught us our value in the marketplace. On the surface this may seem of marginal importance, but on the whole it has had tremendous ramifications for our specialty. First, awareness of financial worth to an employer or contractor relative to services provided has allowed most CRNAs to negotiate salaries that truly reflect their value to patients, not to mention concomitantly sustaining substantial revenue to the institutional or group employer. This fact no doubt also accounts for the substantial salary differential between CRNAs and other advanced practice nurses.

In addition, a clear notion of financial worth has the effect of solidifying professional power, and that, in turn, provides a more formidable basis for negotiating equitable reimbursement rates and policies from both public and private payers and state and federal bureaucrats and policy makers. CRNAs have learned that the vagaries of policy development and implementation have tremendous impact on the structure and function of a work setting, especially in terms of licensure, rights to practice, antitrust protection, scope of practice, protection from antidiscrimination, and guaranteed access to patients, to name only a few.

Finally, our predecessors have taught us the importance of securing and maintaining control of all aspects of our profession, including our scope of practice, accreditation of programs, setting educational and practice standards, certifying and recertifying members to practice, establishing effective systems of professional communication such as the *AANA NewsBulletin* and *AANA Journal,* and maintaining sufficient numbers of CRNAs to meet the manpower needs of the country. History chronicles numerous events that demonstrate how difficult each of these professional functions was to reclaim from organized medicine.

▶ PROFESSIONAL LEADERSHIP

The narrative that follows is divided into five sections, each considered by this author to be fundamental professional responsibilities and values we must each acknowledge to sustain forward momentum. These values are assumed to build on those previously described within the historical context. The reader may recognize that much of what they read currently characterizes their work setting and professional experiences. The information may be new (for others). Regardless, it remains our collective professional responsibility to advance these potentials for ourselves in such a way as to optimally benefit our work efforts and care of patients.

CRNAs as Agents of Change

Doheny and colleagues (1992) maintain that there are certain elements of the nursing role that remain constant, among them the role of change agent. In theory at least, nursing, and especially advanced practice nurses, should be playing the pivotal role in leading and managing change that is characteristic of nearly every facet of our health care delivery system today. One cannot escape the barrage of messages in health care literature and within forums of public debate that change is as inevitable as it is constant; never more so than when dealing with the advent of managed care, attendant corporate mergers, employment restructuring, declining reimbursements, rapidly changing manpower needs, job competition, and perhaps even job loss. Unfortunately most people would rather not deal with change, viewing it as an obstacle or frank threat to normal habits and practice rather than as presenting the challenge of new opportunity. Many CRNAs are no different in their feelings about change than those of the general population of health care providers. This attitude must change; the quality of our future depends on it.

For decades, most CRNAs have appropriately and exclusively concentrated on developing and refining their clinical skills in the operating room, formulating habits and routines that have become comfortable for them and safe for their patients. Many have seen no need to involve themselves outside the arena of service, for instance in local politics at their hospital, community, state, or federal level which would keep them informed of impending change and their role in it. CRNAs have depended too much on the system to protect their interests, including the assumption of secure and continued employment by physician groups or hospitals, generally high salaries as compared with virtually all other nurses (and a significant portion of the medical community), historically high levels of financial reimbursement to employers, and the seemingly unabating demand for anesthesia services. However, all of these historical truths and assumptions are being questioned by policy makers and in many cases are being changed dramatically by law or regulation. There are fewer and fewer professional prerogatives left to any provider. Consequently, every CRNA must be professionally engaged in the issues beyond their clinical role. Although our predecessors taught us that we must lead or be led, current wisdom requires the realization that social engagement is a professional responsibility of not just some of us, but all of us.

What does this mean in terms of our evolution as professional anesthesia providers? On the most basic level, we must become engaged in a new philosophy that has an interdisciplinary focus and shuns the notion that professional isolation will serve us equally well in solving collective problems, especially those that relate to the challenges of managed care or any other proposed change in the delivery system. Society is calling for a renewed commitment to integrated systems, collective communication, mutual cooperation, and above all, a

sense that applying parochial solutions and personal interests to systemic problems will not work. It requires teamwork that utilizes the talents of all providers as critical to problem solving.

This is not an easy task. First, we must become informed participants, professionals who bring accurate and relevant information and/or data to the table. Too often, professional debates center around issues cloaked in rhetoric that is biased and consciously or unconsciously presented as fact when it is not. This situation serves to confuse and complicate the problem-solving process and inflame rather than inform. Second, professional discourse must accommodate other disciplines or specialties who have similar interests but different perspectives. If that is not the case, solutions will be elusive and participants will become frustrated.

Basic to this new perspective is the responsibility each professional has for responsible oral communication, developing competent skills of persuasion, and a reasoned advocacy for positions. It requires skills of negotiation, whether for an employment contract, introduction of new policy, or influence in decision making about patient care or issues affecting employment relationships. Professionals must come to value the skills of rational argument, structured oral and written presentations, and an acute sense of how personal priority must fit within the context of more global issues.

In the final analysis, we must learn that change is inevitable and that we all have a choice of managing it or abdicating that responsibility to others. Successful management of change can only take place in a broader professional forum than that to which we have become accustomed. This fact alone must heighten our awareness of both the personal and professional responsibility we have to exert mature and competent skills of interpersonal communication, civility, and reason to the causes at hand. Above all, we must remain engaged. Excellence in patient care on its own, is no longer a sufficient criteria to meet the challenges that change will inevitably bring.

Preparing Ourselves Educationally

CRNAs have always valued education. Since the first formal programs were begun in the late 1800s and educational standards were initially written at the behest of Helen Lamb in 1934, it was clear that the level of educational preparation for CRNAs would have to keep pace with advancements in the specialty. Consequently, within two decades, the profession moved from the certificate to the graduate level with only a brief interval given to considering the appropriateness of baccalaureate preparation for entry into practice. None of these transitions was easy, as many claimed it would spell the demise of the profession. Clearly change, even within the realm of education, has been an arduous process that will most likely continue to spawn spirited debate.

The level of educational sophistication of entry level programs has increased substantially over the last two decades with a move into colleges and universities and the preparation of more CRNA faculty at the master's and doctoral levels. The next step will likely involve the rather formidable task of preparing both generic students and CRNAs currently in practice with skills for incorporating the increasingly unwieldy body of information required to practice clinically and participate competently in a full range of professional activities. In short, we must all learn new ways of accessing interpreting, and prioritizing information and incorporating valuable portions into clinical practice.

It is likely that education for the next generation will employ new theories of learning. Students will experience new methods of instruction and fulfill requirements that they be fluent in the science of informatics. They will experience less lecture, more clinical simulation; fewer hardcover texts and more electronically relayed sources of literature; less classroom exposure with a live instructor and more experience with distance learning via interactive video, promoting intradisciplinary education. It is likely that student testing will be exclusively simulator or computer based, and clinical progress measured by discrete outcome variables. Students will obtain registration and licenses, and submit assignments and clinical progress reports via computer. Class sizes will be larger and programs fewer as the cost for these innovations and technologies will be substantial. Fluency on the Internet and other electronic databases will be a mandatory skill of all clinicians.

The profession must be mindful that discussions of educational preparation not be limited to debates centered on the appropriate degree level for entry to practice and that we not become mired in controversy over the question of doctoral education for entry to practice. We have hopefully learned the futility of that path from the discipline of nursing at large. In fact, many decisions such as these are made for us, as matters of societal demand, requirements for expanded role responsibilities, or the economic realities of increasing costs of higher education both to the student and the employer. One clear example of that observation is the situation found currently in nursing, where the trend appears to be developing that baccalaureate education may soon be a remnant of an economic and philosophic misstep. It may soon be that the entry to practice professional nursing may be at the master's level. What implications might this have to the future of advanced practice nursing such as CRNAs?

What is clear is that there will be an increasing number of CRNAs prepared at the doctoral level, primarily for the purpose of fulfilling the substantial demand for program faculty. Much to our credit, there are other doctorally prepared CRNAs who fill vital health related roles in business, educational administration, and journalistic pursuits. Regrettably, we still have yet to place any significant numbers of doctorally prepared CRNAs in primary research roles, a requisite for our continued evolution as providers who can contribute credibly to the science of our specialty and discipline.

In addition to filling faculty positions, the profession will rely on doctorally prepared CRNAs to meet the demand for research in educational restructuring and innovation. They will be called on to develop relevant theory to support a rational approach to the preparation and practice of advanced practice nurses, identify relevant educational outcomes, assess educational efficiency and productivity, manage shrinking resources, and move academic ventures to optimal levels of competitiveness. There will also be a place for doctorally prepared clinicians to move the surgical, critical care, or pain populations toward optimal health status; make assessments regarding the quality of clinical practice arrangements; devise clinical pathways; and manage and organize working arrangements within complex, integrated health care systems. All CRNAs of the future, whether they have doctoral degrees or not, must be able to manage clinical data sets for the purpose of planning optimal anesthesia care and make more effective decisions intraoperatively. The demand for a CRNA's doctoral preparation could be substantial when we begin conceptualizing the evolution of our professional role from a much broader perspective.

Realignment With the Discipline of Nursing

In 1931 and 1932, there were a series of formal communications between President Agatha Hodgins, CRNA, and representatives of the American Nurses Association (ANA) in which Hodgins ask the ANA for affiliate status for the newly formed National Association of Nurse Anesthetists (NANA). Her reasons were never really clear in view of the fact that she was often quoted as saying that anesthesia "could not be defined as nursing, but impinges closely upon and is irrevocably attached to the care of the sick" (Bankert, 1989, p. 70). Some purported that she hoped the affiliation would stem the tide of untrained RNs from administering anesthesia. Others suggested that Hodgins felt the affiliation would gain recognition for anesthetists as highly educated nurse specialists.

On the other hand, there were many within the ANA who publicly denied that the practice of anesthesia was within the realm of nursing and viewed nurse anesthetists as mavericks who failed to appreciate, much less revere, the traditional roles and responsibilities of the bedside nurse. Consequently, the mix of Hodgins impatience combined with the pace of ANA decision making, a somewhat questionable philosophical allegiance to nursing on behalf of NANA, and ANA's reticence to accommodate a potentially strong ally in advanced practice, doomed the request. Within six months, after numerous written communications, the ANA ultimately rejected NANA's petition. Regardless of the collective motives, the breech between the ANA and NANA (ultimately, the AANA) was interrupted only occassionally over the next half century by token communication.

Although a cordial relationship between the two groups developed in subsequent decades, several events occurred in the 1980s that would bring the two professional nursing groups closer. First, the health care delivery system was undergoing substantial change that would require nursing to present a united political front for legislative efforts. It was obvious that the success of any political agenda would be much enhanced by a coalition despite the fact that the AANA had experienced significant legislative success at the federal level acting alone. The most important factor prompting a renewed relationship was the movement of programs of nurse anesthesia into colleges and universities that would allow them to offer graduate degrees. More likely than not, programs became housed in academic units of nursing. By the mid-1990s nearly 45% of all nurse anesthesia programs offered a master's degree in nursing, where only a few had exercised that option during the previous decade. Consequently, the nursing community and nurse anesthetists started making more sustained attempts at restoring their relationship.

Efforts toward solidifying this relationship have been challenging, although not so much at the national leadership levels because policy concerns for the most part have been parallel between the organizations. Many of these efforts have dealt with obtaining federal money for the support of nursing education and gaining direct reimbursement for advanced practice nurses. While CRNAs could clearly benefit from their relationship to a larger discipline and the security of nursing's long-standing institutional power structure, nursing and especially advanced nurse practice specialties have benefited from AANA's legislative experience, reimbursement successes, and nationally recognized accreditation and certification programs. The AANA has also been a noted leader in the work of promoting the legislative agenda of advanced practice nursing. The Association also meets regularly and helps financially sponsor the activities of a variety of groups, including the National Federation of Specialty Nursing Organizations. In addition, the Association meets with the American Society of Postanesthesia Nurses, the Association of Operating Room Nurses (AORN), the American College of Nurse Midwives, as well as the ANA.

Efforts at optimizing relationships between CRNAs and academic nursing have presented more formidable challenges. As CRNA educators have long been a rather independent sort, the transition into the culture of organized nursing has been difficult for some, usually in relation to autonomy in budgetary and curricular control. CRNA faculty salaries have also traditionally been higher than other nursing faculty, and in some sectors this has caused difficulties. Most important, few doctorally prepared CRNA faculty held degrees in nursing, which readily highlighted differences in educational philosophy as well as values held about the discipline. Moreover, some CRNAs were denied faculty status in nursing departments because their graduate degrees were not in nursing, regardless of their proven teaching or research expertise.

Nevertheless, it remains clear that the transition is proceeding and nurse anesthesia will and should in the future become a more identifiable specialty within the discipline of nursing. Traditional nursing education departments have provided nurse anesthetists with expanded opportunities to learn the process of collaborative ventures, important in today's changing health care system. They have provided CRNAs with better opportunities to learn and practice skills of research and gain perspectives about the importance of patient care within the context of communities and culturally diverse populations. Nursing has also provided anesthesia education programs with a more secure basis of operation within institutions of higher education, and their efforts will undoubtedly help prepare more CRNAs at the doctoral level. Nursing must, however, also learn to appreciate anesthetists for their strong clinical focus in practice, as well as marketplace, workforce, and reimbursement issues. They will also benefit from the CRNA value of a need for strong and vocal leadership and full engagement in health care issues that make a difference and that will keep nursing economically and professionally viable in tomorrow's health care market.

Claiming and Expanding a Scope of Practice

Organized medicine has frequently accused advanced practice nurses of attempting to expand their scope of practice. This author, for one, is heartened that they have received the message. Their interpretation is in fact correct. It is clearly a professional requisite of nurses and physicians alike to actively expand their clinical scope of services to meet patient need based on the growth of knowledge, emerging technologies, justifiable practice trends, and societal mandates. This expansion however, should always be based on clear evidence of appropriate education, practice standards, and reliable measures of competence. Attempts to maintain the status quo by actively blocking competitive practitioners in any field is merely the residual of failed attempts at professional control and self-serving egoism. It has nothing to do with quality or prerogatives of those who control anesthesia services.

Nurse anesthetists must always value their worth to the health care delivery system. They must transcend the notion that autonomous judgments and actions are beyond their control or capability and expunge the age-old concept that health care services are the exclusive or delegated domain of physicians. Research, legal precedent, and decades of practice successes tell the story otherwise. Clearly, anesthesia is a legitimate function of nursing that can be carried out without physician supervision, medical direction, or arbitrating a nurse's scope of practice; that is a legitimate function of the appropriate state regulatory agency. Patients will be best served when nurses and physicians alike work in a collaborative fashion that exploits the talents of each; where active, respectful and interdependent consultation among colleagues would be commonplace. Collectively, greater effort should be made to examine the unexplored reaches of each discipline's nature, substance, and potentials that would translate into substantively unique contributions to anesthesia care.

Why should the definition and codification of a skill base or scope of practice be so important to nurse anesthetists? The answer lies in careful examination of our past successes as a profession. First, our scope of practice defines and legitimizes our range of services to the public, payers, legislators, bureaucrats, and colleagues. It is discrete and understandable thus providing (1) lawful recognition of practice that translates into expanded and stable employment opportunities, (2) recognition of service by payers as financially reimbursable at market rate, (3) sufficient scope to remain competitive in the marketplace of the same or similar services, (4) recognition of services unique among the specialties of nursing that contributes to the continued role evolution of all advanced practice nurses, and (5) abilities to exert responsible and independent judgments in the care of patients.

As more nurse practice acts open every year (reviewed for potential change or modification), significant effort is being made by many State Boards of Nursing and other professional organizations to accommodate the range of advanced practice nurses, many of whom have lacked formal recognition historically. This is also a time when it is incumbent on CRNAs to reexamine their legitimate function within the context of their work, credentials, and educational preparation to expand their practice scope in a justifiable and responsible manner. Finally, CRNAs must value the importance of maintaining their full scope of practice and continue work to eliminate barriers to practice such as anti-competitive practices and discrimination in the workplace in order that patients may have access to CRNA services of the highest quality.

This position was noted in the Pew Commission Report, *Reforming Health Care Workforce Regulation: Policy Considerations of the 21st Century* (1995). That report stated that "States should base practice acts on demonstrated initial and continuing competence. This process must allow and expect different professions to share overlapping scopes of practices. States should explore pathways to allow all professionals to provide services to the full extent of their current knowledge, training, experience and skills. . . . [States must] eliminate exclusive scopes of practice which unnecessarily restrict other professions from providing competent, effective and accessible care. States should ensure that the training, testing and regulation of health professionals allow different professions to provide the same services when competence—based on knowledge, training, experience and skills—has been demonstrated" (Pew Commission Report, 1995, p. 9).

Designing and Accommodating New Practice Roles

The 1990s will always be remembered as a defining one for health care delivery and be best known for the explosive growth of managed care. It has become obvious that for any professional provider group to survive, they will need to understand the principles of managed care and consequent market pressures brought to bear on employers as well as providers who seek to contract their services. Above all, CRNAs should develop a keen appreciation for the concept and operational principles of competition, as that basic market tenet will become a requisite to success for all types and configurations of providers.

Managed care will substantially reconfigure the workplace. It will require a changed skill mix, change traditional work patterns and roles, and most importantly change how we think about ourselves as professionals, especially in terms of the need for greater collaborative work among providers. How will these changes manifest changes in the CRNA role?

1. CRNAs will need to become experts in information and resource management. Clinical decision making will, in the future, be based on perioperative computer-generated data sets that will predict "best practice" alternatives to particular problems that arise during the course of anesthesia. These clinical guidelines will serve to maximize patient outcome, control cost, and document the quality of care provided. It is also conceivable that provider clinical performance, including the ability to retain liability coverage, will be measured by precise and discrete outcome variables.

2. CRNAs will find new roles for themselves in new environments. It is expected that within the next decade, 80% of all surgeries will be provided on an outpatient basis. Fewer and fewer CRNAs will spend the whole of their time in traditional operating rooms. As the health paradigm moves from acute care to prevention and restoration, CRNAs will find themselves increasingly in physician offices, community-based clinics, and perhaps in patient homes or other community centers providing services. This shift will aid patient access and decrease costs from those associated with tertiary care centers.

3. CRNAs will be expected to broaden their scope of practice by assuming responsibility for functional areas that have not traditionally been part of the CRNA role, for instance, critical care, patient recovery, IV services, and pain management; in other words, "multi-skilling or cross-training" practice. This will result as managed care downsizes the workforce and requires remaining providers to maximize their worth to the employer. There will also be expanded opportunity for CRNAs with graduate credentials to assume increased responsibilities in administration, information management, systems design/flow, perioperative case management, and utilization review. Again, the PEW Commission (1995) speaks to this issue:

> acknowledging that differently trained and differently named professions may deliver the same services—so long as they demonstrate competence. Professionals should be allowed and encouraged to provide services to the full extent of their current knowledge training, experience and skills. A regulatory system that maintains its priority of quality care, while eliminating irrational monopolies and restrictive scopes of practice would not only allow practitioners to offer the health services they are competent to deliver, but would be more flexible, efficient, and effective (p. 10).

Much of what the future will require of providers that mandates changes in role and function can and should be managed and designed by CRNAs themselves because they are the ones who truly understand the potentials of the specialty as it relates to changed service requirements. Furthermore, CRNAs can extrapolate that vision into workable solutions because it is incumbent for all CRNAs to become involved in those discussions.

4. The ultimate success of managed care will be based on whether or not comprehensive health care services can be delivered to all U.S. citizens in a cost-effective manner by competent providers demonstrating quality performance outcomes. This will be no easy task and one which puts onerous yet appropriate responsibilities on the provider to demonstrate competence and acceptable patient outcomes. The basic nature of anesthesia work must exemplify at every juncture, attention to the patient and their needs, examining their expectations and not only meeting but exceeding their expectations for service. Benchmarks of service and quality must be identified and used consistently in practice to measure relevant outcomes, both in terms of physiologic parameters and indices of patient satisfaction.

CRNAs must also learn about and become involved in the continuing debate regarding provider competence, what it means, and how it is measured. It is unlikely that clinical performance will continue to be assessed by outdated measures of minimum competencies though initial certification testing. Pressure will increase to incorporate more formidable measures of competence for recertification such as periodic retesting, actual observed performance on anesthesia simulators, and requirements for data-driven documentation.

▶ CASE STUDY

Despite the fact that CRNAs have been at the forefront of health care for decades, there are many hospital administrators that remain uninformed about our role, scope of practice, liability requirements, and ability to bill for services. Even more unfortunate, there are those outside our profession in leadership positions who promulgate information that is uninformed or patently incorrect.

Assume that you are a CRNA in an environment which has never had CRNAs before. The administrator has heard "good things" about CRNA services, but needs a lot of schooling as to exactly what you do and how your services will be good for the hospital's patients. This could be a likely scenario.

1. The hospital administrator informs you that the medical staff is not sure of how you can become credentialed and have privileges on the medical staff.

   You can and should become a voting member of the regular medical staff to ensure that you have input into issues affecting your patients and the type and scope of care you give. Associate membership may come without voting rights. The AANA maintains prototypes of credentialing documents that you can use as a template to design your own.

2. A surgeon is certain that you need to be supervised by an anesthesiologist. What is your answer?

There is no state that has a legal requirement for CRNA supervision by an anesthesiologist. You need only to have your services requested by a physician who is properly credentialed and privileged by your hospital medical staff. Neither medicare, medicaid, nor the Joint Commission on the Accreditation of Healthcare Organizations require physician supervision, of nurse anesthetists.

3. A surgeon is concerned about vicarious liability. In other words, can the surgeon become liable for your acts?

Again, the AANA maintains voluminous documentation regarding how courts have ruled on this issue. Clearly, the surgeon's liability depends on the amount of involvement he/she maintains in the conduct and management of your anesthesia service at the time of question. This also holds true for anesthesiologists. If the court finds that there has been substantial management or direction imposed on the conduct of the case (whether CRNA or MD anesthesiologist), the court may find reason for the claim of vicarious liability.

4. The surgical staff would like you to make a presentation at their next meeting about your role and scope of practice. Where can you find documents to provide support for your presentation?

The *AANA Clinical Practice Manual,* available from the AANA, is an invaluable guide to such documents. It includes credentialing prototypes, standards of clinical practice in all anesthetizing areas, standards for monitoring, scope of practice statements, and legal precedents on a variety of issues. It will also be helpful for you to provide the audience with their own set of *AANA White Papers* (again, available from the AANA) which succinctly outline issues on scope, safety, quality of care, billing mechanisms, and a variety of other issues. Every practicing CRNA should have these two documents as ready resources available to answer questions of employers, patients, medical staff, and administrators.

▶ SUMMARY

The evolution of the Certified Registered Nurse Anesthetist provides an enviable legacy of vision, strength, commitment to patient care, and tireless work to maintain a leadership role in the world of health care. In addition to clinical practice, for which CRNAs are so prominently noted, many have expanded their work into areas of health related business, research, management, scholarship, and education. Managed care presents new challenges to expand that list in much broader directions with many new opportunities for professional growth.

The professional demands on CRNAs in a new century will require that they broaden their focus well beyond the confines of the operating room. This new individual vision should incorporate not only their view about the scope of their clinical practice but the professional issues that directly impact their ability to practice in any employment setting. The evolutionary process of becoming and maturing as a CRNA involves not only a profound commitment to patient care, but also a commitment to the organizations and institutions that make practice possible, incomes desirous, opportunity at hand, and professional skills a palpable and vibrant commodity in the marketplace. In order to accomplish this goal, all CRNAs need to deliberately examine their history, the values they hold about their professional work, and propose a clear plan to contribute constructively to our collective mission of promoting quality, cost efficiency, market value, and caring.

▶ KEY CONCEPTS

- The strength of the specialty of nurse anesthesia is derived from its commitment to excellence in patient care, cost effective services, and a shared value among its members to maintain national leadership in health care policy development.
- The education of CRNAs has become more advanced with the professional mandate that all programs offer a master's degree in addition to the fact that many teaching faculty are becoming doctorally prepared.
- The profession must be diligent about protecting and expanding its scope of practice to ensure a CRNA's ability to provide a comprehensive range of services and remain marketable.
- CRNA practice scope should be defined by the parameters of state statute, regulation, and educational preparation, rather than from arbitrary and capricious limitations placed on them by other professional groups or bureaucratic agencies.
- The success of the specialty of nurse anesthesia has been greatly enhanced by the efforts of the American Association of Nurse Anesthetists, to which over 92% of all CRNAs belong.
- Each CRNA must acknowledge that professional responsibilities necessarily extend beyond the clinical role to include teaching, leadership, public relations, local community involvement, research, and management.
- CRNAs provide 85% of all anesthesia in the rural United States and manage 65% of the 26 million anesthetics administered annually.

▶ STUDY QUESTIONS

1. What were the two primary legal precedents in the early part of the century that established anesthesiology as the practice of nursing?

2. What are the primary theoretical contructs of a "profession"?

3. Identify factors or reasons why it is important for nurse anesthetists to remain in control of their accreditation and certification mechanisms.

4. Who regulates nursing, including advanced practice nursing, in your state and why is it important for nursing not to abdicate this regulatory responsibility to medicine?

5. What are the legal mechanisms (certifications, licensure, etc) in your state that allow you to practice as a CRNA?

6. List a range of possible professional responsibilities required of CRNAs to keep our profession strong.

KEY REFERENCES

Bankert, M. (1989). *Watchful care: A history of America's nurse anesthetists.* New York, NY: Continuum Publishing Co.
American Association of Nurse Anesthetists, Foster, S. D. &

Jordan, L. J (Eds). (1994). *Professional aspects of nurse anesthesia practice.* Philadephia, PA: F. A. Davis.

REFERENCES

American Association of Nurse Anesthetists. (1997). *AANA white paper, executive summary.* Park Ridge, IL: AANA Publishing.
Bankert, M. (1989). *Watchful care: A history of America's nurse anesthetists.* New York: Continuum Publishing Co.
Chalmers-Francis et al. v. Dagmar Nelson et al. [Calif], 57P [2d] 1312 (1934).
Doheny, M., Cook, C., & Stopper, C. (1992). *The discipline of nursing: An introduction* (3rd ed.). Norwalk, CT: Appleton & Lange.

Frank et al. v. South et al. 175 Kentucky REP:416–428 (1917).
Garde, J. F. (1996). *Nursing Clinics of North America, 31*(3), 568–571.
Pew Commission. (1995, December). *Reforming health care workforce regulation: Policy considerations for the 21st century.* Report of the Taskforce on Health Care Workforce Regulation, pp. 9, 13.

LEGAL FOUNDATIONS OF NURSE ANESTHESIA PRACTICE

Gene A. Blumenreich

Anyone studying the effect of the legal system on nurse anesthesia practice must keep in mind that the legal profession does not understand what Certified Registered Nurse Anesthetists (CRNAs) do. Anesthesia is an area requiring skills, education, and specific knowledge that is not held by either the public or members of the legal profession. Thus, in most matters relating to nurse anesthesia, the legal profession defers to the expertise of nurse anesthetists. Many aspects of the law's expectation and standards are determined not by the legal system, but by CRNAs who in their daily practice set the standards by which all nurse anesthetists are judged.

▶ THE LEGAL SYSTEM

The American legal system was derived from the English. The legal system developed over many centuries as a way for the state to mediate disputes among residents. The first thing needed to solve disputes is some way to determine what the facts are. While in some cases a trial judge acting alone may serve as the finder of fact, the Constitution of the United States guarantees the right of a jury trial in those situations where jury trials were provided under English law at the time of the American Revolution. In feudal times, the jury included persons with actual knowledge of the events for efficient fact finding. In modern times, actual knowledge of the parties or the events of a case are seen as disqualifications for jury members. At trial, the parties have an opportunity to present evidence in an effort to convince a finder of fact who starts off with a blank slate.

Lawyers are taught that although the facts may change from case to case, the law is supposed to stay the same. A goal of the legal system is to provide consistency of legal interpretation. This consistency would be destroyed if juries selected for each case were allowed to determine the law. The determination of the law applicable to the facts is the province of the judge, not the jury. Although everyone knows the distinction between "fact" and "law," there are a number of instances in which it can be less than clear. For example, a determination that a particular act constitutes "medical malpractice" may have aspects of both fact and law. In one case a jury may believe that a dosage of a drug is an overdose while in another, they may be convinced it is normal.

▶ SOURCES OF LAW

There may be several sources of "law." *Statutory law* consists of the laws and statutes enacted by a legislature. They take effect after adoption. That is, when a law is passed it does not affect events that occurred prior to its passage. Statutes may be quite precise and specific. *Case law,* sometimes referred to as *common law,* is a body of law reflecting the interpretation of prior decisions of judges. Common law is a process by which judges attempt to establish principles of fairness which underlie their past decisions. Judges then apply these principles to different factual patterns. It develops gradually, from one case to another. For example, the legal theory known as *res ipsa loquitur* was originally developed as a theory of negligence when a barrel fell out of a warehouse window. Under then existing principles of tort law, it was necessary for the plaintiff to show that the defendant had been negligent. However, the injured plaintiff had not been present in the defendant's warehouse and had not been able to find any evidence of what had occurred other than the fact that a barrel had fallen out of the window. The plaintiff argued that he should not have to present evidence of a specific act of negligence because the mere fact that the barrel had fallen out of the window was in itself evidence that there had been negligence. The judges agreed that "the thing speaks for itself" (or, translated into Latin, *res ipsa loquitur*). From this case developed the modern day principle of *res ipsa loquitur.* If the plaintiff can show that (1) in the ordinary course of events, the injury would not have occurred if someone had not been negligent; (2) the injury was caused by something in the exclusive control of the defendant; and (3) the injury was not due to any voluntary action or contribution on the part of the plaintiff, then the plaintiff need not prove negligence under these circumstances. The burden of proof shifts to the defendant to show that he was not negligent. The principle of *res ipsa loquitur* was originally applied to falling bodies (such as barrels from a warehouse window and in one early English case, a falling cow).

The courts, however, continued to extend the doctrine to more and more cases until eventually it applied to anesthesia. Even though the facts of an anesthesia negligence case are much different than the facts relating to a falling barrel or cow, the courts realized that the underlying principles were the same. Just as the plaintiff hit by a barrel was not present in the warehouse, the anesthetized patient is in no position to monitor his care in an operating room. The doctrine of *res ipsa loquitur* was never enacted by a legislature. Nor could the English courts have realized that the doctrine it adopted for falling barrels would apply to something not yet invented called anesthesia. The doctrine was created, refined, and expanded by the courts in a long process by looking at decided cases and using the arguments and principles in one case to decide disputes in another.

Courts decide only the cases before them. Legislatures, on the other hand, enact laws which are applied generally rather than to specific situations. With a few exceptions, courts defer to the legislature. The legislature may change the common law. When court developed law comes into conflict with a legislative statute, the

statute prevails. Even with statutory law, however, it is the courts who interpret it and decide how it applies to specific statutory situations. Courts are also required to interpret statutes when the statute is ambiguous or internally inconsistent. Under these circumstances, it is up to the court to interpret the statute in such a way as to give as much meaning as it can to what the court believes the legislature meant.

Another area in which a court may interpret a statute is that of constitutional interpretation. In a very early and famous Supreme Court case, Supreme Court Chief Justice John Marshall decided that the Supreme Court of the United States could overturn a statute enacted by Congress if the Supreme Court decided that it violated the terms of the United States Constitution. Up until this case, it was not clear which of the three branches of government was the final arbiter of constitutional decisions.

Regulations are issued by administrative agencies and often provide more specifics than the statute. They set forth additional information to guide the enforcement of statutes. Regulations must be consistent with the statute. They are treated by the court as if they were law as long as they are not arbitrary and do not misinterpret what the court determines the legislature meant.

▶ LAWYERS IN AN ADVERSARIAL SYSTEM

One of the key players in the legal system is the lawyer, who is the expert on the system. Lawyers have several roles in the judicial system. First, they are *advisors.* One of the goals of the legal system is to provide a fair and clear opportunity for parties to mold their behavior so as to avoid risk or loss. It is the lawyer who reviews laws and cases and attempts to advise his client of the legal consequences of certain actions. When court decisions are confusing or inconsistent, parties cannot adjust their behavior. They become dependent on the courts to render decisions to determine their legal rights and obligations. Litigation clogs the system and is unfair to parties who should not have to wait years for a case to be decided to find out what their legal rights and obligations were. Furthermore, if the parties cannot be certain of their rights and liabilities, they may be reluctant to engage in desirable commercial or other activity. The lawyer's training and experience assists him in being able to attempt to predict how the courts will interpret a given set of facts and to describe, in advance, what the party's legal rights and liabilities would be.

In addition to being advisers, lawyers are also *champions.* As experts on the legal system, they become experts at presenting information to make it more understandable by courts and juries. Lawyers learn to make juries see the facts in a light most favorable to their clients. One of the difficulties that has affected all legal systems ever devised is that as human beings, it is difficult for us to determine what is the "truth" and what actually happened in any given event. Each of us sees only our own angle and view of reality. Humans have struggled to develop a system of truth finding since prehistoric times. The English system of justice, adopted by American institutions, gradually became fixed on the *adversary system:* each side to a dispute is allowed to offer testimony and evidence. After viewing both sides, truth is supposed to become apparent to the trier of fact.

Both sides are given extensive tools to investigate in a process known as *discovery*. The parties have the ability to force witnesses to testify under oath and examine documentation. This enables them to carry out their roles as investigators and also permits both sides to learn the other side's case to encourage trials to be complete, to make sure all relevant evidence is collected, and to encourage clients to settle their disputes without having expensive and time-consuming trials. As part of this adversarial approach, lawyers also developed into adversaries. In order to properly present a case, or to assist a client to make the right decision, it is imperative for the lawyer to be taken into the client's confidence and learn at least all of the facts of which the client is aware. This confidential relationship between lawyer and client gives rise to the attorney–client privilege: matters that are expressed to an attorney by a client in the course of representation may not be revealed by the lawyer without the client's permission. One issue that has arisen more frequently since the advent of malpractice insurance is the question of which person the lawyer owes his loyalty to when the lawyer represents a party in litigation but the legal bill is paid by an insurance company.

The *lawyer's code of ethics* provides that lawyers should not represent more than one party at a time if the representation of one client would affect the lawyer's representation of another. In a Massachusetts case (*Tremontozzi v. Safety Insurance Company,* 1991), a lawyer, paid by an insurance company, was defending the driver of a car being sued by a passenger who became a paraplegic in an accident. The driver felt that his claim was improperly handled by his insurance company. The driver ultimately settled with the passenger and assigned to the passenger whatever claim the driver might have against the driver's own insurance company. The passenger's lawyer attempted to obtain documents that the insurance company had provided to the driver's attorney. The insurance company claimed that these documents were entitled to the protection of the attorney–client privilege. The court held that even though the insurance company was paying the lawyer's bill, the lawyer for the driver owed a duty of confidentiality to the driver only. When the insurance company shared confidential documents with the driver's lawyer, it had shared the documents with a third party and information shared with a lawyer (or anyone else) who is not your lawyer is no longer protected by attorney–client privilege.

Similar issues may arise in the health care field. What happens when a single insurance company represents several hospital employees, all of whom are accused of malpractice? What if it is in the interests of some of these defendants to claim that the injury is the fault of another defendant represented by the same attorney? The lawyer's code of ethics requires that each employee retain a separate lawyer.

The adversary system of litigation is not the only model that may be used to arrive at "truth." In some countries, a single judge or tribunal questions witnesses and attempts to determine "truth." In England and the United States, the courts rely on the parties to investigate and report the facts. In some cases involving nurse anesthetists, the adversarial system has caused difficulty. Judges and lawyers are not familiar with nurse anesthesia. If there is no nurse anesthetist as a party (either because the nurse anesthetist has previously settled [*Denton Regional Medical Center v. LaCroix,* 1997] or was never a party [*Jefferson Parish Hospital v. Hyde,* 1984]), the court can be misled by incorrect information.

▶ APPELLATE COURTS

In a typical trial, many legal issues arise and many facts have to be presented to the jury or the finder of fact. What if the judge makes a mistake on a ruling of law or the trier of fact becomes overwhelmed by emotion and renders a judgment which has no relationship to the facts? If one party believes that a decision is in error, the party may *appeal* to a higher court.

In making an appeal, exactly what is being appealed affects the ability of the appellate court to grant relief. If the appeal relates to a ruling of law, the appellate court may decide the issue after listening to arguments by the parties. Although the appellate court may consider the reasoning of the trial court, it is not obligated to give any special attention to it. In factual issues, the appellate court gives substantial deference to the trial court. Humans communicate verbally as well as nonverbally. Courts have learned that a person who does not actually see the party testify is less able to determine whether the party was telling the "truth." Consequently, in factual matters, the courts give substantial deference to the trial court both in determining what weight to place on evidence and whether or not to accept it as "truth." Deferring to the trial court in terms of factual findings avoids giving the parties a sense that nothing is final. Appellate courts can use only facts that were presented to the trial court. If a party neglects to introduce key evidence at trial, that evidence cannot be considered during the appeal.

In some states there may be several levels of appeal. A trial may be held in a trial court, an appeal may be taken to an appellate court, and if one or both of the parties are dissatisfied, the appeal may be taken even further. In the federal system, trials are held in district courts. Appeals may be taken to one of 10 Circuit Courts of Appeal. Appeals can be taken from the circuit courts to the Supreme Court of the United States. When there are intermediate appellate courts, the supreme court limits the number of cases it will hear based on the supreme court's determination as to whether or not a case is important. Certain issues may be so difficult to decide that courts can reach alternative conclusions or there may be inconsistent appellate court cases on a single issue. This is often sufficient reason for the supreme court to hear the appeal.

We have seen that the English system for fact finding established in the United States is adversarial. Each side to a dispute conducts its own investigation and presents the facts in a manner most flattering to its position. Facts change from case to case, and a finding by a jury in one case is binding only in that case. On the other hand, determinations of law by appellate courts are binding on junior courts. Nonetheless, in an adversarial system, the court is also dependent on the parties' lawyers to research the law and present it to the court. Because the appellate court's findings of law affect other cases, courts permit persons who are not parties to provide relevant information to the appellate court on the law to be applied. The procedure used is a brief *amicus curiae,* a brief filed as a "friend of the court."

▶ SOURCES OF LAW CONCERNING NURSE ANESTHESIA

What is the source of law for nurse anesthesia practice? In most states, legal requirements for nurse anesthesia practice begin with the legal requirements for nursing. These are almost always contained in statute. In a typical nursing statute, the legislature creates a board of nursing. Administrative bodies such as boards of nursing combine legislative authority—the power to issue regulations—and judicial authority—the power to hold hearings, assess penalties and remove licenses. Nurse practice acts will frequently provide that, in order to practice nursing, a nurse must meet educational requirements set by the board of nursing and must obtain a license from the board. A license evidences that the nurse has met certain minimum standards such as the completion of a required course of study. The license also serves as a reminder that the nurse is subject to the jurisdiction of the board of nursing.

In some states, CRNAs are in a class of advanced practice nurses. In these states, the licensing statutes provide that certain nurses who have met additional educational requirements and who have met additional certification requirements may be referred to as Advanced Practice Nurses. Nurse anesthetists are an unusual example of advanced practice nurses. Whereas nurse anesthesia clearly requires additional education, the type of functions a nurse anesthetist may perform are the same types of function performed by a registered nurse. For example, some advanced practice nurses may be permitted by their licensing laws to prescribe certain types of medications. In many states, a nurse anesthetist's traditional medication order is not considered a prescription in the sense of a writing that a patient may take to a pharmacy and fill (the laws of each state may differ and whether the types of medication order that a nurse anesthetist writes is a prescription depends on state law). Some advanced practice nurses may have rights to diagnose. Although nurse anesthetists must be keenly aware of a patient's condition and prepared to act promptly if there are changes, what a nurse anesthetist does is considered more similar to "nursing observation" and not diagnosis. [However, many people, including this author, find it impossible to distinguish between "nursing observation" and "medical diagnosis" on a practical level. From the legal standpoint, nurses are expected to perform "nursing observation" and may be held liable in malpractice for failing to do so, while, without statutory authority, it is illegal for a nurse to make a "medical diagnosis."] The powers and functions of the nurse anesthetist are those which are usually associated with nursing. Nevertheless, because of the additional educational requirements that are imposed on CRNAs, nurse anesthetists, are often thought of as one of the four typical examples of advanced practice nurses.

A number of states have statutes specifically identifying nurse anesthetists. Often state statute will require that a nurse anesthetist graduate from a course of study recognized by the Council on Accreditation of Educational Programs of Nurse Anesthesia, be certified by the Council on Certification of Nurse Anesthetists and periodically recertified by the Council on Recertification of Nurse Anesthetists. Sometimes the statute describes the relationship between the nurse anesthetist and other health care professionals. Some statutes may provide for supervision, direction, or collaboration. In addition, statutory references to nurse anesthetists can sometimes be found in hospital licensing or general health care statutes. In a very few states, references to nurse anesthetists can be found as exceptions in medical practice acts. Statutes recognizing nurse anesthetists vary from state to state, and CRNAs must be aware of and act in accordance with these statutes.

In some states, there may be no statutory reference to nurse anesthetists at all. Because of the deference the law gives to health care, in those states where nurse anesthetists are not specifically mentioned in statutes or regulations, the legality of nurse anesthesia practice is based on custom. Nurse anesthetists may and do legally practice in all 50 states. Even if statutes do not specifically require certification as a Certified Registered Nurse Anesthetist, because 97% of all nurses who administer anesthesia are CRNAs, it is a standard of practice that nurses administering anesthesia be CRNAs.

▶ NURSE ANESTHESIA IS A PROFESSION

Because courts do not understand what nurses do, they have held that nurses fall into a special category, that of professionals, who are entitled to set their own standards of care (*Hiatt v. Groce* [1974], *Mohr v. Jenkins* [1981]; but see *Butler v. Louisiana State Board of Education* [1976]; where a nurse who undertook to perform a medical service was subject to the standard of care and liability of a physician). If the court cannot understand what a nurse does, it cannot set the standard of care. Only those with a same or similar education and skill are qualified to do that.

As professionals, nurses engage in the practice of nursing. There are many misperceptions about the practice of nursing and the practice of medicine. Some see these areas as different points on a spectrum of functionality or power. According to this view, advanced practice nurses such as nurse anesthetists, are midway between the practice of nursing and the practice of medicine. Others, just as incorrectly, look at the practice of nursing and the practice of medicine as areas separated by a fence or boundary.

Actually, medicine and nursing are professions that developed independently. There is, and always has been, a great deal of overlap in the functions performed by members of both professions. In legal terms, the practice of nursing is what nurses do and the practice of medicine is what physicians do. When the legislature enacts licensing acts, those acts which it authorizes nurses to perform constitute "the practice of nursing" and those acts which physicians are authorized to perform constitute "the practice of medicine." Where there is overlap, such as in taking histories or vital signs, administering hypodermics and, administering anesthesia, the same functions can be found in both the practice of nursing and the practice of medicine. Even the American Medical Association (AMA) has noted the overlap and pointed out that when an overlapping function is performed by a nurse it is the practice of nursing and when performed by a physician it is the practice of medicine.

Licensing laws do not create monopolies. They are enacted to protect the public, not to protect the professions. In the case of *In re Carpenter's Estate* decided in Michigan in 1917, the court ruled that a dentist who had been treating a cancer of the mouth was not illegally practicing medicine. The legislature permitted both dentists and doctors to treat diseases of the mouth and the fact that the dentist was performing a function which was also permitted to be performed by a physician did not mean that the dentist was illegally practicing medicine.

Two cases established that nurse anesthetists may administer anesthesia without being guilty of the illegal practice of medicine. In *Frank v. South* (1917), a nurse anesthetist was challenged by the Jefferson County, Kentucky Medical Society on the grounds that nurse anesthesia was the illegal practice of medicine. In a very well reasoned decision, the court examined what nurse anesthetists did and compared the types of function carried out by nurse anesthetists with the types of function performed by generic nurses. The court ruled that a nurse anesthetist was not illegally practicing medicine even though anesthesia required great care and education, carried great responsibility, and required the significant exercise of judgement. The last major legal challenge to nurse anesthetists was the case of *Chalmers-Francis v. Nelson* (1936). A nurse anesthetist was again accused of the illegal practice of medicine and once more the court upheld the legality of nurse anesthesia practice.

In *Sermchief v. Gonzales* (1984), the Missouri Supreme Court gave an excellent analysis of the practice of nursing versus the practice of medicine. In 1975, Missouri had expanded its nurse practice act to create nurse practitioners. The Missouri Medical Registration Board challenged a group of nurses operating in a clinic, claiming that they were engaged in the illegal practice of medicine because they were diagnosing and prescribing, functions traditionally limited to physicians. Because the case coincided with the enactment of a number of statutes authorizing advanced practice nursing, there was a great deal of interest in the decision and the court stated that it had been asked to "define and draw that thin and elusive line which separates the practice of medicine from the practice of professional nursing in modern day delivery of health services" (p. 688). The court did not have to draw the line and instead relied on statutory interpretation. The court was satisfied that what the nurse practitioners were doing was within the powers that the legislature had intended nurse practitioners to have. Thus, the court felt that the nurse practitioners were working within their legislative scope of practice; that is, they were providing services the legislature intended as the practice of advanced nursing. The fact that the functions being performed by the nurse practitioners had previously been performed by physicians was irrelevant. What was important was that the nurses were acting within the scope of practice that the legislature had authorized.

This confusion regarding the scope of practice is often seen in anesthesia practice. It is fairly common for an anesthesiologist to begin an attack on nurse anesthesia by stating that "anesthesia is the practice of medicine." The statement is simplistic and irrelevant. The fact that anesthesia is the practice of medicine does not mean that nurse anesthetists cannot administer it (nor does it mean that dentists cannot administer it). What the anesthesiologist may mean is that anesthesia is *exclusively* the practice of medicine which, of course, is incorrect because every state permits nurse anesthetists to administer anesthesia. What may also add to the physician's confusion is that medical practice acts frequently permit physicians to delegate medical functions to nonphysicians. In addition to statutory authorization permitting physicians to delegate, many states have enacted statutes specifically recognizing nurse anesthesia. Even in the most restrictive state, the physician is required only to supervise, not control, the nurse anesthetist. Historically, nurse anesthetists knew more about anesthesia than their supervising physician. The scope of practice of a nurse anesthetist is not dependent on delegation from a physician.

Nurse anesthesia dates back to the 1880s. *Frank v. South* (1917) was one of several cases brought by state medical societies to challenge the practice of nurse anesthesia. *Frank v. South* demonstrated that claims regarding the illegal practice of medicine could be successfully defended on the grounds that administering anesthesia was similar to other generally accepted nursing functions. To the extent that any medical acts were involved, the nurse anesthetist was working with a physician and the physician was "supervising" the nurse anesthetist in any medical aspects. This approach to defending attacks on nurse anesthesia—that the nurse was working under the supervision of, or at the direction of the surgeon— became the cornerstone of a defense to ward off attacks on nurse anesthesia by seeking state legislation. Consequently, after *Frank v. South* a number of statutes recognizing nurse anesthesia were introduced in state legislatures. Sometimes the statute was an amendment to the medical practice act and sometimes it was part of the nursing practice act. But a number of states enacted statutes permitting a nurse anesthetist to administer anesthesia under the supervision or direction of a physician.

▶ SUPERVISION

What is the nature of supervision required in nurse anesthesia practice acts? At the time the statutes were adopted, nurse anesthetists were acknowledged by those who were supervising them to be more knowledgeable, to get better results, and to have better techniques than the physician supervisor. There are very few legal cases that deal with the question of supervision. Because courts tend to defer to the health care system, they seldom disagree with procedures the health care community is comfortable with. In *Brown v. Allen Sanitarium, Inc.* (1978), an intermediate court relied on expert testimony as to custom in the health care community. The plaintiff had argued that the physician was negligent in failing to properly supervise the anesthesia administered by a nurse anesthetist and in permitting the anesthetist to select the drug to be used. There was expert testimony "that after the supervising physician decides the patient is suited for a general anesthetic, it is customary to rely on the anesthetist to decide which drugs are most suited for the particular situation. There is no evidence of any improper selection or administration of drugs...." (p. 664) by the nurse anesthetist. The court held that even though the physician did not specifically direct the nurse anesthetist in the selection and method of application of the drugs used, the physician was, nonetheless, providing the required statutory supervision. "[W]e do not interpret the statute to require the degree of supervision over a person possessing the skill and training of a registered nurse-anesthetist as that contented by appellants," (p. 665).

In *Gore v. United States* (1964), the plaintiff's claim was based in part on the fact that the surgeon was not at the operating table when the anesthetic was administered by a nurse anesthetist. The court determined that under Michigan law, treating physicians, surgeons or nurse anesthetists were responsible for unfortunate results when and only when, it was shown that they departed from the standard in the community of treatment and care by skilled doctors and nurses. The court indicated that there was testimony that it was common practice that a surgeon need not be in the operating room when a nurse anesthetist administered the anesthetic.

The Joint Commission on the Accreditation of Healthcare Organizations (JCAHO) does not require that a supervising physician have any particular substantive knowledge of anesthesia. Under JCAHO requirements, a supervising physician must be responsible for only three things: (1) the anesthesia care of the patient; (2) the determination that the patient is an appropriate candidate to undergo the planned anesthesia; and (3) the decision to discharge the patient after anesthesia.

Statutes recognizing nurse anesthesia practice, some of which placed nurse anesthetists under the supervision of the surgeon, appear to have been successful in stopping medicine's legal attacks on nurse anesthesia as the practice of medicine. But in the mid-1980s competition between anesthesiologists and nurse anesthetists intensified and with it, a renewed attack on nurse anesthesia practice. For a period of time, it became fashionable for some anesthesiologists to market themselves to surgeons by claiming that a surgeon was liable for the negligence of the nurse anesthetist but was not liable for the negligence of an anesthesiologist. Liability of surgeons for the negligence for those with whom they work in an operating room has had a long and complicated history.

Charitable Immunity

In 1876 the Massachusetts Supreme Court decided the case of *McDonald v. Massachusetts General Hospital*. In this case, the patient claimed that he had been damaged by the actions of a doctor on the staff of Massachusetts General Hospital. The patient was receiving free care at a hospital whose funds were derived from grants and charity. The Massachusetts court was concerned that if hospitals were liable for the negligence for those who worked within them, the good that hospitals did would be lost and the benefactors of hospitals would be unwilling to make donations to an institution when their charitable gifts could be used to pay recoveries in malpractice suits. The Massachusetts court reasoned that the hospital was similar to a government and just as the government enjoyed immunity from tort actions (so-called *sovereign immunity*), so should the hospital. This theory became known as *charitable immunity*.

"Captain of the Ship"

If the hospital could not be held liable for negligence of persons on its staff, then who would bear the financial burden of negligence? The choices were the person who was negligent—sometimes a nurse who seldom had the resources to compensate patients, the patient—who was totally innocent, or the surgeon. The courts were reluctant to deny patients any recourse for the damage they incurred and developed a theory that had, as its keystone, the fact that hospitals had been created for the benefit of the surgeon. The surgeon, normally the wealthiest and most controlling person in the operating room, came to be seen as the central figure. He was, in the words of one court "like the captain of a ship." Even though the nurses might be employees of the hospital, they were "borrowed servants" of the surgeon and the surgeon was liable for their negligence because as the "Captain of the Ship" he was liable for anything that occurred "on the ship," that is, in the course of the operation.

The doctrine of "Captain of the Ship" was first introduced into the law of negligence by the case of *McConnell v. Williams* (1949). An obstetrician had asked an intern to care for the newborn. The intern placed too much silver nitrate into the infant's eyes causing damage.

Suit was brought against the obstetrician on behalf of the child, even though there was no evidence that the obstetrician himself was negligent. The incident had occurred during the course of the obstetrician's intended treatment. The obstetrician had chosen the intern, an indication of the obstetrician's control, and finally the obstetrician testified that he had "complete control" of the operating room and of every person within it while the operation was in progress.

Under "Captain of the Ship" there were a number of activities of nurses for which surgeons would not be responsible. In some states, courts began to distinguish between "medical" duties where the physician was liable and "administrative" duties where only the hospital was liable. The surgeon was not liable for the nurse's negligence during preoperative or postoperative procedures. Distinctions between administrative and medical duties, artificial to begin with, did not prove as clear as had been hoped. In 1957 the courts in the state of New York began to move away from the position that surgeons were automatically liable for anything which occurred within the operating room. Gradually, the courts began to see that despite what the surgeon said, and perhaps believed, surgeons did not control everything during an operation. Modern operations are so complicated and the nature of health care personnel in the modern operating room so specialized that surgeons can no longer claim to be in complete control, if indeed they ever were. A recognition that proper health care depends on cooperation and collaboration was the main reason for the decline of the "Captain of the Ship" legal doctrine.

When "Captain of the Ship" prevailed, anesthesiologists, when they were present, were often poorly paid employees of hospitals and themselves not attractive targets for plaintiff's malpractice claims. Surgeons were held liable for the negligence of anesthesiologists just as they were for nurse anesthetists. In fact, the principles that govern the liability of a surgeon for the negligence of an anesthetist are the same whether the anesthetist is an anesthesiologist or a nurse anesthetist. Even as "Captain of the Ship" began to be replaced with a factual *test* of control rather than the *assumption* of control, the principles governing liability continued to be the same whether the anesthetist was a nurse anesthetist or an anesthesiologist.

In those states that require nurse anesthetists to be supervised by a physician, is the physician liable for their negligence? First, the liability of a supervising physician is based on whether the physician controlled the procedure that caused the damage. For example, in *Baird v. Sickler* (1982) the Supreme Court of Ohio held that a surgeon could be liable for injuries attributable to anesthesia. The patient had a number of back problems which made for a difficult intubation. While a nurse anesthetist performed the actual insertion of the tube which caused the damage, the surgeon directed the intubation, helped position the patient and during testimony, admitted that he had the right to control the procedure. Supervision in state statutes does not require control and supervising physicians are not *necessarily* liable for the negligence of nurse anesthetists. In *Baird v. Sickler,* the surgeon was liable because the surgeon was in control of the procedure, not because the statute required the surgeon to supervise. Second, surgeons can also control acts of an anesthesiologist and surgeons have been held liable for the negligence of anesthesiologists under the same principles as they may have liability for the negligence of a nurse anesthetist. If the anesthetist in *Baird v. Sickler* had been an anesthesiologist, the surgeon would have been just as liable. Third, the surgeon's liability depends on the particular facts of the situation. As a practical matter, the surgeon is likely to be included in any law suit whether the surgeon was working with a nurse anesthetist or an anesthesiologist.

Although the principles are the same, the cases have different outcomes depending on how much control the surgeon may have exercised in one case as compared to the amount of control in another. The issue, however, is not the status of the anesthesia provider that determines liability, but the amount of control the surgeon exercises.

▶ MALPRACTICE

Although anesthesia has become safer, it is not risk-free. Anesthesia providers are human and despite extensive monitoring and the constant emphasis on vigilance, sometimes there is a lapse and an anesthetist does something which ought not to have been done or neglects to do something that should have been done. This failure, or "neglect," is referred to as "negligence." In addition to situations where the provider does something wrong, anesthesia has become so safe that when something goes wrong, even without negligence, the injured party sometimes expects the anesthetist to pay for it.

A malpractice case has four elements: duty, breach, cause, and damage.

- **Duty:** What was the duty owed by the practitioner to the patient? First, was the injured a patient? If so, the nurse anesthetist must provide a level of care that other nurse anesthetists would provide in the same situation.
- **Breach:** Did the nurse anesthetist provide the level of care required? In anesthesia, terrible things can happen, even without fault. Just because something happened does not mean there was a breach of the standard of care.
- **Cause:** Was the breach the cause of the injury? The nurse anesthetist has many obligations and

things to keep track of during the administration of an anesthetic. The failure to obtain an adequate history of malignant hypothermia would be a breach of the standard of care but it would be irrelevant if the patient died of massive internal bleeding.
- **Damage:** What damage was caused by the breach?

All of these elements must be proven before the plaintiff will be allowed to recover.

The duty that the health care provider owes to a patient is to at least provide the care that another provider with the same education and background would provide under similar circumstances. How does one go about finding out what this standard is? Anesthesia is unique in the health care field because not only are there two distinct types of practitioners, anesthesiologists and nurse anesthetists, but the practitioners do the same thing and are completely interchangeable. Normally, physician specialties and nursing specialties set their own standards of care. In anesthesia, the standard of care is set by practitioners from both professions. That is, there is only one standard of care in anesthesia and this standard must be adhered to by both anesthesiologists and nurse anesthetists. In *Webb v. Jorns* (1971), an expert was testifying as to whether there had been an overdose of an anesthetic. The testimony that was introduced was not testimony concerning what a nurse anesthetist should have done, it was testimony that there had been an overdose. Thus, the standard by which negligence is judged is what happens in anesthesia, not one which focuses on whether nurse anesthetists follow standards which may be different than those followed by anesthesiologists. There are many malpractice cases in which physicians testify against nurse anesthetists as to the standard of care in anesthesia, not the standard of care to be followed by nurse anesthetists. One can also find cases in which nurse anesthetists are permitted to testify as to the standard of care (see *Young v. Department of Health and Human Resources,* 1981) not only as it applies to nurse anesthetists but as it applies to anesthesiologists as well (*Carolan v. Hill,* 1996).

▶ SOURCES OF THE STANDARD OF CARE

In general, as a profession, nurse anesthetists set their own standard of care. The standard of care is what other nurse anesthetists would do in similar circumstances. There are other sources of the standard of care. The primary source is governmental. Licensing laws are themselves standards of care and often authorize the regulatory body—in the case of nurse anesthetists, the Board of

Nursing—to issue rules and regulations that constitute a part of the standard of care. Criminal statutes regulate the behavior of all citizens. Criminal proceedings may only be enforced by a government. However, a violation of a criminal statute applicable to a professional's practice almost always means that the practitioner has violated the standard of care. If someone violates a standard of care set by a criminal statute, the victim can often use the criminal statute as proof of the standard of care. In many states, indifference to one's obligations or actions which show "reckless" indifference to human safety is criminal. There have been news reports of anesthesia personnel (fortunately, not nurse anesthetists) being prosecuted for repeatedly falling asleep while administering anesthesia or administering anesthesia in settings so ill equipped as to evidence a lack of concern for the patient's safety.

Although nurse anesthetists are advanced practice nurses, they are first nurses and standards applicable to all nurses are, by definition, applicable to nurse anesthetists as well. Perhaps the prime example of a general nursing standard applicable to nurse anesthesia is the requirement that nursing services be rendered to all who are in need without regard to background or illness. Another such standard would be the obligation to maintain the confidentiality of information given in the course of treatment.

Nurses also have a duty to independently exercise their professional judgement within their respective scopes of practice. Nurses are expected to do more than be ordered about by physicians. In *Lunsford v. Board of Nurse Examiners for the State of Texas* (1983), a patient arrived at a hospital complaining of chest pain. He was seen by a nurse who was instructed by a physician to send the patient to another hospital. The nurse established that the patient had not eaten anything unusual but she failed to take the patient's vital signs. She then ordered the patient and the patient's companion to drive 24 miles to the next closest hospital. She understood the seriousness of the patient's condition. She had asked if the patient's companion knew cardiopulmonary resuscitation (CPR) because there was a chance that he would have to use it en route to the hospital. The Texas Board of Nurse Examiners suspended the nurse's license because the Board found that the nurse's conduct was unprofessional and dishonorable. The suspension of the nurse's license was based on her failure to carry out her "duty to evaluate the medical status of the ailing person seeking his or her professional care, and to institute appropriate nursing care to stabilize a patient's condition and prevent further complications of physical and mental harm" (p. 395).

A similar conclusion was reached in *Norton v. Argonaut Insurance Company* (1962). A physician had prescribed a dosage of medication. The nurse was unaware that the medication could be taken orally. She thought it was to be taken by injection and she thought it was a very high dosage. She conferred with another doctor who advised her to follow the prescribing physician's order, which she did. When the patient subsequently died from an overdose, the court held that the nurse should have known that the dosage was incorrect for the method of administering the drug and should have refrained from administering the drug until she had received clarification from the prescribing physician. In this case, even though the nurse believed that she was acting on the doctor's orders, she was held negligent.

The American Association of Nurse Anesthetists (AANA) issues a number of standards affecting practice. Although these standards do not in and of themselves become standards of practice simply because they are issued by the AANA, they reflect the deliberations of nurse anesthetists and purport to set forth what the majority of nurse anesthetists believe. Therefore, they become evidence of the standard of care. Pronouncements by the JCAHO and other accrediting bodies are also evidence of the standard of care because of the expertise of these agencies in the health care field. Hospitals often issue their own requirements and although a hospital requirement does not automatically become a standard of care, it can become binding on hospital personnel and their patients as part of a "contract" between the hospital and the community.

The prime source of the standard of care of nurse anesthetists remains anesthesia personnel themselves. In some cases, health care professionals need only follow practices and procedures observed in their community. In specialty areas, which include anesthesia, practitioners are presumed to be aware of practices and procedures followed across the country. Therefore, in specialty areas such as anesthesia, the standard of care is country-wide.

Practitioners should be aware that although standards are set by practitioners, the standard is part of the facts of a case and is determined by the finder of fact (either the jury or the trial judge). The finder of fact has the benefit of hindsight and may also have sympathy for the injured. In *Washington v. Washington Hospital Center* (1990), the issue became whether end-tidal CO_2 monitors were part of the standard of care in 1987. Many people involved in anesthesia believe that end-tidal CO_2 monitors were *not* the standard of care in 1987. Nonetheless, the plaintiff was able to find an expert who testified that they were part of the standard of care, as well as evidence showing use of end-tidal CO_2 by certain hospitals. The jury decided in favor of the plaintiff and on appeal the court would not overturn the jury decision because the standard of care is factual and, on appeal, courts defer to the jury on factual matters, unless clearly erroneous.

► EXCEPTIONS TO THE NEED TO PROVE NEGLIGENCE

Because of the need to provide expert testimony, an anesthesia malpractice case can be expensive to try and uncertain in outcome. Therefore, malpractice attorneys frequently look for short cuts to avoid the expense and difficulty of presenting a malpractice case. Two of these shortcuts are the doctrines of *res ipsa loquitur* and *negligence per se.*

Res Ipsa Loquitur

Res ipsa loquitur, or "the thing speaks for itself" holds that under certain circumstances the mere fact that the damage occurs is sufficient proof of negligence without requiring the plaintiff to have to prove a specific act of negligence. There are three elements to a *res ipsa loquitur* claim: (1) the injury occurred under circumstances such as in the ordinary course of events the injury would not have occurred if someone had not been negligent; (2) the injury must be caused by something in the exclusive control of the defendant; and (3) the injury must not have been due to any voluntary action or contribution on the part of the plaintiff. Anesthesia cases are prime examples of this doctrine because the plaintiff is unconscious during the procedure, unable to observe the negligence, and incapable of causing his or her own injury.

Negligence Per Se

When the parties fail to comply with a statute designed for the protection of citizens, it is not necessary that actual negligence be proven; negligence is assumed. This doctrine is known as *negligence per se.* In 1985, the Georgia Supreme Court decided the *Worthy* (1985) case. In 1981, a day after giving birth, Ms. Worthy underwent a tubal ligation. Her anesthesia was administered by a student nurse anesthetist being supervised by a physician assistant. Ms. Worthy went into cardiac arrest and although it was never clear that there was any negligence involved, suit was brought against the hospital and anesthesia group. The Georgia statute at the time permitted a CRNA to administer anesthesia only "under the direction and responsibility of a duly licensed physician with training or experience in anesthesia." Whether or not it is good practice to have a student nurse anesthetist supervised by a physician assistant, it is clear that the physician assistant was not "a duly licensed physician with training or experience in anesthesia." Because the hospital had violated a statute designed for the safety and protection of citizens, the Georgia Supreme Court ruled that this was negligence *per se.* The plaintiff did not need further proof of negligence and it was up to the hospital to establish that it was not negligent. The legal principle of negligence *per se* holds that the violation of a statute which creates a standard of conduct is sufficient, by itself, to establish negligence.

Does negligence *per se* apply to a violation of hospital requirements? Although hospital requirements can be used as evidence of negligence, their violation is not negligence *per se* in the same manner that violation of the statute is. However, the courts will consider hospital requirements as part of a hospital's agreement with a patient and a violation of these requirements can be used as evidence that the hospital failed in its duty to a patient. In *Williams v. St. Claire Medical Center* (1983), the hospital had a by-law that provided that anesthesia was to be administered only by a CRNA or a qualified physician. The hospital, contrary to its own policies, permitted a recently graduated nurse anesthetist who had not yet taken the certification exam to administer anesthesia. The patient suffered permanent brain damage even though there was no evidence of negligence. The court held that when a patient consents to and authorizes an operation, the patient accepts the rules and regulations of the particular hospital and should be able to rely on the hospital to follow its own rules. The plaintiff argued that the hospital's violation constituted negligence *per se* but the court refused to extend negligence *per se* to the hospital's policies. However, the plaintiff could introduce the fact that the policies had been violated as evidence of negligence.

In *Harris v. Miller* (1994) and *Denton Regional Medical Center v. LaCroix* (1997), the hospitals' anesthesia departments had adopted policies that restricted the practice of CRNAs. The restrictions, primarily requirements of anesthesiologist supervision, did not improve patient care and were ignored. When an unfortunate event occurred, even though there was no evidence of negligence, the plaintiff's attorney argued that the hospital's failure to comply with its own anesthesia policies was evidence of the hospital's failure to comply with its duty of care.

On the other hand, hospital policies must appear to be for the benefit of patients. In *Herrington v. Hiller* (1989), the United States Court of Appeals for the 5th Circuit sent a case back for a new trial holding that a hospital may be liable to patients for damages when it failed to provide around the clock anesthesia services because of political reasons (the anesthesiologists were following guidelines suggested by the American Society of Anesthesiologists). The court said that a jury should have been allowed to determine whether a hospital's refusal to provide 24-hour anesthesia coverage (because it would have meant that CRNAs would have to give regional anesthesia) was medically sound practice or was motivated by political purposes. Not only do anti-CRNA regulations cause problems in the medical malpractice area when they are not followed, but when they are followed and they keep hospitals from providing proper patient care, the hospital can also be attacked.

▶ OTHER IMPORTANT LEGAL CONCEPTS

Informed Consent

In the law of *torts,* any unconsented touching constitutes a *battery.* Because surgery requires that the patient's body be touched, any surgery must have the patient's consent. Any surgery to which a patient or the patient's legal guardian has not consented is a battery. Justice Cardozo wrote "Every human being of adult years and sound mind has a right to determine what shall be done with his own body; and the surgeon who performs an operation without his patient's consent commits an assault for which he is liable for damages" (*Schloendorff v. The Society of the New York Hospital* 1914, p. 129). This decision was overruled on other grounds in *Bing v. Thunig* (1957). Not every risk must be disclosed; only those which are foreseeable. Although the initial development of the doctrine of informed consent required disclosure only of what other health care professionals disclosed, the more modern view has been to look at informed consent from the viewpoint of the patient. What would a reasonable patient want to know about the proposed operation? Generally, the elements of information that are required for consent are the patient's diagnosis, the general nature of the contemplated procedure, the risks involved, the prospects of success, the prognosis if the procedure is not performed, and alternative methods of treatment available, if any. It is important to note that the duty to disclose is measured by the amount of knowledge the patient needs. The health care professional need not disclose rare or unproven reactions to a procedure, although adverse consequences with a frequency of even less than one percent may not be considered rare. Some reasonable weighing of risk versus reward must be considered.

Informed consent does not protect the practitioner against a practitioner's negligence. Informing patients that a practitioner can be negligent may be valuable in avoiding a charge of a battery but it does nothing to protect the practitioner in a medical malpractice case.

Abandonment

The relationship of health care worker and patient, once initiated, continues until it is ended by the consent of the parties, revoked by the dismissal of the health care worker, or the health care worker's services are no longer needed. Until that point, the health care worker is under a duty to continue to provide necessary care to the patient. A health care worker who *abandons* the patient at a critical stage is guilty of abandonment. Although the concept of abandonment is a fairly new one and is a developing concept, the courts consider a number of factors in determining abandonment. These include a lack of good faith, a lack of justification, and a weighing of the efforts that were made to obtain a competent substitute.

Punitive Damages

Damages based on the "value" of the injury caused, even if difficult to value, are called *compensatory.* If the wrongdoing has been intentional or gives the court a sense of outrage, the courts have permitted juries to award *punitive* or *exemplary damages.* Something more than mere negligence is required to incur punitive damages; there must be circumstances of aggravation, spite or malice, a fraudulent or evil motive, or conscious disregard of the interests of others. Punitive damages are private fines imposed to punish reprehensible conduct and deter its future occurrence. In a case involving a hospital in Georgia, the court overturned a jury award of punitive damages where apparently the jury believed that the nurse anesthetist had permitted the anesthesia machine to run out of anesthetic agent. In *Air Co., Inc. v. Simons First National Bank, Guardian* (1982), the court upheld a jury award against a manufacturer of a ventilator that had been so poorly designed that an anesthesia provider was unaware that a hose had been placed where a bag should have been. The ensuing build up of pressure and lack of oxygen resulted in damage to the patient's lungs and brain. The court reasoned that manufacturers of machines used to administer anesthesia should be careful not to design their machines so that an ordinary user would cause damage.

Statutes of Limitation

All states have statutes that require that lawsuits be brought within a certain period of time. These are referred to as *statutes of limitation.* Their purpose is to reduce the unfairness of defending actions after a substantial period of time has elapsed. With the passage of time, memories fade and documents are lost. A defendant will have greater difficulty defending a law suit 10 to 15 years after an event than within 2 or 3 years. Moreover, the law favors stability. The legal system seeks to avoid the disruption resulting from longstanding threats of legal action. While time periods differ from state to state, a 3-year time period for negligence actions is found in many states. There are exceptions to statute of limitations. One is where the plaintiff is under a disability which keeps the plaintiff from bringing the suit. Typical of these are cases involving children or persons under some kind of legal guardianship. The second exception is where the plaintiff may not have been able to discover that there was an injury caused by negligence before the statute of limitations expired.

Professional Liability Insurance

Every CRNA should have professional liability insurance. The insurance policy should define the risks the company will assume for a specific level of premium paid by the anesthesia provider. Liability insurance may be paid by the CRNA or their employer. In some cases, a hospital or large employer may *self insure*. It is essential for the nurse anesthetist to fully understand the terms of the policy including the policy period and conditions of the policy. Professional liability insurance policies can be "occurrence," which cover all claims arising during the policy period, or "claims made," which provide coverage for only those claims instituted during the policy period. The latter type of policy requires an extended endorsement or, *tail insurance,* be purchased with the insurance carrier to cover claims filed outside of the policy period if the CRNA changes insurance carriers. Most policies grant the insurance carrier the power to effect a settlement whenever it deems necessary. This often requires the consent of the insured CRNA. In addition, legal counsel will be appointed should the CRNA be involved in a litigation. Professional liability policies often require that when the CRNA becomes aware of an incident which may result in malpractice litigation, the insurance carrier should be notified immediately.

► SUMMARY

Because lawyers and judges do not understand what nurse anesthetists do, the courts defer to nurse anesthetists. Nurse anesthetists are professionals who create their own standard of care. They are allowed considerable leeway when statutes affecting them must be interpreted.

On the other hand, because lawyers and judges are not familiar with nurse anesthesia practice, they may make mistakes or come to incorrect conclusions about nurse anesthesia. While lawyers may be helpful, the experts on legal aspects of nurse anesthesia are nurse anesthetists.

► CASE STUDY

Margaret Hatfield is the most popular anesthetist in Jefferson County. Dr. Smith, a successful surgeon, asked her to provide the anesthetic to his wife while she had their second child. The obstetrician was Dr. Brown. Having helped at the birth of their first child, Margaret Hatfield did not bother evaluating Mrs. Smith's health history for the anesthetic complication, malignant hyperthermia. During the scheduled cesarean section, Mrs. Smith's blood pressure reached 200 before decreasing to an acceptable level following appropriate treatment. Dr. Smith, who was present, became visibly upset when Mrs. Smith became hypertensive during delivery and subsequently sued Dr. Brown for pain and suffering.

1. Does Dr. Brown assume more liability depending on whether Margaret Hatfield is an anesthesiologist or a nurse anesthetist?

   The legal principles governing the liability of a surgeon for an anesthetist are the same whether the anesthetist is a nurse anesthetist or an anesthesiologist. Here, the breach in the standard of care—the failure to explore the history of malignant hyperthermia—had no effect on the patient's hypertension and was not the *cause* of the injury, one of four essential elements of any malpractice case. Moreover, Dr. Smith, who suffered the injury, was not the patient and Margaret Hatfield owed no *duty* (a second essential element of malpractice) to him.

► KEY CONCEPTS

- The legal system defers to nurse anesthetists by permitting them to establish their own standard of care.
- The legal system has a variety of methods to regulate nurse anesthetists' conduct through statutes, regulations, criminal law, and tort law.
- Although anesthesia is administered by both nursing and physician specialists, there is only one standard of care in anesthesia.
- When administered by nurse anesthetists, anesthesia is the practice of nursing; when administered by anesthesiologists, anesthesia is the practice of medicine.

- In those states or in those circumstances where nurse anesthetists are supervised by physicians, the physician's liability for the negligence of a nurse anesthetist depends on whether the physician controlled the procedure which caused the damage.
- Control is a level of supervision not required by statutes nor by practice.
- The liability of a surgeon for the negligence of an anesthesiologist is determined by the same legal principles as those governing the liability of a surgeon for the negligence of a nurse anesthetist.

▶ STUDY QUESTIONS

1. In what ways do nurse anesthetists benefit by their treatment in the American legal system and in what ways do they suffer?

2. How does the American legal system differ in its treatment of nurse anesthetists and anesthesiologists?

3. One of the surgeons in your hospital is held liable for a negligent intubation performed by a nurse anesthetist. Will the rest of the surgeons in your hospital also be liable for the negligence of other nurse anesthetists?

4. If nurse anesthetists set their own standard of care, are there circumstances when two nurse anesthetists can do exactly the same thing and yet one be found negligent and the other not?

5. What steps can hospitals and surgeons take to reduce their risks of being sued for anesthesia incidents?

KEY REFERENCES

Blumenreich, G. A. (1983–Present). Legal briefs. In each issue of *AANA Journal.*

Prosser & Keeton. (1984). *The law of torts.* St. Paul, MN: West Publishing Co.

Sermchief v. Gonzales, 660 S.W.2d 683 (Missouri, 1984).

REFERENCES

Air Co., Inc. v. Simons First National Bank, Guardian, (276 Ark. 486, 638 S.W.2d 660, 1982).

Baird v. Sickler, (69 Ohio St.2d 652, 433 N.E.2d 593, Ohio, 1982).

Bing v. Thunig, 143 N.E.2d 3 (New York, 1957).

Brown v. Allen Sanitarium, Inc., 364 So.2d 661 (La. Ct. App. 1978).

Butler v. Louisiana State Board of Education, 331 So.2d 192 (La. Ct. App. 1976).

Carolan v. Hill, 553 N.W. 2d 882 (Iowa, 1996).

In re Carpenter's Estate, 196 Mich. 561, 162 N.W. 963 (Michigan, 1917).

Chalmers-Francis v. Dagmar Nelson, 6 Cal.2d 402 (California, 1936).

Denton Regional Medical Center v. LaCroix, 947 S.W.2d 941 (1997).

Frank v. South, 175 Ky. 416 (Kentucky, 1917).

Gore v. United States, 229 F. Supp. 547 (1964).

Harris v. Miller, 438 S.E.2d 731 (North Carolina, 1994).

Herrington v. Hiller, 883 F.2d 411 (5th Cir. 1989).

Hiatt v. Groce, 523 P.2d 320 (Kansas, 1974).

Jefferson Parish Hospital v. Hyde, 466 U.S. 2 (1984).

Lunsford v. Board of Nurse Examiners for the State of Texas, 648 S.W.2d 391 (Tex. Ct. App. 3Dist. 1983).

McConnell v. Williams, 361 Pa. 355 (1949).

McDonald v. Massachusetts General Hospital, 120 Mass. 432 (Massachusetts, 1876).

Mohr v. Jenkins, 393 So. 2d 245 (La. Ct. App. 1980).

Norton v. Argonaut Insurance Company, 144 So.2d 249 (Louisiana, 1962).

Schloendorff v. The Society of the New York Hospital, 105 N.E. 92 (New York, 1914).

Sermchief v. Gonzales, 660 S.W. 2d 683 (Missouri, 1984).

Tremontozzi v. Safety Insurance Company (Massachusetts, 1991) No citation available.

Washington v. Washington Hospital Center, 579 A.2d 177 (DC Ct. App. 1990).

Webb v. Jorns, 473 S.W.2d 328 (Texas, 1971).

Williams v. St. Claire Medical Center, 67 S.W.2d 590 (Ken. Ct. App. 1983).

Worthy, 333 S.E.2d 829 (Georgia, 1985).

Young v. Department of Health and Human Resources, 405 So. 2D 1209 (La. Ct App. 1981).

Strategies for Learning in Graduate Education

Alfred E. Lupien

This chapter is unusual. While the majority of the book focuses on important clinical and professional topics, the following pages emphasize processes for enhancing learning potential. The body of knowledge we use as anesthesia practitioners grows so quickly that it out paces our ability to stay current. Through metacognition—or learning about learning—the collection, storage, and recall of information can be maximized.

Three themes dominate this chapter: individual characteristics of learners, learning as information processing, and strategies for specific educational activities. Sections and subsections are designed to be read independently. Concentrate on topics that provide the most benefit and skim the others. If nothing else, remember that optimal learning includes three distinct activities: a preparatory period where prior knowledge is activated, the actual learning session, and a postsession synthesis. The time to start is now! Survey the chapter, look at the topics, think about what is already familiar, and what you intend to accomplish as you read this section.

▶ LEARNERS AND LEARNING

Descriptions of learning styles abound in education and health care literature. *Kolb's Learning Inventory* has been used frequently to classify nurse anesthesia students and faculty. Individuals are characterized as *accommodators* who participate actively in the learning process and learn through actual experiences; *assimilators* who create abstract conceptual models; *convergers* who emphasize problem solving based on both conceptualization and experimentation; and *divergers* who use imagination to view situations from multiple perspectives (Kolb, 1976). In 1985 Ramsborg and Holloway reported differences in learning styles based on experience. Beginning anesthesia students were predominantly assimilators, whereas graduating students were mostly accommodators, and staff anesthetists were divergers. Sherbinski (1994) also found differences in learning styles among anesthesia students. Sherbinski reported no predominant learning style among beginning anesthesia students; however, assimilator and converger styles were prevalent among individuals who had completed more than 12 months of anesthesia education. Because neither study was longitudinal, it cannot be concluded directly that an individual's learning style changes over time as a result of anesthesia experience; however, the findings suggest that the process of education may contribute to an evolution of learning styles as an individual progresses from new student to expert clinician.

Less commonly used, but easier to understand, are the learner classifications of Biggs (1985). Biggs described three types of learning styles and motivations for learning: surface, deep, and achieving. *Surface learners* are task-oriented and use learning strategies such as memorization to acquire factual content with little regard for relating the new material to other information. They are characterized as continuously balancing the risk of failing with the reward of meeting minimum standards. The surface learner's motivational factors are external, and include the prospect of earning more money or obtaining a better job (Biggs, 1987). Although the surface learning style is typically "associated with poor academic performance" (Davis, 1988, p. 159), it is not uncommon for any type of learner to exhibit surface behaviors during stressful learning periods (Biggs, 1985).

The surface learner is contrasted sharply by the *deep learner* who studies for the sake of gaining new knowledge. Deep learners have varied interests, read widely, and relate new knowledge to previous knowledge in an attempt to improve understanding (Biggs, 1987). Although it would be expected that the deep learners would be outstanding students, deep learners often struggle to maintain high grades because their pursuit of knowledge is not constrained by the topics that are to be covered in the next lecture or test (Davis, 1988). As students, deep learners need to develop tightly-controlled regimens to assure that required class assignments have been completed. Because the deep learner emphasizes a broader conceptual approach to learning, it is easier to respond to open-ended theoretical issues and more difficult to focus on rote memorization.

Achieving learners seek external recognition for accomplishments. They are naturally competitive and strive to attain high grades regardless of whether they find the material interesting. The achieving learner possesses the learning style characteristics of both surface and deep learners and adopts whichever strategies are most effective in order to receive recognition. Because achieving learners sense teachers' expectations, they typically excel in the classroom (Davis, 1988).

Depending on the nature of a specific learning task, one individual may exhibit surface, deep, or achieving traits. Regardless of the learning situation, a learner is most successful when the individual's learning style and strategy are consistent with the material to be learned.

Beatrice (1995) differentiated between visual, auditory, and kinesthetic learners. Although there are self-tests available to determine an individual's learning style, a general indicator of learning style is how an individual would answer one question:

I learn best how to do something by:
  a) watching a demonstration.
  b) listening to a description.
  c) actually trying it.

Visual learners benefit from colorful written and pictorial study aids including note-taking, highlighting, and drawing. For visual learners, the learning environment should be free from distractions such as frequent movement and windows. *Auditory learners* need a quiet study place. They benefit from attending lectures, recording and replaying lectures, reciting study materials, and talking through steps in problem solving. Study groups where learners share information with others may also

be beneficial. *Kinesthetic learners* benefit from action. They use as many senses as possible when studying and benefit from short concentrated study periods. They may do well when studying with other kinesthetic learners.

The descriptions of learning styles from Biggs (1985) and Beatrice (1995) enable an individual to answer three important questions when entering into a learning situation.

1. What is the purpose of this learning session? Learning efficiency is increased when the learner is able to identify the "end-product" of a study session and devise a study plan specifically tailored to produce the desired result (Brown, Bransford, Ferrara, & Campione, 1983, p. 104).
2. What type of learning strategies are necessary to achieve the desired outcome? If the situation requires rote memorization for recall on an examination in the near future, then the learner should focus on techniques that facilitate memorization. If the situation requires understanding a complex phenomenon then strategies for deep learning are required.
3. Once the learning requirements are identified, what task-specific study strategies can be adopted that are consistent with the individual's personal learning style? For example, the study of volatile anesthetics requires both the memorization of many physical characteristics (such as minimum alveolar concentration, vapor pressure, and various partition coefficients for each agent) and an understanding of how each of the characteristics influences the behavior of that particular anesthetic. To learn the physical characteristics of the agents, a visually-oriented learner might construct flash cards to review the specific values. The auditory learner may create an audio tape or continuously recite the same information. A kinesthetic learner may use some of the same study strategies, but combine study with a physical activity such as walking or riding an exercise bicycle.

Note that assessment of the learning situation precedes the actual time for learning. By the time the learner becomes actively involved in the learning session, the individual must already have an understanding of the outcomes the learning session is to produce.

Motivation

Learning is an active process that requires a substantial commitment to achieve the desired outcomes. Motivation is defined as the initiation and sustainment of goal-directed behavior (Schunk, 1991). In academic settings there are frequently sufficient external influences, such as the fear of failing the next test, to entice a student to study. Even in this situation, however, there is no assurance that the forced study is efficient or maximal. Through a process of self-regulated learning, an individual can activate and sustain behaviors oriented toward accomplishment of academic goals (Schunk, 1991). The myriad of theories and strategies for self-regulation can be condensed into four component activities: monitoring, production, mediation, and reinforcement.

Self-monitoring requires the designation of key activities and then monitoring the actual conduct of the specified activities. For example, an individual who tends to become distracted during designated study sessions may set a timer to ring at frequent random intervals. When the timer sounds, the individual should be engaged in the study task rather than participating in an unrelated activity. Although emphasis is placed on self-monitoring especially for adult learners, monitoring is effective whether it is self-imposed or externally administered. An example of external monitoring would be having a study partner or friend periodically check to see if the student is engaged in the specified study activity.

Advanced self-monitoring techniques require the learner to set specific learning goals and then evaluate whether the goals are achieved. Goal setting is generally more effective than the monitoring of fundamental behaviors such as number of hours of study time; however, results are influenced by the individual's ability to set challenging attainable goals.

Production is the designation of specific activities intended to achieve a particular result. For example, if the goal of a study session is to understand how changes in carbon dioxide and oxygen tensions affect the partial pressure of the other gas at the end organ and alveolus (Bohr and Haldane effects), then production activities focus on evaluation of the educational task, that is, to describe the interrelationship between the two gases. Production activities include reading passages from several texts, drawing pictures, summarizing, and paraphrasing to include the interrelationships. Upon completion of the learning activities, there must be a determination of whether the material is understood. If not, specific new productions are identified.

The ability to accomplish the task-relevant activities is termed *mediation*. In most circumstances, an inability to achieve a desired educational outcome is related to difficulty with either production or mediation (Schunk, 1991). *Reinforcement* is the addition of an event or consequence following an activity that results in an increased likelihood that the original behavior will occur again (Rothstein, 1990). For example, an individual might decide to reward herself with a new pair of jeans if she earns an "A" on a pharmacology test. Although there is am-

ple data to substantiate the benefit of reinforcement, it is less clear whether self-reinforcement is more effective than "externally administered" rewards (Schunk, 1991).

Time Management

Even for the most motivated individual, studying will not be effective unless sufficient time is allocated. It is critical to maximize opportunities for study especially during periods of intense commitments, such as preparing to become a nurse anesthetist.

Beatrice (1995) identifies 12 principles for effective time management. Although directed toward undergraduate college students, the principles have merit for all professionals.

1. Know times for peak performance and study at best times. Some individuals concentrate best in the morning, others in the evening, and so forth.
2. Study in an area that is free from distraction. Depending on an individual's learning style, avoiding particular distractors such as sights or sounds may be particularly important. If there will be distractions at home, find a place to study at work or the university. Equip the environment with appropriate lighting, reference materials, and supplies, as needed.
3. Schedule sufficient time. Allow a minimum of 2 hours of study for every hour of class. Difficult courses may require more time.
4. Study subjects consistently. Schedule the same subject at the same time each day and devote the allotted time to the subject, regardless of whether an actual assignment is pending.
5. Study difficult subjects when rested and better able to concentrate. If it is difficult to get into a study mode, briefly review an enjoyable subject, then concentrate on difficult material.
6. Study similar subjects several hours apart. To avoid the tedium of repetitive tasks, such as copious reading, intersperse with subjects requiring writing or computing. Alternatively, some individuals prefer organizing by activity, concentrating on all the reading, then writing, computing, and so forth.
7. Use study breaks effectively. Every hour take a short (10-minute) break. Take care of something that was distracting during study time, stretch, get something to eat or drink, or do something spontaneous to relieve stress. Avoid involvement in activities that are time consuming such as watching television, playing computer games, or engaging in conversation. After every 2 hours of study, take an hour-long

break to enhance productivity when returning to work.

8. Review before class. Look over previous notes and begin concentrating on lecture subject before class begins.

9. Review new material as soon as possible after class. Recall of information decreases as much as 50% after one hour. Set aside at least 15 minutes to review notes.

10. For ongoing courses, distribute study over the week. Use weekends to even the weekday workload.

11. Use wasted periods efficiently. Prepare short subject packets and review these materials while waiting for an appointment, or between classes and surgical cases.

12. Schedule leisure time daily. Leisure activities reduce stress and facilitate concentration. Through proper planning, there can be time for both study and leisure.

Students may want to construct a term calendar listing academic responsibilities such as exams, papers, projects, and so forth. Use these obligations to develop a study plan for specific activities that will be carried forward to weekly and daily schedules.

On a weekly schedule, note fixed obligations, such as work or class, church, family responsibilities, meals, and so on; then identify blocks of time for study. Schedule specific topics for each study period. Compute study time for each course and assure that time is consistent with course requirements. Place the schedule in a prominent place and use it. Beatrice (1995) admonishes, "you must begin to build your life around your education instead of building education around your life" (p. 38).

A daily "to do" list of home-, school-, and job-related tasks to be accomplished may facilitate the timely completion of all activities and obligations. Large tasks should be divided into smaller parts that can be accomplished on a daily basis. Items that are not completed should be carried over as priorities for the following day. If all requirements to finish a task are not available, avoid doing a task half-way. Wait until all information or materials are available, then act once to complete the activity (Winston, 1994).

Goal Setting

The time management classification system described by Covey, Merrill, and Merrill (1994) facilitates goal setting and the establishment of priorities to be included in the daily and weekly schedules. Activities are divided into four quadrants along two axes: *urgency* and *importance*. In the first quadrant are activities that are both important and urgent. Examples include crises and projects with deadlines such as planning for the following day's anes-

thetics and academic papers. In the second quadrant are important activities that are not urgent. Included in this quadrant are planning for future activities and general personal and professional development. Quadrant three activities are urgent, but not important and include many interruptions such as telephone calls and meetings. Urgency creates an illusion of importance; however, if quadrant three activities are important, it is because they are important to someone else. The misplaced importance creates the illusion that many third quadrant activities are actually first quadrant priorities. The final quadrant consists of activities that are neither important or urgent. The authors term this the "quadrant of waste" (Covey and coworkers, 1989, p. 38). Although we should not dwell in the fourth quadrant, we often escape the turmoil of quadrant one and three activities and retreat to nonproductive behaviors.

From descriptions of the four quadrants, it becomes apparent why Covey, Merrill, and Merrill term the second quadrant "the quadrant of quality" (p. 37). It is in this area of activity that an individual is able to progress beyond absolute requirements and focus on activities for maximal learning and self-promotion. Ideally, quadrant one and three activities are well-managed and controlled so that an individual spends a significant amount of time in quadrant two.

A well-conceived study plan optimizes important activities and minimizes unimportant activities. Covey (1989) describes seven habits of effective individuals. The second habit is to Begin with the End in Mind.™ Applying this principle to study activities suggests that learning will be more effective when specific goals are established for each study session. Although "time on task" is the focus of a scheduling strategy, establishing realistic, attainable goals is necessary to maximize time resources. McLravy (1993b) suggests scheduling study time in terms of assignments rather than fixed time intervals: establishing daily objectives, monitoring for completion, and adjusting time to meet required assignments. Examples of study goals are listed in Table 4–1.

TABLE 4–1. Examples of Study Goals

Range	Activities
Immediate	Review notes after class
	Analyze errors on recent exam(s)
	Complete specific reading assignment
Intermediate	Complete literature review for upcoming paper
	Consolidate lecture notes and reading material on specific lecture topic
	Study for upcoming exam
Long-term	Become involved with state professional organization
	Identify employment opportunities

► LEARNING AS INFORMATION PROCESSING

Cognitive psychologists have used an information processing model to describe the process of learning (Rafoth, Leal, & DeFabo, 1993). Incoming information to be learned first must be perceived and recognized, then used while in short term memory or encoded and stored for recall at a later time.

The initial stage for learning is the *sensory register*. Sensory input is received and held briefly (approximately 1/10 second). Because the register is constantly bombarded with information through each of the five senses, it is necessary to identify and focus on the information selected for retention. The learner can enhance selective retention by preparing in advance for learning activities. Instructors can facilitate retention by focusing students' attention on the most important incoming information.

Once perceived, information is transferred into *short-term memory* where it can be retained through repetition for an unlimited period of time, if uninterrupted. Because the practical limit of short-term memory is 20 to 30 seconds, most information is either disregarded or transferred into long-term memory for permanent storage. *Long-term storage* is accomplished either through memorization or establishing meaningfulness. Information learned through memorization typically is stored in isolation and may have little usefulness by itself. Meaningful learning occurs through the establishment of mental links between newly acquired information and previously acquired concepts.

Storing Information

Beatrice (1995) recommends the following eight principles to facilitate the storage of information.

1. *Review immediately*. The ability to recall information drops by as much as 50% within the first hour after exposure. Frequent and repeated reviews are critical to enhance learning.
2. *Associate new information with previous information*. Because most information is stored with related material, memory may be enhanced by the immediate attachment of meaning. The most effective method for learning new information is to associate it with something about yourself (Ormrod, 1990).
3. *Actively participate in the learning process*. Based on your individual learning style, draw diagrams, visualize presented material, formulate questions, rephrase the material, or participate in projects that demonstrate the information.
4. *Organize carefully selected information*. From the preparatory and actual learning sessions,

there should be a good idea of the most important information. Rather than attempting to learn all the material, concentrate on the most important information.

5. *Chunk information into manageable units*. For example, it is easier to remember one's social security number as three chunks of digits (such as 110–93–7563) rather than a string of nine separate numbers. The ability to process information is generally limited to approximately seven chunks (Miller, 1956); however, an individual's capacity is also influenced by the complexity of the information. In other words, one may be able to retain seven units of simple information, but only four units of complex information (Ormrod, 1990).
6. *Use memory aids such as mnemonics to store information that must be recalled in an exact manner, such as the order of the cranial nerves*. In addition to using superimposed structures like the mnemonic "On old Olympus' towering top . . ." other techniques for remembering include the use of imagery to place new objects in a familiar scene or using keywords to associate new ideas with what is already known. Although books of mnemonics may be available at medical bookstores, construction of unique personalized expressions may be of dual benefit. First, they are helpful as memory aids. Second, the process of constructing the mnemonic involves an active process that facilitates learning. One colleague remembers the composition of Diprivan® through the following mnemonic: each milliliter of Diprivan® contains 10 mg propofol (the perfect 10), 12 mg egg lecithin (a dozen eggs), 100 mg soybean oil (soybeans from the family farm), and 22.5 mg of glycerol (memorized).
7. *See the "Big Picture."* Rather than memorizing intricate details, it is often beneficial to view the entire concept. Because the brain stores information through meaningful relationships, the overall perspective facilitates the eventual integration of finer details.
8. *Distribute study sessions*. As soon as possible after a learning session, construct a set of notes or study cards for future use. Review the notes frequently rather than postponing all study until immediately prior to examinations.

Retrieving and Using Information

The ease with which information is recalled depends on how the information was stored originally. Simply stated, the more organized the storage process, the easier it will be for the information to be located and retrieved for use. Because the storage capacity of the brain is vast, recall is facilitated by cues. According to Ormrod (1990):

1. Information that is memorized without establishing contextual links will be more difficult to recall than information that is processed meaningfully.
2. New knowledge that is linked with previous knowledge will be easier to retrieve because multiple pathways for recall are established.
3. The more frequently information is used, the easier it will be to recall. Consequently, although memorization is generally not considered an effective learning method, its utility can be maximized by practice.
4. Information retrieval is hindered by anxiety and facilitated by relaxation.

Ormrod's observations underscore the significance of a comprehensive planned approach to learning; the ability to recall and use information ultimately will be influenced positively by the learner's effort to store new information in a usable, context-specific fashion.

▶ ACQUIRING NEW KNOWLEDGE

Polit and Hungler (1993) describe five types of human knowledge: tradition, experience, authority, logical reasoning, and the scientific method. Each of the knowledge types is encountered in the clinical practice of anesthesia.

Tradition serves as a basis for practice by providing a common foundation of behaviors or customs that have been accepted by the anesthesia community. Often, the validity of the traditions has never been evaluated.

The second major source of knowledge is *experience*. Whereas the ability to build upon observation is a valuable trait, the representativeness of experiences is limited by the uncertainties from which the observations were made. The introduction of computer-based software such as *Anesthesia Simulation Consultant* (Anesoft Corporation, Issaquah, Washington) and full-body high fidelity anesthesia simulators such as the *Human Patient Simulator* (Medical Education Technologies, Inc., Sarasota, Florida) and *Eagle Patient Simulator* (Eagle Simulation, Inc., Binghamton, New York) offer unprecedented opportunities to gain experience in new anesthesia situations, refine anesthesia skills, practice decision-making, and train for unexpected events.

Authority is the third major source of knowledge. Ideally, authorities have the ability to consolidate scientific evidence, logical reasoning, and experience to serve as a basis for wisdom; however, caution should be exercised to distinguish between the genuine wisdom of an authority and unsubstantiated opinion. *Logical reasoning* combines experience with formal systems of thought. Inductive reasoning is the process of using a series of specific observations to reach a general conclusion. Deductive reasoning draws specific conclusions from a series of generalizations. For both inductive and deductive reasoning, the validity of the conclusion is dependent upon the quality and representativeness of the observations used as a basis for the conclusion.

The *scientific method* is generally accepted as the most rigorous method for knowledge acquisition (Polit & Hungler, 1993). The approach is systematic and controlled, featuring a formal definition of the problem, careful study design, collection of data, and problem solution. Peer-reviewed research-oriented journals are examples of information sources based on the scientific method. Limitations to the scientific method include general investigative design flaws, problems in measurement, complexity of human research, and moral and ethical issues of using humans in research.

One major benefit of the scientific method is the potential for quantification of errors. Investigators typically report the probability of a Type I error; that is, the likelihood of concluding that a relationship existed when, in fact, there was none (Vogt, 1993). It is less common for a researcher to report the probability of a Type II error, the likelihood of concluding that there was no relationship when, in fact, a relationship existed (Vogt, 1993). Other types of decision-making errors have been described, but there is no uniform system for classification. Two of the more common errors are drawing an incorrect conclusion from the correct analysis and applying an inappropriate statistical test.

The Internet is emerging as a new resource containing a wealth of information across the levels of knowledge, from the original text of historical documents through synthesis articles and peer-reviewed essays and investigations. Consolidated anesthesia and perioperative World Wide Web resources are listed in Table 4–2. Discussion groups such as "CRNAtalk" contain useful clinical information that is based on the experience of providers. Participants in the on-line discussions range from new students to experienced providers and international experts. Electronic peer-reviewed journals are appearing on the Internet and provide readers the same assurance of scientific merit as their print counterparts with a more rapid and less expensive distribution process. The quality of material published via the Internet and in traditional media varies widely and "may be contaminated by the author's prejudice" (Rothstein, 1996, p. 317). It is the reader's responsibility to evaluate both the veracity of, and basis for, information presented.

▶ THINKING CRITICALLY

Critical thinking is defined as "the rational examination of ideas, inferences, assumptions, principles, arguments,

TABLE 4–2. Internet Addresses of Anesthesia-Related Resources

Resource	Internet Address	Description
Organizations		
American Association of Critical-Care Nurses	www.aacn.org/	Information about the professional organization for critical care nursing
American Association of Nurse Anesthetists	www.aana.com/	Professional and patient information about anesthesia and nurse anesthetists
Association of Operating Room Nurses	www.aorn.org/	Information about the professional organization for perioperative nursing
American Society of Anesthesiologists	www.asahq.org/	Information for patients and physicians concerning anesthesiology
American Society of PeriAnesthesia Nurses	www.aspan.org/	Information about the organization and history of postanesthesia nursing
Anesthesia references		
Wright's Anesthesia and Critical Care Resources on the Internet	www.eur.nl/cgi-bin/accri.pl	A comprehensive listing of anesthesia-related resources including discussion groups (with subscription information), peer-reviewed journals, e-mail addresses for anesthesia-related organizations, and information on non-Internet electronic resources
Nursing references		
American Nurses Association (ANA)	www.nursingworld.org/rnindex.htm	Includes information about the ANA and a broad listing of nursing-related WWW resources

Note: All Internet addresses begin with http://.

conclusions, issues, statements, beliefs, and actions" (Bandman & Bandman, 1995, p. 7). Critical thinking empowers the individual to question, search for evidence, consider alternatives, and evaluate one's own ideas as well as those of others (Siegel, 1985). Through the application of critical thinking skills, students develop the self-sufficiency and autonomy necessary for ongoing learning.

In the clinical practice of anesthesia, singular clear "textbook" problems and solutions are complicated by the presentation of multiple, and often contradictory, signs and symptoms potentially suggesting a wide variety of intervention strategies. The concepts of critical thinking, as presented in the classroom and applied in the operating room, enable the practitioner to analyze complex problems from multiple perspectives, identify assumptions, test hypotheses, and work toward a reasonable solution.

Critical thinking includes the analysis and evaluation of one's own thought processes. Through the use of logic, conceptually sound patterns of thinking may be developed. Key logical terms and their definitions are presented in Table 4–3. *Argument,* as a logical concept, is considered to be a thoughtful exploration of ideas, as opposed to the confrontational context associated with the word's colloquial use. Two explicit components included in every argument are a substantive contestable claim and supporting evidence that is both reliable and relevant (Booth, Colomb, & Williams, 1995). The claim and its supporting evidence are linked by the argument's premise. Optionally, arguments contain qualifications that serve a variety of purposes including the specification of conditions required for the claim to be true. One method for evaluating an argument is to explore a series of questions (Bandman & Bandman, 1995; Brookfield, 1987).

1. What assumptions are being made?
2. What are the premises of the argument?
3. What is the context of the argument?
4. What are the alternative explanations or actions?
5. What conclusions will require action?
6. What are the consequences of the actions?

These questions serve as an excellent starting point for the extension of critical thinking into decision making in clinical practice. A formal process of decision making includes problem definition; collection of relevant data; considering, testing and evaluating possible conclusions; and reaching decisions (Moore, McCann, & McCann, 1985). Refer to the case study at the end of this chapter, which demonstrates how the concepts of critical thinking and

TABLE 4–3. Key Terms Used in Logic

Term	Definition
Proposition	A statement that is verifiable as either true or false
Premise	A proposition that is assumed, affirmed, or denied
Argument	A formal structure of propositions so that the conclusion is supported by the premises
Fallacy	An error in reasoning

decision making are combined to guide the practice of a clinician encountering an unanticipated clinical problem.

To avoid errors in decision making, different types of fallacies should be recognized and avoided. Bandman and Bandman (1995) describe five types of fallacies pertinent to nursing. Examples of these fallacies are presented in Table 4-4. It is important to recognize that a logical fallacy is not necessarily incorrect. Simply stated, a *fallacy* is an error in reasoning that occurs when the conclusion cannot be substantiated by the stated or implied premises. For example, in Table 4-4, a researcher was criticized for concluding that drug A was more ef-

fective than drug B. In reality, drug A may be the more effective drug; however, until sufficient data is collected to substantiate the position statistically, it is fallacious to report the drug's superiority.

Rogerian rhetoric is a distinct rhetorical model that minimizes the adversarial approach to argumentation and provides specific strategies for understanding and cooperation. Young, Alton, and Pike (1970) describe the general components of a written Rogerian argument:

1. Problem introduction to include a demonstration that the opponent's position is understood.
2. Statement of the contexts in which the opponent's position may be valid.
3. Statement of the writer's position and the contexts in which it is valid.
4. Description of how the opponent's position would benefit if elements of the writer's position were adopted.

For clinical practitioners, a softer persuasive strategy such as Rogerian rhetoric, which includes an acknowledgment of alternative positions, may create a stronger basis for understanding and result in a more persuasive and effective discussion (Brent, 1996).

▶ SPECIFIC KNOWLEDGE ACQUISITION STRATEGIES

Two popular study techniques are the SQ3R (Cherney, Dickinson, Hammond, & McLravy, 1993) and PPR (Beatrice, 1995) methods. Each of these techniques illustrates how the learning process extends from prior to the actual "learning" period to after the session has been completed. The SQ3R method as illustrated in Table 4-5 describes how to use the method to prepare for a reading assignment; however, its application extends into all study areas.

Generalizability of the SQ3R method as a knowledge acquisition strategy can be illustrated using an ex-

---

TABLE 4–4. Illustrations of Fallacies Pertinent to Nursing

Irrelevant Grounds

The stated (or implied) premise does not lead to the conclusion.

Example: A healthy-appearing patient during a pre-anesthetic interview denies asthma and shortness of breath. The practitioner summarizes the patient's pulmonary status as "within normal limits."

Analysis: The absence of evidence to support one conclusion (presence of pulmonary disease) does not assure that the opposing conclusion is true.

Inadequate Grounds

The stated (or implied) premise is inadequate to support the conclusion.

Example: A researcher compares the effects of two different antisialogogues and concludes that "there is insufficient evidence to reject the null hypothesis: however, there appears to be a statistical trend toward the conclusion that drug A is more effective."

Analysis: There is insufficient evidence to support the claim that drug A is the better drug.

Faulty Grounds or Unjustified Assumptions

The stated (or implied) premise may be relevant, but cannot support the conclusion.

Example: A critic claims that morphine increases the incidence of nausea and vomiting in postoperative knee arthroscopy patients.

Analysis: The statement implies that there is a greater than expected frequency of nausea and vomiting among postoperative knee arthroscopy patients.

Inconsistency

The stated (or implied) premise is simultaneously asserted and denied.

Example: A practitioner is an outspoken advocate of regional anesthesia for all Cesarian deliveries, then consistently administered general anesthesia for cesarean deliveries between midnight and six in the morning.

Analysis: Actions of the practitioner contradict the practitioner's stated position.

Ambiguity

The stated (or implied) premise is subject to different interpretations.

Example: A pair of researchers report on the incidence of hypoxemia. One investigator considers hypoxemia to be present if the patient's oxyhemoglobin saturation falls below the baseline value. The other investigator defines hypoxemia as an oxyhemoglobin saturation below 90%.

Analysis: The differing definitions confuse the interpretations of research results.

TABLE 4–5. Components of the SQ3R Study Technique

Component	Description
Survey	Skim the assignment looking for key words and points
Question	Formulate a series of questions that should be answered by completing the assignment
Read	Complete the assigned material specifically looking to answer questions and locate the important points in the material
Recite	Recite, write out, or illustrate the answers to questions without using the textbook
Review	Periodically review notes looking for relationships between concepts

ample from clinical practice. A patient requires the administration of a general anesthetic to include the use of a neuromuscular blocking agent. Unsure of which agent to select, the student surveys the literature (or perhaps the hospital formulary) to identify the possible blocking agents for use and then compiles a series of questions about the drugs such as, how long does the drug last? how is it metabolized? are there any contraindications? and so forth. Information is sought to answer the questions posed by the student. Once the reading is completed, a chart is constructed comparing the characteristics of each of the neuromuscular blocking agents. Finally, the student looks for relationships between this new knowledge and existing concepts such as the patient's medical history, surgical requirements for skeletal muscle relaxation, the length of the proposed surgical procedure, and airway management priorities.

The PPR system is a three-step method incorporating many subactivities. The first stage of the PPR system is *preparation*. During this initial phase, the individual eliminates distractors in order to concentrate on the tasks, establishes a purpose for the activity, and activates prior knowledge that may contribute to the current study session. The second stage is the *processing stage* during which information is acquired, organized, and associated with what is already known. In the final phase, *recall*, stored information is reactivated. Because information is usually retrieved in a manner consistent with the format in which it has been stored, anticipation of how information is intended to be used will dictate storage formats. General patterns of organization include simple lists, ordered lists, definitions and examples, cause and effect relationships, and comparisons (Beatrice, 1995).

The SQ3R and PPR strategies illustrate that the process of learning is not a "one time" phenomenon occurring only during a lecture or reading assignment. Learning is an ongoing process requiring preparation prior to the session and a significant mental commitment after the session in order to optimally store and recall newly acquired information.

Reading

An efficient reader can save considerable amounts of time compared to a slow, inefficient reader. Reading speed is hindered by concentrating on one word at a time, subvocalizing each word, lapsing concentration, and looking back over what has just been read. Speed is enhanced by reading words as blocks and continuously moving forward through the material (Cherney & McLravy, 1993). Five different rates of reading speed have been described (Table 4–6). From the fastest scanning rates of up to 1500 words per minute to the slow-

TABLE 4–6. Characterizations of Reading Rates

Description	Purpose	Example
Scanning	Locate specific information	Finding answer to specific question
Skimming	Provide overview	Pre-reading study materials for general concepts
Speeded	Identify central themes	Reading article for main ideas and supporting facts
Study	Attain maximal understanding	Reading study materials to retain information
Careful	Reflect on content	Complex philosophical works

est and most careful reading at 74 words per minute, the pace of reading is determined by the purpose of the activity. The pace of study reading, 250 words per minute, is significantly faster than pensive reflective reading. Rather than slow plodding, the student may use study time more effectively by reading at an accelerated pace and then working to identify questions that remain unanswered and developing relationships between what has just been read and what is already known.

Beatrice (1995) compared college-level reading with high school and pleasure reading materials. College reading introduced many new words and concepts, required the readers to supply their own interest, obtain the necessary background information, and recognize, organize and store the most important information. Reading at the graduate level is even more dependent on the reader's initiative. Prior to a reading session, the individual should preview the material to evaluate the type of information presented and consider the purpose for undertaking the reading assignment. During the session, an ongoing monitoring process includes reflecting on what the writer is attempting to convey, how persuasive the text is, and optimal methods for organizing the information for later recall. Following the session, reflection on the reading should include recalling the main themes and headings, relating the new information to what is already known, and identifying what was not understood as well as areas where additional information is needed (Beatrice, 1995).

Listening and Note Taking

Used correctly, note taking serves two functions. First, note taking is used to facilitate the encoding of new information to be used at a later time. Secondly, the finished notes serve as a storage medium for important information (Rafoth, Leal, and DeFabo, 1993). The process of note taking during a class session can be difficult because it requires both the identification of important information and the ability to accurately record the information in an organized fashion. Kiewra and Frank (1988) found that university students were able to record only 24% of the important ideas presented in a videotaped lecture.

Although notetaking may be viewed as a physical task, the process is accompanied by intense mental activity over an extended period of time. Prior to the lecture, the student prepares by completing assigned readings, analyzing the nature of the material, relating the new material to what is already known, and preparing questions to clarify difficult concepts. During the lecture, the listener monitors what the instructor is saying and why it is being said, organizational patterns in the material being presented, key words and relationships, points that are not understood, questions that arise, the nature of the material being presented, other sources for information (such as reading assignments), discrepancies between what is already known and the new information, and particular points emphasized by the lecturer. Following the lecture, the student reviews the material identifying themes, monitoring understanding, and relating the new information to previous information (Beatrice, 1995; McLravy, 1993a).

Leaving a 2″ to 3″ margin on one side of the note paper facilitates postlecture review. In this space, the learner can classify the organizational structure of the material (simple list, cause-and-effect relationship, examples, etc.); define unfamiliar terms; identify areas that require additional development or clarification; list key words, concepts, and main and supporting ideas; and provide cross-references. If a lecturer closely follows the format of the reading assignment, some individuals prefer to take notes in the margin of the text. Ideally, following the lecture, information from all available sources, including the reading assignment, handouts, and notes, are consolidated for future study.

Written Communication

Consistent with other learning activities, writing is amenable to application of study methods such as PPR and SQ3R. During the preparatory phase, the writer should develop a clear understanding of the purpose for the writing, what the writer is intending to convey, the audience, and the type of work involved with development of the paper (Beatrice, 1995). Common types of writing projects include descriptions of personal experiences, reaction papers, position papers, critical analyses of theory or research, topic summaries, factual reports, and communication of original research (Beatrice, 1995).

Often, the transition from planning to actual writing is facilitated by the "pre-writing" and "free-writing" of ideas. During the pre-write process, the author lists or diagrams ideas, concepts, and words that should be included in the final paper. The prewrite could be a list or an illustration connecting words and ideas such as spokes emanating from a central wheel hub. The free-write is a 5 to 10 minute session where the writer writes quickly and continuously about the topic at hand without regard for grammar, punctuation, or spelling. The purpose of free-writing is to initiate and sustain an outpouring of ideas. Both pre- and free-writing are creative processes (Dickinson, 1993). From the pre- and free-writes, the author constructs a logical outline for the development of the paper.

General Principles of Writing

The general structure of all papers includes three main parts: an introduction, body, and end. Dickinson (1993) describes the introductory portion of the paper as an inverted triangle (∇) where the author attracts the reader's attention and progressively narrows the focus of attention to the purpose of the paper. In the body of the paper, specific points are developed sequentially supporting and strengthening the argument. The concluding section of the paper resembles an upright triangle (Δ) with a restatement of the paper's purpose, a summary of the support for the position, and, in some cases, a discussion of new ideas or applications emanating from the paper.

The finishing process for a completed paper can be divided into four steps. During the first step, the paper is reread for general structure. Key points are highlighted or underlined. The purpose of this initial review is to compare the final paper with the intended structure. The statement of purpose, development of ideas, and clarity of the conclusion should receive particular attention.

The second step of the finishing process includes reading the paper for overall clarity of expression. Clarification strategies include reading the paper sentence by sentence from the end of the document to the beginning. The purpose of this exercise is to determine whether each sentence communicates effectively without the support of previous writing. A second technique is to read the paper slowly and out loud, as if giving a speech. Frequently, use of the second (auditory) sense identifies errors that were overlooked during rapid reading.

A search for errors is the third step in the finishing process. Common mistakes include changing between present and past tenses, grammatical errors, punctuation, and agreement in structure between subject and verb. Spelling and grammar checkers included in word-processing programs facilitate this step, but they should not be relied on as the sole source for proofreading a paper.

The final step of the finishing process is "external review" by another reader. Ideally, the individual should be familiar with the content; however, even someone unfamiliar with the subject matter often can identify areas in the paper needing refinement. It may be helpful to watch the external reader review the paper. Following the eyes and watching facial expressions may indicate areas of the paper where the reader has struggled to read or understand.

Writing for Publication

Publication is an essential element in the process of communication for a profession. Traditional writing formats include books, book chapters, and journal articles. Although a wide variety of forums are available to nurse anesthetists, two of the most common are the *AANA Journal* and *CRNA: The Clinical Forum for Nurse Anesthetists*. Each journal routinely publishes information about the journal and its publication requirements to include instructions for manuscript preparation and a description of the types of submissions that will be considered for publication. As an example, the *AANA Journal* accepts manuscripts pertinent to the specialty of anesthesia and the practice of nurse anesthetists within six broad categories: research, case reports, clinical episodes (abbreviated case report), review articles, professional issues, and letters to the editor ("Information for Authors," 1997). The *AANA Journal* uses the *American Medical Association Manual of Style* as a guide for scientific references. Additional information provided includes instructions for manuscript format and submission instructions. Some journals include background information for prospective authors, such as the general philosophy and target audience of the journal.

Not all manuscripts are accepted for publication. However, many are selected following a resubmission of the manuscript once the author has addressed queries from the reviewers. To be selected for publication, an article must be well written, unique, timely, consistent with the journal's style, and attractive to the readers. When in doubt about an editor's interest in a manuscript, a query letter may be submitted. The letter should be limited to one page. Components of the letter include a short introduction to the subject describing why the topic is important and the author's qualifications for writing the article. A second paragraph summarizes the paper and describes the focus of the article. The query is concluded with a request to submit the article for consideration (Tornquist, 1986). Responses to query letters generally are returned by the editor within a few weeks.

Other factors to consider in selecting a journal for publication include its peer-review process, size of circulation, frequency of citation in other works, and prestige (Thyer, 1994). Three sources of information about specific nursing journals are the extensive *Cabell's Directory of Publishing Opportunities in Nursing* (Cabell Publishing Company; Beaumont, TX), which was last published in 1993, and summaries of publishing opportunities compiled by McConnell (1995) and Swanson, McCloskey, and Bodensteiner (1991).

Testing and Test Taking

Preparation for test taking can be divided into two main components: knowing the material to be tested and knowing the process by which the material will be tested (Cherney & Hammond, 1995). Preparatory strategies include identifying the material to be tested and establishing a schedule and plan for comprehensive study to include specific goals for each study session. As the test date nears, information about the length of the test, time for completion of the examination, and types of test items will facilitate development of a strategy for completing the testing session.

Understanding how a test is weighted and scored will influence test taking strategies. Because most traditional examinations give credit for correct answers and no credit for incorrect answers, it is usually recommended to answer all test questions. As the testing session begins, survey the entire test to identify the overall length, number of items, types of questions, and relative point allocations. Decide how much time can be spent on each item based on its relative worth.

Whereas some individuals are content to start from the beginning of a test and answer items consecutively until the test is complete, other students employ a variety of strategies to determine the sequence in which test items are completed. Common systems include answering all the easy questions first, then returning to more difficult items; starting at a predetermined point in the exam (such as the third page) and working forward from that point; or answering all of one item type (eg, multiple choice), then moving to a second type of item (eg, short answer), and continuing until all item types are answered.

Essay items, because they are frequently worth a significant number of points on an examination, deserve particular attention. Keys to successful completion of essay questions include a clear statement of main points, the addition of supporting detail, and an organized, error-free presentation of the information (Cherney & Hammond, 1993). Care must be taken not to spend a disproportionate amount of time on any essay question if the result is sacrificing valuable time that could be used to answer many questions with lesser point values.

Following a testing session, the examination should be reviewed to gain a better understanding of the items missed and conduct an error assessment (Beatrice, 1995). Common sources of error in test taking can be classified as *mental errors* such as anxiety, fear, or anger; *tactical errors,* such as a lack of preparation for the format of test item, focusing on the wrong material, or not studying in sufficient depth; and finally, *implementation errors* such as not allowing sufficient time to answer all questions, misreading or misinterpreting items, and second guessing. Recognizing patterns in testing errors enables the individual to prepare a strategy for future testing sessions.

In recent years, the use of computers for test administration has become more common. Computerized tests may be either computer "administered," meaning that the examination is identical in structure to a traditional pencil and paper test, but administered with the aid of a computer; or computer "adaptive" which uses algorithms to select test items interactively based on the responses to previous test items. Computer adaptive tests may be of fixed or variable length. Advantages of adaptive testing include more frequent and convenient scheduling of examinations, decreased frustration for some test takers, minimization of the effects of guessing, rapid reporting of scores, increased assessment accuracy, improved test security, reduced administration costs, and improved data management (Hambleton, Swaminathan & Rogers, 1991; Lunz & Bergstrom, 1994; Sax, 1989; Weiss, 1982). The certification examination for nurse anesthetists has been administered in a computer adaptive format since April, 1996.

Clinical Learning

The practice of anesthesia cannot be learned solely by reading textbooks, listening to lectures, or completing classroom exercises. The clinical portion of anesthesia education focuses on the refinement of both technical skills and thought processes. Clinical decision making is often required to solve problems that include a degree of uncertainty and conflicting values. Solutions to problems are sought using specialized knowledge and judgement (Harris, 1993). Two key components to clinical learning are the establishment of clear, obtainable daily goals and the maximal utilization of clinical experts.

As a student progresses through the clinical phase of the education process, it is easy to fall into the trap of establishing a daily "routine" of administering anesthesia as each clinical experience is viewed as one of the 500 to 600 experiences required for certification. Instead of looking for opportunities to learn something new with each anesthetic, the tendency is to focus on practical matters of getting patients asleep, awake, and to the recovery room. Optimal learning occurs in the clinical portion of anesthesia education when clinical is approached similarly to classroom learning. Beatrice's (1995) PPR method provides an effective method for maximizing the educational benefit of each clinical experience. During the preparatory phase, educational objectives are identified. Objectives may be as simple as timely and complete documentation of the anesthetic process or more complex, such as learning to manage multiple simultaneous continuous infusions of intravenous anesthetic agents.

Objectives may be ongoing or immediate, such as learning to implement an efficient sequence for the induction of anesthesia.

Clinical learning goals may be determined solely by the student or by the student in collaboration with faculty and clinical preceptors. Most importantly, the learning objectives should be communicated and negotiated with the clinical preceptor prior to the beginning of the clinical experience. Clinical experiences may become overly stressful and ineffective when the student and preceptor have differing expectations for what should be occurring during the conduct of an anesthetic. Clarification and mutual acceptance of learning objectives promote a productive clinical learning experience.

During the process phase of clinical learning, the preceptor and student work together as a team. Preceptor roles vary with the experience level of the learner. Initially, the preceptor may model procedures and thought processes. The behaviors of a preceptor are invaluable as mental templates for the student to reference at a later time. As the student progresses, instructor involvement gradually fades into the background, progressing from demonstration to coaching and verbal cueing, then to interpreting confusing phenomenon. With increasing student proficiency, the preceptor may serve only as a passive supporter (McLellan, 1996; Rogoff, 1990; Tharp & Gallimore, 1988). Even at these advanced stages, observation of expert practitioners should not be dismissed by students eager to get involved. The opportunity to observe experienced practitioners provides a mechanism for self assessment and revision of previous mental templates.

In the review phase, the learner may use a variety of techniques to review clinical learning experiences in an effort to improve performance. Techniques include written and verbal feedback from instructors, self-evaluation, and completion of a journal noting clinical activities with questions, traps, and ideas for future clinical opportunities. Periodic performance reviews include a candid assessment of the student's abilities. Although identification of activities that have never been experienced is straightforward, individuals should also consider how capable or comfortable they feel in completing previously obtained experiences. For example, a student's case log may indicate that she has performed 10 oral fiberoptic intubations. Depending on the time lapsed since the last procedure was performed, the student may currently feel less proficient despite overall progress as a clinician. Another opportunity to perform fiberoptic intubations may be necessary to maintain or regain previous skills. Figure 4–1 illustrates a portion of a clinical skills self-assessment instrument that can be completed by students for both self-appraisal and to provide information to clinical coordinators. Open, honest dialogue between students, clinical coordinators, and program faculty can facilitate optimal clinical learning for beginning practitioners.

Procedure	Never done	Limited experience	Comfortable	Need to review
Direct laryngoscopy				
Oral				
Nasal				
Fiberoptic laryngoscopy				
Oral				
Nasal				
Indirect laryngoscopy				
Blind nasal				
Lighted stylet				
Bullard intubating Laryngoscope				
Laryngeal mask airway				
Combitube				

Figure 4–1. Example of student self-assessment worksheet for airway management procedural skills.

▶ CASE STUDY

Unexplained Increase in Heart Rate under General Anesthesia

A previously healthy 26-year-old female weighing 55 kg has been receiving general anesthesia with isoflurane 1.0% and nitrous-oxide 69% in oxygen 30% for a diagnostic laparoscopy (which requires insufflation of the abdomen with carbon dioxide to enhance operative conditions). The anesthetic state was induced with a standard dose of sodium pentothal. Placement of an oro–tracheal tube was facilitated by the administration of succinylcholine. Skeletal muscle paralysis is maintained with a continuous infusion of cisatracurium.

The patient has been placed in low lithotomy position and the procedure began approximately 30 minutes ago. Over the past 15 minutes, the patient's heart rate has gradually increased from baseline of 60 beats per minute (BPM) to 90 BPM. All other vital signs have remained essentially unchanged from baseline. The electrocardiograph tracing suggests a normal sinus rhythm. Observable blood loss has been negligible.

▶ ARGUMENT FUNDAMENTALS

1. *Claim:* The patient is experiencing a significantly elevated heart rate which may have potentially deleterious physiologic consequences.

2. *Evidence:* Heart rate has increased by 50% (from 60 to 90 BPM) over the past 15 minutes.

3. *Premise:*
   A. Tachycardia is a sign of hypoxia which could result in damage to internal organs, most significantly, the brain; and
   B. Tachycardia increases the likelihood of myocardial infarction because the amount of time the heart spends in diastole, which is when the heart receives its coronary blood flow, is reduced.

4. *Qualifiers:*
   A. Other causes of tachycardia include inadequate general anesthesia, hypercarbia, hypovolemia, drug reaction, drug side effect, and various pathologies.
   B. The heart rate, although elevated significantly from baseline, remains in the range of rates that can be tolerated for an extended period of time by a young healthy patient.

▶ SUPPLEMENTAL QUESTIONS

1. What assumptions are being made?

   The implications of cerebral anoxia, myocardial infarction, and inadequate anesthesia are of sufficient magnitude to warrant investigation of the problem.

2. What are the premises of the argument?

   See Argument Fundamentals.

3. What is the context of the argument?

The patient is a young healthy subject capable of tolerating a moderate increase in heart rate, especially in the absence of changes in blood pressure and hemoglobin saturation, as measured by pulse oximetry. Conversely, she is unable to communicate symptoms she may be experiencing as a result of the general anesthetics and muscle relaxant.

4. What are the alternative explanations?

Potential explanations for elevated heart rate in a healthy patient receiving general anesthesia for a laparoscopic procedure include pain; endobronchial intubation from the cephalad displacement of abdominal contents as a result of abdominal insufflation and Trendelenburg position; hypoventilation from the intraperitoneal absorption of insufflated carbon dioxide; hypovolemia from either inadequate fluid replacement or acute occult blood loss; decreased venous return from the increased intra-abdominal pressure associated with insufflation; side effect of isoflurane; and pathophysiologic conditions such as malignant hyperthermia.

5. What conclusions will require action?

Aside from verifying placement of the endotracheal tube, assuring adequate ventilation, ruling out inadequate anesthetic depth, evaluating current fluid status, and monitoring intra-abdominal insufflation pressures, no other actions are warranted as long as other vital signs (specifically blood pressure, hemoglobin saturation, end-tidal carbon dioxide, and ST segments on ECG) remain stable.

6. What are the consequences of the actions?

There are no untoward consequences of the monitoring actions. Increasing anesthetic depth to rule out inadequate anesthesia may result in hypotension and potential exacerbation of the tachycardia, depending on the specific agent selected.

▶ DECISION-MAKING PROCESS

1. *Problem:* Unexplained increase in heart rate under general anesthesia.
2. *Relevant data:* heart rate, blood pressure, heart and lung sounds, temperature, minute ventilation, ECG pattern, hemoglobin saturation, end-tidal carbon dioxide and oxygen levels, estimated blood loss, NPO status, fluid replacement received, abdominal insufflation pressure.
3. *Considerations and evaluation of possible conclusions.*
   A. Oxygenation and ventilation status, excluding arterial blood gas analysis, can be completed quickly with no patient risk.
   B. Effect of increasing depth of anesthesia can be evaluated with minimal risk to the patient. Increasing concentration of isoflurane is not an option because tachycardia is a side effect of the agent.
   C. Volume status could be evaluated using fluid bolus with minimal patient risk.
   D. The actions listed in considerations A–C above address the most likely causes of the tachycardia.
4. *Decisions*
   A. Confirm adequacy of oxygenation and ventilation.
   B. In the absence of signs such as dilated pupils, tearing, patient movement, or an elevation in end-tidal CO_2; maintain current concentrations of anesthetic agents because the delivered concentration of isoflurane exceeds the minimum alveolar concentration of isoflurane with nitrous oxide.
   C. Administer 250 to 500 mL bolus of isotonic crystalloid solution. Recompute fluid status.
   D. Administer small dose of analgesic (eg, fentanyl) or hypnotic (eg, thiopental).
   E. Reevaluate if condition persists.

▶ SUMMARY

Learning potential can be maximized through the process of metacognition as we achieve a better understanding of ourselves as learners. Key components in all learning situations include advance preparation to activate prior knowledge and set goals, in-context processing of new information, and post-session review to assure that intended outcomes have been achieved.

► **KEY CONCEPTS**

- Each individual has a personal learning style, including learners as accommodators, assimilators, convergers, and divergers (Kolb); learning strategies as surface, deep, or achieving (Biggs): or visual, auditory, and kinesthetic (Beatrice).
- The three most important questions to be asked in every learning session are: what is the purpose of the learning session; what types of learning strategies are necessary to achieve the desired outcome; and what learning strategies will be most effective.
- The most common causes of failure to achieve desired learning outcomes are production and mediation deficiencies.
- The information processing model of cognition is

used to describe how information is perceived, recognized, stored, and recalled.
- Critical thinking involves the rational examination of ideas, arguments, and conclusions. The main components of a logical argument are the claim, evidence, premise, and qualifications.
- Effectiveness of clinical learning is enhanced when the student and preceptor have established educational goals that are mutually clear and agreeable.
- Techniques such as SQ3R (*s*urvey, *q*uestion, *r*ead, *r*ecite, and *r*eview) and PPR (*p*repare, *p*rocess, and *r*eview) are general study strategies that can be applied in educational endeavors.

► **STUDY QUESTIONS**

1. Define the learner descriptions by Kolb, Biggs, and Beatrice. How would you describe your personal learning style?

2. Evaluate your current weekly time schedule. What are your fixed time obligations and how would you arrange the schedule to maximize study opportunities?

3. Find an interesting journal article. What argument is the writer proposing? Describe the claim, evidence,

premise, and qualifiers. Which aspects of the premise are verifiable?

4. Use one of the provided Internet addresses to locate an anesthesia resource and find one piece of information that interests you. What is the source of knowledge for the information?

5. You have been given an assignment to write a 15-page paper on if, and how, the information presented in this chapter will facilitate your future learning. Prepare a prewrite and free-write for an essay that would serve as a basis for the essay.

KEY REFERENCES

Bandman, E. L., and Bandman, B. (1995). *Critical thinking in nursing* (2nd ed.). Stamford, CT: Appleton & Lange.

Beatrice, J. A. (1995). *Learning to study through critical thinking.* Chicago: Irwin.

Brookfield, S. D. (1987). *Developing critical thinkers.* San Francisco: Jossey-Bass.

Cherney, E., Dickinson, E., Hammond, G., & McLravy, Y.

(Eds.). (1995). *Achieving academic success* (2nd ed.). Dubuque, IA: Kendall/Hunt.

Covey, S. R. (1989). *The 7 habits of highly effective people.* New York: Simon & Schuster.

Thyer, B. A. (1994). *Successful publishing in scholarly journals.* Thousand Oaks, CA: Sage.

Winston, S. (1994). *The organized executive.* New York: Warner.

REFERENCES

Bandman, E. L., & Bandman, B. (1995). *Critical thinking in nursing* (2nd Ed.). Stamford, CT: Appleton & Lange.

Beatrice, J. A. (1995). *Learning to study through critical thinking.* Chicago: Irwin.

Biggs, J. B. (1985). The role of metalearning in study processes. *British Journal of Educational Psychology, 55,* 185–212.

Biggs, J. B. (1987). *Study process questionnaire manual.* Hawthorn, Australia: Australian Council for Educational Research.

Booth, W. C., Colomb, G. G., & Williams, J. M. (1995). *The craft of research.* Chicago: University of Chicago Press.

Brent, D. (1996). Rogerian rhetoric. In B. Emmel, P. Resch, &

D. Tenney (Eds.) *Argument revisited; Argument redefined* (pp. 73–94). Newbury Park, CA: Sage.

Brookfield, S. D. (1987). *Developing critical thinkers.* San Francisco: Jossey-Bass.

Brown, A. L., Bransford, J. D., Ferrara, R. A., & Campione, J. C. (1983). Learning, remembering, and understanding. In J. H. Flavell & E. M. Markman (Eds.), *Handbook of child psychology: Vol. 3 Cognitive development* (pp. 77–166). New York: Wiley.

Cherney, E., Dickinson, E., Hammond, G., & McLravy, Y. (Eds.), (1993). *Achieving academic success* (2nd Ed.). Dubuque, IA: Kendall/Hunt.

Cherney, E., and Hammond, G. (1993). Preparation and strategies for test taking. In E. Cherney, E. Dickinson, G. Hammond, & Y. McLravy (Eds.), *Achieving academic success* (2nd Ed., pp. 73–91). Dubuque, IA: Kendall/Hunt.

Cherney, E. & McLravy, Y. (1993). Speed reading and strategies for memory and concentration. In E. Cherney, E. Dickinson, G. Hammond, & Y. McLravy (Eds.), *Achieving academic success* (2nd Ed., pp. 93–104). Dubuque, IA: Kendall/Hunt.

Covey, S. R. (1989). *The 7 habits of highly effective people.* New York: Simon & Schuster.

Covey, S. R., Merrill, A. R., & Merrill, R. R. (1994). *First things first.* New York: Simon & Schuster.

Davis, A. R. (1988). Developing teaching strategies based on new knowledge. *Journal of Nursing Education, 27,* 156–160.

Dickinson, L. (1993). Writing as process. In E. Cherney, E. Dickinson, G. Hammond, & Y. McLravy (Eds.), *Achieving academic success* (2nd Ed., pp. 105–114). Dubuque, IA: Kendall/Hunt.

Hambleton, R. K., Swaminathan, H., & Rogers, H. J. (1991). *Measurement methods for the social sciences: Fundamentals of item response theory.* Newbury Park, CA: Sage.

Harris, I. B. (1993). New expectations for professional competence. In L. Curry & J. F. Wergin (Eds.), *Educating professionals: Responding to new expectations for competence and accountability* (pp. 26–27). San Francisco: Jossey-Bass.

Information for Authors. (1997). *AANA Journal, 65,* 72.

Kiewra, K. A. & Frank, B. M. (1988). Encoding and external storage effects of personal lecture notes, skeletal notes, and detailed notes for field-independent learners. *Journal of Educational Research, 81,* 143–48.

Kolb, D. A. (1976). *Learning style inventory: Technical manual.* Boston: McBer.

Lunz, M. E., & Bergstrom, B. A. (1994). An empirical study of computerized adaptive test administration conditions. *Journal of Educational Measurement, 31,* 251–263.

McConnell, E. A. (1995). Journal publishing characteristics for 42 nursing publications outside the United States. *Image, 27,* 225–9.

McLellan, H. (1996). Situated learning: Multiple perspectives. In H. McLellan (Ed.), *Situated learning perspectives* (pp. 5–17). Englewood Cliffs, NJ: Educational Technology Publications.

McLravy, Y. (1993a). Listening and lecture note-taking. In E. Cherney, E. Dickinson, G. Hammond, & Y. McLravy (Eds.), *Achieving academic success* (2nd Ed., pp. 61–72). Dubuque, IA: Kendall/Hunt.

McLravy, Y. (1993b). Scheduling time. In E. Cherney, E. Dickinson, G. Hammond, & Y. McLravy (Eds.), Achieving academic success (2nd Ed., pp. 11–29). Dubuque, IA: Kendall/Hunt.

Miller, G. A. (1956). The magical number seven, plus or minus two: Some limits on our capacity to process information. *Psychology Review, 63,* 81–97.

Moore, W. E., McCann, H., & McCann, J. (1985). *Creative and critical thinking* (2nd Ed.). Boston: Houghton Mifflin.

Ormrod, J. E. (1990). *Human learning: Theories, principles, and educational applications.* New York: Merrill.

Polit, D. F., & Hungler, B. P. (1993). *Essentials of nursing research: Methods, appraisal, and utilization* (3rd Ed.). Philadelphia: Lippincott.

Rafoth, M. A., Leal, L., & De Fabo, L. (1993). *Strategies for learning and remembering.* Washington, DC: National Education Association.

Ramsborg, G. C., & Holloway, R. L. (1985). Learning style analysis: A comparison of CRNA clinical instructors and student nurse anesthetists. *AANA Journal, 53,* 439–444.

Rogoff, B. (1990). *Apprenticeship in thinking: Cognitive development in social context.* New York: Oxford.

Rothstein, P. (1996). Learning from the literature. In C. L. Lake, L. J. Rice, & R. J. Sperry (Eds.), *Anesthesia* (Vol. 14, pp. 317–337). St. Louis: Mosby.

Rothstein, P. R. (1990). *Educational psychology.* New York: McGraw-Hill.

Sax, G. (1989). *Principles of educational and psychological measurement and evaluation* (3rd Ed.). Belmont, CA: Wadsworth Publishing.

Schunk, D. H. (1991). *Learning theories: An educational perspective.* New York: Merrill.

Sherbinski, L. (1994). Learning styles of nurse anesthesia students related to level in a master of science in nursing program. *AANA Journal, 62,* 39–45.

Siegel, H. (1985). Critical thinking, informal logic, and the philosophy of education, part two. Philosophical questions underlying education for critical thinking. *Informal Logic, 7*(2&3), 69–81.

Swanson, E. A., McCloskey, J. C., & Bodensteiner, A. (1991). Publishing opportunities for nurses: A comparison of 92 U.S. journals. *Image, 23,* 33–8.

Tharp R. G., & Gallimore R. (1988). *Rousing minds to life.* Cambridge, England: Cambridge University Press.

Thyer, B. A. (1994). *Successful publishing in scholarly journals.* Thousand Oaks, CA: Sage.

Tornquist, E. M. (1986). *From proposal to publication: An informal guide to writing about nursing research.* Menlo Park, CA: Addison-Wesley.

Vogt, W. P. (1993). *Dictionary of statistics and methodology.* Newbury Park, CA: Sage.

Weiss, D. J. (1982). Improving measurement quality and efficiency with adaptive testing. *Applied Psychological Measurement, 6,* 473–492.

Winston, S. (1994). *The organized executive.* New York: Warner.

Young, R. E., Alton, L., & Pike, K. L. (1970). *Rhetoric: Rediscovery and change.* New York: Harcourt.

Environment

Surgical Environments for the Twenty-First Century

Christine S. Zambricki

Predicting the future is risky business. The anesthesia community, along with other health professionals, has experienced significant uncertainty in recent years as everything from models of patient care to payment systems have undergone a metamorphosis. Looking to the long term makes one think of what lies ahead—challenges, conflicts, and possibilities. There are two predominant questions about the future changes in health care for the twenty-first century. What will happen? And when will it happen? Although the first question can be answered with some educated speculation and reasonable predictability, few experts in the health care field would be willing to commit their predictions to a timeline. Aggressive change is taking place in some areas of the country but not in others; in some portions of a given state while others remain the same; and even in some local hospitals and not others. This chapter provides the reader with some thoughts on what anesthesia care will look like in the twenty-first century based on analysis of present trends. Fortunately the twenty-first century is sufficiently long to accommodate the uncertainty of saying exactly "when."

Our health care industry is undergoing massive evolution that has been described as truly revolutionary. These changes are taking place at the federal, state, and local levels and have had the effect of producing tremendous anxiety in the anesthesia community as well as a flurry of activity among hospital administrators and payers. In the health care world, transformation is not without opportunity. Modification of existing conventions of practice and payment is not, of itself, a positive or negative phenomenon.

Examples abound in nature, which demonstrate that for every significant evolutionary change, there are some beneficiaries as well as some who fare poorly. If our health care system can be compared to the dinosaurs of old, we can see that as the dinosaurs disappeared, man evolved. Thus, the same phenomenon had both a positive and a negative effect, depending on whose perspective is considered. The same can be said for health care reform. As our health care system changes, our practice, patients and work environment will be dramatically different in the twenty-first century. Will these changes have a positive or negative effect? The answer is both.

As cataclysmic change occurs in the health care industry, what lessons can be learned from similar occurrences in nature? In the case of human evolution, conditions that lead to the death of the dinosaurs allowed an optimum environment for man's development. Pessimism and optimism can exist simultaneously, as both are different sides of the same event. The challenge for certified registered nurse anesthetists (CRNAs) is in finding the opportunity in the changes that the future brings.

Anticipating future changes are the best we can do. Today, scientists can predict that a volcano will erupt or an earthquake will occur. No one makes claims about the timing, which of course, is the crucial element to the success of the prediction. Changes in the health care industry are sweeping the country; however, the timing of these changes will be unique to each state, community, and even to each practice setting. Predicting the complexion of anesthesia care in the twenty-first century is speculative at best, and based on trends on the horizon today. How long will it take us to get there is an even more difficult question; to answer factors such as government regulation, advancement in technology, and changes in patient demographics all play a role. The best approach to facing anesthesiology practice in the twenty-first century is to be ready with an open mind and flexibility. Some of the changes discussed in this chapter may be less than a decade away.

► THE TWENTY-FIRST CENTURY PATIENT

What characteristics will our patients possess in this future practice world? How should we plan for these changes as we design future anesthesia care delivery systems? Demographic shifts such as extended life spans, decentralization of care, increasing ethnicity diversity, and increased patient access to health care information have far-reaching implications that will affect every health care facility and every health care provider.

Increasing Life Span

There is no doubt that the future population of the United States will be far different than it is today. Projections for demographic shifts are made with certainty. These changes will have major implications for anesthesiology as it relates to quality initiatives and patient care.

The aging of the "baby boomers" is a major event that is rapidly approaching. Early in the twenty-first century it is anticipated that for the first time in the history of this country, senior citizens will outnumber the general population. When one considers that the elderly have always experienced a higher rate of surgical procedures, it is easy to project that over the next decades our senior patients will constitute an ever-increasing percent of anesthesia practice. This increase in the elderly population, along with their greater percent of surgical procedures relative to the population as a whole, will balance out the pressures to reduce surgical procedures in a managed care environment well into the twenty-first century. Surgical volumes in the United States will remain the same or slightly increase.

How will this change in demographics affect the nurse anesthetist's daily practice environment? Quality initiatives will have to take this demographic shift into account, focusing on new technologies to create a physically comfortable environment for these patients which address their special concerns.

The entire perioperative process will have to be designed to facilitate the movement of large numbers of aged patients throughout complex health care systems, both in terms of physical access as well as system mobility. Large numbers of patients who are living alone, with physical, hearing or vision disabilities, will need to get to our operating rooms and safely home afterwards. Once in our system, transportation methods will be developed such as moving walkways and motorized mini transport vehicles, to assist our patients in reaching the operating room area.

There will be an explosion in the development of pharmaceuticals and technology that promote the safe care and unique physiologic conditions of the elderly patient. Structural modifications to everything from pulse oximetric probes to stretchers will be developed and tailored to the physiologic changes associated with aging. Anesthetic agents will be developed which have advantages for this population in light of their altered pharmacodynamic profile.

These improvements will be demanded by a population that will constitute the majority of patients. As government programs require more financial contribution by the patient, our ability to deliver care in a manner that patients judge to be convenient and of high quality will be the essential key to success. Patients may elect to pay for their proposed care, shift to lower-cost alternatives, or elect no treatment at all. This patient involvement in priority setting and evaluation represents a major shift away from provider-focused quality assurance programs which are commonplace today. The customer will be king and that customer will be more than 65 years old.

► DECENTRALIZATION AND ALTERNATIVE SITES OF CARE

Another population that will continue to rise as a percent of overall surgeries performed is the outpatient population. The movement towards non-hospital sites of surgical service will accelerate as managed care becomes the dominant delivery model for all patients, including those insured by Medicare and Medicaid. Even today, health maintenance organizations (HMOs) have brought about fundamental changes in surgery. Inpatient procedures have fallen rapidly in areas where there is great HMO activity, setting a trend for shifting cases to the outpatient setting across the country.

Outpatient sites are common today; however, nontraditional sites of surgical care will develop as access to health care procedures is taken to the patient. Nursing homes, factories, and even schools and churches, may become satellite sites for providing health care services. With continued economic pressure to reduce utilization of expensive resources such as hospitals, alternative sites of care will be sought for minor surgical procedures. This shift will be further fueled by concerns about access to care for the uninsured population. Is there a point of diminishing return of decentralization of care as related to costs of manpower and technology?

Length-of-stay reductions will be a serious issue for the majority of patients, based on age and inability to care for themselves in the home, transferred to alternate sites of care for recovery from their surgery. In the twenty-first century, more and more surgery will be done in nursing homes and extended care facilities, bringing perioperative services to the patient's location. Regardless of site of care, postoperative pain management will be critical to the early healing of elderly patients with minimal complications. Acute pain management of the surgical patient will expand outside of the hospital, to extended care facilities and into the home.

Cultural Diversity

A third demographic shift that will impact the anesthesia environment is the increasing number of patients of different ethnicity and cultures. Based on their own cultural background, these patients will approach the U.S. healthcare system with their own perspective on surgery and anesthesia care, pain control, and educational needs. The field of transcultural nurse anesthesia practice will expand as expertise develops related to the special needs of patients.

Patient Access to Health Information

Another trend relative to patient attributes is the knowledge and involvement of patients living in the twenty-first century. Health care information will become more personally accessible. Patients will pull medical knowledge from the Internet in their homes. In some ways, medicine will become a commodity product, with patients, or customers, deciding when and how they will have their surgery and anesthesia. Patients will make more informed choices driven by new technology, new techniques, and cost.

There will be an increasing interest in alternative therapies and treatments as patients are exposed to "global" health care ideas via computer access. There will be a mainstreaming of alternative forms of medicine such as chiropractic services and herbal medicines. In response to consumer demand, modalities such as acupuncture, aroma therapy, and therapeutic touch will be employed in the perioperative environment for anxiolysis and pain management.

Cognizant of these shifts in patient characteristics, how will the anesthesia provider deliver better outcomes and safer anesthetic techniques? Despite their diversity, patient satisfaction will continue to be a key driver of value. Health care systems will rely on patient satisfaction data for the assessment and demonstration of quality. Patients will drive the system: a knowledgeable, culturally diverse group of elderly patients with a financial interest in selecting the anesthesia provider who can best meet their needs. Patient satisfaction data will assume a role equally important to objective outcome measures.

▶ INFORMATICS IN ANESTHESIA CARE

The Department of Labor estimates that by the year 2000 at least 44% of all workers will be in data services—for example, gathering, processing, retrieving or analyzing information (Pritchett, 1997). Health care systems of the future will be less likely to spend money on bricks and mortar, shifting their investments toward information technology and other infrastructure needs. Capital will be used for technology that enables electronic communication across multiple inpatient and outpatient sites, as well as between caregivers throughout the system.

Information systems will be integrated into all aspects of anesthesia practice, from the preanesthetic assessment to the postoperative phase of care. A national data dictionary will be developed that lists conventions of medical terms agreed on for use in health care institutions across the country. With uniformity of language, standardization of hardware and software, and lightweight notebook computer technology, computer access will be available to health care providers everywhere.

One likely application for information systems technology in the patient planning to undergo anesthesia is the development of a "smart card." The preanesthetic health history could be obtained from the patient's "smart card," a credit-card-like device with the patient's medications, previous hospitalizations and surgeries, diagnostic information, and systems review encoded on a microchip. On admission to hospital, the patient will present their card, and all "smart card" information will be downloaded into the hospital information system and updated throughout the duration of the patient's visit. Network technology will exist which will allow a patient to go to a neighborhood health care information station, not unlike a bank ATM site, to update their health information on a computer terminal networked with the community health care system. One week prior to surgery, the patient will be instructed to update their health history at a local health care information station, and bring their smart card on the day of surgery! User concerns about computer literacy, on the part of both patients and health care professionals, will be eliminated as voice recognition and security measures evolve to a high level of sophistication.

Computer technology will have application in multiple operating room (OR) processes such as intraoperative charting, sponge counts, and surgical notes. Wireless technology, basically an extension of the existing wired network environment that uses radio-based systems to transmit data signals through the air, will be available in notebook or laptop computer format. This will greatly increase efficiency and communication between perioperative areas as nurse anesthetists use bedside documentation modalities that can later be added to by registered nurses in the postanesthesia care unit using handheld computers.

Telemedicine will expand by linking remote sites with specialty sites. Information support, on-line through world-renowned medical libraries, will be at the nurse anesthetist's fingertips in the OR. Consultation with required specialists will be immediately available in the operating room, complete with on-line review of ECG, radiographic, and other diagnostic data.

Information systems will play a critical role in response to the impact of capitation and managed care to the operating room. Efficient patient flow processes, scheduling optimization, materials management, and surgical staffing will depend on information systems that can quickly reevaluate information based on new cases added on a real-time basis. Information systems will also be used for physician and CRNA profiling, monitoring quality and outcome performance as well as economic performance case-by-case. This information will be fed on an ongoing basis to accreditation bodies and federal/state government entities with responsibility for the approval of reimbursement to providers in health care facilities.

Numerous financial and cost reports will be provided on a continuous basis, including reports of revenue per case, surgeon-specific cost per procedure, and microcosting of labor and supplies for each case. Clinical reports detailing quality indicator performance, variance and complications reports, blood usage, and implant logs will be automated. Information systems will reveal where costs are higher and how health care workers, including nurse anesthetists, can be more efficient. This information can give the leading edge in managed care contracting situations, as key insurance information, utilization review data, and quality assurance files will be managed in a consolidated way.

Bar coding technology will allow for real-time entry of time, supplies, and equipment usage. This information will be interfaced with hospital financial systems in order to pass case-specific charges to the billing system. Inventory management will be improved due to automated supply requests, product inventory reports, and supply usage data. Systems will monitor and track equipment usage and maintenance/repair costs, track manufacturers and vendors, and look at historic supply utilization for budget projections.

Informatics will have application in the field of nurse anesthesia education as well. University systems will be fundamentally changed, as high quality compressed video and computers bring the university to the student. Nurse anesthesia students in the twenty-first century may never set foot in a classroom. Even in the clinical arena, informatics can provide a safe learning laboratory with real life situations involving drugs, equipment, and concomitant patient responses to those interventions. These simulator laboratories will be regionalized, and offer learning opportunities to generic students as well as experienced CRNAs who want to increase their skill level. Simulations in anesthesia will replace clinical study in the initial phases of the student's educational preparation. The next generation of CRNAs must be prepared to practice in more intensely managed and integrated systems. Nurse anesthetists of the future will be required to use sophisticated information and communication technology in the perioperative environment.

► PHYSICAL ENVIRONMENT

The physical environment within the operating rooms of the twenty-first century will be dramatically different than that of today. Surgical suites will be quieter, safer, and more technologically advanced than that presently functioning. The noise associated with the gas machine and other pieces of operating room equipment will be gone, as electronics replace pneumatically powered devices such as drills and ventilators. Alarms will be silenced as equipment technology develops feedback systems that are self-correcting.

Fewer people will be in the operating room, some having been replaced by "intelligent" machines. Many surgical procedures will be performed using highly sophisticated robotic devices, either controlled by a remote operator or programmed for precision in cases such as ophthalmology. In an off-site location, the surgeon will control the movements of the robotic device utilizing a virtual reality environment whereby he can feel the discrete movements of the surgical maneuvers through hand controls as he views the surgical site on a computer screen. The anesthesia provider may be the only health care professional in the operating room, as cost containment strategies, coupled with technologic developments, have replaced the circulating nurse in every operating room with technicians. The professional registered nurse now freed from the operating room will assume a broader role in assuring that patient care conforms to perioperative clinical pathways in the continuum of care.

Anesthesia technology will continue to advance exponentially as we move into the twenty-first century. Anesthesia machines will change dramatically, as components such as flowmeters and ventilator bellows are replaced with electronics. Tidal volume and gas flows will be digitally displayed and the integration of these devices with the physiologic monitoring systems and information recording device will be complete.

Anesthetic agents will still need to be administered and adjusted in response to patient conditions. Electronic infusion pumps and electronic vaporizers will be used in manner not unlike physiologic biofeedback mechanisms. Intravascular electronic sensors will be inserted prior to anesthetizing the patient to determine blood levels of pharmaceutical agents on a continual basis. This information will be charted automatically and analyzed along with other physiologic data. The results of this analysis will be integrated into an automated feedback system to the administration devices. Adjustments will be made in order to maintain a steady state of anesthesia throughout the case, and the resultant changes in dosage and patient response recorded on the automated record keeper. Using this technology, the nurse anesthetist may be responsible for several anesthetized patients at once, with a radiofrequency beeper response system managed by the biofeedback computer.

Operating rooms will be safer places to work following a heightened awareness and remedy of hazards to employees. The hospital environment will be latex-free. Nurse anesthetists will have developed sensitivity to a wide range of chemicals and environmental toxins in the operating room, resulting in the development of additional protective clothing. As we saw scavenging systems become routine in the late twentieth century, advanced understanding of the dangers of laser plume and surgical smoke will result in similar attention to smoke evacuation.

▶ SURGICAL TECHNOLOGY

Hallmarks of change in the twenty-first-century operating room are beginning at the end of this century, as new surgical techniques are developed. Some of these changes are brought about by payment changes. For example, it is estimated that endoscopic surgery, thought to represent about 5% of surgical cases in early stage managed care markets, will progressively increase as managed care penetrates the market. In the mature managed care market of the future, endoscopic procedures will comprise 40% of all cases.

Innovations in surgery will continue to abound. Transplant technology will continue to advance. Biogenetics and cloning applications will allow animal organs to be developed, which are ideally suited for transplant in the numbers required to meet the needs of the aging population. Transplant of everything from bowel to certain central nervous system components will be advanced.

Genetic technology, or the use of hormones to treat disease, will have application in the OR. Surgical techniques will be developed to place these agents close to the intended site of action. Genetic technology introduces the idea that human beings will be partly man made for the first time in history. The rules regarding rendering care and the price of that care in these situations is still to be determined.

Operating rooms of the future will take advantage of "smart" materials, remote sensing and advanced imaging technologies that will enhance the safety of increasingly complex procedures. The surgical environment will be automated including temperature, lighting, evacuation systems, and airflow controls.

Telemedicine will extend access to new imaging techniques and immediate consultation from specialists. Surgical simulators will offer physical properties such as the stretching of organs, contracting of muscles, bleeding, and leaking bile. These three dimensional images will be programmed with patient-specific data, allowing a distant operator to interact with the image of a specific patient.

Innovations in imaging technology will become commonplace in the next millenium. In the future, holographic x-ray systems will allow surgeons to look at a hologram of a patient's skull to determine how far into the brain to place instruments or test sizes of screws for an orthopedic procedure by waving the hardware through life-size holograms. These virtual reality devices will give the surgeon an opportunity to rehearse a complex surgical procedure before attempting it.

Minimally invasive procedures will continue to develop as improvements to traditional surgical methods. Some of these procedures will be done in alternate locations. For example, placement of a stent in the colon of a patient using endoscopic assistance may be done in the endoscopy suite, with conscious sedation as the anesthetic. Minimally invasive techniques will continue to change the face of heart surgery. The minimally invasive direct coronary artery bypass (MIDCAB) procedure and the port-access approach for not only coronary arterial bypass grafting (CABG) but mitral valve replacement are gaining in popularity. The MIDCAB procedure incorporates a 3 to 4 inch incision rather than a 15 inch incision and does not require cardiopulmonary bypass—both changes having immense implications for anesthesia management. A variety of new methods, including ways to graft arteries through tiny incisions, place stents, and apply laser to break up clots, will move out of the operating room and into the cardiac catheritization lab.

Endovascular cardiopulmonary bypass systems will permit a patient's heart to be stopped, placed on bypass, and operated on without a sternal incision. Mini-bypasses will become available, not just for single graft, but also for double and triple mini-bypass procedures also. New laser technology, such as transmyocardial revascularization (TMR), is promoted as an alternative to both angioplasty and cardiac bypass surgery. TMR uses laser energy to drill through the heart muscle, allowing blood to flow to ischemic regions. Where will these cases be done and what are the anesthetic requirements? Alternative surgical techniques for all specialties will grow substantially as the quest for shortened lengths of stay and rapid functional return escalates.

► ANESTHESIA WORKFORCE IN THE TWENTY-FIRST CENTURY

In a time of rapid change in the anesthesia marketplace, there are both great opportunities and substantial risks for CRNAs. Because managed care models emphasize such things as patient satisfaction, quality care, and lowering costs, nurse anesthetists will be well-positioned to provide this care. The need for good data that can be related to both cost of anesthesia care and patient outcomes with nurse anesthetist practice is critical. Some of the risks that are inevitable with managed care include the turbulence of the marketplace and the resultant dislocation that occurs as a result of hospital downsizing, mergers, and other dramatic changes in the health care environment. CRNAs, as individuals and as a profession, will need to develop the self-confidence and political expertise necessary to assume a position of leadership in the perioperative world.

Anesthesia care in the twenty-first century will be highly competitive, with remaining players in the market at discounted fee-for-service pricing. Capitated managed care programs will have driven costs down, and payers will subsequently demand that they make payments only for services rendered rather than for a covered life. This will result in an environment where reimbursement for anesthesia services is deeply discounted, and quality becomes the primary competitive factor.

Advanced practice nurses, including CRNAs, will continue to have real opportunities as long as they provide cost effective, quality service. The evolution of managed care will force health care institutions to enter into capitated contracts of significantly discounted fee-for-service arrangements to provide anesthesia care. Hospitals will opt for the most efficient anesthesia work force mix of CRNAs and anesthesiologists.

Nurse anesthetists will find themselves consulting with other advanced practice nurses on a regular basis, as nurse practitioners function as primary care providers preoperatively and acute care practitioners postoperatively. Repetitive, technical tasks such as endoscopic procedures and minor surgery will be performed by advanced practice nurses. In the future, as now, the CRNA will need to deliver high-quality anesthesia care at the lowest reasonable price. What will be different is that everyone, from the accrediting body, to the payer, to the health care institution, will continuously monitor the nurse anesthetist's performance in this regard. These entities will make no assumptions; rather, they will know, through clinical data systems, the quality of anesthesia care and how much it costs.

The improvement of anesthesia and operating room efficiency is integral to controlling costs; thus greater emphasis will be placed on professional staffing of these areas. Typically, personnel costs constitute 40% to 70% of all health care expenditures. Improved process efficiency of surgical patient throughput will be built into systems to allow for additional cases to be done during the day. Productivity will be measured by each minute spent in the operating room with a focus on how much "nonproductive" time per hour is spent preparing or waiting for surgery. Management engineering reports will become as commonplace as monthly financial reports, as professional nurse anesthetists are required to monitor productivity improvements on an ongoing basis.

Utilization of high capital investments, such as operating rooms, will improve significantly as they become cost centers rather than revenue centers. Vertical scheduling of surgical cases will result in valuable operating room space being used 24 hours per day, 7 days per week. This economically motivated approach allows technologic resources to be used continuously rather than sitting idle for the majority of hours during the week. It will also contribute to reducing the patient's length of stay, as patients will not have to remain in the hospital overnight or over the weekend to be placed on the surgical schedule.

In response to these changes, anesthesia departments, mimicking trends in other industries, will be more inclined to hire anesthesia providers when they are needed for hours when there are surgeries to be done, rather than on a straight shift basis. This may even be done on a case-by-case or contract basis. CRNAs may come in for a specific case and be paid a case rate based on the length of time and complexity of the case. This system has the advantage of eliminating benefit costs while maintaining productivity by not having to pay staff salaries during times of work shortage.

As an alternative to contract arrangements, a hospital may find it preferable to employ anesthesiologists and CRNAs due to high case volumes or twenty-four hour coverage demands. Anesthesia professionals can expect to function in a multidisciplinary, cross-trained, multifunctional manner. Beyond the obvious perioperative role as specialist in the preoperative preparation, intraoperative care, and postoperative phase of the patient's experience, CRNAs and anesthesiologists will find themselves providing expertise in the intensive care units, postoperative surgical floors, and emergency departments.

Breaking away from the traditional and expensive day, afternoon, and evening shift system, OR workers, including CRNAs, will be scheduled based on the needs of the institution. For example, 4-hour shifts, weekends only and late schedules will be commonplace as institutions fine-tune the coordination of resources and surgical cases.

Anesthesia personnel in the twenty-first century will no longer have the luxury of being relegated to the operating room. Productivity per paid hour of professional time is enhanced when skills related to airway maintenance, medical management, and pharmaceutical titration are employed in areas other than the OR during times of reduced volume. In addition, administrative duties with concomitant responsibility for other areas within the hospital, which may be related or unrelated to anesthesia practice, will become more common for anesthesia providers, as management layers are consolidated.

▶ CLINICAL PRACTICE CHANGES

Clinical pathways or care maps, commonly used in health care institutions today, will be expanded to include the perioperative environment. Many of the choices available to anesthesia practitioners will be gone, as the continuous flow of information through quality data systems continues. Anesthetic management will be refined according to the national standard of care, which will continue to evolve on a minute by minute basis. Nurse anesthetists will be required to follow anesthesia "clinical pathways" which have been shown to deliver the best outcome at the lowest cost.

Traditionally, clinical pathways have been used to standardize patient care using guidelines for common diagnosis related groups. This standardization is expected to offer consistent quality while minimizing costs through elimination of unnecessary laboratory tests and reducing length of stay. Development of clinical pathways by clinicians in hospitals will be superseded by those developed by insurance companies, managed care organizations, and other payers based on a national patient care data base. Despite standardization of care for the majority of patients, anesthetists will remain challenged to care for patient "outliers"—those patients who do not respond in typical fashion to surgery or anesthesia. This population will account for the highest percentage cost of anesthesia services and require a focused look at pathways for managing specific clinical problems, similar to the Malignant Hyperthermia Association of the United States (MHAUS) protocols for malignant hyperthermia.

The majority of hospitals in the United States are presently using these interdisciplinary clinical paths developed for specific diagnoses or surgical procedures. These tools typically leave out the operating room experience, and focus on more global patient outcomes, associated care provider interventions, and expected length of stay. The goal of clinical paths is to decrease rates of patient complications and readmissions, reduce resource utilization, decrease errors, reduce legal liability, and contribute to the overall betterment of the patient's care.

As one of the last bastions of "provider preference" based practice, the anesthesia providers of the future will be required to comply with practice guidelines that have been shown, through national studies, to provide consistent quality at a low cost and early discharge from the recovery areas.

Length-of-stay reductions in these areas will be serious business. Implications for nurse anesthetists include more involvement in preoperative treatments, education, and postoperative pain management, all with the objective of allowing the patient to go home, safely, as soon as possible.

Emphasis on control of anesthesia care costs will lead to dramatic changes in the perioperative course of the patient. There will continue to be close scrutiny of routine preoperative laboratory testing. Tests will be evaluated for aggregate cost and yield of positive results. Routine preoperative testing without clinical indication will be eliminated, with tests ordered only on the basis of findings from the history and physical examination. All preoperative testing will be point of service based, using low-cost bedside testing devices that provide immediate results. These results will be downloaded into the information system and displayed on the anesthesia computer terminal.

Anesthetic agents will be developed that are fast-acting with minimal residual effects in order to meet the needs of the outpatient population. Patients will be able to walk out of the operating room, get dressed, and prepare for discharge home, eliminating the post anesthesia care unit (PACU) and Phase II recovery experience.

▶ SUMMARY

CRNAs in the future will be required to be more customer or consumer focused, respond to outcome information using sophisticated information and communication technology, and readily move into new roles that strike an equitable balance between resources and patient requirements. The new millennium brings both fears and forecasts in the face of uncertainty. Nurse anesthetists need to develop creativity and innovation in order to benefit from the changes to come in the twenty-first century. New models of care will extend beyond the anesthesia delivery system, permeating the entire health care environment, and these changes will impact the profession and its patients. Empowerment will come through CRNAs using their knowledge and experience to change processes in order to increase clinical effectiveness and control costs.

► KEY CONCEPTS

- Operating environments in the twenty-first century will be scheduled much more tightly and the workforce will be smaller, including the use of more technical support staff. Some staff, including the surgeon, may be managing the OR via robotics from remote sites.
- Anesthesia providers will be making clinical decisions based on critical pathways or maps that are largely data driven. Assessment of provider performance will be determined by objective performance data amassed by computer technology.
- Although the penetration of managed care will continue, it is projected that the number of surgical cases will increase. However, much more surgery will be done with noninvasive techniques.
- Instructional techniques for students enrolled in nurse anesthesia programs will be centered around simulation technology at the expense of traditional lecture.

► STUDY QUESTIONS

1. Describe three informatics applications that will become part of the nurse anesthetist's practice environment in the next century.

2. Analyze the impact of clinical pathways on anesthesia practice in the future.

3. List three trends projected for future patient populations and their impact on perioperative care of the patient.

4. Describe anticipated changes in the nurse anesthesia educational environment in the twenty-first century.

5. Discuss the overall impact of managed care on the evolution of the anesthesia work environment.

KEY REFERENCES

Anonymous. 3-D, virtual reality, and robotics are nearing OR application (1994). *OR Manager, 10*(6), 10.

Anonymous. Profiles of four new surgical suites. (1992). *OR Manager, 8*(7), 10–13.

Breen, P. T., Grinstein, G. G., Leger, J. R., Southard, D. A., & Wingfield, M. A. (1996). Virtual design prototyping applied to medical facilities. *Studies in Health Technology and Informatics, 29,* 388–399.

Daft, R. & Lengel, R. H. (1986). Organizational information requirements, media richness and structural design. *Organization Science, 32,* 554–571.

Davis, R. N. (1993). Cross functional clinical teams: Significant improvement in operating room quality and productivity. *Journal of the Society for Health Systems, 4*(1), 34–47.

Jolesz, F. & Kinkinis, R. (1992). The role of imaging in the operating room of the future. *Administrative Radiology, 11*(11), 43–46.

Mathias, J. M. (1994c). Telepresence lets surgeons operate from remote sites. *OR Manager, 10*(6), 11.

Mathias, J. M. (1995a). Ahead . . . robots, digital surgeons, and virtual reality. *OR Manager, 11*(1), 1, 6–7.

Mathias, J. M. (1995b). OR of the future to be less complicated, more efficient. *OR Manager, 11*(1), 7.

Mathias, J. M. (1996c). Surgeons operate across miles with remote system. *OR Manager, 12*(2), 11, 14.

Pritchett, P. (1997). *New work habits for a radically changing world.* Dallas, TX: Pritchett & Associates, Inc.

Rotondi, A. J., Brindis, C., Cantees, K. K., Deriso, B. M., Ilkin, H. M., Palmer, J. S., Gunnerson, H. B., & Watkins, W. D. (1997). Benchmarking the perioperative process. I. Patient routing systems: A method for continual improvement of patient flow and resource utilization. *Journal of Clinical Anesthesia, 9*(2), 159–169.

SUGGESTED READINGS

Borzo, G. (1997). 24 hour videotaping in OR raises questions. *OR Manager, 13*(8), 17–18.

Buchanan, D. & Wilson, B. (1996). Re-engineering operating theatres: The perspective assessed. *Journal of Management in Medicine, 10*(4), 57–74.

Buckingham, R. A. & Buckingham, R. O. (1995). Robots in operating theatres. *BMJ—Clinical Research Edition, 311*(7018), 1479–1482.

Call, C. A. & Maloney, J. P. (1993). Utilizing field medical equipment to support fixed facilities during major renovation projects. *Military Medicine, 158*(5), 326–333.

Dartmouth, a pioneer in computerizing the OR. (1996). *OR Manager, 12*(5), 18–9, 22.

DeVos, C. B., Abel, M. D., & Abenstein, J. P. (1991). An evaluation of an automated anesthesia record keeping system. *Biomedical Sciences Instruments, 27,* 219–225.

Fiala, D., Grady, K. P., & Smigla, R. (1993). Continued cost justification of an operating room satellite pharmacy. *American Journal of Hospital Pharmacy, 50*(3), 467–469.

Fogg, D. (1991). Operating room construction requirements, disinfecting floors, floating nurses. *AORN, 53*(2), 496–498.

Humphreys, H. (1993). Infection control and the design of a new operating theatre suite. *Journal of Hospital Infection, 23*(1), 61–70.

Important trends to watch in surgical technology. (1995). *OR Manager, 11*(4), 17.

Kanich, D. G. & Byrd, J. R. (1996). How to increase efficiency in the operating room. *Surgical Clinics of North America, 76*(1), 161–173.

Liner, E. R. (1996). Panel targets operating room management for the future. *Today's Surgical Nurse, 18*(2), 11–14.

Lynch, W. (1993). Understanding health care utilization: Health promotion as a tool within demand management. *Wellness Management, 9*(2), 2–5.

Maihot, C. B. (1996). The operating room of the future. *Nursing Management, 27*(12), 28E, 28H.

Marmarinou, J. (1990). The autonomous endoscopy unit. *AORN, 51*(3), 764–773.

Mathias, J. M. (1994a). Robotic assistant for laparoscopic surgery. *OR Manager, 10*(1), 1, 9–10.

Mathias, J. M. (1994b). Innovative devices expanding laparoscopy. *OR Manager, 10*(6), 1, 9–10.

Mathias, J. M. (1996a). Remote surgery and virtual endoscopy on the horizon. *OR Manager, 12*(2), 1, 9–10.

Mathias, J. M. (1996b). High-tech borrows from B-2 bomber. *OR Manager, 12*(2), 10–1.

Meyer-Witting, M. & Wilkinson, D. J. (1992). A safe haven or a dangerous place—Should we keep the anesthetic room? *Anesthesia, 47*(12), 1021–1022.

Patterson, P. (1990). Stockless inventory: Supplies of the future. *Today's OR Nurse, 12*(12), 26.

Patterson, P. (1992). Shift to OP surgery key issue in redesign. *OR Manager, 8*(4), 1, 7.

Patterson, P. (1996). OR technology decisions shift to outcomes. *OR Manager, 12*(4), 16.

Patterson, P. (1997). Meeting airs differences on need for smoke evacuation. *OR Manager, 13*(4), 1, 10, 12–13.

Rea, C. M. & Walker, G. J. (1990). Designing a state-of-the-art operating room complex. *Today's OR Nurse, 12*(3), 28–32.

Routledge, J. D. & Henderson, L. J. (1996). Testing prototype products in the operating room. *AORN 63*(2), 450–451.

Satava, R. M. (1995). Virtual reality, telesurgery, and the new world order of medicine. *Journal of Image Guided Surgery, 1*(1), 12–16.

Shortell, S. M., Gillies, R.R., Anderson, D. A., Mitchell, J. B., & Morgan, K. L. (1993). Creating organized delivery systems: The barriers and facilitators. *Hospital and Health Services Administration, 38,* 447–466.

Siker, D., Sprung, J., Escorcia, E., Koch, R., & Vukcevich, M. (1997). Effects of gas flow management on postintubation end-tidal anesthetic concentration and operation room pollution. *Journal of Clinical Anesthesia, 9*(3), 228–232.

Zomiska, M. (1991). Computers and the future: Increasing efficiency. *Today's OR Nurse, 13*(4), 28–31.

Occupational Health and Safety

Brent Sommer

Certified registered nurse anesthetists (CRNAs) experience particular job-related risks that are inherent to both the specialty and their immediate working environments. Federal, state, regional, and local statutes, standards, and policies mandate several practice-specific and safety-related requirements that govern the health care workplace. While the CRNA maintains a current state nursing license, maintaining professional practice standards and adhering to particular statutes become a dual responsibility for which all providers are accountable. Health care organizations and facilities that provide anesthesia care services as well as the CRNA are responsible for meeting or exceeding standards and rules mandated by the Occupational Safety and Health Administration (OSHA) and the U.S. Environmental Protection Agency (EPA). These agencies require compliance to standards that they promulgate and are mandated by Federal laws. The U.S. OSHA regulates practice standards and recommendations provided by the Centers for Disease Control and Prevention (CDC) which serves to protect citizens and all persons who receive health care in this country (1988).

The Occupational Safety and Health Act of 1970 provides protection to cover nearly 6.5 million health care workers from work related injury and illness. Professional accountabilities and responsibilities are outlined in the *Professional Practice Manual for the Certified Registered Nurse Anesthetist* of the American Association of Nurse Anesthetists (AANA) (1996). The manual contains an *Infection Control Guide* that is maintained according to current standards and recommendations for implementing and maintaining effective infection control programs for anesthetizing locations.

▶ NOSOCOMIAL INFECTION AND PRACTICE COMPLIANCE

All health care facilities that are accredited by the Joint Commission on the Accreditation of Health Care Organizations (JCAHO) are required to maintain and promote infection control standards, yet Bauer (1997) and others have questioned the compliance of many institutions where nosocomial infections are not uncommon. Hand washing studies conducted in large teaching institutions reflect a failure of health care workers to comply with recommended infection control practices nearly half of the time (Griffin, 1996). Concern regarding noncompliance with such basic infection control practice standards should stress the importance of maintaining basic nursing practices that adhere to policies while minimizing nosocomial infection rates. Hospital and other health care facility environmental control measures are the primary means to maintaining the safest environment for both patients and providers.

▶ OCCUPATIONAL ILLNESS AND INJURY

The National Safety Council reported an average occupational injury and illness rate of approximately 9% for all documented cases during a 1992 insurance reporting survey (National Council on Compensation Insurance, 1992). Garb and Dockery (1995) reported a high incidence of employee back injuries for those working in the operating room. Programs designed to improve body mechanics and incorporate ergonomically efficient work stations have been successful, although several factors that contribute to anesthesia provider safety and well-being are somewhat more difficult to quantify. Work-related particulars and concomitant factors associated with anesthesia provider stress are recognized, but no easy process to identify or influence such concerns has been discovered. Stress-associated conditions were found by Seeley (1996) to be more common in anesthesia providers, yet practice-specific data continues to be limited. Provider well-being and related concerns of a profession-specific nature should be addressed and expert consultation sought when indicated. Employee assistance and professional support programs and networks should be consulted whenever possible.

Physical Risk

Documentation and knowledge regarding physical and environmental threats that present during the practice of anesthesia are clearer and more easily calculated than some of those previously mentioned. Because anesthesia practice requires close contact between patients and providers and the areas that they share, a majority of provider risks for occupationally acquired disease and illnesses evolves from direct contact and resultant transmission.

Environmental Exposure

Contact exposure in and around the operating room (OR) and general health care environment poses some degree of risk for transmission of various viral and bacterial strains that can range from insignificant to serious (see section on drug-resistant organisms). Herpes simplex, type I or oral lesions frequently referred to as "cold sores" can be easily transferred as a result of contact transmission. Herpetic Whitlow, a lesion of the distal phalanx, occurs when the virus enters opened skin or cuticles. Antiviral agents are used to treat these often difficult to cure conditions that are exposure driven. Strict adherence to recommended infection control practices will prevent such transmission. Avoidance of transfer to face and hands following contact is essential to maintaining an exposure-free workspace.

Viral Exposure

Infectious hepatitis and human immunodeficiency viruses (HIV) present serious risk for occupational exposure with detrimental and potentially fatal outcomes.

Knowledge of these disease processes, their modes and routes of transmission, and preventative strategies are the individual responsibility of every provider and his or her employer.

Drug-Resistant Organisms

First reported in Europe several decades ago, a presence of microorganisms resistant to conventional antibiotic agents such as methicillin, nafcillin, and cephalosporins has emerged in this country. *Staphylococcus* is the bacteria responsible for a majority of nosocomial infections seen in hospitals and institutions where patients are housed. Drug-resistant strains of staphylococcus and certain strains of enterococci are resistant to traditional treatment with potent preparations such as vancomycin. These organisms have continued to present on a more frequent basis. Preventing transmission of these microorganisms in facilities including perioperative areas requires meticulous adherence to recommended infection control practices and potent chemotherapeutic intervention.

Patients exhibiting clinical symptoms of these infections are frequently debilitated and immunocompromised. Standard precautions and disease-specific contact control measures to prevent cross-contamination include reverse isolation and thorough disinfection of all equipment and adjacent environmental surfaces. Planning care for these patients should include appropriate case management that permits terminal disinfection of equipment used for these cases.

Provider caution to apply appropriate barrier precautions and avoid direct contact with patients who are known or suspected to be harboring these highly virulent microorganisms is an absolute necessity. Universal precautions and an approach that assumes that all body fluids are of an infectious nature as described by CDC guidelines (1995) should consistently be applied throughout all patient care areas.

Product- and Equipment-Related Injury

Several products, some equipment, and some procedures specific to surgery, obstetrics, and other areas where anesthesia care occurs, pose some degree of risk for provider injury. Injuries range from the more frequent, such as hand lacerations resulting from broken drug ampules, described by Parker (1995) to be as high as a 6% incidence, to the rarer, yet significant dangers such as penetrating injuries resulting from broken air-driven power tools used in the OR.

Blood-Borne Pathogens

Blood-borne pathogens include all infectious agents that are transmittable by accidental exposures. Body fluids ca-

TABLE 6–1. Body Fluids Capable of Transmitting Blood-Borne Pathogens

- **Absolute**
  - Blood
  - Body fluids containing blood
- **Possible**
  - Cerebrospinal fluid
  - Pericardial fluids
  - Amniotic fluids
  - Semen, vaginal secretions
  - Synovial fluid
  - Pleural fluid
- **Remote**
  - Feces
  - Saliva
  - Sputum
  - Sweat
  - Tears
  - Urine
  - Wound drainage
  - Nasal secretions
- **Not implicated in health care settings**
  - Human breast milk

pable of transmitting blood-borne pathogens of a more serious consequence (including hepatitis B virus [HBV] and HIV) and the likelihood of their transfer capabilities are depicted in Table 6–1. Although isolated reports of transmission of blood-borne pathogens from infected providers to their patients have been reported, a much greater degree of risk exists for the provider to contract infectious pathogens from infected patients.

The overall workplace risk of seroprevalence has consistently been shown by Bell (1996) and others to be very low and directly reflective of the prevalence of HIV infection in patient populations with whom the provider is involved. Nearly 5% of adults infected with HIV or diagnosed with acquired immunodeficiency syndrome (AIDS) or advanced HIV disease have reported some history of employment within the health care industry. Determining risk factors and careful case review is necessary to determine the likelihood of occupation-related transmission.

Disease Surveillance and Occupational Exposure

The CDC has consistently calculated the risk of acquiring HIV from a needlestick exposure to HIV-infected blood at approximately 0.3%. Over 2000 health care workers are reported as having sustained exposures from the blood of HIV-infected persons. Fifty-two health care workers have contracted HIV by exposure solely attributable to occupational exposures that have resulted in seroconversion. Independent risk factors for HIV in-

fection after an occupational percutaneous exposure to infected blood include depth of penetration, visibility of contaminant present on the device used, direct vessel (vein/artery) cannulation, virility and disease stage of the source patient, and influence of postexposure chemoprophylaxis.

Needlestick Injury

The majority of needlestick injuries that have been reported have occurred following the actual use of a needle or device wherein improper handling after use and before or during disposal has occurred. Because needles and sharp devices are responsible for the majority of injuries sustained by health care providers, intensified efforts to develop products that eliminate or minimize this risk are being promoted by professional experts and industry leaders who develop these items.

Needlestick injuries are associated with recapping of used needles in approximately one third of reported incidents. Tait and Truffle (1994) reported an even higher incidence in reviews of over 400 needlestick injuries reported by anesthesia providers. Noncompliance with standard precautions and recommended practice for disposal of contaminated sharps continue to be observed more often than not throughout many institutions where patient populations have considerable risk for hepatitis B and C (HCV) and HIV.

Appropriate application of barrier precautions during procedures wherein some degree of exposure risk exists is another area where anesthesia providers have been noncompliant with recommended practice guidelines. Table 6–2 lists anesthesia-related procedures associated with potential exposures to blood-borne pathogens.

The Training for Development of Innovative Control Technology (TDICT) project is an example of the current focus on developing efforts to prevent needlestick and sharp injuries through the use of safer medical devices. The TDICT project brings together health care workers, designers, and manufacturers to formulate standards by which the safety of medical devices can be judged

TABLE 6–2. Anesthesia Procedures Associated with Exposure to Blood-Borne Pathogens

- Laryngoscopy and intubation
- Oral, endotracheal, bronchial, and gastric suctioning
- Emergency, trauma, neonatal resuscitation
- Regional anesthesia procedures
- Induction and maintenance of general anesthesia
- Administration of blood products
- Bodily output/discharge collection
- Invasive monitoring system

(J. Fisher, personal communication, August, 1997). The project has been successful in guiding both manufacturers and providers to be more critically involved with the development and selection of medical devices used in their practice. Nurse anesthetists are encouraged to participate in such design projects and similar efforts that facilitate such workplace changes. These developmental efforts contribute to device design, implementation of workplace practice guidelines, and standards that improve both quality and safety for patients and providers.

OSHA Blood-Borne Pathogen Standard

The Occupational Safety and Health Administration issued its *Occupational Exposure to Blood-Borne Pathogens Standard* in 1991 to minimize and eliminate occupational exposure to HBV, HCV, HIV, and other contagious pathogens. The standard requires the following components that must be incorporated into the infection control program in every health care facility:

- Training and education of all employees
- Record keeping to document compliance
- Control methods that include:
    Standard precautions
    Engineering controls
    Work practice controls
    Personal protective clothing and equipment
- HBV vaccination (at no charge to employees)
- Exposure determination program
- Postexposure evaluation and follow-up
- Infectious waste disposal
- Tags, labels, and bags
- Housekeeping practices
- Laundry practices

Failure to comply with these requirements has resulted in significant fines and threats to institutional licensure and funding capabilities.

Exposure Prevention and Management

Prevention of occupationally acquired blood-borne diseases depends on critical strategies that include exposure avoidance, immunizations, and postexposure management including chemoprophylaxis. Immunoprophylaxis has made significant progress toward eradicating HBV as an occupational threat, yet occupational exposures continue that progress to fatal outcomes. As the pathogenesis of both HCV and HIV are better understood and management strategies result in continued progress to combat and prevent infection by these serious viruses, efforts to prevent their transmission remain the primary defense against their spread. Speculative prophylactic treatments for all viral infections continue to be researched for their effectiveness in preventing disease progression and insult, while potentially eradicating these serious health care practitioner threats.

Postexposure Prophylaxis

Those not previously vaccinated for HBV should seek immediate counseling to include laboratory determination of hepatitis status and appropriateness of HBV vaccination. Human immunodeficiency virus testing should be done to establish baseline parameters. The CDC has recommended a chemoprophylaxis protocol to treat occupational exposure to known or suspected HIV based on reported experiences resulting from previous postexposure treatments. The recommended regimen for chemoprophylaxis is a combination therapeutic approach that includes multiple antiretroviral agents and is based on current theory and experience. Recent reports indicate that use of zidovudine and additional agents, including various antiretroviral agents and protease inhibitors available to treat HIV disease, is associated with nearly a 79% reduction in risk following an exposure.

Blood Exposure Management

Immediate response to an occupational exposure to potential blood-borne pathogens should include the steps outlined in Figure 6–1. Exposed body parts should be cleansed with an appropriate antimicrobial soap; eye splashes should be irrigated with an appropriate sterile rinse agent; and persistent bleeding should be controlled. The source object should be evaluated for contamination if possible.

Risk determination to calculate the potential that an exposure might incur detrimental sequelae should be made when specific information is gathered. A source person known to be infected with a form of hepatitis or HIV or to be at risk from either social or health history should be considered as high or probable risk for transmission. Once triage efforts have calculated the degree of risk that the exposure carries, the appropriateness of further treatment and management strategies should be decided and initiated.

Tuberculosis

A resurgence in the prevalence of *Mycobacterium tuberculosis* (TB) in recent years, following nearly three decades of declining morbidity, has given rise to considerable concern throughout all areas of health care. The World Health Organization (WHO) estimates that nearly 20 000 new TB cases are reported annually. Experts state that the majority of currently diagnosed TB cases have resulted from inadequate initial treatment of previous TB disease, increased prevalence of TB in various populations, and drug-resistant strains that have evolved.

One in 10 persons infected with TB actually experiences TB disease without intervention, which includes appropriate preventative therapy. Persons infected with HIV are six times more likely to develop active TB disease when compared with the general population according to Castro (1992) and others. Nearly 3% of those infected with TB harbor a strain that is resistant to at least

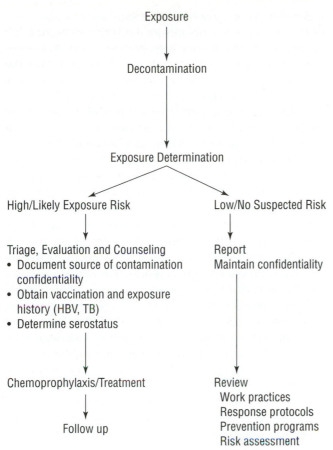

Figure 6–1. Basic components of an exposure management program.

one or more of the drugs commonly used to treat the disease. In many areas, particularly those with a high incidence of HIV disease, as many as one third of those infected may be infected with a multidrug resistant (MDR) strain.

Health care workers are at risk for contracting TB through the airborne route; droplet nuclei can remain airborne for several hours. Tuberculosis transmission is dependent on several factors, including the following:

- Rate and concentration of infectious organisms
- Physical status of the airborne discharge
- Volume and rate of air exchange in the exposed area
- Length of time that TB-contaminated air is shared

Exposure likelihood increases during cough-inducing procedures such as bronchoscopy, endotracheal intubation, sputum induction, and the administration of aerosolized medications. Because these procedures are routine in areas where anesthesia care is provided, it is essential that the CRNA monitor the environment for potential transmission and diminish the risk whenever possible. Education and early intervention to identify suspected TB cases

is the responsibility of all health care providers. Those involved with patients who are accessing health care institutions for initial treatment are at particular risk. Departments such as emergency and urgent care units, where patients tend to cluster and share the same air for prolonged periods of time, maintain the greatest risk for TB transmission. Persons most likely to experience exposure to TB are those living in environments where TB transmission has been documented, including: prisons, jails, hospitals, congregate living sites, centers for persons infected with HIV, nursing homes, drug treatment programs, shelters for the homeless, and migrant camps.

Tuberculosis Prevention

Prevention of TB transmission involves protection from infected air expelled from a host to those in the immediate physical area. Engineering guidelines and regulations for TB isolation and treatment rooms require a negative-pressure room that exhausts air to the outside environment and contains greater than 10 air exchanges per hour. Although most ORs and areas where anesthesia is provided do not necessarily meet these standards, administrative and practice controls must prevail.

All providers who care for patients at risk or those suspected or known to be infected with TB should be test-fitted for masks that are suitable for preventing airborne transmission of TB. OSHA recommendations for TB masks require a minimum efficiency rate of 95% in filtering environmental air which will inhibit inhalation of infectious particles. Confirmation that a person has been exposed to TB is obtained by the administration of the Mantoux skin test of purified protein derivative (PPD). This intradermal test is read between 48 to 72 hours following administration and confirms an infection with TB if it results in an induration exceeding 5 mm. Table 6–3 lists the recommended guidelines for administering the Mantoux skin test for health care workers. The Occupational Safety and Health Administration is currently developing an occupational standard for TB control that will mandate testing and recommend disease prevention measures.

Health care workers who exhibit a positive TB test should be immediately evaluated by their local occupational health department and begin treatment as soon as possible. Those who do not have direct access to such services should be seen by their personal physician or health care professional or access their local Department of Public Health. Anesthesia providers who exhibit a positive response to a PPD test or are known or suspected of having been exposed to active TB should refrain from direct patient contact until evaluation has been completed. High efficiency particulate (HEPA) filters can be incorporated into ventilatory systems and used to filter air in areas where the potential for TB transmission is high. Ultraviolet (UVA) lighting systems are another method used to deactivate TB in air where transmission

TABLE 6–3. OSHA Guidelines for Occupational Exposure to Tuberculosis

Recommend Mantoux skin test administration.
Guidelines:
- All employees must be offered the skin test free of charge.
- All tests must be in accordance with standard medical practices.
- Frequency of testing should be
  - At the time of initial employment.
  - Every 6 months if the health care worker has frequent exposure to patients with TB, or is involved with high-hazard procedures for TB risk.
  - Annual testing for all other health care workers.
  - After suspected TB exposure.

risk exists. Infection control guidelines applied to ORs (see section on blood-borne pathogens) should be applied to all areas where a risk for TB transmission might exist.

Latex

An increasing incidence of sensitivity and allergy to products containing latex has occurred throughout recent years. Nutter first described an allergic reaction to rubber products in 1979. Since then, documented cases of type IV or delayed hypersensitivity to latex products in the form of eczematous contact dermatitis has proliferated. Increasing numbers of reports of type I or anaphylactic allergic responses to latex-containing products have been consistent throughout most areas of health care.

Latex occurs naturally in the rubber tree *Hevea brazilienses* and consists of a terpene polymer found in many products used across the medical field. Siegel, Rich, and Brock (1993) explained a strong response to specific IgE antibodies found in a histamine release assay due to a low molecular weight protein within rubber. All adaptive immune responses occur in a more exaggerated form when resulting tissue damage causes a hypersensitivity. Such reactions are classified into four specific responses or types (I through IV). Types I and IV are most commonly seen. A type I response hypersensitivity occurs following initial contact with the responsible antigen. True anaphylaxis follows repeated exposure to the allergen and potentially detrimental results ensue.

Health care workers who develop a sensitivity to latex-containing products must determine the seriousness of their reactivity and decide to continue, limit, or avoid exposure. Testing, including intradermal injections of the allergen (similar to tuberculin testing), is available, yet carries a considerable risk for anaphylactic reaction. Less invasive scratch or patch tests, wherein limited exposures to latex are applied and evaluated, are another option. To date no specific FDA-approved latex skin testing materials are available. The radioimmunoassay test (RAST) tests plasma for latex-included IgE antibodies that are specific to the allergic response yet produces a somewhat arbitrary result. Kelly and coworkers (1994) site the RAST as only 53% sensitive, compared to a 99% sensitivity with a skin prick test.

Recently researchers (Charon, 1995) have quoted an 8% to 17% incidence of latex sensitivities among health care workers. Asthma-induced allergy due to latex exposure in this group has been noted to be as high as 2% (Charons, 1995). Continued efforts to reduce and eliminate, whenever possible, products used in health care that contain latex allergens are widespread; however, access to quality products and incurred expenses continue to hinder these efforts. Table 6–4 lists products used in anesthesia equipment and supplies that are likely to contain latex. Products such as gloves that contain powder can be responsible for allergic reactions when residue from the powder dissipates in the atmosphere and on surrounding surfaces. Chapter 7 describes signs and symptoms of latex allergic reactions. The American Association of Nurse Anesthetists (AANA) has published a *Latex Allergy Protocol*. Providers who experience latex allergy that impairs their ability to practice should obtain referral and placement according to institutional and local policy. Legislation that protects employee rights and disabilities guarantees provider protection with appropriate accommodation and placement.

Workplace Violence

The health care and social service industries report the highest risk for violent incidents according to the Bureau of Labor Statistics. Public service institutions such as hospitals are believed to carry a higher risk for violent crime due to positioning in central urban areas and provision of around-the-clock services. Additional factors that place

TABLE 6–4. Anesthesia Equipment Containing Latex

• Rubber masks	• Rubber ventilator bellows
• Electrode pad, (eg, electrocardiogram, peripheral stimulator)	• Rubber endotracheal tubes
• Head straps	• Latex cuffs on plastic tracheal tubes
• Rubber tourniquets	• Latex injection ports on intravenous tubing
• Rubber nasal–pharyngeal airways	• Multidose vial stoppers
• Rubber oral–pharyngeal airways	• Patient-controlled analgesia systems
• Teeth protectors	• Rubber suction catheters
• Bite blocks	• Injection ports on intravenous bags and infusion circuits
• Blood pressure cuffs	• Certain epidural catheter injection adapters
• Rubber breathing circuits	
• Reservoir breathing bags	
• Rubber ventilator hoses	

providers at risk for workplace violence include interacting with the public, exchanging money, delivering services or goods, working late at night or during early morning hours, working alone, guarding valuable goods or property, and dealing with violent people and volatile situations. Throughout the general population approximately 50% of all murder victims were related to their assailants; the majority of workplace homicides, however, are believed to occur among people who are unacquainted.

Predictive factors and warning signs of potential or threatened violent acts include the following:

- History of violent behavior
- Substance abuse (recent escalation in use)
- Unabated anger; inability to control anger
- Paranoia
- Persistent threatening physical actions
- Boundary-crossing approach
- Irrational violent statements and threats
- Depression
- Isolation; lack of desire to join in with others
- Significant personal, family, or financial problems
- Romantic obsession; persistent attention or stalking behaviors
- Weapons possession, proficiency, or obsession
- Strong sense of entitlement to job
- Verbal threats (direct or veiled) to hurt or kill someone
- Recent changes in behavior, moods, and approach to others
- Recent changes in work habits (attendance, punctuality, quality, appearance)
- Increasing conflicts with co-workers

Anecdotal reports from the American Emergency Nurses Association (ENA) and the AANA have cited incidents where nurse providers have been victims of hostile acts and violent crime while on duty. Providers must be alert to environmental cues and behavioral patterns that are suggestive of impending violence and respond quickly, safely, and appropriately.

Subtle clues that a violent act is imminent include provocative behavior, an angry demeanor, manic responses, intoxication, and delirium or confusion. More overt signs of impending violence are motor restlessness, loud and angry speech, actual threats, agitation, and obvious weapons. Any and all clues that suggest violence should be taken seriously, and immediate response should include physical separation and activation of a violence response program. Trained and qualified persons should be responsible for managing and preventing workplace violence.

Hostility and belligerent behavior can be a precursor to violent crime and should elicit appropriate responses. If at any time providers feel threatened or in danger, they should excuse themselves from the immediate area and summon assistance. No one should be expected to tolerate repeated personal, abusive comments or threatening actions.

Violence Prevention

A number of environmental, administrative, and behavioral strategies can potentially reduce the risk of workplace violence. Examples of prevention strategies include good visibility within and outside the workplace, policies for managing desired goods and property, physical separation of providers from patients, good lighting, security, escort services, and employee in-service training. No single strategy is appropriate for all workplaces, but all providers and employers should assess the risk of violence in their workplaces and take appropriate action to reduce those risks. A workplace violence prevention program should include a system for documenting incidents, procedures to be taken in the event of an incident, and open communication between providers and administrators.

Stress

Any job that involves accountability for the life or well-being of an individual inevitably carries a considerable degree of stress. Stress is a recognized potential health hazard of the anesthetist. A hectic or excessive work schedule, the process of making difficult decisions, the constant vigilance required in the OR, night duty, varying schedules, fatigue, increasing reliance on technology, and interpersonal tensions cause stress for anesthesia and surgery personnel. Areas of stress that are specific to the practice of anesthesia are (1) the induction of anesthesia; (2) overlapping realms of responsibility with the surgeon; and (3) dealing with uncertainty, the critically ill, and the dying patient. Recognition of factors that cause or contribute to job-related stress is essential for all providers. Professional counseling and guidance is available from qualified practitioners and employee assistance programs and should be used to address such concerns when they are present. Qualified programs are available from employers and state and national professional organizations.

▶ VIGILANCE

Vigilance is one of the most critical functions performed by the anesthetist, yet is not in itself sufficient for avoiding anesthetic mishaps. A vigilance task is defined as one requiring the detection of changes in stimulus during long monitoring periods when the subject has little or no prior knowledge of the sequence of changes. Baker and Ware (1966) described that the ability to perform a vigilance task varies inversely with its complexity. Factors that diminish the ability to sustain concentration are important considerations. Ergonomic considerations such as poor design of monitor displays, inappropriate equipment positioning in both the vertical and horizontal planes, and alarm artifacts are examples of factors that contribute to distraction from the primary vigilance task and can cause fatigue from excessive and unnecessary energy expenditure.

► ERGONOMICS

The consideration of human factors in equipment design is the area of ergonomics, long recognized by health care industry experts as important to overall provider performance and well-being. A move toward modernizing anesthetic equipment and the operating room environment to ergonomic standards has begun. Although OSHA does not directly mandate workplace ergonomic standards, the General Duty clause provides direction for employers to accommodate these environments to provider needs. Particular goals for ergonomic control plans usually include efforts to reduce large body and repetitive movements that contribute to work-related injuries. Elimination of acute injuries while reducing chronic disorders resulting from poor task and physical movements are basic responsibilities of such programs. Health care organization safety officers and industrial engineering specialists are responsible for evaluating workspace dynamics and coordinating modifications and design changes that improve workplace environments. Provider participation in these processes are essential to the development of ergonomically efficient workstations and programs that control and prevent work-related injuries. Computer technology for data integration to provide trending information and "intelligent" warnings of potential difficulties as well as automation in anesthetic delivery is a promising area of research. Comprehensive anesthesia simulation environments such as those developed by Gaba and DeAnda (1988) and others have contributed to increased provider comfort in managing stress and related consequences in the anesthesia setting.

► WASTE ANESTHETIC GASES

The literature and research on waste anesthetic gases (WAG) have failed to define a "safe" level of occupational exposure based on currently available data. It is, therefore, reasonable that every effort be made to keep OR exposure of WAG as low as possible.

Scavenging or waste gas evacuation systems in today's anesthetizing locations should contain the following components:

- Gas-collecting assembly
- Transfer system that connects the gas-collecting

assembly to the ventilator or adjustable pressure-limiting valve in the breathing circuit
- Gas disposal tubing that connects the gas-collecting assembly to the disposal system

Scavenging systems are characterized by the way in which gas is removed from the circuit. Vacuum types use either a negative-pressure relief valve or an open port to the atmosphere to prevent the negative pressure from affecting the anesthesia circuit.

The National Institute for Occupational Safety and Health (NIOSH) recommends air monitoring of all ORs at least annually, when new equipment is used, and if complaints suggest a problem. Scavenging systems must comply with the American Society of Testing and Materials (ASTM) standards as outlined in other areas of this text. These specific standards should be available from the facility biomedical engineering department. Reports should be made available to all providers who work with, in, and around anesthesia machines. Suspected problems should be reported immediately and the suspect equipment should be removed from the practice setting pending repair and checkout.

Multiple investigations over several decades have been conducted in an attempt to calculate the potential risk from provider exposure to anesthetic gases. Several studies reviewed the impact with regard to hemopoietic impact, behavioral assessment, cellular influence, and animal responses. Concerns regarding WAG and fertility, carcinogenicity, teratogenicity, and reproduction continue to be explored. Research validity and conclusions continue to be questioned and challenged.

► CASE STUDY

W.W., a 39-year-old CRNA, was exposed to blood while on duty in a large inner-city teaching hospital. Responding to a cardiac arrest "code blue" situation, W.W. sustained a puncture in her left dorsal palm from a large-bore guide needle used to establish a subclavian access line during the resuscitation.

The patient, an unidentified male, approximately 30 years old, was admitted to the intensive care unit (ICU) 3 hours prior to arrest. He was unresponsive on arrival to the emergency department (ED) but began to respond to verbal commands, remaining lethargic following the administration of naloxone 1.0 mg once intravenous access was accomplished in the ED. His temperature was 95.8°; heart rate 48; respiratory rate 58; and blood pressure 92/54 on admission.

Paramedics responded to a call in the warehouse district where they found the victim on the ground, discovered by a freight dock loader reporting for work at 0400 Sunday morning. The paramedics were unable to initiate venous access in the field due to "poor visualized potential" and "marked scarring over all extremities." W.W. reported her exposure to the administrative supervisor on duty immediately following the occurrence.

1. What steps should W.W. and the supervisor take to manage this exposure? List the individual steps and their priority, including follow-up management and treatment, interventional options, and counseling.

   - **Step 1: Treatment.** Cleanse wound and control bleeding. Isolate needle.
   - **Step 2: Triage and Risk Determination.** Evaluate the risk related to this incident and determine the appropriate intervention that should occur. The source patient in this case presents with considerable risk factors that include the following:

     1. Situation at discovery including hypothermia, unresponsiveness, and physical environment: Physical findings such as extremity scarring could suggest a potential intravenous drug use history, and unstable vital signs could support the above potential.
     2. Determination of suspected degree or amount of innoculum that was potentially transmitted: A large-bore hollow needle used in this case could contain a sufficient concentration to support a potential blood-borne pathogen transmission.

   This scenario is representative of a significant high-risk exposure.

   - **Step 3: Counseling.** The provider should be informed of the risks and options available to respond to such an event. High-risk exposures such as this should include the option and availability of immediate (within 24 hours) exposure response including chemoprophylaxis of the provider should she choose to participate in a recommended treatment program. Current chemoprophylaxis regimen should consist of agents and schedules as described previously in this chapter. The exposed provider should be told of all related risks including the questionable

efficacy and potential side effects of such therapy. Institutional policies and procedure may alter such steps as described.

   - **Step 4: Serologic Markers.** Determine laboratory serologic parameters including HBV, HCV, and HIV status. If the provider is immune to HBV due to prior exposure or vaccination, additional titers are not necessary. Human immunodeficiency virus status should be documented regardless of prior tests unless the provider is previously documented as HIV positive. Serologic determinations from the source patient should be obtained for HBV, HCV, and HIV following appropriate counseling and informed consent. These baseline studies should be repeated in 6 to 12 weeks and again in 6 months to establish further treatment guidelines. Institutional policies and procedures may alter such steps as described.
   - **Step 5: Follow-up Management.** Medical treatment and management should be coordinated by the provider's personal physician or provider of choice. Some institutions may offer an occupational medicine source for continuation of care and follow-up treatment. Worker compensation claim processes, quality management, and institutional safety programs should be contacted, and appropriate processing should be initiated and information maintained according to institutional protocols and policies. Future counseling, treatment, and management should be mutually planned and agreed on by both the exposed person and primary care provider. Confidentiality should remain a top priority.

▶ SUMMARY

Many hazards exist in the anesthesia workplace that can threaten the well being of the nurse anesthetist. The CRNA must be alert to these hazards and take precautions to assure maximum workplace safety. It is incumbent on the nurse anesthetist to review current literature on occupational safety and to incorporate the recommendations into practice.

► **KEY CONCEPTS**

- Needlestick injuries continue to be a major cause of anesthesia provider workplace exposures to potential infection by blood-borne pathogens. Practice behaviors, technique, and consistent application of standard and needle precautions while handling sharps influence and prevent needlestick injuries during anesthesia practice.
- Cough-inducing procedures such as laryngoscopy, intubation, and bronchoscopy increase the probability of transmission of droplet nuclei that are responsible for the transmission of TB.
- A patient infected with HIV is at greater risk of

contracting drug-resistant strains of TB and organisms that fail to respond to conventional antibiotic treatment.
- Exposure to harmful levels of WAG are prevented by compliance with standards that control leakage, including a functional gas scavenging system that is appropriately used and receives preventative maintenance, and waste gas monitoring programs.
- Violent acts in the health care setting are more likely to occur in isolated areas, where persons are working alone, and maintain immediate access to desirable commodities such as controlled substances.

► **STUDY QUESTIONS**

1. Who should determine provider risk when an occupational exposure to potential blood-borne pathogens occurs?

2. What laboratory tests or results are necessary to properly manage an occupational exposure and determine future intervention strategies?

3. What information will be most beneficial in determining

if chemoprophylaxis is indicated and the appropriate follow-up of an occupational exposure?

4. What agents, dosage, and schedule are appropriate for chemoprophylaxis in response to a significant, high-risk occupational exposure to blood?

5. What intervention steps should be taken to manage a blood exposure following initial decontamination, source, and exposure determination?

KEY REFERENCES

American Association of Nurse Anesthetists (AANA). (1996). *Professional practice manual for the certified registered nurse anesthetist* (5th ed.). Park Ridge, IL: AANA.

American Society of Anesthesiologists (ASA). (1994). *Recommendations for infection control for the practice of anesthesiology.* Park Ridge, IL: ASA.

Centers for Disease Control and Prevention (CDC), National Center for Injury Prevention and Control. (1996). *National summary of injury mortality data, 1988–1994.* Atlanta, GA: CDC.

National Institute of Occupational Safety and Health. (1997). NIOSH Home Page [on-line]: http://www.cdc.gov/niosh/homepage.html.

REFERENCES

American Association of Nurse Anesthetists (AANA). (1996). *Professional practice manual for the certified registered nurse anesthetist* (5th ed.). Park Ridge, IL: AANA.

Baker, R. A. & Ware, J. R. (1966). The relationship between vigilance and monotonous work. *Ergonomics, 9,* 109.

Bauer, J. (1997). Is it really a secret? *Journal of Perianesthesia Nursing, 12,* 67–68.

Bell, D. (1996). Occupational risk of HIV Infection in health care workers: Improving the managment of HIV disease. *International AIDS Society—USA, 4*(2), 7–10.

Castro, K. G. (July, 1992). *HIV infection and tuberculosis.* Pa-

per presented at the meeting of the American Medical Association: Chicago, IL.

Centers for Disease Control and Prevention. (1995). Guidelines for isolation precautions in hospitals. *Infection Control & Hospital Epidemiology, 17,* 1.

Charons, B. L. (1995). Latex-induced asthma among health care workers. Medical news & perspectives. *Journal of the American Medical Association, 273,* 10.

Gaba, D. M. & DeAnda, A. (1988). A comprehensive anesthesia simulation environment: Recreating the operating room for research and training. *Anesthesiology, 69,* 387.

Garb, J. & Dockery, C. (1995). Reducing employee back injuries in the perioperative setting. *Journal of the Association of Operating Room Nurses, 61*(6), 1046-1052.

Griffin, K. (1996). They should have washed their hands. *Health, Nov./Dec.,* 82–91.

Kelly, K. J., Pearson, M. L., Kurup, V. P., Havens, P. L., Byrd, R. S., Setlock, M. A., Butler, J. C., Slater, J. E., Grummer, L. C., & Resnick, A. (1994). A cluster of anaphylactic reactions in children with spina bifida during general anesthesia Epidemiologic features, risk factors, and latex hypersen-sitivity. *Journal of Allergy & Clinical Immunology, 94,* 53–61.

National Council on Compensation Insurance (NCCI). (1992). *Issues report.* Boca Raton, FL: NCCI.

Nutter, A. F. (1979). Contact urticaria to rubber. *British Journal of Dermatology, 1012,* 597–598.

Parker, M. (1995). The use of protective gloves, the incidence of ampoule injury and the prevalence of hand laceration amongst anesthetic personnel. *Anaesthesia, 50*(8), 726–729.

Seeley, H. (1996). The practice of anesthesia—A stressor for the middle-aged? *Anaesthesia, 51*(6), 571–574.

Short, L. J. & Bell, D. M. (1993). Risk of occupational infection with blood-borne pathogens in operating and delivery room settings. *American Journal of Infection Control, 21,* 343-350.

Siegel, J. F., Rich, M. & Brock, W. A. (1993). Latex allergy and anaphylaxis. *International Anesthesiology Clinics, 31,* 141–145.

Tait, A. & Tuffle, D. (1994). Prevention of occupational transmission of human immunodeficiency virus and hepatitis B among anesthesiologists: A survey of anesthesiology practice. *Anesthesia & Analgesia, 79,* 623–628.

U.S. Department of Labor, Occupational Safety and Health Administration. (1991). Occupational exposure to blood-borne pathogens [Final Rule, 29 CFR Part 1910, 1030]. *Federal Register 56*(235): 64003–64182.

Patient Health and Safety

Brent Sommer

Those unfamiliar with anesthesia practice often question the degree of risk and related anxiety regarding inherent dangers that present during management of anesthesia. A usual response would include reference to the thoroughness and degree of education involved in preparing a professional to legally qualify to practice anesthesia. Additionally, application of sophisticated monitoring technologies, operator vigilance, and accountability are required to ensure all patients the safest possible experience.

Commitment to the safety and well being of patients in our care is a proper expectation of all anesthesia providers based on both patient rights and inherent professional obligations. This chapter explores the potential risks that patients incur while in our care as well as methodologies, practice standards, and techniques appropriate to ensure the safest environment possible. This topic demands our attention and constant commitment to assure the appropriate application and maintenance of accepted practice guidelines and standards.

Practice safety has long been the focus of anesthesia providers in this country as evidenced by early educational programs of study that have evolved over the past 60 years. The first formal symposium on anesthesia morbidity and mortality was held in 1983 when representatives of the Harvard Medical School and the Royal Society of Medicine of England met jointly to develop future studies and strategies for the promotion of anesthesia safety. The Anesthesia Patient Safety Foundation (APSF) was established in 1984 to assure that "no patient shall be harmed by the effects of anesthesia (1996)" (p. 2). The APSF continues to investigate numerous factors influencing the perianesthetic environment and periodically provides published information to all practitioners that describes specific concerns and recommended management strategies.

The International Committee for Prevention of Anesthesia Mortality and Morbidity (ICPAMM) meets annually to explore the processes used to study issues related to anesthesia safety. Although these programs continue to promote research and new technologic applications regarding practice safety, there remains no substitution for constant vigilance to each patient.

Adverse outcomes directly attributable to anesthesia care are uncommon in healthier patients and rarely present as the singular cause of related morbidity or mortality. These risks increase proportionately in relation to the degree of system involvement and patient acuity. Studies by Cooper and colleagues (1978, 1979, 1984) calculating anesthesia-related mishaps estimate that over 80% of those cases reported are directly attributable to human error and are preventable. The challenge for each Certified Registered Nurse Anesthetist (CRNA) is to be able to protect the patient from any source of harm that might exist or emerge during the perianesthesia period.

▶ ANESTHESIA SAFETY

Derrington and Smith (1987) report that anesthesia-related injuries are most often associated with hypoxia, hypoventilation, airway obstruction, drug overdosage, airway mismanagement, inadequate patient preparation, student/resident supervision issues, and crisis management. Most studies examining these situations, which are commonly referred to as *critical incidents,* are often considered preventable. Such incidents are a result of human error and equipment malfunction or failure that ultimately results in some degree of morbidity and mortality.

Cooper and colleagues (1978, 1979, 1984) found that accidental circuit disconnection was a frequently reported problem during anesthesia via critical incident surveys. Poor retention of some plastic fittings received the majority of blame for these incidents. The problem of accidental disconnection became so widespread and troublesome that the Food and Drug Administration (FDA) funded a study to determine the cause and, if possible, a solution to this problem. As a result, current standard gauges and test methods specially designed to allow for the variable characteristics of plastics are available. An antidisconnect fitting designed to prevent disconnection of the 15-mm male tube connector fitting from the grooved 22-mm male Y-piece fitting is in general use throughout U.S. health care institutions.

The practice of anesthesia in America is significantly influenced by a multitude of statutes, associated regulations, accrediting standards, standards of professional associations, and rules and regulations promulgated by a myriad of governmental and nongovernmental agencies. These established practice standards and guidelines require that providers properly and consistently apply appropriate safety interventions or appliances in all patient care practices. Environmental standards in health care settings are mandated by regulatory agencies such as the National Electrical Code (NEC) and National Fire and Protection Agency (NFPA). These bodies maintain the recommended parameters of environmental standards and establish necessary guidelines to ensure compliance.

▶ EXPOSURE RISK

Risk of infection and exposures to communicable disease accounts for a majority of patient care morbidity. Nosocomial infection rates in the United States have remained steady for several years. The American Association of Nurse Anesthetists (AANA; 1996) Practice Standard IX states that "precautions shall be taken to minimize the risk of infection to the patient, the CRNA, and other health care providers" (p. 5). Most professional health care organizations that represent patient care specialists maintain similar practice standards as a commitment to patient protection and well-being.

U.S. surveillance data reports that the rate of cases of sepsis exceed 400 000 and that associated health care costs exceed $10 billion annually. Quartin and associates (1997) noted that, as the thirteenth most frequent cause of death, more than 25% of septic patients succumb while hospitalized. Although the documented incidence of direct relationships between anesthesia care and septicemia is difficult to determine, the need for meticulous

aseptic technique during this vulnerable period is obvious. It is crucial that an appreciation for patients both identified and suspected to be at risk for sepsis and appropriate application and management of infection control strategies be a constant focus.

▶ ASEPSIS

Nosocomial infection rates have been shown to be decreased by consistent and improved hand-washing techniques. Hand-washing is thought to be the single most important step in preventing the transmission of infections, yet it is often minimized, neglected, or performed inappropriately. Although no specific frequency or hand-washing during routine patient care is recommended, standard universal precautions call for providers to wash their hands after performing any "at-risk" tasks and in between their contact with patients. Hands should also be washed after removing gloves and on completion of any patient care task or procedure.

The Centers for Disease Control and Prevention (CDC) and Public Health Service recommend that an adequate hand-wash—lasting from 10 to 15 seconds up to 2 minutes—be performed with liquid antimicrobial soaps. Whenever adequate hand-washing facilities and supplies are not readily available, such as in the immediate anesthetizing location, an appropriate antiseptic hand cleanser and clean towels should be available and used.

As many patients present with preexisting disease and pathophysiologic conditions that challenge their safety, the CRNA should have a thorough appreciation of such states and be able to formulate and implement a plan of care that will lead to an improved and sustained condition, one that minimizes further physiologic compromise. Infection control in health care settings has evolved historically from the nursing profession and developed as an integral part of virtually all present health disciplines.

▶ ENVIRONMENTAL RISK

Basic infection control practices and adherence to recommended environmental safety measures will serve to maintain safe surroundings during the paranesthesia period. The American Association of Operating Room Nurses (AORN) practice standards recommend environmental strategies for minimizing risks that increase the likelihood of contamination and infection transmission in and around the operating room (OR). In addition to the strict application of aseptic technique during both preparation and maintenance of surgery, the following recommendations reduce the likelihood of OR bacterial contamination:

- Limited numbers of persons in the actual OR suite
- Traffic control and maintenance in and around the OR
- Doors that are kept closed and separate vulnerable areas from cross-contamination
- Disposable surgical garb, drapes, gloves, and personal protective equipment that will prevent and minimize transmission.

The American Association of Operating Room Nurses (1989) has been instrumental in providing continued research and education, surveillance information, and practice standards for the surgical arena. The Association of Women's Health, Obstetrical, and Neonatal Nurses (AWHONN) provides similar resources for the obstetrical practice areas. Recommended standards of practice regarding environmental hygiene and maintenance have been effective in containing and preventing infection throughout the workplace. Published AORN standards are used routinely in most U.S. hospitals and health care agencies to ensure compliance with infection control requirements and standardization of practice.

Principles guiding infection control during anesthesia have evolved from the profession as a combination of safety guidelines and recommended practice standards. In recent years the AANA Occupational Safety and Hazard Committee has updated the association's *Infection Control Guide* (see AANA, 1996) which serves as a practice reference for the design, implementation, and maintenance of infection control programs wherever anesthesia is administered. The guide is an integral component of the *Professional Practice Manual* for the CRNA and is available from the AANA.

▶ ENVIRONMENTAL RESPONSIBILITY AND PROTECTION

The frequently unfamiliar surroundings to which our patients are exposed during their surgical or obstetrical experience contain a multitude of potentially harmful components. Fortunately, current technology and equipment safeguards provide an inherent degree of protection. There is, however, no substitution for an alert and vigilant provider. Failure to properly apply and operate the varieties of machinery and ancillary equipment found in today's operative suites intensifies patient risk of harm and injury while increasing provider liability. Industrial hygiene and biomedical engineering specialists often work in conjunction with facility operations, administrative, and professional staff to ensure that a safe physical environment exists throughout the health care facility.

The equipment and products used to deliver anesthesia care and adjunct therapies should always be main-tained, operated, and administered according to the manufacturer's recommendations. A suspected malfunction or obvious problem with equipment or a product should result in its immediate discontinuation and removal from the OR. All personnel who are likely to use the same or similar device or product should be alerted to any malfunction.

▶ PROVIDER RESPONSIBILITY AND ACCOUNTABILITY

The CRNA should be knowledgeable and trained to appropriately prepare, apply, and manage all products, equipment, and accessories contained within anesthesia and ancillary delivery systems. The maintenance of anesthesia equipment requires the absolute attention of the provider to ensure appropriate application and performance while ensuring its integrity, performance, and safety.

Every institution and anesthesia department should maintain a process whereby such incidents are reported as soon as possible. A program sponsored by the FDA known as *MedWatch* is available for prompt reporting of product or medication problems regarding their quality, performance, or safety. Programs like these serve as a direct line to report potential dangers and obtain the necessary support and direction to appropriately intervene and prevent further problems.

Disease Prevention

The evolution of current infection control standards has resulted largely from the progressive refinement of recommended practice standards from the CDC. The CDC is responsible for disease surveillance and epidemiologic investigation that results in recommended practice guidelines. Known or suspected threats to patient safety and disease control are thoroughly investigated by CDC experts before standardized guidelines are formulated and published to all concerned disciplines in health care.

Surveillance

Hospital-based epidemiology programs use a surveillance process that calculates nosocomial infection rates and adverse occurrence events to identify changes and distributions that influence environmental health and safety. Information obtained by these processes are then used to institute control measures and determine interventional effectiveness. Useful information including compliance rates and notable trends for future studies are identified through this process. Practice guidelines published by the CDC address all areas of clinical practice and related infection control elements for maintaining the safest practice environment possible. These guidelines are available from the CDC Injury Prevention and Control Directory (CDC Injury Prevention and Control Directory: 888-232-3299).

Equipment and Instrumentation Management

Effective strategies for operating and maintaining anesthesia machine systems, ancillary instrumentation, and medical devices come under the purview of the nurse anesthetist. As previously mentioned, the provider is responsible for the appropriate operation and application of these items. Effective infection control practices include the application of recommended standards and intervention to prevent the spread of disease and cross-contamination.

Concern regarding possible cross-infection from anesthesia equipment has been stimulated by a dramatic increase in nosocomial infections, particularly those caused by gram-negative bacilli. Studies by Pace and coworkers (1979) and Garibaldi and associates (1981) clearly showed a link between the use of respiratory therapy equipment, particularly nebulizers, and the incidence of necrotizing pneumonia. Although no strong clinical studies demonstrated that anesthesia equipment was the direct cause of the infections, disposable breathing systems with bacterial filters have been advocated as the answer to the problem. Most surveillance studies have reported that bacterial filters failed to reduce the incidence of pneumonia following inhalation anesthesia.

Many argue that the incidence of postoperative atelectasis and pneumonia is more directly influenced by the patient's preoperative pulmonary condition, the location and duration of surgery, and the amount of postoperative pain and narcotics given than by the presence of a small number of skin or surface contaminants found on breathing circuitry. There is a tendency, because filters are expensive, to use them for more than one patient, thus increasing the chance that bacteria may accumulate in condensation trapped within the filter. The filter may therefore become a bacterial accumulator rather than a bacterial eliminator. Preventive maintenance for all anesthesia, ventilatory, and monitoring equipment at the recommended 3- or 6-month intervals is currently the usual practice in most departments of anesthesia.

Several key steps are crucial in minimizing the risk of exposure to infection from patient to patient, provider to patient, patient to provider, or other personnel in or around the anesthetizing location. Figure 7-1 depicts the general conditions and classification of risks for equipment, devices, and instruments used in providing anesthesia care and the levels of cleaning, disinfection, and preparation required to prevent the transmission of infection. This classification scheme recommended by the

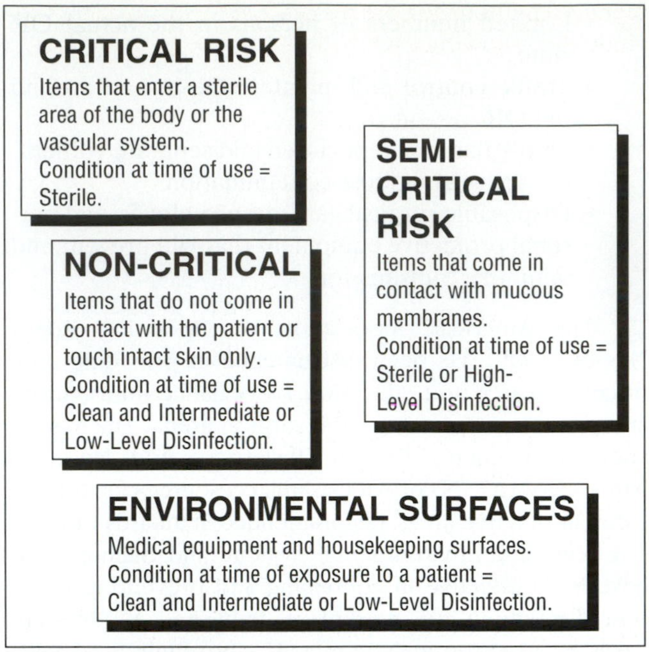

CRITICAL RISK
Items that enter a sterile area of the body or the vascular system.
Condition at time of use = Sterile.

SEMI-CRITICAL RISK
Items that come in contact with mucous membranes.
Condition at time of use = Sterile or High-Level Disinfection.

NON-CRITICAL
Items that do not come in contact with the patient or touch intact skin only.
Condition at time of use = Clean and Intermediate or Low-Level Disinfection.

ENVIRONMENTAL SURFACES
Medical equipment and housekeeping surfaces.
Condition at time of exposure to a patient = Clean and Intermediate or Low-Level Disinfection.

Figure 7-1. Classification of risks for transmitting infection in anesthesia applications.

AANA separates equipment, instruments, and other devices according to the degree of risk involved with their use. Recommendations provided by the equipment manufacturer should be followed to ensure that the proper method of cleaning, disinfection, and sterilization is applied for each instrument, device, or surface that is being processed.

Disposable equipment can be reused if it is carefully handled, cleaned, tested, repackaged, and resterilized by recommended methods. The FDA guidelines (1987) mandate the reuse of disposables by requiring that (1) the device can be adequately cleaned and sterilized, (2) the physical characteristics or quality of the device will not be altered or adversely affected, (3) the device remains safe and effective for its intended use, and (4) the user accepts full responsibility for the device's safety and effectiveness. Decontamination of equipment and items to be reused during anesthesia care are first cleaned according to recommended practice standards. The appropriate disinfectant and cleaning process will vary according to the nature and degree of contaminant and intended reuse of the item. Cleansing with an appropriate germicidal detergent is sufficient for OR environmental surfaces, furniture, and items that do not penetrate the integument or mucosal membranes. Invasive items require high-level disinfection and/or sterilization. Current infection control nomenclature separates patient care/equipment into three general categories: critical, semicritical, and noncritical (Fig. 7-1). Recommended methods for processing reusable equipment include the following (AORN, 1989):

1. Sterilization
   - Steam autoclaving
   - Ethylene oxide gas autoclaving
   - Sterilant concentrate agents (eg, peroxyacetic acid)
2. Disinfection
   - Alkaline glutaraldehyde (eg, Cidex)
   - Phenolic solution (eg, Wexcide)
   - Sodium hypochlorite (chlorine bleach)
3. Antisepsis
   - Idophor preparation (eg, Betadine)
   - Chlorhexidine gluconate (eg, Hibiclens)
   - Hexachlorophene
   - 70% alcohol

Cross-Contamination

Controversies continue over the incidence of cross-contamination from equipment to patient and vice versa. Tactile, airborne, and blood-borne pathogens are proven sources of infectious contamination and transmission and will be addressed individually. As gases flow throughout the anesthesia patient circuit, moisture accumulates and can harbor infectious bacteria within the system. Anesthesia machines have been shown to harbor such organisms as *Pseudomonas aeruginosa* following administration exceeding 1 hour (Garibaldi and coworkers, 1981). Prevention of bacterial spread and cross-contamination can be maintained by changing the breathing circuit and rebreathing bag or incorporating an appropriate bacterial filter into the system at the Y-piece.

Du Moulin and Saugermann (1977) found that the anesthesia machine is rarely a source of bacterial contamination. Research continues to address the relationship between benefits of bacterial filtration and patient morbidity secondary to infection transmitted from this source. However inconclusive, nosocomial infection rates and the inability to identify an immunocompromised host from clinical presentation when adequate information is unavailable supports the use of filters as recommended by their manufacturers. The APSF continues to entertain arguments for and against the use of bacterial filtration as a component of anesthesia breathing circuitry and reuse of disposable products.

Microbial Resistance

Resistance to chemotherapeutic agents commonly used to combat microorganisms has been documented from several strains of bacteria, viruses, fungi, and parasites. These cases of resistance inevitably result in longer, more serious illnesses that carry significant sequelae, greater incidences of mortality, and the need for therapeutic agents that are expensive and tend to complicate patient response to traditional medical treatments. Inadequate application or absence of aseptic techniques during patient care has been implicated in various reported cases.

Reported cases of microbial resistance in hospitals have been documented as early as the 1950s when penicillin-resistant *Staphylococcus aureus* was identified. Nosocomial infections today are most often caused by organisms, such as coagulase-negative staphylococci, *S. aureus,* enterococci, candida speuer, *Escherichia Coli, Pseudomonas aeruginosa,* and other gram-negative rods. Research continues to determine the appropriate management strategies of such conditions.

Product Labeling

Disposable items that are labeled as *single-use* devices or for *one-time use* should not be applied to more than one patient. Decontamination, sterilization, or use beyond the manufacturer's label would constitute violation of suggested application and could incur patient harm and provider liability.

Waste Containment and Disposal

Current OSHA regulations (1988) require practices that prevent the transmission of blood-borne pathogens in any health care setting. Biohazardous waste and used laundry contain many potentially infectious materials that could cause disease in humans, most notably, blood-borne pathogens. These wastes should be placed in closed containers that are designed to prevent fluid leakage during handling, storage, transport, and shipping. Containers should be color coded and labeled as *biohazardous waste* in accordance with OSHA regulations concerning blood-borne pathogens. Employees handling biohazardous waste should use appropriate personal protective equipment provided by the employer.

Tuberculosis

The resurgence of infectious *Mycobacterium tuberculosis* (TB) in recent years has caused particular concern in health care facilities. After 30 years of decreasing TB prevalence, the clinical incidence of this disease has begun to rise over the past decade. An advanced strain of multidrug resistant (MDR) TB has caused serious threats to those susceptible to exposure, particularly those in an already immunocompromised state such as HIV infection or posttransplantation. The World Health Organization (WHO) has estimated that nearly 100 000 persons are coinfected with HIV and TB, further complicating their course and increasing their likelihood of developing active disease by 50% or more. Nearly 50% of those afflicted with the MDR strains will die as a result of their disease.

Conditions that increase the likelihood of TB infectivity include the concentration and rate of expelled organisms, physical properties of discharged material into the air, air volume, and rate of exchange and length of time exposure of exchange in expelled air. Hospitalized patients are at risk for TB exposure when undergoing or adjacent to cough-inducing procedures such as bronchoscopy, endotracheal intubation, and aerosolized inhalational therapeutic treatments. Preventing the spread of TB is most effective in systems maintaining reliable surveillance and early detection programs. It is crucial for all health care workers and ancillary staff to suspect that a patient may be infected with TB if they exhibit one or more of the suspicious signs, symptoms, or characteristics listed in Table 7-1. Some medical conditions are consistent with increased TB risk including silicosis, intravenous drug abuse, diabetes mellitus, corticosteroid therapy, immunosuppressive therapy, or renal disease.

Tuberculosis Diagnosis and Prevention Strategies

An intradermal Mantoux skin test is indicative of TB infectivity if it results in an induration at the test site of 5 mm or larger in diameter within 48 to 72 hours and in conjunction with specific criteria regarding risk factors such as a significant health history and known or suspected exposure. Maintenance of an active TB surveillance program includes early detection and intervention that serves to decrease the spread of TB infection and active disease progression. Early treatment with recommended anti-TB agents will diminish and eliminate infectivity of the disease.

Environments with adequate air flow and appropriate exchange rates are most effective in preventing the spread of TB. Measures that prevent the spread of droplet nuclei will support this process. Commercially prepared face masks that comply with the National Institute for Occupational Health and Safety (NIOSH) recommendations of appropriate design, fit, and filtration efficiency (95% or greater) are necessary to prevent spread of the disease. Areas where potentially infectious droplet contamination has occurred should be thoroughly cleaned according to suggested recommendations. Disposable equipment should be used and appropriately discarded whenever possible. Reusable equipment and environmental furniture and fixtures should be processed according to suggested guidelines as recommended by the CDC and outlined in the *AANA Infection Control Guide.*

Disease Transmission and Safeguards

The CDC (1983) has published a *Guideline for Isolation Precautions in Hospitals* that categorizes distinct methods for infection control practice that are based on known routes of infection transmission. *Standard precautions* include the primary strategies for nosocomial infection control of blood-borne pathogens and body fluids that are known to transmit disease. These precautions replace former isolation categories that were disease-specific. Standard precautions exist to reduce the risk of transmission of microorganisms from both recognized and undiagnosed sources of infection in the health care setting.

Transmission-based precautions are used to prevent the transmission of pathogens that are known or suspected to be a source of infection or colonization within the host. These precautions apply to airborne, droplet, and contact transmission and are designed to further complement standard precautions while applied on an empiric and temporary basis pending a definite diagnosis. These guidelines are based on sound epidemiologic research and contain recommended precautions for the prevention and transmission of nosocomial pathogens.

► BLOOD-BORNE PATHOGENS

Infectious pathogens that are transmitted via the bloodstream and in body fluids containing blood constitute a significant risk for both patients and providers. Although exhaustive efforts have been made to predict the actual risk of patient exposure to nosocomial blood-borne disease, calculations repeatedly reflect a minuscule likelihood of such an occurrence in the health care setting. Blood-borne pathogens include all hepatitis strains and human immunodeficiency virus (HIV). Chapter 6 describes provider risk and strategies for managing blood-borne pathogens during anesthesia care.

The OSHA blood-borne pathogen standard (1991) mandates the application of universal precautions, engineering controls, work practices, and personal protective equipment while caring for patients in the health care setting. Appropriate application of these standards (McMillan-Jackson, 1993) should be determined by the provider when risks are calculated and compared to patient presentation and individual practice history. Potentials for related morbidity and mortality are markedly increased.

TABLE 7–1. Clinical Characteristics and Manifestations of Infectious Tuberculosis

Cough	Laboratory or chest x-ray abnormality
Hemoptysis	Recent exposure to clinically active TB
Weight loss	Known or documented history of TB in the past

Needlestick Injury

An estimated 80% of all occupational blood exposures are due to needlestick injuries sustained by health care workers as noted by the Prevention Services Division of the California Department of Health Services when comparing national reporting data. Strict adherence to protocols and programs that are designed to prevent needlestick injury in health care settings are applicable to patient safety in reducing nosocomial risk and transmission.

The CDC has recommended practice alterations to decrease the incidence of needlestick injuries. To prevent needlestick injuries, needles should not be recapped by hand using a two-handed recapping technique, nor should they be purposely bent or broken by hand, removed from disposable syringes, or otherwise manipulated by hand. Following use, disposable syringes, needles, and other sharp items should be placed in puncture-resistant containers for disposal. The puncture resistant containers should be located as close as practical to the area in which they are used.

Exposure Management and Prevention

The fact that patient exposures to infectious blood-borne pathogens are highly unlikely in the hospital setting does not detract from the seriousness and necessity of maintaining immaculate infection control and universal precaution practices during all aspects of patient care. Immunization against hepatitis B virus (HBV) has markedly influenced the prevalence and incidence for the patient in recent years. The HBV vaccine is genetically engineered and contains no human tissue, blood, or blood product that would harbor HBV that could potentially infect a recipient of such products. Unfortunately, no passive or active immunization products are yet available to prevent transmission of hepatitis C. In the unlikely event that a patient would sustain an exposure to blood or blood-containing fluids, an immediate risk determination should follow initial efforts to eliminate the exposure and minimize transmission (see Chapter 6).

Airborne Pathogens

Aerosolization and transmission of infectious agents occur when invisible particles less than 10 microns in diameter are carried across air currents. This type of transmission requires considerable energy to generate a force adequate to diffuse such particles, a situation that is uncommon in most health care settings. Procedures that are capable of producing forces sufficient to cause such transfer are well documented and placed under airborne precautions recommended by the CDC. Some researchers have evaluated the likelihood of transmission of HBV via the airborne route, and research continues to explore the potential of HIV being carried in similar situations. To date, studies remain inconclusive.

Prevention of airborne pathogen transmission begins with environmental safety and risk-reduction programs. Appropriate isolation techniques should be initiated when appropriate. High-efficiency particulate aspirators (HEPA) filters are used to isolate known respiratory contaminants (see Chapter 6).

▶ FIRE AND ELECTRICAL SAFETY

The widespread use of electrically powered equipment in the OR presents a potential for hazardous conditions and related mishaps. An appreciation of this potential danger combined with a working knowledge and appropriate application of equipment best serve as the primary preventative measures against these hazards. Fire and explosions in the OR have become rare since the abandonment of flammable anesthetic agents in the 1970s. Fires that do occur in the surgical suite can, however, be of devastating consequence with significant morbidity and mortality. The National Electrical Code (NEC) and the National Fire Protection Association (NFPA) have developed standards that address electrical safety and the use of anesthetic and therapeutic gases (both explosive and nonexplosive) and other substances capable of sustaining fires. Testing and grounding parameters are included in safety standards for application to health care facilities.

A most critical element in sustaining OR electrical safety is appropriate grounding. Proper grounding will dissipate static electrical charges and divert dangerous currents that might develop. Ungrounded charges can cause serious injury and death as noted by Norris (1994) and others. Areas in which anesthesia is administered require an isolation transformer that separates any connection between the power source and electrical outlets by preventing current flow through a grounded patient. Auxiliary systems that use what is known as line isolation monitoring are incorporated into devices applied to patients as a further safeguard against inadvertent electrical shock. In the unlikely event of an electrical accident wherein a person is a victim of electrocution, the immediate response and treatment should be as follows:

1. Discontinue the electrical source. If unable to do so, separate the victim from the electrical contact by using a nonconductive material (eg, rubber, wood). Do not touch a victim until he or she is separated from the source.
2. Summon help and emergency services.
3. Initiate cardiopulmonary resuscitation, when indicated.
4. Defibrillate as soon as possible, when indicated.

5. Transport to an appropriate facility for medical care as soon as possible.

Fire prevention in the OR begins with provider vigilance and attention in avoiding and eliminating potential hazards that exist. The three components necessary to start a fire are fuel, oxygen, and an ignition source. The ignition source or some form of heat serves as the impetus for a fire and presents as open flames, static sparks, or an electrical arc within the OR. Certain chemical reactions can also serve as an ignition source. Once the ignition source combines with the fuel source or flammable material and oxygen, a fire is sustained.

The ignition source is the easiest component of a fire to control. Flashpoint is the initial temperature required for the fire to ignite and also for it to cease when the ignition source is removed. Ignition temperature is reached when the fire is sustained following removal of the ignition source. Detonation point is that temperature at which a mixture will explode. Fire and explosion usually occur when flashpoint temperatures increase to 500°C. Static electricity is frequently a major ignition source of fires in the OR. The removal of static charges and resistance provided by conductive flooring combined with air moisture sustained at the relative humidity of 55% to 60% will divert static charges to a ground before fire erupts. These important OR environmental parameters are consistently monitored according to hospital standards.

Adiabatic compression or expansion occurs when volume changes of gases occur under conditions whereby environmental heat gain or loss is restricted. These volume changes occur too rapidly for normal temperatures to accommodate the concomitant pressure changes and a flash fire results. Adiabatic compression is unique to compressed gas cylinders that entrain foreign particulate matter or are opened or *cracked* too quickly prior to the attachment of regulating valves.

A concise fire prevention and control plan should be incorporated into departmental and facility safety programs and reviewed by all providers on a regular basis. Immediate response to a fire or explosion in the OR should involve the following steps:

1. **Notification**
   - Alert all personnel.
   - Sound fire alarms.
   - Eliminate traffic.
   - Close all doors.
2. **Initiation**
   - Gather and operate fire fighting equipment.
   - Extinguish visible flames.
   - Discontinue all possible electric circuitry.
   - Remove flammable agents, items that will burn.

- Discontinue anesthetic gases; maintain low flow of oxygen.
- Prepare evacuation and necessary equipment for transport.
3. **Implementation**
   - Extinguish fire or evacuate immediate (threatened) areas.
   - Disconnect all main electrical and gas lines.
   - Transport to safe area.

Routine planning and preparedness to respond appropriately to a threatened or actual fire is an absolute necessity of any department where surgery is performed. Fire drills should include all staff members who are trained to be proficient at recognizing and responding to a fire or explosion in a timely fashion. All participants should be required to understand and operate firefighting apparatus such as a fire extinguisher approved for use in combating all three classes of fire: *A,* wood or paper; *B,* liquid or grease; and *C,* electrical. The Halon® extinguisher is an example of such apparatus. Routine participation and appropriate documentation should be incorporated into the departmental quality management program.

Explosion Hazards

Although battery-operated equipment is typically at low voltage, malfunction under certain conditions can be dangerous and result in hazardous outcomes. Biomedical clearance of any apparatus used in patient care areas should be examined and cleared for operation by a qualified technician prior to use. Endoscopic equipment has been responsible for detonating explosions within patient body cavities. Fuel for such explosions can be flammable anesthetics sequestered in a body cavity or natural organic by-products. Arcing or heat caused by malfunction of an endoscope can ignite volatile substances. Laparoscopy involves insufflation of gas into an abdominal cavity to allow passage of the laparoscope. Carbon dioxide or nitrous oxide, when used as the insufflating gas for laparoscopy, can contribute to an explosion and fire. Nitrous oxide supports combustion and readily diffuses into the gut to mix with the highly explosive methane and hydrogen gases contained there. Heat generated by electrocautery forceps, if misapplied, can ignite the gases resulting in explosion.

Another potential hazard in the OR is burns caused by passage of an electric current through an area of electrolyte solution. If physiologic saline is pooled under an electrode or on a surface in contact with the patient's skin, passage of the current will ionize the solution to sodium hydroxide and chlorine gas. Contact of these substances with the skin for an extended period can result in caustic burns of a significant magnitude. The anesthetist should always examine the patient's skin for evidence of such burns, particularly beneath electrode or grounding pads when they are removed or become suspect. Without the presence of an electrolyte solution, leakage of current applied to the skin for a long period can produce a thermal injury as current is carried through the patient's body to a grounding site.

▶ ENVIRONMENTAL POLLUTION

Concerns regarding the biologic effects of trace anesthetic gases have been debated for several decades. Current standards recommended by NIOSH are available (see Chapter 6) and should be applied to all areas where anesthesia is administered. While conflicting evidence supports trace anesthetic gas exposure as a health hazard, the vigilant anesthetist is responsible for patient protection from inadvertent and unnecessary exposure by ensuring functional scavenging systems and avoiding spillage or leakage of volatile agents.

Radiation Safety

Ionizing radiation in and around the OR is a source of potential biologic damage for both patients and providers. Protecting the patient from unnecessary exposure with techniques of isolation and protection of exposed body parts should be carefully managed when x-rays are involved in a procedure. Provider exposure to radiation is monitored by *roentgen equivalent man* or *REM units* as a measurement of biologic damage from radiation that is administered to various body parts. A maximum yearly occupational exposure limit mandated by NIOSH is rarely reached when routine exposure management and prevention strategies are maintained. Radiation protection policies as described by Voelz (1988) should include education and monitoring programs that protect patients and providers from unnecessary and threatening levels of radiation exposure.

Lasers

Exposure to nonionizing radiation occurs when lasers are used in the OR. Tissue damage results as the heat generated by the laser beam penetrates tissues. Laser stands for *light amplifications by stimulated emission of radiation*. Lasers emit either infrared, visible, or ultraviolet light depending on the medium used to generate the beam. Burns caused by laser contact and inadvertent fires present the greatest risk to patients undergoing such procedures. Hayes, Graba, and Goode (1986) described characteristics necessary for laser-restraint endotracheal tubes used to deflect leaser beams. Protection afforded by shielding body parts that are not targets for laser exposure with adequate covering, such as moistened sponges and appropriate eyewear that resists the

particular laser used, should afford appropriate protection.

Hazardous Materials

Various materials and their particular compounds and by-products present as environmental hazards in the perioperative area. Identification of every product, agent, or apparatus considered to be hazardous according to OSHA definition is the responsibility of the health care employer. A Material Safety Data Sheet (MSDS) is required for each material identified as being potentially hazardous. An MSDS lists the product's trade name, ingredients, physical data, and information regarding its appropriate handling and disposal. An MSDS for each hazardous material must be readily available in the health care workplace. Hazardous materials particular to anesthesia practice are presented and discussed in Chapter 6.

Chemical Exposure

Exposure to various types of chemicals present during surgery is inevitable. Patient protection from hazards associated with various chemicals to which they are exposed is consistent with precautions to be taken by providers and is addressed in Chapter 6. Significant and serious sequelae can result from exposure to many chemicals, therefore emphasizing the necessity to control patient contact and minimize exposure.

Latex Exposure

An increasing incidence of allergy to latex-containing products has evolved over recent years. Latex derives from the sap of the rubber tree and contains low molecular weight proteins that are soluble and thought to cause the allergic response. These soluble proteins are most prevalent in medical products that are either produced or coated with a latex covering. Powder from gloves and balloons attracts latex and causes inhalational absorption once airborne. Gloves used in anesthesia care are a common vector for transmission of latex protein from both tactile and airborne routes (powder inhalation). Latex-free gloves are commercially available and should be kept in stock when suspected or known latex sensitive or allergic patients present or staff members exhibit reactions. All latex-containing products should be removed from the immediate patient care areas, and direct patient care items should be replaced with latex-free products.

Populations at high risk for latex allergy include children with myelodysplasia (spina bifida) and genitourinary malformations such as bladder exstrophy. These children are thought to become sensitized to latex through repeated exposure via multiple surgical procedures, bladder catheterization, and bowel preparations.

TABLE 7–2. Signs and Symptoms of Allergic Reactions to Latex

Awake Patient	Anesthetized Patient[a]
Itchy eyes	Tachycardia
Generalized pruritus	Hypotension
Shortness of breath	Wheezing
Feeling of faintness	Bronchospasm
Feeling of impending doom	Cardiorespiratory arrest
Nausea	Flushing
Vomiting	Facial edema
Abdominal cramping	Laryngeal edema
Diarrhea	Urticaria
Wheezing	

[a] Symptoms usually occur within 30 minutes following induction of anesthesia.

Certain health care workers have shown a similar sensitivity to latex products or chemicals used in the processing of latex. However, reported cases from patients outside of these known risk groups are not common.

A definitive and predictable test for latex allergy is not currently available. Therefore, a patient's complete medical history is key to isolating one who might maintain a latex allergy (AANA, 1992). Persons found to be sensitive to latex often have allergies to certain foods, including bananas, chestnuts, avocados, and kiwi fruit. Allergic manifestations of latex range from a localized erythema, urticaria, and pruritus to life-threatening reactions including angioedema and anaphylaxis. Table 7–2 shows signs and symptoms of allergic reactions to latex in both the awake and anesthetized patients. Latex allergy precautions continue to be refined, and current recommendations are provided when a threat exists (AANA, 1992).

Management of a latex allergy reaction includes removing the latex agent(s) if known and possible and initiation of emergency therapies including airway support, vascular expansion, and intravenous epinephrine. Considerable time and planning is required to accommodate the latex-sensitive patient, and a departmental protocol and latex–free supply of necessary products should be maintained in the department. The AANA provides a published *Latex Allergy Protocol* (1992) designed to prevent and manage such situations.

▶ CASE STUDY

J.B., a 13-year-old boy, is undergoing a posterior spinal rod placement for scoliosis repair. His anesthesia interview revealed an occasional sinusitis that appeared to be seasonal and was last treated approximately 3 months prior with an over-the-counter antihistamine. His medical history is otherwise unremarkable. Family history was negative for any anesthesia-related specifics. His development

is normal and according to his mother, his teachers report that he excels in most of his classes at school yet talks a lot, eliciting a "C" grade in conduct. His physical activities are becoming somewhat more restricted as a result of his scoliosis. He weighs 44 kg, and is 61 inches tall.

Surgical history revealed a tonsillectomy and adenoidectomy at age 5 that was uneventful. His history and physical findings were noncontributory. Airway examination revealed a I–MP scale, and he has no limitation to neck extension or oral opening. His teeth are in good repair and intact. He has no known allergies to medication, but his mother notes that he developed mild generalized itching after attending a family picnic where he ate a hot dog, beans, and fruit salad and drank orange soda. She was unclear as to which food item may have caused the symptoms if indeed it was the food; he also spent the afternoon playing with his cousins in a field of grass where there might have been poison ivy, yet none of the children developed a rash. He is scheduled with his parents' consent for general anesthesia in 3 days for the rod placement. He has two units of donor-specific blood in the bloodbank that was drawn from his uncle.

J.B. was premedicated with midazolam 1 mg IV in the OR holding area after an intravenous (IV) infusion (18-gauge catheter) was initiated in his left forearm. He was given 15 mL of Bicitra in 15 mL of water. In the OR routine monitors (electrocardiogram, ECG; blood pressure, BP; precordial stethoscope, and oximeter) were applied. He was given another 1 mg of midazolam IV and began breathing 100% oxygen via circle system mask. Blood pressure was 98/60, heart rate (HR) was 88 (NSR), respiratory rate (RR) was 14, Sao_2 was 100%, and temperature (T) was 36°C (skin).

Induction consisted of sufentanil 35 μg (divided) followed by propofol 60 mg. He was intubated with a 7.0 cuffed endotracheal tube following rocuronium 30 mg. His vital signs remained stable and were recorded as BP = 96/54, HR = 70, Sao_2 = 100%, and T = 37.1°C (esophageal probe) 5 minutes postinduction while the resident inserted a foley catheter. An orogastric tube (18 gauge) was inserted and his eyes were taped closed.

As the team began to turn the OR table (ortho frame) into the prone position, the CRNA noted a reddened flush across J.B.'s head, neck, and thorax. His heart rate had increased to 122 (sinus tachycardia) and BP was now 84/50. Sao_2 dropped to 97% and T was 36.9°C. The turning process was stopped. Auscultation of the chest revealed a loud expiratory wheeze with positive inspiratory pressures increasing to 30 cm H_2O (up from a previous range of 18–20 cm H_2O).

1. What should the CRNA do?

The CRNA suspects that some adverse response is evolving. Because he frequently works in the orthopedic OR and recently attended a state association conference on the hazards of anesthesia, he recognizes these symptoms as latex allergy. Subsequent review of J.B.'s history could reveal a sensitivity to various fruit items (ie, salad at the picnic) which is common in those who possess an allergy to latex.

J.B. was wheezing, displayed a generalized reddened flush, had dropped his blood pressure, exhibited saturation, and developed a tachycardia. He had been handled by several persons in the OR who wore latex gloves. He also had an inserted angiocath, esophageal probe, blood pressure cuff, EKG pads, and tape that could all potentially contain latex. The breathing circuit could potentially contain latex, frequently in the rebreathing bag.

2. What is the primary response and treatment?

Apply cardiovascular support with increased IV fluids (lactated ringers) and vasopressors if indicated. Discontinue anesthesia agents, administer oxygen 100%, and postpone surgery. Remove all latex-containing products including foley catheter, orogastric tube, and eye tapes. Change blood pressure cuff and IV catheter to nonlatex products when feasible. Administer epinephrine 30 μg to 50 μg bolus (10 mcg/mL dilution) IV, repeated in 5 minutes if symptoms continue and hypotension persists.

3. What would the secondary treatment include?

Use aminophylline or aerosolized bronchodilator such as albuterol, diphenhydramine (1 mg/kg), methylprednisolone (2 mg/kg), or selected amnestic agent, as indicated. Stabilize following resuscitation then transfer to an appropriate monitored area.

4. What should the follow-up care for this patient include?

Obtain referral from allergy service. Explain the events to J.B. and his parents. Document the event extensively. Prepare for his return and know which products contain latex and which do not. Review in morbidity and mortality conference. Report to appropriate institutional departments.

▶ SUMMARY

Patient safety requires strict attention to potential risks, prevention, and management strategies. It also requires that the provider be knowledgeable of current epidemiologic standards regarding blood and airborne transmission of disease. An informed provider can deliver quality anesthesia in a safe environment when he or she is well informed, prepared, vigilant, and dedicated to patient well being and quality outcomes. In today's surgical environment, we must continue to care for both ourselves and the patient. Safety should always be our first priority.

▶ KEY CONCEPTS

- Studies calculating anesthesia-related mishaps estimate that over 80% of those cases reported and reviewed are directly attributable to human error and are preventable.
- Fire prevention in the OR begins with provider vigilance and attention to avoiding and eliminating the potential hazards that exist. Once an ignition source such as open flames, an electrical arc, or static sparks combines with a fuel source or flammable material and oxygen, a fire is sustained.
- Reusable patient care items that enter a sterile area of the body or vascular system require a process that insures sterility prior to their reuse. Processing that renders items sterile includes steam autoclaving, ethylene oxide gas autoclaving, or sterilant-concentrated washing.
- The OSHA Blood-borne Pathogen Standard mandates the application of universal precautions, engineering controls, work practices, and personal protective equipment while caring for patients in a health care setting.
- A tuberculin skin test is used to identify persons who are infected with *M. tuberculosis.* Most infected persons will display a positive reaction to the tuberculin skin test within 2 to 10 weeks following infection. Persons infected with *M. tuberculosis* who do not have TB disease are not infectious to others.

▶ STUDY QUESTIONS

1. What professional resource does the CRNA have to use as a guide for maintaining appropriate infection control standards and where can it be found?

2. During a laser case for vaporization of a vocal cord lesion a flame exits the oral cavity. What steps should be taken and why?

3. What is the significance of the Mantoux skin test relative to a diagnosis of tuberculosis?

4. What food allergies might alert the anesthetist that a patient may possess a latex sensitivity?

5. What is the most common cause of blood-borne pathogen transmission and how can it best be prevented?

KEY REFERENCES

American Association of Nurse Anesthetists (AANA). (1996). *Professional practice manual for the certified registered nurse anesthetist* (5th ed.). Park Ridge, IL: AANA.

American Society of Anesthesiologists (ASA). (1994). Recommendations for infection control for the practice of anesthesiology. Park Ridge, IL: ASA.

REFERENCES

American Association of Nurse Anesthetists (AANA). (1992). Latex allergies: Anesthesia concerns. *AANA Newsbulletin/Anesthesia Quality Plus, 48*(9)(suppl.), 3.

American College of Allergy and Immunology (ACAI). (1992). *Interim recommendations to health care professionals and organizations regarding latex allergy precautions.* Chicago, IL: ACAI.

Centers for Disease Control. (1983). Guideline for isolation precautions in hospitals. *Infection Control, 4,* 245–235.

Centers for Disease Control. (1988). Update: Universal precautions for prevention of transmission of HIV, HBV, and other blood-borne pathogens in health-care settings. *Morbidity and Mortality Weekly Report, 37,* 378–388.

Cooper, J. B., Long, C. D., *et. al.* (1979). Multi-hospital study of preventable anesthesia mishaps [Abstract]. *Anesthesiology, 51,* 5348.

Cooper, J. B., Newbower, R. S., & Kitz, R. J. (1984). An analysis of major errors and equipment failures in anesthesia: Considerations for prevention and detection. *Anesthesiology, 60,* 34–42.

Cooper, J. B., Newbower, R. S., Long, C. D., & Mcpeele, B. (1978). Preventable anesthesia mishaps: A study of human factors. *Anesthesiology, 49,* 399–406.

Derrington, M. C. & Smith, G. (1987). A review of studies of anesthetic risk, morbidity and mortality. *British Journal of Anaesthesia, 59,* 815–833.

Du Moulin, G. C. & Saugermann, A. J. (1977). The anesthesia machine and circle system are not likely to be sources of bacterial contamination. *Anesthesiology, 47,* 353–358.

Food & Drug Administration. (1987). Reuse of medical devisces. *FDA Compliance Policy Guide 7124–16.* Washington, DC: U.S. Government Printing Office.

Garibaldi, R. A., Britt, M. R., Webster, C., & Pace, N. L. (1981).

Failure of bacterial filters to reduce the incidence of pneumonia after inhalation anesthesia. *Anesthesiology, 54,* 364.

Haney, P. E., Raymond, B. A., & Lewis, L. C. (1989). Ethylene oxide: An occupational health hazard in the surgical environment. *Journal of the Association of Operating Room Nurses, 50,* 396.

Hayes, D. M., Gaba, D. M., & Goode, R. I. (1986). Incendiary characteristics of a new laser-resistant endotracheal tube. *Otolaryngology and Head Neck Surgery, 95,* 37.

Historical perspective of APSF shows safety advocacy. (1996). *APSF Newsletter, 11*(3), 26.

McMillan-Jackson, M. (1993). Infection precautions: What works and what does not. *The Clinical Forum for Nurse Anesthetists, 4,* 77–82.

Norris, J. L. (1994). Fire safety in the operating room. *Journal of the American Association of Nurse Anesthetists, 62,* 342–345.

Pace, N. L., Webster, B., Epstein, S., Matsumiya, M., Coleman, M. S., Britt, M. R., & Garibaldi, R. A. (1979). Failure of anesthetic circuit bacterial filters to reduce postoperative pulmonary infections. *Anesthesiology, 51,* 5362.

Quartin, A. A., Scheim, R. M., Kett, D. H., & Peduzzi, P. N. (1997). Effects of sepsis on survival. *Journal of the American Medical Association, 277,* 1058–1063.

U.S. Department of Labor, Occupational Safety and Health Administration. (1991). Occupational exposure to bloodborne pathogens: Final rule [29 CFR Part 1910.1030]. *Federal Register 56,* (235):64003–64182.

U.S. Department of Health and Human Services. *Med Watch, The FDA Medical Products Reporting Program.* Rockville, MD.

Voelz, G. L. (1988). Ionizing radiation. In C. Zenz (Ed.), *Occupational medicine: Principles and practical applications* (2nd ed., p. 426). Chicago: Year Book Medical.

Anesthetic Delivery Systems

Wynne R. Waugaman

The anesthesia machine is a sophisticated life-support system that relies on the principles of mechanics, pneumatics, and electronics to manage pressure, flow, and volume as it delivers anesthetic gases to provide ventilation and oxygenation. Fresh gas sources, the internal machine circuitry, flowmeters, vaporizers, the patient circuit, and the waste gas evacuation systems are major components that require study and understanding because problems can arise at any time. To detect, prevent, or minimize the effects of machine system problems, the anesthetist must be able to verify that all components are functioning properly.

The ability to make an appropriate differential diagnosis of what is happening in the machine system is a learned set of tasks that evolves from a student's work in mastering basic gas flow pathways through the machine. For this reason, the text and figures used in this chapter are generic and may be applied, in principle, to all anesthesia machines manufactured after 1979.

The fundamentals of machine operation are introduced in this chapter to enable students to appreciate and understand the instruction and operations manual, cautions, and warnings that accompany each unique machine and accessory device manufactured for use with an anesthesia delivery system.

The scope of this chapter is limited to the discussion of gas flow, proper function of major system components, normal machine operations, and related concepts of chemistry and physics. Recognition of the major parts of the machine and their performance is mandatory preparation for understanding how the system ultimately affects the clinical signs and symptoms exhibited by both the patient and the machine. Without the benefit of understanding these basics, the daily and preuse testing procedures are apt to be inadequate, incomplete, misapplied, and misinterpreted.

Constant vigilance has always been the foundation for accurate and timely assessment of the machine's function and its minimum performance. Vigilance is not adequate, however, unless the user knows how the system is designed to operate and has personally checked and verified its proper working condition. Routine use of appropriate monitoring devices and techniques, an integral part of machine system operation, is also required to ensure that life-sustaining information is accurate, complete, and available.

▶ PRINCIPLES OF GAS DELIVERY

Anesthesia machine systems are basically designed to deliver the right amount of gas, at the right time, and at the right pressure to ensure an appropriate level of surgical anesthesia and to manage ventilation and oxygenation of the patient. Oxygen (O_2) and nitrous oxide (N_2O) enter the machine from two sources: the wall supply and the cylinder supply (Fig. 8–1).

Machine Components that Manage Oxygen

Oxygen Supply and Regulation of Pressure

Oxygen, the dominant gas, flows into the machine through the pipeline inlet check valve (Fig. 8–2) at a pressure of approximately 50 pounds per square inch gauge (psig). Oxygen also provides pressure to the power outlet accessory, where the ventilator may be con-

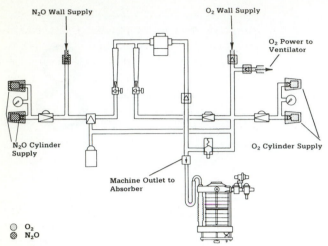

Figure 8–1. Sources of oxygen and nitrous oxide supply within the flow diagram of a basic anesthesia machine. *(Redrawn with permission granted by Ohmeda, a division of BOC Health Care, Inc.)*

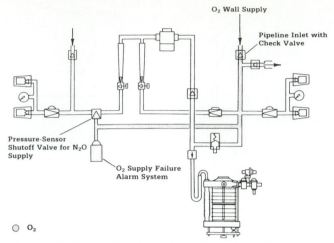

Figure 8–3. Oxygen flow from the wall supply to the pressure-sensor shutoff valve and the oxygen supply failure alarm system. *(Redrawn with permission granted by Ohmeda, a division of BOC Health Care, Inc.)*

nected. At the same time, oxygen travels from the machine inlet to pressurize the oxygen flush valve. As soon as oxygen is connected to the machine, the oxygen flush valve is able to deliver oxygen to the patient circuit. The flow rate delivered by an open flush valve should range from 35 L/min to 75 L/min (Fig. 8–2) (ASTM, 1988).

Aside from pressurizing the power outlet and the flush valve, oxygen flow opens the pressure-sensor shutoff valve (Fig. 8–3), permitting nitrous oxide to be delivered. This sensor is placed in-line, between the nitrous oxide supply and the nitrous oxide flowmeter. When oxygen supply is adequate and is being delivered to the

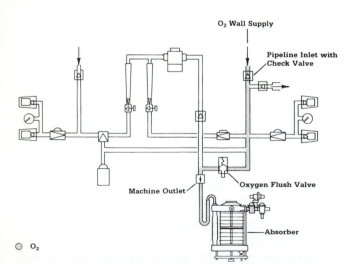

Figure 8–2. Flow pathway of oxygen from the wall supply to the patient circuit. Note that the oxygen flush valve is immediately usable once the hose has been connected. *(Redrawn with permission granted by Ohmeda, a division of BOC Health Care, Inc.)*

machine at 50 psig, the pressure-sensor shutoff valve opens to direct nitrous oxide to the flowmeter. This valve will remain open as long as the oxygen supply pressure stays above 25 psig. If the oxygen supply pressure falls below this pressure, the shutoff valve closes and stops the flow of nitrous oxide. This mechanical action is responsible for limiting the delivery of nitrous oxide whenever the oxygen pressure is less than appropriate.

The pressure-sensor shutoff valve is essential, but it does not warn the practitioner that it has terminated nitrous oxide flow. The clinician may visually note that the nitrous oxide float is dropping in the flowmeter; however, the oxygen supply failure alarm system is the component that sounds an alarm to provide a warning. This alarm, adjacent to the shutoff valve, contains a reservoir filled with oxygen pressure at 50 psig. When oxygen pressure falls below a predetermined setting of approximately 28 psig, the alarm is activated. It whistles loudly to alert the practitioner that the oxygen pressure in the machine is falling. The alarm begins to sound before the oxygen pressure has fallen to 25 psig, the pressure at which nitrous oxide flow will cease. Whether the alarm is momentary or prolonged, it indicates that the clinician needs to reestablish an adequate oxygen supply by turning on the reserve oxygen cylinder.

Oxygen pressure is usually, but not always, delivered from the wall supply at 50 psig. Fluctuations do occur, and the pressure may decrease to 40 psig, based on the delivery system and the hospital's demand for oxygen. The second-stage regulator (Fig. 8–4) eliminates the need to continuously adjust the flowmeter based on fluctuations in the wall supply pressure. A constant pressure of approximately 16 psig is maintained by the second-stage regulator at the flow control valve to eliminate changes

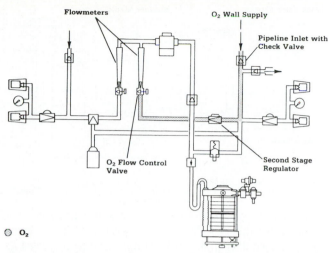

Figure 8–4. Oxygen flows from the wall supply through the second-stage regulator before flowing to the base of the flowmeter. *(Redrawn with permission granted by Ohmeda, a division of BOC Health Care, Inc.)*

in oxygen flow resulting from changes in the oxygen supply pressure. This ensures that oxygen is the last gas to cease flowing to the patient if an oxygen supply failure occurs.

Oxygen that is supplied by cylinders instead of the wall system passes through the hanger yoke check valve(s) and the cylinder pressure regulator before it reaches the second-stage regulator. Because the approximate pressure in a full E-size cylinder of oxygen is 2200 psig, it is too high to be easily controlled by the flow control valve. Therefore, it too must be regulated or reduced to 40 psig to 50 psig. Regardless of the source of oxygen, gas travels the same course within the machine circuitry once it passes through the second-stage regulator.

Check Valves, Flush Valve, and Flowmeters

CHECK VALVES. All anesthesia machines come from the manufacturer with a pipeline inlet consisting of one of two general types of fittings and an enclosed check valve. These fittings are either the diameter-indexed safety system (DISS) type or the *quick-connect* type. Both fittings are indexed to a specific gas and are noninterchangeable between specific gases (Fig. 8–5) so that the appropriate gas flows through the correct inlet. Oxygen and nitrous oxide gas inlet check valves permit gas to flow only into the machine. The check valve in the power outlet permits gas to flow from the machine to a gas-powered accessory such as a ventilator. If the ventilator hose is not attached, the outlet check valve will close to prevent oxygen from flowing into the atmosphere. The mechanical force of attaching the ventilator hose opens the power outlet.

In contrast, pneumatic pressure from the wall supply opens the check valve in the pipeline inlets. The inlet check valve stays in the open position as long as adequate gas pressure is exerted from the wall supply. Gravity and any existing pressure within the gas machine, or the pneumatic pressure from the reserve cylinder supply, close the check valve (Bowie & Huffman, 1985; Rice & Kolek, 1996).

If the pipeline inlet check valve was not present, gas from a reserve cylinder could escape through the machine and rapidly empty into the piping system in the wall. This would occur any time the pressure in the hospital pipeline was interrupted or dropped below the pressure being supplied to the machine from the reserve cylinder pressure regulator.

Some clinicians feel that when this check valve is present, it is good practice to turn on one cylinder and leave it on as an automatic backup to the wall supply system (Bowie & Huffman, 1985; Rice & Kolek, 1996). Considering the fact that wall supply pressure changes from time to time, this practice is not acceptable. If a cylinder of oxygen is turned on at the same time that the oxygen pipeline supply is in use, the cylinder could be depleted without warning. The machine will always use oxygen from the source that has the higher pressure. Most cylinder regulators are set lower than the typical wall supply pressure, but the wall pressure can fall even lower than the cylinder regulator's set point during times of peak oxygen demand. In this situation, the higher reserve cylinder pressure closes the inlet check valve, stopping the wall supply and consuming the gas in the reserve cylinder. Because there is no loss of oxygen pressure to trigger the alarm, the reserve supply is depleted without warning. If both reserve cylinders are

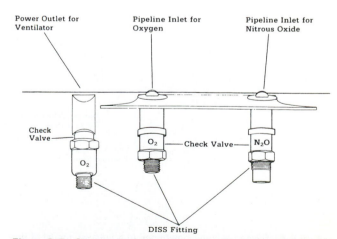

Figure 8–5. Gas supply inlets equipped with noninterchangeable diameter-indexed fittings on the back of the anesthesia machine. *(Redrawn with permission granted by Ohmeda, a division of BOC Health Care, Inc.)*

in use at the same time, the cylinder with the higher pressure will supply the gas machine system until its pressure drops to that of its companion cylinder. At this time, both cylinders will begin to supply the system, ultimately causing both reserve cylinders to become empty at the same time. For this reason, it is not appropriate to have both reserve cylinders turned on at the same time.

The reserve cylinders are connected to the gas machine by means of pin-indexed hanger yokes. The pin-indexed configuration for oxygen is readily visible, permitting the pins on the yoke to be inserted into the matching holes located on the cylinder valve (Fig. 8–6). The location of the pins in the hanger yoke is designed to ensure that only cylinders filled with oxygen can be seated on the oxygen yoke (Fig. 8-7). Although the pin system is quite durable, it can be altered or damaged. Therefore, it is important to state that if the cylinder does not attach easily, it should not be forced. Also, never use more than one cylinder valve gasket on the yoke mechanism. The use of a second gasket may defeat the pin index and permit the wrong gas to be mounted in the yoke (Bowie & Huffman, 1985; Dorsch & Dorsch, 1994; Rice & Kolek, 1996).

Once the cylinder is turned on, oxygen enters the yoke and passes through a strainer nipple, a filter that removes dust particles that may be present on the cylinder valve or the contact surface of the yoke (Fig. 8–7). Oxygen flow pushes the check valve off its seat, while the pressure of the gas holds the valve against its retainer

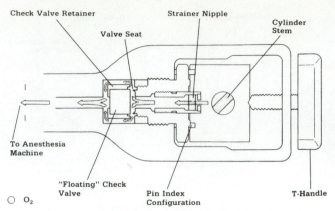

Figure 8–7. Oxygen hanger yoke, cut away to demonstrate the location of the PISS in relation to its placement on the yoke and the flow of oxygen through it. *(Redrawn with permission granted by Ohmeda, a division of BOC Health Care, Inc.)*

and keeps it open. Gas flows around the check valve and retainer into the machine.

When the first cylinder in a double-yoke, two-cylinder assembly is turned on, the flow of gas that enters the machine from the cylinder in one hanger, yoke A, opens the check valve, and its pressure is indicated by the cylinder pressure gauge (Fig. 8-8). Pressure is exerted on the check valve in yoke B, forcing it onto its seat and closing it. With the valve in hanger yoke B closed, the possibility of gas leaving cylinder A and filling cylinder B is minimized. These hanger yoke valves are intended to

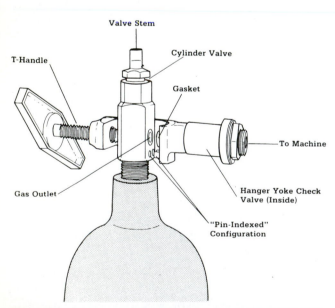

Figure 8–6. Oxygen cylinder positioned in a cutaway model of the hanger yoke. Note the location of the gas outlet and the single gasket. *(Redrawn with permission granted by Ohmeda, a division of BOC Health Care, Inc.)*

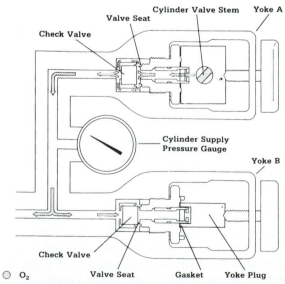

Figure 8–8. Oxygen flow through a double yoke when one cylinder is turned on and a yoke plug is present. *(Redrawn with permission granted by Ohmeda, a division of BOC Health Care, Inc.)*

reduce cross-filling, the condition in which gas from one cylinder fills the other. Note, however, that the hanger yoke check valve is designed to limit flow, but it is not a leak-free seal. This is another reason that only one cylinder should be opened at a time. Likewise, when only one cylinder is connected to a double-yoke system, the vacant yoke should be sealed with a standard yoke plug and gasket. Without the yoke plug in place, gas from the cylinder in yoke A could slowly leak from yoke B into the ambient air (Bowie & Huffman, 1985; Petty, 1987; Rice & Kolek, 1996).

OXYGEN FLUSH VALVE AND OXYGEN SUPPLY FAILURE ALARM.   The oxygen flush valve receives its gas supply at approximately 50 psig from the wall or the cylinder and is ready to be used whenever oxygen is present in the machine's system (Fig. 8–9). The flush valve stays in the closed position until the operator opens the valve by pressing the button. Manual depression of this valve moves the pin, which forces the valve off of its seat and creates a path for immediate flow to the machine outlet. The ball valve retaining spring is the opposing force that moves the ball back onto its seat once manual pressure is removed. This spring automatically closes the valve.

The flush valve is used any time more oxygen needs to be added to the rebreathing bag. Flushing the system to add volume results in dilution of the mixture contained in the rebreathing bag and can prolong inhalation inductions. When a poor mask fit is the cause of decreasing volume in the rebreathing bag, using the flush valve is not the preferred method to supplement the loss. Higher flows to the patient circuit can easily be provided by temporarily increasing the liter flow at the flowmeter(s). This will not dilute the agent concentration being delivered when using an integrated calibrated vaporizer.

Indiscriminate, repeated use of the flush valve at the start of the case is generally disruptive to the smooth course of anesthesia. Furthermore, holding the valve in the open position can deliver an unnecessarily high flow, up to 75 L/min (Dorsch & Dorsch, 1994) of positive-pressure gas to the patient circuit. This maneuver may overinflate the patient's lungs and lead to increased intrathoracic pressure and potential barotrauma (Dorsch & Dorsch, 1994).

The pressure-sensor shutoff valve also receives its oxygen supply at approximately 50 psig, and it operates by using the lack of adequate oxygen pressure to shut off the nitrous oxide. Oxygen delivered to the machine exerts its pressure on the diaphragm and moves the piston, pin, and valve off the valve seat. This force holds the valve open. As long as at least 25 psig of oxygen pressure is exerted on the diaphragm, the valve will remain open and allow the flow of nitrous oxide from its supply source to the flow control valve (Fig. 8–10). The purpose of this valve is to shut off nitrous oxide or any other gas, for example, medical air, helium, or carbon dioxide, whenever the oxygen pressure drops below 25 psig, as when the wall or cylinder supply fails. Historically, this valve was called a *fail-safe* valve by clinicians who relied on cylinder supply oxygen as the primary source of gas. Before central gas supply systems were common, losing oxygen pressure was a constant aggravation. As a result, this component was a welcome machine monitor and typically the assumption was made that a machine so equipped was fail-safe and could not be used to adminis-

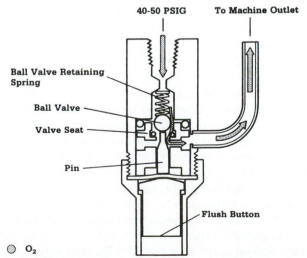

Figure 8–9. Oxygen flow through the activated flush valve. *(Redrawn with permission granted by Ohmeda, a division of BOC Health Care, Inc.)*

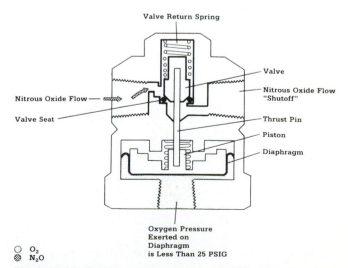

Figure 8–10. Oxygen pressure-sensor shutoff valve closed to prevent nitrous oxide from flowing. *(Redrawn with permission granted by Ohmeda, a division of BOC Health Care, Inc.)*

ter a hypoxic mixture. This is a myth and continues to be misleading.

The so-called fail-safe valve is a pressure-sensor valve only. It cannot determine flow, volume, ventilation, or fractional inspired oxygen concentration. It is designed to sense the pressure of oxygen in the machine, and it must be checked daily to ensure its proper operation. To test the pressure-sensor shutoff valve, select a midrange flow for oxygen and nitrous oxide. Verify that flow by looking at the position of the floats in the flowmeter tubes. Then disconnect the oxygen wall supply hose and turn off the oxygen cylinder supply. As the oxygen supply is depleted, the nitrous oxide float should fall to the bottom of the flow tube before the oxygen float descends (Bowie & Huffman, 1985; Rice & Kolek, 1996).

The alarm assembly (Fig. 8–11) warns when a condition of low oxygen pressure develops. It is aptly called the oxygen supply failure alarm system. Oxygen enters this assembly from the wall or cylinder supply through its inlet check valve and flows into the reservoir at approximately 50 psig. This creates a balance between the pressure inside the reservoir and the supply pressure. When oxygen supply pressure fails and the pressure in the reservoir is slowly depleted to its present level, oxygen rushes out of the reservoir, passes through the relief

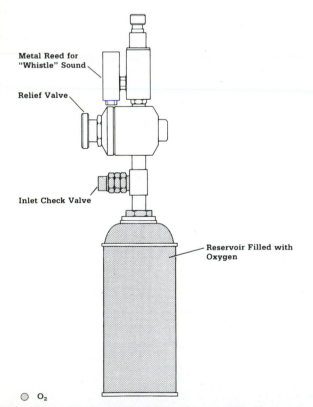

Metal Reed for "Whistle" Sound

Relief Valve

Inlet Check Valve

Reservoir Filled with Oxygen

O₂

Figure 8–11. Oxygen supply failure alarm system warns when oxygen pressure falls. *(Redrawn with permission granted by Ohmeda, a division of BOC Health Care, Inc.)*

valve, vibrates a metal reed, and causes the alarm to sound. This event occurs at the same time as, or slightly before, the pressure-sensor shutoff valve terminates the flow of nitrous oxide. The alarm will continue to sound until the reservoir is depleted, or for a minimum period of approximately 7 seconds. This time interval may vary with different models, but the presence of the alarm condition means the same thing. Oxygen pressure must be reestablished and verified. Unlike smart monitors that cease sounding when the alarm condition is corrected or passed, the ending of the warning tone does not necessarily mean that the low-pressure condition has ended. Whenever the alarm is activated, simply turn on the reserve oxygen cylinder before beginning to analyze the cause of the problem.

The second-stage regulator receives a pressure of approximately 50 psig from the wall or reserve cylinder, reduces it to 16 psig, and delivers this constant pressure to the flow control valve. This regulator serves to isolate any pressure changes in either the pipeline or cylinder supply from the flow control valve and ensures that the oxygen supply failure alarm is activated before the falling oxygen pressure affects the oxygen flowmeter.

FLOWMETERS. Although many components that manage oxygen pressure are not visible, the oxygen flowmeter is immediately recognized for its role in the delivery of oxygen flow through the machine to the patient circuit (Fig. 8–12). Turning the knob counterclockwise moves the needle back and away from its seat, allowing oxygen to flow into the tube. Turning the knob clockwise closes the space between the needle and its seat, reducing oxygen flow. In addition to operating the on and off functions, this control is used to adjust the flow delivered to the patient circuit. Each turn makes a precise adjustment in the opening that carefully measures and meters the oxygen flow.

The control knob is designed to be readily identified as the oxygen flowmeter by both touch and sight. The knob is fluted, larger in diameter than other gas knobs, and color- and symbol-coded for oxygen (Dorsch & Dorsch, 1994). The valve stops on the knob indicate when the valve is closed and oxygen flow has ceased. The stop position feels like an abrupt resistance and is designed to remind the user not to rotate this valve any further (Bowie & Huffman, 1985; Rice & Kolek, 1996).

Two float stops are present in the flow tube itself. The one at the top of the tube prevents the float from colliding with the surface of the gas outlet, where it could potentially lodge and obstruct gas flow to the common manifold (Waugaman & Bradshaw, 1985). The stop at the bottom of the tube provides the float with a place to rest in the center of the flow tube when the oxygen flow is turned off. When the flow control valve is opened, this style of float is centered by the flow of the

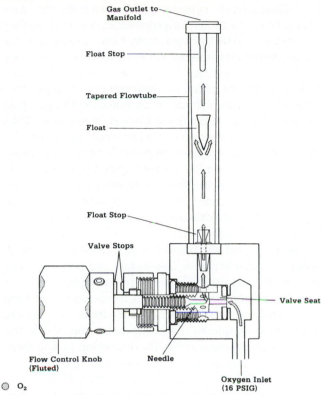

Figure 8–12. Oxygen flowmeter, cut away to illustrate the needle valve in relation to its valve seat. Note the valve and float stops within the component. *(Redrawn with permission granted by Ohmeda, a division of BOC Health Care, Inc.)*

gas and is read at the point where the top of the float corresponds to the scale.

The flowmeter is a hand-calibrated system that includes a tapered glass tube, a float, and a scale. No two flow tubes are exactly alike. To compensate for differences, the flowmeter scales are individually calibrated to provide a high degree of accuracy over the full range of the scale. The float is inserted into the tube, and the scale is engraved to correspond with each measured flow of the specific gas that passes through that particular tube. After this, the scale becomes specific for that tube and its float, and all parts are regarded as an inseparable unit (Bowie & Huffman, 1985; Rice & Kolek, 1996). As a result, whenever any flow tube, float, or scale for any gas needs replacement, the complete set must be replaced.

The oxygen flowmeter is always positioned closest to the manifold outlet and to the right of all other flow tubes, as one faces the machine (Bowie & Huffman, 1985; Petty, 1987; Rice & Kolek, 1996). This is a requirement for all American and Canadian machines. With oxygen on the right, it is always downstream of all other gases that flow into the common manifold. Should a crack or leak develop in a nitrous oxide or a third gas

flowmeter, oxygen would be the last gas to escape to the atmosphere.

Some older machines and models that do not meet current American Society for Testing and Materials (ASTM) standards may have oxygen flowmeters positioned to the left or in the center of a group of flow tubes (Ward, 1985; Petty, 1987; Dorsch & Dorsch, 1994). This configuration may be present from time to time when a substitute machine is brought out of storage and placed into service temporarily. Therefore, it is important to examine every machine closely and be aware of this possibility to prevent the unfortunate experience of reaching for the oxygen flow control valve on the right and later discovering that the adjustment made was in the flow of nitrous oxide (Dorsch & Dorsch, 1994).

Machine Components that Manage Second and Third Gas Options

Nitrous Oxide Supply and Regulation of Pressure

Nitrous oxide delivery is less involved in the overall function of the anesthesia machine. Nitrous oxide enters the machine from the wall supply through the nitrous oxide inlet and its check valve at the nominal pressure of 50 psig. It flows freely through the pressure-sensor shutoff valve, providing the machine system is pressurized with more than 25 psig of oxygen. From this point, nitrous oxide travels directly to its flow control valve (Fig. 8–13). When the supply hose for nitrous oxide is connected between the wall source and the machine inlet and the machine system has been pressurized with oxygen, nitrous oxide can be turned on at the flowmeter,

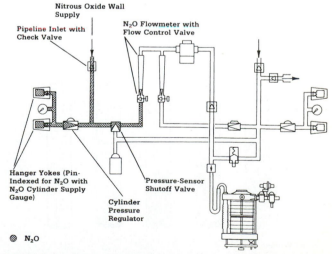

Figure 8–13. Nitrous oxide flows from the wall or cylinder supplies through the cylinder pressure regulator and the pressure-sensor shutoff valve to the base of the flowmeter. *(Redrawn with permission granted by Ohmeda, a division of BOC Health Care, Inc.)*

even though the oxygen flowmeter remains off. Oxygen pressure needs only to be present to keep the pressure-sensor shutoff valve open; oxygen does not have to be flowing.

Although nitrous oxide is not a gas that is in high demand in other hospital departments, its supply pressure can also fluctuate above or below the usual 50-psig level (Bowie & Huffman, 1985; Rice & Kolek, 1996). This is caused by the peculiarities of the hospital's central system and the current demand on all of the supply outlets in the surgery suite, as well as any other anesthetizing areas connected to the same supply source.

Unlike cylinder oxygen, which is a compressed gas at room temperature, nitrous oxide is contained in a full cylinder primarily as a liquid, and exerts a gas pressure of about 745 psig (Fig. 8–14). As nitrous oxide is withdrawn from the cylinder, some of the remaining liquid vaporizes to a gas and replaces the withdrawn gas. The pressure is maintained until all of the liquid has vaporized. As a result, the nitrous oxide pressure gauge will read 745 psig, even though the weight and volume of the contents are both decreasing. For this reason, an additional full cylinder of nitrous oxide should always be available when using nitrous oxide. Once all of the liquid has evaporated, the cylinder gauge will then reflect actual pressure changes of the remaining gas. A nitrous oxide cylinder can be considered empty when the pressure gauge reads significantly lower than 745 psig. When the cylinder is in use and the pointer on the nitrous oxide pressure gauge is falling, be prepared to replace the cylinder immediately.

Nitrous oxide cylinder yoke assemblies also have check valves to minimize cross-filling, but they too are not designed to be leak-tight seals. Nitrous oxide may still escape to the atmosphere and expose health care workers to excess trace gas (Petty, 1987) unless a standard yoke plug and its gasket are installed in the empty yoke whenever a single cylinder is mounted on the two-yoke assembly (Bowie & Huffman, 1985; Rice & Kolek, 1996).

Nitrous oxide reserve cylinders must be managed in the same way as oxygen reserve cylinders. They should be turned on during the machine checking procedure or when the wall supply gas is unavailable. They should not be left on at the same time the wall supply is in use. Although it may be reassuring to have them on and ready to switch over automatically if the wall supply fails, the fact remains that the reserve supply is silently depleted when the wall pressure falls below the pressure delivered by the nitrous oxide pressure regulator.

A nitrous oxide cylinder has its own dedicated regulator that reduces the pressure to about 50 psig. The regulator is simply an automatic balancing device that balances all gas pressures—those coming in and those going out—against a spring load. The pressure-relief valve will vent to the atmosphere when an excessive level of pressure (above 75 psig) develops on the low-pressure side of the regulator (Bowie & Huffman, 1985; Rice & Kolek, 1996).

The nitrous oxide flowmeter (and flow control valve) is similar to the oxygen flowmeter in its functional role—measuring the flow of gas delivered to the patient circuit. This knob feels different from the oxygen knob and can also be distinguished by sight. Unlike the oxygen control knob, the nitrous oxide knob has a knurled surface and is smaller in diameter.

Operations Using Medical Air, Helium, Carbon Dioxide, and Nitrogen

When another medical gas is supplied to the anesthesia machine such as air, helium, or carbon dioxide, the attachment is similar to nitrous oxide. Supply pressure gauges are provided for each supply source, and a valve control for the flow of each gas to the flowmeter based on the oxygen pressure of the machine is inherent in the system. There may be specific indications for the use of the adjunct gases. For example, helium may be used as a diluent for other gas mixtures. Because it diffuses more rapidly than oxygen, it facilitates oxygen delivery when combined with O_2 and is administered to patients with respiratory obstruction from airway narrowing. Medical air is often selected as the gas to combine with oxygen for surgical cases where nitrous oxide may be contraindicated, for example, in cases where the trapping of nitrous oxide in closed spaces would be detrimental, including patients with pulmonary blebs or pneumothorax; during middle ear surgery like tym-

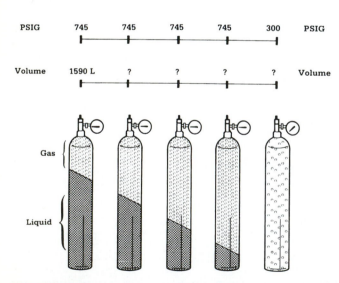

Figure 8–14. Nitrous oxide is stored as a liquid and its pressure gauge does not reflect the volume in the cylinder until all the liquid has been used. *(Redrawn with permission granted by Ohmeda, a division of BOC Health Care, Inc.)*

panoplasty; or in patients who may be undergoing extensive bowel surgeries where gas trapping of nitrous oxide in the intestines may make the surgical procedure more difficult.

Calibrated Vaporizers

An agent-specific calibrated vaporizer is a device that controls the concentration of a volatile anesthetic agent delivered through the common gas outlet. It is dedicated to one agent only, precisely calibrated, and automatically compensated to perform over the usual range of temperatures and variations in gas flow. For example, if one sets the concentration control knob to deliver 1% of anesthetic agent, the vaporizer will make adjustments for temperature and flow to keep its output at 1%, plus or minus the small variation (tolerance) specified by the manufacturer. This holds true as the liquid agent warms and cools, whether the room is hot or cold and whether the total flow rate is high or low.

In the Ohio calibrated vaporizer (Fig. 8–15), gas flows from the flowmeters through the common manifold to the vaporizer inlet, passes through a filter, and moves on toward the relief valve. Under normal conditions, this relief valve remains closed. It opens only when the rate of gas flow is greater than that which will deliver the concentration set on the concentration control valve. In this situation, the relief valve opens to shunt this gas over to the vaporizer outlet instead of permitting it

to flow into the vaporizing chamber (Bowie & Huffman, 1985; Rice & Kolek, 1996).

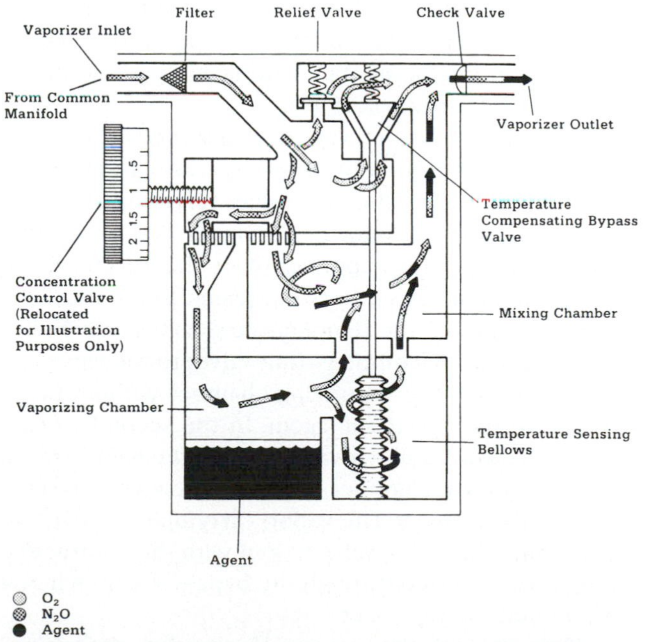

A portion of the gas moves up and around the temperature-compensating bypass valve and out through the check valve (Fig. 8–15). Not all of the gas travels to the depths of the vaporizer. The proportion of the gas that goes through the channel at the bypass valve is adjusted according to the temperature. Changes in ambient temperature and cooling caused by vaporization are continuous. The temperature-compensating bypass valve is connected to the temperature-sensing bellows, next to the vaporizing chamber. When energy is lost in the form of heat during vaporization, this sensor responds. It increases in height when the vapor is warm and pushes on the stem, which elevates the bypass valve to increase the size of its opening. As this space enlarges, a greater proportion of the incoming gas can flow to the outlet, reducing the total amount of gas available to the other routes. When the vapor cools, the bellows contracts, and the stem and the funnel-shaped bypass valve move down and partially close the channel around the bypass valve. This causes more gas to flow through the pathways of the concentration control valve, where the flow is divided between the mixing chamber and the vaporizing chamber. In this manner, the vaporizer continually compensates for temperature to maintain the desired concentration.

The desired percentage of agent is obtained by turning the concentration control valve. This valve alters the ratio of flow through the calibrated pathways (orifices) and splits the stream of gas between the two chambers. When a higher concentration is selected, more gas flows into the vaporizing chamber and less gas flows into the mixing chamber.

Once in the vaporizing chamber, gas passes over a series of wicks saturated with liquid anesthetic agent and becomes saturated with anesthetic vapor. High-concentration settings require more flow to pass over the agent. Low concentrations require less gas flow through the chamber. The saturated gas leaves the vaporizing chamber and joins the unsaturated gas in the mixing chamber. From here it moves up to the top of the vaporizer, where it meets the gas that was diverted through the temperature-compensating bypass valve. The gas mixture carrying the desired concentration of vaporized anesthetic agent passes through the check valve and flows through the vaporizer outlet to the machine outlet.

The vaporizer outlet is equipped with a check valve to prevent reverse flow into the vaporizer. This minimizes the effects of downstream pressure fluctuations on anesthetic agent concentration. The reason for concern about pressure fluctuations and backflow into the vaporizer is simple. This could cause the patient to receive the desired percentage of agent plus additional

Figure 8–15. Nitrous oxide and oxygen flow through the Ohio calibrated vaporizer. Note that the control knob has been graphically moved to the left to better illustrate the gas pathway. *(Redrawn with permission granted by Ohmeda, a division of BOC Health Care, Inc.)*

agent picked up by the gas that went back into the vaporizer. Thus, the outlet check valve on this type of vaporizer protects the patient from receiving a higher percentage of agent than dialed on the concentration control valve. It must be noted, however, that all vaporizers do not necessarily require a check valve.

In general, a vaporizer should never be tilted beyond 45° when it contains liquid agent because a dangerously high output of agent may result (Waugaman & Bradshaw, 1985; Dorsch & Dorsch, 1994). Should this happen, the vaporizer must not be used until it has been drained and dried in order to purge it. Liquid agent may have spilled into the area above the vaporizing chamber, and when fresh gas flows through it, the agent will vaporize without compensation for temperature and flow. A vaporizer that is calibrated and labeled as agent specific is not designed to be used with any other agent, regardless of molecular similarity (Petty, 1987). Never introduce any agent other than the designated agent into any vaporizer. If a vaporizer is inadvertently filled (or charged) with the wrong agent, draining the liquid will not eliminate the agent; some of the agent will have been absorbed by the wick. As a result, the vaporizer must be removed from service and purged of agent by flushing it with 100% oxygen or medical air, while the concentration control valve is turned to its maximum setting. This drying procedure must continue until the odor of the agent can no longer be detected at the vaporizer outlet. It should be noted that drying procedures will not remove thymol, the preservative present in halothane, once it is introduced into a nonhalothane vaporizer. In this situation, the vaporizer should be completely serviced in accordance with the manufacturer's recommendation.

When filling a vaporizer, carefully examine the labels on both the bottle and the vaporizer. Cap, adapter, and bottle labels are usually color coded to help prevent mixing of agents when the liquid is poured into the vaporizer. Vaporizers may have either a funnel-filling system with a screwcap or a keyed-filling receptacle located on the front. Unlike the funnel-filling type, the keyed filler helps prevent the wrong agent from being used in the vaporizer. The TEC 4 vaporizer (Fig. 8–16) was one of the first vaporizers to meet the appropriate ASTM standard, published in 1988. This is also true for the later modification TEC 5. However, the TEC 5 is available with either the keyed-filling device or a screwcap with a drain plug. The TEC 4 and 5 vaporizers are temperature and flow compensated and have a special manifold that completely isolates the vaporizer from the flow of gases to the patient when the vaporizer is in the off position. Unlike the Ohio calibrated vaporizers (Fig. 8–15), the manifold is not *common* to oxygen, nitrous oxide, and anesthetic vapor. Gas supply to the TEC 4 is directed around the device when the vaporizer is turned off. The TEC 6

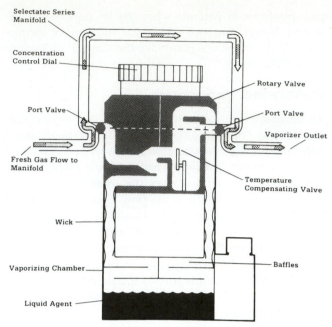

Selectatec Series Manifold

Concentration Control Dial

Port Valve

Fresh Gas Flow to Manifold

Wick

Vaporizing Chamber

Liquid Agent

Rotary Valve

Port Valve

Vaporizer Outlet

Temperature Compensating Valve

Baffles

○ O₂
⊗ N₂O
● Agent

Figure 8–16. Flow of gases through an isolated manifold routes oxygen and nitrous oxide around the vaporizer when it is turned off. Note the location of the port valves in this TEC 4 vaporizer. *(Redrawn with permission granted by Ohmeda, a division of BOC Health Care, Inc.)*

vaporizer is for desflurane and, unlike the TEC 4 and 5, heats the agent and keeps it pressurized (Fig. 8–17). Desflurane boils near room temperature, and the higher controlled temperature state of the TEC 6 vaporizer keeps desflurane in the vapor state during mixing within the vaporizer (Rice & Kolek, 1996).

When the TEC 4 or 5 vaporizer is turned on, the port valves are pushed open to permit gas flow to enter the vaporizer (Fig. 8–18). The port valves serve a dual role by allowing gas to flow into the vaporizer and preventing gas from reaching the vaporizer. Once the gas enters the vaporizer, it is divided into two streams. In the first one, gas passes through the temperature-sensitive valve (also called temperature-compensating valve) to the vaporizer outlet, bypassing the vaporizing chamber without being exposed to the anesthetic agent. In the second stream, gas flow is diverted downward through the wick portion of the vaporizing chamber where it becomes saturated with anesthetic agent. The vapor- carrying gas moves up and through the rotary valve to join with the unsaturated gas that was diverted through the bypass stream when it first entered the vaporizer.

Flow through the vaporizing chamber determines the concentration of anesthetic agent delivered to the vaporizer outlet. The greater the flow, the larger the amount of vapor is produced. Flow is regulated by turn-

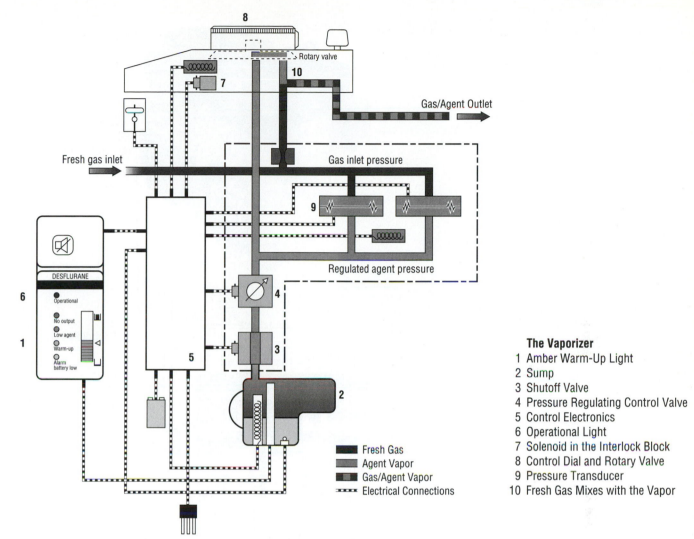

Fresh gas inlet

Gas/Agent Outlet

Gas inlet pressure

Regulated agent pressure

DESFLURANE

- Operational
- No output
- Low agent
- Warm-up
- Alarm battery low

■ Fresh Gas
■ Agent Vapor
▨ Gas/Agent Vapor
┅ Electrical Connections

The Vaporizer
1 Amber Warm-Up Light
2 Sump
3 Shutoff Valve
4 Pressure Regulating Control Valve
5 Control Electronics
6 Operational Light
7 Solenoid in the Interlock Block
8 Control Dial and Rotary Valve
9 Pressure Transducer
10 Fresh Gas Mixes with the Vapor

Figure 8–17. Flow diagram of the TEC 6 vaporizer for desflurane illustrating the heating supply. *(Redrawn with permission granted by Ohmeda, a division of BOC Health Care, Inc.)*

ing the dial, which positions the rotary valve and in-creases or decreases resistance in the stream. Contrac-tion and expansion of the temperature-sensitive valve also increase or decrease the flow of unsaturated gas within the vaporizer.

This vaporizer and its manifold have a safety inter-lock system that prevents more than one vaporizer from being turned on at any given time. Another advantage of this design is a release mechanism located adjacent to the control dial that ensures that the vaporizer cannot be turned on unless it is correctly mounted.

A system of baffles (Fig. 8–19) inside the vaporizer as shown in the TEC 4 schematic helps minimize the risk of liquid agent spilling into the rotary valve mechanism when the vaporizer is unintentionally tilted. However, should such tilting occur, it is still necessary to check the vaporizer output with an agent analyzer prior to return-

ing the vaporizer to use. Although baffles minimize the chance of an overdose, they do not prevent liquid agent from flowing out of the vaporizing chamber.

Liquid anesthetic agent corresponding to the label on the vaporizer is poured directly from the bottle into a funnel-fill receptacle, or it is poured into the vaporizer through a keyed-filling adapter or screwcap filler. The keyed-filling adapter has an agent-specific configuration that must match on both ends. On one end the adapter must correspond to the keyed collar on the bottle of the agent. The other end must correspond to the keyed-filling receptacle on the vaporizer. The keyed-filling sys-tem assists in preventing the error of pouring an agent into the wrong vaporizer; however, it is imperative that one always check that the label on the bottle of liquid agent corresponds to the label on the vaporizer. It is equally important to note that any filling system can be

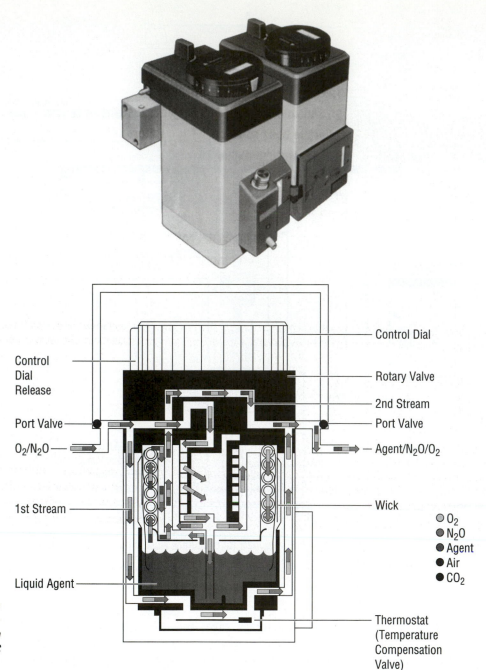

Figure 8–18. Fresh gas flow through the TEC 5 vaporizer and into the vaporizing chamber. *(Redrawn with permission granted by Ohmeda, a division of BOC Health Care, Inc.)*

Labels in figure:
Control Dial Release
Port Valve
O_2/N_2O
1st Stream
Liquid Agent
Control Dial
Rotary Valve
2nd Stream
Port Valve
Agent/N_2O/O_2
Wick
Thermostat (Temperature Compensation Valve)
O_2
N_2O
Agent
Air
CO_2

defeated if one drains unused agent from the vaporizer back into a bottle. If an agent is drained into the wrong bottle, the risk of pouring unknown agent into a subsequent vaporizer exists (Bowie & Huffman, 1985; Petty, 1987; Rice & Kolek, 1996).

Common and Isolated Manifolds

Oxygen and nitrous oxide leave their respective flowmeters and enter the space just above the flow tubes called the common manifold (Fig. 8–20). Here gases mix to-

gether as they travel to the vaporizer, where they become the carrier of a volatile anesthetic agent. Gases may also flow through an isolated manifold, one that directs gas around the vaporizer so none of the gas passes over the vaporizing chamber. There are several kinds of manifolds and a vaporizer can be mounted within them in a variety of ways. To understand how the particular manifold on each machine is connected to the flowmeters and vaporizer(s) and what characteristics each configuration presents, the operations manual must be reviewed for each model of anesthesia machine.

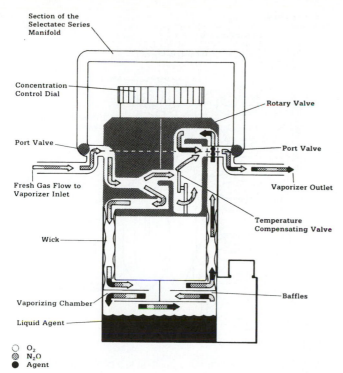

Figure 8–19. Fresh gas flow through the TEC 4 vaporizer and into the vaporizing chamber. *(Redrawn with permission granted by Ohmeda, a division of BOC Health Care, Inc.)*

Gas Flow Through the Patient Circuit and Absorber

Oxygen flows upward through the flowmeter once the flow control valve is turned on. It then enters the com-

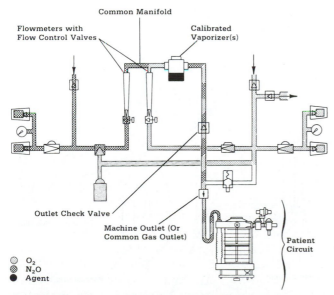

Figure 8–20. Oxygen and nitrous oxide enter the manifold, pass through a vaporizer that is turned off, and flow to the absorber. *(Redrawn with permission granted by Ohmeda, a division of BOC Health Care, Inc.)*

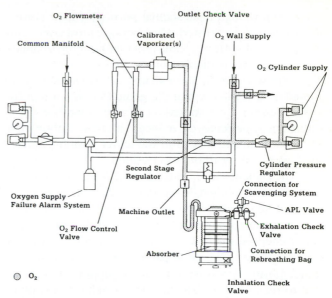

Figure 8–21. Oxygen flow from the wall supply or the cylinder supply through the second-stage regulator, flowmeter, and "in-line" vaporizer to the absorber. *(Redrawn with permission granted by Ohmeda, a division of BOC Health Care, Inc.)*

mon manifold, passes through the vaporizer, and proceeds through the machine outlet check valve. This valve, when present, ensures flow in only one direction. The gas mixture continues from the machine outlet through the absorber's inhalation check valve before flowing to the patient (Fig. 8–21). Exhaled gases pass from the patient through the exhalation check valve and enter the rebreathing bag. When the exhaled gases have filled the bag, excess gas will flow through the adjustable pressure-limiting (APL) valve into the scavenging system that removes waste gases. On the next inspiration, gas remaining in the rebreathing bag passes through the absorber canister(s), where carbon dioxide is removed, before joining the fresh gas flowing into the inspiratory limb of the breathing circuit.

This pattern of gas flow is typically described as a semiclosed breathing system or a circle-with-absorber system. Closed breathing systems have the same flow pattern, but the APL valve is not opened or regularly adjusted as with semiclosed breathing circuits.

Carbon Dioxide Absorber

Oxygen, nitrous oxide, and anesthetic agent flow into the absorber from the common gas outlet. The absorber selectively eliminates carbon dioxide from the exhaled gases without affecting the composition of other gases or used agents in the mixture. If the absorbent granules have been exhausted, the absorber cannot effectively remove carbon dioxide. Therefore, the condition of the granules must be checked at the end of each case. Absorbent granules change color at rest and may return to their original color, even though a substantial portion of their absorption capacity is exhausted. Absorbers are most commonly manufactured with two canisters that hold the granules. The top canister is the first one to be exhausted because it is exposed first to the exhaled gases. The absorbent should be discarded when the granules in the top of the lower canister have started to change color. The upper canister may be removed, refilled with fresh carbon dioxide absorbent, and placed in the lower position, moving the lower canister to the top position.

The patient circuit must be checked for leaks after the canister is refilled. Even though a machine was leak-tight before the absorbent was changed, failure to realign the canisters properly can produce a leak. If the system is not checked for leaks before starting a case, the leak produced may become apparent just as the patient requires positive-pressure ventilatory support. It is important to reemphasize that the entire machine must be inspected and tested daily, and the patient circuit must be tested before every case (Appendix A).

Gases from the flowmeters and anesthetic agent from the vaporizer leave the machine outlet, enter the fresh gas inlet on the absorber, and flow through the inhalation check valve into the breathing circuit, where they pass through the inspiratory limb. When the patient inhales, gas is supplied from the fresh gas flow and from the rebreathing bag via this inspiratory limb of the breathing circuit.

When inhalation is manually assisted, the flow pattern is the same. As the rebreathing bag is squeezed, positive pressure is exerted within the circuit and the flow of gases opens the inhalation check valve. Gas from the rebreathing bag moves down through the absorber canisters and absorbent granules and then flows up the return tube, where it joins the fresh gas going to the patient (Bowie & Huffman, 1985; Rice & Kolek, 1996). The exhalation check valve is closed and the weight of the disc keeps it closed.

When the patient exhales (Fig. 8-22), gases enter the breathing circuit, open the exhalation check valve, and fill the rebreathing bag. Excess gas exits from the APL valve. Fresh gas continues to flow from the common gas outlet into the absorber throughout inspiration and expiration. This characteristic makes the anesthesia machine a continuous-flow gas delivery system.

Once the oxygen flush valve is manually opened, a high flow of oxygen (35–75 L/min) immediately enters the absorber (Fig. 8–23) (ASTM, 1989). Most of this supplemental flow takes the path of least resistance and flows through the top of the absorber and inhalation check valve, on to the patient, and back to the rebreathing bag until the pressure rises sufficiently to cause the APL valve to vent the excess. The rest of the flush flow travels down the return tube, up through the absorbent, and into the rebreathing bag (Bowie & Huffman, 1985; Rice & Kolek, 1996).

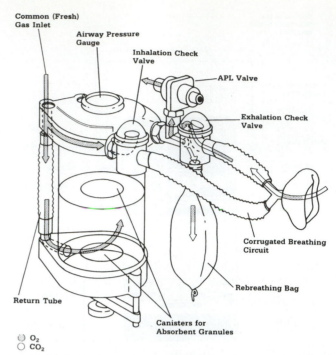

Figure 8–22. Gas flow during exhalation in a continuous-flow circle system. As the patient exhales, gas flows into the rebreathing bag until it fills; excess gas escapes through the APL valve. Fresh gas continues to flow into the circle. *(Redrawn with permission granted by Ohmeda, a division of BOC Health Care, Inc.)*

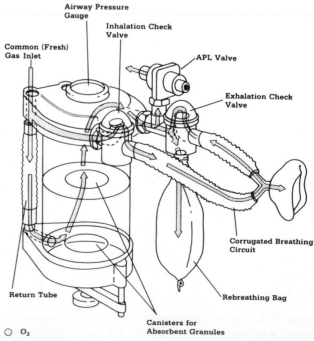

Figure 8–23. Flow of gas during oxygen flush. *(Redrawn with permission granted by Ohmeda, a division of BOC Health Care, Inc.)*

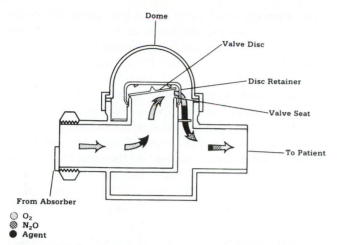

Figure 8–24. Gas flow through the inhalation check valve during inspiration. Note the location of the valve disc and the disc retainer, which maintains alignment with the valve seat. *(Redrawn with permission granted by Ohmeda, a division of BOC Health Care, Inc.)*

The inhalation check valve permits flow of gases to the patient during inspiration (Fig. 8–24). When the patient inhales, the valve disc is lifted off its seat. While the inhalation check valve is open, the exhalation check valve is closed. The barrier ring prevents the valve disc from being dislodged and potentially creating an obstruction to inhaled or exhaled gases (Fig. 8–25).

Exhaled gases flow to the rebreathing bag first. The

remaining or excess gas exits from the APL valve. Exhaled gases flow from the bag to the absorber during the next inspiration. While exhaled gases are opening the valve on the exhalation side of the breathing circuit, the inhalation check valve rests on its seat. This check valve prevents exhaled gas from flowing in a reverse pattern and entering the absorber from the inhalation side; however, fresh gas from the common gas outlet continues to flow into the system.

Also located on the absorber is the APL valve located in the expiratory side of the absorber (Fig. 8–26). The APL valve is adjusted so that the right amount of pressure is applied to assist ventilation. Gas in excess of that needed to achieve the required airway pressure is discharged into the waste gas scavenging system. The APL valve has been commonly called the *pop-off* valve, but this is a misnomer. The term *pop-off* implies a pressure-relief function only, as in basic relief valves found in the ventilator and the waste gas scavenger system. The APL valve adjusts the limit of positive pressure attained within the rebreathing bag and vents excess gas once the preset pressure is reached. The knob controls the adjustment by loading the spring with tension. This tension translates into force exerted against the diaphragm, and each turn of the knob alters this force. The circuit pressure gauge reflects the force as pressure delivered to the patient's airway, not the specific pressure within the patient's thorax.

The function of the APL valve is checked daily to be sure that it opens and closes smoothly. In this absorber,

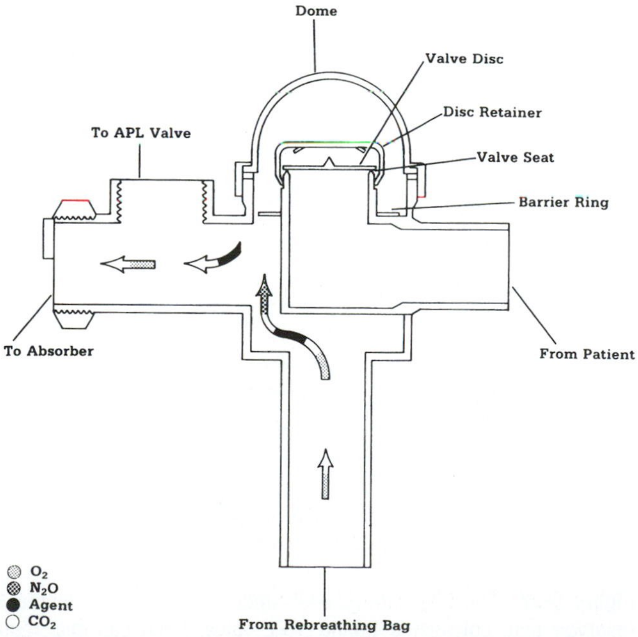

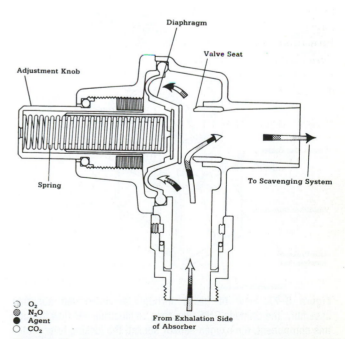

Figure 8–25. Gas flow through the exhalation check valve during inspiration. The barrier ring is designed to reduce the risk of the valve disc becoming lodged in the flow pathway. *(Redrawn with permission granted by Ohmeda, a division of BOC Health Care, Inc.)*

Figure 8–26. Flow of gases through the APL valve. *(Redrawn with permission granted by Ohmeda, a division of BOC Health Care, Inc.)*

the APL valve is attached to the exhalation check valve. The APL valve should be precisely adjusted so that volume intended for the patient is not exhausted into the scavenging system.

An integrated absorber has all the necessary valves and mechanisms built into it, rather than added onto it (Fig. 8–27). Included in its housing are the bag-to-ventilator switch, the APL valve, the oxygen monitor sensor, the circuit pressure-sensing port, a breathing circuit pressure-sensing gauge, and a drain valve to remove water. When the bag-to-ventilation selector switch is present, the APL valve is usually out of circuit and is not closed. With all other absorbers, the APL valve must be closed during mechanical ventilation.

An oxygen sensor is found in the inhalation chamber of this absorber. If a nonintegrated absorber is used, a T-piece adapter is usually employed to attach a fractional inspired oxygen sensor between the inhalation check valve and the inspiratory limb of the circuit.

Systems Without Absorber Components

Nonrebreathing systems do not use an absorber and employ a specific nonrebreathing valve and appropriate delivery hose attached to the common gas outlet.

Mapleson A, B, C, D, E, and F Systems. Mapleson breathing systems have no valves to direct gas flow to or from the patient. Because there is no carbon dioxide (CO_2) absorber within this system, the fresh gas flow must wash carbon dioxide out of the system. Mapleson systems have six classifications as illustrated in Figure 8–28. Modifications E and F involve the Ayre's T-piece or a modification of the T-piece. These two techniques are less popular than they were prior to the advent of waste gas scavenging. However, the Mapleson F (Jackson–Rees modification of the T-piece) system can be scavenged. Only Mapleson A to D systems including the Bain modification are described in this chapter. The Mapleson A system and similar variations are the most efficient for spontaneous unassisted ventilation, and Mapleson D, E, and F systems, including the Bain and Jackson–Rees modifications, are the most efficient for assisted or controlled ventilation (Ehrenwerth & Eiskenkraft, 1993).

The Mapleson A system is also known as the Magill attachment. It differs somewhat from the other Mapleson systems in that fresh gas does not enter the system near the patient connection, but rather near the reservoir bag at the opposite end of the system. Corrugated tubing con-

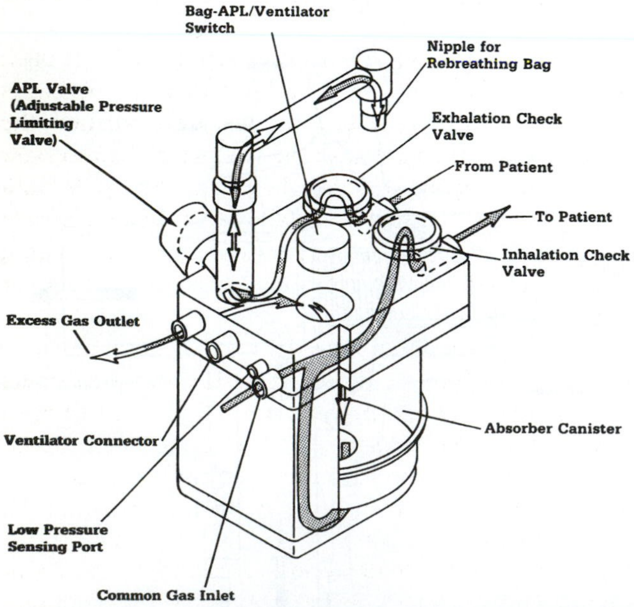

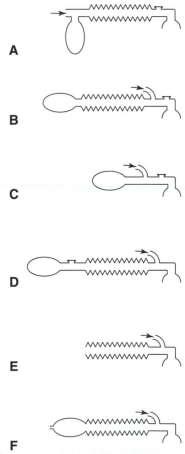

Figure 8–28. The Mapleson classification. Components include a reservoir bag, corrugated tubing, APL valve, fresh gas inlet, and patient connection. *(Redrawn from Mapleson, W. W. [1954]. The elimination of rebreathing in various semiclosed anesthetic systems. British Journal of Anaesthesia, 26, 323–332. With permission from Dorsch, J. A. & Dorsch, S. E. [1994]. Understanding anesthesia equipment [3rd ed.] [p. 168].)*

Figure 8–27. Flow of gases through an integrated absorber assembly: the Ohmeda GMS absorber. To illustrate gas flow through this component, the oxygen-sensor socket, the locking lever on the canisters, and the mechanism that attaches it to the machine are not shown. *(Redrawn with permission granted by Ohmeda, a division of BOC Health Care, Inc.)*

Labels for Figure 8–27: Bag-APL/Ventilator Switch; Nipple for Rebreathing Bag; APL Valve (Adjustable Pressure Limiting Valve); Exhalation Check Valve; From Patient; To Patient; Inhalation Check Valve; Excess Gas Outlet; Ventilator Connector; Absorber Canister; Low Pressure Sensing Port; Common Gas Inlet

nects the reservoir bag to the APL valve at the patient end of the system. This system can be used for spontaneous, controlled, or assisted ventilation, but use of a ventilator with the Mapleson A is not recommended. Fresh gas flow is generally high and computed on a minute volume.

The Mapleson B to F modifications have the fresh gas flow entering the system near the patient's face. Corrugated tubing connecting the reservoir bag to the patient is used with all systems except C, and an APL valve is placed near the patient system in Mapleson B and C. In order to avoid rebreathing completely with these systems, the fresh gas flow must be equal to the peak inspiratory flow rate. A fresh gas flow more than double the minute volume is sometimes recommended, although flows as low as $1\times$ the minute volume have been shown to be sufficient (Conway, 1985).

Bain Circuit: Modified Mapleson D System.

The Bain circuit uses a small-bore fresh gas delivery tube within the corrugated tube between the patient and the reservoir bag (Conway, 1985). This features departs from the Mapleson D system where the fresh gas inflow port is close to the patient's face as was seen in other variations already described. Fresh gas flow is recommended to be equal to the minute volume to minimize rebreathing (Meakin & Coates, 1983). Fresh gas flow can also be computed based on ventilatory requirements. Adequate carbon dioxide removal has been demonstrated with a fresh gas flow of 70 mL/kg/min during assisted or controlled ventilation (Bain & Spoerel, 1972; Bain & Spoerel, 1975; Spoerel, 1980). Spontaneous ventilation using a Bain circuit for long periods of time is not recommended because greater fresh gas flows of up to 150 mL/kg/min are required (Byrick, Janssen, & Yamashita, 1977; Byrick, 1980; Spoerel, 1983). This circuit can malfunction if the central fresh gas delivery tube becomes disconnected, either where it enters the corrugated outer tube or at the patient end. Either type of disconnection increases the dead space and, for any given minute volume, reduces alveolar ventilation (Foex & Crampton Smith, 1977). The patency of these systems should be evaluated prior to each use.

Waste Gas Management

A waste gas scavenging system includes the interface manifold valves (Fig. 8–29) and the hospital's central evacuation system, which receives waste gases from the anesthesia machine and vents them outside the operating room (OR). The interface valve is essentially a manifold with four ports and two relief valves. As gas is pulled into the hospital vacuum system, it flows through the manifold past the two relief valves. One relief valve is for positive pressure and one is for negative pressure. A 3-L reservoir bag is attached. When more flow is passing into the valve than the vacuum can remove, the gas is tem-

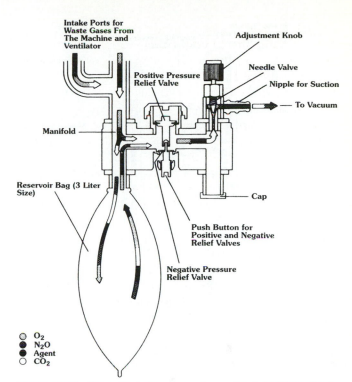

Figure 8–29. Flow of waste gases from the breathing circuit (machine) and the ventilator. The waste gases enter the intake ports of the interface valve, travel to the reservoir, and exit through the vacuum in an active scavenging system. *(Redrawn with permission granted by Ohmeda, a division of BOC Health Care, Inc.)*

porarily stored in the bag. When a waste gas scavenging system is attached to a vacuum source, it is called an active scavenging system.

The rate of flow through the manifold is controlled by adjusting the needle valve so that the reservoir bag is not allowed to become filled. In the ideal situation, the rate of flow is maintained so the volume in the reservoir lies between being empty and half-full (Bowie & Huffman, 1985; Rice & Kolek, 1996). Adjusting the needle valve alters the flow of waste gases into the vacuum source. This adjustment does not regulate the vacuum or suction level.

If the vacuum flow is insufficient and the reservoir bag is allowed to distend, the positive-pressure relief valve on the interface manifold opens and vents exhaled gases into the room. Exposure to trace gas is minimized by adjusting the needle valve to increase the flow of waste gas to the vacuum. If the flow is too high and the bag collapses, the negative-relief valve opens and pulls in room air to satisfy the needs of the vacuum. These valves are installed to protect the patient circuit from extremes in pressure. The positive-pressure relief valve will not be activated if the flow is properly adjusted. In active scavenger systems, any unused nipple must be capped or the vacuum will draw room air, instead of waste gases, into the central system.

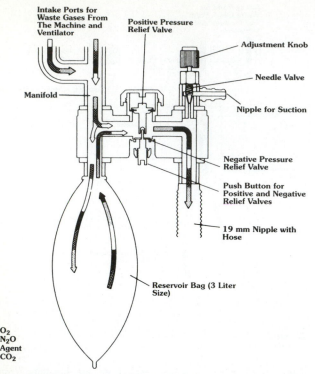

Figure 8–30. Flow of waste gases through the manifold in a passive scavenging system. Note that the cap has been replaced by a 19-mm hose and the adjustment knob for the vacuum is closed. *(Redrawn with permission granted by Ohmeda, a division of BOC Health Care, Inc.)*

A passive waste gas system (Fig. 8–30) uses the hospital ventilation ducts to exhaust the gas through the air circulation system. Waste gases enter the manifold in the same way and the flow is similarly controlled by the relief valves; however, the needle valve is closed and a 19-mm corrugated hose is connected between the interface valve and the exhaust grille of the air-conditioning system.

A waste gas scavenging interface valve is required on every anesthesia machine (Huffman, 1991). The clinician is responsible for verifying that it is properly adjusted to protect OR personnel from exposure to waste gases. Because the anesthesia machine continually receives a supply of fresh gas and the flow is usually more than the patient uses, an efficient means of disposal must be provided. To understand fully how each waste gas system functions and how to adjust it properly, consult the specific manufacturer's operation manual.

Anesthesia Ventilators

An anesthesia ventilator replaces the function of the reservoir bag in the breathing system. Ventilators are accessories to the patient circuit and must be checked, prior to use, according to the manufacturer's recommen-

dations. Ventilator and machine hoses and tubing must be visually examined to verify appropriate connections. If a selector valve is present, its function must be tested in both bag and ventilator modes. Ventilator function should be tested using the breathing system and a test lung at the patient end of the breathing circuit (Waugaman & Bradshaw, 1985).

After setting an appropriate flow on the anesthesia machine, close the APL valve and turn on the ventilator and any accompanying monitors. This will simulate the patient's breathing, permitting tidal volume and respiratory rates to be set, and will allow for assessment of the system for pressure and leaks. Check the volume delivered by the ventilator with a mechanical or electronic volume monitor located in the exhalation limb of the circuit. The difference between the volume set on the ventilator and the volume measured at the expiratory limb is the result of compliance and resistance in the patient circuit. Tidal volume settings marked on any ventilator bellows, its housing, or any accessory scale are estimates of volume and are not patient measurements.

All anesthesia ventilators are equipped with a bellows that communicates directly with the breathing circuit and moves gases via pressure fluctuations in the housing surrounding it. Two types of bellows exist in anesthesia ventilators: (1) the type that rises during inspiration and falls with gravity during exhalation, and (2) the type in which the bellows falls or descends during inspiration and ascends during exhalation. Both types fill during exhalation.

A ventilator that ascends during inspiration and falls during exhalation is called a *hanging bellows* and will continue to cycle even in the presence of a disconnection in the patient circuit. A *standing bellows* ventilator which ascends during exhalation will not appear to be operating normally in the event of a disconnection because exhaled gases from the patient as well as fresh gas flow, are required to fill the bellows. An incomplete or interrupted cycle is a visual image that helps warn the anesthetist of a disconnection; however, the bellows configuration does not appropriately substitute for the use of ventilator low-pressure sensors, a volume monitor, an airway pressure monitor, and all analysis monitors for oxygen and carbon dioxide (Roth, Tweedie, & Sommer, 1986).

Most anesthesia ventilators are volume-controlled ventilators. These ventilators can deliver an elevated tidal volume during oxygen flush that can result in barotrauma and potential patient morbidity unless the ventilator has an adequate pressure-relief system. Most anesthesia ventilators used today have a pressure-limiting valve built into each ventilator in order to vent the driving gas when a given pressure is reached (usually 65–80 cm) (Dorsch & Dorsch, 1994).

Regardless of the type of ventilator used, the nurse anesthetist must understand the expected operation and performance of each model of ventilator and routinely use all appropriate monitors to verify the adequacy of both mechanical and manual ventilation.

▶ PHYSICS OF ANESTHESIA DELIVERY

Medical Gases

Medical gases can be stored in either metal cylinders or in reservoirs of bulk gas storage and supply systems as previously identified. Cylinders can be directly attached to the anesthesia machine. Bulk supply systems use pipelines to transport the gases from the storage supply to the anesthesia machine.

Cylinders

Generally, two sizes of cylinders are used in anesthesia practice. The E cylinder is most commonly used both on anesthesia machines and as a portable cylinder for transport. H cylinders are large and are used as a source of gas for infrequently used gases or those in which a large bulk supply is not needed. These cylinders may be used in the OR to power instruments such as drills. They can also serve as a reserve supply of gas should the pipelines fail.

Oxygen cylinders (E) are filled to a pressure of approximately 1900 psig and H cylinders to 2200 psig. One atmosphere (atm) of pressure [760 mmHg = 0 psig = 14.7 psia (pounds per square inch absolute pressure)]. When full, these cylinders contain a fixed number of molecules. Oxygen exists only as a gas at room temperature so the cylinder gauge will accurately reflect the contents. If the temperature is held constant, the contents of the cylinder can be computed using Boyle's Law, which states that at a constant temperature, the volume of a gas varies inversely with its pressure or $P_1V_1 = P_2V_2$. The internal volume of an E cylinder equals 5 L (V_1). Using this formula, the contents of a full E cylinder can be found by using $V_2 = (P_1 \times V_1)/P_2 = (1900 \text{ psig} \times 5 \text{ L})/14.7$ psia $\simeq$ 660 L. To compute the length of time the cylinder will last, divide the total volume in liters of the cylinder by the liter flow rate of oxygen eg, 660 L/6 L/min = 110 min). A full E cylinder of oxygen will last approximately 110 minutes using a 6 L/min flow. If the cylinder is not full, for example, the gauge reads 1100 psig, then one must divide the remaining oxygen by the amount in the full cylinder to identify the percentage of oxygen in the cylinder (1100 psig/1900 psig $\simeq$ 58% and 660 L $\times$ 58% = 382.2 L of oxygen available).

As was previously mentioned, nitrous oxide exists in cylinders as a liquid at room temperature. E cylinders are filled to 90% to 95% capacity with liquid nitrous oxide and the remaining space contains the gaseous nitrous oxide (Ehrenwerth & Eisenkraft, 1993). The pressure exerted by the nitrous oxide vapor is its saturated vapor pressure (SVP) at room temperature because the liquid is in equilibrium with its vapor phase. A full nitrous oxide

E cylinder will produce approximately 1590 L of gaseous nitrous oxide at 1 atm of pressure (14.7 psia) (Ehrenwerth & Eisenkraft, 1993). Because nitrous oxide is stored as a liquid rather than a gas, the pressure gauge on the cylinder will remain at 745 psig (the SVP of N_2O at 20°C) until all the liquid has vaporized. Therefore, the pressure gauge of a nitrous oxide cylinder does not reflect the contents, and Boyle's Law may only be used to calculate the amount of nitrous oxide remaining in the cylinder when all the liquid has been vaporized. The contents of a liquid nitrous oxide cylinder can be determined by weighing it and then subtracting from that value the weight of an empty cylinder (tare weight), which is stamped on each cylinder. This will yield the cylinder's volume of nitrous oxide. Then by using Avogadro's law [1 g molecular weight of any gas or vapor occupies 22.4 L at standard temperature and pressure (STP)], the volume can be computed. If 44 g N_2O occupies 22.4 L at 0°C (273°K) and 1 atm of pressure, at 20°C (293°K), the volume increases to 22.4 L $\times$ 293°K/273°K = 24 L. Hence, each gram weight of nitrous oxide equals 0.55 L of gas at 20°C.

It would be impractical and inconvenient to try to weigh a nitrous oxide cylinder to determine the contents. If the use of nitrous oxide cylinders is anticipated, the nurse anesthetist should begin the procedure with a full cylinder. A full E cylinder of nitrous oxide will last about 9 hours when administered at a flow rate of 3 L/min (Ehrenwerth & Eisenkraft, 1993). Once only gas remains, the cylinder contents can be computed using Boyle's law where V_1 = 5 L. When the cylinder gauge begins to fall, there is only about 250 L N_2O remaining: $V_2 = (P_1 \times V_1)/P_2$ or (745 psig $\times$ 5 L)/14.7 psia $\simeq$ 253 L.

There is an international color coding for cylinders. The United States deviates from this in two gases: oxygen and compressed air. The international color code for oxygen is white, but the United States uses green. The international color for compressed air is black and white; the United States uses yellow. Other important cylinder colors in anesthesia practice include carbon dioxide (gray), nitrous oxide (blue), cyclopropane (orange), helium (brown), and nitrogen (black).

All medical gas cylinders contain certain markings and codes. Each cylinder in the United States is stamped with the code for the U.S. Department of Transportation (DOT). This is the agency that regulates cylinders and their transfer. Each cylinder has a serial number and commercial designation, the last date of inspection with the inspector's mark, and the service pressure (psig) indicated. Medical gas cylinders are inspected at least once a decade by testing the structural integrity of the cylinder. This is accomplished by filling the cylinder to 1.66 the normal service pressure indicated on the cylinder (Ehrenwerth & Eisenkraft, 1993). All gas cylinders should have a tag perforated in three sections and marked as *empty, in use,* or *full.* The certified nurse anesthetist

(CRNA) should remove the *full* perforation when a cylinder is placed in service. When a cylinder is emptied, the perforation should be removed to reveal *empty,* and the cylinder returned for filling.

All cylinders have a pressure-relief mechanism to vent the cylinder contents and prevent it from exploding from excessive pressure (Compressed Gas Association, 1989). This pressure relief can occur in one of three different forms (or a combination): a fusible plug made of a metal alloy with a low melting point that will melt in a fire, allowing the gas to escape; a frangible metal disc assembly that will break when a certain pressure is exceeded, permitting the gas to escape through a vent; and the safety-relief valve, which is a spring-loaded mechanism that will open as the pressure rises and remain open until the pressure falls below the valve's opening threshold (LeBel, 1992).

Connectors between the cylinder valve and yoke, where it is attached to the anesthesia machine or other apparatus, are made gas specific by a pin-indexing system as previously mentioned. The placement of the pins is different for each agent. The pins are located on the yoke of the anesthesia machine. The corresponding ports for these pins match a particular gas cylinder. The purpose of this pin-indexing system is to prevent cylinders from being attached to the wrong yoke, possibly leading to administration of the wrong agent.

Other laws of physics apply to gases used in anesthesia besides Boyle's and Avodgadro's laws. If a substance (gas) is heated, the molecular movement is increasd and there is a tendency for the volume to expand. It was found experimentally by Charles that if equal volumes of gases were kept at a constant pressure, they would expand by equal amounts of volume for each degree rise in temperature (centigrade). Charles' law can be written as a formula: $T_1V_1 = T_2V_2$ (pressure constant). Gay-Lussac corroborated Charles' findings, but he used volume as the constant. He found that if volume is kept constant, pressure increases incrementally as temperature increases, or $T_1P_1 = T_2P_2$ (volume constant). The three gas laws of Boyle, Charles, and Gay-Lussac can be combined to become the ideal or combined gas law which states that $PV = nRT,$ where pressure (P) multiplied by volume (V) is equal to the number of molecules (n) times a constant R, which is the same for all ideal gases, times the absolute temperature (T) (LeBel, 1992).

A modified version of this formula can be used in clinical anesthesia practice to determine the effects of changes in volume, temperature, or pressure. The modified formula is $P_1V_1A_2 = P_2V_2A_1$, where P_1 is the initial pressure, V_1 is the initial volume, A_1 is the initial temperature (Kelvin), P_2 is the new pressure, V_2 is the new volume and A_2 is the new temperature (Kelvin). For example, if there is a 100 L volume of gas at 273°K (0°C), which exerts a pressure of 1000 pounds per square inch

(psi) and doubling the temperature (273°K × 2 = 546°K) causes a fourfold increase in pressure, what is the new volume of gas?

$$100 \text{ L} \times 1000 \text{ psi} \times 546°\text{K} = V_2 \times 4000 \text{ psi} \times 273°\text{K}$$
$$54\,600\,000 \text{ L} \cdot \text{psi} \cdot °\text{K} = V_2 \times 1\,092\,000 \text{ psi} \cdot °\text{K}$$
$$V_2 = \frac{54\,600\,000 \text{ L} \cdot \text{psi} \cdot °\text{K}}{1\,092\,000 \text{ psi} \cdot °\text{K}}$$
$$V_2 = 50 \text{ L}$$

According to Charles' law, doubling the temperature could be expected to double the volume, making it 200 L; but by Boyle's law, a quadrupling of pressure would decrease volume to one quarter of the initial volume. The net change in volume then must be ¼ of 200 or 50 L. This simple example serves to illustrate how the formula can be used to solve practical problems in the clinical setting, such as calculating the volume of a gas in a cylinder transported from a cold outdoor environment to a warm indoor one (LeBel, 1992). When using these formulae, all temperatures must be converted to Kelvin, and all volumes and pressures must be in the same measurement units.

The Anesthesia Machine

Pressure and Flow

The basic functions of any anesthesia machine are to receive compressed gases from their supplies (either cylinder or bulk) and to create a mixture of identified composition and flow rate at the machine's common gas outlet. The relationship between pressure and flow is stated in Ohm's law:

$$\text{Flow} = \frac{\text{Pressure}}{\text{Resistance}}$$

In order for the flow of gases from high-pressure sources through the machine to exit the common gas outlet at pressures approximating atmospheric requires changes in pressure, resistance, or both to achieve this goal of gas administration. This is most often accomplished with the use of a variety of pressure regulators within the system.

The flowmeters in the anesthesia machine use a physical property of the gas to measure flow. When low flows are employed, the gas flow is laminar, and the property used is the viscosity of the gas. At low flow rates when gas flow is laminar, Poiseuille's law applies:

$$\text{Flow} = \frac{\pi p r^4}{8vl}$$

where π = a constant, 3.142; p = pressure drop across the bobbin; r = radius of the tube; v = viscosity of the gas; and l = length of the bobbin or float. At high flows, gas flow is usually turbulent. In this instance gas density is used to measure the flow of the gas. With turbulent flow,

$$\text{Flow} \simeq p \simeq r^2 \simeq l^{-1} \simeq \frac{1}{\sqrt{d}}$$

where d = the gas density.

Carbon Dioxide Absorption

Hypercarbia and respiratory acidosis develop when the body is unable to rid itself of end products of metabolism, or when a patient is allowed to breathe from an atmosphere high in carbon dioxide content. The latter situation can develop when a person rebreathes from an anesthesia circuit unless means are taken to disperse exhaled carbon dioxide or remove it by chemical means. With circuits that allow rebreathing of exhaled gases, such as a circle system, chemical removal provides a means of eliminating excess carbon dioxide. The amount chemically removed depends on whether the circuit is fully closed, allowing rebreathing of all exhaled gases, or partially closed, allowing only a fraction of exhaled gases to be rebreathed (semiclosed system). The rate of fresh gas inflow relative to production of exhaled carbon dioxide is also a factor.

Chemical absorption depends on the fact that carbon dioxide is a gaseous, nonmetal oxide, forming carbonic acid when in contact with water, and is capable of reacting with metal oxides. Metal oxides in contact with water form hydroxides (bases), which can neutralize acids. How effective a metal oxide will be in neutralizing acids depends on the metal's reactivity (position on the periodic table). Alkali metals are the most active. Of this group, potassium and sodium hydroxides are most commonly used. Alkaline earth metals are less reactive than alkali metals, but may also be used. Of this group, barium and calcium hydroxides are used most often. As neutralization occurs, the reaction produces water and the carbonate of the metal hydroxide evolves; for example, calcium hydroxide becomes calcium carbonate. Additional exposure of the carbonate to the acid produces a bicarbonate. Sodium, potassium, calcium, and barium hydroxides can all eventually be converted to bicarbonates. Although some bicarbonate may form in carbon dioxide absorption canisters, complete conversion is usually not seen because canister efficiency is depleted before the conversion is complete. The canister must then be changed to maintain efficient carbon dioxide absorption. The carbonates formed are quite stable, with decomposition occurring only under unusual conditions. As neutralization proceeds, the canister emits heat because of exothermic reactions produced by the hydroxides dissolving in water (heat of solution). Hydroxides have such affinity for water that they are termed hygroscopic; that is, they are substances that absorb, even become dissolved in, water from the surrounding environment. Yet a small amount of water is added as a film to soda lime granules to allow for ionization. The amount of water has to be controlled because too much water reduces absorption efficiency.

Size, shape, and consistency of absorbent granules are important in maximizing efficiency. Granules are of a size termed *4 to 8 mesh* because they must pass through a mesh screening having four to eight openings per inch. Because hydroxides are normally soft and easily pulverized, a small amount of silica is added to increase hardness. Granules should have a hardness number greater than 75, a number determined by agitating the granules with steel ball bearings prior to passing them through the sizing mesh. The shape of each granule, which looks like a small piece of lava rock with many indentations, maximizes the surface area available for chemical reactions.

Soda lime is composed of 4% sodium hydroxide, 1% potassium hydroxide, and 14% to 19% water, the balance being calcium hydroxide. This is known as the *wet* variety and is the most commonly used absorbent today. Silica may be added in small amounts to increase hardness. The amount of sodium hydroxide is limited to prevent caking caused by hygroscopic absorption of water. Caking reduces absorption efficiency and increases resistance to gas flow within the circuit. With older forms of soda lime, a phenomena known as *peaking* or *regeneration* occurred. After prolonged use, the soda lime efficiency would fall. Removing the canister from use allowed for some carbonate to be reconverted to soda lime. The canister could be reused with high efficiency but only for short periods. With modern canisters, peaking is of little clinical importance.

Because soda lime is used in the presence of dry gases, one might think that absorption efficiency is reduced. This is not the case, provided the moisture content for granules is high (about 14%). Besides water adhered to granules, additional water for chemical reactions is provided by exhaled moisture and by chemical release of hydrogen and hydroxyl ions, which combine to form water. Production of water by chemical reactions liberates heat, 13 700 calories per mole (cal/mol) of carbon dioxide absorbed, which warms gases within the absorber. If excessive heat develops, the canister may feel warm to the touch. Excessive temperatures may have an adverse impact on patients by preventing dissipation of body heat.

Barium hydroxide granules are not as widely used. These granules differ in some respects from those of soda lime. Because barium hydroxide is an octahydrate [$Ba(OH)_2 \times 8H_2O$], additional water is not required. The barium hydroxide type of absorbent also contains calcium (about 80%) and potassium hydroxide (1%). It too is 4 to 8 mesh in size, but no hardening material is added. The water of crystallization keeps dust formation to a minimum. Heat production and additional water formation are essentially the same as with soda lime. As with soda lime, a color indicator is used to indicate expenditure of the granules; however, barium hydroxide does not regenerate to any appreciable extent.

Color indicators or dyes are added to both soda lime and barium hydroxide to indicate the extent to which the absorbent has been exhausted. Those indicators are themselves either acids or bases that react with hydrogen ions and produce a color change. With regeneration, dye color disappears. But any change in absorbent coloration indicates reduced efficiency with further use, and one should consider replacing the canister. A number of indicator dyes are used including ethyl violet, Clayton yellow, ethyl orange, mimosa Z, and phenolphthalein. Package inserts generally describe the color change to be expected from a particular brand of absorbent. Indicators are not absolutely reflective of the extent to which absorbent has been used because a number of factors may impact dye color changes.

Absorbers used today have a dual-canister configuration. Fresh canisters come packaged in airtight containers to prevent moisture contamination prior to use. Each has a baffle at the top and bottom, which some manufacturers seal with an adhesive label. Failure to remove the label will obstruct gas flow within the absorber. Typically, modern absorbers are designed to allow a flow of gas exceeding expected tidal volumes breathed by patients. They also minimize mechanical resistance to breathing. A number of factors influence the efficiency of absorbers including the rate and pattern of ventilation, amount of carbon dioxide produced by the patient, rate of fresh gas flows used, and pattern of gas flow through the absorber. This last factor results in what is termed channeling. As gases pass through the canister, they take the path of least resistance. This path is usually along the sides of the canister where granules are less tightly packed. The effect is to funnel flows over the same areas of absorbent. Because of channeling, absorbent around the walls of the container is used up first, one factor responsible for rapid indicator dye changes along easily visible canister outer walls.

The chemical steps involved in carbon dioxide absorption may be summarized as follows:

1. Exhaled carbon dioxide combines with available water to form carbonic acid:

$$CO_2 + H_2O \rightarrow H_2CO_3$$

2. Carbonic acid dissociates into hydrogen and bicarbonate ions:

$$H_2CO_3 \rightarrow H^+ + HCO_3^-$$

3. The metal oxides dissociate to their respective ions. Soda lime absorbent includes sodium, calcium, and potassium hydroxides. Barium hydroxide lime includes calcium, potassium, and barium hydroxides.

Sodium	NaOH	$\rightarrow Na^+ + OH^-$
Calcium	$Ca(OH)_2$	$\rightarrow Ca^{2+} + 2OH^-$
Potassium	KOH	$\rightarrow K^+ + OH^-$
Barium	$Ba(OH)_2 \times 8H_2O$	$\rightleftarrows Ba^{2+} + 2OH^-$ $+ 8H_2O$

4. Hydroxides react with carbonic acid to produce carbonates:

Sodium	$2NaOH + H_2CO_3 \rightarrow Na_2CO_3 + 2H_2O$ $+ \, heat$
Calcium	$Ca(OH)_2 + H_2CO_3 \rightarrow CaCO_3 + 2H_2O$ $+ \, heat$
Potassium	$2KOH + H_2CO_3 \rightarrow K_2CO_3 + 2H_2O$ $+ \, heat$

Barium   Here four reactions are involved:

a. Barium hydroxide directly reacts with carbon dioxide:

$$Ba(OH)_2 \, 8H_2O + CO_2 \rightarrow BaCO_3 + 9H_2O + heat$$

b. Water from step a combines with carbon dioxide to form carbonic acid:

$$9H_2O + 9CO_2 \rightarrow 9H_2CO_3 + heat$$

c. The carbonic acid reacts with the available calcium and potassium hydroxides:

$$9H_2CO_3 + 9Ca(OH)_2 \rightarrow 9CaCO_3 + 18H_2O + heat$$
$$2KOH + H_2CO_3 \rightarrow K_2CO_3 + 2H_2O + heat$$

When regeneration reactions are allowed to occur, only sodium and potassium carbonates are reconverted to their respective hydroxides by reacting with unused calcium hydroxide. This is because both carbonates are soluble. Barium carbonate and calcium carbonate, being insoluble, cannot be reconverted to hydroxides. Thus, two regenerative reactions are possible:

$$K_2CO_3 + Ca(OH)_2 \rightarrow CaCO_3 + 2KOH$$
$$Na_2CO_3 + Ca(OH)_2 \rightarrow CaCO_3 + 2NaOH$$

Regenerative reactions further deplete available calcium hydroxide and contribute to additional formation of calcium carbonate.

Anesthesia Vaporizers

Inhaled anesthetic agents are often referred to as volatile anesthetics, meaning they vaporize readily. When potent anesthetic agents are placed in a closed container at atmospheric pressure (760 mmHg) and room temperature (20°C), they are in liquid form. Some of the molecules will escape from the surface of the liquid and vaporize. At constant temperature, there is equilibrium between the molecules in the vapor phase and those in the liquid phase. The molecules in the vapor phase are in constant motion, striking the walls of the container to exert a vapor pressure (Ehrenwerth & Eisenkraft, 1993). As temperature increases, more molecules enter the vapor phase (through evaporation), which increases the vapor pressure. The gas phase above the liquid is saturated when it contains all the anesthetic vapor it can hold at a given temperature. The pressure from this anesthetic vapor is referred to as its SVP at a particular temperature (Ehrenwerth & Eisenkraft, 1993).

The saturated pressure exerted by the vapor phase of a volatile agent depends only on the agent and the ambient temperature. The agent's boiling point is the temperature at which vapor pressure equals ambient pressure and at which all of the liquid changes to vapor. The more volatile the agent, the lower the boiling point and the higher the SVP (Ehrenwerth & Eisenkraft, 1993). The boiling point will decrease as barometric pressure decreases, as occurs at high altitudes.

Anesthetic vapor is often quantified in the terms of volumes percent (volumes of vapor per 100 volumes of total gas). Using Dalton's law, the volumes percent can be calculated as the partial pressure of the agent from its vapor compared to the total ambient pressure. This is then multiplied by 100. Dalton's law states that the pressure exerted by a mixture of gases enclosed in a given space is equal to the sum of the pressures that each gas or vapor would exert if it alone occupied the container (Davis, Parbrook, & Kenny, 1995). For example, oxygen is 21% of dry ambient air at atmospheric pressure so the partial pressure exerted by oxygen is 21% × 760 mmHg or ~160 mmHg. If this air is not saturated with water vapor at normal body temperature (37°C), what is the pressure of oxygen? Because vapor pressure depends on temperature, the SVP for water at 37°C is 47 mmHg, so the pressure due to oxygen is now 21% × (760 − 47) or 713 mmHg. The partial pressure of oxygen for this computation is ~150. The student should remember that volumes percent is a relative ratio of proportion of gas molecules in a mixture and partial pressure is an absolute value. This becomes critical when considering anesthetic uptake and potency because they are related directly to partial pressure and only indirectly to volumes percent (Ehrenwerth & Eisenkraft, 1993).

Energy is required to convert molecules from liquid to vapor. This energy is called the latent heat of vaporization and is defined as the amount of heat (calories) required to convert a unit mass (grams) of liquid into vapor (Davis, Parbrook, & Kenny, 1995). The practical aspects of this are that at lower temperatures, more heat is required for vaporization. This was particularly important when vaporizers used in anesthesia practice were not temperature compensated. When the room temperature was cold first thing in the morning, vaporizers had to be adjusted for this temperature and later in the day if the room warmed, particularly if a pediatric patient is present and the room temperature is manually increased, the

CRNA would have to recalibrate the vaporizer settings so as not to deliver a concentration higher than anticipated.

Specific heat is the quantity of heat in calories required to raise the temperature of a unit mass (grams) of a substance by one degree centigrade (Davis, Parbrook, & Kenny, 1995). Specific heat and thermal conductivity play important roles in vaporizer construction material. Temperature changes are more gradual for materials with a high specific heat. Thermal conductivity is the rate at which the heat is transmitted through a substance. Therefore, vaporizers should be constructed from materials with a high specific heat and a high thermal conductivity (Ehrenwerth & Eisenkraft, 1993). Most vaporizers used today are constructed from bronze and stainless steel.

Nearly all vaporizers in current anesthesia practice are concentration calibrated and of the variable bypass design, for example, the TEC series of Ohmeda previously described. Nonconcentration-calibrated vaporizers are often referred to as measured flow vaporizers. These include the Copper Kettle (Foregger/Purtian-Bennett) or Verni-Trol (Ohmeda, formerly Ohio Medical). A measured flow of oxygen is selected on a separate flowmeter to pass to the vaporizer from which vapor emerges saturated. The oxygen is bubbled through the liquid agent. These bubbles increase the surface area which creates a liquid–gas interface over which evaporation of the agent occurs quickly (Ehrenwerth & Eisenkraft, 1993). The flow is then diluted by an additional measured flow of gases, usually oxygen and nitrous oxide from the other flowmeters on the anesthesia machine. To deliver the correct percentage of anesthetic vapor, a calculation must be performed to determine the anesthetic vapor concentration in the mixture.

At a room temperature of 20°C, the saturated vapor pressures of the commonly used inhaled agents are (in mmHg) halothane = 243; enflurane = 175; isoflurane = 238; sevoflurane = 160; and desflurane = 664. If atmospheric pressure (ambient) is 760 mmHg, then the SVP represents 32% halothane, 23% enflurane, 31% isoflurane, 21% sevoflurane, and 87% desflurane. When calculating the vaporizer concentration, the student must remember that the volume of carrier gas that flows from the machine into the vaporizer is the same volume of carrier gas that exits the vaporizer. However, because of the additional vaporized anesthetic agent, the total volume exiting the vaporizer is actually greater than that entering. The volume of carrier gas is the difference between 100% of the atmosphere in the vaporizing chamber and that due to anesthetic vapor (Ehrenwerth & Eisenkraft, 1993). In the vaporizing chamber, anesthetic vapor at its SVP constitutes a fractional volume of the atmosphere. When administering isoflurane through this type of vaporizer, 31% of the agent is in the vaporizer as saturated vapor at 20°C and 760 mmHg. If 100 mL of carrier gas flows per minute through a vaporizing chamber containing isoflurane, the carrier gas represents 69% (100%–31%) of the atmosphere, and the remaining 31% is the isoflurane vapor (Ehrenwerth & Eisenkraft, 1993). This can be expressed as (100 mL/69%) × 31%, which equals 45 mL of isoflurane vapor per minute. This concept can be translated to a calculation:

$$\frac{\text{SVP agent (mmHg)}}{\text{Total pressure (mmHg)}} = \frac{\text{Agent vapor } (x \text{ mL})}{\text{Carrier gas } (y \text{ mL}) + \text{Agent vapor } (x \text{ mL})}$$

$$= \frac{\text{Volume of agent vapor}}{\text{Total volume leaving the vaporizer}}$$

If isoflurane is used in this example and the carrier gas flow is 100 mL/min (y), then:

$$\frac{238 \text{ mmHg}}{760 \text{ mmHg}} = \frac{x}{100 \text{ mL/min} + x}$$

$$x = 44 \text{ mL}$$

The reader will note that there is a slight difference in the answer when it is computed exactly as illustrated in the longer formula than when using the more approximate measurement of SVP as a percentage of the total gas flow. If x is known, the carrier gas flow y can be calculated. At a steady state the total volume of gas leaving the vaporizing chamber is larger than the total volume that entered. The additional vapor is the saturated vapor concentration. If administration of 1% of isoflurane is desired with a total fresh gas flow rate of 5 L/min, the vaporizer will have to evolve 50 mL of isoflurane per minute or 1% × 5 000 mL (Ehrenwerth & Eisenkraft, 1993). If 50 mL represents 31% isoflurane, then oxygen (the carrier gas) must represent the other 69%:

$$\frac{50 \text{ mL}}{31\%} = \frac{x}{69\%}; \quad x = \frac{50}{31\%} \times 69\%; \quad x = 111 \text{ mL}$$

This can also be computed using y as the carrier (oxygen) flow:

$$\frac{238 \text{ mmHg}}{760 \text{ mmHg}} = \frac{50 \text{ mL}}{y + 50 \text{ mL}} = 110 \text{ mL}$$

Once again, the reader will note that there is a slight difference in the answer when it is computed exactly as illustrated in the longer formula than when using the more approximate measurement of SVP as a percentage of the total gas flow.

▶ REGULATIONS AND STANDARDS

All anesthesia machine and patient breathing systems must meet or exceed the minimum standard for safety and performance, as published by the American Society of Testing and Materials (1989; 1990). The set of standard specifications for the anesthesia machine, published in 1989, replaced the previous anesthesia machine standard document known as the American National Standards Institute (ANSI) Z.79.8, *Standard for Safety and Performance of Anesthesia Machines for Human Use*. The ANSI Z.79.8 document was the first full consensus standard that defined minimum performance and safety specifications developed by representatives from all sectors of anesthesia practice and interests: CRNAs, physicians, professional engineers, and representatives of manufacturing, government, academic, and consumer groups. Full consensus standards are comprehensively sound and credible because all participants must concur on every aspect of the standard, including words, phrases, terminology, performance specifications, and testing protocols. The standard is also submitted for ballot and vote prior to approval and publication.

The currently applicable ASTM standard document is designated as F1161-88 and is officially titled *Standard Specification for Minimum Performance and Safety Requirements for Components and Systems of Anesthesia Machines*. This standard is under the jurisdiction of the ASTM Committee on Anesthetic and Respiratory Equipment and is the direct responsibility of Subcommittee F29.01.01 on Continuous Flow Anesthesia Gas Machines. The ASTM F1161-88 document, like its predecessor, is a full-consensus standard, and is the foundation for ongoing standards writing aimed at ensuring that anesthesia machines purchased in the future will meet the minimum expectations for safety.

Manufacturing anesthesia machines requires compliance with this standard and numerous other standards' specifications relating to circuits, accessories, ventilators, regulators, compressed gases, monitors, and alarms. Each standard is a set of rules established by authority, expertise, custom, and general consensus as a model to be followed. Standards also serve as the basic elements by which quality is defined as part of the overall commitment to public safety. Therefore, it is inappropriate for a clinician or hospital to modify, alter, refine, redesign, or manufacture anesthesia equipment components. Changes and alterations in select equipment configuration are acceptable providing the original product manufacturer describes the intended alteration in the appropriate operations and maintenance manual(s) required for the specific model of machine, component, or accessory used in the anesthesia system.

The Safe Medical Devices Act of 1990, also known as Public Law 101-629, assures that devices entering the market are safe and effective and that serious problems are reported to the Food and Drug Administration (FDA) expediently so the device can quickly be removed from the market. Health care institutions are required to report within 10 working days all incidents that reasonably suggest that there is a probability that a medical device caused or contributed to the death or serious illness or injury of a patient (Dorsch & Dorsch, 1994). Deaths must be reported to both the FDA and the manufacturer. Health care institutions should provide inservice education on the responsibility of anesthesia providers to report problems with medical devices. In addition, policies, procedures and record-keeping systems must be established to document, store, and retrieve data submitted to the FDA and/or manufacturers concerning equipment or devices.

▶ CLINICAL CONSIDERATIONS

Problems with oxygen supply have historically been the cause of anesthetic morbidity and mortality, and these problems remain today. The most common problem associated with external pipeline systems is insufficient oxygen pressure (Waugaman & Bradshaw, 1985). As a result, pipeline pressure gauges are positioned on the front of each machine that meets the current ASTM machine safety and performance standard. Nurse anesthetists should regularly monitor the pipeline gauges to verify adequate pressure before and during the anesthetic course.

If a pipeline source is used, at least one reserve cylinder must be present on the machine. Cylinder contents should be checked to ensure adequate gas supply and then closed so the reserve oxygen is not depleted. If a central pipeline gas source is not available, a machine with a double-yoke assembly for oxygen and nitrous oxide permits the use of one cylinder and the readiness of a reserve cylinder at all times. The pin-indexed safety system (PISS) and the diameter-indexed safety system (DISS) are designed to minimize the risk of making an incorrect connection to a cylinder or pipeline source. Specifically, the gas-specific pin configuration serves to prevent placement of the wrong cylinder into a yoke. The diameter-specific fittings help prevent placement of the wrong gas supply hose into a machine inlet or a wall supply outlet.

The oxygen supply failure alarm system is a pressure-related audible alarm component that warns when oxygen pressure is decreasing or has fallen below the machine's predetermined nominal requirement. This alarm always implies that the reserve cylinder should be immediately turned on before the cause of the problem is evaluated and corrected. When the oxygen supply failure alarm is sounding, the pressure-sensor shutoff valve is activated to stop the flow of nitrous oxide or any other gas. This component senses pressure and does not deal with oxygen flow or oxygen concentration.

The airway pressure alarm should also be checked prior to the start of the workday. Numerous models of airway pressure monitors exist and the routine preuse inspection and testing should be conducted according to the manufacturer's instructions. This simple device is able to warn of disconnection in the patient circuit, often before other clinical evidence of change is apparent.

The precision flowmeter requires careful handling and should receive respectful attention during the preuse checking procedure. Forceful closure of this valve should be avoided to prevent wear and tear on the valve seat, which may lead to inaccurate flow readings. The float should be visually inspected to be certain it moves freely within the flow tube. Halting, irregular, or erratic movement of the float may signal the possibility of inaccurate readings. In addition, care should be exercised when turning the flowmeter on to avoid propelling the float to the top of the flow tube where it may lodge, obstructing the flow of gas into the manifold (Dorsch & Dorsch, 1994).

Always verify that the oxygen flush valve is operational to ensure that a supplement of 100% oxygen can be delivered to the patient circuit without delay. Monitor the effects of the flush maneuver on the airway pressure manometer or monitor located within the circuit. Indiscriminate use of the flush valve is not appropriate because it can significantly increase the patient's airway pressure. Unintentional opening of the flush valve is also a concern, now minimized by a recessed casing in machines that meet current ASTM standards for machine safety and performance (Dorsch & Dorsch, 1994).

Calibrated vaporizers play an important role in the integrity of gas flow through the machine. Machine function should be tested with the vaporizers both closed and opened to ensure their proper alignment within the manifold and to detect potential leaks. Anesthetic agent should be carefully poured into the vaporizer, following the manufacturer's recommendation for funnel-filling and key-filling procedures. Liquid agent drained from a vaporizer should never be poured back into a bottle, and the liquid agent should be disposed of in an appropriate manner to minimize the exposure of trace gas to health care workers.

Vaporizers should be mounted upstream from the common gas outlet and properly placed within their integrated, isolated manifold. It is unacceptable to install a vaporizer downstream from the common gas outlet. Not only is this practice out of date and unnecessary, it fails to meet the minimum ASTM (1988) standard of safety and performance for vaporizers. Downstream vaporizers are prone to be tilt and may be readily misconnected to the fresh gas flow. Both of these conditions lead to overdose. Use of the flush valve is also problematic with a downstream vaporizer because an oxygen flow up to 75 L/min may be flushed through the head of the vaporizer without the safeguard of appropriate flow compensation to minimize the risk of uncontrolled vaporization and patient overdose.

Vaporizers are instruments that need periodic maintenance, regardless of the stability of their performance and the apparent clinical verification of their output. The goal of every equipment maintenance program is to minimize the possibility that a device or component will fail or malfunction. These efforts are undertaken with all medical equipment to detect evidence of wear or deterioration long before it causes a problem for a patient or results in financial loss. For this reason, the basic foundations of preventive maintenance and equipment safety apply to mechanical vaporizers in the same way as they do to all other mechanical or pneumatic components of the anesthesia system.

Depending on the specific model of vaporizer, manufacturers recommend service on a regular basis, for example, every 1 to 2 years, so that all parts can be inspected, new parts can be installed if there is any doubt about wear, and calibration can be verified with a precision refractometer. This procedure is not to be confused with the practice of spot-checking a vaporizer's output, a routine that is only one phase of a regular maintenance program. Using a portable gas indicator, an agent analyzer, or an agent monitor to follow trends in vaporizer output is not a sufficient reason to justify operating vaporizers that are clearly performing outside the limits of their specifications (Huffman, 1990). A calibration spot check can detect a malfunction but it cannot predict one. In addition, a spot check can determine the concentration of an agent, but it cannot verify that the temperature-compensating system is operating at its mechanical best.

When a temperature-compensating mechanism fails, the resultant increase in vaporizer output does not cause a gradually changing reading. Instead, the change is usually sudden and develops without subtle indicators. The agent monitor can demonstrate the sudden overdose and sound an alarm, but it cannot protect the patient from exposure to this problem.

Vaporizers may not perform as intended when they suffer from abuse, misuse, or improper maintenance. Currently, all calibrated models are mechanical and prone to the same risks of wear and tear as any other component of the anesthesia machine system. When funnel-filling vaporizers are used instead of key-filling vaporizers, the risks of contamination by dust and particulate matter increase. Dust, when introduced into the vaporizer, contributes to wear on its moving parts. Thymol, normally present in halothane vaporizers, is another example of particulate matter that adds to the problem of mechanical deterioration. Filling errors continue to be a problem, as the halothane preservative thymol continues to be discovered inside enflurane and isoflurane vaporizers (Dorsch & Dorsch, 1994).

The patient circuit includes all components located between the common gas outlet and the patient's airway, and every component must be checked daily in accor-

dance with the manufacturer's recommendations. Testing for unacceptable leaks in the patient circuit is only one of the concerns that needs clinical attention. The gas delivery tube should be inspected to be sure it is not kinked and is, in fact, a high-pressure medical gas delivery hose. Hospital-grade rubber tubing and plastic tubes should not be used as gas delivery hoses when administering anesthesia. The inhalation and exhalation check valves should also be inspected to be certain that the dome is intact, the disc is present, and the guard and the barrier ring are properly positioned.

The patency of the breathing circuit and rebreathing bag should be inspected and functionally tested (along with the entire patient circuit) prior to each case. The absorber must be filled with soda lime or an equivalent absorbent, firmly packed in canisters, and mounted in the absorber with correct alignment. Failure to check absorber alignment and canister placement may result in an undetected leak within the patient circuit.

The color indicator in the absorbent granules signifies when a fresh supply is needed. When the granules in the top canister change color in a two-chamber absorber, place the bottom canister in the upper position and add fresh granules to the bottom canister. This check must be done at the end of a case, as the granules can return to their original color between cases.

Test the APL valve daily to be sure it can be fully opened and closed and that the airway pressure gauge corresponds to these adjustments. Correct function of this valve is necessary for appropriate management of pressure within the patient circuit and for control of gas flow to the waste gas scavenging system.

The needle valve on the waste gas manifold must be adjusted when excess flow from the patient circuit increases or decreases. The needle valve on this component does not regulate the vacuum (suction) level, but alters the amount of flow allowed to leave the manifold and enter the evacuation system. The vacuum level remains *constant* except for fluctuations that occur when heavy demand decreases the level of vacuum available to the wall outlet or when lower demand increases the vacuum.

The reservoir bag on the waste gas scavenger serves as a temporary storage site so that one does not need to adjust the waste gas flow minute-by-minute. Changes in total flow of fresh gas do occur, however, and the waste gas needle valve setting must be appropriately adjusted to prevent overinflation or underinflation of the reservoir bag. Visual monitoring of the contour of this bag offers a valuable reminder to the clinician when flow needs to be altered. Should a higher level of vacuum exist than is needed, the negative-pressure relief valve on the manifold will open to allow room air to enter the evacuation system. If an inadequate vacuum supply occurs, the positive-pressure relief valve will open and exhaust the excess gas into the room. This prevents and accumulation of undesirable high pressure within the manifold that could be referred to the patient circuit.

▶ CASE STUDY

At 6:30 AM, the CRNA performed a machine check on the Ohmeda Excel anesthesia machine in OR 7 according to the FDA checklist. After finishing two rather short general surgical cases, the CRNA is ready for her third surgical case, a 60-kg, 37-year-old female patient undergoing a breast reduction. Prior to starting this case, the anesthesia technician changed the patient circuit and prepared the machine for use. There was very little time between the second and third case, and after the CRNA saw the technician checking the machine, she brought the patient into the room and proceeded with the induction of anesthesia. Anesthesia induction was uneventful and general endotracheal anesthesia using oxygen and nitrous oxide (1 : 2 L flows), and isoflurane 0.75% to 1% through a TEC 4 vaporizer was initiated.

Approximately 1-½ hours into the surgical procedure an earthquake of 4.7 magnitude occurs. Although there was substantial movement of the equipment within the room and electricity was lost momentarily, there appeared to be no visible damage in the OR. The emergency generators began functioning immediately and power was restored. The patient's vital signs remained stable and the surgery continued. During the conduct of the regular assessment of equipment function and patient monitoring parameters 10 minutes after the earthquake, the CRNA notes that the oxygen supply pressure has dropped from 50 psig to 15 psig. At the same time, the OR supervisor comes to the OR to inform the CRNA that there appears to be damage to the hospital bulk oxygen supply and confirms that pressure is falling within the pipeline system. Within a few seconds, the oxygen supply failure alarm begins to sound.

1. What will happen within the anesthesia machine when this alarm sounds?

   When the oxygen supply pressure drops below 25 psig to 30 psig, an alarm is triggered. The Ohmeda Excel machine alarm is a canister pressured with oxygen. This canister emits an audible alarm for at least 7 seconds when the pressure falls below the threshold. Because the oxygen pressure has fallen below 20 psig to 25 psig, the flow of nitrous oxide and other gases to their flowmeters is interrupted. The alarm stops within 10 seconds.

2. Does this mean the supply pressure has returned to normal?

   Once the pressurized alarm has been exhausted, the oxygen supply problem will still exist unless the cause of the failure of the oxygen supply has been identified and remedied.

3. Does the oxygen supply failure alarm also warn of problems with oxygen flow?

   No, the oxygen supply failure alarm only responds to pressure changes; it is not a flow-sensitive alarm.

4. What should the CRNA do?

   The reserve cylinders of oxygen and nitrous oxide should be turned on immediately. There are two reserve cylinders on the machine. The amount of gas and/or liquid in both cylinders placed in use should be evaluated. The CRNA notes that the nitrous oxide cylinder tags are both marked full. One oxygen cylinder tag reveals that it is "in use," while the other cylinder is full. The partially full oxygen cylinder shows 1000 L remaining.

5. How long will this cylinder last?

   Using Boyle's law, $P_1 V_1 = P_2 V_2$ (temperature constant), $V_2 = (P_1 \times V_1)/P_2 = 1900$ psig (full E cylinder of O_2) $\times$ 5 L/14.7 psia $\approx$ 660 L (5 L is the internal volume of the E cylinder). 1000 L/1900 psig = 52% full or 340 L O_2. If the oxygen flow rate is 2 L/min, it will empty in (340 L/2 L/min) 170 minutes. Because there is a second full cylinder of oxygen, there is ample cylinder oxygen supply to complete the surgery.

   The surgery was completed and the patient awakened successfully. The CRNA should have completed an equipment check herself on the anesthesia machine between cases even if it meant a slight delay in the start of the next case. She should not have permitted another person to do this task for her. Because the CRNA did not perform the equipment check, she would have had an extremely difficult time demonstrating that all component machine parts were functioning properly prior to the earthquake, particularly if the loss of oxygen pressure in the anesthesia machine was not from a problem with the oxygen supply. Vigilance is essential in all aspects of anesthesia practice to assure patient safety.

▶ SUMMARY

The anesthesia machine is a complex piece of equipment that requires a thorough comprehension of the components, functions, and related concepts of physics. Although standards are set for the production of the equipment, it is incumbent on the nurse anesthetist to thoroughly check the functioning of all machine components prior to its use in the anesthetic management of patients. The CRNA should have a comprehensive system to assess and troubleshoot all aspects of machine function in order to avoid preventable mishaps.

ACKNOWLEDGMENT

The author acknowledges Linda M. Huffman for her original contribution to this chapter.

▶ KEY CONCEPTS

- The anesthesia machine is a sophisticated life-support system that relies on the principles of mechanics, pneumatics, and electronics to manage pressure, flow, and volume as it delivers anesthetic gases to provide ventilation and oxygenation.
- Fresh gas sources, the internal machine circuitry, flowmeters, vaporizers, the patient circuit, and the waste gas evacuation systems are the major components of the anesthesia delivery system.
- Oxygen, the dominant gas, flows into the machine through a pipeline inlet check valve at a pressure of 50 psig where it provides pressure to the power outlet accessory for the ventilator; travels from the machine inlet to pressurize the oxygen flush valve, which can deliver a flow rate of 35 L/min to 75 L/min of oxygen; and opens the pressure-sensor shutoff valve permitting nitrous oxide to be delivered.
- Pipeline inlet and cylinder fittings are either DISS or PISS, which are gas specific to prevent attachment of the wrong gas to a yoke.
- The oxygen supply failure alarm system warns of low oxygen pressure when sounded and requires the anesthetist to turn on the reserve oxygen supply and then investigate the cause of the problem.
- An agent-specific calibrated vaporizer is dedicated to one agent only, is precisely calibrated and automatically compensated to perform over the usual range of temperatures and variations in gas flows, and controls the concentration of a volatile anesthetic delivered through the common gas outlet.
- The APL valve controls the flow of excess gas within the patient circuit and allows this excess to enter the scavenging system that removes waste gases.
- Breathing systems are classified according to rebreathing (primarily those using a CO_2 absorber) of exhaled gases or nonrebreathing (primarily those systems that do not use CO_2 absorption, such as the Mapleson systems including the Bain modification).
- Anesthesia ventilators with a hanging bellows that ascends during inspiration and falls during exhalation will continue to cycle even in the presence of a disconnection in the patient circuit, whereas those with a standing bellows that ascends during exhalation will not appear to be operating normally in the event of a disconnection because exhaled gases from the patient, as well as the fresh gas flow, are required to fill the bellows.
- All anesthesia machine and patient breathing systems must meet or exceed the minimum standard for safety and performance as published by the ASTM in 1989.

▶ STUDY QUESTIONS

1. How are the flows and pressure of oxygen and nitrous oxide regulated from the external supply at the wall outlet or cylinder to the patient circuit?

2. What are the safety features of the anesthesia machine that alert the anesthetist to problems with the oxygen delivery system?

3. What principles or laws of chemistry and physics apply to components and utilization of parts of the anesthesia machine and vaporizer and how are these principles applied?

4. What different breathing systems manage gas flow to the patient and how do they differ in form and function?

5. How do anesthesia vaporizers transform liquid anesthetic to saturated anesthetic vapor?

6. How does the waste gas scavenging system work and how is it incorporated into the anesthesia machine?

KEY REFERENCES

American Society for Testing and Materials (ASTM). (1989). *Standard specification for minimum performance and safety requirements for components and systems of anesthesia gas machines* (F1161-88). Philadelphia: The society.

Bowie, E. & Huffman, L. M. (1985). *The anesthesia machine: Essentials for understanding.* Madison, WI: BOC Group.

Dorsch, J. A. & Dorsch, S. E. (1994). *Understanding anesthesia equipment: Construction, care and complications* (3rd ed., pp. 1–225, 255–281, 693–718). Baltimore, MD: Williams & Wilkins.

Ehrenwerth, J. & Eisenkraft, J. B. (1993). *Anesthesia equiment: Principles and applications* (pp. 3–171, 521–536). St. Louis, MO: Mosby.

Huffman, L. M. (1990). Calibrated vaporizers: Maintaining clinical performance. *AANA Journal, 58,* 119–120.

Huffman, L. M. (1991). Common problems in waste gas management. *AANA Journal, 59,* 109.

Petty, C. (1987). *The anesthesia machine.* New York: Churchill Livingstone.

Rice, J. R. & Kolek, R. (1996). *Explore! The anesthesia system.* Madison, WI: Ohmeda, Inc.

Waugaman, W. R. & Bradshaw, H. (1985). Monitoring in anesthesia: Clinical application of monitoring gas and vapor delivery. *AANA Journal, 53,* 446–452.

REFERENCES

American Society for Testing and Materials (ASTM). (1989). *Standard specification for minimum performance and safety requirements for components and systems of anesthesia gas machines* (F1161-88). Philadelphia: The society.

American Society for Testing and Materials (ASTM). (1990). *Standard specification for minimum performance and safety requirements for anesthesia breathing circuits* (F20.01.02). Philadelphia: The society.

Bain, J. A. & Spoerel, W. E. (1972). A streamlined anaesthetic system. *Canadian Anaesthetists' Society Journal, 19,* 426–435.

Bain, J. A. & Spoerel, W. E. (1975). Prediction of arterial carbon dioxide tension during controlled ventilation with a modified Mapleson D system. *Canadian Anaesthetists' Society Journal, 22,* 34–38.

Bowie, E. & Huffman, L. M. (1985). *The anesthesia machine: Essentials for understanding.* Madison, WI: BOC Group.

Byrick, J. J., Janssen, E., & Yamashita, M. (1977). Rebreathing and co-axial circuits. *Anaesthesia, 32,* 294.

Byrick, R. J. (1980). Respiratory compensation during spontaneous ventilation with the Bain circuit. *Canadian Anaesthetists' Society Journal, 27,* 96–104.

Compressed Gas Association (CGA). (1989). *Pressure relief device standards: Part 1, cylinders for compressed gases* (publication S-1.1, 7th ed.). Arlington, VA: CGA.

Conway, C. M. (1985). Anaesthetic breathing systems. *British Journal of Anaesthesia, 57,* 649–657.

Davis, P. D., Parbrook, G. D., & Kenny, G. N. (1995). *Basic physics and measurement in anaesthesia* (4th ed., pp. 125–133). Oxford, Great Britain: Butterworth, Heineman.

Dorsch, J. A. & Dorsch, S. E. (1994). *Understanding anesthesia equipment: Construction, care and complications* (3rd ed. pp. 1–225, 255–281, 693–718). Baltimore, MD: Williams & Wilkins.

Ehrenwerth, J. & Eisenkraft, J. B. (1993). *Anesthesia equipment: Principles and applications* (pp. 3–171, 521–536). St. Louis, MO: Mosby.

Foex, P. & Crampton Smith, A. (1977). A test for co-axial circuits. *Anaesthesia, 32,* 294.

Huffman, L. M. (1990). Calibrated vaporizers: Maintaining clinical performance. *AANA Journal, 58,* 119–120.

Huffman, L. M. (1991). Common problems in waste gas management. *AANA Journal, 59,* 109.

Le Bel, L. A. (1992). Principles of chemistry and physics in anesthesia. In W. R. Waugaman, S. D. Foster, & B. M. Rigor (Eds.), *Principles and practice of nurse anesthesia* (2nd ed., pp. 57–84). Norwalk, CT: Appleton & Lange.

Meakin, G. & Coates, A. L. (1983). An evaluation of rebreathing with the Bain system during anaesthesia with spontaneous ventilation. *British Journal of Anaesthesia, 55,* 487–495.

Ohmeda. (1985). *Modulus II anesthesia system: Operation and maintenance manual* (p. 8). Madison, WI: BOC Group.

Ohmeda. (1990). *Modulus anesthesia system: Operation and maintenance manual* (p. 19). Madison, WI: BOC Group.

Petty, C. (1987). *The anesthesia machine* (pp. 39–47, 119–139). New York: Churchill Livingstone.

Rice, J. R. & Kolek, R. (1996). *Explore! The anesthesia system.* Madison, WI: Ohmeda, Inc.

Roth, S., Tweedie, E., & Sommer, R. M. (1986). Excessive airway pressure due to a malfunctioning anesthesia ventilator. *Anaesthesia, 65,* 532–534.

Spoerel, W. E. (1980). Rebreathing and carbon dioxide elimination with the Bain circuit. *Canadian Anaesthestists' Society Journal, 27,* 357–361.

Spoerel, W. E. (1983). Rebreathing and end-tidal CO_2 during spontaneous breathing with the Bain circuit. *Canadian Anaesthestists' Society Journal, 30,* 148–154.

Ward, C. S. (1985). *Anesthetic equipment: Physical principles and maintenance* (2nd ed., p. 48). London: Bailliere Tindall.

Waugaman, W. R. & Bradshaw, H. (1985). Monitoring in anesthesia: Clinical application of monitoring gas and vapor delivery. *AANA Journal, 53,* 446–452.

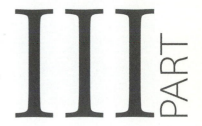

Assessment Across the Life Span

Perianesthetic Assessment in a Health Model

Wynne R. Waugaman

Assessment is the collection of data about an individual's state of health. In nurse anesthesia practice, this collection of data concerning the individual patient's health status is focused on the perianesthetic period. This period is defined as the first interaction with the patient in the preanesthetic phase through the intra-anesthetic phase and ending with the postanesthetic phase which generally concludes within the first 24 to 48 hours following the anesthetic. Although anesthesia providers are concerned with a finite portion of the patient's health as it relates to the anesthetic process, this portion cannot be accurately assessed without fully considering the whole person and the implications for a return to wellness. Indeed, the role of the anesthesia provider in the perianesthetic assessment process is critical, because the responsibility for authorizing the surgical team to proceed with the planned operation rests with the health care provider administering the anesthetic (Zambricki, 1996). Zambricki (1996) affirmed that the American Association of Nurse Anesthetists (AANA) has validated the importance of patient assessment and perianesthetic planning by promulgating three standards of care related to this evaluation process in their *Standards for Nurse Anesthesia Practice* (Table 9–1).

Health promotion and disease prevention form the core of advanced practice nursing. Certified registered nurse anesthetists (CRNAs), as advanced practice nurses, must focus their care toward this goal. Many factors must be considered when assessing the health of the patient including his or her position in the life span; physical and emotional factors; cultural, religious, and socioeconomic factors; patterns of coping and interaction with others; and environmental factors. The assessment process involves collecting these data related to the overall health status and the implications for the anesthetic experience. Data collection can be categorized into subjective data obtained during the history taking, objective data from the physical examination, and diagnostic data from laboratory studies. These data are evaluated in terms of the patient's disease state and impending surgery or procedure, and a judgement is made regarding the anesthesia care. Different data may be required depending on the clinical situation. It is unlikely that the anesthesia provider would be responsible for collecting the complete database on the patient's health. In most situations, the data collected are episodic or problem centered (Jarvis, 1996) and are for a short-term situation such as a surgical procedure. Anesthesia providers may also provide data for follow-up of any identified problems that may arise during the perianesthetic process, such as a prolonged response to a neuromuscular blocking agent or a difficult airway. This follow-up database may be used during the postanesthetic period and may be referred to if the patient returns for subsequent surgery. Data can also be collected during an emergency when a trauma victim presents to the operating room (OR). This type of

TABLE 9–1. Selections from the AANA Standards for Nurse Anesthesia Practice

Standard	Interpretation
I. A thorough and complete preanesthetic assessment shall be performed.	The responsibility of the CRNA begins with the preanesthetic assessment. Except in emergency situations, the CRNA has an obligation to determine that relevant tests have been obtained and reviewed and a thorough evaluation of the patient has been made.
II. Informed consent for the planned anesthetic intervention shall be obtained from the patient or legal guardian.	The CRNA shall obtain or verify that an informed consent has been obtained by a qualified provider. Anesthetic options and risks should be discussed with the patient and/or legal guardian in language the patient and/or legal guardian can understand. Documentation in the patient's medical record should reflect that informed consent was obtained.
III. A patient-specific plan for anesthesia care shall be formulated.	The plan of care developed by the CRNA is based on comprehensive patient assessment, problem analysis, anticipated surgical or therapeutic procedure, patient and surgeon preferences, and current anesthesia principles.

From Standards for Nurse Anesthesia Practice, *p. 3. Copyright 1996 by the American Association of Nurse Anesthetists. Adapted with permission.*

assessment requires rapid collection of client data, often coupled with lifesaving measures (Jarvis, 1996). A thorough assessment is essential to provide client-specific care in any clinical situation.

▶ PERIANESTHETIC ASSESSMENT IN A MULTICULTURAL ENVIRONMENT

The concept of culture has only recently received attention in the anesthesia community. Many anesthesia providers have been confronted with the inability to communicate with patients as a result of language barriers. In fact, CRNAs report the inability to communicate with a patient in his or her native language as the primary problem in providing care to individuals from diverse cultures (Horton & Waugaman, 1996). However, beyond language and certain socioeconomic issues, anesthesia providers often do not consider the broader concept of culturally competent care in preparing clients for anesthesia.

The National Academy of Nursing has defined culturally competent care as "care that takes into account issues related to diversity, marginalization and vulnerability due to culture, race, gender, and sexual orientation" (Meleis, Isenberg, Koerner, Lacey, & Stern, 1995, p. 4). This definition includes not only issues related to ethnicity but other issues that may isolate individuals further, even within a given ethnic group. For example, a female may have certain health issues because of her age and gender as part of an Asian American ethnic culture. In addition, if she is poor, this may further disenfranchise her from the center of her cultural society (Meleis, 1996). This separation is known as *marginalization* and may deprive the patient of voice, power, and the right to resources (Hall, Stevens, & Meleis, 1994). Marginalization illustrates how people are treated and how their culture contributes to this separation whether it be by gender, sexual orientation, or socioeconomic factors (Meleis, 1996).

Dreher (1996) proposes that the complex concept of culture may be the core of what differentiates nursing from medicine. When a surgeon performs a cholecystectomy or prescribes an antibiotic, the ethnic background or social culture of the patient is seldom considered because pathophysiology and treatment of a disease process are subject to much less variation than human behavior. The advanced practice nurse's focus is not on the disease or treatment but rather on the patient receiving the treatment. The manner in which advanced practice nurses interact with patients is profoundly affected by the patient's culture and other issues related to diversity. Assessment must not only consider physiologic considerations of the patient's disease state, but also cultural terms, conditions, and behaviors that must be explored to deliver effective culturally appropriate anesthesia care (Cooper, 1996) (Table 9–2). In order to assist patients in negotiating the changing health care environment, nurse anesthetists must develop cultural strategies that will facilitate the perianesthetic process and continuity of care across the health care continuum.

Culture, Values, and Beliefs

Culture encompasses four characteristics: (1) It is learned from birth through language and socialization; (2) it is shared by all members of the same cultural group; (3) it adapts to specific environmental conditions and is influenced by the availability of resources; and (4) it is dynamic and changing (Andrews, 1996). Differences may occur within cultures because of ethnicity, religion, education, occupation, age, and gender (Andrews, 1996). These differences may themselves produce a subculture if they distinguish a particular group from the larger culture. Subcultures based on ethnicity may include Hispanic Americans, African Americans, or Native

TABLE 9–2. Cultural Behaviors Relevant to Health Assessment

Cultural Group	Cultural Variations (Common Belief/Practice)	Nursing Implications
African Americans	Dialect and slang terms require careful communication to prevent error (eg, "bad" may mean "good").	Question the client's meaning or intent.
Arab/Muslim Americans	Admiration may be viewed as the "evil eye." Admiring a child must be accompanied by touch. Touching from members of the opposite sex is offensive. A female client may request a female relative to be present for exams.	Refrain from overt expressions of admiration. Care should be provided by nurses who are the same gender as the client.
Mexican Americans	Eye behavior is important. An individual who looks at and admires a child without touching the child has given the child the "evil eye."	Always touch the child you are examining or admiring.
Native Americans	Eye contact is considered a sign of disrespect and is thus avoided.	Recognize that the client may be attentive and interested even though eye contact is avoided.
Appalachians	Eye contact is considered impolite or a sign of hostility. Verbal patter may be confusing.	Avoid excessive eye contact. Clarify statements.
American Eskimos	Body language is very important. The individual seldom disagrees publicly with others. Client may nod yes to be polite, even if not in agreement.	Monitor own body language closely as well as client's to detect meaning.
Jewish Americans	Orthodox Jews consider excess touching, particularly from members of the opposite sex, offensive.	Establish whether client is an Orthodox Jew and avoid physical contact with opposite sex.
Chinese Americans	Individual may nod head to indicate yes or shake head to indicate no. Excessive eye contact indicates rudeness. Excessive touch is offensive.	Ask questions carefully and clarify responses. Avoid excessive eye contact and touch.
Filipino Americans	Offending people is to be avoided at all cost. Nonverbal behavior is very important.	Monitor nonverbal behaviors of self and client, being sensitive to physical and emotional discomfort or concerns of the client.
Haitian Americans	Touch is used in conversation. Direct eye contact is used to gain attention and respect during communications.	Use direct eye contact when communicating.
East Indian/Hindu Americans	Women avoid eye contact as a sign of respect.	Be aware that men may view eye contact by women as offensive. Avoid eye contact.
Vietnamese Americans	Avoidance of eye contact is a sign of respect. The head is considered sacred; it is not polite to pat the head. An upturned palm is offensive in communication.	Limit eye contact. Touch the head only when mandated and explain clearly before proceeding to do so. Avoid hand gesturing.

From Kozier, B., Erb, G., Blaise, K., Johnson, S., & Smith-Temple, J. Techniques in clinical nursing (2nd ed.). Copyright 1993 by Addison-Wesley. Adapted with permission.

Americans. Subcultures based on occupation may include nursing, medicine, or law. Some of these subcultures may be further defined. Certified registered nurse anesthetists are nurses but may have characteristics that differentiate them from the general nursing culture, making nurse anesthesia a subculture of nursing.

Cultures possess different value orientations. These value orientations develop from early common experiences and can be focused in a variety of ways. One aspect of value orientation relates to the time dimensions—past, present, and future. Many cultures have a strong association with the past through traditions. It may be very important for these clients to consult with elder family members when an illness or the need for surgery occurs. Relationships with others also play a critical role in the development of value orientations. These relationships often impact the patient's decision-making

process when faced with surgery. Some patients may value the counsel of a family member such as a grandparent and may look to this individual to make decisions concerning health matters. Other patients may value the influence of the entire family or even the community when facing a health care decision. In other situations, the patient may consider this decision making an individual matter, and he or she may not consult with others concerning care. Family relationships may be critically important to identify in the assessment process. This is particularly true when assessing pediatric patients preoperatively. The primary care provider may or may not be the child's biologic parent (Andrews, 1996). For example, in some Asian American families, the mother may be the care provider but the father may make decisions regarding the welfare of the child (Cooper, 1996). This may contrast with some African American families where the grandmother may be both the decision maker and the primary caretaker of children (Morris, 1996).

Religious and spiritual beliefs may significantly influence a patient presenting for surgery. An individual's religious beliefs can provide insight into the patient's understanding of the illness and its cause, perception of the severity of the disease process, as well as choice of healer (Andrews, 1996). It is important to distinguish between religion, an organized system of beliefs including belief in God or gods, and spirituality that develops from an individual's unique life experiences in determining the meaning and purpose of life (Andrews, 1996). Both religion and spirituality play important roles in how a patient views and responds to therapies surrounding illness and surgery, particularly life-threatening illnesses. Some religious practices may directly influence health care practices. For example, organ donation in a Jewish trauma victim is acceptable within Jewish law if the organs are harvested with the highest standard of dignity (Rosenberg, 1991). Providing anesthesia care in this situation would require the CRNA to ensure that the body is treated with respect once all organs have been harvested, which includes straightening the limbs rather than crossing them, closing the eyes, binding the lower jaw, and appropriately covering the body (Abraham, 1990). The CRNA may request that a rabbi be consulted to provide counsel to the OR team.

Some other religious practices may also influence perianesthetic care. In Orthodox Judaism and Islam, women and men may not touch each other, even to shake hands. This belief would preclude a female CRNA from conducting a physical exam on a male patient. Scientologist patients do not permit music to be played in the OR, nor do they allow the anesthesia provider to provide any suggestive comments to them concerning surgical process or outcome, (eg, "you're doing fine") during the entire anesthetic process. Religious beliefs and practices can play a significant role in the patient's perianesthetic experience, and it is extremely important for the anesthesia provider to be sensitive to these cultural issues.

Culture, Health, and Healing

In order to evaluate and understand a patient's cultural practices and responses to health and illness, the CRNA must be sensitive to and aware of his or her own cultural beliefs and values. Although these are important for all health care providers to be aware of, advanced practice nurses as a group seem to espouse middle-class American values, beliefs, and attitudes while typically providing health care to multiethnic Americans from low socioeconomic groups (Cooper, 1996). Therefore, it is extremely important for CRNAs to set aside any biases or judgmental attitudes that may negatively affect the anesthesia care by promulgating any stereotypical images. Members of a cultural group can best articulate what constitutes appropriate care for them. The better that nurse anesthetists can integrate the patient's perception of care into the anesthesia care plan, the more accepted and appropriate this care will be for the patient.

Nurse anesthetists must be able to identify the meaning of health to the patient and differentiate this from illness. The causes of illness may be identified in various ways by different cultures. European Americans may believe in a scientific theory of illness, or cause and effect. Other cultures may explain illness in terms of nature. These cultures believe that the forces of nature must be kept in natural balance or harmony (Andrews, 1996). Asian Americans often believe in the philosophy of Tao, the theory of Yin and Yang, and the proper proportion of the five elements (metal, wood, water, fire, and earth) which stipulate that health exists when these elements are in proper balance (Chan, 1992). Native Americans believe that disease results from the body being out of balance or from a *disturbed spirit* and may seek a spiritual approach to healing (Kutenai, 1996). Proponents of the naturalistic perspective believe that the laws of nature create imbalances, chaos, and disease and that there is healing power in nature. Herbs and other natural therapies are often the chosen treatments for the imbalance.

Some cultures may believe the forces of good and evil are responsible for health and disease. The oldest and most widespread of these superstitious beliefs is illness caused by the *evil eye* (Spector, 1991). This belief has been found to exist in many cultures throughout the world and is often described in folklore. Some practices thought to prevent the evil eye include wearing charms, amulets, medals, or colored ribbons.

Religious beliefs play a vital role not only in the perception of health and illness, but also in the healing process. Many religions profess the power of prayer in the healing process. Some religions have a *healer* who has received the gift of healing from a divine source, perhaps through a vision. The healer then uses his or her powers to heal the individual by removing the evil spirit that caused the illness. Healers have been active since ancient times and still exist today, as can be observed through television evangelism. Folk healers and medicine men or women are present in many cultures including Hispanic American, African American, Native American, and Asian American cultures. It is important to query patients in the preanesthetic interview concerning their beliefs or utilization of folk healers and therapies. The CRNA should know the herbs and therapies being used, and also if the patient's use of these folk remedies is in lieu of prescriptive therapy. Some patients refuse medications and treatments based on their belief in faith and/or folk healing (Kutenai, 1996).

Culture and Anesthesia

Nurse anesthetists are often challenged to develop rapport with their patients in a very short period of time. The preoperative interview may take place in a clinic or hospital setting where the anesthesia provider may spend 15 to 30 minutes with the patient. However, these interviews often occur in the preoperative holding area under less-than-ideal circumstances, perhaps prior to emergency surgery. Developing rapport under such circumstances is at best difficult, but when the patient's culture and language differ from those of the CRNA, this can impact the anesthetic process.

Horton and Waugaman (1996) reported that European Americans were the dominant patient group in nurse anesthesia practice. African Americans were the most frequently identified culturally diverse patient group, followed by Hispanic Americans, Asian Americans, and Native Americans (Table 9-3). As previously identified, the major barrier to the provision of patient-centered anesthesia care in a diverse cultural environment is the inability to communicate in the patient's native language (Horton & Waugaman, 1996). Although interpreters can be used to overcome this barrier, this service may not be accessible in all locations and throughout the entire perianesthetic period. Every attempt should be made to learn the patient's history and communicate the anesthetic plan in his or her native language. Both verbal and nonverbal communication can be interpreted differently according to culture. An understanding of the culture will facilitate verbal and nonverbal communication approaches. Postanesthetic assessments should also be conducted using an interpreter if the CRNA cannot communicate in the patient's native language.

Clinical observations reveal that anesthetic requirements may vary among cultural groups. Asian Americans exhibit an increased sensitivity to inhalation anesthetics and narcotics (Horton & Waugaman, 1996). The response to pain has been studied among cultures and research suggests that the way a person experiences pain is culturally prescribed (Ludwig-Beymer, 1995).

TABLE 9-3. Culture Distribution of Clients in Nurse Anesthesia Practice

Culture	Percent
European American	58
African American	21
Hispanic American	9
Asian American	5
Native American	1
Others	6

From Horton, B. J., & Waugaman, W. R. (1996). Nurse anesthesia and multiculturalism. Advanced Practice Nursing Quarterly, 2, 24. Copyright 1996 by Aspen Publishers, Inc. Adapted with permission.

TABLE 9-4. Template for Cultural Assessment in Nurse Anesthesia Practice

What is the client's primary language and method of communication?
What is the language that is usually spoken in your home?
How well do you speak, read, and write English?
Are there special rituals of communication in your family?
To whom should questions be directed during this interview?
What are the client's personal beliefs about health and illness?
How do you define health and illness?
Do you believe that you have control over your health?
Are there any practices or rituals that you believe will improve your health?
Do you or have you used any alternative healing methods, such as acupuncture, healing touch, or herbs? How was this treatment effective for you?
Are there particular practices or rituals that you believe should be used to treat your health problem? Are there any practices that you believe should be used prior to surgery and anesthesia?
What are your attitudes toward undergoing surgery to treat your illness? Pain? Having an anesthetic? Recovery? Death and dying?
Are you the one who makes the health decisions in your family? If not, who is the decision maker?
What are the religious influences and special rituals that affect the client?
Is there a religion that you observe.
Is there a significant person to whom you look for guidance and support?
Are there any special religious practices or beliefs that are likely to feel supportive before, during, or after your surgery?
Are there any special rituals or ceremonies that are important as you prepare for your surgery?
What are the roles of individual people in the family?
Who makes the decisions in the family?
What is the composition of your family? How many generations or family members live in your household?
If you are divorced, separated, or widowed, what is the attitude toward this as it relates to your surgical experience?
What is the role of and attitude toward children in the family?
Do you or the members of your family have special beliefs and practices surrounding the surgical or obstetrical experience?

From Thompson, J., & Wilson, S. F. (1996). Ethnic and cultural considerations. Health assessment for nursing practice (pp. 28–29). Copyright 1996 by Mosby. Adapted with permission.

A direct assessment of health beliefs and practices that may reflect that cultural heritage should be part of the assessment process in nurse anesthesia practice. The purpose of a cultural assessment is to identify culture care patterns, expressions, and meanings that reflect individual needs or influence the patterns of illness, disability, or death (Leininger, 1995). Because the cultural assessment goes beyond traditional physical and psychologic parameters, attention is focused on the particular needs of patients. The CRNA must be an active listener, learner, and reflector in order to encourage sharing of ideas and beliefs. The data gathered during the assessment can provide valuable insight into planning culturally appropriate care. A suggested template for cultural assessment is provided in Table 9-4.

Phase V   Develop a culturally-based client-nurse care plan as a
             co-participant for decisions and actions for culturally
             congruent care.

             ↑

Phase IV   Synthesize themes and patterns of care derived from
             the information obtained in phases I, II, and III.

             ↑

Phase III   Identify and document recurrent client patterns and
             narratives (stories) with client meanings of what has
             been seen, heard, or experienced.

             ↑

Phase II   Listen to and learn from the client about cultural values,
             beliefs, and daily (nightly) practices related to care and
             health in the client's environmental context. Give
             attention to generic (home or folk) practices and
             professional nursing practices.

             ↑

Phase I   Record observations of what you see, hear or
             experience with clients (includes dress and appearance,
             body condition features, language, mannerisms and
             general behavior, attitudes, and cultural features).

             ↑

             Start Here

Figure 9–1. Leininger's short culturalogic assessment guide
(Model B). [From Leininger, M. (1995). Culture care assessment to
guide nursing practices. In M. Leininger (Ed.), Transcultural nursing:
Concepts, theories, research and practices (2nd ed., pp. 115–134).
New York: McGraw-Hill. Reprinted with permission of the author.]

Leininger's *Short Cultural Assessment Guide* (1995, p.
142) is an alternative tool that has been used in short-
term, emergency, and acute care settings in order to obtain culturally appropriate information to guide clinical
decision making (Figure 9-1). Each patient should be
treated as an individual regardless of race, gender, ethnicity, or sexual orientation. Prior to conducting the
physical assessment, the CRNA should take time to develop a patient profile from the history. The cultural assessment is an important prelude to the collection of
subjective data.

▶ SUBJECTIVE DATA COLLECTION

The personal interview is often the first and most important component of data collection. The interview provides data about what the patient says or believes about
him or herself. The interview tells the anesthesia
provider what the patient believes about the state of
health and current health problem or situation for which
he or she presents. The interview establishes a trusting
relationship between the anesthetist and the patient that

is critically important to how the perianesthetic process
is perceived and experienced.

The interview should be the first opportunity for a
positive interaction between the anesthesia provider and
the patient. To accomplish this, the anesthetist must control the environment in which the interview is conducted. The location of the interview should be quiet,
private, and free from interruption. If the patient is an inpatient, the interview should not be conducted during a
time when treatments are being conducted or during
mealtime. If visitors are present, they should be asked to
leave the patient's room during the interview unless the
visitor is serving as an interpreter or a history provider
for pediatric patients or other patients who are unable to
provide this reliable historic information. Preanesthetic
interviews for patients requiring surgery as an outpatient
or as a *same-day admission* may also be conducted in a
clinic or via telephone rather than in the traditional hospital setting. When the interview is conducted by telephone, the anesthetist should ascertain that the time
of the interview is convenient. Language interpreters
should be used if the anesthesia provider is unable to communicate with the patient in his or her native tongue. If
the anesthesia provider finds him or herself in a situation
where no interpreter is available, be polite and formal.
Try to use simple words and gestures to obtain information (Table 9-5). Medical phrase books are often available in different languages. These language aids can
greatly assist in obtaining basic information, particularly
in an emergency situation.

It is important for the anesthetist to make a favorable
impression by appearing professional, empathetic, and unhurried. Clothing should be neat, clean, and professional.
The anesthetist should never approach a patient wearing
soiled or bloodstained clothing. Adult patients should be
addressed formally using surnames, such as Mrs. Green,
rather than informally using first names. Pediatric patients
may be addressed on a first name basis. Under no circumstances should patients be addressed in any manner that
could be perceived as disrespectful, such as referring to
them as "honey" or "dear" or an elderly person as
"Grandpa." The anesthesia provider should indicate who
he or she is by title and the role he or she will play in the
perianesthetic care. Patients have a right to be informed
whether the anesthesia provider is a student nurse anesthetist, CRNA, anesthesiologist, or resident in anesthesiology. The anesthesia care setting should be described particularly in situations where the provider is part of an
anesthesia care team. Patients should also be informed if
the anesthesia provider conducting the preoperative interview will not be the person providing anesthesia care.
It is optimal for the anesthesia provider to conduct the
preoperative interview on all patients with whom he or
she will participate in the perianesthesia care.

TABLE 9–5. Overcoming Language Barriers: What to Do When No Interpreter Is Available

1. Be polite and formal.
2. Greet the person using the last or complete name. Gesture to yourself and say your name. Offer a handshake or nod. Smile.
3. Proceed in an unhurried manner. Pay attention to any effort by the patient or family to communicate.
4. Speak in a low, moderate voice. Avoid talking loudly. Remember that there is a tendency to raise the volume and pitch of your voice when the listener appears not to understand. The listener may perceive that you are shouting and/or angry.
5. Use any words that you might know in the person's language. This indicates that you are aware of and respect his or her culture.
6. Use simple words, such as "pain" instead of "discomfort." Avoid medical jargon, idioms, and slang. Avoid using contractions (eg, don't, can't, and won't). Use nouns repeatedly instead of pronouns. Example:
   Do not say: "He has been taking his medicine, hasn't he?"
   Do say: "Does Juan take medicine?"
7. Pantomime words and simple actions while you verbalize them.
8. Give instructions in the proper sequence. Example:
   Do not say: "Before you rinse the bottle, sterilize it."
   Do say: "First wash the bottle. Second, rinse the bottle."
9. Discuss one topic at a time. Avoid using conjunctions. Example:
   Do not say: "Are you cold and in pain?"
   Do say: "Are you cold (while pantomiming)? Are you in pain?
10. Validate whether the person understands by having him or her repeat instructions, demonstrate the procedure, or act out the meaning.
11. Write out several short sentences in English and determine the person's ability to read them.
12. Try a third language. Many Indo-Chinese speak French. Europeans often know more than one language. Try Latin words or phrases.
13. Ask who among the person's family and friends could serve as an interpreter.
14. Obtain phrase books from a library or bookstore; make or purchase flash cards; contact hospitals for a list of interpreters; and use both a formal and an informal network to locate a suitable interpreter.

From Jarvis, C. (1996). The interview. Physical Examination and Health Assessment (2nd ed., p. 76). Copyright 1996 by W. B. Saunders. Reprinted with permission of the author.

The Health History

A significant amount of information is needed from the patient's health history to formulate the anesthesia care plan. Communication techniques that encourage patient response should be used. Direct questioning should proceed from general to specific information. Questions should be formulated to encourage patient verbalization rather than a yes or no response. For example, "How many pillows do you sleep with?" should be asked rather than, "Do you sleep with your head up?" (Zambricki, 1996). Ask questions clearly, one at a time, allowing the patient to completely respond. Do not use medical jargon that may distance the provider from the patient pre-

cluding access to accurate information. Speak in lay terms: "Has your doctor ever told you that you had a heart attack?" rather than, "Have you ever had a myocardial infarction?" Bear in mind that during the interview, the CRNA may encounter culturally acceptable sick role behavior ranging from aggressive, demanding behavior to silent passivity. Complaining, demanding behavior has been reported to be rewarded with attention among Jewish American and Italian American groups, whereas Native Americans and Asian Americans may be quiet and compliant during the interview (Andrews & Boyle, 1997). Pediatric patients will be socialized from an early age into the behavior of the respective cultural group and may respond similarly to the adult.

Oral health history data should be collected in an organized fashion, usually by organ system (Table 9-6).

TABLE 9–6. The Preanesthetic Health History

General health history
General state of health
Age, height, weight
Current vital signs
Activities of daily living/work
Previous hospitalization/ surgery/anesthesia
Medications/dosage/efficiency
Allergies
Alcohol intake/drug use
Nutrition

Personal or family history of surgical or anesthetic complications
Postoperative bleeding
Perioperative cardiac arrest
Cancellation of surgery
Postoperative jaundice
Prolonged apnea
High fevers or malignant hyperthermia
"Allergies" to anesthesia
Inability to awaken quickly after anesthesia

Respiratory history
Dyspnea/orthopnea
Exercise tolerance
Asthma/bronchitis
Tuberculosis
Pneumothorax
Smoking history
Cough/wheezing
Colds
Epistaxis
Hoarseness

Neuromuscular history
Headaches
Seizures
Transient ischemic attacks
Paralysis/paresis/neuropathies
Muscular disorders
Back pain
Syncope/paresis

Cardiovascular history
Hypertension or hypotension
Myocardial infarction
Heart failure
Anemia
Angina
Exercise tolerance
Paroxysmal nocturnal dyspnea
Coagulopathy
Peripheral vascular disease

Gastrointestinal tract
Most recent intake
Hiatal hernia
Ulcers

Endocrine history
Diabetes
Liver disease/jaundice
Thyroid disease

Renal history
Kidney disease
Genitourinary disease

Gynecologic history
Vaginal bleeding
Pregnancy
Menstrual history

From Zambricki, C. (1992). Preoperative Assessment and Evaluation. In W. R. Waugaman, S. D. Foster, & B. M. Rigor (Eds.), Principles and Practice of Nurse Anesthesia (2nd ed., p. 183). Copyright 1992 by Appleton & Lange. Adapted with permission.

Subsequent chapters orient the reader to detailed information required in the assessment of each system as well as special considerations for pediatric, obstetric, and geriatric patients. General information should be obtained first, including health and nutrition status, activities, previous surgeries and/or anesthetics, current medication regime, allergies, and recreational drug/alcohol and smoking history. Some patients may be reticent to provide complete information on drug and alcohol use. The necessity of collection of this data must be communicated to the patient to provide a clear understanding of the physiologic effects of chronic drug or alcohol abuse on the organ systems and its implications for a safe anesthetic.

An accurate assessment of the patient's medication regime must be conducted, and the anesthetist must consider any potential interactions of drug therapy with the proposed anesthetic. The assessment of nutritional status plays an important role in assessing drug dose and response. Patients who are malnourished may have diminished protein stores and an altered response to protein-bound drugs such as sodium thiopental. Patients who are obese should have a lean body weight calculated for computation of appropriate drug doses. Recent surgery, trauma, burns, or infection will also impact the patient's nutritional status.

A patient-centered and family history of surgical or anesthetic complications should be elicited to include adverse effects or allergies to anesthetic agents, prolonged apnea, bleeding problems, and airway difficulties. Any history of allergic response to environmental allergens or food products, such as eggs, should also be noted. Some patients may have increased risk for developing an anaphylactic response to latex products because of frequent exposure to these products. Patients at risk include those who have a daily exposure to latex products in the workplace such as medical or dental offices; history of chronic conditions requiring continuous or intermittent catheterization; or other risk factors including a history of allergies and asthma; reactions to latex products such as balloons, condoms, or gloves; and allergies to bananas, avocados, tropical fruits, kiwi, and chestnuts (Jackson, 1995).

Females should be queried concerning their reproductive history. Pregnancy testing may be indicated for any female patient of childbearing years who has not been sterilized. Drugs and anesthetic agents commonly utilized in anesthesia practice have been implicated in the production of teratrogenic fetal effects in women with unrecognized pregnancies. Collection of accurate health and anesthetic history information is critically important for a complete assessment and for assigning anesthetic risk according to a physical status ranking based on effect of disease processes on the patient's health status.

Assessment of Anesthetic Risk and Physical Status

One essential element of the preanesthetic assessment is the evaluation of the patient's chance of survival or risk involved in undergoing anesthesia. The risk of anesthesia has been greatly reduced over the past 20 years with the advent of new surgical and anesthetic techniques and technologies, enhanced monitoring capabilities, and improved drugs available for anesthetic use. Although no system to calculate the anesthetic risk exists per se, evaluation of the physical status provides a common language and method for anesthesia practitioners to evaluate the patient's health and disease status. The current system used for evaluating physical status by both nurse anesthetists and anesthesiologists was adopted by the American Society of Anesthesiologists (ASA) in 1962 and has been modified slightly since then (ASA, 1963). The system for evaluation of the patient's physical condition is a medical model, based on the presence of disease and its affect on the patient's ability to participate in activities of daily living (Table 9–7). The planned operation is not a consideration when assigning physical status. However, a separate class now exists for patient's diagnosed as brain dead undergoing organ harvest (Morgan & Mikhail, 1996). The classification lacks scientific precision and much inconsistency, and variation is found among anesthesia providers who assign the ratings. Often this variation in physical status assignment reflects the experience of the provider; it is, therefore, a subjective assessment. Although inconsis-

TABLE 9–7. American Society of Anesthesiologists (ASA) Physical Status Classification

Class	Definition
1	Normal healthy patient without systemic disease.
2	A patient with mild to moderate systemic disease without functional limitations (eg, controlled hypertension).
3	A patient with moderate to severe systemic disease that results in limitation of function and affects the ability to carry out the activities of daily living (eg, chronic congestive heart failure).
4	A patient with severe systemic disease that is life-threatening and functionally incapacitating (eg, renal failure and widespread cardiovascular disease).
5	A moribund patient who is not expected to live 24 hours with or without surgery (eg, head injury complicated by a stroke).
6	A brain-dead patient whose organs are being harvested.
E	The patient is in one of the classes listed above and is having surgery on an emergency basis. The physical status is followed by an "E" designation (eg, "2E").

tencies in assignment of physical status may exist among providers, the rating system is universal and provides a basis for comparisons of morbidity and mortality in anesthesia practice.

▶ OBJECTIVE DATA COLLECTION

Objective data are collected by the anesthesia provider through the physical examination. The anesthetist must use all senses (sight, touch, smell, and hearing) to gather this data. Skills requisite for the conduct of the physical exam include inspection, palpation, percussion, and auscultation. *Inspection* is concentrated observation and scrutiny of the patient. First, an overall inspection of the patient's physical status is conducted. Following a general inspection, the assessment of each system begins with inspection. A focused inspection takes time and often yields significant data important to the anesthetic process. The anesthesia provider should not be rushed or hurried to allow sufficient time to conduct a thorough inspection of the patient. Inspection of the airway, for example, is critical to the anesthetic plan.

Palpation provides information on skin temperature, texture, and moisture. The anesthetist can assess swelling or edema, pulsation, crepitation, and presence of pain and masses through palpation techniques. *Percussion* involves tapping the skin of the patient with short, sharp strokes to assess underlying structures (Jarvis, 1996). This technique can be performed with either one or two hands in order to elicit a vibration. Percussion is often used by anesthetists to assess the resonance of the lungs or presence of air in the stomach. The principle underlying this technique is that a structure containing air, such as the lungs, produces a louder, deeper, and longer sound because it vibrates freely when contrasted with percussion of a more solid structure, such as the liver, which does not vibrate as freely (Jarvis, 1996).

Auscultation is accomplished by listening through a stethoscope to sounds produced by the body, such as heart or breath sounds. Anesthesia providers become quite adept at the skill of auscultation because it is done continually during the anesthetic process. The minimum physical assessment required prior to the anesthetic includes evaluation of the cardiopulmonary system through auscultation of heart and lung sounds. The anesthetist notes any abnormal heart sounds, murmurs, or dysrhythmias (Zambricki, 1996). The quality of breath sounds must also be described. The patient's overall physical condition must be considered in the conduct of the physical exam to ensure that minimum distress is produced by this procedure.

▶ DIAGNOSTIC DATA COLLECTION

Over the last few decades preanesthetic diagnostic testing has shifted from general health screening to specific clinical indications. According to Kaplan and associates (1985), 60% of routinely ordered tests are performed without specific indication, and less than 1% of any revealed abnormalities influence preoperative management of the patient. In the current climate of cost containment in health care, unnecessary diagnostic testing cannot be justified. Current minimum laboratory testing may vary from institution to institution and should be based on the patient's individual needs. Some institutions may still require evaluation of the hematocrit and hemoglobin on a routine basis, whereas others may reserve this test for surgeries where either blood loss is expected or the patient's medical history warrants the screening. Electrocardiograms and chest x-rays may not be evaluated routinely unless indicated by the patient's history or age. The anesthesia provider should recommend preoperative diagnostic testing not ordered by the attending physician based on the health history, physical assessment, and anesthetic considerations of the impending surgery.

▶ PERIANESTHETIC CARE PLAN

The anesthesia provider must collate all information obtained during the assessment process, both objective and subjective, in order to formulate the anesthesia care plan. The patient's specific needs and overall health status should be the primary consideration in planning the anesthetic, not the intended surgery. Restoration to health must be the goal following anesthesia. The anesthetist must provide education and instructions to the patient and family during the preanesthetic assessment to optimize patient safety. Expectations prior to and after surgery should be discussed including instructions for fasting, continuance or discontinuance of drug therapy, and postanesthetic discharge precautions such as no driving, operating equipment, or signing legal documents for 24 to 48 hours after anesthesia (Zambricki, 1996). The goal of developing a patient-specific anesthetic plan is to tailor perianesthetic care to meet the specific health care needs throughout the surgical process and return the patient to a state of health.

▶ CASE STUDY

A 4-year-old Chinese American male is evaluated in the preoperative clinic prior to surgery scheduled for elective tonsillectomy. The child's medical history includes asthma related to exposure to pollen and certain foods, namely bananas and eggs. His treatment for asthma includes episodic use of an albuterol inhaler. No other health problems are reported. The child speaks and understands English and Chinese but his parents have limited command of English.

1. What cultural considerations are important in the perianesthetic assessment?

Because the child is from an Asian culture, it is appropriate to direct the questioning to the father. Speak slowly and use gestures when necessary to explain the anesthetic and elicit health history information. Ascertain that the parents understand, and request the services of an interpreter if there is a communication problem. It is important to assess whether the child is on any herbal or other natural therapy for his asthma or current tonsillar inflammation.

2. What are the anesthetic/surgical implications for this patient who has a history of allergic response to eggs and bananas?

Allergy to eggs indicates that the child may have an adverse response to certain anesthetic agents such as propofol, which is prepared in an emulsion containing soybean oil and purified egg phosphatide. Propofol should be avoided in clients with allergies to eggs. Because the child has a history of allergic response to bananas, he may be susceptible to latex allergy. Care should include reducing the child's exposure to latex-containing products. Drug therapy should be available to treat allergic response. The anesthetist should be vigilant for symptoms of anaphylaxis.

3. Are any diagnostic laboratory studies needed, and what objective data from the physical examination are important to the anesthetic care plan?

No laboratory tests are needed unless oxygen saturation is reduced abnormally when measured with the peripheral oxygen saturation monitor. The anesthetist should auscultate breath sounds and evaluate for wheezing or other adventitious signs. The chest should be percussed as part of the physical examination to assess any vibration that deviates from normal. Exercise tolerance should be assessed during the history.

▶ SUMMARY

Perianesthetic assessment is integral to successful execution of the anesthetic plan. The anesthesia provider is responsible for fully evaluating the health of the patient prior to anesthesia. This includes a complete and thorough history and physical examination and evaluation of diagnostic data critical to the anesthetic process. In addition, other factors that play a significant role in the patient's response to surgery and anesthesia, such as culture, must be considered. By evaluating the whole patient through accurate assessment of subjective, objective, and diagnostic data, the CRNA can formulate and deliver individualized perianesthesia care that will return the patient to the optimum state of health following anesthesia.

▶ KEY CONCEPTS

- Assessment involves the collection of individualized subjective, objective, and diagnostic data related to overall health status and the implications for the anesthetic experience.
- Assessment for an emergency surgery may provide only critical information such as NPO status, allergies, current medications, and presenting health problems.
- The patient's culture, values, beliefs, and health practices must be evaluated to provide culturally appropriate care and avoid cultural sterotyping.
- Communication techniques during the interview should encourage patient response and verbalization, proceeding from gathering general to specific information.

- General information obtained during the history should culminate in an ASA physical status assignment on the basis of health and nutrition status, physical activities, social history, previous surgeries and/or anesthetics, current medications, allergies, recreational drug/alcohol use, smoking history, and preexisting disease.
- Objective data are assessed during the physical exam and diagnostic data should be collected based on the patient's individual needs, age, physical condition, and impending surgery rather than standardized laboratory testing.
- The goal of developing a patient-specific anesthetic plan is to tailor care to meet the specific needs and return the patient to a state of optimal health.

▶ Study Questions

1. What types of data are collected as part of the perianesthetic assessment process?

2. What cultural values, beliefs, and health practices must be assessed when planning the anesthetic?

3. How might cultural beliefs influence the perianesthetic process?

4. How can the anesthesia provider effectively overcome communication barriers in non-English speaking patients?

5. What type of information is elicited during the interview to obtain the health history and how is physical status evaluated?

6. What skills are used to collect objective data through the physical examination?

KEY REFERENCES

Andrews, M. M. & Boyle, J. S. (1995). *Transcultural concepts in nursing care* (2nd ed.), (Appendix A). Philadelphia: Lippincott.

Giger, J. N. & Davidhizar, R. E. (1995). *Transcultural nursing: assessment and intervention* (2nd ed.). St. Louis: Mosby.

Helperin, S. W. (Ed.) (1994). *Spanish phrase book for anesthesia.* Santa Monica, CA: Wordsworth.

Jarvis, C. (Ed.) (1996). *Physical examination and health assessment* (2nd ed.). Philadelphia: Saunders.

Leininger, M. (1995). Culture care assessment to guide nursing practices. In M. Leininger (Ed.), *Transcultural nursing: Concepts, theories, research and practices* (2nd ed., pp. 115–143). New York: McGraw-Hill.

McLeod, R. P. (Issue Ed.) (1996). Approaches to cultural diversity. *Advanced Practice Nursing Quarterly, 2*(2), 1–86.

Thompson, J. M. & Wilson, S. F. (1996). *Health assessment for nursing practice.* St. Louis: Mosby.

Zambricki, C. (1996). Clinical aspects of the preanesthetic evaluation. *Nursing Clinics of North America, 31,* 607–621.

REFERENCES

Abraham, S. A. (1990). *Comprehensive guide to medical halachah.* Jerusalem, Israel: Feldheim.

American Society of Anesthesiologists House of Delegates. (1963). New classification of physical status. *Anesthesiology, 24,* 111.

Andrews, M. M. (1996). Transcultural considerations in assessment. In C. Jarvis (Ed.), *Physical examination and health assessment* (2nd ed., pp. 48–57). Philadelphia: Saunders.

Andrews, M. M. & Boyle, J. S. (1997). Competence in transcultural nursing care. *American Journal of Nursing, 97*(8), 16AAA–16DDD.

Chan, S. (1992). Families with Asian roots. In E. W. Lynch & M. J. Hanson (Eds.), *Developing cross-cultural competence* (pp. 181–257). Baltimore: Brookes.

Cooper, T. P. (1996). Culturally appropriate care: Optional or imperative. *Advanced Practice Nursing Quarterly, 2,* 1–6.

Dreher, M. C. (1996). Nursing: A cultural phenomenon. *Reflections, 22,* 4.

Hall, J. M., Stevens, P. E., & Meleis, A. I. (1994). Marginalization: A guiding concept for valuing diversity in nursing knowledge development. *Advances in Nursing Science, 16,* 23–41.

Horton, B. J. & Waugaman, W. R. (1996). Multiculturalism and nurse anesthesia. *Advanced Practice Nursing Quarterly, 2,* 23–30.

Jackson, D. (1995). Latex allergy and anaphylaxis: What to do? *Journal of Intravenous Nursing, 18,* 33–52.

Jarvis, C. (1996). Assessment for health and illness. In C. Jarvis (Ed.), *Physical examination and health assessment* (2nd ed., pp. 4–10). Philadelphia: Saunders.

Jarvis, C. (1996). Assessment techniques and approach to the clinical setting. In C. Jarvis (Ed.), *Physical examination and health assessment* (2nd ed., pp. 162–173). Philadelphia: Saunders.

Kaplan, E. B., Sheiner, L. B., Boeckmann, A. J., Roizen, M. F., Beal, S. L., Cohen, S. N., & Nicoll, C. D. (1985). The usefulness of preoperative laboratory screening. *Journal of the American Medical Association, 253,* 3576–3581.

Kutenai, K. (1996). A Native-American nurse's view. *Advanced Practice Nursing Quarterly, 2,* 59–61.

Leininger, M. (1995). *Transcultural nursing: Concepts, theories, research and practices* (2nd ed., pp. 115–143). New York: McGraw-Hill, Inc.

Ludwig-Beymer, P. (1995). Transcultural aspects of pain. In M. M. Andrews & J. S. Boyles (Eds.), *Transcultural concepts in nursing care* (2nd ed., pp. 301–322). Philadelphia: Lippincott.

Meleis, A. I. (1996). Culturally competent scholarship: Substance and rigor. *Advances in Nursing Science, 19,* 1–16.

Meleis, A. I., Isenberg, M., Koerner, J. E., Lacey, B., & Stern, P. (1995). *Diversity, marginalization and culturally competent health care: Issues in knowledge development* (monograph). New York: American Academy of Nursing Press.

Morgan, G. E. & Mikhail, M. S. (1996). Clinical Anesthesiology (2nd ed., pp. 1–12). Stamford, CT: Appleton & Lange.

Morris, R. I. (1996). Bridging cultural boundaries: The African American and transcultural caring. *Advanced Practice Nursing Quarterly, 2,* 31–38.

Rosenberg, S. (1991). Organ donation: The ultimate tzedakah. *Jewish Exponent, 190,* 2x–3x.

Spector, R. E. (1991). Healing: Magico-religious traditions. In R. E. Spector (Ed.), *Cultural diversity in health and illness* (pp. 117–153). Norwalk, CT: Appleton & Lange.

Zambricki, C. (1996). Clinical aspects of the preanesthetic evaluation. *Nursing Clinics of North America, 31,* 607–621.

Assessment of the Cardiovascular System of the Adult

Debra A. Barber and J. L. Reeves-Viets

Assessing the cardiovascular system involves collecting data about the heart, arteries, and veins to develop a perianesthetic plan. This data is collected by recording the patient history, conducting a physical examination, and evaluating laboratory and cardiac diagnostic studies. This data must be analyzed by an anesthetist who has a thorough understanding of the cardiovascular anatomy, physiology, and pathophysiology. Heart disease and stroke are leading causes of death among Americans, particularly those from culturally diverse backgrounds. Therefore, it is imperative that anesthetists be highly skilled in perianesthetic assessment of the cardiovascular system.

▶ ANATOMY OF THE CARDIOVASCULAR SYSTEM

The heart is a four-chambered organ that functionally consists of a right and left pump, each of which contains an atrium and a ventricle. The atria serve primarily as conduits and primer pumps to the ventricles, which act as the major pumping chambers. The cardiovascular system is separated into a low-pressure right ventricle and pulmonary vascular system and a high-pressure left ventricle and systemic vascular system. These two systems function parallel to each other and share a coronary vascular and conductive system (Fig. 10–1).

The right ventricle receives deoxygenated systemic venous blood that is directed to the pulmonary circulation. The left atrium receives oxygenated pulmonary venous blood that is directed to the systemic circulation. The atrioventricular (AV) valves (mitral on the left and tricuspid on the right) are large-bore valves permitting high flow at lower pressures. Papillary muscles are attached to the mitral and tricuspid valves by chorda tendineae. The ventricular outflow valves (aortic and pulmonic) are smaller in diameter, permitting equal flow with the higher ventricular pressures generated. The cardiac muscle is striated and contains actin and myosin filaments that interact with each other similar to skeletal muscle.

Special conducting fibers are present throughout the heart allowing for rapid transmission of impulses. These fibers initiate the normal rhythmic heartbeat and coordinate contraction of the four chambers. The sinoatrial (SA) node is located in the wall of the right atrium. It is a specialized collection of cardiac muscle fibers or nodal tissue. The SA node functions as the natural pacemaker of the heart. The AV node is a smaller collection of nodal tissue found in the interatrial septum, on the ventricular side of the orifice of the coronary sinus. The AV bundle or Purkinge fibers originate in the AV node and run through the membranous part of the interventricular septum. The AV bundle is the only bridge between the atrial and ventricular myocardium.

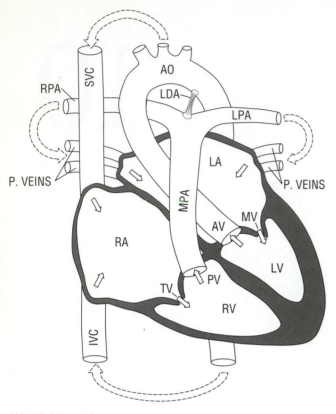

Abbreviations used:
AO—Aorta
AV—Aortic valve
IVC—Inferior vena cava
LA—Left atrium
LPA—Left pulmonary artery
LV—Left ventricle
MPA—Main pulmonary artery
MV—Mitral valve

LDA—Ligamentum ductus arteriosus
PV—Pulmonary valve
P. VEIN—Pulmonary vein
RA—Right atrium
RPA—Right pulmonary artery
RV—Right ventricle
SVC—Superior vena cava
TV—Tricuspid valve

Figure 10–1. The normal heart. *(Used with permission of Ross Products Division, Abbott Laboratories, Columbus, OH 43216 from CEA #7, ©1970 Ross Products Division, Abbott Laboratories.)*

The vascular system is made up of arteries and veins. The aorta carries oxygenated blood to the arteries that supply the peripheral tissues. The pulmonary artery takes unoxygenated blood to the lungs for gas exchange. Arteries are composed of several tissue layers: endothelium, elastic tissue, smooth muscle, and fibrous tissue. As the systemic arterial branches progress toward the periphery, they become smaller and more muscular. The arterioles have a dominant muscular layer and serve as the principle points of resistance to blood flow in the circulatory system.

Blood flows from the arterioles into capillaries where it enters the venous system via small vessels known as venules. From the venules, the blood passes into veins that increase in size as they approach the heart. As the heart is approached, the number of veins decrease and the walls become thicker. Valves located throughout the veins allow for forward flow of blood to the heart. The superior and inferior vena cavae transport blood back into the right atrium of the heart.

There are three brachiocephalic branches that extend from the aorta. These include the left subclavian artery, the left common carotid, and the right brachiocephalic, which branches into the right subclavian and the right common carotid. The blood supply of the brain arises from of the internal carotid artery from which the ophthalmic artery also branches. The internal carotid then passes inferior to the optic nerve and branches into the anterior and middle cerebral arteries.

The vertebral arteries begin in the root of the neck as a branch of the first part of the subclavian artery. The right and left vertebral arteries join to form the basilar artery which gives off the superior cerebellar and posterior cerebral arteries. The posterior communicating arteries connect the branches of the basilar artery with the internal carotid. As the internal carotid arteries branch into the anterior cerebral arteries, these two branches are joined by the anterior communicating arteries. The connecting arteries form what is known as the Circle of Willis. The circle is an important means of collateral blood flow in the event of unilateral obstruction of the cerebral vascular tree (McMinn, Hutchings, Pegington, & Abrahams, 1993).

Distally the aorta extends into the thorax and abdomen forming intercostal branches at each intercostal space. The abdominal aorta has many branches including the superior mesenteric artery which supplies blood to the gut. Large dual branches from the abdominal aorta give rise to the right and left renal arteries. The abdominal aorta continues as a single unit until it bifurcates into the two common iliac arteries. The iliacs divide into the internal iliac and femoral arteries which supply blood to the lower portion of the body and lower extremities.

Coronary Circulation

The myocardium is supplied entirely by the right and left coronary arteries. Blood flows from epicardial to endocardial vessels at a rate of 225 mL/min, which constitutes about 5% of the total cardiac output. The left and right coronary arteries arise from the sinuses of Valsalva which are located behind the cusps of the aortic valve at the root of the aorta. Blood return to the right atrium is via the coronary sinus and the anterior cardiac veins, with a small amount being returned into the chamber of the heart by way of the thebesian veins. The distribution of the coronary arteries is noted in Table 10–1.

The left ventricular wall has a 12-mm to 15-mm thickness as opposed to the 3-mm to 5-mm thickness of the right ventricular wall. The increased thickness, greater chamber pressure, and increased wall tension during normal function produce a greater oxygen de-

TABLE 10–1. Coronary Artery Distribution

Area	Blood Supply
Sinus node	SA nodal artery off proximal RCA (55%) or circumflex (45%)
Atrioventricular node	AV nodal artery off distal RCA (90%) or distal circumflex (10%)
Right bundle branch	Septal branches of LAD and PDA
Left anterior bundle branch	Septal branches of LAD
Left posterior bundle branch	Septal branches of LAD
Left anterior papillary muscle	LAD
Left posterior papillary muscle	Distal positions of RCA and LCA
Intraventricular septum	
Anterior superior two-thirds	Septal branches of LAD
Posterior inferior one-third	PDA off RCA (or LCA)
Apical portion	Acute marginal branch off RCA
Left ventricle	
Anterior	LAD
Anterolateral	Anterolateral obtuse marginal off the circumflex
Posterolateral	Posterolateral obtuse marginal off the circumflex
Posterior	Posterolateral termination of circumflex
Inferior (basal)	PDA is most distal portion of RCA or circumflex artery
Apex	Most distal portion of LAD

Abbreviations: SA, sinoatrial; RCA, right coronary artery; AV, arteriovenous; LCA, left coronary artery; LAD, left anterior descending artery; PDA, posterior descending artery; (%) refers to proportion of patients.
From Miller, R. D. (1986). *Anesthesia* (2nd ed., p. 168). New York: Churchill Livingstone. Reprinted with permission.

mand in the left ventricle that can lead to ischemia, infarction, or failure. In contrast, the thin-walled right ventricle generates greater changes in wall tension when distended.

▶ PHYSIOLOGY OF THE CARDIOVASCULAR SYSTEM

Electrophysiology

Cardiac muscle cells have a unique organization that allows the action potential generated by one cell to spread to all of them along special excitatory and conductive fibers. The impulses generated by the pacemaker cells in the SA node are transmitted throughout conductive pathways to effect sequential contraction of the atria and ventricles. The SA node functions as the dominant pacemaker of the heart with an intrinsic rate of 60 to 100 beats per minute (bpm). The impulse then passes to the AV node, which has an intrinsic rate of 40 to 60 bpm, and on to the Purkinje fibers and the ventricles themselves (rate < 40 bpm). Figure 10–2 notes the single-cell voltage recordings initiated from the electrical activity of the heart.

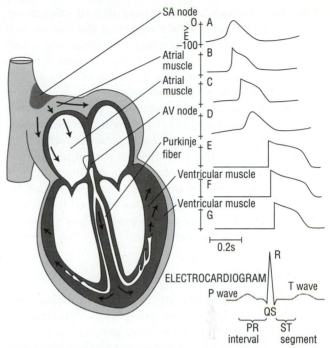

Figure 10–2. Electrical activity of the heart. *(From Mohrman & Heller [1986]. Cardiovascular physiology [2nd ed., p. 167]. Reprinted with permission from The McGraw-Hill Companies.)*

Cardiac Action Potential

The resting membrane potential of a normal cardiac muscle cell is about −90 mV. The myocardial cell membrane is normally permeable to potassium ions (K^+), but relatively impermeable to sodium ions (Na^+). Intracellular sodium concentration is kept low, whereas intracellular potassium concentration is high. Changes in this gradient determine the cardiac cycle. The action potential of a cardiac pacemaker cell is divided into phases 0 through 4 (Fig. 10–3). Phase 0 is the phase of rapid depolarization generated by the movement of sodium ions into the cell. Phase 1 is a brief phase of initial rapid repolarization. Phase 2 is a plateau phase in which closure

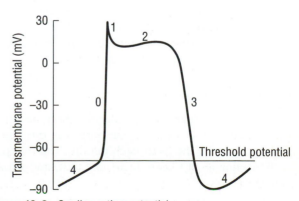

Figure 10–3. Cardiac action potential.

of sodium channels and an inward flux of calcium occurs. Phase 3 results from a return of the cardiac cell membrane's normal permeability to sodium and a sudden increase in permeability to potassium ions. A return to the resting transmembrane potential of -90 mV describes phase 4 depolarization. Propagation of an action potential occurs when the membrane potential reaches -70 mV (Reeves-Viets, 1992). Following depolarization, the cells are refractory to normal depolarizing stimuli until phase 4. During phases 1 through 3, another depolarization cannot occur regardless of the stimulus intensity. This is referred to as the *absolute refractory period*. Between phases 3 and 4, the stimulus required to elicit an action potential is larger than normal. This is known as the *relative refractory period*.

Automaticity

The atria are innervated by the parasympathetic and sympathetic nervous systems, whereas the ventricles are supplied principally by the sympathetic nervous system. Intrinsic sympathetic pathways and cardioaccelerators arise in the cervical chain; these fibers terminate in discrete nerve terminals in the conductive pathways and the myocardium (Viets, Martin, Heaton, & Biddle, 1987). Norepinephrine activates alpha-receptor sites, creating an increase in automaticity, inotropy, and arrhythmogenicity. There is also a humoral mediated route in which epinephrine, released from the adrenal medulla, produces the same physiologic effects at the beta-receptors which are located diffusely throughout the heart (Viets, Martin, Heaton, & Biddle,1987). The parasympathetic innervation, which invokes opposing responses, is provided by branches of the vagus nerve.

Cardiac Cycle

The cardiac cycle is defined by both electrical and mechanical events (Ganong, 1993). *Systole* describes the phase of contraction while *diastole* refers to the relaxation phase. The majority of ventricular filling occurs during diastole in a passive manner prior to atrial contraction. Atrial contraction generally is responsible for 20% to 30% of ventricular filling in the normal heart, but may represent up to 50% of ventricular filling in a noncompliant heart.

Hemodynamics

Cardiac output (CO) and ventricular function are often seen as parallel processes. Cardiac output is the blood volume pumped by the heart each minute. The two primary determinants of CO are heart rate (HR) and stroke volume (SV).

$$CO = HR \times SV$$

Cardiac output is generally calculated based on thermodilution techniques utilizing a pulmonary artery catheter.

$$CI = \frac{CO}{BSA}$$

A number of variables may affect CO calculation based on temperature gradients, necessitating a thorough understanding of the principles that control CO. Cardiac index (CI) is a measure of ventricular function that allows for variations in body size by dividing the CO by the body surface area (BSA). Cardiac output is normally directly proportionate to the HR when preload is constant (Fig. 10-4). Stroke volume is the volume of blood ejected in one systolic beat, and cannot be directly measured in the clinical setting.

Stroke volume is determined by three variables: preload, afterload, and contractility. *Preload* is the ventricular muscle distention at the end of diastole and immediately prior to contraction (systole). *Afterload* is the tension that the muscle must contract against to initiate the ejection phase of systole. *Contractility*, or *inotropy*, may be defined as the work performed during the cardiac cycle.

Ventricular preload correlates with the end-diastolic volume of the heart, which is the primary determinant of SV in the presence of normal ventricular function. This relationship is described by the Frank–Starling curve (Fig. 10-5), which illustrates the association between resting tension (preload) and peak-induced tension (contractility). Cardiac output is directly proportionate to preload, if the heart rate is constant, until excessive end-diastolic volumes are reached (Ganong, 1993). When the ventricle becomes overly distended, CO may cease to change or even decrease. Venous return is the most important determinant of preload in the normal heart. Variations from normal HR and alterations in the electrical mechanism may also act to decrease preload.

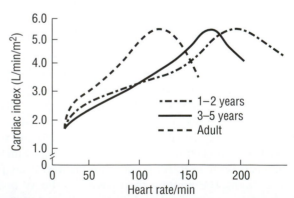

Figure 10–4. Relationship between heart rate and cardiac output. *(From Morgan, G. E. & Mikhail, M. S. [1996]. Clinical anesthesiology [2nd ed., p. 292]. Philadelphia: Lippincott-Raven. Reprinted with permission.)*

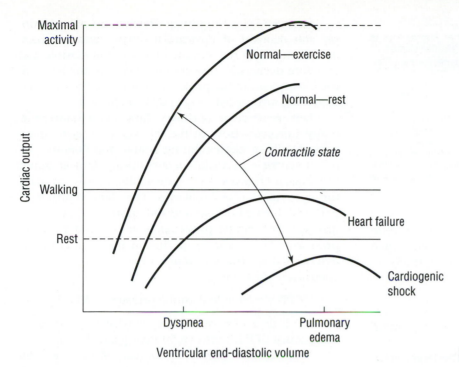

Figure 10–5. Starling curve.

Ventricular compliance is defined as an index of change assessed by volume status changes and pressure changes in the chamber or the ventricle. The left ventricular end-diastolic pressure (LVEDP) is often used as a means of evaluating preload and estimating compliance. Ventricular compliance is proportional to changes in volume, but inversely proportional to changes in pressure, as described by the formula:

$$C = \frac{\Delta V}{\Delta P}$$

Figure 10–6 illustrates normal and abnormal compliance curves. The relationship between ventricular compli-

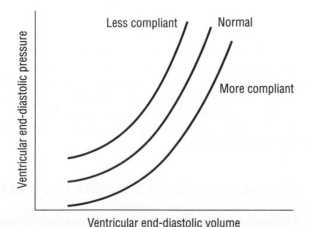

Figure 10–6. Compliance curve. *(From Morgan, G. E. & Mikhail, M. S. [1996]. Clinical anesthesiology [2nd ed., p. 293]. Philadelphia: Lippincott-Raven. Reprinted with permission.)*

ance and volume is normally nonlinear, which creates difficulties in estimating preload, as many factors may alter LVEDP. Some of the causes of decreased compliance are myocardial ischemia, scarring, overdistention of the ventricle, and ventricular hypertrophy (Morgan & Mikhail, 1996). Other factors besides ventricular compliance may affect the relationship between preload and contractility such as AV valve stenosis, peak airway pressures, and pulmonary vascular resistance.

Left ventricular afterload is often equated or used interchangeably with the term *resistance,* though the two should be recognized as separate phenomena (Reeves-Viets, 1992). Afterload is the force that the ventricle must overcome to initiate ejection during systole. A reduction in forward flow may occur if the force against which the ventricle operates increases beyond a physiologic range. Resistance is a reflection of vasomotor tone. Resistance shares a linear relationship with the arterial pressure when the CO is constant and may be calculated for the systemic or pulmonary circulations. Blood pressure will increase as the systemic vascular resistance (SVR) increases if the CO remains constant, as demonstrated by the formulas in Table 10–2. Therefore, resistance is primarily a vascular phenomenon, whereas afterload is a reflection of the ventricle itself.

In a patient without a normal left ventricular outflow tract obstruction, the SVR is the primary determinant of mean systemic blood pressure when CO is constant:

$$MAP = CO \times SVR$$

where MAP is the mean arterial pressure. This relationship, which is applied to circulation, is relative to Ohm's

TABLE 10–2. Hemodynamic Formulas

Equation	Normal Values (dynes/sec cm^{-5})
$SVR = \dfrac{(MAP - CVP) \times 80}{CO}$	900–1500
$PVR = \dfrac{(MPAP - PCWP) \times 80}{CO}$	50–250

Abbreviations: SVR, systemic vascular resistance; MAP, mean arterial pressure; CVP, central venous pressure; CO, cardiac output; PVR, pulmonary vascular resistance; MPAP, mean pulmonary artery pressure; PCWP, pulmonary capillary wedge pressure; 80 represents the constant factor.

law, whereby, blood flow (amperes) is directly proportional to the pressure drop across two points (voltage) and inversely proportional to resistance (Stoelting, 1995).

$$Q = \frac{\Delta P}{R}$$

where Q is the blood flow, P is the pressure drop, and R is the resistance.

Systemic blood flow is pulsatile in the larger arteries, which have a normal MAP of about 95 mmHg. The flow becomes laminar or continuous by the time the blood reaches the capillaries. The largest decrease in pressure occurs across the arterioles which account for the majority of the SVR. An increase in resistance in either the pulmonary or systemic circulation translates as an increase in afterload by increasing diastolic pressure.

Coronary blood flow is the result of vascular responses to the needs of the cardiac muscle for oxygen and metabolic substrates. The normal coronary blood flow is generally parallel to the myocardial oxygen demand. The heart's metabolic oxygen requirements utilize 65% of the total oxygen transported in the arterial blood. Increased coronary flow is the only mechanism available to meet an increased oxygen demand by the heart. Myocardial oxygen demand is the most important determinant of myocardial blood flow. Table 10–3 outlines the factors that affect myocardial oxygen supply and demand.

TABLE 10–3. Factors Affecting Myocardial Oxygen Supply and Demand

Supply	Demand
Heart rate	Basal requirements
Diastolic time	Heart rate
Coronary perfusion pressure	Wall tension
Aortic diastolic blood pressure	Preload (ventricular radius)
Ventricular end-diastolic pressure	Afterload
Arterial oxygen content	Contractility
Arterial oxygen tension	
Hemoglobin concentration	
Coronary vessel diameter	

From Morgan, G. E. & Mikhail, M. S. (1996). Clinical anesthesiology (2nd ed., p. 302). Philadelphia: Lippincott-Raven. Reprinted with permission.

Heart rate is an important determinant of both supply and demand of myocardial oxygen and coronary flow. Tachycardia reduces the time spent in diastole and therefore decreases coronary blood flow to the left ventricle, especially in the presence of atherosclerosis, while increasing myocardial oxygen demand linearly.

Left ventricular coronary flow occurs intermittently. Coronary flow to the left ventricle is reduced substantially or ceases during systole and 60% to 70% of left ventricle perfusion occurs during diastole when the muscle relaxes and allows blood flow to pass through ventricular capillaries. The right ventricle is perfused during both systole and diastole because normal right ventricular pressures never exceed systemic pressures. The coronary perfusion pressure (CPP) is determined by the difference in aortic pressure and ventricular pressure:

CPP = Systemic diastolic pressure − VEDP

where VEDP is the ventricular end-diastolic pressure. The normal CPP is between 50 mmHg and 120 mmHg.

Wall tension may limit coronary flow when increased beyond the normal physiologic range as described previously. Ventricular wall tension can be expressed by the law of Laplace:

Circumferential stress = [P] × [R/2] = [H]

where P is the ventricular pressure, R is the radius of the ventricle, and H is the wall thickness. Therefore, the larger the ventricular radius and chamber pressure, the greater the wall tension. The wall tension decreases as the wall thickness increases.

An increase in wall tension may mechanically impede forward flow. Three factors determine wall tension: pressure, diameter of the chamber, and wall thickness. Ventricular hypertension and dilation will produce an increase in wall tension. If the heart is continually subjected to pressure or volume overload, the sarcomeres will begin to increase in length and, over time, the ventricular muscle mass will enlarge. Ventricular hypertrophy is a compensatory mechanism that reduces wall tension while permitting an increase in contractile force. In the volume-overloaded ventricle, the sarcomeres will replicate in series, which produces *eccentric hypertrophy* where the wall thickness is unchanged. In the pressure-overloaded ventricle, the sarcomeres will replicate in parallel, resulting in *concentric hypertrophy* with an increased wall thickness.

▶ CARDIOVASCULAR SYSTEM HISTORY

A thorough and detailed history of the cardiovascular system is crucial for any patient undergoing surgery. Limitations related to cardiovascular disease can lead to an increase in morbidity and mortality if not determined preoperatively.

The presence and quality of angina should be determined. The following information should be ascertained when collecting data on cardiovascular history:

- Do you have any pain or tightness in your chest, especially running to your neck or arms? Where did it first occur? Is it increasing in frequency or relatively stable?
- Describe the location and character of the pain.
- What activity brings on the pain?
- With what duration of this activity does the pain occur?
- What relieves this pain?
- Do you become short of breath when you have the pain?
- Do you become short of breath when you lie flat?

The above questions will aid in determining the severity of the angina. Also, the presence of congestive heart failure can be determined from this information.

The vascular system should be assessed by determining the presence of claudication in the extremities. A reported history of syncope, vertigo, transient ischemic attacks, or stroke can provide evidence of carotid disease.

► CARDIOVASCULAR PHYSICAL ASSESSMENT

General Cardiovascular Physical Assessment

When performing a physical assessment of the cardiovascular system, it should include (1) the heart and circulation; (2) the chest and abdomen; and (3) signs of coexisting diseases that may affect the cardiovascular system (Perloff, 1994). The assessment of the heart and circulation should include physical appearance, arterial pulses, jugular pulse and peripheral veins, heart movements, and auscultation.

The general appearance of the patient should be noted with attention to details such as edematous legs, ascites of abdomen, and muscle weakness. The breathing pattern should be observed and signs of respiratory distress such as dyspnea, diaphoresis, and tachypnea when the patient is sitting up at rest should be noted. The patient's overall weight and body mass should be noted because obesity is associated with coronary artery disease. The patient with long-standing congestive heart failure may develop cachexia.

The extremities should be examined for cyanosis and clubbing. The degree and distribution of these findings should be noted. The presence of petechiae on the skin may be an early indicator of infective endocarditis (Perloff, 1994).

The arterial pulses should be palpated and compared to include radial, brachial, femoral, posterior tibial, dorsalis pedis, and carotid pulses. The rate and rhythm of the various pulses should be noted. Blood pressure should be taken on both upper and lower extremities with the patient in the sitting and supine positions. The neck should be examined for thrills with palpation over both carotid arteries, subclavian arteries, and substernal notch. Thrills commonly arise from the presence of atherosclerotic plaques in the arteries.

The jugular veins should be examined for distention with the patient lying supine and then slowly raised to the sitting position. Venous distention that persists when upright may indicate the presence of congestive heart failure. Venous distention and edema in the extremities are also indicators of possible heart failure.

The chest and abdomen should be observed for respiratory patterns and appearance. The presence of scoliosis, kyphosis, pectus carinatum, or excavatum should be noted. Auscultation of the chest should be performed to assess for rales, rhonchi, or decreased breath sounds on one or both sides. The presence of crepitant rales can indicate pulmonary edema. Thoracic percussion should also be performed during the cardiac assessment as discussed in Chapter 11.

Assessment of the abdomen in the cardiac patient should include observation of general appearance, palpation, percussion, and auscultation. Palpation may identify an enlarged liver or the presence of aortic aneurysms below the umbilicus. Auscultation allows for the assessment of murmurs in the abdominal aorta which may indicate obstruction of flow.

The chest wall should be observed for heart movements and also palpated for thrills and vibrations. Sites routinely palpated and observed include apex, left and right sternal borders, subxiphoid area, suprasternal notch, and the right sternoclavicular junction.

The point of maximal impulse (PMI) should be noted. Normally the left ventricle occupies the apex of the heart and is best identified with the patient in a left lateral decubitus position. In the normal heart, the left ventricle should yield a gentle, sustained anterior systolic movement. In the presence of left ventricular hypertrophy, the left ventricle will occupy the apex, but will yield a more sustained pressure or dynamic impulse. With right ventricular enlargement, the right ventricle may occupy the apex and yield a left sternal edge systolic impulse (Perloff, 1994).

Heart Sound Analysis

Audible sounds may be heard when auscultating the heart as the valves close. The first heart sound (S1) is produced by closure of the mitral and tricuspid valves at the onset of ventricular systole. This sound is the loudest and longest of the heart sounds and is a series of mixed low frequencies that is the result of blood oscillating in the ventricular chambers. The first heart sound is best heard over the apical region of the heart and occurs when the atrioventricular valves suddenly tense and recoil.

The second heart sound (S2) is a high-frequency vibration that occurs with the closure of the aortic and pulmonic valves. This sound has more of a snapping quality than the first heart sound which occurs as the semilunar valves abruptly close. The second heart sound is of greater intensity in the presence of systemic or pulmonary hypertension, as this sound is determined by the rate of decrease in ventricular pressure at the end of systole (Stoelting, 1995).

A third heart sound (S3) is noted primarily in children as a normal phenomenon or in patients with left ventricular failure. This sound is best heard in the apex region and occurs early in diastole. It is the result of vibrations of the ventricular walls caused by abrupt cessation of ventricular distention and deceleration of blood entering the ventricles (Berne & Levy, 1990). This sound is of such low frequency that it is rarely detected by a stethoscope. A fourth heart sound (S4) is the result of atrial contraction as blood rapidly flows into the ventricles. This sound is also difficult to auscultate with a stethoscope due to the low frequency.

The optimal area for auscultating the aortic valve is on the right side of the chest just lateral to the sternum at the second intercostal space. The pulmonic valve is best heard on the left side of the chest in the second intercostal space lateral to the sternum. The tricuspid valve is heard best over the right ventricle, and mitral valve is heard best over the apex of the heart. Valve deformities or asynchronous valve closure may produce heart murmurs.

► CARDIOVASCULAR DIAGNOSTIC STUDIES

Electrocardiogram Analysis

The electrocardiogram (ECG) is a recording of the transmission of the cardiac impulse, created by the electrical currents of the heart. The information provided by ECG analysis allows for the assessment of a variety of parameters. Heart rate is measured directly as well as electrical rhythm disturbances. The ECG may also be used to detect myocardial ischemia and/or infarction, electrolyte abnormalities, and toxic responses to anesthetic agents.

The normal ECG tracing in Fig. 10-7 (Reeves-Viets, 1992) consists of the P wave, the QRS complex, and the T wave. The P wave occurs as the atria depolarize prior to atrial contraction. The QRS complex is created by the electrical currents that are generated during ventricular depolarization. The T wave is a reflection of ventricular repolarization. The normal P-R interval is 0.12 to 0.20 second. The QRS complex is normally 0.5 to 0.10 second. The Q-T interval is normally 0.26 to 0.45 second. The S-T segment is a valuable tool in detecting myocardial ischemia. Elevation or depression of the S-T segment greater than a 1-mm difference from the baseline indi-

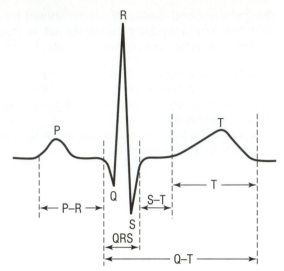

Figure 10–7. Normal ECG.

cate ventricular muscle ischemia. Table 10-4 illustrates the correlation between areas of infarct in the heart and the affected ECG leads.

Normal sinus rhythm (NSR) reflects a synchronous depolarization of the atria, followed by the ventricles. Normal sinus rhythm is characterized by a rate of 60 bpm to 100 bpm with a regular rhythm. Beat-to-beat variations may occur in relation to the respiratory cycle. Sinus tachycardia (ST) is defined as a normal rhythm with a HR greater than 100 bpm. Sinus tachycardia is often related to stimulation such as that produced during light anesthesia. Fever and reflex stimulation from vasodilator drugs can also produce ST.

Sinus bradycardia (SB) is a normal rhythm with a HR less than 60 bpm. This slowing of the heart may be the result of parasympathetic nervous system stimulation. An SB rhythm in athletes is not uncommon or considered abnormal because the conditioned heart is able to eject a greater SV with each heartbeat.

Atrial dysrhythmias may present as premature beats, tachycardias, flutter, or fibrillation. Premature atrial contractions (PACs) are characterized by an abnormal P

TABLE 10–4. Area of Infarct Associated with ECG Leads

Area of Infarct	Affected ECG Leads
Anterior	I, aV_L, V_3, V_4
Inferior	II, III, aV_F
Lateral	I, aV_L, V_5, V_6
Posterior	Reciprocal changes in V_1, V_2
Anterolateral	V_{1-6}
Anteroseptal	V_{1-4}
Inferolateral	Inferior + V_5, V_6
Right Ventricle	V_{4R}–V_{6R}

wave and a shortened P–R interval. The QRS has a normal configuration. Atrial tachycardias present with a 1 : 1 ratio between the P wave and QRS complex. The rhythm of the ECG is regular with abnormal P waves. Atrial flutter generally presents with a regular rhythm and conduction of only a fraction of the atrial beats to the ventricle. The atrium may be contracting as rapidly as 300 bpm, with only one out of two (1 : 2), one out of three (1 : 3), or one out of four (1 : 4) reaching the ventricles. Atrial fibrillation presents with the appearance of numerous small depolarization waves that are irregular in both form and frequency. There are no visible P waves, only high-frequency, low-voltage waves. The rhythm is generally irregular as conduction across the AV node is inconsistent.

Atrioventricular conduction abnormalities may occur as either dissociation, junctional, or nodal dysrhythmias. Nodal contractions are characterized by the absence of a P wave preceding the QRS complex, or the P wave may follow the QRS complex. The nodal beats may appear as premature complexes or as escape beats in the presence of severe SB. Junctional escape beats are generally noted with severe SB when the sinus mechanism fails to maintain a HR above the normal AV nodal rate of 40 bpm to 60 bpm (Foster & Reeves-Viets, 1992).

Several AV conduction abnormalities may occur. A first-degree AV block is defined as a P–R interval that exceeds 0.2 seconds in the presence of a normal HR. A second-degree block is classified as either a Wenckebach (Type I) or a Mobitz (Type II) heart block. A Wenckebach block is identified by a progressive lengthening of the P–R interval until conduction of the atrial impulse is completely blocked, and a P wave will be recorded that is not followed by a QRS complex. A Mobitz heart block occurs when there is spontaneous failure to propagate an atrial impulse without a prior change in the P–R interval. A third-degree block (complete AV block) is a complete dissociation of the atrial and ventricular mechanisms. The P waves are dissociated from the QRS–T complexes as each chamber beats at its own intrinsic rhythm without any coordination of conduction. The rates of ventricular response depends on the site of origin of the ventricular mechanism. Third-degree heart block can create an interval of ventricular immobility that may be fatal; therefore, insertion of a pacemaker is the treatment for this conduction abnormality.

Ventricular arrhythmias appear in four primary forms: premature ventricular contractions (PVCs), ventricular tachycardia (VT), ventricular fibrillation (VF), and bundle branch blocks (BBB). Premature ventricular contractions are the result of an ectopic pacemaker in the ventricles. A ventricular contraction will occur prior to a normally conducted complex. The QRS complex is generally prolonged and abnormal in conformation, reflecting the transmission of the cardiac impulse through the slow-conducting ventricular muscle rather than the Purkinje system. The T wave following a PVC has an electrical potential opposite to that of the QRS complex as the slow conduction of the impulse through the cardiac muscle causes the area first depolarized to repolarize first.

A compensatory pause follows a PVC, indicating a refractory pause in the AV node. The first impulse from the SA node reaches the ventricle when the ventricle is in a refractory period. The second impulse from the atria does reach the ventricle and conduction is normal. When a PVC occurs, the ventricle may be unable to adequately fill in order for the SV to produce a detectable pulse. Fixed, unifocal PVCs are generally benign, whereas multiform PVCs, multiple PVCs in sequence, or PVCs occurring near the T wave can be of more serious consequence. Premature ventricular contractions often occur in the presence of cardiac disease. Myocardial ischemia may lead to initiation of a PVC from an irritable site in a hypoxic ventricular muscle.

Ventricular tachycardia is defined as a sequence of three or more PVCs with a rapid, regular rate (>100 bpm) and without normal beats interspersed. Stroke volume may be severely depressed, resulting in a lack of transmission of arterial pressure due to decreased ventricular filling time. Drugs or cardioversion may be required to terminate the dysrhythmia if there is no spontaneous termination.

Ventricular fibrillation is characterized by a highly irregular rhythm with no discernible pattern. The ventricles are unable to contract and arterial pressure is not obtainable in the presence of VF. The only effective treatment for VF is defibrillation with an electrical current through the heart. Defibrillation causes the ventricular muscle to depolarize and reestablishes the cardiac pacemaker at a site other than the irritable focus responsible for the fibrillation.

Bundle branch blocks are the result of abnormal conduction of the impulse to the ventricles. Depolarization occurs in a retrograde fashion from the point distal to the block. The QRS is broad and atypical as a result (Foster & Reeves-Viets, 1992). A single BBB is usually benign, as are those involving the right bundle and left anterior branch. Right BBBs and left posterior hemiblocks carry a 90% incidence of progression to complete AV block.

Laboratory Analysis

Standard preoperative laboratory values should be obtained for the patient with cardiovascular disease who is to undergo surgery. These values include serum electrolytes, renal function tests, complete blood count, clotting studies, and glucose levels.

Serum creatine kinase (CK) levels are indicated for confirmation of the diagnosis of acute myocardial infarction. Creatine kinase is released within 4 hours after a myocardial ischemic event, and peak levels rise between 12 and 24 hours. The higher the peak CK level, the more extensive the infarct. This enzyme is rapidly cleared from the body and will generally return to normal limits after 72 hours. The skeletal muscle holds the largest reservoir of CK. In the event of trauma or intramuscular injections prior to a suspected myocardial infarction, the MB isoenzyme fraction of CK must be relied on (Perloff, 1990). An elevated MB–CK level is highly specific for confirmation of the diagnosis of myocardial infarction. MB–CK clears more rapidly from the circulation (Perloff, 1994) and therefore, must be determined early in the course of evaluation (within 36 to 48 hours).

Lactic dehydrogenase and its subfractions are released slowly from the infarcted area over a period of 7 to 10 days after an acute myocardial infarction. These enzyme levels, particularly the myocardial subfraction of the enzyme, may be useful in confirming the diagnosis in the late phase. The myocardial subfraction of lactic dehydrogenase is contained in red blood cells, so hemolysis of the sample or red cell breakdown will skew the results (Perloff, 1994).

Cardiac Angiography

Cardiac catherization is considered the gold standard for diagnosing cardiac pathology. This invasive procedure provides assessment of the following findings: coronary anatomy, left ventricular function, regional ventricular function, valvular function, and pulmonary compliance. Radiopaque dye is injected through a catheter placed in the coronary ostia to allow visualization of both the right and left coronary arteries. The degree of stenosis in each vessel is assessed as a percent reduction in diameter of the vessel. Lesions that reduce vessel diameter by more than 50% are considered significant (Hensley & Martin, 1995).

Echocardiography

Echocardiography and nuclear imaging are noninvasive studies that may precede or complement cardiac catherization for complete assessment of the cardiovascular system. The clinical information obtained from these studies include wall motion abnormalities, ejection fraction, valvular function, and anatomic defects.

► CARDIAC PATHOPHYSIOLOGY

Coronary Artery Disease

Myocardial ischemia is often signified by the presence of angina pectoris which is most frequently described as a heavy, aching sensation in the chest, tightness in the chest, or chest pressure. The pain may radiate to the neck, jaw, either arm, back, or abdomen (Hensley & Martin, 1995). Ischemia occurs when metabolic oxygen demand exceeds oxygen supply. Angina often occurs after physical exertion, eating, or when emotionally stressed. Causes of ischemia include hypertension, tachycardia, severe hypotension, hypoxemia, anemia, aortic valvular disease, and obstruction of the coronary arteries; of these, coronary atherosclerosis is the most common cause of myocardial ischemia.

Coronary artery disease contributes to over one third of the deaths in all Western societies and is a major cause of morbidity and mortality (Morgan & Mikhail, 1996). Risk factors for coronary artery disease include hypertension, hyperlipidemia, diabetes mellitus, cigarette smoking, aging, male sex, and a family history of the disease. Obesity, peripheral vascular disease, menopause, sedentary lifestyle, and oral contraceptive use in women who smoke may also contribute to coronary disease.

Angina can be characterized as exercise induced, occurring at rest, or unstable. Exercise-induced angina will occur in the presence of physical obstruction as the working myocardium's oxygen demand is increased. An atherosclerotic lesion will gradually obstruct blood flow, leading to angina noticed first during exercise. Table 10–5 notes the level of exercise producing angina and provides an important guide for predicting the risk of operative mortality (Hensley & Martin, 1995).

Angina that occurs at rest indicates subtotal ob-

TABLE 10–5. Classification of Angina

Functional Class	New York Heart Association Classification	Canadian Cardiovascular Society Classification
I	Cardiac disease without limitation of physical activity	No angina with ordinary physical activity (walking or climbing stairs); angina with strenuous or prolonged exertion
II	Slight limitation of physical activity Ordinary physical activity results in fatigue or angina	Slight limitation of ordinary activity; limitation of walking or climbing stairs rapidly, walking uphill, after meals, in cold wind
III	Marked limitation of physical activity Comfortable at rest	Marked limitation of physical activity; walking 1 to 2 blocks on level
IV	Angina at rest, increased with activity	Unable to carry on any physical activity without discomfort; angina may be present at rest

struction of the coronary artery, either by atherosclerotic plaque, vasospasm, or a combination of both. Unstable angina describes the onset of new angina or recent progression of existing symptoms, such as an increase in frequency, severity, or duration of anginal attacks. Unstable angina is often referred to as crescendo or preinfarction angina. Patients presenting with unstable angina have a higher incidence of myocardial infarction and operative mortality.

Patients with diabetes mellitus often have silent or asymptomatic angina. The ischemic changes may be noted only on the ECG. More than half of perioperative infarctions associated with all types of surgery are thought to be precipitated by silent ischemia (Hensley & Martin, 1995).

Myocardial infarction is a serious complication of ischemic heart disease and can be fatal. Overall mortality is about 25%, with over half of the deaths occurring within the first hour. Most myocardial infarctions occur in patients with more than one severely stenosed coronary artery and are generally the result of thrombosis from an atherosclerotic plaque. The size of the infarct depends on the distribution of the occluded artery and the presence or absence of collateral circulation. A thrombosis of the left anterior descending coronary artery will typically lead to infarction in the anterior, apical, and septal regions of the heart. Occlusion of the left circumflex system will typically result in lateral and posterior left ventricular infarcts. Right coronary blockage is typically associated with infarcts of the right ventricle.

Ventricular Hypertrophy

Ischemic heart disease may occur secondary to ventricular hypertrophy. The hypertrophy may result from aortic stenosis, long-standing outflow obstruction such as idiopathic hypertrophic subaortic stenosis (IHSS), chronic hypertension, or any condition that increases resistance and therefore increases the workload of the left ventricle. When the heart is subjected to a pressure or volume overload, over time the end result will be replication of the sarcomeres and an increased muscle mass.

Ischemia is the result of the additional metabolic demands placed by the enlarged ventricular muscle mass. Blood flow must increase in order to supply the extra metabolic substrates required by the hypertrophied ventricle. This increase in demand will often exceed the supply required to maintain myocardial oxygen requirements. This leads to a chronic state of mild myocardial ischemia early in the disease.

The ischemia of hypertrophy is global in nature (Reeves-Viets, 1992). The entire ventricle is subjected to ischemia, as the reduction in myocardial flow is not limited to discrete areas from stenotic lesions in the coronary vessels. The ischemia is life threatening and measures to halt its progress must be instituted.

The ischemia is subendocardial as a result of the in-

creased ventricular mass and frequent accompaniment of hypertension and ventricular dilation. There is a requirement of increased filling pressure to dilate the hypertrophied ventricle, which translates to an increase in LVEDP. The increases in the wall tension and filling pressures lead to reductions in the efficacy of subendocardial coronary perfusion (Reeves-Viets, 1992).

Congestive Heart Failure

Heart failure occurs when the heart is unable to provide sufficient CO to meet metabolic demands. Diminished ventricular function may be the single greatest risk factor for patients undergoing cardiac surgery (Hensley & Martin, 1995). Clinical symptoms include fatigue, weight loss, weakness, venous congestion that manifests as edema in the lower extremities, jugular venous distention, and pulmonary congestion. The clinical manifestations generally reflect a low CO state and the vascular congestion behind the failing ventricle.

Left ventricular failure occurs most commonly, often with subsequent right ventricular failure. Left ventricular failure usually is the result of coronary artery disease, but may also occur secondary to valve disorders, arrhythmias, or pericardial disease. Advanced pulmonary pathology is generally associated with isolated right ventricular failure.

Sympathetic vascular tone, circulating catecholamines, and blood volume all increase in an attempt to compensate for the failing ventricle. Hypertrophy may also occur as a compensatory measure. The ventricular ejection will remain depressed, but the increased end-diastolic volume may maintain a normal SV and CO at rest. Untreated congestive heart failure correlates with a 5-year, 50% mortality rate (Mangano, 1990).

Congestive heart failure is generally associated with a low CO state. High CO states also exist, though less commonly. A high CO failure is generally associated with sepsis or any hypermetabolic state in which the SVR is low (Stoelting & Dierdorf, 1993).

Valvular Heart Disease

The major valvular disorders are discussed in this section. Only the left-sided lesions are discussed because management of valvular lesions is similar for both sides of the heart. The right-sided hemodynamics should be considered when applying these principles to valvular disorders of the right heart.

The severity of the lesion, hemodynamic alterations, ventricular function, and other organ systems affected should be determined regardless of which valve is involved. Coronary artery disease may coexist with valvular dysfunction and should be carefully evaluated.

Mitral regurgitation may develop acutely or chronically. Acute mitral regurgitation is usually secondary to myocardial ischemia that affects the papillary muscles or chorda tendinea, chest trauma, or infective endocarditis. The most common cause of chronic mitral regurgitation is rheumatic fever. Mitral regurgitation that follows rheumatic disease develops slowly over an asymptomatic period lasting 20 to 40 years. Once symptoms begin to occur (fatigue, dyspnea, orthopnea), the disease progresses rapidly with death usually occurring within 5 years if left untreated. Atrial fibrillation occurs in about 75% of the cases. The survival rate for patients with mitral regurgitation is improved if surgical correction is performed before ventricular dysfunction occurs. All patients with valvular heart disease should receive prophylactic antibiotics for infective endocarditis as stated by the American Heart Association (Table 10–6).

In mitral regurgitation, forward SV is reduced as retrograde flow directs blood into the left atrium as a result of an incompetent mitral valve. Initially, the left ventricle attempts to compensate by dilating and increasing end-diastolic volume. Over time, eccentric hypertrophy occurs in the left ventricle. The CO is maintained even though forward ejection fraction decreases as a result of the increasing end-diastolic volume. Chronic left atrial volume overload eventually produces impairment in contractility and a decrease in ejection fraction.

The regurgitant volume that enters the left atrium is dependent on the size of the mitral valve orifice, HR, and the pressure gradient across the mitral valve during systole. Mild increases in HR improve SV, whereas bradycardia decreases the CO as a result of left atrial overload. Left atrial compliance and SVR are the major factors in determining the pressure gradient across the left ventricle and left atrium. A decrease in SVR or an increase in left atrial pressure will decrease the amount of regurgitant volume through the mitral valve. The decrease in vascular resistance can be accomplished with vasodilator drugs, which may be very effective in improving the CO. Patients with increased atrial compliance, as seen in long-standing mitral regurgitation, often have a large, dilated left atrium, reduced CO, and signs of pulmonary congestion. A regurgitant fraction of less than 30% of the total SV results in mild symptoms. A 30% to 60% regurgitant fraction will produce moderate symptoms, whereas patients with fractions greater than 60% are considered to have severe mitral regurgitation (Stoelting, 1995).

Mitral stenosis generally occurs secondary to rheumatic fever. The stenosis of the valve occurs as a result of fusion and calcification of the valve leaflets. The prognosis for a patient with mitral stenosis is a 50% mortality rate in 10 years without surgical intervention (Hensley & Martin, 1995). Surgery to repair or replace the valve should be performed before irreversible ventricular dysfunction or pulmonary vascular changes occur.

Symptoms usually do not develop until 20 to 30 years after the initial episode of rheumatic fever. The size

TABLE 10–6. Prophylaxis for Subacute Bacterial Endocarditis

I. Dental, oral, nasal, pharyngeal or upper airway procedures
   A. Standard regimen:
      1. Adults:
         a. Penicillin V, 2 g PO 1 hour before and 1 g 6 hours after; or—
         b. Penicillin G, 2 million units IV or IM 0.5 hour before and 1 million units 6 hours after.
      2. Children < 60 lb:
         a. Penicillin V, 1 g PO 1 hour before and 500 mg 6 hours after; or—
         b. Penicillin G, 50 000 units/kg IV or IM 0.5 to 1 hour before and 25 000 units/kg IV or IM 6 hours after.
   B. Penicillin allergy:
      1. Adults: Erythromycin, 1 g PO 1 hour before and 500 mg 6 hours after.
      2. Children < 60 lb: Erythromycin, 20 mg/kg PO 1 hour before and 10 mg/kg 6 hours after.
   C. High-risk patients:
      1. Adults:
         a. Ampicillin, 2 g IM or IV, plus gentamicin, 1.5 mg/kg IM or IV, 0.5 hour before, and penicillin, 1 g PO 6 hours after; or—
         b. The same combination once 8 hours after.
      2. Children < 60 lb:
         a. Ampicillin, 50 mg/kg IM or IV, plus gentamicin, 2 mg/kg IM or IV, 0.5 hour before, and penicillin, 500 mg PO 6 hours after; or—
         b. The same combination once 8 hours after.
   D. High-risk patients with penicillin allergy:
      1. Adults: Vancomycin, 1 g slowly IV 1 hour before.
      2. Children < 60 lb: Vancomycin, 20 mg/kg slowly IV 1 hour before.

II. Genitourinary or gastrointestinal procedures
   A. Standard regimen (high-risk procedures):
      1. Adults: Ampicillin, 2 g IM or IV, plus gentamicin, 1.5 mg/kg IM or IV, 1 hour before, and the same combination once again 8 hours after.
      2. Children < 60 lb: Ampicillin, 50 mg/kg IM or IV, plus gentamicin, 2 mg/kg IM or IV, 1 hour before, and the same combination once again 8 hours after.
   B. Alternative regimen (low-risk procedures):
      1. Adults: Amoxicillin, 3 g PO 1 hour before and 1.5 g 6 hours after.
      2. Children < 60 lb: Amoxicillin, 50 mg/kg PO 1 hour before and 25 mg/kg PO 6 hours after.
   C. Penicillin allergy:
      1. Adults: Vancomycin, 1 g slowly IV, plus gentamicin, 1.5 mg/kg IM or IV, 1 hour before, and the same combination 8 to 12 hours after.
      2. Children < 60 lb: Vancomycin, 20 mg/kg slowly IV, plus gentamicin, 2 mg/kg IM or IV, 1 hour before, and the same combination 8 hours after.

From Morgan, G. E. & Mikhail, M. S. (1996). Clinical anesthesiology (2nd ed., p. 325). Philadelphia: Lippincott-Raven. Reprinted with permission.

of the valvular orifice determines the severity of the symptoms. A normal mitral valve orifice is 4 cm^2 to 6 cm^2. When the valve orifice has decreased to about 50% of its normal size, symptoms may begin to occur. A valve area of 1.5 to 2.0 cm^2 may be asymptomatic or have mild symptoms with exertion. When the valve area is less than 1 cm^2, the patient is considered to have severe mitral stenosis and will present with symptoms even at rest. Symptoms include varying degrees of dyspnea, paroxysmal nocturnal dyspnea, fatigue, chest pain, palpitations, hemoptysis, atrial fibrillation, and pulmonary edema. The symptoms are the result of a distended left atrium with pulmonary congestion. The onset of atrial fibrillation often causes the symptoms to be more apparent. These patients have an increased risk of thrombus formation as a result of atrial fibrillation and low CO in progressive stages. Left ventricular diastolic filling is mechanically obstructed by the stenotic mitral valve. Stroke volume and left ventricular filling pressures can usually be maintained due to the increased left atrial pressure if the mitral stenosis is mild. Tachycardia or loss of a sinus rhythm can decrease SV.

Aortic regurgitation may be acute or chronic. Acute aortic valve regurgitation usually occurs secondary to infective endocarditis, trauma, or dissection of the aorta. Chronic aortic valve regurgitation is slow, progressive, and due to a variety of causes such as rheumatic fever or diseases affecting the ascending aorta and connective tissue (eg, syphilis, Marfan's syndrome, ankylosing spondylitis). Most patients with chronic aortic regurgitation remain asymptomatic for 10 to 20 years. After the development of symptoms, survival time is about 5 years if left untreated.

Symptoms of aortic regurgitation include dyspnea, fatigue, and palpitations. Angina is a late and ominous sign that may occur without the presence of coronary artery disease (Stoelting & Dierdorf, 1993). Symptoms generally become severe when the regurgitant fraction of the SV exceeds 60%. The symptoms result from progressive volume overload of the left ventricle (Stoelting & Dierdorf, 1993). Stroke volume is reduced as a result of regurgitant flow into the left ventricle. A decreased systemic vascular resistance and an increased HR will aid in improving SV by increasing it and reducing the interval of diastolic regurgitant flow. As a result, patients with aortic regurgitation may improve with exercise and exhibit signs of pulmonary edema at rest.

Left ventricular eccentric hypertrophy develops with chronic aortic regurgitation from the increased volume load. Mild aortic regurgitation is often accompanied by an increased ejection fraction and chronic peripheral vasodilation. With moderate aortic regurgitation, the continued dilation and hypertrophy of the left ventricle lead to irreversible left ventricular myocardial damage and left ventricular dysfunction. Signs and symptoms of congestive heart failure may be noted. Severe aortic regurgitation is often accompanied by coronary artery disease due to the increased myocardial oxygen demand of the hypertrophied left ventricle. Cardiac output is decreased at this stage with compensatory sympathetic vasocon-

striction in the peripheral vessels, which serves to further decrease the CO.

Aortic stenosis causes the outflow obstruction of blood from the left ventricle to the aorta as the result of a calcified or degenerated valve. Aortic stensois can be classified as valvular, subvalvular, or supravalvular depending on the anatomic location of the stenotic lesion. Pure valvular aortic stenosis is the most common defect and may be due to a congenital bicuspid valve that calcifies, rheumatic valvular degeneration, or senile degeneration of the valve with aging.

Patients who develop aortic stenosis secondary to rheumatic fever may remain asymptomatic for more than 30 years. Congenital bicuspid valve calcification usually occurs after the age of 30 and in the seventh and eighth decades of life. The onset of symptoms is an ominous sign and indicates a life expectancy of less than 5 years. The normal adult aortic valve area is 2.6 cm^2 to 3.5 cm^2, which represents a normal valve index of 2 cm/m^2. Critical aortic stenosis is noted with a valve index less than 0.5 cm/m^2.

Advanced aortic stenosis usually presents with a classic triad of symptoms: angina, dyspnea on exertion, and syncope (Stoelting & Dierdorf, 1993). The left ventricle becomes hypertrophied and noncompliant as the muscle mass increases due to pressure overload. Eventually, with progression of the disease, the left ventricle will dilate as well as hypertrophy from increases in volume. When this occurs, contractility may be compromised, leading to a decrease in ejection fraction. The onset of dyspnea usually signals the beginning of congestive heart failure in the patient with aortic stenosis. Once heart failure occurs, the prognosis is very poor, with life expectancy of only 1 to 2 years (Hensley & Martin, 1995). The development of atrial fibrillation often is associated with the onset of other symptoms, as the loss of atrial systole can expedite heart failure or hypotension in the patient with aortic stenosis.

Idiopathic hypertrophic subaortic stenosis is characterized by a left ventricular outflow obstruction that usually results from asymmetric hypertrophy of the interventricular septum. Hyperdynamic ventricular function exists in spite of elevated left ventricular end-diastolic pressures, resulting in diastolic wall stiffness. The obstruction is variable, instead of fixed as seen in aortic stenosis. The hypertrophied outflow tract often narrows during systole to obstruct left ventricular ejection (Reich, Brooks, & Kaplan, 1990).

Symptoms include dyspnea on exertion, fatigue, syncope, and angina. Most patients will be asymptomatic and the disease may manifest as sudden death in persons under the age of 30 (Kaplan, 1993). Ventricular arrhythmias and supraventricular arrhythmias may occur. The ECG will demonstrate left ventricular hypertrophy and deep, broad Q waves. The obstruction is exacerbated by increased contractility, decreased preload, and decreased left ventricular afterload.

Treatment consists of beta-blockers and calcium channel blockers to decrease contractility. Calcium channel blockers may aid in relaxing the ventricle and improving compliance. Amiodarone is an effective treatment for the arrhythmias (Morgan & Mikhail, 1996). Vasodilators, digoxin, and diuretics should be avoided because these agents may worsen the left ventricular obstruction. Surgical intervention in the form of a left septectomy or myotomy may be needed for patients exhibiting moderate to severe symptoms.

Volatile agents have myocardial depressant effects that are desirable for the patient with IHSS. Regional anesthesia should be avoided, as the resulting sympathectomy will decrease preload and afterload. Vasoconstrictors such as phenylephrine should be utilized because these agents have no positive inotropic effects.

Conduction Defects Requiring Pacemakers

The patient with cardiac disease may present with an artificial pacemaker in place, or the need may arise during surgery for temporary pacing. If the patient has a pacemaker in place, the adequacy of the device should be confirmed prior to surgery. The indications for artificial pacing include symptomatic bradyarrhythmias, a new BBB, type II second-degree AV block, third-degree AV block, chronic bifascicular and trifascicular block, sinus node dysfunction, carotid sinus syndrome, and refractory supraventricular tachyarrhythmias (Hensley & Martin, 1995). Pacing systems may be either temporary or permanent. Basically, the purpose of the pacemaker is to initiate electrical–mechanical activity in a heart that is unable to maintain its own automaticity (Baller & Kirsner, 1995).

Pacing sites include the atrium, ventricle, or both. Pacemakers are expected to monitor and react to the intrinsic activity of either or both chambers (Moses, Schneider, Miller, & Taylor, 1991). Some pacemakers are also able to sense the patient's physiologic state and adjust to the increasing CO requirements (Baller & Kirsner, 1995).

A five-letter code of nomenclature is used to define pacemaker types, as indicated in Table 10–7 (Hensley & Martin, 1995). The first letter is the chamber that is sensed. The second letter indicates the paced chamber. The third letter indicates the response to sensing. The fourth letter relates to programmability of the pacemaker, and the fifth letter identifies whether the pacemaker possesses antiarrhythmic functions.

Temporary ventricular pacing may be indicated for the treatment of short-term conduction defects until symptoms are abolished. Temporary pacing can be established with transvenous pacing electrodes inserted into the subclavian, jugular, and basilic veins to the right atrium via the superior vena cava and then through the tricuspid valve into the right ventricle. Permanent ventricular pacing is indicated for patients who suffer from congestive heart failure with associated dysrhythmias, conduction defects, postmyocardial infarction, symptomatic sinus bradycardia, and fascicular block.

▶ PERIANESTHETIC PLAN FOR THE CARDIOVASCULAR SYSTEM

General Considerations of the Cardiovascular System

The patient with cardiovascular disease presenting for surgery has many unique considerations. Risk factors associated with cardiovascular disease need to be identified and prepared for appropriately. Standard anesthesia monitoring is needed and in some cases, invasive hemodynamic monitors must be inserted. An arterial line may be beneficial in patients with cardiovascular disease for

TABLE 10–7. Pacemaker Codes

	I	II	III	IV	V
Category	Chamber(s) paced	Chamber(s) sensed	Response to sensing	Programmability, rate modulation	Antitachyarrhythmia function(s)
	O = None	O = None	O = None	O = None	O = None
	A = Atrium	A = Atrium	T = Triggered	P = Simple programmable	P = Pacing (antitachyarrhythmia)
	V = Ventricle	V = Ventricle	I = Inhibited	M = Multiprogrammable	S = Shock
	D = Dual (A + V)	D = Dual (A + V)	D = Dual (T + I)	C = Communicating	D = Dual (P + S)
				R = Rate modulation	
Manufacturer's designation	S = Single (A or V)	S = Single (A or V)			

From Hensley, P. A. & Martin, D. E. (1995). The practice of cardiac anesthesia (p. 394). Philadelphia: Lippincott-Raven. Reprinted with permission.

beat-to-beat blood pressure regulation. Placement of the arterial catheter may be difficult in the presence of atherosclerosis, necessitating the need to cannulate larger arteries such as the femoral, brachial, or axillary arteries rather than the radial artery. The brachial artery is associated with a higher risk of ischemic complications due to the lack of collateral blood supply. If the axillary artery must be used for cannulation, the left is preferable because the risk of carotid artery obstruction or embolization is lower.

A central venous line may allow for appropriate management of fluids in the patient with heart disease. If a large blood loss is anticipated, the central venous line will aid in assessing replacement of volume. If the use of inotropic agents is a possibility, a central venous line will also allow for rapid administration of these drugs.

The use of a pulmonary artery catheter has been considered controversial, although there is some data that support a reduction in perioperative complications in high-risk patients (ASA, 1993). Cardiac indices, volume status, and the mixed venous oxygenation are all valuable tools for management of a critically ill patient, particularly one with cardiac disease.

Certain positions, such as the lateral decubitus or prone position, are associated with ventilatory and hemodynamic changes that may impact the patient with cardiovascular disease. These effects should be carefully monitored and may necessitate the need for more extensive hemodynamic monitoring. Positions that involve rotation of the neck should be used with caution in the patient with carotid occlusion, as cerebral blood flow may be severely limited or obliterated.

Preoperative Considerations Related to the Cardiovascular System

Risk factors for surgery such as a recent myocardial infarction (within 6 months) or evidence of congestive heart failure should be identified in the preoperative period. Conditions such as hypertension need to be carefully evaluated. A patient with uncontrolled hypertension (diastolic pressure greater than 110 mmHg) may need to be treated and possibly have elective surgery delayed to permit better control of the blood pressure. Table 10–8 summarizes the minimal preoperative studies needed to evaluate the cardiac patient preoperatively.

The decision to administer premedication should be based on the patient's cardiac condition, level of preoperative anxiety, and the patient's coexisting diseases. The risks and benefits of a premedication should be carefully weighed. Anxiety may contribute to tachycardia which can increase myocardial oxygen consumption (Hug, 1994). If this is the case, allaying the patient's anxiety is beneficial. A premedication may increase patient comfort during the placement of invasive lines. Care should

TABLE 10–8. Minimal Preoperative Studies Used in Evaluating the Cardiac Patient

Function	Factors to Consider
Angina	Type Severity Medication Dosage
Electrocardiogram	Presence of arrythmias Myocardial ischemia Cardiac catheterization report
Left ventricular	Ejection fraction Left ventricular end-diastolic pressure Cardiac output Cardiac index
Peripheral vascular	Carotid stenosis Aortic disease Renal vascular disease
Respiratory	Pulmonary function studies Arterial blood gas analysis Chest x-ray
Renal/hepatic	Blood urea nitrogen Serum creatinine Prothrombin time Partial thromboplastin time Platelet and bleeding times
Fluid compartment volume	State of hydration Electrolyte values Pulmonary artery pressure Pulmonary wedge pressure Pulmonary mean pressure
Chronic medications	Type Dosage Side effects
General appearance	Dyspnea Exercise tolerance Retinopathy Xanthoma

be taken not to compromise the patient's cardiac or respiratory condition with excessive or inappropriate medications.

An understanding of the patient's daily medications and how these may interact with the drugs to be given during the procedure is necessary. A thorough evaluation of the cardiac disease is necessary, including exercise tolerance, previous myocardial infarction and the date on which it occurred, hypertension, congestive heart failure, peripheral vascular disease, cerebral vascular disease, smoking history and its effects, recent laboratory tests, and previous anesthesia records if this is a reoperation. Cardiac catherization data, including coronary artery status and ejection fraction, will increase the anesthetist's understanding of the individual patient's needs.

Appropriate prophylaxis for bacterial endocarditis should be employed. The patient with heart disease may not be a candidate for outpatient surgery, depending on the nature of the surgery and patient's physical condition.

The patient should be evaluated to determine what type of anesthetic technique will be utilized. Regional anesthesia may be an option if appropriate for the procedure, allowing the patient to avoid such stimulating events as endotrachial intubation and exposure to higher levels of medications that may induce myocardial depression. For a patient with congestive heart failure, regional anesthesia may not be a good choice because the induced sympathectomy may be poorly tolerated. Vasodilation may be beneficial in some cases as a result of the increased forward blood flow if the patient tolerates regional anesthesia.

The patient's routine medications should be administered on the day of surgery. Particularly, the cardiac-related medications, such as antihypertensives and digoxin, should be administered. Antihypertensive agents, if neglected, may result in rebound hypertension (Wray, Rothstein, & Thomas, 1997).

Excessive blood loss is often associated with cardiac and vascular surgery. If the patient is undergoing a cardiovascular procedure, a type and cross for blood should be done and blood should be readily available in the OR.

A patient with a history of carotid disease should be carefully evaluated for the presence of preexisting neurologic deficits. Preoperatively, the patient should turn his or her head to each side for evaluation of neurologic changes associated with head position.

The anesthetist needs to thoroughly understand the pathophysiology of the patient's disease. Maintenance or improvement of the patient's hemodynamic status should be the overall goal when formulating the anesthetic plan (Lake, 1985).

Intraoperative Considerations Related to the Cardiovascular System

Induction of Anesthesia

Induction of anesthesia is always a critical period. The patient with cardiovascular disease has special needs that must be considered. The cardiac status of the patient will dictate what agents should be used for induction and how the case will be managed. Agents that produce myocardial depression should be used carefully, especially in the presence of ventricular failure. These agents include sodium pentothal, dipravan, and, to some degree, all the inhalational agents. Etomidate is associated with less myocardial depressant effects than other agents, but may produce hypotension in a hypovolemic patient or if depressed ventricular function exists.

Fentanyl is an opioid that does not exhibit myocardial depressant effects, even at high doses, although it may exaggerate the cardiovascular effects of other agents (diazepam, nitrous oxide). For the patient with ventricular dysfunction, high doses of opioids (50 µg/kg to 100 µg/kg) for induction and maintenance of anesthesia is a widely accepted practice. Due to the climate of managed care and the need to expedite a patient's discharge from intensive care, lower doses of opioids (10 µg/kg to 25 µg/kg) have been used in conjunction with inhalation agents, propofol, and benzodiazepines without patient compromise. Other opioids, primarily sufentanil, are often used for induction and maintenance of cardiac surgical cases.

Benzodiazepines (diazepam and midazolam) have been used for the induction of anesthesia with minimal myocardial depressant effects, although midazolam may decrease SVR when combined with opioids at high doses. These agents do not have analgesic effects and must be combined with analgesic agents.

Ketamine is generally avoided for induction in patients with cardiac disease due to its sympathomimetic effects that can be detrimental to the patient with heart disease. Dipravan and sodium pentathol can be used for induction if titrated carefully, but should probably be reserved for patients with good ventricular function.

Muscle relaxants should be chosen with regard to their cardiovascular effects and the time interval of the surgery. Pancuronium has a vagolytic effect that may not be desirable in the patient with cardiac disease as the increase in HR can increase myocardial oxygen consumption. Vecuronium, pipercuronium, and doxacurium are associated with cardiac stability. Agents such as atracurium, which may cause histamine release, may be avoided.

Endotracheal intubation is a highly stressful time during an anesthetic, but is particularly critical in patients with cardiovascular disease. The stress response should be attenuated with appropriate levels of narcotics and/or other agents before attempting to intubate the trachea. The release of catecholamines in response to stressful stimuli will cause tachycardia and hypertension, which will increase myocardial oxygen consumption.

Maintenance of Anesthesia

Once the induction of anesthesia is safely accomplished, the patient can generally be maintained on a combination of inhalation agent, opioids, benzodiazepines, and a muscle relaxant. As mentioned previously, caution should be used with these agents when the patient has depressed myocardial function.

Prior to surgery, all invasive lines and monitors should be connected when indicated. The decision to connect these monitors before or after induction will be made based on the patient's cardiac status. Once hemodynamic monitoring begins, the values should be accurately interpreted and treated accordingly.

The basic principles of anesthesia, such as proper airway maintenance and positioning, should be attended to in addition to the patient's special cardiovascular needs. The surgical incision stimulus should be prepared for and attenuated with an adequate level of anesthesia. The anesthetist should be aware of what the surgeon is doing and be prepared for the various phases of the surgery.

Based on the patient's condition, a baseline arterial blood gas may be obtained, as well as serum electrolytes and hemoglobin/hematocrit. If large volume shifts are expected, this data will be useful in managing the patient. It is wise to notify other persons in the room that an arterial sample is being drawn from the line to avoid alarm when it is noticed that the arterial waveform has disappeared from the screen.

Cardiopulmonary Bypass

Cardiopulmonary bypass (CPB) will typically be utilized for heart cases and some aortic surgeries. Total CPB is obtained when the lungs and heart are completely bypassed and the entire systemic venous return to the heart is collected and delivered to an oxygenator via gravity drainage, and when oxygenated blood is pumped at arterial pressure into one of the great arteries. Cardiopulmonary bypass is able to sustain systemic blood flow, oxygenation, and ventilation with nonpulsatile flow.

The CPB circuit works by draining blood from the vena cava by gravity through the venous cannula into the venous reservoir. Blood from the surgical field is suctioned into a cardiotomy reservoir and then drained into the venous reservoir. A ventricular venting device also is used during aortic cross-clamping to remove blood from the heart. The venous blood travels through the oxygenator and the heat exchanger, and is then filtered through the bubble catcher and pumped back into the arterial return line, delivering oxygenated blood to the body (Gravlee, Davis, & Utley, 1993). Refer to Figure 10–8 for a diagram of the CPB circuit.

Once full CPB is initiated, the ventilator and any inhalation agents on the anesthesia machine should be discontinued. The patient should be well relaxed and anesthetized. Supplemental doses of muscle relaxants and intravenous (IV) anesthetics may be needed prior to bypass. Intravenous infusions such as inotropes should be discontinued. The MAP should be monitored and generally is maintained between 50 torr and 80 torr. Pump flow is generally maintained at 2 L/min to 2.5 L/min per square meter of BSA. An initial decrease in MAP may occur as a result of the hemodilution that occurs when cardiopulmonary bypass is begun and the patient receives a 2-L crystalloid dilution of his or her blood volume. Vasoconstricting agents may be needed to maintain MAP at desirable levels. Mean arterial pressures greater than 150 mmHg are associated with cerebral hemorrhage and aortic dissection, and should be avoided.

Hematocrit generally should not be allowed to fall below 20%. Packed red blood cells can be added if the hematocrit decreases to this level. Temperature should be monitored in at least two locations during bypass. A core temperature, obtained with a nasopharyngeal probe, reflects brain temperature. A shell temperature obtained with a rectal probe will reflect the temperature of the body's muscle and fat tissues that constitute the majority of the body's mass.

Inotropic support may be needed for the patient

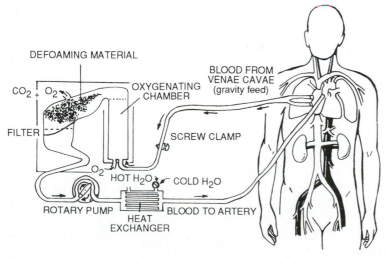

A   **B**

Figure 10–8. Cardiopulmonary bypass circuit.

with cardiac disease intraoperatively. Indications include decreased CO and poor contractility. Often inotropic support is needed to aid in weaning a patient undergoing heart surgery from cardiopulmonary bypass. A patient with a decreased ejection fraction may benefit from the addition of a phosphodiesterase inhibitor such as amrinone or milrinone. These agents have inotropic and vasodilator properties. When used in conjunction with a catecholamine, a synergistic positive inotropic effect is created.

Intraoperative Management of the Patient with Ischemic Heart Disease

For patients undergoing surgery with a previous history of myocardial infarction, there is an increased risk of reinfarction during the perioperative period. The risk of a reoccurring myocardial infarction is greatest within 3 months after the previous infarct (Hensley & Martin, 1995). With advances in anesthesia management and monitoring, including aggressive intervention to maintain hemodynamic stability, the risk of perioperative infarction has decreased (Estafanous, Barash, & Reves, 1994).

A critical factor in managing patients with coronary artery disease is avoidance of increased myocardial oxygen demand. This can be accomplished by preventing tachycardia and hypertension with appropriate levels of anesthesia during the perioperative period. Hypotension, especially decreases in diastolic blood pressure, should be avoided to maintain adequate coronary perfusion.

The management of patients with ischemia associated with hypertrophy focuses on the reduction of the hyperdynamic state. Coronary flow must be maintained because it may already be insufficient to meet the myocardial oxygen demands. Filling pressures must be maintained to aid in dilation of the hypertrophied, noncompliant ventricle in order to maintain CO. As in all types of ischemic heart disease, maintenance of diastolic blood pressure is critical for maintenance of the coronary perfusion pressure.

Myocardial depressants, if used cautiously, may be beneficial for the patient with a hypertrophied ventricle. These agents, such as enflurane, beta-blockers, and sodium thiopental, may suppress ventricular contractility without deleterious effects on CO.

Intraoperative Management of the Patient with Congestive Heart Failure

The anesthetist must aggressively monitor the patient who presents for surgery with heart failure. This includes monitoring with a pulmonary artery catheter and possibly transesophageal echocardiography. Drugs that decrease the sympathetic tone should be administered with caution. Hypotension and low CO should be

treated carefully. Fluids should be minimized and guided by hemodynamic parameters. Dilators and inotropic agents may be needed to increase CO.

If inotropic support is inadequate to maintain CO, an intra-aortic balloon pump (IABP) may be placed in the patient with a low CO state or in the patient with myocardial ischemia. The IABP may be inserted preoperatively but is often inserted during cardiac procedures to aid in weaning from CPB. The IABP is generally placed by way of the femoral artery, with the balloon in the descending thoracic aorta to prevent occlusion of the carotid artery. The balloon inflates during diastole, displacing blood from the thoracic aorta and increasing aortic root pressure. This increases diastolic filling pressure and subsequently results in increased coronary artery perfusion.

The inflation of the balloon must be timed with the dicrotic notch of the arterial blood pressure tracing to prevent the balloon from impeding ventricular ejection (Figs. 10–9 and 10–10). The ECG may also be utilized for timing of IABP inflation as illustrated in Figure 10–11. Deflation should occur when the arterial pressure reaches its lowest level at the onset of the next ventricular pulse. This results in an abrupt reduction in left ventricular afterload and improved SV. The ratio of native beats to IABP varies depending on the patient. However, the IABP should never be left in place when off, as it represents a thrombogenic source.

Intraoperative Management of the Patient with Valvular Disease

The anesthetic management of the patient with mitral regurgitation should include the avoidance of factors that exacerbate the regurgitation such as bradycardia and increased vascular resistance. Preload should be maintained with care taken to avoid excessive volume overload, as this may worsen the regurgitation. Mitral regurgitation often results in an enlarged V wave on the pulmonary capillary wedge pressure tracing that may resemble the pulmonary artery pressure tracing. Care must be taken to differentiate the two waves to prevent leaving the pulmonary artery catheter in a permanent wedge position.

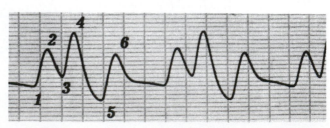

Figure 10–9. Intra-aortic balloon pump tracing.

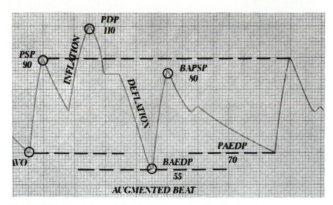

Figure 10–10. Intra-aortic balloon pump tracing.

The goals of management for the patient with mitral stenosis include increasing left atrial pressure to increase forward flow across the stenotic valve and to maintain left ventricular preload, avoid tachycardia, maintain contractility, maintain the SVR, and decrease pulmonary vascular resistance (Hensley & Martin, 1995). Fluids should be guided carefully with appropriate hemodynamic monitoring to avoid overloading an already distended left atrium. Hypoxia should be avoided, as this condition will increase pulmonary vascular resistance.

Anesthetic management goals for the patient with aortic regurgitation include increasing or maintaining left ventricular preload, increasing the HR to reduce diastolic regurgitant flow, maintaining contractility, reducing SVR to increase forward flow, and maintaining pulmonary vascular resistance (Hensley & Martin, 1995).

The anesthetic management goals for the patient presenting with aortic stenosis should include increasing or maintaining an appropriate left ventricular volume, a decreased HR to allow adequate filling time of the left ventricle, maintenance of contractility, increasing SVR to maintain CPP, and maintaining pulmonary vascular resistance. Many patients with advanced aortic stenosis appear to have a fixed SV, therefore, CO is rate dependent

and must be maintained. The patient is very sensitive to changes in intravascular volume, necessitating the need for volume management guided by a pulmonary artery catheter (Hensley & Martin, 1995). One must keep in mind that patients with aortic stenosis will have higher pulmonary artery and wedge pressures than the normal patient and must guide fluids by the patient's baseline pressures. Agents with vasodilator properties should be used only with extreme caution, as a loss of vascular resistance is poorly tolerated, and systemic hypotension can result in global left ventricular hypoperfusion and severe ischemia.

Intraoperative Management of the Patient with a Pacemaker

Anesthetic considerations for the patient with a pacemaker include a careful history and understanding of the type of pacemaker involved. The ECG should be observed at all times for signs of pacemaker malfunction. If a pacemaker is being inserted, the patient should be made comfortable, and dysrhythmias resulting from insertion should be controlled. When a temporary pacemaker is in place, the patient needs to be protected from microshock with the use of a rubber sheet or gloves over the exposed pacing leads (Mastropietro, 1992).

Electrical cautery can interfere with a permanent pacemaker's function if the pacer is set in a demand mode because the electrical interference from the cautery may be interpreted as myocardial electrical activity by the pacemaker sensor. Placing a magnet over the chest will convert the demand pacemaker to a fixed, asynchronous mode. Competing rhythms may develop, resulting in dysrhythmias. The characteristics of the pacemaker should be known before applying a magnet; different generators respond to magnets in different ways. If a magnet is used during the surgical procedure, the patient's cardiologist should be informed so the pacemaker can be checked and reprogrammed if needed.

Intraoperative Management for Vascular Disease and Surgery

Peripheral vascular surgery is often associated with substantial blood loss. Methods to rapidly warm and infuse blood and blood products should be available. Patients with peripheral vascular disease often have coexisting diabetes, or cardiac, renal, and cerebral vascular diseases. The considerations for these disease processes and other coexisting diseases should be part of the anesthetic plan.

Aortic surgery represents one of the greatest anesthetic challenges. The procedure is often complicated by large, intraoperative blood loss and aortic cross-clamping. Indications for aortic surgery include aortic dissection, aneurysms, occlusive disease, trauma, and coarctation (Morgan & Mikhail, 1996).

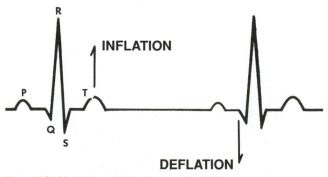

Figure 10–11. Intra-aortic balloon pump tracing.

Aortic dissection occurs when there is a tear in the intimal wall of the aorta, allowing blood to penetrate the wall of the vessel producing a false lumen (Kaplan, 1991). Aortic aneurysms most commonly involve the abdominal aorta, but may occur at any point along the aorta. Aneurysms greater than 4 cm to 5 cm in diameter have an increased incidence of spontaneous rupture and should be electively resected.

Aortic cross-clamping acutely increases left ventricular afterload and compromises organ perfusion distal to the point of occlusion. Paraplegia and renal failure may occur as a result of ischemia to the spinal cord and kidneys. Release of the aortic cross-clamp often results in severe hypotension that must be treated with volume replacement. Metabolic acidosis also occurs with cross-clamp release. An infusion of sodium bicarbonate or boluses of the drug may be used to counteract the acidosis. Venous access with large-bore catheters is essential for aortic surgical procedures because the blood loss associated with this type of surgery can be massive. Pulmonary artery catheters are invaluable for intraoperative management of fluids.

The patient with myocardial disease represents an additional challenge to the anesthetist during aortic surgery. The aortic cross-clamp imposes an additional workload on the heart. The patient may develop myocardial ischemia or increased pulmonary artery pressures during cross-clamping. Vasodilators that decrease left ventricular afterload also may decrease these complications. Left ventricular assist devices may be used when the aortic cross-clamp is to be placed very high on the thoracic aorta or if the patient has severe myocardial dysfunction.

Surgery involving the ascending aorta and aortic arch usually requires CPB and hypothermic circulatory arrest. The patient is cooled to about 15°C or when a flat electrocardiogram (ECG) is obtained. Cardiopulmonary bypass is terminated briefly while the aortic repair is performed. This type of surgery is associated with postbypass coagulopathy due to the excessive hypothermia and long rewarming phase. Renal protection with mannitol and possibly a low-dose infusion of dopamine should be considered.

Intraoperative Management of the Patient with Carotid Disease

The patient with carotid disease often presents to the OR with uncontrolled hypertension and hypovolemia. Hypotension on induction may occur as a result, with exaggerated hypertensive responses to stimulation. A careful induction with adequate fluid volume replacement can minimize these problems. The hypertension is controlled more effectively if the patient receives the appropriate antihypertensives as scheduled prior to surgery.

Many of these patients also present with diabetes, requiring monitoring and control of blood glucose levels.

Regardless of the anesthetic agents utilized, MAP should be maintained at or slightly above the patient's normal range to ensure adequate blood flow to the brain via collateral perfusion. Normocapnia is preferable, as hypercapnia may induce intracerebral steal and excessive hypocapnia will decrease cerebral perfusion.

Manipulation of the carotid area can result in severe bradycardia as a result of the carotid baroceptor reflex. Removing the stimulation will generally cause the HR to return to normal. If this is not effective, atropine should be administered.

Postoperative Considerations Related to the Cardiovascular System

The control of postoperative pain is extremely important because pain can result in an increased myocardial oxygen consumption. The amount of pain medication must be carefully considered as opioids may cause respiratory depression and interfere with a timely extubation.

The decision to extubate the patient should be based on the hemodynamic stability during the procedure, the amount of blood loss and fluid volume administered during surgery, and the type of surgery that was performed. Often a patient with heart disease will benefit from a delayed extubation if excessive postoperative pain is expected or if the blood loss was considerable.

The decision to send the patient to the PACU or the intensive care unit (ICU) also should be weighed based on the above criteria. If a delay in extubation is expected, sending the patient to the ICU may be desirable.

For the patient undergoing cardiac or vascular surgery, there is the risk of postoperative bleeding from graft sites. The patient's hemodynamic status should be carefully monitored for signs of fluid loss.

▶ CASE STUDY

A 61-year-old woman with a left lung mass presents for a left thoracotomy. The patient has a 30-year history of smoking, hypertension, and adult-onset diabetes that is well-controlled with insulin. She denies angina, but becomes short of breath when cleaning her house. A cardiac catherization was done and revealed 90% stenosis of the left anterior descending artery. Her lab values are within normal ranges. Her blood pressure is 150/90, with a HR of 89 bpm. Her preoperative medications include insulin and enalapril for blood pressure control.

1. What is the most important aspect of induction for this patient?

Controlling HR to avoid tachycardia to prevent an increase in myocardial oxygen demand.

2. What is one possible explanation for the lack of chest pain?

   Diabetic patients frequently have silent ischemia.

3. What are some possible intraoperative or postoperative complications this patient may encounter?

   Control of blood glucose and pulmonary complications such as difficulty in weaning from mechanical ventilation due to the history of smoking may occur in this patient.

4. Which of the following infusions may be beneficial for this patient? Nitroglycerin or dopamine?

   Nitroglycerin can contribute to coronary artery dilation and may be beneficial. Unless the patient becomes hemodynamically unstable, inotropic agents should be avoided because they will increase myocardial oxygen demand.

5. Why would hypovolemia from blood loss be detrimental to this patient?

   The coronary arteries are perfused during diastole. If the patient is hypovolemic, there will be inadequate filling pressures for perfusion of the coronary arteries.

► SUMMARY

The anesthetist must have a thorough understanding of cardiac anatomy, physiology, and pathophysiology to provide a thorough assessment and develop an anesthetic plan. The patient's history can provide important information concerning the stability of the cardiovascular system and key information essential to a safe anesthetic. Objective data obtained from the physical exam should focus on physical appearance, evaluation of pulses and peripheral veins, and analysis of heart sounds. Diagnostic studies to evaluate the cardiovascular system should be appropriate to the surgical procedure intended and the patient's history of cardiac disease. Twelve-lead ECG analysis is indicated in all patients with a history of cardiac disease or in those patients where it may be necessary to verify historical findings. Other diagnostic studies should be evaluated as needed, including cardiac angiography and echocardiography. The anesthetic plan should be tailored for the procedure and be appropriate to provide maximum cardiovascular stabilization. Hemodynamic stability is the anesthetic goal throughout the perioperative period. Although managing the patient with cardiovascular disease can be challenging, maintenance of hemodynamic stability is important for all patients with or without a history of cardiac disease.

► KEY CONCEPTS

- Maintenance or improvement of the patient's hemodynamic status should be the overall goal of the anesthetic plan.
- Limitations related to cardiovascular disease can lead to an increase in morbidity and mortality if not determined preoperatively. For example, patients presenting with unstable angina may have a higher incidence of myocardial infarction and operative mortality.
- A critical factor in managing patients with coronary artery disease is to avoid increased myocardial oxygen demand by preventing tachycardia and hypertension and maintaining appropriate levels of anesthesia.
- Electrical cautery can interfere with a permanent pacemaker's function if the pacer is set in a demand mode, as the electrical interference from the cautery may be interpreted as myocardial electrical activity by the pacemaker sensor.
- Agents producing myocardial depression should be used judiciously, especially in the presence of ventricular failure.
- During carotid surgery, MAP should be maintained at or slightly above the patient's normal range to ensure adequate blood flow to the brain via collateral perfusion.
- Aortic vessel surgery represents one of the greatest anesthetic challenges because the procedure is often complicated by large, intraoperative blood losses and the physiologic sequelae of aortic cross-clamping.
- The control of postoperative pain is extremely important, as pain can result in an increased myocardial oxygen consumption.

► STUDY QUESTIONS

1. What relationship is demonstrated by the Frank–Starling curve?

2. What is an important determinant of both supply and demand to the myocardium and coronary blood flow?

3. Venous distention in the jugular veins when a patient is in the sitting position may indicate the presence of which cardiovascular disorder?

4. Name the classic triad of symptoms seen with aortic stenosis.

5. Why is the stress response, which is evoked with such stimuli as endotracheal intubation, potentially harmful to the patient with coronary artery disease?

KEY REFERENCES

Estafanous, F. G., Barash, P. G., & Reves, J. G. (Eds.) (1994). *Cardiac anesthesia: Principles and clinical practice.* Philadelphia: Lippincott.

Hensley, F. A. & Martin, D. E. (Eds.) (1995). *A practical approach to cardiac anesthesia* (2nd ed.). Boston: Little, Brown & Company.

Kaplan, J. A. (Ed.) (1993). *Cardiac anesthesia* (3rd ed.). Philadelphia: Saunders, pp. 90–117

REFERENCES

Baller, M. R. & Kirsner, K. M. (1995). Anesthetic implications of implanted pacemakers. *AANA Journal, 63*(3), 209–216.

Berne, R. M. & Levy, M. N. (1990). Cardiovascular system. In R. M. Berne & M. N. Levy (Eds.), *Principles of physiology* (pp. 188–300). St. Louis: Mosby.

Bernstein, A., Camm, A. J., Fletcher, R. D., Gold, R. D., Rickards, A. F., Smyth N. P., Spielman, S. R., & Sutton, R. (1987). The NASPE/BPEG generic pacemaker code for antibradyarrhythmia and adaptive-rate pacing and antitachyarrhythmia devices. *PACE Pacing Clinics in Electrophysiology, 10*(1), 794–799.

Braunwald, E. (Ed) (1988). *A textbook of cardiovascular medicine* (3rd ed., pp. 53–61). Philadelphia: Saunders.

De Hert, S. G., Rodrigus, I. E., Haenen, L. R., De Mulder, P. A., & Gillebert, T. C. (1996). Recovery of systolic and diastolic left ventricular function early after cardiopulmonary bypass. *Anesthesiology, 85*(5), 1063–1075.

Despostis, G. J., Filos, K. S., Zoys, T. N., Hogue, C. W., Jr., Spitznagel, E., & Lappas, D. G. (1995). Factors associated with excessive postoperative blood loss and hemostatic transfusion requirements: A multivariate analysis in cardiac surgical patients. *Anesthesia & Analgesia, 82,* 13–21.

Estafanous, F. G., Barash, P. G., & Reves, J. G. (Eds.) (1994). *Cardiac anesthesia: Principles and clinical practice* (pp. 3–7, 241–248, 294–299). Philadelphia: Lippincott.

Ferraris, V. A. & Ferraris, S. P. (1996). Risk factors for postoperative morbidity. *Journal of Thoracic and Cardiovascular Surgery, 111*(4), 731–739.

Foster, S. D. & Reeves-Viets, J. L. (1992). Perioperative monitoring. In W. R. Waugaman, S. D. Foster, & B. M. Rigor (Eds.), *Principles and practice of nurse anesthesia* (2nd ed., pp. 195–220). Norwalk, CT: Appleton & Lange.

Ganong, W. F. (1993). *Review of medical physiology* (pp. 524–530). Norwalk, CT: Appleton & Lange.

Gravlee, G. P., Davis, R. F., & Utley, J. R. (Eds.) (1993). *Cardiopulmonary bypass: Principles and practice* (pp. 44–48). Baltimore: Williams & Wilkins.

Guyton, A. & Hall, J. (Eds.) (1997). *Human physiology and mechanics of disease* (6th ed., pp. 85–110). Philadelphia: Saunders.

Hensley, F. A. & Martin, D. E. (Eds.) (1995). *A practical approach to cardiac anesthesia* (2nd ed., pp. 5–605). Boston: Little, Brown & Company.

Hug, C. C. (1994). Anesthesia for adult cardiac surgery. In R. D. Miller (Ed.), *Anesthesia* (4th ed., pp. 1759–1809). New York: Churchill Livingstone.

Kaplan, J. A. (Ed.) (1993). *Cardiac anesthesia* (3rd ed., pp. 243–248). Philadelphia: Saunders.

Kaplan, J. A. (Ed.) (1991). *Vascular anesthesia* (pp. 107–179, 363–394). New York: Churchill Livingstone.

Karp, R. B., Hillel, L., & Wechsler, A. S. (Eds.) (1996). *Advances in cardiac surgery* (Vol. 7, pp. 32–54). St. Louis: Mosby.

Kirklin, J. W. & Barrett-Boyes, B. G. (Eds.) (1993). *Cardiac surgery* (2nd ed., pp. 61–80, 167–172). New York: Churchill Livingstone.

Lake, C. L. (Ed.) (1985). *Cardiovascular anesthesia* (pp. 181–185). New York: Springer-Verlag.

Lema, G., Meneses, G., Urzua, J., Jalil, R., Canessa, R., Moran, S., Irarrazaval, M. J., Zalaquett, R., & Orellana, P. (1995). Effects of extracorporeal circulation on renal function in coronary surgical patients. *Anesthesia & Analgesia, 81,* 446–451.

Mastropietro, C. (1992). Anesthesia for cardiac and peripheral vascular surgery. In W. R. Waugaman, S. D. Foster, & B. M. Rigor (Eds.), *Principles and practice of nurse anesthesia* (2nd ed., pp. 705–748). Norwalk, CT: Appleton & Lange.

Mangano, D. T. (1990). Perioperative cardiac morbidity. *Anesthesiology, 72*(1), 153–177.

Maurer, G. (Ed.) (1994). *Transesophageal echocardiography* (pp. 10–11). New York: McGraw-Hill.

McMinn, R. M. H., Hutchings, R. T., Pegington, J., & Abrahams, P. (1993). *Color atlas of human anatomy* (pp. 81–92). London: Mosby-Wolfe.

Morgan, G. E. & Mikhail, M. S. (Eds.) (1996). *Clinical anesthesiology* (pp. 317–395). Stamford, CT: Appleton & Lange.

Moses, H. W., Schneider, J. A., Miller, B. D., & Taylor, G. J. (Eds.) (1991). *A practical guide to cardiac pacing* (3rd ed., pp. 1–88). Boston: Little, Brown & Company.

Perloff, J. K. (1994). Physical examination of the cardiovascular system. In J. H. Stein (Ed.), *Internal medicine* (3rd ed., pp. 15–27). Boston: Little, Brown & Company.

Practice guidelines for pulmonary artery catherization: A report by the American Society of Anesthesiologists task force on pulmonary artery catherization. (1993). *Anesthesiology, 78,* 380.

Reeves-Viets, J. L. (1992). Cardiovascular physiology. In W. R. Waugaman, S. D. Foster, & B. M. Rigor (Eds.), *Principles and practice of nurse anesthesia* (2nd ed., pp. 313–327). Norwalk, CT: Appleton & Lange.

Reich, D. L., Brooks, J. L., & Kaplan, J. A. (1990). Uncommon cardiac diseases. In J. Katz, J. L. Benumof, & L. B. Kadis (Eds.), *Anesthesia and uncommon diseases* (3rd ed., pp. 333–377). Philadelphia: Saunders.

Schwartz, D. S., Ribakove, G. H., Grossi, E. A., Stevens, J. H., Siegel, L. C., St. Goar, F., Peters, W. S., McLoughlin, D., Baumann, F. G., Coluin, S. B., & Galloway, A. C. (1996). Minimally invasive cardiopulmonary bypass with cardioplegic arrest: A closed chest technique with equivalent myocardial protection. *Journal of Thoracic and Cardiovascular Surgery, 111*(3), 556–566.

Shiono, M., Noon, G. P., Coleman, C. L., & Nose, Y. (1993). Overview of ventricular assist devices. In S. J. Quaal, (Ed.), *Cardiac mechanical assistance beyond balloon pumping* (pp. 25–35). St. Louis: Mosby.

Stoelting, R. K. & Dierdorf, S. F. (Eds.) (1993). *Anesthesia and co-existing diseases* (3rd ed., pp. 1–80). New York: Churchill Livingstone.

Stoelting, R. K. (Ed.) (1991). *Pharmacology and physiology in anesthetic practice* (2nd ed., pp. 692–718). Philadelphia: Lippincott-Raven.

Viets, J. L., Martin, P. D., Heaton, D. A., & Biddle, C. (1987). AANA Journal Course: Advanced scientific concepts: Update for nurse anesthetists—Part 1—The cardiovascular system. *AANA Journal, 55*(2), 165–177.

Wray, D. L., Rothstein, P., & Thomas, S. J. (1997). Anesthesia for cardiac surgery. In P. G. Barash, B. F. Cullen, & R. K. Stoelting (Eds.), *Clinical anesthesia* (3rd ed., pp. 835–869). Philadelphia: Lippincott.

Respiratory Assessment in the Adult

Michael Kremer

The management of the airway, ventilation, and uptake and distribution of volatile anesthetic agents all entail knowledge of respiratory anatomy, physiology, and pathophysiology. Anesthesia providers must have strong physical assessment skills with respect to the respiratory system so that pulmonary pathology impacting anesthesia and ventilation can be identified and anesthesia care appropriately modified.

Anesthetic management goals regarding the respiratory system, especially in those patients with respiratory disease should be as follows:

1. Avoid perioperative hypoxemia.
2. Avoid perioperative bronchospasm.
3. Prevent lobar collapse.
4. Minimize postoperative pulmonary complications that may be related to the surgical site.
5. Avoid postoperative mechanical ventilation.

Changes in vital capacity as measured via pulmonary function testing best predict individuals who may be at risk for developing postoperative pulmonary complications. Patients undergoing upper abdominal or thoracic surgery are at the greatest risk for developing postoperative pulmonary complications. Whenever possible, a laparoscopic surgical approach is the preferred alternative because this technique produces less pulmonary compromise than an abdominal incision (Domino, 1996).

Discussion of respiratory assessment necessitates understanding of pulmonary anatomy, physiology, and pathophysiology. Pulmonary physical assessment includes inspection, palpation, percussion, and auscultation. Diagnostic data, such as pulmonary function testing, is particularly important in patients with known chronic respiratory diseases, such as chronic obstructive pulmonary disease (COPD), or patients at high risk for perioperative pulmonary complications. For example, an obese elderly man with a history of tobacco use scheduled for elective repair of an abdominal aortic aneurysm may require postoperative mechanical ventilation. Careful preoperative assessment of the pulmonary system enables the anesthetic and surgical teams to optimize pulmonary function preoperatively and intraoperatively to minimize postoperative pulmonary sequelae.

▶ ANATOMY OF THE RESPIRATORY SYSTEM

The anatomy of the respiratory system entails the pathway for airflow from the mouth or nose down to the alveolar sacs. As gases flow toward the alveoli, the oropharynx or nasopharynx, larynx, trachea, bronchi, and bronchioles are traversed. The trachea divides at the carina into right and left mainstem bronchi that branch into lobar bronchi. There are three lobar bronchi on the right and two on the left. The bronchi then arborize into segmental, subsegmental, and smaller bronchi. These conducting airways divide approximately 15 to 20 times down to the level of terminal bronchioles, the smallest units that do not participate in gas exchange (Slonim & Hamilton, 1987; Weinberger, 1992).

Beyond the terminal bronchioles, further divisions include respiratory bronchioles, alveolar ducts, and alveoli. The smallest units, from the respiratory bronchioles on, form the portion of the lung concerned with gas exchange and comprise the terminal respiratory unit, known as the acinus. The acinus includes structures distal to a terminal bronchiole: respiratory bronchioles, alveolar ducts, and alveolar sacs. At this level, inhaled gas comes into contact with alveolar walls (septae), and pulmonary capillary blood loads oxygen and unloads carbon dioxide as it courses through the septae (Weinberger, 1992).

The network of pulmonary capillaries and the blood within provide the other major requirement for gas exchange: a transportation system for oxygen and carbon dioxide to and from other body tissues and organs. After blood arrives at the lungs via the pulmonary artery, it courses through a widely branching system of smaller pulmonary arteries and arterioles to the major locale for gas exchange, the pulmonary capillary network. The capillaries generally allow red blood cells to flow through only in single file so that gas exchange between each cell and alveolar gas is facilitated. On completion of gas exchange and travel through the pulmonary capillary bed, oxygenated blood then flows through pulmonary venules and veins, arriving at the left side of the heart, where flow to the systemic circulation is initiated (Slonim & Hamilton, 1987; Weinberger, 1992).

The trachea, bronchi, and bronchioles down to the level of the terminal bronchioles comprise the conducting airways because their function is to provide transport. Beyond the terminal bronchioles are the respiratory bronchioles that mark the beginning of the respiratory zone of the lung, where gas exchange actually occurs. With successive generations of respiratory bronchioles, more alveoli appear along the walls to the site of the alveolar ducts (Weinberger, 1992).

The airways are made up of several tissue layers. Adjacent to the airway lumen is the mucosa, beneath which is a basement membrane separating the epithelial cells of the mucosa from the submucosa. Within the submucosa are mucous glands whose contents are extruded through the mucosa, smooth muscle, and loose connective tissue with nerves and lymphatic vessels. Surrounding the submucosa is a fibrocartilaginous layer that contains the cartilage rings supporting several generations of airways. Finally, a layer of peribronchial tissue with fat, lymphatics, vessels, and nerves encircles the rest of the airway wall (Weinberger, 1992).

The surface layer or mucosa consists of psuedostratified, columnar epithelial cells that appear to be several cells thick in the trachea and large bronchi. The ciliated cells, which are mostly superficial, are responsible for protecting the deeper airways by propelling tracheobronchial secretions toward the pharynx. The cilia have the characteristic ultrastructure seen in other ciliated cells, namely a central pair of microtubules and an outer ring of nine double microtubules. Scattered between the ciliated epithelial cells are secretory cells called goblet cells that produce and discharge mucous into the airway lumen. However, the largest portion of mucous in the respiratory tract is generated by the bronchial mucous glands in the submucosa (Weinberger, 1992).

The surface epithelium has other vital functions that can be altered by various clinical conditions. Because of the tight junctions between epithelial cells at the luminal surface, the epithelium prevents access of inhaled foreign material to deeper levels of the airway wall. Another important function of the surface epithelium is the active transport of ions, especially chloride, to maintain ionic balance in the mucous layer lining of the airway wall. In cystic fibrosis, an abnormality in chloride transport by surface epithelial cells is believed to play a crucial role in the pathogenesis of the disease (Weinberger, 1992).

The deepest layer of epithelial cells, which abuts the basement membrane, includes cells known as basal cells. The function of the basal cells is to differentiate into and replenish the more superficial cells of the mucosa. Another important cell type found in the basal layer of the surface epithelium is the Kulchitsky or K cell, which is thought to have a neuroendocrine function. These different cell types are important not only because of their normal physiologic roles but also because of the way they respond to airway irritation and their potential for becoming neoplastic (Weinberger, 1992).

The submucosal layer has two principal components: bronchial mucous glands and bronchial smooth muscle. The mucous glands are the main source of bronchial secretions: A duct transports the secretions through the mucosa and discharges them into the airway lumen. Airway smooth muscle is present from the trachea to the bronchiolar level and also appears in the alveolar ducts. Disturbances in the quantity and function of the smooth muscle are important in disease, especially in bronchial asthma (Weinberger, 1992).

The fibrocartilaginous layer is important because of the structural support that cartilage provides to the airways. The configuration of cartilage varies significantly at different levels of the tracheobronchial tree, but the function at all levels is probably similar.

Neural Control of Airways

The neural control of airways affects not only the contraction and relaxation of bronchial smooth muscle but also the activity of bronchial mucous glands. An understanding of the innervation, receptors, and mediators involved in neural control of airway function is important because of the potential role that neural control may have in the pathogenesis of asthma and because of the established role of pharmacotherapy that is based on agonism or antagonism of airway receptors. The following discussion focuses on three components of the neural control of airways: the parasympathetic (cholinergic) system, the sympathetic (adrenergic system), and the nonadrenergic inhibitory system (Barnes, 1986).

The parasympathetic nervous system provides the primary bronchoconstrictor tone to the airways. This innervation comes from branches of the vagus nerve, and stimulation of these branches causes contraction of smooth muscle in the airway wall. Additionally, vagal fibers innervate bronchial mucous glands and goblet cells, resulting in increased secretions from both components of the mucous-secreting apparatus. The receptors on smooth muscle and on the mucous-secreting apparatus are muscarinic cholinergic receptors with acetylcholine as the neurotransmitter. These cholinergic receptors are more dense in central versus peripheral airways (Barnes, 1986).

The role of the sympathetic nervous system in controlling airway tone is less clear. Adrenergic beta$_2$-receptors (β_2-receptors) reside in bronchial smooth muscle. These receptors are stimulated by circulating catecholamines. When stimulated, the β_2-receptors activate adenyl cyclase, increasing the intracellular concentration of cyclic adenosine monophosphate (cAMP), causing relaxation of bronchial smooth muscle. In contrast, stimulation of the less important alpha-adrenergic receptors results in bronchoconstriction. Receptor density for the β_2-adrenergic receptors is opposite that of the cholinergic receptors. β_2-adrenergic receptors are more dense in peripheral than in central airways (Barnes, 1986).

There are airway receptors with sensory nerve innervation. These include irritant or cough receptors that are located in the airway epithelial layer and are responsive to various chemical and mechanical stimuli. Neural traffic is carried from these sensory endings in afferent fibers of the vagus nerve. This sensory information is not only communicated to the central nervous system via the afferent vagal fibers but also is responsible for activation of local reflexes causing release of mediators called tachykinins from nerve endings in the airway wall. The tachykinins, which include substance P, can cause bronchoconstriction, increased submucosal gland secretion, and increased vascular permeability (Barnes, 1986).

Anatomy of the Pulmonary Parenchyma

For the lung to function effectively as a gas-exchanging organ, a large surface area must be available for oxygen uptake and carbon dioxide release. At the alveolar wall, where gas exchange occurs, an extensive network of capillaries facilitates this exchange. In the normal lung the capillaries are closely apposed to the alveolar lumen (Taylor, Rehder, Hyatt, & Parker, 1989).

The surface of the alveolar walls is lined by a continuous layer of epithelial cells. Two different types of epithelial cells have been identified: type I and type II cells. Type II cells predominate and produce surfactant, which acts like a detergent, reducing alveolar surface tension. Type I cells act as a barrier preventing the free movement of material such as fluid from the alveolar wall into the alveolar lumen (Taylor, Rehder, Hyatt, & Parker, 1989).

Pulmonary capillaries course through the alveolar walls as part of an extensive network of intercommunicating vessels. Unlike the alveolar epithelial cells, which are normally impermeable, junctions between capillary endothelial cells permit passage of small molecular weight proteins.

Both the alveolar epithelial and capillary endothelial cells rest on a basement membrane. At some regions of the alveolar wall, nothing stands between the epithelial and endothelial cells other than their basement membranes. At other regions a space called the interstitial space, consisting of relatively acellular material, intervenes.

Within the alveolar lumen a thin layer of liquid covers the alveolar epithelial cells. This extracellular alveolar lining layer is composed of an aqueous phase immediately adjacent to the epithelial cells, covered by a surface layer of lipid-rich surfactant produced by type II epithelial cells (Taylor, Rehder, Hyatt, & Parker, 1989).

Anatomy of the Pulmonary Vasculature

In contrast to systemic arteries that carry blood from the left ventricle to the rest of the body, the pulmonary arteries are thin-walled vessels. The pulmonary trunk, which is the outflow from the right ventricle, divides into the right and left main pulmonary arteries, which divide into progressively smaller branches. Throughout these progressive divisions, the pulmonary arteries and their branches travel with companion airways, following the course of the successively dividing bronchial tree (Murray, 1986; Taylor, Rehder, Hyatt, & Parker, 1989).

The pulmonary capillaries form an extensive network of communicating channels coursing through alveolar walls. The capillary system has been described as a continuous meshwork or sheet bounded by alveolar walls on each side and interrupted by *posts* of connective tissue. The capillaries are close to alveolar gas, separated only by alveolar epithelial cells and a small amount of interstitium present in some regions of the alveolar wall. The pulmonary veins, responsible for transporting oxygenated blood from the pulmonary capillaries to the left atrium, combine into sequentially larger vessels, culminating into four major pulmonary veins that enter the left atrium (Taylor, Rehder, Hyatt, & Parker, 1989).

The bronchial arteries, which are part of the systemic circulation, provide nutrient blood flow to a variety of nonalveolar structures, such as the bronchi and the visceral pleural surface. Generally, a single bronchial artery of variable origin supplies the right lung. Two bronchial arteries, usually arising from the thoracic aorta, supply the left lung. Venous blood from the large, extrapulmonary airways drains via bronchial veins into the azygous vein and eventually into the right atrium. In contrast, venous blood from intrapulmonary airways drains into the pulmonary venous system, providing a small amount of anatomic shunting of desaturated blood to the systemic arterial circulation (Weibel, 1984).

An extensive network of lymphatic channels is also located primarily within the connective tissue sheaths around small vessels and airways. Although these channels do not generally course through the interstitial tissue of the alveolar walls, they are in close enough proximity to be effective at removing liquid and some solutes that constantly pass into the interstitium of the alveolar wall (Weinberger, 1992).

► PHYSIOLOGY OF THE RESPIRATORY SYSTEM

Mechanical Aspects of the Lungs and Chest Wall

Both the lungs and the chest wall have elastic properties. These structures have a particular resting volume that they would assume if no internal or external pressure were exerted on them; any deviation from this volume requires some additional influencing force (Taylor, Rehder, Hyatt, & Parker, 1989). If the lungs were removed from the chest and no longer had the external influences of the chest wall and the pleural space acting on them, they would be almost airless. To expand these isolated lungs, positive pressure would have to be exerted on the air spaces, as could be done by putting positive pressure through the airway (Taylor, Rehder, Hyatt, & Parker, 1989).

The alternative to alveolar positive pressure for ventilation is exertion of negative pressure from outside the lungs to cause their expansion. What increases the volume of the isolated lungs from the resting, airless state is the application of a positive transpulmonary pressure, or pressure inside the lungs relative to pressure outside. Either internal pressure can be made positive or external pressure can be made negative—the net effect is the same (Murray, 1986).

Transpulmonary pressure is defined as alveolar pressure (P_{alv}) minus pleural pressure (P_{pl}). The presence of air in the lungs requires that pleural pressure be relatively negative compared with alveolar pressure (Taylor,

Rehder, Hyatt, & Parker, 1989). The relationship between transpulmonary pressure and lung volume can be described for a range of transpulmonary pressures. This relationship is depicted in the compliance curve of the lung. As transpulmonary pressure increases, lung volume naturally increases. The relationship is curvilinear: At high lung volumes, the lungs reach their limit of distensibility, and even rather large increases in transpulmonary pressure do not result in significant increases in lung volume (West, 1995).

Function of the lungs and chest wall involves the elastic properties of each, acting in opposite directions. At the normal resting end-expiratory position of the respiratory system, called functional residual capacity (FRC), the lung is expanded to a volume greater than the resting volume it would have in isolation. However, the chest wall is contracted to a volume smaller than it would have in isolation. At FRC, the tendency of the lung to become smaller (the elastic recoil of the lung) is exactly balanced by the tendency of the chest wall to expand (the outward recoil of the chest wall). The transpulmonary pressure at FRC is equal in magnitude to the pressure across the chest wall but acts in an opposite direction. Therefore, pleural pressure is negative, a consequence of the inward recoil of the lungs and the outward recoil of the chest wall (West, 1995).

The chest wall and lungs are considered as a unit, comprising the respiratory system. The respiratory system has its own compliance curve, which is a combination of the individual compliance curves of the lungs and chest wall. The transrespiratory system pressure, defined as internal minus external pressure, is therefore airway pressure minus atmospheric pressure (Weinberger, 1992).

Two additional lung volumes require discussion along with their determinants. The first, total lung capacity (TLC), is the volume of gas within the lungs at the end of a maximal inhalation. At this point the lungs and chest wall are stretched beyond their resting positions. Muscles of inspiration exert an outward force to counterbalance the inward elastic recoil of the lung and, at TLC, the chest wall. The primary determinants of TLC are the expanding action of the inspiratory musculature balanced by the inward elastic recoil of the lung (West, 1995).

At the other extreme, exhalation produces residual volume (RV). At this point, there is still a significant amount of gas remaining within the lungs. It is not possible to exhale sufficiently to entirely empty the lungs of gas. The chest wall becomes so stiff at low volumes that additional effort by the expiratory muscles cannot further decrease pulmonary volume. Residual volume is determined primarily by the balance of outward recoil of the chest wall and the contracting action of the expiratory musculature. This model for RV applies only to the young individual with normal lungs and airways. With age or disease of the airways, further expulsion of gas during expiration is limited not by the outward recoil of the chest wall but rather by the tendency for the airways to close during expiration and for gas to be trapped behind these closed airways (West, 1995; Weinberger, 1992).

Ventilation

To maintain normal gas exchange, an adequate volume of air must pass through the lungs for provision of oxygen (O_2) to and removal of carbon dioxide (CO_2) from the blood. A normal person under resting conditions typically breathes approximately 500 mL of air per breath 12 to 16 times per minute, resulting in ventilation of 6 L/min to 8 L/min, termed the minute ventilation (V_E). The volume of each breath, or the tidal volume, is not used entirely for gas exchange. A portion of the tidal volume stays in the conducting airways and does not reach the distal part of the lung capable of gas exchange. This portion of the tidal volume that is wasted relative to gas exchange is termed *dead space* (V_D); the volume that reaches the gas-exchanging portion of the lung is called the alveolar volume (V_A). The dead space, which includes the larynx, trachea, and bronchi down to the level of the terminal bronchioles, is approximately 150 mL in a normal person, so that 30% of a tidal volume of 500 mL is wasted (Weinberger, Schwartzstein, & Weiss, 1989).

Carbon dioxide is eliminated as a function of V_A that is equal to the breathing frequency (f) multiplied by V_A. The partial pressure of CO_2 in arterial blood ($Paco_2$), is inversely proportional to V_A so that as V_A increases, $Paco_2$ decreases. Additionally, $Paco_2$ is affected by the body's rate of CO_2 production (Vco_2); if Vco_2 increases without any change in V_A, $Paco_2$ also shows a proportional increase (Weinberger, Schwartzstein, & Weiss, 1989).

Dead space comprises the amount of each breath going to parts of the tracheobronchial tree not involved in gas exchange. The *anatomic dead space* consists of the conducting airways and generally is about 150 mL in a normal person. In disease states, areas of lung that normally participate in gas exchange, such as parts of the terminal respiratory unit, may not receive normal blood flow even though they continue to be ventilated. In these areas, some of the ventilation is wasted; such regions contribute additional volume to the dead space (West, 1995).

A more useful concept than anatomic dead space is physiologic dead space, which accounts for the volume of each breath not involved in gas exchange, whether at the level of the conducting airways or the terminal respiratory units. In certain disease states where there may be areas with normal ventilation but decreased or no perfusion, the physiologic dead space is larger than the anatomic dead space (West, 1995).

Quantitation of the physiologic dead space, or the fraction of the tidal volume that is represented by the dead space (V_D/V_T) can be made by measuring $Paco_2$ and expired Pco_2, ($PEco_2$), and by using the Bohr equation for physiologic dead space:

$$V_D \, Paco_2 - PEco_2 = V_T + Paco_2$$

For gas coming directly from alveoli that have participated in gas exchange, the Pco_2 approximates that of arterial blood. For gas coming from the dead space, the Pco_2 is 0 because the gas never came into contact with pulmonary capillary blood (Weinberger, Schwartzstein, & Weiss, 1989).

Each normal or tidal volume breath can be divided into alveolar volume and dead space, just as the total minute ventilation can be divided into alveolar ventilation and wasted (or dead space) ventilation. Elimination of CO_2 by the lungs is proportional to alveolar ventilation; therefore $Paco_2$ is inversely proportional to alveolar ventilation, not to minute ventilation. The wasted ventilation can be quantitated by the Bohr equation, with use of the principle that increasing amounts of dead space ventilation augment the difference between Pco_2 in arterial blood and expired gas (Weinberger, 1992).

Circulation

Because the entire cardiac output flows from the right ventricle to the lungs and back to the left side of the heart, the pulmonary circulation handles a blood flow of approximately 5 L/min. If the pulmonary vasculature were similar in structure to the systemic vasculature, large pressures would need to be generated because of the thick walls and high resistance offered by systemic arteries. Pulmonary arteries are quite different structurally from systemic arteries, with thin walls that provide much less resistance to flow. Despite equal right and left ventricular outputs, the normal mean pulmonary artery pressure of 15 mmHg is strikingly lower than the normal mean aortic pressure of approximately 95 mmHg (West, 1985).

One important feature of blood flow in the pulmonary capillary bed is the distribution of flow observed in different areas of the lung. The pattern of flow is due to the effects of gravity and the need for blood to be pumped upward to reach the apices of the lungs. In the upright position, the apex of each lung is approximately 25 cm higher than the base, so that the pressure in pulmonary vessels at the apex is 25 cm H_2O (19 mmHg) lower than in pulmonary vessels at the bases. Because flow through these vessels depends on the perfusion pressure, the capillary network at the bases receives much more flow than do capillaries at the apices (West, 1985).

West uses a model of pulmonary blood flow that divides the lung into zones, based on the relationships among pulmonary arterial, venous, and alveolar pressures. The pulmonary arterial and venous pressures depend partly on the vertical location of the vessels in the lung because of the hydrostatic effect (West, 1985). At the apex of the lung (West's zone 1), alveolar pressure exceeds both arterial and venous pressures, and no flow results. In West's zone 2, arterial but not venous pressure exceeds alveolar pressure, and the driving force for flow is determined by the difference between the arterial and alveolar pressures. In West's zone 3, both arterial and venous pressures exceed alveolar pressure, and the driving force is the difference between arterial and venous pressures, as seen in the systemic vasculature (West, 1985; West, 1995).

When cardiac output is increased, the normal pulmonary vasculature is able to handle the increase in flow both by recruiting previously unperfused vessels and by distending previously perfused vessels. The ability to expand the pulmonary vascular bed and decrease vascular resistance allows major increases in cardiac output with exercise to be accompanied by only small increments in mean pulmonary artery pressure. In disease states that affect the pulmonary vascular bed, the ability to recruit additional vessels with increased flow may not be available, and significant increases in pulmonary artery pressure may result (West, 1985).

Diffusion

For oxygen and carbon dioxide to be transferred between the alveolar space and blood in the pulmonary capillary, diffusion through several compartments must take place: alveolar gas, alveolar and capillary walls, plasma, and membrane and cytoplasm of the red blood cell. Under normal circumstances, the process of diffusion of both gases is rapid, and full equilibrium occurs during the transit time of blood flowing through the pulmonary capillary bed. The Po_2 in capillary blood rises from the mixed venous level of 40 torr to the end-capillary level of 100 torr in approximately 0.25 seconds, or one third of the total transit time (0.75 seconds) that an erythrocyte spends within the pulmonary capillaries (West, 1995). Although the diffusion of oxygen is normally a rapid process, it is not instantaneous. The resistance to diffusion comes primarily from the alveolar–capillary membrane and by the reaction that forms oxygenated hemoglobin within the erythrocyte (West, 1995).

Even though limitations on diffusion rarely contribute to hypoxemia, an abnormality in diffusion may be a useful marker for diseases of the pulmonary parenchyma that affect the alveolar–capillary membrane or the volume of blood in the pulmonary capillaries, or both. Rather than using oxygen to measure diffusion within the lung, clinicians generally use carbon monoxide (CO), which also combines with hemoglobin and provides a technically easier test to perform and interpret (Weinberger, 1992).

Oxygen Transport

The eventual goal of tissue oxygenation requires transport of O_2 from the lungs to the peripheral tissues and organs. Therefore, any discussion of oxygenation is incomplete without considering transport mechanisms.

The partial pressure of any gas is the product of the ambient total gas pressure and the proportion of total gas composition made up by the specific gas of interest. For example, air is composed of 21% O_2. Assuming a total pressure of 760 mmHg at sea level and no water vapor pressure, the partial pressure of O_2 is 0.21 × 760 mmHg, or 160 mmHg. If the gas is saturated with water vapor at body temperature (37°C), the water vapor has a partial pressure of 47 mmHg. The partial pressure of O_2 is then calculated on the basis of the remaining pressure, or 760 mmHg − 47 mmHg = 713 mmHg. Therefore, when room air is saturated at body temperature, the Po_2 is 0.21 × 713 mmHg = 150 mmHg. Because inspired gas normally is humidified by the upper airway, it becomes fully saturated by the time it reaches the trachea and bronchi, where inspired Po_2 is approximately 150 mmHg (West, 1990).

Almost all O_2 transported in the blood is bound to hemoglobin. A small fraction is dissolved in plasma. Hemoglobin is 90% saturated with O_2 at a Pao_2 of 60 mmHg (West, 1995). Oxygen content in arterial blood depends on Pao_2 and the hemoglobin level (Fig. 11-1). Tissue O_2 delivery depends on Pao_2, hemoglobin, and cardiac output (Weinberger, 1992).

Carbon Dioxide Transport

Carbon dioxide is transported through the circulation in three different forms as (1) bicarbonate (HCO_3^-), the quantitatively largest component; (2) CO_2 dissolved in plasma; and (3) carbaminohemoglobin, bound to terminal amnio groups on hemoglobin. The first of these, HCO_3^-, results from the combination of CO_2 with H_2O to form carbonic acid (H_2CO_3), catalyzed by the enzyme carbonic anhydrase, and the subsequent dissociation to hydrogen ion (H^+) and HCO_3^-. This reaction takes place primarily within the red blood cell, but HCO_3^- then diffuses out into the plasma in exchange for chlorine ion (Cl^-) (West, 1995).

Although dissolved CO_2, the second form in which CO_2 is transported, comprises only a small portion of the total CO_2 transported, it is quantitatively more important for CO_2 transport than dissolved O_2 is for O_2 transport, because CO_2 is approximately 20 times more soluble in plasma than O_2. Carbaminohemoglobin, formed by the combination of CO_2 with hemoglobin, is the third trans-

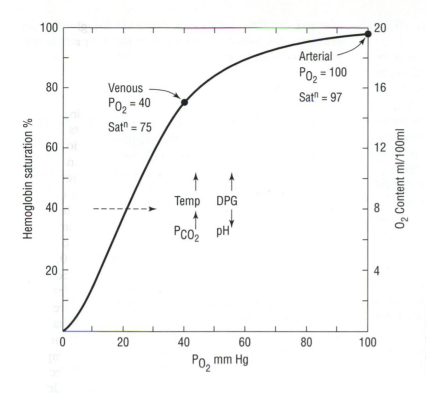

Figure 11–1. Anchor points of the oxygen dissociation curve. The curve is shifted to the right by an increase in temperature, P_{CO_2}, and 2,3-diphosphoglucose (2,3-DGP) and a fall in pH. The oxygen content scale is based on a hemoglobin concentration of 14.5 g/100 mL.

port mechanism available for CO_2. The oxygenation status of hemoglobin is important in determining the quantity of CO_2 that can be bound, as deoxygenated hemoglobin has a greater affinity for CO_2 than oxygenated hemoglobin. This is known as the Haldane effect. Therefore, oxygenation of hemoglobin in the pulmonary capillaries decreases its ability to bind CO_2 and facilitates the elimination of CO_2 by the lungs (West, 1995).

The P_{CO_2} in mixed venous blood is approximately 46 mmHg, whereas normal Pa_{CO_2} is approximately 40 mmHg. This decrease of 6 mmHg in going from mixed venous to arterial blood, combined with the effect of oxygenation of hemoglobin on release of CO_2, corresponds to a change in CO_2 content of approximately 3.6 mL per 100 mL of blood. Assuming a cardiac output of 5 L/min to 6 L/min, the CO_2 production can be calculated as the product of the cardiac output and the arteriovenous CO_2 content difference, or approximately 200 mL/min (West, 1995).

Ventilation–Perfusion Relationships

The topics of ventilation, blood flow, and diffusion and their relationship to gas exchange (O_2 uptake and CO_2 elimination) actually are more complicated. Effective gas exchange depends on the relationship between ventilation and perfusion in individual gas-exchanging units. A disturbance in this relationship, even if the total amounts of ventilation and blood flow are normal, frequently is responsible for markedly abnormal gas exchange in disease states (Weinberger, 1992; West, 1985).

The optimal efficiency for gas exchange would be provided by an even distribution of ventilation and perfusion throughout the lung, so that a matching of ventilation and perfusion is always present. Blood flow is largely determined by hydrostatic forces, so the dependent regions of the lung receive a disproportionately large share of the perfusion. The uppermost regions of the lung are relatively underperfused. There is a gradient of ventilation through the lung with greater amounts also going to the dependent areas. Even though ventilation and perfusion are both greater in the gravity-dependent regions of the lung, the gradient is more marked for perfusion than for ventilation. Consequently, the ratio of ventilation to perfusion (V/Q) is higher in apical regions of the lung than in basilar regions. Gas exchange throughout the lung varies depending on the ventilation and perfusion of each region (Weinberger, 1992; West, 1985).

To understand the effects on gas exchange of altering the V/Q ratio it is necessary to consider the individual alveolus and then a more involved model with multiple alveoli and variable V/Q ratios. In a single alveolus a continuous spectrum exists for the possible relationships between V and Q. At one extreme, where V is maintained and Q approaches 0, the ventilation is wasted as far as gas exchange is concerned. The alveolus in such a case is part of the dead space. At the other extreme, V approaches 0 while Q is preserved, and the V/Q ratio approaches 0. When there is no ventilation, a shunt exists; oxygenation does not occur during transit through the pulmonary circulation; and the hemoglobin is still desaturated when it leaves the pulmonary capillary (Weinberger, 1992; West, 1985).

Alveolar-capillary units may fall anywhere along the continuum of V/Q ratios. The higher the V/Q ratio in an alveolar-capillary unit, the closer the unit comes to behaving like an area of dead space. The lower the V/Q ratio, the closer the unit comes to behaving like a shunt, and the more the P_{O_2} and P_{CO_2} of blood leaving the capillary approach the gas tensions in mixed venous blood (40 torr and 46 torr, respectively) (Weinberger, 1992).

When multiple alveolar-capillary units are considered, the net P_{O_2} and P_{CO_2} of the resulting pulmonary venous blood depend on the total O_2 or CO_2 content and the total volume of blood collected from each of the contributing units. Considering P_{CO_2} first, areas with relatively high V/Q ratios contribute blood with a lower P_{CO_2} than do areas with low V/Q ratios (West, 1985).

A high P_{O_2} in blood coming from a region with a high V/Q ratio cannot compensate for blood with a low P_{O_2} from a region with a low V/Q ratio. The difference stems from the shape of the oxyhemoglobin dissociation curve. Once hemoglobin is nearly saturated with O_2, the rising P_{O_2} does not boost O_2 content. Blood with a higher than normal P_{O_2} does not have a correspondingly higher O_2 content and cannot compensate for blood with a low P_{O_2} and low O_2 content (West, 1985).

In the normal lung, regional differences in V/Q ratio affect gas tensions in blood coming from specific regions, as well as gas tensions in the resulting arterial blood. The net P_{O_2} and P_{CO_2} of the combined blood coming from the apices, the bases, and the areas in between are a function of the relative amounts of blood from each of these areas and the gas content of each (Weinberger, 1992).

In disease states, ventilation-perfusion mismatch is often more severe, resulting in clinically significant gas exchange abnormalities. When an area of the lung behaves as a shunt or even as a region of very low V/Q ratio, blood coming from this area has a low O_2 content and saturation, which cannot be compensated for by blood from more preserved areas of the lung. If V/Q mismatch is severe, particularly with areas of high V/Q, this can produce dead space, decreasing alveolar ventilation to other areas of the lung carrying a disproportionate share of the perfusion. Because CO_2 excretion depends on alveolar ventilation, P_{CO_2} may rise unless there is an overall increase in the minute ventilation to restore effective alveolar ventilation (West, 1985).

Abnormalities in Gas Exchange—Hypoxemia

Blood that has traversed pulmonary capillaries leaves with a P_{O_2} that should be similar to the P_{O_2} in the companion alveoli. It is difficult to measure O_2 tension in alve-

olar gas, but this can be calculated via the alveolar gas equation. According to this formula, the alveolar O_2 tension ($P_{A_{O_2}}$) can be calculated by the following equation:

$$P_{A_{O_2}} = F_{IO_2} (P_b - P_{H_2O}) - \frac{P_{A_{CO_2}}}{R}$$

where F_{IO_2} is the fractional content of inspired O_2, P_b is barometric pressure, P_{H_2O} is the vapor pressure of water in the alveoli, $P_{A_{CO_2}}$ is alveolar CO_2 tension, and R is the respiratory quotient. In practice, for the patient breathing room air, the equation is often simplified to a less cumbersome form. When constant numbers are substituted for F_{IO_2}, P_b, and P_{H_2O}, and when $P_{A_{CO_2}}$ is used instead of $P_{A_{CO_2}}$, the resulting equation at sea level is

$$P_{A_{O_2}} = 150 - (1.25 \times P_{A_{CO_2}}).$$

By calculating the alveolar O_2 content, the expected arterial O_2 content can be determined. In a physiologically normal person, alveolar O_2 content is greater than arterial oxygen content by an amount that is called the alveolar-arterial O_2 difference or gradient, commonly abbreviated $A_aD_{O_2}$. Gradients exist in normal people because a small amount of the cardiac output behaves as a shunt, without ever going through the pulmonary capillary bed. This includes venous blood from the bronchial circulation, a portion of which drains into the pulmonary veins, and coronary venous blood draining via thebesian veins directly into the left ventricle. Desaturated blood from these sources lowers the O_2 tension in the resulting arterial blood. Another reason for alveolar-arterial gradients is that ventilation-perfusion gradients from the top to the bottom of the lung result in less oxygenated blood from the bases combined with better oxygenated blood from the apices (Weinberger, 1992; West, 1997).

The $A_aD_{O_2}$ is normally less than 15 torr, although it increases with age. $A_aD_{O_2}$ may be elevated in disease states for several reasons. First, a shunt may be present so that some desaturated blood combines with fully saturated blood and lowers the P_{O_2} in the resulting arterial blood. The following are common causes of a shunt:

1. Intracardiac lesions, with a right to left shunt at the atrial or ventricular level.
2. Structural abnormalities of the pulmonary vasculature that result in direct communication between pulmonary arterial and venous systems, such as pulmonary arteriovenous malformations.
3. Pulmonary diseases that result in filling of the alveolar spaces with fluid, such as pulmonary edema or alveolar collapse. Either process can result in complete loss of ventilation to the affected alveoli, while some perfusion through the associated capillaries may continue (Weinberger, 1992).

Another cause of an elevated $AaDo_2$ is ventilation–perfusion mismatch. Even when total ventilation and perfusion to both lungs is normal, if some areas receive less ventilation and more perfusion while others receive more ventilation and less perfusion, then the $AaDo_2$ increases and hypoxemia results. The reason for this phenomenon is that areas of low V/Q provide relatively desaturated blood with a low O_2 content. Blood coming from regions with a high V/Q ratio cannot compensate for this problem because the hemoglobin is already fully saturated and cannot increase its O_2 content by increasing ventilation (West, 1997).

True shunt (V/Q = 0) and V/Q mismatch (V/Q low but not 0) can be distinguished by having the patient breathe 100% O_2. True shunt will not be affected by a high concentration of inspired O_2 because increasing the inspired Po_2 does not add further O_2 to the shunted blood and O_2 content does not increase significantly. In the case of V/Q mismatch, however, the alveolar and capillary Po_2 rise considerably with additional O_2, fully saturating the blood coming from regions with a low V/Q ratio, and arterial Po_2 rises substantially (West, 1997).

Lung disease can result in hypoxemia for multiple reasons. Shunting and ventilation–perfusion mismatch both are associated with an elevated $AaDo_2$, and often can be distinguished if necessary by inhalation of 100% O_2, which markedly increases Pao_2 with V/Q mismatch but not with true shunting. In contrast, both hypoventilation (identified by a high $Paco_2$), and a low inspired Po_2 lower alveolar Po_2 and cause hypoxemia, although $AaDo_2$ remains normal (West, 1997).

Hypercapnia

Alveolar ventilation is the prime determinant of arterial Pco_2, assuming CO_2 production remains constant. It is clear that alveolar ventilation is compromised either by decreasing the total minute ventilation (without changing the relative proportions of dead space and alveolar ventilation) or by keeping the total minute ventilation constant and increasing the relative proportion of dead space to alveolar ventilation (Weinberger, 1992).

If significant ventilation–perfusion mismatching occurs, well-perfused areas may be underventilated, while underperfused areas receive a disproportionate amount of ventilation. The net effect of having a large proportion of ventilation go to poorly perfused areas is similar to that of increasing the dead space. By wasting this ventilation, the remainder of the lung with the large share of the perfusion is underventilated, and the net effect is to decrease the effective alveolar ventilation. In many disease conditions, when such significant V/Q mismatch exists, any increase in the Pco_2 stimulates breathing, increases the total minute ventilation, and compensates for the effectively wasted ventilation (Weinberger, 1992).

Several causes of hypercapnia can be defined, all of which share a decrease in the effective alveolar ventilation. A decrease in the minute ventilation, an increase in the proportion of wasted ventilation, and significant ventilation–perfusion mismatch can all result in CO_2 retention. By increasing the total minute ventilation, a patient is often capable of compensating for hypercapnia due to V/Q mismatch, increased wasted ventilation, and decreased minute ventilation of various etiologies, so that CO_2 retention does not result (Weinberger, Schwartzstein, & Weiss, 1989).

Function

With each breath, air flows from the mouth, through the bronchial tree, to the regions of the lung responsible for gas exchange. In order to generate this flow of air during inspiration, the pressure must be lower in the alveoli than at the mouth because air flows from a region of higher pressure to one of lower pressure. The diaphragm and inspiratory muscles of the chest wall cause expansion of the chest and lungs, producing negative pressure in the pleural space and in the alveoli, which initiates airflow (Weinberger, 1992).

Flow in the airways is analogous to flow in an electrical system. Rather than a voltage drop when electrons flow across a resistance, airways have a pressure difference between two points of airflow, and resistance to flow is provided by the airways themselves. The rate of airflow depends partly on this pressure difference between the two points and partly on the airway resistance. During inspiration, alveolar pressure is negative relative to mouth pressure (which is atmospheric), and air flows inward. During expiration, alveolar pressure is positive relative to mouth pressure and air flows outward from alveoli toward the mouth (Weinberger, 1992).

Airway Resistance

Normal airway resistance is 0.5 cm H_2O/L/s to 2 cm H_2O/L/s. Because resistance to airflow in the tracheobronchial tree depends on the total cross-sectional area of the airways, large- and medium-sized airways provide greater resistance than do the more numerous small airways (West, 1997).

Maximal Expiratory Effort

There is a distinction between normal breathing and forced or maximal respiratory efforts. Much information can be gleaned from looking at flow during a forced expiration. Forced expiration involves breathing out from total lung capacity down to RV as hard and as fast as possible. The flow–volume curve illustrates these principles. A series of expiratory curves show the kind of flow rates generated by progressively greater expiratory efforts (West, 1992). Greater expiratory efforts cause a continuing increase of expiratory flow rates, which results from increased pleural pressure and an increased force for expiratory airflow. The region of the vital capacity during maximal expiratory flow is often termed the *effort-dependent portion* (West, 1997).

During most of a forced expiration, flow is limited by critical narrowing of the airway; further effort does not result in augmented flow. Airway diameter depends on the level of the airway in the tracheobronchial tree, airway smooth muscle tone, traction on the airway from surrounding lung tissue, and internal and external pressures on the airway (West, 1997).

At the equal pressure point, internal and external pressures on the airway are equal. The net driving pressure from the alveolus to the equal pressure point is the elastic recoil pressure of the lung. The equal pressure point moves peripherally toward smaller airways as lung volume decreases during a forced expiration. Therefore, the resistance of small airways limits maximal expiratory flow more at low than at high lung volumes (West, 1997).

Flow through the tracheobronchial tree reflects a combination of factors: airway size, support or radial traction exerted by the surrounding lung parenchyma, and driving pressure provided by the elastic recoil of the lung. Although pleural pressure contributes to the driving pressure for airflow, it also exerts a counterbalancing external pressure on the airway, promoting airway collapse (Weinberger, 1992).

Physiology of the Pulmonary Parenchyma

Gas exchange between the alveolus and the capillary bed depends on the passive diffusion of gas from a region of high partial pressure to one of lower partial pressure. The P_{O_2} in the alveolus is normally about 100 torr, whereas the blood entering the pulmonary capillary has a P_{O_2} of approximately 40 torr. This difference gives rise to a driving pressure for O_2 to diffuse from the alveolus to the pulmonary capillary, where it binds with hemoglobin in the erythrocyte. The barrier to diffusion includes a thin (0.5 μm) cytoplasmic extension of the type I cell (Weinberger, 1992).

Although the rate of gas transfer across the alveolar–capillary interface depends on the thickness of the barrier, O_2 uptake by the blood is usually complete early during the transit time through the capillaries. The total period of time spent by a red blood cell traveling through the pulmonary capillaries is approximately 0.75 second, and equilibration with O_2 occurs within the first third of this time period. Therefore, extra time is available for diffusion should there be disease affecting the alveolar–capillary interface and impairing the normal process of diffusion. Carbon dioxide diffuses even more readily than does O_2, so that there is also reserve time available for its diffusion (Weinberger, 1992).

Oxygen uptake and CO_2 elimination at the alveolar–capillary interface are completed early during transit of an erythrocyte through the pulmonary vascular bed. The compliance curve of the lung in interstitial lung disease is shifted downward and to the right; that is, lung volume falls and transpulmonary pressure increases (Weinberger, 1992).

Pulmonary Vascular Resistance

Although the pulmonary circulation handles the same cardiac output from the right ventricle as the systemic circulation handles from the left, the former operates under much lower pressures and has substantially less resistance to flow than the latter. The systolic and diastolic pressures in the pulmonary artery are normally approximately 25 mmHg and 10 mmHg, respectively, in contrast with 120 mmHg and 80 mmHg in the systemic arteries. The pulmonary resistance can be calculated according to the following formula:

$$R = \frac{\text{Change in pressure}}{\text{Change in flow}}$$

The change or drop in pressure across the pulmonary circuit is the mean pulmonary artery pressure minus the left atrial pressure (Weinberger, 1992).

Assuming mean pulmonary artery and left atrial pressures of 15 mmHg and 6 mmHg, respectively, along with a cardiac output of 6 L/min, the pulmonary resistance would be $(15 - 6)/6$ mmHg/L/min, or 1.5 mmHg/L/min. This resistance is approximately one tenth that found in the systemic circulation.

Under conditions of increased cardiac output such as exercise, the pulmonary circulation is actually able to decrease its resistance and handle the extra flow with only a minimal increase in pulmonary artery pressure. Two mechanisms appear to be responsible: recruitment of new vessels and, to a lesser extent, distension of previously perfused vessels. With a means for increasing the total cross-sectional area of the pulmonary vasculature on demand, the pulmonary circulation is capable of lowering its resistance when the need for increased flow arises (Weinberger, 1992).

Another factor that affects pulmonary vascular resistance is lung volume. In discussing the nature of this effect, it is useful to distinguish two categories of pulmonary vessels on the basis of size and location. One category, called *alveolar vessels,* includes the capillary network coursing through the alveolar walls. When alveoli are expanded and lung volume is raised, these vessels are compressed in the stretched alveolar walls, and their contribution to pulmonary vascular resistance is increased. In contrast, when alveoli are emptied and lung volume is lowered, the resistance of these alveolar vessels is diminished. However, the larger vessels, called *extra-alveolar vessels,* are not compressed by air-filled alveoli. The supporting structure that surrounds the walls of these vessels has attachments to alveolar walls, and the elastic recoil of the alveolar walls provides radial traction to keep these vessels open. When lung volume is increased, elastic recoil of the alveolar walls is increased, and the extra-alveolar vessels become larger. When lung volume is decreased, the resistance of the extra-alveolar vessels increases (Weinberger, 1992).

Pulmonary vasoconstriction occurs in response to alveolar hypoxia. This protective mechanism reduces blood flow to poorly ventilated alveoli, minimizing ventilation–perfusion mismatch. A low pH value in blood is an additional stimulus for pulmonary vasoconstriction.

▶ HISTORY OF THE RESPIRATORY SYSTEM

Subjective Data

The patient with a pulmonary problem generally comes to the attention of the clinician for one of two reasons: (1) a complaint of a symptom that can be traced to a respiratory cause or (2) an incidental finding of an abnormality on a chest radiograph. Although the former presentation is more common, the latter can be seen when an x-ray is obtained as either part of a routine examination or for evaluation of a seemingly unrelated problem (Weinberger, 1992).

To elicit information on the respiratory system, the clinician needs to ask about recent illnesses involving the respiratory system, such as upper respiratory infections (URIs). If the patient experienced a recent URI, its course and manifestations need to be determined. Relevant questions include:

1. Was a fever associated with the URI?
2. Did the patient have a productive cough?
3. Was purulent, colored sputum present?

The current status of respiratory system patients with URIs needs to be ascertained. A resolving nonproductive cough without associated fever would be less likely to lead to postoperative pulmonary complications, such as pneumonia, than would fever with productive cough.

Chronic respiratory diseases such as asthma or COPD need to be explored in depth preoperatively. In asthmatic patients, it is important to determine the frequency of wheezing episodes, sometimes described by patients as feeling *tight.* The precipitants of airway reactivity, such as environmental irritants or exercise, need to be elucidated. Current treatment for asthma may range from occasional use of a β_2 agonist inhaler, to use of multiple inhalers and other medications. Treatment history is important because patients who have never been hospitalized for asthma are at lower risk for perioperative bronchospasm than are patients who have required hospitalization, especially in intensive care with mechanical ventilation. Patients need to be reminded to bring their bronchodilating inhalers to surgery with them on the day of their procedure.

It is also important to determine the course of disease and treatment for patients with COPD. Clinicians should ask about activity tolerance, need for supplemental O_2, dyspnea, and orthopnea, especially at rest. If patients are dyspneic, orthopneic, and tachypneic at rest, it is clear that advanced COPD is present. With advanced COPD, postoperative ventilation may be more likely following general anesthesia, and patients need to be counseled about this possibility.

Four particularly common symptoms bring patients with lung disease to health care providers: dyspnea (and its variants), cough (with or without sputum production), hemoptysis, and chest pain. Each of these symptoms may result from nonpulmonary disorders, especially cardiac disease. For each symptom, a discussion of some of the important clinical features is followed by the pathophysiologic features and the differential diagnosis (Weinberger, 1992).

Dyspnea

Dyspnea, or shortness of breath, frequently is a difficult symptom for the clinician to evaluate because it is a subjective feeling experienced by the patient. Patients may describe this complaint in a variety of ways, including shortness of breath, difficulty in getting air, or difficulty catching their breath. To a large degree, the symptom of dyspnea reflects an uncomfortable awareness of one's own breathing, which is normally something we pay little attention (Cherniack & Altose, 1987). Not only is the symptom highly subjective, but the patient's appreciation of it and its importance to the clinician depend heavily on the stimulus or amount of activity required to precipitate it. Clinicians must also account for how the stimulus, when quantified, compares with the patient's usual level of activity (Tobin, 1990).

Tachypnea and Hyperventilation

It is important to distinguish dyspnea from several other signs or symptoms that may have an entirely different

TABLE 11–1. Differential Diagnosis of Dyspnea

Respiratory	Cardiovascular
Airways disease	Elevated pulmonary venous
Asthma	pressure
Chronic obstructive lung disease	Left ventricular failure
Upper airway obstruction	**Mitral stenosis**
Parenchymal lung disease	Decreased cardiac output
Adult respiratory distress syndrome	Severe anemia
Pneumonia	**Anxiety/psychosomatic**
Interstitial lung disease	
Pulmonary vascular disease	
Pulmonary emboli	
Pleural disease	
Pneumothorax	
Pleural effusion	
"Bellows" disease	
Neuromuscular disease, eg,	
polymyositis, myasthenia gravis,	
Guillain–Barré syndrome	
Chest wall disease, eg, kyphoscoliosis	

From Tobin, M. (1990). Dyspnea: Pathophysiologic basis, clinical presentation, and management. Archives of Internal Medicine, 150, 1604–1613.

significance. First, the term *tachypnea* refers to a rapid respiratory rate and may be present with or without dyspnea. *Hyperventilation* refers to ventilation that is greater than the amount required to maintain normal CO_2 elimination. A decrease in P_{CO_2} in arterial blood is the hallmark of hyperventilation. The symptom of exertional fatigue must be distinguished from dyspnea. Fatigue may be due to cardiovascular, neuromuscular, or other nonpulmonary diseases, and the implication of this symptom is different from that of true shortness of breath (Tobin, 1990).

Orthopnea

There also are some variations on the basic theme of dyspnea. *Orthopnea,* or shortness of breath when supine, often is quantitated by the number of pillows or the angle of elevation necessary to relieve or prevent the sensation. One of the main causes of orthopnea is an increase in venous return and central intravascular volume when supine. Orthopnea frequently suggests cardiac disease and some element of congestive heart failure (Raffin & Theodore, 1977).

There is a broad differential diagnosis of disorders resulting in dyspnea, and it is best to separate them into the major categories of respiratory, cardiovascular, and anxiety-related or psychosomatic (Table 11–1). Disorders at many levels of the respiratory system—airways, pulmonary parenchyma, pulmonary vasculature, pleura, and bellows—cause dyspnea (Cherniack & Altose, 1987).

► REACTIVE AIRWAY DISEASE

Cough

Cough usually is initiated by stimulation of irritant receptors at multiple locations (Table 11–2). These irritant receptor nerve endings are found primarily in the larynx, trachea, and major bronchi, particularly at points of bifurcation. There are also sensory receptors located in other parts of the upper airway, on the pleura, the diaphragm, and the pericadium. Irritation of these nerve endings initiates an impulse that travels via afferent nerves to a poorly defined cough center in the medulla. The efferent signal is then carried in the recurrent laryngeal nerve that controls closure of the glottis, and in phrenic and spinal nerves, which effect contraction of the diaphragm and the expiratory muscles of the chest and abdominal wall. The initial part of the cough sequence is a deep inspiration to a high lung volume, followed by closure of the glottis, contraction of the expiratory muscles, and opening of the glottis. When the glottis suddenly opens, contraction of the expiratory muscles and relaxation of the diaphragm produce an explosive rush of air at high velocity, which transports airway secretions or foreign material out of the tracheobronchial tree (Braman & Corrao, 1987).

The symptom of cough generally is characterized by whether it is productive or nonproductive of sputum. Virtually any cause of cough may be productive at times of small amounts of clear or mucoid sputum. Thick yellow or green sputum indicates the presence of numerous leukocytes in the sputum (Braman & Corrao, 1987).

TABLE 11–2. Differential Diagnosis of Cough

Airway irritants	**Parenchymal disease**
Inhaled smoke, dusts, fumes	Pneumonia
Aspiration	Lung abscess
Gastric contents	Interstitial lung disease
Oral secretions	**Congestive heart failure**
Foreign body	**Miscellaneous**
Postnasal drip	Drug-induced (angiotensin
Airways disease	converting enzyme
Upper respiratory tract infection	inhibitors)
Acute or chronic bronchitis	
Bronchiectasis	
Neoplasm	
External compression by a node	
or mass lesion	
Reactive airways disease (asthma)	

From Braman, S. & Corrao, W. (1987). Cough: Differential diagnosis and treatment. Clinical Chest Medicine, 8, 177–188.

TABLE 11–3. Differential Diagnosis of Hemopytsis

Airways disease	**Vascular disease**
Acute or chronic bronchitis	Pulmonary embolism
Bronchiectasis	Elevated pulmonary venous
Bronchogenic carcinoma	pressure
Bronchial carcinoid tumor	Left ventricular failure
Parenchymal disease	Mitral stenosis
Tuberculosis	Vascular malformation
Lung abscess	**Miscellaneous/rare causes**
Pneumonia	Impaired coagulation
Mycetoma ("fungus ball")	Pulmonary endometriosis
Miscellaneous	
Goodpasture syndrome	
Idiopathic pulmonary	
hemosiderosis	

From Israel, R. & Poe, R. (1987). Hemoptysis. Clinical Chest Medicine, 8, 197–205.

Hemoptysis

Hemoptysis is defined as coughing or spitting up blood derived from airways or the lung itself (Table 11–3). When the patient complains of coughing or spitting up blood, it is not always apparent whether the blood originates from the respiratory system. Other sources of blood include the nasopharynx, mouth, and upper gastrointestinal tract. The major causes of hemoptysis fall into three categories by location: airways, pulmonary parenchyma, and vasculature. Airways disease is the most common cause, with bronchitis, bronchiectasis, and bronchogenic carcinoma heading the list. Bronchial carcinoid tumor, a less common neoplasm, also originates in the airway and falls within this category (Israel & Poe, 1987).

Chest Pain

Chest pain as a reflection of respiratory disease does not originate in the lung itself, which is free of sensory fibers. When chest pain occurs in this setting, its origin is usually in the parietal pleura, the diaphragm, or the mediastinum (Branch & McNeil, 1983). Assessment of chest pain needs to include the potential for coronary artery disease or an inflammatory process such as costochondritis.

▶ EVALUATION OF THE PATIENT WITH PULMONARY DISEASE

Physical Examination

The most accessible method for evaluating the patient with respiratory disease is the physical examination. Objective data on the respiratory system are gathered with a stethoscope and the eyes, ears, and hands of the examiner. Skill in eliciting and recognizing abnormal findings develops with guided mentoring (Weinberger, 1992; Domino, 1996).

Palpation and Percussion

Apart from general observation of the patient, the respiratory rate, and the pattern and difficulty of breathing, the examiner relies primarily on palpation and percussion of the chest, and auscultation with a stethoscope. Palpation is useful for comparing the expansion of the two sides of the chest; the examiner can determine if the two lungs are expanding symmetrically or if some process is affecting aeration much more on one side than the other. Palpation of the chest wall also is useful for feeling the vibrations created by spoken sounds. When the examiner places his or her hand over an area of lung, vibration normally should be felt as the sound is transmitted to the chest wall. This vibration is called vocal or tactile fremitus. Some disease processes improve transmission of sound, and they will augment the intensity of the vibration. Other conditions diminish transmission of sound and reduce the intensity of the vibration or eliminate it altogether (Weinberger, 1992).

When percussing the chest, the clinician notes the quality of sound produced by tapping a finger of one hand against a finger of the opposite hand pressed closely to the patient's chest wall. The principle is similar to that of tapping a surface and judging whether what is underneath is solid or hollow. Normally, percussion of the chest wall overlying air-containing lungs gives a resonant sound; in contrast, percussion over a solid organ such as the liver produces a dull sound. This contrast allows the examiner to detect areas with something other than air-containing lung beneath the chest wall, such as fluid in the pleural space, or airless lung, each of which is dull to percussion. At the other extreme, air in the pleural space or a hyperinflated lung may produce a hyperresonant or more *hollow* sound, approaching what one hears when percussing over a solid viscus, such as the stomach (Weinberger, 1992).

Auscultation

Auscultation of the lungs with a stethoscope has two functions: assessment of the quality of the breath sounds and detection of any abnormal, or adventitious, sounds. As the patient takes a deep breath, the sound of airflow can be heard through the stethoscope. When the stethoscope is placed over normal lung tissue, sound is heard primarily during inspiration, and the quality of the sound is relatively smooth and soft. These normal breath sounds heard over lung tissue are called *vesicular* breath sounds. There is not general agreement about where these sounds originate, but the source is presumably somewhere distal to the trachea and proximal to the alveoli (Weinberger, 1992).

When the examiner listens over consolidated lung, or lung that is airless and filled with liquid or inflammatory cells, the findings are different. The sound is louder and harsher, more hollow or tubular in quality, and expiration is at least as loud and long as inspiration. Such breath sounds are called *bronchial* breath sounds, as opposed to the normal vesicular sounds. This difference in quality of the sound is due to the ability of consolidated lung to transmit sound better than normally aerated lung. As a result, sounds generated by turbulent airflow in the central airways (trachea and major bronchi) are transmitted to the periphery of the lung and can be heard through the stethoscope. Normally these sounds are not heard in the lung periphery; they can be demonstrated only by listening near their site of origin (Weinberger, 1992; Martin & Khalil, 1990).

Better transmission of sound through consolidated rather than normal lung also can be demonstrated when the patient whispers or speaks. The enhanced transmission of whispered sound results in more distinctly heard syllables and is termed *whispered pectoriloquy*. Spoken words can be heard more distinctly through the stethoscope placed over the involved area, a phenomenon known as bronchophony. When the patient says the vowel *E,* the resulting sound through consolidated lung has a nasal *A* quality; the E to A change is termed *egophony*. All these findings are variations on the same theme—altered transmission of sound through an airless lung—and have similar significance (Martin & Khalil, 1990).

Two qualifications are important in interpreting the quality of breath sounds. First, the normal transmission of sounds depends on patency of the airway. If a relatively large bronchus is occluded such as by tumor, secretions, or a foreign body, airflow into that region of lung is diminished or absent, and the examiner hears decreased or absent breath sounds over the affected area. A blocked airway proximal to consolidated or airless lung also eliminates the increased transmission described previously. Second, either air or fluid in the pleural space acts as a barrier to sound, so that either a pneumothorax or a pleural effusion causes a diminution of breath sounds (Hansen-Flaschen & Nordberg, 1987).

The second major task of the examiner is to listen for adventitious sounds (Table 11–4). The terminology for these adventitious sounds varies. Only the most commonly used terms will be considered here: *crackles, wheezes,* and *friction rubs.* A fourth category, *rhonchi,* is used inconsistently by different examiners, thus decreasing its clinical usefulness for communicating abnormal findings (Weinberger, 1992).

Crackles, also called rales, are a series of individual clicking or popping noises heard with the stethoscope over an involved area of lung. Their quality can range from the sound produced by rubbing hairs together to that generated by opening a Velcro fastener or crumpling a piece of cellophane. These sounds are *opening* sounds of small airways or alveoli that have been collapsed or decreased in volume during expiration because of fluid, inflammatory exudate, or poor aeration. On each subsequent inspiration, opening of these distal lung units creates the series of clicking or popping sounds heard either throughout or at the latter part of inspiration. The most common disorders producing rales are pulmonary edema, pneumonia, interstitial lung disease, and atelectasis. Although some clinicians believe the quality of the crackles helps to distinguish the different disorders, others think that such distinctions in quality are of little clinical value (Hansen-Flaschen & Nordberg, 1987).

Wheezes are high-pitched continuous sounds that are generated by airflow through narrowed airways. The causes of such narrowing include airway smooth muscle constriction, edema, secretions, or collapse because of poorly supported walls (Hansen-Flaschen & Nordberg, 1987).

Although clinicians most commonly use the term rhonchi in referring to sounds generated by secretions in airways, different examiners use the term in different ways. It is sometimes used to describe low-pitched continuous sounds that are somewhat coarser than high-pitched wheezing. Rhonchi also refer to the very coarse crackles that often result from airway secretions. The term rhonchi is frequently used to describe the variety of

TABLE 11–4. Typical Chest Examination Findings in Selected Clinical Conditions

Condition	Percussion	Fremitus	Breath Sounds	Voice Transmission	Crackles
Normal	Resonant	Normal	Vesicular at lung bases	Normal	Absent
Consolidation or atelectasis with patent airway	Dull	Increased	Bronchial	Bronchophony, whispered pectoriloquy, egophony	Present
Consolidation or atelectasis with blocked airway	Dull	Decreased	Decreased	Decreased	Absent
Emphysema	Hyperresonant	Decreased	Decreased	Decreased	Absent
Pneumothorax	Hyperresonant	Decreased	Decreased	Decreased	Absent
Pleural Effusion	Dull	Decreased	Decreased	Decreased	Absent

From Weinberger, S. (1992). Principles of pulmonary medicine (p. 33). Philadelphia: Saunders.

noises and muscial sounds that cannot be readily classified within the more generally accepted categories of crackles and wheezes but that all appear to have airway secretions as an underlying cause (Weinberger, 1992).

A friction rub is the term for sounds generated by inflamed or roughened pleural surfaces rubbing against each other during respiration. A rub is a series of creaky or rasping sounds heard during both inspiration and expiration. The most common causes are primary inflammatory diseases of the pleura or parenchymal processes that extend out to the pleural surface, such as pneumonia or pulmonary infarction (Martin & Khalil, 1990).

Nonthoracic Manifestations of Pulmonary Disease

Clubbing and cyanosis are two of the more common nonthoracic manifestations of pulmonary disease (Hansen-Flaschen & Nordberg, 1987). Clubbing is a change in normal configuration of the nails and the distal phalanx of the fingers or toes. Several features may be seen: (1) loss of the normal angle between the nail and the skin; (2) increased curvature of the nail; (3) increased sponginess of the tissue below the proximal part of the nail; and (4) flaring or widening of the terminal phalanx. Although several nonpulmonary disorders can result in clubbing, such as congenital heart disease with right to left shunting, endocarditis, chronic liver disease, or inflammatory bowel disease, the most common causes are pulmonary. Occasionally clubbing is familial and of no clinical significance. Carcinoma of the lung is the single leading etiologic factor. Other pulmonary causes of clubbing include chronic pulmonary infection with suppuration, such as bronchiectasis or lung abscess, and interstitial lung disease. Uncomplicated chronic obstructive lung disease is not associated with clubbing, and its presence in such a patient should suggest unsuspected malignancy or suppurative disease (Hansen-Flaschen & Nordberg, 1987).

Clubbing may also be accompanied by hypertrophic pulmonary osteoarthropathy, characterized by periosteal new bone formation, particularly in the long bones, and arthralgias and arthritis. When there is coexistent pulmonary osteoarthropathy, either pulmonary or pleural tumor is the likely cause of the clubbing because pulmonary osteoarthropathy is relatively rare with the other causes of clubbing (Hansen-Flaschen & Nordberg, 1987).

The mechanism of clubbing and hypertrophic pulmonary osteoarthropathy is not clear. It has been observed that clubbing is associated with an increase in digital blood flow, whereas osteoarthropathy is characterized by an overgrowth of highly vascular connective tissue. Why these changes occur is a mystery (Hansen-Flaschen & Nordberg, 1987).

Cyanosis, the second extrapulmonary physical finding arising from lung disease, is a bluish discoloration of the skin, particularly under the nails and mucous membranes. Whereas saturated hemoglobin gives the skin its usual pink color, a sufficient amount of unsaturated hemoglobin produces cyanosis. Cyanosis may be either generalized, due to low Po_2 or low systemic blood flow resulting in increased extraction of O_2 from the blood, or localized, owing to low blood flow and increased O_2 extraction from the localized area. With lung disease, the common factor causing cyanosis is low Po_2, and several types of lung disease may be responsible. It is also important to remember that the total amount of hemoglobin affects the likelihood of detecting cyanosis. In the anemic patient, if the total quantity of desaturated hemoglobin is less than the amount needed to produce the bluish discoloration, even a very low Po_2 may not be associated with cyanosis. In the patient with polycythemia, much less depression of the Po_2 is necessary before sufficient unsaturated hemoglobin exists to produce cyanosis (Martin & Khalil, 1990).

▶ DIAGNOSTIC DATA FROM NONINVASIVE AND INVASIVE MODALITIES

Chest Roentgenography

The chest x-ray, which is largely taken for granted in health care today, is used not only in evaluating patients with suspected respiratory disease but also frequently in the routine evaluation of asymptomatic patients. Of all the viscera, the lungs are best suited for radiographic examination. Air in the lungs provides an excellent background against which abnormalities can be seen. The presence of two lungs allows each to serve as a control for the other, so that unilateral abnormalities may be more easily recognized (Fraser, Pare, Pare, & Genereux, 1988).

The appearance of any structure on a radiograph depends on its density; the denser it is, the whiter it appears on the film. At one extreme is air, which is radiolucent and appears black on the film. At the other extreme are metallic densities, which appear white. In between, there is a spectrum of increasing density from fat to water to bone. The viscera and muscles fall within the realm of water density tissues and cannot be distinguished in their radiographic density from water or blood (Fraser, Pare, Pare, & Genereux, 1988).

In order for a line or an interface to appear between two adjacent structures on a radiograph, the two structures must differ in density. For example, within the cardiac shadow the heart muscle cannot be distinguished from the blood within its chambers because both are of water density. In contrast, the borders of the heart are visible against the lungs because the water density of the heart contrasts with the density of the lungs, which is closer to that of air. However, if the lung adjacent to a normally denser structure such as the heart or diaphragm is airless, either because of collapse or consolidation, the neighboring structures are now both of the same density, and no visible interface or boundary separates them. This principle is the basis of the silhouette sign: If an expected border with an area of lung is not visualized or is not distinct, the adjacent lung is abnormal and lacks full aeration (Fraser, Pare, Pare, & Genereux, 1988).

Chest x-rays are usually taken in two standard views—posteroanterior (PA) and lateral (Figure 11-2). For a PA film, the roentgen beam goes from the back to the front of the patient, and the patient's chest is adjacent to the film. The lateral view is taken with the patient's side against the film, and the beam is directed through the patient to the film. If a film cannot be taken with the patient standing with chest to the film, as in the case of a bedridden patient, then a PA view is taken (Weinberger, 1992).

Knowledge of the radiographic anatomy is fundamental for the interpretation of consolidation or collapse (atelectasis) and for localization of other abnormalities on the chest film. Lobar anatomy and the locations of fissures separating the lobes are shown in Figure 11-3. It is important to realize that location of an abnormality often requires information from both the PA and lateral views. The major fissure separating the upper and middle lobes

from the lower lobe runs obliquely through the chest. Thus, it is easy to be misled about location on the PA film alone—a lower lobe lesion may appear in the upper part of the chest, whereas an upper lobe lesion may appear much lower in position (Weinberger, 1992).

When a lobe becomes filled with fluid or inflammatory exudate, as can be seen with pneumonia, it is full of water rather than air density and therefore is easily delineated on the chest film. With pure consolidation the lobe does not lose volume, and it occupies its usual position, retaining its usual size (Fraser, Pare, Pare, & Genereux, 1988). However, when a lobe has airless alveoli and collapses, it becomes more dense and has features of volume loss characteristic for each individual lobe. Such features of volume loss include change in the position of a fissure or the indirect signs of displacement of the hilum, diaphragm, trachea, or mediastinum in the direction of the volume loss. A common cause for atelectasis is occlusion of the airway leading to the collapsed region of lung, for example, by a tumor, an aspirated foreign body, or a mucous plug. All of the preceding examples reflect either pure consolidation or pure collapse. In practice, a combination of these processes often occurs, leading to consolidation accompanied by partial volume loss (Fraser, Pare, Pare, & Genereux, 1988).

With relatively diffuse abnormalities on the chest film, it is necessary to determine whether the process is primarily interstitial, affecting the alveolar walls and in-

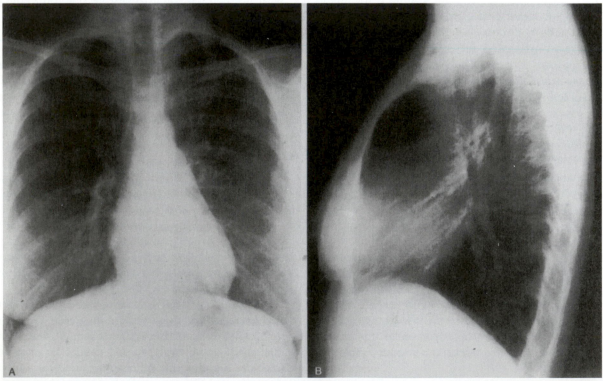

Figure 11-2. Normal chest roentgenogram. **A.** Posteroanterior (PA) view. **B.** Lateral view. *(From Weinberger, S. [1992]. Principles of Pulmonary Medicine. Philadelphia: Saunders.)*

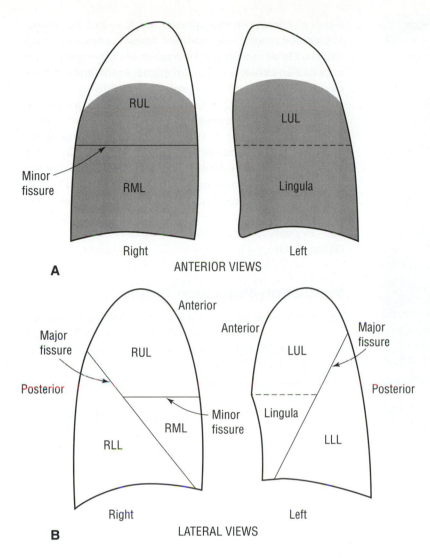

Figure 11–3. Lobar anatomy as seen from anterior (**A**) and lateral (**B**) views. RUL, right upper lobe; RML, right middle lobe; RLL, right lower lobe; LUL, left upper lobe; LLL, left lower lobe. In anterior views, shaded regions represent lower lobes and are behind upper and middle lobes. Lingula is part of LUL, and dotted line between the two does not represent an actual fissure. *(From Weinberger, S. [1992].* Principles of Pulmonary Medicine. *Philadelphia: Saunders.)*

terstitial tissue, or alveolar, filling the alveolar spaces. This distinction frequently is important because of the clues it gives about etiologic factors; many diffuse disorders of the lung are characterized by one or the other roentgenographic pattern. An interstitial pattern generally is described as reticulonodular, consisting of an interlacing network of linear and small nodular densities. In contrast, an alveolar pattern appears more fluffy, and the outlines of air-filled bronchi coursing through the alveolar densities are often seen. This latter finding is called an air bronchogram and is due to air in the bronchi being surrounded and outlined by alveoli that are filled with fluid. This finding does not occur with a purely interstitial pattern (Weinberger, 1992).

When viewing a chest x-ray, the clinician assesses for aeration, symmetry of lung expansion, appearance of the vessels, such as the aorta and pulmonary artery, and areas of consolidation and effusion. Additionally, the cardiac silhouette reflects appropriate organ size versus cardiomegaly, or rare conditions such as dextrocardia.

Computed Tomography

Tomography provides views at different planes through the lung, rather than a summation of all areas the beam passes through. This method may be used to give better definition to small or questionable lesions, and is useful in determining if a lesion has calcification within it (Fig. 11–4) (Zerhouni, 1989). With computed tomography (CT), a narrow beam of x-rays passes through the body and is sensed by a rotating detector on the other side of the patient. The beam is partially absorbed within the patient. Computer analysis of the information received by the detector allows a series of cross-sectional images to be constructed.

The CT scan is particularly useful in detecting subtle differences in tissue density that cannot be distinguished by conventional radiography. In addition, the cross-sectional views obtained from the slices provide very different information from that provided by the vertical orientation of plain films or conventional tomogra-

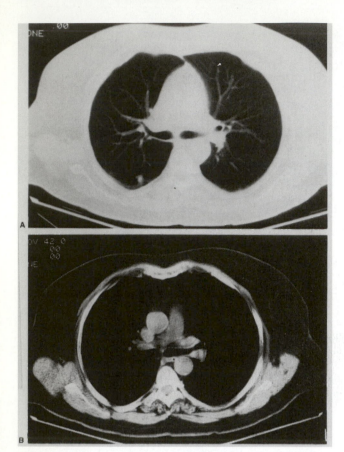

Figure 11–4. Cross-sectional "slice" from a computed tomography (CT) scan performed for evaluation of a solitary peripheral pulmonary nodule. Nodule can be seen in posterior portion of right lung. The two images were taken using different "windows" at the same cross-sectional level. On the top view (**A**), settings were chosen to optimize visualization of the lung parenchyma. On bottom view (**B**), settings were chosen to distinguish between different densities of soft tissues, such as structures within the mediastinum. *(From Weinberger, S. [1992]. Principles of Pulmonary Medicine. Philadelphia: Saunders.)*

phy techniques. The greatest utility of chest CT has been in evaluating pulmonary nodules and the mediastinum, but it also has been useful in characterizing chest wall and pleural disease (Zerhouni, 1989).

Magnetic Resonance Imaging

Magnetic resonance imaging (MRI) is a technique that depends on the way nuclei within a stationary magnetic field change their orientation and release energy delivered to them by a radio frequency pulse. The time required to return to the baseline energy state can be analyzed by a complex computer algorithm, and a visual image can be created (Fisher, 1989).

In the evaluation of intrathoracic disease, MRI provides several important features. First, flowing blood pro-

duces a *signal void* and appears black, so that blood vessels can be readily distinguished from nonvascular structures without needing intravenous contrast agents. Images can be constructed in any plane, so that information can be displayed as sagittal, coronal, or transverse (cross-sectional) views. Differences can be seen between normal and diseased tissues that are adjacent to each other, even when they are of the same density and therefore could not be distinguished by routine radiography or CT scanning (Fig. 11–5). An MRI can be a valuable tool in the evaluation of hilar and mediastinal disease, as well as in defining intrathoracic disease that extends into the neck, although it appears to be less useful than CT scanning in the evaluation of pulmonary parenchymal disease (Fisher, 1989).

Ventilation–Perfusion Scans

Injected or inhaled radioisotopes readily provide information about pulmonary blood flow and ventilation. Imaging of the gamma radiation from these isotopes produces a picture showing the distribution of blood flow and ventilation throughout both lungs (Fig. 11–6). Perfusion and ventilation scans are performed for two reasons: detection of pulmonary emboli and assessment of regional lung function. When a pulmonary embolus occludes a pulmonary artery, blood flow ceases to the lung region normally supplied by that vessel, and a corresponding *perfusion defect* results. Generally, ventilation is preserved and a ventilation scan does not show a corresponding *ventilation defect.* In practice, many pieces of information are considered in the interpretation of the scan, including the appearance of the chest x-ray and the size and distribution of defects on the perfusion scan (Spies, Spies, & Mintzer, 1983).

Ventilation and perfusion lung scans to assess regional lung function often are performed before surgery involving resection of part of the lung, usually one or more lobes. By visualizing which areas of the lung receive ventilation and perfusion, clinicians can determine how much of the area to be resected is contributing to overall lung function (Spies, Spies, & Mintzer, 1983).

Pulmonary Angiography

Pulmonary angiography is a radiographic technique in which a catheter is guided from a peripheral vein through the right atrium and ventricle and into the main pulmonary artery or one of its branches. A radiopaque dye is then injected, and the pulmonary arterial tree is visualized on a series of rapidly exposed chest films. A clot

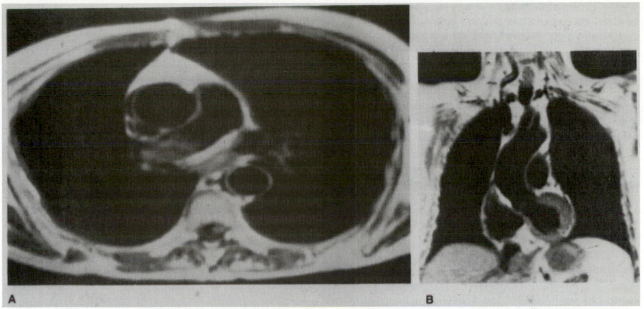

Figure 11–5. Magnetic resonance images of normal chest: cross-sectional (**A**) and coronal (**B**) views. Lumen of structures that contain blood appears black because flowing blood produces "signal void." *(From Weinberger, S. [1992].* Principles of Pulmonary Medicine. *Philadelphia: Saunders.)*

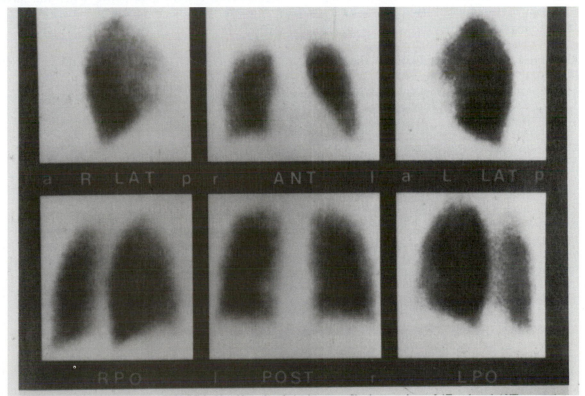

Figure 11–6. Normal perfusion lung scan. Six views are shown. LAT, lateral; ANT, anterior; POST, posterior; RPO, right posterior oblique; LPO, left posterior oblique; a, anterior; p, posterior; r, right; l, left. *(From Weinberger, S. [1992].* Principles of Pulmonary Medicine. *Philadelphia: Saunders.)*

in a pulmonary vessel appears either as an abrupt termination of the vessel or as a filling defect within its lumen (Fedullo & Shure, 1987).

Bronchoscopy

Direct visualization of the airways is possible using bronchoscopy, which was originally performed with a rigid bronchoscope (a hollow metal tube). More recently, flexible fiberoptic bronchoscopy has been used. The flexible instrument has fiberoptic bundles, the fibers of which transmit light even when they are bent or curved. Because of the flexible nature of the scope, the bronchoscopist can bend the tip at will with a control lever and maneuver into the airways at least down to the subsegmental level (Shure, 1987). The bronchoscopist not only can obtain an excellent view of the airways, but also can obtain a variety of samples for cytologic, pathologic, and microbiologic examination. There are many indications for bronchoscopy, including (1) evaluation of a suspected endobronchial malignancy; (2) sampling an area of parenchymal disease either by bronchoalveolar lavage, brushings, or biopsy; (3) evaluation of hemoptysis; and (4) removal of a foreign body (Shure, 1987).

The simplest test of lung function is a forced expiration. The majority of patients with lung disease have an abnormal forced expiration, and the information obtained from this test is useful in their management. In spite of this, the test is not used as often as it should be (Weinberger, 1992).

► TESTS OF VENTILATORY CAPACITY

Forced Expiratory Volume

The forced expiratory volume (FEV) is the volume of gas exhaled in 1 second by a forced expiration from full inspiration. The vital capacity is the total volume of gas that can be exhaled after a full inspiration (West, 1997). To assess FEV, the patient is comfortably seated in front of a spirometer having a low resistance. The patient breathes in maximally and then exhales as hard and as far as possible. As the spirometer bell moves up, the kymograph pen moves down, thus indicating the expired volume against time (Fig. 11-7). Forced expiratory volume tracings for normal, obstructive, and restrictive airway diseases are shown in Figure 11-8 (West, 1997).

In a normal tracing, for example, the volume exhaled in 1 second was 4 L and the total volume exhaled was 5 L. These two volumes are the FEV in 1 second (FEV_1) and the vital capacity (VC). The VC measured with a forced expiration may be less than that measured with a slower exhalation, so the term *forced vital capacity* (FVC) is generally used. Note that a normal ratio of FEV_1 to FVC is about 80% (West, 1997). The FEV can be measured over other times, such as 2 or 3 seconds, but the 1-second value is most informative. When the subscript is omitted, it is understood that the period is 1 second (West, 1997).

Figure 11-9 shows the type of tracing obtained from a patient with COPD. Note that the rate at which air was exhaled was much slower, so that only 1.3 L were

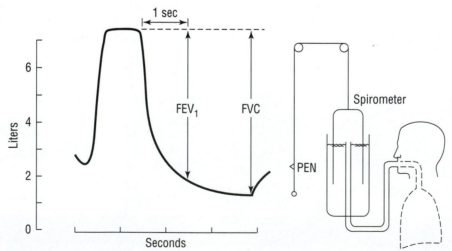

Figure 11-7. Measurements of forced expiratory volume (FEV_1) and vital capacity (FVC). *(From West, J. B. [1997]. Pulmonary pathophysiology—the essentials [5th ed.]. Baltimore: Williams & Wilkins.)*

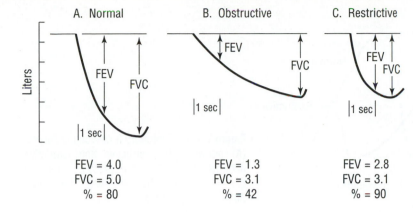

Figure 11–8. Normal, obstructive, and restrictive patterns of a forced expiration. *(From West, J. B. [1997]. Pulmonary pathophysiology—the essentials [5th ed.]. Baltimore: Williams & Wilkins.)*

blown out in the first second. In addition, the total volume exhaled was only 3.1 L, and FEV_1/FVC was reduced to 42%. These figures are typical of an obstructive pattern (West, 1997). Contrast this pattern with that of Figure 11-10 which shows the type of tracing obtained from a patient with pulmonary fibrosis. Here the VC was reduced to 3.1 L, but a large percentage (90%) was exhaled in the first second. These figures mean restrictive disease is present (West, 1997).

Forced Expiratory Flow

The forced expiratory flow ($FEF_{25-75\%}$) index is calculated from a forced expiration as shown in Figure 11-11. The middle half (by volume) of the total expiration is marked and its duration is measured. The $FEF_{25-75\%}$ is the volume in liters divided by the time in seconds (West, 1997). The correlation between $FEF_{25-75\%}$ and FEV_1 is generally close in patients with obstructive pulmonary disease. The changes in $FEF_{25-75\%}$ are often more striking, but the range of normal values is greater (West, 1997).

Interpretation of Tests of Forced Expiration

In some respects, the lungs and thorax can be regarded as a simple air pump. The output of such a pump depends on the stroke volume, the resistance of the airways, and the force applied to the piston. The last factor is relatively unimportant in a forced expiration (West, 1995).

The VC (or FVC) is a measure of the stroke volume, and any reduction in it will affect the ventilatory capacity. Causes of stroke volume reduction include diseases of the thoracic cage, such as kyphoscoliosis, ankylosing spondylitis, and acute injuries; diseases affecting the nerve supply to the respiratory muscles or the muscles themselves, such as poliomyelitis or muscular dystrophy; abnormalities of the pleural cavity, such as pneumothorax or pleural thickening; pathology in the lung itself, such as fibrosis, which reduces its distensibility; space-occupying lesions, such as cysts; or an increased pulmonary blood volume, as in left heart failure. In addition, there are diseases of the airways that cause them to close prematurely during expiration, thus limiting the volume that can be exhaled. This occurs in asthma and bronchitis (West, 1995).

The FEV and related indices such as the $FEF_{25-75\%}$ are affected by the airway resistance during forced expiration. Any increase in resistance will reduce the ventilatory capacity. Causes include bronchoconstriction as in asthma or following the inhalation of irritants, such as cigarette smoke; structural changes in the airways, as in chronic bronchitis; obstruction within the airways, such as an inhaled foreign body or excess bronchial secre-

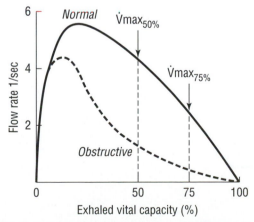

Figure 11–9. Example of an expiratory flow–volume curve in chronic obstructive pulmonary disease. Note the scooped-out appearance. The arrows show the maximum expiratory flow after 50% and 75% of the vital capacity have been exhaled.

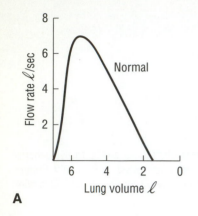

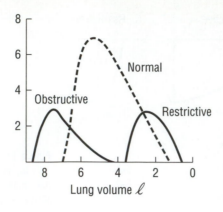

A

B

Figure 11–10. Expiratory flow–volume curves: **(A)** normal; **(B)** obstructive and restrictive patterns. *(From West, J. B. [1997]. Pulmonary pathophysiology—the essentials [5th ed.]. Baltimore: Williams & Wilkins.)*

tions; and destructive processes in the lung parenchyma, which interfere with the radial traction that normally supports the airways (West, 1995).

Expiratory Flow–Volume Curve. Flow rate and volume during maximal forced expiration yield a pattern that is similar to the one shown in Figure 11-12. A curious feature of the flow–volume curve is that it is virtually impossible to get outside it (West, 1997). In obstructive diseases such as chronic bronchitis and emphysema, the maximal expiration typically begins and ends at abnormally high lung volumes and the flow rates are much lower than normal. In addition, the curve may have a scooped-out appearance. By contrast, patients with restrictive disease such as interstitial fibrosis operate at low lung volumes. Their flow envelopes are flattened compared with normal ones, but if flow rate is related to lung volume, the flow is seen to be higher than normal (West, 1997).

To understand these patterns, consider the pressures inside and outside the airways. Before inspiration, the pressures in the mouth, airways, and alveoli are all atmospheric because there is no flow. Intrapleural pres-

sure may be 5 cm H_2O below atmospheric pressure, and it is assumed that the same pressure exists outside the airways. Thus, the pressure difference expanding the airways is 5 cm H_2O. At the beginning of inspiration, all measures fall and the pressure difference holding the airways open increases to 6 cm H_2O. At the end of inspiration, this pressure is 8 cm H_2O (West, 1997).

Early in a forced expiration, both intrapleural and alveolar pressures rise greatly. The pressure at some point in the airways increases, but not as much as alveolar pressure because of the pressure drop caused by flow. Under these circumstances, we have a pressure difference of 11 cm H_2O tending to close the airways. Airway compression occurs, and now flow is determined by the difference between alveolar pressure and the pressure outside the airways at the collapse point (West, 1997).

In the patient with chronic bronchitis and emphysema, the low flow rate in relation to lung volume is caused by several factors. There may be thickening of the walls of the airways and excessive secretions in the lumen because of bronchitis; both increase the flow resistance. The number of small airways may be reduced be-

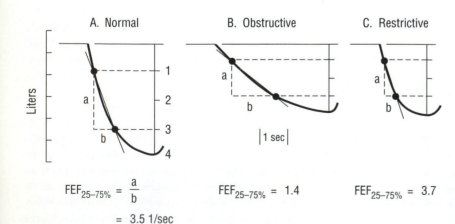

$$FEF_{25-75\%} = \frac{a}{b}$$

$$= 3.5 \; 1/sec$$

$$FEF_{25-75\%} = 1.4$$

$$FEF_{25-75\%} = 3.7$$

Figure 11–11. Calculation of forced expiratory flow $(FEF_{25\%-75\%})$ from a forced expiration. *(From West, J. B. [1997]. Pulmonary pathophysiology—the essentials [5th ed.]. Baltimore: Williams & Wilkins.)*

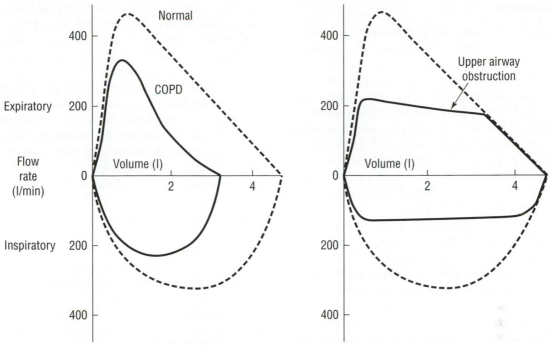

Figure 11–12. Expiratory and inspiratory flow–volume curves. In normal subjects and patients with chronic obstructive pulmonary disease, inspiratory flow rates are approximately normal. In fixed upper airway obstruction, both inspiratory and expiratory flow rates are reduced. *(From West, J. B. [1997]. Pulmonary pathophysiology—the essentials [5th ed.]. Baltimore: Williams & Wilkins.)*

cause of destruction of lung tissue. Also, the patient may have a reduced static recoil pressure because of breakdown of elastic alveolar walls. Finally, the normal support offered to the airways by the traction of the surrounding parenchyma is probably impaired because of loss of alveolar walls, and the airways collapsing more easily than they should (West, 1997).

The patient with interstitial fibrosis has normal or high flow rates in relation to lung volume because static lung recoil pressures are high and the caliber of airways must be normal (or even increased) at a given lung volume. However, because of the greatly reduced compliance of the lung, volumes are very small and absolute flow rates are therefore reduced (West, 1997).

Closing Volume. Toward the end of the VC expiration there is an abrupt rise in nitrogen (N_2) concentration, which signals the onset of airway closure or phase 4. The lung volume during the beginning of phase 4 is called the closing volume, and the closing volume plus the RV is known as the closing capacity. In practice, the onset of phase 4 is obtained by drawing a straight line through the alveolar plateau (phase 3) and noting the last point of departure of the nitrogen tracing from this line (West, 1997). Unfortunately, the junction between phases 3 and 4 is seldom clear-cut, and there is considerable variation of this volume when repeated measure-

ments are made on the same patient. The test is most useful in the presence of small amounts of disease, because severe disease distorts the tracing so much that the closing volume cannot be identified (West, 1997).

The mechanism of the onset of phase 4 is still disputed, but much evidence suggests that it is caused by closure of small airways in the lowest part of the lung. At RV just before the single breath of O_2, the N_2 concentration is virtually uniform throughout the lung, but the basal alveoli are much smaller than the apical alveoli in the upright subject because of distortion of the lung by its weight. Indeed, the lowest portions are compressed so much that small airways in the region of the respiratory bronchioles are closed. However, at the end of a VC inspiration, all the alveoli are approximately the same size. Thus, the N_2 at the base is diluted more than that of the apex by the breath of oxygen (West, 1997).

The volume at which airways close is very age dependent, being as low as 10% of the VC in young normal subjects but increasing to 40%, or about the functional residual capacity (FRC), at approximately 65 years of age. There is some evidence that the test is sensitive to small amounts of disease. For example, apparently healthy cigarette smokers sometimes have increased closing volumes when their ventilatory capacity is normal (West, 1995).

Gas Exchange

It is often essential to know the partial pressure of O_2 in the arterial blood of acutely ill patients. With modern blood gas electrodes, the measurement of arterial P_{O_2} is relatively simple, and the test should be available in all hospitals where patients with respiratory failure are managed (West, 1995). Arterial blood is usually taken by puncture of the radial artery or from an indwelling radial artery catheter. The dead space of the syringe should be filled with dilute heparin, and ideally the blood should be analyzed within a few minutes. If this is not possible, the syringe should be placed in a beaker of ice to slow the metabolism of the blood (West, 1995).

Arterial P_{O_2} is measured with a polarographic O_2 electrode. The principle is that if a small voltage (0.6 V) is applied to a platinum electrode immersed in a buffer solution, the current that flows is proportional to the P_{O_2}. Oxygen is consumed by the electrode; consequently, the measured P_{O_2} falls with time (West, 1997).

The normal value for P_{O_2} in young adults averages 95 mmHg, with a range of about 85 to 100 mmHg. The normal value falls steadily with age, and the average is about 85 mmHg at age 60. The cause of the fall in P_{O_2} with age is probably increasing ventilation–perfusion inequality (West, 1997).

The oxygen–hemoglobin dissociation curve should be considered when interpreting an arterial P_{O_2}. Figure 11–1 is a reminder of two anchor points on the normal curve—arterial blood (P_{O_2} 100, O_2 saturation 97%) and mixed venous blood (P_{O_2} 40, O_2 saturation 75%). Above 60 mmHg, the curve is fairly flat and cyanosis is probably undetectable. The curve is shifted to the right by an increase in temperature and P_{CO_2} and a fall in pH. These all occur in exercising muscle where enhanced unloading of O_2 is advantageous. The curve is also shifted to the right by an increase in 2,3-diphosphoglycerate (DPG) inside the red blood cells, which occurs as a result of prolonged hypoxia, for example, in chronic pulmonary disease or cyanotic heart disease. An increased concentration may also occur in anemia (West, 1995, 1997).

Causes of Hypoxemia

There are four primary causes of a reduced P_{O_2} in arterial blood: hypoventilation, diffusion impairment, shunt, and ventilation–perfusion inequality.

Hypoventilation. Hypoventilation occurs when the volume of fresh gas going to the alveoli per unit of time (alveolar ventilation) is reduced. If the resting O_2 consumption is not correspondingly reduced, this results in hypoxemia. Hypoventilation always causes a rise in the P_{CO_2} and this is a valuable diagnostic feature. Hypoxemia can be abolished by increasing the inspired P_{O_2} by increasing inspired O_2 (West, 1995).

The causes of hypoventilation include (1) depression of the respiratory center by drugs (especially barbiturates and opioids) or anesthesia; (2) diseases of the medulla, including encephalitis, trauma, hemorrhage, or neoplasm; (3) abnormalities of the spinal conducting pathways, such as following high cervical dislocation; (4) anterior horn cell diseases, such as poliomyelitis; (5) diseases of the nerves to the respiratory tract, including Guillain-Barré syndrome and diptheria; (6) diseases of the myoneural junction, such as myasthenia gravis and anticholinesterase poisoning; (7) disease of the respiratory muscles, such as progressive muscular dystrophy; (8) thoracic cage abnormalities, such as crushed chest; and (9) upper airway obstruction, such as tracheal compression by a thymoma (West, 1997).

Sleep apnea is a condition that is understood better today than in the past. Sleep apnea can be either central or obstructive in origin. Central sleep apnea occurs in patients with hypoventilation because respiratory drive is depressed during sleep. It is known that during random eye movement (REM) sleep, breathing is often irregular and unresponsive to chemical and vagal drives. An exception is hypoxemia, which usually remains a powerful stimulus to breathing (West, 1997).

Obstructive sleep apnea occurs much more commonly than was once thought. The first reports were in extremely obese patients, but it is now recognized that the condition is not confined to such patients. Airway obstruction can be caused by backward movement of the tongue, collapse of the pharyngeal walls, greatly enlarged tonsils or adenoids, and other anatomical causes of pharyngeal narrowing. During obstructive sleep apnea, loud snoring often occurs and the patient may awaken violently after an apneic episode. There is sometimes chronic sleep deprivation and the patient may have daytime somnolence, impaired cognitive function, chronic fatigue, morning headaches, and other personality disturbances (West, 1997).

A condition affecting infants is sudden infant death syndrome (SIDS). Here the child is typically found dead in bed without apparent cause. The etiology of this problem is still obscure. One hypothesis is that in these infants, the nervous control of ventilation is not fully developed and the respiratory muscles are poorly coordinated.

Diffusion Impairment. Equilibrium does not occur between the P_{O_2} in the pulmonary capillary blood and alveolar gas in diffusion impairment. Under normal resting conditions, the capillary blood P_{O_2} almost reaches that of alveolar gas after about one third of the total contact time of 0.75 second available in the capillary. Diseases in which diffusion impairment may contribute to hypoxemia include asbestosis; sarcoidosis; diffuse interstitial fibrosis; interstitial pneumonia; and connective tissue diseases affecting the lung, including scleroderma, lupus erythematosus, and Goodpasture syndrome. In all these conditions, the diffusion path from the alveolar gas to the red blood cells may be increased, at least in some regions of the lung, and the time course for oxygenation may be affected.

Any hypoxemia caused by diffusion impairment can be corrected by administering 100% O_2 to the patient. This is because the resultant large increase in alveolar P_{O_2} of several hundred mmHg can easily overcome the increased diffusion resistance of the thickened alveolar membrane. Carbon dioxide elimination is thought to be unaffected by diffusion abnormalities (West, 1997).

Shunt. With a shunt, some blood reaches the arterial system without passing through ventilated regions of the lung. Intrapulmonary shunts can be caused by arterial–venous fistulas, although these are uncommon. In addition, a completely unventilated but perfused area of lung, such as a consolidated pneumonic lobule, constitutes a shunt. Very large shunts are often seen in adult respiratory distress syndrome (ARDS). Many shunts are extrapulmonary, including those that occur in congenital heart disease through atrial or ventricular septal defects or a patent ductus arteriosus. In such patients there must be a rise in right heart pressure; otherwise the shunt is from left to right.

If a patient with a shunt is given pure O_2 to breathe, the arterial P_{O_2} fails to rise to the level seen in normal subjects. Although the end-capillary P_{O_2} may be as high as that in alveolar gas, the O_2 content of the shunted blood is as low as in venous blood. When a small amount of shunted blood is added to arterial blood, the O_2 content is depressed. This causes a large fall in arterial P_{O_2} because the O_2 dissociation curve is so flat in its upper range. As a result, it is possible to detect small shunts by measuring arterial P_{O_2} during 100% O_2 breathing.

The magnitude of shunt during O_2 breathing can be determined from the shunt equation:

$$\frac{\dot{Q}_s}{\dot{Q}_T} = \frac{C_c' - C_a}{C_c' - C_v}$$

where $\dot{Q}_s$ and $\dot{Q}_T$ refer to the shunt and total blood flows and C_c', C_a, and C_v refer to the O_2 contents of end-capillary, arterial, and mixed venous blood. The O_2 content of end-capillary blood is calculated from the alveolar P_{O_2} assuming complete equilibration between the alveolar gas and the blood. Mixed venous blood can be sampled via a pulmonary artery catheter (West, 1997).

Ventilation–Perfusion Inequality. Ventilation and blood flow are mismatched in various regions of the lung in ventilation–perfusion inequality, with the result that all gas transfer becomes inefficient. This mechanism of hypoxemia is extremely common; it is responsible for

most if not all of the hypoxemia of COPD, interstitial lung disease, and vascular disorders such as pulmonary embolism. It is generally identified by excluding the other three causes of hypoxemia: hypoventilation, diffusion impairment, and shunt.

All lungs have some ventilation–perfusion inequality. In the normal upright lung this takes the form of a regional pattern, with the ventilation–perfusion ratio decreasing from apex to base. But as disease occurs and progresses, this pattern becomes disorganized until the normal relationships between ventilation and blood flow are destroyed at the alveolar level. The severity of a ventilation–perfusion inequality can be assessed from arterial blood gases. The arterial P_{O_2} is a useful guide. A patient with an arterial P_{O_2} of 40 mmHg is likely to have more ventilation–perfusion inequality than a patient with an arterial P_{O_2} of 70 mmHg.

Alveolar P_{O_2} covers a wide spectrum of potential values. An ideal alveolar P_{O_2} can be calculated. The alveolar-arterial difference for P_{O_2} makes an allowance for the effect of any under- or overventilation on the arterial P_{O_2} and is a purer measure of ventilation–perfusion inequality. The normal value for physiologic dead space is about 30% of the tidal volume at rest and less during exercise, and it consists almost completely of anatomical dead space. In chronic pulmonary disease it may rise to 50% or more due to the presence of ventilation–perfusion inequality.

Mixed causes of hypoxemia frequently occur. For example, a patient who is being mechanically ventilated because of acute respiratory failure following an automobile accident may have a large shunt through unventilated lung in addition to severe ventilation–perfusion inequality. A patient with interstitial lung disease may have some diffusion impairment, and this will be accompanied by ventilation–perfusion inequality, and possibly a shunt (West, 1997).

Arterial P_{CO_2}

A P_{CO_2} electrode is a glass pH electrode surrounded by a HCO_3^- buffer, which is separated from the blood by a thin membrane through which CO_2 diffuses. The CO_2 alters the pH of the buffer, and this is measured by the electrode which gives a direct reading of the P_{CO_2} (West, 1995). The normal arterial P_{CO_2} is 37 mmHg to 43 mmHg and is unaffected by age. It tends to fall slightly on heavy exercise and rise slightly during sleep.

There are two major causes of CO_2 retention: hypoventilation and ventilation–perfusion abnormality. Hypoventilation must cause hypoxemia and CO_2 retention. The alveolar ventilation equation emphasizes the inverse relationship between the ventilation and the alveolar P_{CO_2}. In normal lungs the arterial P_{CO_2} closely follows the alveolar value. The hypoxemia of hypoventilation can be easily relieved by increasing inspired P_{O_2}; the CO_2

retention can only be treated by increasing the ventilation.

Some patients with ventilation–perfusion inequality increase their ventilation and some do not. Many patients with emphysema hold their P_{CO_2} at the normal level even when their disease is far advanced. Patients with asthma generally do the same (West, 1997).

Arterial pH

The acid–base status of the blood is closely linked to the arterial P_{CO_2} through the Henderson–Hasselbalch equation. Acidosis means a decrease in arterial pH or a rocess that does this. Respiratory acidosis is caused by CO_2 retention, which increases the denominator in the Henderson–Hasselbalch equation and so depresses the pH. Both hypoventilation and ventilation–perfusion ratio inequality contribute to respiratory acidosis (West, 1995).

It is important to distinguish between acute and chronic CO_2 retention. A patient with hypoventilation following an overdose of barbiturate is likely to develop acute respiratory acidosis. There is little change in HCO_3^- concentration, the numerator in the Henderson–Hasselbalch equation, and the pH falls rapidly as the P_{CO_2} rises. Typically a doubling of the P_{CO_2} from 40 mmHg to 80 mmHg in such a patient reduces the pH from 7.4 to 7.2.

By contrast, a patient who develops chronic CO_2 retention over a period of many weeks as a result of increasing ventilation–perfusion inequality caused by chronic pulmonary disease typically has a smaller fall in pH. This is because the kidneys retain HCO_3^- in response to the increased P_{CO_2} in the renal tubular cells, increasing the numerator in the Henderson–Hasselbalch equation.

Metabolic acidosis is caused by a fall in the numerator (HCO_3^-) in the Henderson–Hasselbalch equation, an example being diabetic ketoacidosis. The fall in arterial pH stimulates the peripheral chemoreceptors, increasing ventilation and lowering the P_{CO_2}.

Respiratory alkalosis is seen in acute hyperventilation where the pH rises. If hyperventilation is maintained, for example, at high altitude, compensated respiratory alkalosis is seen. The pH returns toward normal as the kidney secretes HCO_3^-. Metabolic alkalosis is seen in disorders such as severe prolonged vomiting, when the plasma HCO_3^- concentration rises. The arterial P_{CO_2} typically increases a little because of slight respiratory depression. Metabolic alkalosis also occurs when a patient with long-standing lung disease and compensated respiratory acidosis is mechanically overventilated, bringing the P_{CO_2} rapidly to nearly 40 mmHg (West, 1997).

Diffusing Capacity

A common test of gas exchange is the diffusing capacity of the lung for carbon monoxide (CO). The most popu-

lar method of measuring the diffusing capacity (D_{CO}) is the single breath method. The patient takes a VC breath of 0.3% CO and 10% helium, holds the breath for 10 seconds, and then exhales. On the assumption that the CO lost from alveolar gas in proportion to the P_{CO} during breathholding, the D_{CO} is calculated as the volume of CO taken up per minute per mmHg alveolar P_{CO}.

Carbon monoxide is used to measure diffusing capacity because when it is inhaled in low concentrations, the partial pressure in the pulmonary capillary blood remains extremely low in relation to the alveolar volume. As a result, CO is taken up by the blood all along the capillary. The uptake of CO is determined by the diffusion properties of the blood-gas barrier and the rate of combination of CO with blood.

The diffusion properties of the alveolar membrane depend on its thickness and area. Thus, the diffusing capacity is reduced by diseases in which the thickness is increased, including diffuse interstitial fibrosis, sarcoidosis, and asbestosis. It is also reduced when the surface area of the blood-gas barrier is reduced, for example, by pneumonectomy. The rate of combination of CO with blood is reduced whenever the number of red cells in the capillaries is reduced. This occurs in anemia and also diseases that reduce the capillary blood volume, such as pulmonary embolism (West, 1995).

Microscopic Examination of Pulmonary Function

Tracheobronchial secretions are provided by three sources: (1) expectorated sputum, (2) tracheobronchial aspiration, or (3) fiberoptic bronchoscopy. Lung biopsies can be obtained by fiberoptic bronchoscopy, percutaneous needle aspiration, or an open surgical procedure. Specimens can be processed for staining and culture of microorganisms and for cytologic and histopathologic examinations (Shure, 1989).

▶ FUNCTIONAL RESPIRATORY ASSESSMENT

Pulmonary evaluation on either a microscopic or macroscopic level aims at a diagnosis of lung disease, but neither can determine the extent to which normal functions of the lung are impaired. Functional assessment determines how much lung disease may limit a patient's daily activities. The two most common ways to view a patient's functional status are by pulmonary function tests and measurement of arterial blood gases (Bates, 1989).

Pulmonary Function Tests

Pulmonary function testing provides an objective method for assessing functional changes in a patient with known or suspected lung disease. With the results of screening tests that are available at most hospitals, clinicians are able to determine the following: (1) Does the patient have significant lung disease sufficient to cause respiratory impairment and to account for his or her symptoms? and (2) What functional pattern of lung disease does the patient have—restrictive or obstructive disease (Mahler, 1989)?

Three main categories of information can be obtained with *screening* or routine pulmonary function testing:

1. Lung volumes, which provide a measurement of the size of the various compartments within the lung
2. Flow rates, which measure maximal flows within the airway
3. Diffusing capacity, which indicates how readily gas transfer occurs from the alveolus to the pulmonary capillary blood (Zibrak, O'Donnell, & Marton, 1989)

Although the lung can be subdivided into compartments in different ways, four volumes in particular need to be evaluated:

1. *Total lung capacity* (TLC): the total volume of gas within the lungs after a maximal inspiration
2. *Residual volume* (RV): the volume of gas remaining within the lungs after a maximal expiration
3. *Vital capacity* (VC): the volume of gas expired when going from TLC to RV
4. *Functional residual capacity* (FRC): the volume of gas within the lungs at the resting state, that is, at the end of expiration during the normal tidal breathing pattern

The VC can be easily measured by having the patient breathe into a spirometer from TLC down to RV. By definition, the volume expired in this manner is the VC. Because RV, FRC, and TLC all include the amount of gas left within the lungs even after a maximal expiration, these volumes cannot be determined simply by having the patient breathe into a spirometer. Lung volumes are determined by spirometry and either gas dilution or body plethysmography.

The measurement of flow rates on routine pulmonary function testing involves assessing airflow during maximal forced expiration, for example, with the patient breathing as hard and as fast as possible from TLC down to RV. The volume expired during this maneuver is the FVC, whereas the amount expired during the first second is the FEV_1. In interpreting flow rates, it is common to use the ratio between these two measurements, (FEV_1/FVC), as an index of obstruction to airflow. Another parameter often calculated from the forced expira-

tory maneuver is the maximum midexpiratory flow rate (MMEFR) which is the rate of airflow during the middle half of the expiration, that is, between 25% and 75% of the volume expired during the FVC. It is also frequently called the FEF between 25% and 75% of the VC ($FEF_{25-75\%}$). The MMEFR or $FEF_{25-75\%}$ is a sensitive index of airflow obstruction and may be abnormal when the FEV_1/FVC ratio is still preserved (Zibrak, O'Donnell, & Marton, 1989).

Interpretation of Pulmonary Function Tests

Interpretation of pulmonary function tests necessarily involves a qualitative judgment about normality or abnormality on the basis of the quantitative data obtained from these tests. To arrive at a relatively objective way to make such judgments, normal standards have been established for each test by using large numbers of normal, nonsmoking control subjects. Regression lines have been constructed to fit the data obtained from these normal control subjects. A *normal* or predicted value for a test in a given patient can then be found by putting the patient's age and height into the regression equation. The standards for determining what constitutes the *lower limits of normal* for a particular test may vary from laboratory to laboratory. Some laboratories use *95% confidence intervals,* based on standard errors around the regression line, whereas others consider the observed value to be normal if it is greater than 80% of the predicted value. No matter what criteria are used, it is important to take all data into consideration to see if certain patterns are consistently present. Interpretation of any test in isolation, with the assumption that a patient value of 79% has lung disease while one with a value of 81% is disease free, obviously is dangerous (Weinberger, 1992).

Interpretations of the FEV_1/FVC ratio is the only exception to the general rule that a normal value is greater than 80% of the predicted value. If this ratio is compared with the predicted ratio, this ratio of the ratios should be greater than 95%. It is important to emphasize that this 95% value does not refer to the actual FEV_1/FVC ratio, but rather to the comparison of this observed ratio with the predicted ratio (Mahler, 1989).

Patterns of Pulmonary Function Impairment

In the analysis of pulmonary function tests, abnormalities usually are categorized into one of two patterns (or a combination of the two): (1) an obstructive pattern characterized mainly by obstruction to airflow and (2) a restrictive pattern, with evidence of decreased lung volumes but no airflow obstruction (Mahler, 1989).

An obstructive pattern, as seen in patients with asthma, chronic bronchitis, or emphysema, consists of a decrease in rates of expiratory airflow and usually mani-

TABLE 11–5. Further Analysis of Pulmonary Function Tests

Examination of the Lung Volumes

- A decrease in TLC generally indicates the presence of a restrictive pattern. However, it is important to remember that TLC measured by helium dilution may also be artificially depressed when there are poorly communicating or noncommunicating regions within the lung (eg, in bullous lung disease).
- Are the lung volumes symmetrically reduced? Are TLC, RV, FRC, and VC all decreased to approximately the same extent? If so, this suggests interstitial lung disease as the cause of the restrictive pattern. A low diffusing capacity also supports the diagnosis of interstitial lung disease as the cause of the restrictive pattern.

Interpretation of the FEF$_{25\%-75\%}$

- FEF$_{25\%-75\%}$ is subject to more variability than most other measurements obtained during a forced expiration, so that guidelines for normal values are less established.
- When lung volumes are low, FEF$_{25\%-75\%}$ can also be decreased without necessarily indicating coexisting airflow obstruction. Therefore, in the presence of decreased lung volumes, a low FEF$_{25\%-75\%}$ is out of proportion to the decrease in lung volumes.

Interpretation of Diffusing Capacity for CO

- Make sure the value has been corrected for the patient's hemoglobin level. If not, the value will be falsely low if the patient is anemic.
- A decrease in the diffusing capacity reflects disease affecting the alveolar–capillary membrane (decreased surface area for gas exchange and/or abnormal thickness of the membrane) or a decrease in pulmonary capillary blood volume.

Interpretation of the Flow–Volume Curves

- An obstructive pattern is reflected by decreased flow relative to lung volume, generally accompanied by a scooped-out or coved appearance to the descending part of the expiratory curve.

- A relatively preserved RV and a normal diffusing capacity suggest another cause of restrictive disease, such as neuromuscular chest wall disease. Poor effort from the patient may also create this type of pattern.
- Examination of the mechanics or the flow rates measured from the forced expiratory spirogram: A decrease in the FEV$_1$/FVC ratio indicates obstruction. In some cases of airflow obstruction, both the FEV$_1$ and the FVC are reduced by approximately the same extent, and the FEV$_1$/FVC ratio may be preserved. Clues to the presence of obstructive disease in this setting are a low FEF$_{25\%-75\%}$, a normal to high TLC with a high RV/TLC ratio, and the configuration of the flow–volume curve.

- Taking into account the aforementioned qualifications, FEF$_{25\%-75\%}$ is a sensitive measurement for airway obstruction (Shapiro, Harrison, Cane, & Templin, 1989).

- An increase in diffusing capacity can reflect increased pulmonary capillary blood volume or erythrocytes within alveolar spaces, for example, pulmonary hemorrhage (Shapiro, Harrison, Cane, & Templin, 1989).

- A restrictive pattern is characterized by decreased volumes, that is narrowing of the curve along the volume or x-axis, and preserved flow rates. The flow rates often appear increased relative to the small lung volumes, producing a tall, narrow curve (Shapiro, Harrison, Cane, & Templin, 1989).

---

fests as a decrease in MMEFR and the FEV$_1$/FVC ratio. Diffusing capacity tends to be decreased in those patients who have loss of alveolar–capillary bed (eg, emphysema), but not in those without loss of surface area for gas exchange (eg, chronic bronchitis or asthma) (Mahler, 1989).

The hallmark of restrictive disease is a reduction in lung volumes. Expiratory outflow is normal; therefore, TLC, RV, VC, and FRC all tend to be reduced, whereas MMEFR and FEV$_1$/FVC are preserved. In some patients with significant loss of volume from restrictive disease, the MMEFR is decreased because of less volume available to generate a high flow rate. It is, therefore, difficult to interpret a low MMEFR in the face of significant restrictive disease unless it is clearly decreased out of proportion to the decrease in lung volumes (Mahler, 1989).

A wide variety of parenchymal, pleural, neuromuscular, and chest wall diseases can demonstrate a restrictive pattern. Certain clues often are useful in distinguishing among the causes of restriction. For example, a decrease in the diffusing capacity of CO suggests loss of alveolar–capillary units and points toward interstitial dis-

ease as the cause of the restrictive pattern. However, the finding of a relatively high RV can indicate either expiratory muscle weakness or a chest wall abnormality that makes the thoracic cage particularly stiff (noncompliant) at low volumes (Mahler, 1989).

Although lung diseases often occur with one or the other of these patterns, a mixed picture of obstructive and restrictive disease can be present, making interpretation of tests more complex. It should be noted that these tests do not directly reflect a patient's overall capability for O_2 and CO_2 exchange, which is assessed by measurement of arterial blood gases (Bates, 1989). Further analysis of pulmonary function tests is described in Table 11-5.

▶ PULMONARY PATHOPHYSIOLOGY

Chronic Obstructive Pulmonary Disease

The term *chronic obstructive pulmonary disease* (COPD) refers to chronic disorders that disturb airflow, whether the most prominent process is within the airways or within the lung parenchyma. The two disorders generally included within this category are chronic bronchitis and emphysema. Although the pathophysiology of airflow obstruction is different in these two disorders, patients frequently have features of both.

Chronic bronchitis is a diagnosis based on chronic cough and sputum production. Patients with chronic bronchitis frequently have periods of worsening symptoms, often precipitated by respiratory tract infection. Chronic bronchitis is characterized by enlargement of the mucous-secreting glands and an increased number of goblet cells. Pathologic changes from smoking often start in small airways, predating the advanced findings associated with chronic bronchitis and emphysema (Habib & Burrows, 1990).

Emphysema is a diagnosis based on dilatation and destruction of air spaces distal to the terminal bronchiole. Because chronic bronchitis and emphysema coexist to a variable extent in different patients, the broader term *chronic obstructive pulmonary disease* is frequently more accurate. Cigarette smoking, a single etiologic factor, is primarily responsible for both processes. Inflammation produced by cigarette smoke, from the large airways down to the alveolar walls of the pulmonary parenchyma, is believed to be the common link for the various manifestations of COPD (Habib & Burrows, 1990).

Smoking is the key etiologic factor for chronic bronchitis. Air pollutants and respiratory tract infection cause exacerbations but have no significant etiologic role. Cigarette smoking is responsible for most cases of emphysema. Deficiency of serum alpha$_1$ antitrypsin is a predisposing factor for emphysema in a small proportion of cases (Weinberger, 1992). Current theories claim that proteolytic enzymes (especially elastase) are balanced by alpha$_1$ antitrypsin. Disturbance of this balance in favor of proteolytic enzymes, either due to smoking or to a deficiency of alpha$_1$ antitrypsin may result in emphysema.

Pathophysiology and Functional Abnormalities in Chronic Obstructive Pulmonary Disease

In emphysema, decreased expiratory flow rates are largely due to loss of elastic recoil of the lung, resulting in (1) lower driving pressure for expiratory airflow and (2) loss of radial traction on the airways provided by supporting alveolar walls, thus promoting airway collapse during expiration.

In obstructive lung disease, nonuniformity of the disease process results in V/Q mismatch and hypoxemia. Mechanisms that contribute to alveolar hypoventilation and CO_2 retention in obstructive lung disease include (1) increased work of breathing, (2) abnormalities of the

ventilatory drive, and (3) V/Q mismatch (Habib & Burrows, 1990).

The major cause of pulmonary hypertension in COPD is hypoxia. Additional factors include hypercapnia, polycythemia, and destruction of the pulmonary vascular bed. Two types of clinical presentation are possible for patients with COPD.

Clinical Presentation of Chronic Obstructive Pulmonary Disease

Two presentations of obstructive lung disease are the *pink puffer* (type A) and the *blue bloater* (type B). A clear distinction between their underlying processes is an oversimplification. The precipitating factor in an exacerbation of COPD is often a viral infection. Continuation of smoking is a major risk factor affecting the prognosis in COPD.

Characteristic radiographic findings in the more frequently recognized arterial deficiency pattern of COPD are (1) large lung volumes, (2) flat diaphragms, (3) increased anteroposterior diameter, and (4) loss of vascular markings (Burrows, Bloom, Traver, & Cline, 1987). Pulmonary function tests in COPD show (1) airflow obstruction with decreased FVC, FEV$_1$, FEV$_1$/FVC, and MMEFR; (2) air trapping, with increased RV, FRC, and often TLC; and (3) a generally decreased diffusing capacity in emphysema, normal in chronic bronchitis (Burrows, Bloom, Traver, & Cline, 1987). The clinical distinctions between type A and type B pathophysiology are shown in Table 11–6. Type B patients are more hypoxemic than type A patients and often have hypercapnia.

Modalities available for treatment of COPD include bronchodilators, chest physiotherapy, antibiotics, corti-

TABLE 11–6. Clinical Distinctions Between Type A and Type B Pathophysiology

Feature: Commonly Used Name	Type A: Pink Puffer	Type B: Blue Bloater
Disease association	Predominant emphysema	Predominant bronchitis
Major symptom	Dyspnea	Cough and sputum
Appearance	Thin, wasted, not cyanotic	Obese, cyanotic
Po$_2$	Low	Very low
Pco$_2$	Normal or low	Normal or high
Elastic recoil of lung	Low	Normal
Diffusing capacity	Low	Normal
Hematocrit	Normal	Often high
Cor pulmonale	Infrequent	Common

From Burrows, B., Bloom, J., Traver, G., & Cline, M. (1987). The course and prognosis of different forms of chronic airways obstruction in a sample from the general population. New England Journal of Medicine, 317, 1309–1314.

costeroids, and supplemental O_2 (Faling & Snyder, 1989). An important adjunct to therapy is the administration of supplemental O_2 to those patients with significant hypoxemia (eg, arterial Po_2 of 55 mmHg or less). The Po_2 of hypoxemic patients with COPD usually responds well to even small amounts of supplemental O_2 (eg, Fio_2 of 0.24 L to 0.28 L). A low flow rate of O_2 (eg, 1 L/min to 2 L/min) given by nasal prongs is an effective and well-tolerated method for achieving these concentrations of inspired O_2 (Faling & Snider, 1989).

The goal of O_2 therapy is to shift the Po_2 into the range in which hemoglobin is almost fully saturated, that is a Po_2 of greater than 60 mmHg to 65 mmHg. Ideally, O_2 saturation should be well maintained on a continuous basis throughout the day and night. In some patients with COPD who are not significantly hypoxemic during the day, a substantial drop in their Po_2 and O_2 saturation can occur at night; in these patients, noctural O_2 is beneficial (Faling & Snider, 1989).

Asthma

Asthma is characterized by hyperreactivity of the airways and reversible episodes of bronchoconstriction. Although some asthmatic patients have allergies, many do not, and the overall relationship between allergies and asthma is not clear. Airway inflammation and epithelial injury may contribute to nonspecific bronchial hyper-responsiveness. One theory suggests that autonomic nervous system abnormalities contribute to the pathogenesis of asthma. Common stimuli that precipitate bronchoconstriction in asthmatics are discussed in Table 11–7.

In asthma and other diseases associated with the obstruction of intrathoracic airways, airflow is most compromised during expiration. Pulmonary function tests with asthma generally show a decreased FEV_1, FVC, and FEV_1/FVC ratio. Air trapping and hyperinflation are demonstrated by increases in RV, FRC, and sometimes TLC. The most common pattern of arterial blood gases in asthma is a low Po_2, due primarily to V/Q mismatch, and a low Pco_2.

Epidemiology of Asthma

A linear increase in asthma cases worldwide has been demonstrated. Reasons for this increase are multifactorial; certainly environmental contaminants have a role (Lapin & Cloutier, 1995). Asthma affects more than 3 million people worldwide, and is currently the most common chronic respiratory disease. Between 1981 and 1988, the prevalence of asthma increased 39%. Asthma deaths increased 31% between 1980 and 1987. In terms of morbidity, over 2 million individuals are limited in their daily lives because of asthma. There has been a

TABLE 11–7. Potential Chemical Mediators in Asthma

Common stimuli that precipitate bronchoconstriction in the asthmatic patient include

1. **Exposure to an allergen**—house dust, especially antigens from the house dust mite
   - Histamine
   - Leukotrienes (SRS-A)
   - Platelet-activating factor
   - Eosinophil chemotactic factor of anaphylaxis
   - Neutrophil chemotactic factor of anaphylaxis
   - Prostaglandins
   - Bradykinin
   - Serotonin
   - Kallikrein

2. **Inhaled irritants**—for example, cigarette smoke, dust, environmental pollutants

3. **Respiratory tract infection**—viral infection most common

4. **Exercise**—can provoke bronchoconstriction in patients with hyperreactive airways; airway drying and cooling important in exercise-induced bronchoconstriction

From Sheller, J. (1987). Asthma: Emerging concepts and potential therapies. American Journal of Medical Science, 293, *298–308.*

worldwide increase in the rate of asthma-related hospitalizations (Lapin & Cloutier, 1995).

The understanding of the pathophysiologic basis for asthma has evolved to include an increased emphasis on the inflammatory component of the disease. An increased emphasis on anti-inflammatory treatment has occurred, coupled with the understanding that mortality may rarely accompany the use of β_2 agonists (Lapin & Cloutier, 1995). A recent definition of asthma emphasized that this is a chronic lung disease with (1) usually reversible airway obstruction, (2) airway inflammation, and (3) increased airway responsiveness to multiple stimuli (Lapin & Cloutier, 1995).

In the United States, children are increasingly affected by asthma; it is the most common childhood disease, and is the leading cause of school absence. In 1990, asthma-related expenses were $6.2 billion. Of that amount, $3.2 billion was in health care costs, and $2.5 billion was in time lost from school or work (Lapin & Cloutier, 1995).

Clinical Features of Asthma

The major symptoms seen during an acute asthma attack include cough, dyspnea, wheezing, and chest tightness. Patients do not necessarily have a classic presentation with several or all of these complaints, but may have unexpected cough or breathlessness on exertion. Despite its prominence, the presence of wheezing is not synonymous with asthma and only reflects airflow through narrowed airways. Severe asthma may be associated with no wheeze if airflow is too impaired to generate an audible wheeze.

Classic asthmatic symptoms, especially in children, include cough, wheezing, dyspnea, and tachypnea. A cough of several weeks' duration may be the sole symptom. Nocturnal, posttussive emesis, triggered by smoke, fumes, laughing, or crying, is frequently confused with bronchitis (Lapin & Cloutier, 1995).

Diagnostic and Treatment Approaches

A diagnosis of asthma includes a history of episodic dyspnea, wheezing, or cough, along with reversible airflow obstruction documented by pulmonary function testing. Sympathomimetic agents increase intracellular cAMP by activating adenyl cyclase. Newer agents preferentially stimulate β_2-receptors and decrease potential adverse cardiac effects caused by stimulation of β_1-receptors. Findings and recommendations from the National Heart, Lung, and Blood Institute recognized the inflammatory component of asthma and the role of selective β agonists (Murphy, 1995).

Methylxanthines (aminophylline, theophylline) increase cAMP by inhibiting the enzyme phosphodiesterase, which degrades cAMP. This mechanism arguably is responsible for bronchodilation. Systemic and inhaled cortico-steroids now have an important role in acute therapy and preventive management, respectively (Murphy, 1995).

Treatment Guidelines

Current treatment guidelines for asthma emphasize the use of peak expiratory flow rates (PEFR) to monitor air-way reactivity (Table 11-8). Family involvement in the monitoring and treatment of asthmatic patients also helps maximize home care options. The best approach to asthmatic exacerbations is felt to be early treatment. Moderately to severely asthmatic children need to perform regular peak flow measurements at home. When available, oximetry helps to rapidly assess the severity of acute asthma exacerbations (Table 11-9). Fatal asthma can occur and etiologic factors are presented in Table 11-10.

Assessment of Asthma Severity

When asthma is mild, associated symptoms do not interfere with sleep or lifestyle. Mild asthma does not require daily drug therapy. Moderate asthma involves attacks occurring more than once a week. Patients will have coughing or wheezing with acute episodes, sometimes at night. Moderate asthmatics require urgent treatment one to three times annually. Treatment for these patients includes daily anti-inflammatory medication and bronchodilators.

Individuals with severe asthma experience daily symptoms of reactive airways disease. Asthmatic exacerbations for these people are frequent and severe in nature. Wheezing is present in severe asthma most days or nights. Urgent care, possibly requiring hospitalization, may be required more than three times per year. Some

---

TABLE 11–8. Correlation of Clinical Findings with Treatment

- PEFR green zone should be 80% to 100% personal best value recorded to date/predicted value for patient.
- No asthma symptoms are present, so continue current therapies.
- Yellow PEFR zone represents 50% to 80% personal best/predicted values.
- With an acute exacerbation, extra bronchodilator doses and possibly steroids are indicated.
- Performance in the red PEFR zone means the patient is at less than 50% of his or her personal best/predicted pulmonary performance. At this point, a medical alert should be initiated (eg, calling the primary health provider and/or emergency medical services, immediate bronchodilator therapy with back-to-back breathing treatments).
- Asthma exacerbation treatment includes albuterol 0.1 mg/kg to 0.15 mg/kg via nebulizer, with a minimum dose of 1.25 mg of albuterol 2 to 4 puffs via multidose inhaler using a spacer device, every 20 minutes for up to 1 hour, or 3 back-to-back treatments.
- Spacer devices maximize drug delivery and decrease the cough reflex (Marley, 1995).
- If a good response to aerosol therapy results, continue treatments every 3 to 4 hours with frequent reassessment of pulmonary status for the presence of wheezing (Lapin & Cloutier, 1995).

TABLE 11–9. Assessing Adequacy of Response to Therapy

Good response
- PEFR > 70% baseline
- Decreased heart rate and respiratory rate
- No wheezing
- Minimal to no dyspnea
- Pulsus paradoxus < 10 mmHg
- Spo_2 > 95% on room air

Incomplete or inadequate response
- PEFR > 50%, < 70% baseline
- Increased heart rate and respiratory rate
- Mild wheezing
- Moderate use of accessory muscles
- Moderate dyspnea
- Pulsus paradoxus ≥ 10 mmHg to 15 mmHg
- Spo_2 91% to 95% on room air

Poor response
- PEFR < 50% baseline
- Increased heart rate and respiratory rate
- Decreased air movement
- Major use of accessory muscles
- Severe dyspnea
- Pulsus paradoxus > 15 mmHg
- Spo_2 < 91%

From Lapin, C. & Cloutier, M. (1995). Outpatient management of acute exacerbations of asthma in children. Journal of Asthma, 32(1), 5–20.

TABLE 11–10. Risk Factors for Fatal Asthma

Age
   Late teens, early 20s
Ethnicity
   African American males
Previous life-threatening asthma exacerbations
Hospital admissions for asthma in previous year
Poor appreciation of disease severity
Psychosocial problems, lack of access to care

From Lapin, C. & Cloutier, M. (1995). Outpatient Management of acute exacerbations of asthma in children. Journal of Asthma, 32(1), 5–20.

suggested steps in the management of asthma are in Table 11–11.

Current recommendations emphasize treating asthma with steroids in all but the mildest cases due to the central role of airway inflammation in this disease process. If bronchodilators are needed more than every 3 to 4 hours, patients probably need corticosteroids such as prednisone, 1 to 2 mg/kg/day (Murphy, 1995).

There is little to recommend the use of theophylline preparations for acute asthma exacerbations. Theophylline is of less benefit in acute asthma than inhaled β agonists, and theophylline adds little to combined aerosol and steroid therapy. The side effects of theophylline toxicity outweigh its potential benefits (Murphy, 1995).

The use of subcutaneous epinephrine or terbutaline is recommended only for patients with altered levels of consciousness who would be unable to use MDI or

TABLE 11–11. Management of Asthma

- Decrease exposure to triggering agents such as allergens and upper respiratory infections.
- Use a treatment to reverse bronchospasm, reduce airway inflammation, and airway wall edema.
- Decrease dyspnea.
- Ensure adequate oxygenation and ventilation.
- Family members should know how to recognize asthma exacerbations and be able to gauge their severity.
- Patients and families need to know how to use the zone system of peak expiratory flow (PEFR) meters.
- Written guidelines for asthma maintenance therapy have to be available to the patient and family.
- Patients and family members need to understand when to call their primary care provider for additional treatment guidelines during exacerbations of asthma

From Lapin, C. & Cloutier, M. (1995). Outpatient Management of acute exacerbations of asthma in children. Journal of Asthma, 32(1), 5–20.

aerosol therapy. Because epinephrine has significant alpha, β_1, and β_2 activity, it is a less desirable treatment option than selective β_2 agonists (Murphy, 1995).

Anesthesia Implications of Asthma

It is worth noting that 3.5% of 10 000 surgical patients are asthmatic. When these patients develop perioperative complications, 75% of those complications involve the pulmonary system. Of those asthmatics who were previously asymptomatic, 5.6% will develop intraoperative bronchospasm. Perioperative cardiac arrest is reported to be twenty times more frequent in asthmatic than in nonasthmatic patients. Although it is counterintuitive, no correlation appears to exist between severity of asthma and the frequency of perioperative complications (Geiger & Hedley-Whyte, 1993).

Lung Cancer

Anesthesia providers will encounter patients with lung cancer presenting for diagnostic and therapeutic procedures. Potential clinical problems with lung cancer include symptoms from an endobronchial tumor (eg, cough, hemoptysis), problems of bronchial obstruction (postobstructive pneumonia, dyspnea), pleural involvement (chest pain, pleural effusion, dyspnea), involvement of the adjacent structures (eg, heart, esophagous), complications of mediastinal involvement (phrenic or recurrent laryngeal nerve paralysis, superior vena cava obstruction), distant metastases (brain, bone or bone marrow, liver, adrenals), ectopic hormone production (ACTH, ADH, parathyroid hormone), other paraneo-plastic syndromes (neurologic, clubbing, hypertrophic osteoarthropathy), and nonspecific systemic effects (anorexia, weight loss) (Gazdar & Linnoila, 1988).

Although bronchial carcinoid tumors occur less frequently than lung lesions, it is important to understand factors that contribute to their etiology. Common features of bronchial carcinoid tumors are (1) common appearance in young adults; (2) hemoptysis; and (3) pneumonia distal to an obstructing endobronchial mass (Gazdar & Linnoila, 1988). The basis for the staging of lung cancer involves the following factors: (1) size, location, and local complications of the primary tumor; (2) hilar and mediastinal lymph node involvement; and (3) distant metastasis (Gazdar & Linnoila, 1988).

The utility and cost-effectiveness of preoperative pulmonary function testing are debated for some patient populations. However, assessment of pulmonary function helps determine whether surgical resection can be tolerated in the patient with compromised pulmonary function (Ginsberg, Ross, & Field, 1989).

Tuberculosis

It has been estimated that there are 8 to 10 million new cases of tuberculosis (TB) and approximately 3 million tuberculosis deaths worldwide each year. In recent decades until the early 1980s, this staggering number of cases was a public health problem primarily in developing countries. However, this is no longer the case; TB is now on the rise in the United States, particularly in indigent and immigrant populations and in patients with acquired immunodeficiency syndrome (AIDS) (Dutt & Stead, 1990).

The transmission of TB is by inhalation of small aerosol droplets containing the organism. The majority of active TB cases involve reactivation of a previously dormant focus within the lungs. After development of delayed hypersensitivity, the pathologic hallmarks of TB are granulomas and caseous necrosis, often with cavity formation (Dutt & Stead, 1990). The common presenting problems with TB include (1) systemic symptoms such as weight loss, fever, and night sweats; (2) pulmonary symptoms including cough, sputum production, and hemoptysis; and (3) abnormal chest x-ray findings (Dutt & Stead, 1990). Common features of the chest x-ray in primary TB are (1) nonspecific infiltrates, often involving the lower lobes; (2) hilar and paratracheal node enlargement; and (3) pleural effusion (Dutt & Stead, 1990).

A common treatment for pulmonary TB is isoniazid (INH) and rifampin given for 6 months, supplemented by pyrazinamide for the first 2 months. Isoniazid alone for 6 to 12 months is frequently given to patients without currently active tuberculosis who are at high risk for active disease. Resistant strains of tuberculosis require longer courses of drug therapy and may require additional antimicrobial agents (Davidson, 1990).

Acquired Immune Deficiency Syndrome

The human immunodeficiency virus (HIV) binds to the CD41 receptors of helper-inducer T lymphocytes. In full-blown AIDS, the major pulmonary infections seen are Pneumocystis carinii pneumonia (PCP), cytomegalovirus infections, and mycobacterial and fungal infections. P. carinii pneumonia often has an indolent onset in AIDS. Diagnosis of PCP is made most commonly on samples obtained by induction of sputum or bronchoalveolar lavage. Standard therapy for PCP is trimeothoprim–sulfamethoxazole or pentamidine. Atypical presentations of PCP infections commonly are seen in patients receiving aerosolized pentamidine (Edelson & Hyland, 1990).

Pulmonary infiltrates, often accompanied by fever, dyspnea, and cough, present a common problem in the patient known to have either HIV infection or risk factors for exposure to HIV. Although typical radiographic presentation of some of the aforementioned diseases may suggest a particular diagnosis, often the findings are nonspecific (Murray & Mills, 1990). Recent advances in the treatment of AIDS with protease-inhibiting drugs and combinations of antiretroviral agents may delay or lessen the frequency of opportunistic infections associated with this disease.

▶ PERIANESTHETIC PULMONARY SYSTEM PLAN

Patients who smoke should be encouraged to stop smoking for at least 2 months preoperatively, to minimize airway reactivity associated with smoking. Any existing respiratory infection should be treated (Domino, 1996).

For asthmatics, treatment with steroids for 3 days prior to elective surgical cases may reduce perioperative bronchospasm. The administration of β_2 agonists in the preoperative holding area is also recommended (Domino, 1996). Further administration of β_2 agonists may be necessary intraoperatively if bronchospasm refractory to anesthetic agents develops.

Patients at high risk for pulmonary complications, such as those who are obese or who are undergoing upper abdominal or thoracic surgical procedures, or patients with histories of respiratory disease, should be taught incentive spirometry preoperatively. Those patients at risk for postoperative pulmonary complications should have chest physiotherapy to mobilize secretions and enhance pulmonary toilet postoperatively.

Patients at risk for postoperative pulmonary complications include those with chronic respiratory diseases such as asthma, bronchitis, COPD, and TB. Surgical factors also contribute to the potential for postoperative pulmonary complications: The right subcostal incisions used for open cholecystectomies, sternotomies, thoracotomies, or the xiphoid to symphysis pubis incisions made in patients undergoing major surgical procedures compromise ventilation. Aggressive postoperative pain management in these patients coupled with early mobilization and vigorous pulmonary toilet measures help minimize the potential for atelectasis, hypoxia, hypercapnia, or pneumonia.

Elective surgeries should be delayed in the face of recent or uncontrolled pulmonary infection. There should be a lower threshold for delaying upper abdominal or thoracic surgery in patients with ongoing pulmonary infection owing to the higher risk of pulmonary

TABLE 11–12. Recommended Intraoperative Respiratory System Monitoring

Ventilation
- Intubation of the trachea shall be verified by auscultation, chest excursion, and confirmation of carbon dioxide in the expired gas.
- Controlled or assisted ventilation during the anesthetic shall be monitored continuously with an end-tidal carbon dioxide monitor.
- Additionally, spirometry and ventilatory pressure alarms may also be used.
- Breathing system disconnect monitor: When the patient is ventilated by an automatic mechanical ventilator, the integrity of the breathing system must be monitored by a device that is capable of detecting disconnection of any component of the breathing system. Such a device shall be equipped with an audible alarm which is activated when its limits are exceeded.

Oxygenation
- Adequacy of patient oxygenation shall be monitored continuously with pulse oximetry.
- In addition to pulse oximetry, oxygenation shall also be monitored by observations of skin color, the color of the blood in the surgical field, and arterial blood gas analysis when indicated.
- During general anesthesia, the oxygen concentration delivered by the anesthesia machine shall be monitored continuously with an oxygen analyzer with a low oxygen concentration limit alarm.
- An oxygen supply failure alarm system shall be operational to warn of low oxygen pressure to the anesthesia machine.

From The American Association of Nurse Anesthetists (AANA) (1996). Scope & standards for nurse anesthesia practice (p. 3). Park Ridge, IL: AANA. Adapted with permission.

complications such as pneumonia in these patients (Domino, 1996). Recommendations for intraoperative monitoring of the respiratory system are provided in the AANA *Scope and Standards for Nurse Anesthesia Practice* (1996). These recommendations are summarized in Table 11–12.

Nurse anesthetists are responsible for thorough assessment of all body systems, including the respiratory system. It is incumbent on individual nurse anesthetists to synthesize data obtained through physical assessment and take appropriate actions (AANA, 1996). These actions may include ordering additional diagnostic testing or delaying surgery. Assessing room O_2 saturation prior to the administration of sedatives provides a baseline indication of oxygenation.

General Considerations

Intraoperative respiratory monitoring involves oximetry, capnography, spirometry, peak inspiratory pressure, and monitoring of inspired and end-tidal gas concentrations. Baseline oximetry values can help determine the degree of existing respiratory compromise. Capnography, in addition to demonstrating adequacy of ventilation, can also show prolonged expiratory times in COPD, and spontaneous breaths taken during controlled ventilation. Peak inspiratory pressures demonstrate airway resistance, and can be modified by adjustment of the inspiratory : expiratory (I : E) ratio. Spirometry is essential to monitor adequacy of ventilation.

The anesthetist needs to be aware of the effects of positioning on ventilation. Recall that the lateral position, used in procedures such as nephrectomies, thoracic surgeries, and total hip arthroplasties, leads to increased perfusion and decreased ventilation in the dependent lung. The nondependent lung is less perfused and better ventilated. This altered physiology mandates careful patient monitoring and adjustment of ventilatory parameters to maintain adequate minute ventilation and oxygenation. Another problematic position for ventilation is the Trendelenburg (head-down) position used during procedures such as laparoscopies. The combination of pneumoperitoneum and viscera pressing against the diaphragm can compromise ventilation and oxygenation. Monitoring of oximetry and capnography can lead the anesthetist to increasing minute volume as necessary and maintaining adequate oxygenation.

Drugs to avoid in patients with respiratory compromise include substances that produce respiratory depression. Narcotics, especially when combined with medications known to potentiate their respiratory depressant effects such as benzodiazepines or barbiturates, are best administered in the preoperative holding area or the operating room. In such locations, positive-pressure O_2, suction, and oximetry should be available. Histamine-releasing drugs, such as morphine, meperidine, and curanform muscle relaxants, should be avoided in patients with reactive airways as histamine release can lead to bronchospasm.

Regional anesthesia is commonly advocated for patients with chronic respiratory disease for several reasons. Well-managed regional anesthesia preserves normal respiratory muscle activity. General anesthesia produces decrements in pulmonary function that may lead to hypoxia. Extubation may be difficult in patients with pulmonary disease because airway reactivity predisposes them to bronchospasm. General anesthesia depresses mucociliary function, compromising oxygenation and ventilation. Stimuli such as intubation can lead to bronchospasm, especially with an inadequate anesthetic depth (Domino, 1996).

It is interesting to note that no research findings to date show that regional anesthesia produces more optimal outcomes than general anesthesia in patients with asthma or COPD. Analysis of closed malpractice insurance claims involving anesthesia providers has not demonstrated a statistically significant association between damaging anesthetic events and the type of anesthetic technique used (general or regional anesthesia) (Caplan, 1995; Kremer, Crawforth, Golinski, Jordan, Larson, Mahinger, Moody, Nagelhout, Shott, Williams, & Bulau, 1996).

▶ CASE STUDY

A 76-year-old male patient with end-stage COPD who has a chronically productive cough and requires O_2 therapy at home presents for an elective transurethral resection of the prostate for benign prostatic hypertrophy. In the preanesthetic interview, the patient expresses displeasure at the prospect of regional anesthesia for this procedure because of a headache following a previous spinal anesthetic.

1. How might the anesthesia provider approach this patient when discussing alternatives for anesthesia care and their associated risks and benefits?

   Establishing a rapport with a patient who is resistant to regional anesthesia would help to develop a trusting relationship between the anesthesia provider and the patient. Without resorting to scare tactics, the anesthetist could indicate that general anesthesia could lead to prolonged postoperative ventilation because COPD would make weaning from the ventilator difficult. The anesthetist could allay anxiety regarding spinal anesthesia by describing the low risk for a postdural puncture headache in this patient.

2. If the patient continues to refuse regional anesthesia, how would one plan a general anesthetic for this procedure?

Knowing that V/Q mismatch and hypoxemia accompany COPD resulting in a hypoxic respiratory drive should influence the planned anesthetic. One option would be to use a mask anesthetic technique with a volatile agent, maintaining spontaneous ventilation. Disruption of the hypoxic ventilatory drive in this patient with large doses of narcotics, muscle relaxants, or high-inspired O_2 concentrations can delay weaning and extubation in COPD patients who undergo intubation and mechanical ventilation.

▶ SUMMARY

This chapter has described essential pulmonary anatomy and physiology necessary for anesthesia practice. Suggestions on how to obtain a pulmonary history in terms of both subjective and objective data have been provided. The role of diagnostic data in the process was discussed. Pertinent pulmonary pathophysiologic entities were reviewed. Management of the airway, ventilation, and the uptake and distribution of volatile anesthetic agents all entail knowledge of respiratory anatomy, physiology, and pathophysiology. Anesthetic management goals regarding the respiratory system include (1) avoiding perioperative hypoxemia and bronchospasm; (2) preventing lobar collapse; (3) minimizing postoperative pulmonary complications related to the surgical site; and (4) avoiding postoperative mechanical ventilation.

Changes in VC as measured by pulmonary function testing best predict individuals who may be at risk for developing postoperative pulmonary complications. Patients undergoing upper abdominal or thoracic surgery are at the greatest risk for developing postoperative pulmonary complications.

▶ KEY CONCEPTS

- Changes in vital capacity (by pulmonary function testing) best predict individuals at risk for postoperative pulmonary complications, especially for surgeries involving the upper abdomen or thorax.
- Recent upper respiratory infections are best evaluated by (1) associated fever, (2) presence of a productive cough, and (3) presence of purulent, colored sputum.
- Management of asthmatic patients should include questions regarding (1) frequency of wheezing, (2) precipitants of airway reactivity, and (3) treatment history.

- Surgical patients with COPD should be assessed preoperatively by activity tolerance, presence of supplemental oxygen, and presence of dyspnea, orthopnea, or tachypnea at rest.
- Orthopnea, which may suggest some element of congestive heart failure, is often quantified by the angle of elevation necessary to relieve or prevent the sensation.
- A chronic nonproductive cough is often related to reactive airway disease. Hemoptysis is often associated with bronchitis, bronchiectasis, and bronchogenic carcinoma. The origin of

noncardiac chest pain is usually in the parietal pleura (eg, pleuritis), the diaphragm, or the mediastinum.
- Assessment of the pulmonary system involves observation of the patient, respiratory rate, pattern and difficulty of breathing, and presence of any abnormal or adventitious sounds (rales, rhonchi, and wheezes).

- The ratio of forced expiratory volume in 1 second to forced vital capacity (FEV_1/FVC) is the only exception to the general rule that a normal value is greater than 80% of the predicted value.
- Obstructive patterns of disease are characterized by obstruction to airflow, while a restrictive pattern shows decreased lung volumes, but no airflow obstruction.

▶ Study Questions

1. With cost constraints imposed by managed care, how can one justify obtaining preoperative pulmonary function tests today?

2. What kinds of postoperative respiratory outcomes can be predicted by pulmonary function tests?

3. What types of subjective and objective data would an anesthetist want to gather on a 45-year-old, 5′4″-tall, 90-kg female with a 25-year smoking history scheduled for an open cholecystectomy procedure?

4. How is neural control of respiration related to asthma?

5. In the preoperative holding area, a patient complains to the anesthetist about feeling short of breath. The patient indicates that he or she occasionally uses an inhaler for asthma. What are the considerations involved in the differential diagnosis of dyspnea?

6. In the recovery room following a general anesthetic, a patient with COPD who has a patent airway is receiving O_2 with an FiO_2 of 0.4 via mask. The SpO_2 readings fall to the upper 80s. What are reasonable diagnostic and therapeutic interventions for the anesthetist to take?

7. What are some of the potential chemical mediators in asthma?

8. How are obstructive and restrictive pulmonary disease differentiated using flow–volume curves?

KEY REFERENCES

Geiger, K. & Hedley-Whyte, J. (1993). Preoperative and postoperative considerations in bronchial asthma. In E. Weiss & M. Stein (Eds.). *Bronchial asthma—mechanisms and therapeutics* (3rd ed., pp. 1099–1112). Boston, MA: Little, Brown & Co.

Lapin, C. & Cloutier, M. (1995). Outpatient management of acute exacerbations of asthma in children. *Journal of Asthma, 32*(1), 5–20.

Marley, R. (1995). Administration of inhaled drugs. *AANA Journal, 63,* 173–178.

Shapiro, B., Harrison, R., Cane, R., & Templin, R. (1989). *Clinical application of blood gases* (4th ed.). Chicago: Year Book Publishers.

Weinberger, S. (1992). *Principles of pulmonary medicine.* Philadelphia: Saunders.

West, J. (1995). *Respiratory physiology—the essentials* (5th ed.). Baltimore: Williams & Wilkins.

West, J. (1997). *Pulmonary pathophysiology—the essentials* (5th ed.). Baltimore: Williams & Wilkins.

REFERENCES

American Association of Nurse Anesthetists (AANA). (1996). *Scope and standards for nurse anesthesia practice* (pp. 1–4). Park Ridge, IL: AANA.

Barnes, P. (1986). Neural control of human airways in health and disease. *American Review of Respiratory Disease, 134,* 1289–1314.

Barnes, P. (1989). A new approach to the treatment of asthma. *New England Journal of Medicine, 321,* 1517–1527.

Bates, D. (1989). *Respiratory function in disease* (3rd ed., pp. 110–115). Philadelphia: Saunders.

Berkin, K. & Ball, S. (1988). Cough and angiotensin converting enzyme inhibition. *British Medical Journal, 296,* 1279–1280.

Braman, S. & Corrao, W. (1987). Cough: Differential diagnosis and treatment. *Clinical Chest Medicine, 8,* 177–188.

Branch, W. & McNeil, B. (1983). Analysis of the differential diagnosis and assessment of pleuritic chest pain in young adults. *American Journal of Medicine, 75,* 671–679.

Burrows, B., Bloom, J., Traver, G., & Cline, M. (1987). The course and prognosis of different forms of chronic airways obstruction in a sample from the general population. *New England Journal of Medicine, 317,* 1309–1314.

Caplan, R. (1995). Adverse outcomes in anesthesia practice. *1995 Annual Refresher Course Lectures, 254,* pp. 1–7. Park Ridge, IL: The American Society of Anesthesiologists.

Cherniack, N. & Altose, M. (1987). Mechanisms of dyspnea. *Clinical Chest Medicine, 8,* 207–214.

Corrao, W., Braman, S., & Irwin, R. (1979). Chronic cough as the sole presenting manifestation of bronchial asthma. *New England Journal of Medicine, 300,* 633–637.

Davidson, P. (1990). Treating tuberculosis: What drugs, for how long? *Annals of Internal Medicine, 112,* 393–395.

Djukanovic, R., Roche, W., Wilson, J., Beasley, C., Twentyman, O., Howarth, P., & Holgate, S. (1990). Mucosal inflammation in asthma. *American Review of Respiratory Disease, 142,* 434–457.

Domino, K. (1996). The patient with respiratory disease. *Audio-Digest Anesthesiology, 38*(6), 1–3.

Donat, W. (1987). Chest pain: Cardiac and noncardiac causes. *Clinical Chest Medicine, 8,* 241–252.

Dutt, A. & Stead, W. (1990). In D. Simmons (Ed.). *Current pulmonology* (Vol. 11, pp. 333–355). Chicago: Year Book Medical Publishers.

Edelson, J. & Hyland, R. (1990). The pulmonary complications of acquired immunodeficiency syndrome (AIDS). In D., Simmons (Ed.). *Current pulmonology* (Vol. 11, pp. 273–311). Chicago: Yearbook Medical Publishers.

Faling, L. & Snider G. (1989). Treatment of chronic obstructive pulmonary disease. In D. Simmons (Ed.). *Current pulmonology* (Vol. 10, pp. 209–263). Chicago: Year Book Medical Publishers.

Fedullo, P. & Shure, D. (1987). Pulmonary vascular imaging. *Clinical Chest Medicine, 8,* 53–64.

Fisher, M. (1989). Magnetic resonance imaging for evaluation of the thorax. *Chest, 95,* 166–173.

Fraser, R., Pare, J., Pare, P., & Genereux, G. (1988). *Diagnosis of diseases of the chest* (Vol. 1, 3rd ed., pp. 21–37). Philadelphia: Saunders.

Gazdar, A. & Linnoila, I. (1988). The pathology of lung cancer—changing concepts and newer diagnostic techniques. *Seminars in Oncology, 15,* 215–225.

Geiger, K. & Hedley-Whyte, J. (1993). Preoperative and postoperative considerations in bronchial asthma. In E. Weiss & M. Stein (Eds.). *Bronchial asthma—mechanisms and therapeutics* (3rd ed., pp. 1099–1112). Boston: Little, Brown & Co.

Ginsberg, R., Ross, R., & Field, R. (1989). Fifth world congress on lung cancer. *Chest, 96,* 1S–107S.

Habib, M. & Burrows, B. (1990). Chronic airway obstruction: The importance of certain risk factors for its development. In D. Simmons (Ed.). *Current pulmonology* (Vol. 11, pp. 247–272). Chicago: Year Book Medical Publishers.

Hansen-Flaschen, J. & Nordberg, J. (1987). Clubbing and hypertrophic osteoarthropathy. *Clinical Chest Medicine, 8,* 287–298.

Israel, R. & Poe, R. (1987). Hemoptysis. *Clinical Chest Medicine, 8,* 197–205.

Johnston, H. & Reisz, G. (1989). Changing spectrum of hemoptysis: Underlying causes in 148 patients undergoing diagnostic flexible fiberoptic bronchoscopy. *Archives of Internal Medicine, 149,* 1666–1668.

Kremer, M., Crawforth, K., Golinski, M., Jordan, L., Larson, S., Mahinger, L., Moody, M., Nagelhout, J., Shott, S., Williams, J., & Bulau, J. (1996). Abstract: An analysis of closed malpractice claims filed against nurse anesthetists. *AANA Journal, 64*(5), 440.

Lapin, C. & Cloutier, M. (1995). Outpatient management of acute exacerbations of asthma in children. *Journal of Asthma, 32*(1), 5–20.

Lemanske, R. & Kaliner, M. (1990). Autonomic nervous system abnormalities and asthma. *American Review of Respiratory Disease, 141,* S157–S161.

Mahler, D. (1989). Pulmonary function testing. *Clinical Chest Medicine, 10,* 129–296.

Marley, R. (1995). Administration of inhaled drugs. *AANA Journal, 63,* 173–178.

Martin, L. & Khalil, H. (1990). How much reduced hemoglobin is necessary to generate central cyanosis? *Chest, 97,* 182–185.

Murphy, K. (1995). Acute exacerbation of asthma in children: A role for prevention and education. *Journal of Asthma, 32*(1), 1–3.

Murray, J. (1986). *The normal lung: The basics for diagnosis and treatment of pulmonary disease* (2nd ed., pp. 202–218). Philadelphia: Saunders.

Murray, J. & Mills, J. (1990). Pulmonary infectious complications of human immunodeficiency virus infection. *American Review of Respiratory Disease, 141,* 1582–1598.

Nelson, H. (1986). Adrenergic therapy of bronchial asthma. *Journal of Allergy Clinical Immunology, 77,* 771–785.

Petty, T., Rollins, D., Christopher, K., Good, J., & Oakley, R. (1989). Cromolyn sodium is effective in adult chronic asthmatics. *American Review of Respiratory Disease, 139,* 694–701.

Raffin, T. & Theodore, J. (1977). Separating cardiac function from pulmonary dyspnea. *Journal of the American Medical Association, 238,* 2066–2067.

Reider, H., Cauthen, G., Kelly, G., Bloch, A., & Snider, D. (1989). Tuberculosis in the United States. *Journal of the American Medical Association, 262,* 385–389.

Shapiro, B., Harrison, R., Cane, R., & Templin, R. (1989). *Clinical application of blood gases* (4th ed., pp. 50–60). Chicago: Year Book Publishers.

Sheller, J. (1987). Asthma: Emerging concepts and potential therapies. *American Journal of Medical Science, 293,* 298–308.

Shure, D. (1987). Fiberoptic bronchoscopy—diagnostic applications. *Clinical Chest Medicine, 8,* 1–13.

Shure, D. (1989). Transbronchial biopsy and needle aspiration. *Chest, 95,* 1130–1138.

Slonim, N. & Hamilton, L. (1987). *Respiratory physiology* (5th ed., pp. 8–12). St. Louis: Mosby.

Spies, W., Spies, S., & Mintzer, R. (1983). Radionuclide imaging in diseases of the chest. *Chest, 83,* 122–127.

Taylor, A., Rehder, K., Hyatt, R., & Parker, J. (1989). *Clinical respiratory physiology* (pp. 50–60). Philadelphia: Saunders.

Tobin, M. (1990). Dyspnea: Pathophysiologic basis, clinical presentation, and management. *Archives of Internal Medicine, 150,* 1604–1613.

Wasserman, K. (1982). Dyspnea on exertion: Is it the heart or the lungs? *Journal of the American Medical Association, 248,* 2039–2043.

Wasserman, K. & Casburi, R. (1988). Dyspnea: Physiological and pathophysiological mechanisms. *Annual Review of Medicine, 39,* 503–515.

Weibel, E. (1984). *The pathway for oxygen: Structure and function in the mammalian respiratory system* (pp. 110–118). Cambridge, MA: Harvard University Press.

Weinberger, S., Schwartzstein, R., & Weiss, J. (1989). Hypercapnia. *New England Journal of Medicine. 321,* 1223–1231.

Weinberger, S. (1992). *Principles of pulmonary medicine* (pp. 21–71). Philadelphia: Saunders.

West, J. (1985). *Ventilation/blood flow and gas exchange* (4th ed., pp. 35–45). Oxford, UK: Blackwell Scientific Publications.

West, J. (1997). *Pulmonary pathophysiology—the essentials* (5th ed., pp. 3–76, 137–140). Baltimore: Williams & Wilkins.

West, J. (1995). *Respiratory physiology—the essentials* (5th ed., pp. 8–50). Baltimore: Williams & Wilkins.

Wilkins, R., Sheldon, R., & Krider, S. (1990). *Clinical assessment in respiratory care* (2nd ed., pp. 115–120). St. Louis: Mosby.

Zerhouni, E. (1989). Computed tomography of the pulmonary parenchyma: An overview. *Chest, 95,* 901–907.

Zibrak, J., O'Donnell, C., & Marton, K. (1989). Indications for pulmonary function testing. *Annals of Internal Medicine, 112,* 763–771.

CHAPTER

12

Assessment of the Neurologic System of the Adult

Steve L. Alves and Stephen J. Yermal

▶ OVERVIEW OF THE PERIOPERATIVE ASSESSMENT AND MANAGEMENT OF THE NEUROLOGIC SYSTEM OF THE ADULT

The intent of this chapter is to present essential information in the perioperative assessment and management of patients with neurologic dysfunction to the novice nurse anesthesia student. Patients presenting with neurologic disease are challenging to the nurse anesthetist. Integration of a knowledge of anatomy, physiology, and pathophysiology is essential to the perianesthetic plan. The major emphasis in this chapter is related to the evaluation of the neurologic system of the adult patient. Within the assessment phase, the focus is on the history, physical examination, level of consciousness, pupillary signs, motor and sensory function, and vital signs. These factors are critical to the neurologic assessment and management of the adult patient.

▶ ANATOMY AND GENERAL ORGANIZATION OF THE CENTRAL NERVOUS SYSTEM AND PERIPHERAL NERVOUS SYSTEM

Central Nervous System

Neuronal Transmission

The neuron is the basic structural and functional unit of the nervous system. The human nervous system is an ex-

tensive network of billions of interconnected neurons supported by glial cells (Rando, 1992; Harrigan, 1997). The cell body is an essential component and is also referred to as the *soma* or the *perikaryon* (Fig. 12-1). The cell bodies contain structures called Nissl bodies which are critical to normal cell function, protein synthesis, and neuronal repair. Very little chromatin (a deoxyribonucleic acid) is found within the cell body, possibly reflecting its inability to regenerate. The functions of the cell body are to receive nerve endings that convey excitatory or inhibitory stimuli generated in other nerve cells and to transmit these stimuli to the remainder of the neuron.

Another component of the neuron is the dendrite. As many as 4000 dendrites have been identified in some neurons. This widespread innervation by the proliferation of axons and dendrites allows an extensive relay of stimuli. The function of a dendrite is to conduct excitatory or inhibitory impulses to the cell body.

A third component of the neuron is the axon. It originates from a broadened area of the cell body known as the hillock, and only one axon arises from each cell body. The axon is longer and narrower than the dendrite and constitutes the bulk of the white matter in the nervous system. Many of the axons are covered with a layer of fat and protein material known as myelin. The myelin is secreted by cells that surround all peripheral axons. Schwann cells originate from an outer layer that covers the axon, also known as the neurilemma. In contrast to the myelin, the neurilemma is a thin, delicate, nucleated, fatty substance. Axons with a diameter greater than 2 μm are usually myelinated; those smaller than 2 μm are not. The gap between two adjacent Schwann cells wrapped

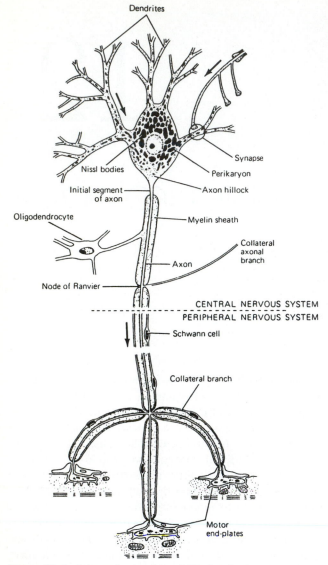

Figure 12–1. Schematic drawing of Nissl-stained motor neuron. *(Reprinted, with permission, from Junqueria, L. C., Carneiro, J., & Long, J. A. [1986]. Basic histology [5th ed.]. Norwalk, CT: Appleton & Lange.)*

around the axon is called the node of Ranvier. It is from these gaps, or nodes of Ranvier, that collateral axons extend from the main axon, usually at a 90° angle. The axon functions to conduct stimuli away from the cell body of its neuron.

Neurons have been typically classified in three ways (Katz, 1997): (1) by the number and processes; (2) by the diameter of the axon; and (3) by the length of the axon. Classification of neurons based on diameter is commonly referred to by both clinicians and academicians (Table 12-1). The first group of neurons is referred to as A type. They are myelinated and are the axons with the largest diameter, ranging from 2 μm to 20 μm. Because the ve-

locity of neuron conduction varies directly with the diameter of the axon, this group has the greatest velocity of conduction, 12 m/s to 120 m/s. A-type neurons are further subdivided into (1) alpha neurons, which conduct impulses of the innervation of skeletal muscles and proprioception; (2) beta neurons, which conduct impulses of touch and pressure; (3) gamma neurons, which innervate impulses of muscle tone; and (4) delta neurons, which conduct impulses of fast pain, touch, and temperature. The second group of neurons classified according to axonal diameter is known as B type. They are also myelinated, having a diameter of 1 μm to 3 μm and a conduction velocity of 3 m/s to 15 m/s, and function as preganglionic autonomic fibers. The third classification is the C type. These neurons are usually unmyelinated or only lightly myelinated with a diameter of 0.4 μm to 1.2 μm and a conduction velocity of 0.5 m/s to 2 m/s. These fibers serve four functions: to conduct slow pain impulses, touch, and temperature, and to make up the postganglionic autonomic fibers.

Brain

The brain is the enlarged, convoluted, and highly developed rostral portion of the central nervous system (CNS). The average adult human brain weighs about 1500 g, or approximately 2% of the total body weight. The composition and function of the brain include the brain stem, the cerebellum, and the cerebrum as described and analyzed by Rando (1992), Harrigan (1997), and Katz (1997).

The brain stem is continuous with the spinal cord within the foramen magnum and lies on the basioccipital bone in the posterior cranial fossa. The brain stem contains the medulla oblongata and the pons, which regulate bodily functions such as respiration. The brain stem also contains the reticular activating system, which is responsible for maintaining the conscious, alert state. Lesions that occur within the brain stem may have serious consequences. The cerebellum extends dorsally from the brain stem and fills the posterior cranial fossa. The cerebellum is primarily responsible for the coordination of motor activity. The cerebrum occupies the greater portion of the middle and anterior cranial fossae. The cerebrum is divided into right and left cerebral hemispheres that are separated by a deep cleft, the longitudinal cerebral fissure, and connected in the midline by the corpus callosum. The cerebrum is divided into a number of lobes named by the overlying bone, including frontal, parietal, occipital, temporal, central, and limbic lobes.

Substructures of the brain include gray matter, white matter, and the basal ganglia. Gray matter covers the surface of the brain and consist of cell bodies (neurons) arranged in vertical functional columns with a complex circuitry. White matter lies deeper in the brain and consists of tracts or fascicles of axons. The basal ganglia lies

TABLE 12–1. Classification of Neurons

	Myelinated	Fiber Diameter (μm)	Conduction Velocity (m · sec^{-1})	Function	Sensitivity to Local Anesthetic (Subarachnoid, procaine) (%)
A					
A-alpha	Yes	12–20	70–120	Innervation of skeletal muscles Proprioception	1
A-beta	Yes	5–12	30–70	Touch Pressure	1
A-gamma	Yes	3–6	15–30	Skeletal muscle tone	1
A-delta	Yes	2–5	12–30	Fast pain Touch Temperature	9.5
B	Yes	3	3–15	Preganglionic autonomic fibers	0.25
C	No	0.4–1.2	0.5–2	Slow pain Touch Temperature Postganglionic sympathetic fibers	0.5

deep within the base of the cerebral hemispheres. The basal ganglia is comprised of the caudate nucleus, the lenticular nucleus (consisting of the putamen and globus pallidus), the subthalamic nucleus, and the substantia nigra (important in motor function).

The entire blood supply to the brain arises from the internal carotid and vertebral arteries (Fig. 12–2). Venous drainage is completed by the superior sagittal sinus and the sigmoid sinuses into the internal jugular veins. The internal carotid arteries extend up the neck, enter the area of the temporal bone without branching, supplying the anterior cerebral circulation, which accounts for 80% of total cerebral blood flow (Fig. 12–3). The vertebral artery network is somewhat less complex and supplies 20% of the cerebral blood flow directed toward the posterior cerebral circulation.

The network of anastomosing blood vessels, known as the circle of Willis, surrounds the optic chiasm and allows for collateral circulation of the brain. It provides a union of blood vessels supplying the brain by way of the carotid and vertebral arteries.

Vertebral Column and Spinal Cord

The vertebral column is composed of five regions: cervical, thoracic, lumbar, sacral, and coccygeal regions (Rando, 1992; Katz, 1997). The spine curves in a double "C" formation. The cervical and lumbar curves are convex in a ventral direction, whereas the thoracic and sacral curves are convex dorsally. This curvature has clinical implications because it influences the spread of local anesthetics during subarachnoid blockade.

The structure of a typical vertebrae is similar at all levels (Fig. 12–4). The base of the vertebrae is the body

which forms the major supportive portion of the vertebrae and consists of two pedicles anteriorly and two laminae posteriorly. The transverse processes are formed by the junction of the two pedicles and laminae. The spinous processes are formed by joining each lamina. The foramina of the vertebrae contain the spinal cord, its coverings, blood supply, and allows spinal nerves to exit.

The spinal cord is located in the upper two thirds of the vertebral canal of the bony vertebral column and is a continuation of the brain stem (Fig. 12–5). It extends from the foramen magnum at the base of the skull to its termination as the conus medullaris. The spinal cord enlarges in those segments that innervate the extremities. The cervical (brachial) enlargement, C5 to T1, innervates the upper extremities, while the lumbosacral enlargement, L3 to S2, innervates the lower extremities. In the adult, the spinal cord usually ends at the level of L1 and in the infant usually at L3. The cauda equina ("horse's tail") is formed by the long roots from the lumbar and sacral nerves.

The spinal meninges are three individual membranes that surround the spinal cord and are fundamentally similar to those of the brain. The pia mater is highly vascular, continues beyond the termination of the spinal cord as the filumterminale, and contains the blood supply to the spinal cord. The arachnoid is a thin, avascular, membranous layer external to the pia mater and connected by web-like trabeculations. The subarachnoid space, which is located between the arachnoid and pia mater, contains the spinal nerves and cerebrospinal fluid (CSF). The subarachnoid space extends caudally to the level of S2. Spinal anesthesia is accomplished by infusing the anesthetic around the nerve roots (usually every site between L1 and S2).

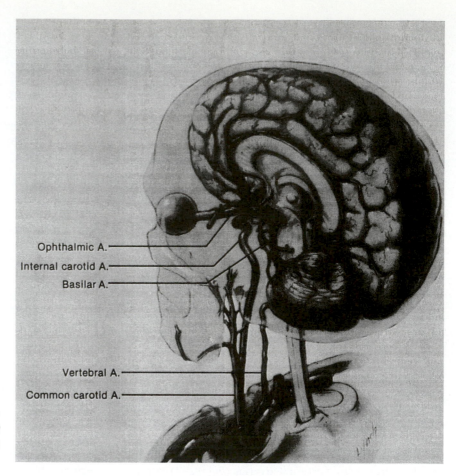

Ophthalmic A.
Internal carotid A.
Basilar A.

Vertebral A.
Common carotid A.

Figure 12–2. Normal cerebral circulation (lateral view). *(Reprinted, with permission, from Toole, J. F. [1990]. Cerebrovascular disorders [4th ed., p. 4]. New York: Raven Press.)*

The dura mater is a tough, fibrous, single-layered membrane external to the arachnoid that extends from the foramen magnum superiorly to the lower border of S2 anteriorly. The subdural space is a potential space located between the arachnoid and dura that does not contain CSF. The epidural space lies between the dura mater and the periosteum of the vertebral column and contains profuse venous plexuses, along with fat. Epidural anesthesia is conducted by perfusing the anesthetic agent about the spinal nerves.

The blood supply to the spinal cord consist of two distinct systems, the anterior spinal artery and the paired posterior spinal arteries. The anterior spinal artery lies in the anterior median sulcus and is formed at the level of the foramen magnum on the union of the two vertebral arteries. The anterior spinal artery supplies the anterior two thirds of the spinal cord with segmental blood supply from contributions of the two vertebral arteries as well as three radicular branches. These include the cervical, thoracic, and the radicularis magna of the thoracolumbar region (also known as the artery of Adamkiewicz, which has a variable origin along the cord but arises on the left 80% of the time). Anterior spinal artery syndrome results from spinal cord lesions and may render anterior central cord ischemia. The two posterior

spinal arteries arise from the vertebral or posterior inferior cerebellar arteries and descend as two branches, one anterior and the other posterior to the dorsal nerve root. The posterior spinal arteries supply the posterior third of the spinal cord and, because of its rich collateral contributions from the subclavian, intercostal, lumbar, and sacral arteries, the posterior spinal arteries are not segmented like the anterior spinal artery.

Peripheral Nervous System

Cranial Nerves

The cranial nerves can be thought of as peripheral nerves arising from the brain. They consist of 12 pairs of nerves numbered in reference to their points of origin on the brain stem, anteriorly to posteriorly or superiorly to inferiorly. Each nerve is represented by a name and a Roman numeral. Cranial nerves enter or exit the brain by way of foramina in the base of the cranium. Because of the higher level of development of cephalic structures, cranial nerves are more complex than spinal nerves. Cranial nerves are involved primarily in innervation of structures of the head and neck and are differentiated on the basis of input or output to special senses. The cranial nerves consist of either sensory or motor fibers, with

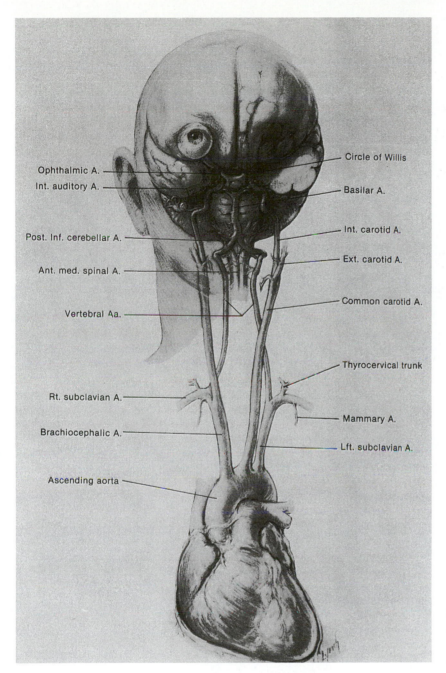

Ophthalmic A.

Int. auditory A.

Post. Inf. cerebellar A.

Ant. med. spinal A.

Vertebral Aa.

Rt. subclavian A.

Brachiocephalic A.

Ascending aorta

Circle of Willis

Basilar A.

Int. carotid A.

Ext. carotid A.

Common carotid A.

Thyrocervical trunk

Mammary A.

Lft. subclavian A.

Figure 12–3. Normal cerebral circulation (frontal view). *(Reprinted, with permission, from Toole, J. F. [1990]. Cerebrovascular disorders [4th ed., p. 2]. New York: Raven Press.)*

some nerves containing both types. All of the cranial nerves are summarized with respect to type, course, function, and pathology in Table 12–2.

Spinal Nerves

The spinal nerves are part of the peripheral nervous system and are composed of 31 pairs exiting from the spinal cord, including 8 cervical, 12 thoracic, 5 lumbar, 5 sacral, and 1 coccygeal. Each spinal nerve has a dorsal root from which afferent impulses enter the cord and a ventral root from which efferent impulses leave. The first pair of cervical spinal nerves leaves the cord above the C1 vertebra, and spinal nerves of C2 through C7 leave by way of

the intervertebral foramina, above their corresponding vertebrae. Because there are seven vertebrae and eight pairs of spinal nerves, the C8 spinal nerve leaves the cord by way of the intervertebral foramina below the C7 vertebra. All spinal nerves from T1 to the caudal end of the cord leave by way of the foramina immediately below the corresponding vertebrae.

The dorsal roots convey sensory input (afferent impulses) from specific areas of the body known as *dermatomes*. Afferent impulses are directed from the dermatomal area by way of the dorsal root to the dorsal root ganglia, in which the cell bodies of the sensory component are located. There are two types of sensory fibers:

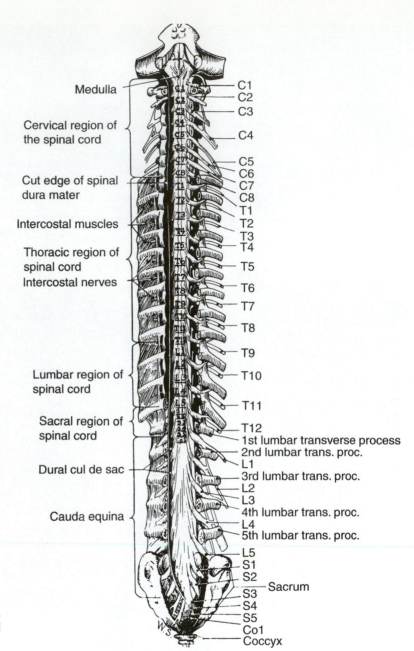

Medulla

Cervical region of the spinal cord

Cut edge of spinal dura mater

Intercostal muscles

Thoracic region of spinal cord
Intercostal nerves

Lumbar region of spinal cord

Sacral region of spinal cord

Dural cul de sac

Cauda equina

C1
C2
C3
C4
C5
C6
C7
C8
T1
T2
T3
T4
T5
T6
T7
T8
T9
T10
T11
T12
1st lumbar transverse process
2nd lumbar trans. proc.
L1
3rd lumbar trans. proc.
L2
L3
4th lumbar trans. proc.
L4
5th lumbar trans. proc.
L5
S1
S2
Sacrum
S3
S4
S5
Co1
Coccyx

W.S.

Figure 12–4. Dorsal view of the spinal cord. *(Reprinted, with permission, from Buchanan, A. R. [1961]. Functional neuroanatomy [p. 24]. Malvern, PA: Lea & Febiger.)*

general somatic afferent (GSA) fibers, which carry sensory impulses for pain, temperature, touch, and proprioception from the body wall, tendons, and joints; and general visceral afferent (GVA) fibers, which carry sensory impulses from the organs within the body. Table 12–3 identifies sensory nerve roots and the areas that they innervate (dermatome).

The ventral motor roots convey efferent impulses from the spinal cord to the body. There are two types of motor fibers: general somatic effernet (GSE) fibers, which innervate voluntary striated muscles and have axons originating from the alpha and gamma motor neu-

rons of lamina IX (Hickey, 1997); and general visceral efferent (GVE) fibers, include the preganglionic and postganglionic autonomic fibers that innervate smooth and cardiac muscle and regulate glandular secretion. Table 12–4 describes the motor nerve roots (myotones) and the areas innervated.

Plexuses

A plexus is a network of interlacing nerves. The cervical, brachial, lumbar, and sacral plexuses are formed by their primary branches. The cervical plexus is formed from the ventral branches of the first four cervical nerves of the

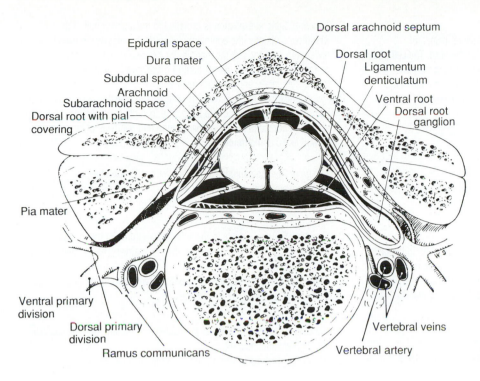

Dorsal arachnoid septum
Epidural space
Dura mater
Subdural space
Arachnoid
Subarachnoid space
Dorsal root with pial covering
Dorsal root
Ligamentum denticulatum
Ventral root
Dorsal root ganglion
Pia mater
Ventral primary division
Dorsal primary division
Ramus communicans
Vertebral veins
Vertebral artery

Figure 12–5. Cross section of the spinal cord in the spinal canal. *(Reprinted, with permission, from Buchanan, A. R. [1961]. Functional neuroanatomy (p. 25). Malvern, PA: Lea & Fabiger.)*

TABLE 12–2. The Cranial Nerves

I. Olfactory Nerve
A. *Type:* Sensory.
B. *Course:* Receptors are modified; exposed dendrites are located in the nasal cavity and are sensitive to a variety of vapors. Cell bodies are embedded in respiratory mucosa covering the cribriform plate of the ethmoid bone. Axons terminate in the primary area of smell in the temporal bone.

C. *Function:* Sense of smell is relatively poorly developed in humans compared with lower animals.
D. *Pathology:* Usually, local dysfunction is due to respiratory mucosal inflammation leading to anosmia (loss of sense of smell). Pathology may be caused by intracranial tumors or head injuries.

II. Optic Nerve
A. *Type:* Sensory.
B. *Course:* The dendrites and cell bodies are in the retina and are not directly stimulated by light; rather, the stimulus causes a release of hemical transmitters—rhodopsin in the rods and iodopsin and photopsin in cones. From the retina, the optic nerve travels to the optic chiasm, where medial fibers from each eye decussate. Each tract from the optic chiasm to the visual cortex of the occipital lobe carries fibers from both eyes. The visual cortex is necessary for conscious perception of an upright image. Collateral fibers of this nerve also extend to the cranial nerves involved in extraocular movement o coordinate globe movement with visual perception.

C. *Function:* Vision.
D. *Pathology:* Prechiasmic involvement produces ipsilateral blindness; chiasm or postchiasm pathology produces varieties of hemianopsia (absence of half of the normal field of vision).

III. Oculomotor Nerve
A. *Type:* Somatic and visceral motor.
B. *Course:* Somatic fibers originate in the Edinger–Westphal nucleus of the midbrain and synapse with all extraocular muscles except superior oblique and lateral rectus muscles, in addition to muscles elevating eyelids. Visceral fibers share their origin with the preganglionic fibers terminating in the ciliary muscle of the lens and the sphincter muscle of the iris.

C. *Function:* Somatic fibers innervate levator palpebral, inferior oblique, inferior rectus, medial rectus, and superior rectus extraocular muscles to provide conjugate globe movement. The visceral nerves provide accommodation for far vision and for constriction of the iris.
D. *Pathology:* Disjunctive eye movements, ptosis, and loss of accommodation.

IV. Trochlear Nerve
A. *Type:* Somatic motor.
B. *Course:* Fibers originate in the midbrain at the floor of the cerebral aqueduct, at the junction of the upper pons and cerebellar peduncles. These fibers terminate in the superior oblique extraocular muscle.

C. *Function:* Allow conjugate globe movement medially.
D. *Pathology:* Inability to turn eyes downward and outward with vertical diplopia.

(Continued)

TABLE 12–2. The Cranial Nerves *(Continued)*

V. Trigeminal Nerve

A. *Type:* Sensory and somatic motor.

B. *Course:* Sensory receptors for touch, pressure, pain, and temperature originate in the anterior half of the head. The cell body is in the gasserian ganglion and fibers terminate in the pons. The somatic motor fibers originate in the pons and terminate in the muscles of mastication and the tympanic membrane.

C. *Function:* General sensation is provided to the anterior half of the face with three divisions: the ophthalmic division is sensory, the maxillary division is sensory, and the mandibular division is both sensory and motor. The motor components control mastication, swallowing, movement for the soft palate, and eardrum tension.

D. *Pathology:* Injury to the sensory root results in anesthesia to the anterior half of the face, dryness of the nose, and loss of sense of taste. Motor root involvement results in loss of mastication and paralysis of facial muscles, as well as tic douloureux.

VI. Abducens Nerve

A. *Type:* Somatic motor.

B. *Course:* The multipolar neurons of this nerve originate in the pons and innervate the lateral rectus extraocular muscle.

C. *Function:* Operate conjugate globe movement temporally.

D. *Pathology:* Internal or convergent squint.

VII. Facial Nerve

A. *Type:* Sensory, somatic, and visceral motor.

B. *Course:* Sensory unipolar neurons have their receptors in the taste buds of the anterior two thirds of the tongue. Somatic motor fibers course from the pons to the facial muscles. Visceral fibers synapse in parasympathetic ganglia and terminate in salivary glands.

C. *Function:* Sensory—taste to the anterior two thirds of the tongue; somatic motor—facial expression; visceral motor—salivary, nasal, lacrimal, and oral secretions.

D. *Pathology:* Loss of sensation of taste to anterior two thirds of the tongue, Bell's palsy, and inability to grimace.

VIII. Vestibulocochlear Nerve

A. *Type:* Sensory.

B. *Course:* The vestibular portion has receptors and cell bodies in the otoliths and semicircular canal of the inner ear and terminates in the cerebellum.

The dendrites of the cochlear portion of this nerve originate as dendrites in the organ of Corti of the inner ear and terminate in the primary auditory area of the temporal lobe.

C. *Function:* The vestibular division ensures equilibrium, and the cochlear division ensures hearing.

D. *Pathology:* Results in vertigo and perceptive deafness.

IX. Glossopharyngeal Nerve

A. *Type:* Sensory, somatic, and visceral motor.

B. *Course:* Sensory neurons originate in the taste buds in the posterior third of the tongue, the chemoreceptors in the carotid bodies, the pressoreceptors in the carotid sinuses, as well as general sensory receptors in the oropharynx, hypopharynx, and middle ear. They erminate in the medulla oblongata. Somatic and visceral motor fibers originate in the medulla, with somatic efferent fibers innervating the pharyngeal constrictor muscles and the visceral efferent fibers terminating in the salivary glands.

C. *Function:* Taste, general sensation to the throat, swallowing, salivation, and monitoring of blood pressure, Pao_2, and $Paco_2$.

D. *Pathology:* Loss of taste in posterior third of the tongue, inability to swallow, and loss of gag reflex.

X. Vagus Nerve

A. *Type:* Visceral sensory and motor.

B. *Course:* Sensory fibers originate in abdominal and thoracic viscera, as well as in chemoreceptors and pressoreceptors. They terminate in the medulla. The motor fibers originate as preganglionic parasympathetic fibers in the medulla and, after synapsing, innervate smooth muscles, cardiac muscle, and glands.

C. *Function:* Sensory components provide general visceral afferent sensations and monitor blood pressure, Pao_2, $Paco_2$, left-sided heart filling, and lung inflation. Motor components provide the characteristic parasympathetic autonomic excitatory effects.

D. *Pathology:* Sensory dysfunction ranges from anesthesia of the larynx to overdistention of the lungs. Motor dysfunction results in paralysis of laryngeal function, absence of bowel activities, and generalized decrease in daily anabolic functions.

XI. Spinal Accessory Nerves

A. *Type:* Somatic motor.

B. *Course:* The cell bodies originate in the medulla and the anterior horn gray matter of the first five cervical spinal cord segments. The cranial fibers terminate in pharyngeal and laryngeal muscles; the spinal fibers innervate muscles of the neck and shoulders.

C. *Function:* The cranial segment aids in swallowing and phonation; the spinal segments in movement of head and shoulders.

D. *Pathology:* Dysphagia, hoarseness, and weakness of head and shoulder muscles.

XII. Hypoglossal Nerve

A. *Type:* Somatic motor.

B. *Course:* Cell bodies originate in the medulla and terminate in the tongue.

C. *Function:* Movement of the tongue.

D. *Pathology:* Inability to extend the tongue or weakness in movement of the tongue.

Adapted with permission from Rando, J. T. (1992). Neurophysiology. In W. R. Waugaman, S. D. Foster, & B. M. Rigor (Eds.), Principles and practice of nurse anesthesia (2nd ed.). Norwalk, CT: Appleton & Lange.

TABLE 12–3. Sensory Nerve Roots and the Areas Innervated (Dermatome)

Spinal Nerves	Dermatome
C2	Back of head (occiput)
C3	Neck
C4	Neck and upper shoulder
C5	Lateral aspect of shoulder
C6	Thumb; radial aspect of arm; index finger
C7	Middle finger; middle palm; back of hand
C8	Ring and little fingers; ulnar forearm
T1–T2	Inner aspect of arm and across shoulder blade
T1	Nipple line
T7	Lower costal margin
T10	Umbilical region
T12–L1	Inguinal (groin) region
L2	Anterior thigh and upper buttocks
L3–L4	Anterior knee and lower leg
L5	Outer aspect of lower leg; dorsum of foot; big toe
S1	Sole of foot and small toes
S2	Posterior medial thigh and lower leg
S3	Medial thigh
S4–S5	Genitals and saddle area

Adapted from Hickey, J. V. (1997). The clinical practice of neurological and neurosurgical nursing (4th ed.). Philadelphia: Lippincott.

spine. The resulting branches innervate the muscles of the shoulders and neck. The cervical plexus also gives rise to the phrenic nerve (C3, C4, C5) which supplies the diaphragm. The brachial plexus is composed of the ventral branches of the lower four cervical and the first tho-

TABLE 12–4. Motor Nerve Roots (Myotones) and the Areas Innervated

Spinal Nerves	Muscles
C1–C4	Neck (flexion, lateral flexion, extension, rotation)
C3–C5	Diaphragm (respirations)
C5–C6	Shoulder movement and flexion of elbow
C5–C7	Forward thrust of shoulder
C5–C8	Adduction of arm from front to back
C6–C8	Extension of forearm and wrist
C7, C8, T1	Flexion of wrist
T1–T12	Control of thoracic, abdominal, and back muscles
L1–L3	Flexion of hip
L2–L4	Extension of leg; adduction of thigh
L4, L5, S1, S2	Abduction of thigh; flexion of lower leg
L4–L5	Dorsal flexion of foot
L5, S1, S2	Plantar flexion of foot
S2, S3, S4	Perineal area and sphincters

Adapted from Hickey, J. V. (1997). The clinical practice of neurological and neurosurgical nursing (4th ed.). Philadelphia: Lippincott.

racic spinal nerves. The radial, medial, and ulnar nerves emerge from this plexus. The lumbar plexus originates from the ventral branches of the twelfth thoracic and the first four lumbar nerves. The femoral nerve arises from this plexus. Finally, the sacral plexus arises from the ventral branches of the last two lumbar and first four sacral nerves. The sciatic nerve arises from this plexus.

Autonomic Nervous System

As part of the peripheral nervous system (PNS), the autonomic nervous system (ANS) is made up of only motor neurons, collectively called the GVE system. The ANS regulates the activities of the viscera, which includes all smooth (involuntary) muscles, cardiac muscles, and glands. The purpose of the ANS is to maintain a relatively stable internal environment for the body. The two major divisions are the sympathetic and parasympathetic systems.

Sympathetic System. The sympathetic system is activated during stressful situations such as fright, fight, or flight phenomena. During the stressful event, there is vasoconstriction of the peripheral blood vessels, increased heart rate, and elevated blood pressure. The sympathetic system is also called the thoracolumbar system because its preganglionic fibers emerge from cell bodies that extend through the thoracic and upper two lumbar levels (T1 to L2). The neurotransmitters released by the postganglionic fibers is norepinephrine (NE); hence, the term adrenergic. Some blood vessels in skeletal muscles and most sweat glands in the palms of the hands have adrenergic postganglionic neurons.

Parasympathetic System. The parasympathetic system is also called the craniosacral system because its preganglionic fibers emerge with cranial nerves III, VII, IX, and X. The sacral portion of the parasympathetic system arises from cell bodies of sacral segments S2 through S4. The parasympathetic system secretes acetylcholine at the postganglionic neuron. This is why the parasympathetic system is called the cholinergic system. Acetylcholine is secreted at the preganglionic terminal and quickly deactivated by cholinesterase. Figure 12–6 explains the autonomic effects of the nervous system.

▶ PHYSIOLOGY

Neurophysiologic knowledge is centered on the relationships between cerebral blood flow (CBF), cerebral metabolic rate for oxygen ($CMRo_2$), and intracranial pressure (ICP). Physiologic and pharmacologic influences that are under the control of the nurse anesthetist may alter this fragile relationship.

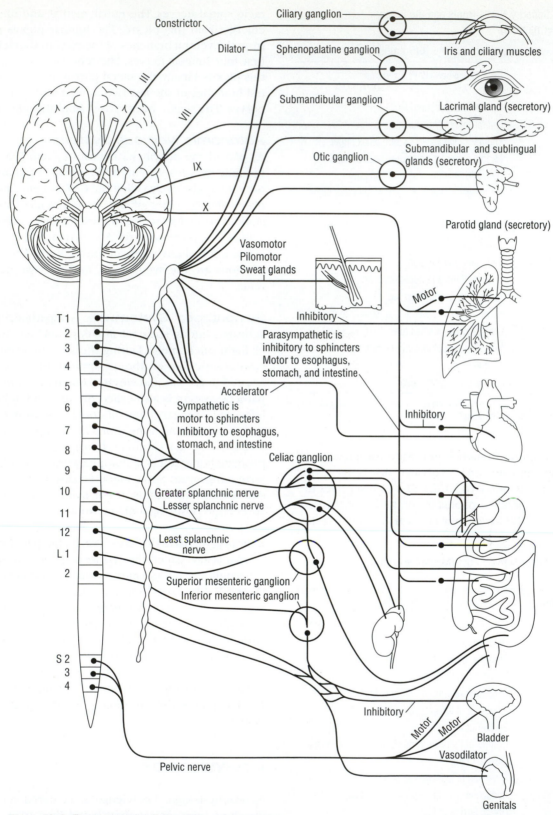

Figure 12–6. The autonomic effects of the nervous system.

Cerebral Blood Flow and Intracranial Pressure Dynamics

Cerebral blood flow is maintained relatively constant at the rate of 45 to 50 mL/100 g of tissue weight per minute (Donegan, 1991; Rando, 1992; Todd & Warner, 1993). The CBF is approximately 665 mL/min, or 15% of the cardiac output. The regional distribution of CBF results in the white matter receiving only 20 mL/100 g of tissue, and the gray matter 80 mL/100 g. This shows that gray matter receives a proportionately greater amount of blood flow owing to its greater metabolic rate. The overall CMR_{O_2} is 3.3 mL of oxygen (O_2) per 100 g of tissue per minute. The ratio of CBF to CMR_{O_2} is approximately 15 : 1. Despite the disproportionately high ratio, there is minimal basal O_2 reserve in the brain, and the interruption of adequate blood flow for as little as 10 seconds can lead to loss of consciousness.

The constancy of CBF is ensured by maintaining a stable, effective cerebral perfusion pressure (CPP). Cerebral perfusion pressure is the difference between mean arterial pressure (MAP) and ICP or cerebral venous pressure, whichever is greater. If the cerebral venous pressure exceeds the ICP, CPP becomes the difference between MAP and cerebral venous pressure: CPP = MAP − ICP. The use of central venous pressure, (CVP) if available, is a reasonable indirect measure of cerebral venous pressure when ICP is not being monitored. Venous pressure is relatively low (less than 10 mmHg) in the internal jugular vein. Cerebral perfusion pressure is normally about 100 mmHg. A decrease of CPP to 50 mmHg is associated with slowing of the electroencephalogram (EEG). At pressures of 25 mmHg to 40 mmHg, the EEG becomes flat; and when CPP falls below 20 mmHg, irreversible tissue damage takes place if body temperature is normal. Because ICP remains relatively constant in the healthy individual (less than 15 mmHg), MAP is the major factor affecting CPP. Intracranial pressure will be discussed later in this chapter.

Control of Cerebral Blood Flow

Autoregulation. In the healthy individual, CBF remains almost constant despite wide variations in the CPP (Fig. 12–7). This phenomenon, referred to as autoregulation, occurs not only in the vasculature of the CNS, but also in the vessels of many other organs, including the kidneys and the heart (Donegan, 1991; Farnsworth, Johnson, & Sperry, 1996). Autoregulation is an active vascular response. During increases in MAP, the cerebral vessels constrict (cerebrovascular resistance increases), and during decreases in MAP, the cerebral vessels dilate (cerebrovascular resistance decreases). The lower limit of autoregulation is a MAP between 50 mmHg and 60 mmHg and the upper limit is about 150 mmHg. When MAP ex-

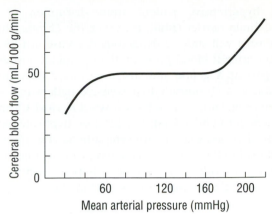

Figure 12–7. Cerebral autoregulation.

ceeds 150 mmHg, autoregulatory breakthrough occurs. This breakthrough, according to Donegan (1991) is associated with an increase in CBF, disruption of the blood–brain barrier at many sites, and formation of cerebral edema.

The mechanism of cerebrovascular autoregulation is not completely understood. Both myogenic and metabolic mechanisms have been proposed to explain cerebral autoregulation. The myogenic hypothesis states that autoregulation is an intrinsic response of the smooth muscle of the arterial wall. When the smooth muscle is stretched by increasing pressure, it contracts, producing vasoconstriction. The response of the smooth muscle to a reduction in systemic arterial tension is relaxation, thus producing vasodilatation. According to the metabolic theory, blood flow is regulated by the metabolic activity of the tissue. Therefore, anything that interferes with oxygen delivery to the tissue (eg, hypotension) results in the liberation of acid metabolites, which produce vasodilatation and increased blood flow.

Causes of loss of autoregulation include hypoxia, ischemia, hypercapnia, trauma, and some anesthetic agents. The autoregulatory curve may be shifted in either direction. A shift to the right, increasing the lower and upper limits of autoregulation, occurs with chronic hypertension and sympathetic activation (eg, stress or shock). With chronic hypertension, this shift is caused by hypertrophy of the vessel walls and is established over about 4 to 8 weeks. A right-shifted curve means that a greater perfusion pressure is necessary to maintain CBF, but it also allows for a greater perfusion pressure to be continued before autoregulatory breakthrough and disruption of the blood–brain barrier occur. A left-shifted autoregulatory curve is produced by hypoxia, hypercarbia, and vasodilators. A left-shifted curve allows CBF to be maintained at a lower than normal perfusion pressure. It is key according to Farnsworth, Johnson, & Sperry (1996), that pressure containment protects the chronically hypertensive patient from disruption of the blood–brain barrier (BBB). However, the chronically hypertensive will suffer a dangerous decrease in CBF at a greater arterial blood pressure than would a normotensive patient. A gentle and sustained blood pressure reduction in a chronically hypertensive patient may shift the autoregulatory curve back toward normal. Clearly, it is essential to understand that, because hypovolemic hypotension is associated with sympathetic activation and a right-shifted autoregulatory curve, CBF will be better maintained with pharmacologic hypotension (rather than only reducing intravenous fluid intake).

Carbon Dioxide Tension. Alterations in carbon dioxide tension (Pa_{CO_2}) can profoundly affect CBF. Cerebral blood flow varies linearly with Pa_{CO_2} from 20 mmHg to 80 mmHg in normocapnic persons. This variation produces direct changes in CBF of about 2% for every 1 mmHg change in Pa_{CO_2} (Fig. 12–8). The exact mechanism by which carbon dioxide (CO_2) exerts its effect on cerebral vessels is not completely understood. The prevailing theory is that changes in CO_2 produce changes in the pH of the CSF surrounding the vessels and in the walls of the arterioles. Although this is still controversial, Donegan (1991) and Todd & Warner (1993) purport that this alteration occurs because CO_2 crosses the blood–brain barrier freely, whereas bicarbonate crosses more slowly. Thus, increases in Pa_{CO_2} decrease pH in the CSF and arteriolar walls. Because bicarbonate ions do cross the blood–brain barrier, changes in CSF pH and CBF resulting from alterations in Pa_{CO_2} last only a few hours. After this time, CBF returns to normal despite continuing hypocapnia or hypercapnia.

Oxygen Tension. Measurable increases in CBF do not occur until the oxygen tension (Pa_{O_2}) is reduced below 50 mmHg. If CBF as a function of arterial O_2 content (Ca_{O_2}) rather than Pa_{O_2} is examined, the resultant curve does not demonstrate a threshold. According to Donegan (1991), the reason that some studies have failed to demonstrate an increase in CBF at Pa_{O_2} above 50 mmHg may be that in most species substantial reductions in Ca_{O_2} do not occur until Pa_{O_2} falls below 50 mmHg. When Pa_{O_2} is less than 50 mmHg, there is a rapid linear increase in CBF to compensate for reduced O_2 delivery. The mechanism for the increase in flow with hypoxia is not completely understood. However, hyperoxia, produced by inhalation of 80% to 100% O_2 in the normal individual, is associated with a 10% to 12% decrease in CBF.

Cerebral Metabolism. Total CBF generally parallels overall cerebral metabolism (CMR_{O_2}). The CMR_{O_2} and consequently CBF are closely correlated with brain activity. When the level of activity is lowest, as in coma, metabolism and CBF are lowest. When overall brain activity is high, as in a grand mal seizure, metabolism and CBF are high. According to Donegan (1991), the same is true of activity, metabolism, and CBF at the regional level (rCBF). For example, when stereognostic test objects are placed in a subject's hand, there is an increase in rCBF of the hand area of the contralateral postcentral gyrus.

Body Temperature. A decrease in body temperature lowers cerebral metabolism, resulting in a decrease in CBF. The depression in metabolism is about 5% per degree centigrade reduction in body temperature. Similarly, raising body temperature increases CBF and cerebral metabolism.

Intracranial Pressure Dynamics and Cerebral Spinal Fluid

Intracranial contents including the brain, intra-, and extracellular water, CSF, blood, and meninges, generate an average ICP of 8 mmHg to 12 mmHg (Rando, 1992; Morgan & Mikhail, 1996). Because the skull is relatively rigid, a change in volume of one of the intracranial constituents must be accompanied by a reciprocal change in one of the other constituents if increased ICP is to be avoided. If these reciprocal changes do not occur, the craniospinal compartment is said to be noncompliant or *tight*. Normal intracranial compliance permits limited expansion of intracranial volumes without increasing ICP. Patients with low compliance poorly tolerate increases in intracranial volume (Fig. 12–9).

Cerebrospinal fluid is located in the cerebral ventricles, the cisterns, and the subarachnoid space surrounding the brain and spinal cord. Its major function is to protect the CNS against trauma. Most of the CSF is formed by the choroid plexuses of the cerebral ventricles (mostly the lateral ventricles). In adults, normal total CSF

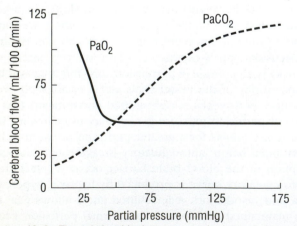

Figure 12–8. The relationship between cerebral blood flow and arterial respiratory gas tensions.

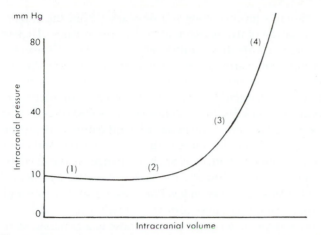

Figure 12–9. Intracranial compliance curve. *(Adapted, with permission, from Shapiro, H. M. [1975]. Intercranial hypertension: Therapeutic and anesthetic considerations.* Anesthesiology, *43, 445.)*

volume is about 120 mL to 150 mL. The rate of CSF production is approximately 0.35 mL/min (ie, 450 mL/day); turnover is three times per day. The CSF flows from the lateral ventricles through the interventricular foramina (of Monro) into the third ventricle, through the cerebral aqueduct (of Sylvius) into the fourth ventricle, and through the medium opening of the fourth ventricle (foramen of Magendie) and the lateral opening of the fourth ventricle (foramina of Luschka) into the cerebellomedullary cistern (cisterna Magna). The CSF enters the subarachnoid space, circulating around the brain and spinal cord before absorption takes place in the arachnoid villi and spinal venous plexi. Normally, the rate of formation equals the rate of absorption ($V_f = R_a$). If the rate of formation increases faster than the rate of absorption ($V_f > R_a$) or absorption is obstructed ($R_a < V_f$), an increase in CSF volume will occur. Increases in CSF production occur in hyperthermia, cervical sympathectomy, low serum osmolarity, functioning tumors, and from some anesthetic agents (eg, enflurane and halothane). Decreases in CSF production occur in hypothermia, acetazolamide, higher serum osmolarity, raised ICP, and during steroid therapy.

Blood–Brain Barrier

The BBB was conceived in an attempt to explain the different rates of permeability of most substances between the capillary bed and interstitial fluids of the brain compared with the more rapid equilibration between these two compartments, as seen in other organ systems (Rando, 1992; Morgan & Mikhail, 1996). Permeability in the CNS is limited by pericapillary glial cells and endothelial cell-tight junctions, which constitute the BBB. This lipid barrier allows the passage of lipid-soluble substances but restricts the movement of those that are ion-ized or have large molecular weights. Thus, the movement of a given substance across the BBB is governed simultaneously by its size, charge, lipid solubility, and degree of protein binding in the blood. Carbon dioxide, oxygen, and lipid-soluble substances (such as most anesthetic agents) freely enter the brain, whereas ions, such as Na^+, K^+, Mg^{2+}, Cl^-, HCO_3^-, and HPO_4^{2-}, proteins, and large substances, such as mannitol, penetrate poorly.

Water moves freely across the BBB as a consequence of bulk flow, whereas movement of small ions (eg, Na^+) is impeded to some extent. As a result, rapid changes in plasma electrolyte concentrations produce a transient osmotic gradient between plasma and the brain. Acute hypertonicity of plasma results in net movement of water out of the brain, whereas acute hypotonicity causes a net movement of water into the brain. These effects are short lived (Morgan & Mikhail, 1996) because equilibration eventually occurs, but when marked they can cause rapid fluid shifts in the brain. Thus, correcting marked abnormalities in serum sodium and glucose concentrations should be instituted slowly. Some areas of the brain are more impregnable than others. The pineal gland, posterior pituitary, and areas surrounding the ventricular structures are most susceptible to substances circulating in the plasma.

The clinical implications associated with knowledge of the permeability of the BBB to drugs focuses on anesthetics with a high solubility coefficient that generally cause unconsciousness more quickly. For example, atropine, a tertiary amine, readily crosses the BBB, whereas glycopyrrolate, a quaternary ammonium, does not. Mannitol, an osmotically active substance, causes a sustained decrease in brain water content and is often used to decrease brain volume.

▶ PERIANESTHETIC EVALUATION OF THE NEUROLOGIC SYSTEM IN ADULTS

History

The neurologic examination is preceded by a complete history and general physical examination. The circumstances surrounding the examination of a patient can vary greatly. At the time of the examination, patients may be alert, oriented, and conversant, or they may have an altered level of consciousness with significant neurologic deficits. The patient's condition and ability to cooperate will influence the skill of the practitioner to collect a complete database.

Hickey (1997) points out that many parts of the mental status examination are integrated into the history-taking portion of the interview. In a screening examination, the following areas should be evaluated: orientation, appearance and behavior, mood, speech pattern, and thoughts and perceptions.

The patient must be awake, alert, able to understand questions, and able to respond. A patient who presents as neat and clean reflects good grooming and personal hygiene habits. An unkept appearance might suggest chronic organic brain disease or a depressed state. Ask the patient about the perception of his or her mood. Questions that are useful include "How are your spirits?", "What makes you angry?", and "What makes you sad?". Observing the patient's speech pattern is important; the examiner should listen for quality, quantity, pace, tone, and spontaneity of the flow of words.

Thought processes, content, perception, insight, and judgement are evaluated throughout the interview to identify deviations (Hickey, 1997). Thought processes refer to subjective responses to life experiences and how they are verbally expressed. Be alert for flight of ideas, incoherence, confabulation, and other disorders of thought. Thought content refers to abnormal themes in content. By listening and reflecting, the examiner can evaluate flaws in content. These include compulsive behaviors, indecision, feelings of unreality, delusions, illusions, and hallucinations. Hickey (1997) defines perception as a person's subjective interpretation of real or perceived stimuli. Insight is the act of seeing the inner nature of things or seeing intuitively. "What seems to be the problem?" and "Why are you here today?" are good questions to uncover insight into a situation. Judgement is the process of forming an opinion or evaluation of a situation or problem. "How are you going to manage at home following this hospitalization?" is an example of a way the examiner can determine how accurate and reasonable judgements are based.

Cognitive functions, sometimes referred to as higher-level functions, should also be examined. In the examination, the focus proceeds from general to special functions (Hickey, 1997). General cognitive functions include orientation to time, place, and person; attention and concentration; memory; calculations; general fund of information; and abstract thinking. Special functions include naming objects, construction ability, and language.

Physical Examination

A complete neurologic assessment should include level of consciousness, motor and sensory function, cerebellar function, vital signs, and cranial nerves. An abbreviated neurologic assessment, sometimes referred to as *neuro signs,* provides a global overview of the patient's condition. These signs include level of consciousness, pupillary signs, and motor function.

Level of Consciousness

Consciousness is defined as a state of general awareness of oneself and the environment. Challenges in evaluating a patient's level of consciousness arise from the subjective nature of the assessment skill. Consciousness, Hickey (1997) reports, has traditionally been divided into two components: arousal, which is concerned with the patient's appearance of wakefulness, and content or cognition, which includes the sum of cerebral mental functions. As consciousness cannot be measured directly, it is estimated by observing behavioral indicators in response to stimuli. Consciousness is the most sensitive indicator of neurologic change; as such, a change in the level of consciousness is usually the first to be noted in neurologic signs. A change in level of consciousness can occur rapidly (within minutes), or very slowly, over a period of hours, days, or weeks. Consciousness is a dynamic state that is subject to change. When an assessment is conducted, the patient's arousability and behavior merely provide an estimate of consciousness at a given point in time. The level of consciousness is assessed by applying stimuli and observing the response (verbal or motor). Auditory and tactile stimuli are the two stimuli used to assess level of consciousness and must be considered on a continuum. Auditory stimuli such as a normal speaking voice are used initially. If the patient responds, then the observer can talk to him or her and ask questions to assess the level of orientation. If the patient does not respond to a normal voice volume, a louder voice or a loud noise, such as that produced by clapping the hands, is utilized. Tactile stimuli may be attempted if there is no response to auditory stimuli. The patient's arm is gently shaken while calling his or her name. If no response is elicited by these measures (the patient appears unconscious), painful (noxious) stimuli are applied.

Pupillary Signs

Evaluating the pupils is an extremely important part of patient assessment that provides vital information about CNS function. The general points to consider when assessing the pupils include their size, shape, and reaction to light. The finding in the one pupil is always compared with the finding in the other pupil, and differences between the two are noted. Normally, the pupils are equal in size, measuring about 2 mm to 6 mm in diameter with an average diameter of 3.5 mm (Table 12-5). Two methods are used to record pupillary size: the millimeter scale (most common) which is objective, and the descriptive method which is subjective (Table 12-6). When the millimeter scale is used, the nurse anesthetist compares the patient's individual pupillary size to a standard pupillary gauge. Subjective evaluation of pupil size includes terms such as *pinpoint, small, midpoint, large,* and *dilated.* Pupil shape needs to be assessed concurrently with size.

When light is directed into the eye, the pupil should immediately constrict. Withdrawal of the light should produce an immediate and brisk dilation of the pupil. Introducing the light into one pupil should cause similar constriction to occur simultaneously in the other

TABLE 12–5. Nursing Assessment of Pupillary Size

In assessing pupillary size using either descriptive terms or a gauge, each pupil is assessed individually and then the findings for each pupil are compared. This is very important because pupils are normally equal (see note on anisocoria).

Descriptive Term	Definition	Findings
Pinpoint	The pupil is so small that it is barely visible or appears as small as a pinpoint.	Seen with opiate overdose, pontine hemorrhage, ischemia.
Small	The pupil appears smaller than average but larger than pinpoint.	Seen normally if the person is in a bright room; also seen with miotic ophthalmic drops, opiates, pontine hemorrhage, Horner's syndrome, bilateral diecephalic lesions, and metabolic coma.
Midposition	When the pupil and iris are observed, about half of their diameter is iris and half is pupil.	Seen normally; if pupils are midposition and nonreactive, midbrain damage is the cause.
Large	The pupils are larger than average, but there is still an appreciable amount of iris visible.	Seen normally if room is dark; may be seen with some drugs, such as amphetamines; glutethimide (Doriden) overdose; mydriatics; cycloplegic agents; and some orbital injuries.
Dilated	When the pupil and iris are observed, one is struck by the largeness of the pupil with only the slightest ring of iris, which is barely visible.	Abnormal finding; bilateral, fixed, and dilated pupils are seen in the terminal stage of severe anoxia–ischemia or at death.

Note: **Anisocoria** is the term used to describe inequality in size between the pupils. About 17% of the population has slight anisocoria without any related pathological process. It is, therefore, important to make a baseline assessment of pupillary size and compare subsequent assessments with the baseline. If pupillary inequality is a new finding, it should be reported. If the patient is admitted with slight pupillary inequality and no other abnormalities are detected on the neurological assessment, the pupil inequality may not be significant.

From Hickey, J. V. (1997). The clinical practice of neurological and neurosurgical nursing (4th ed., p. 147). Philadelphia: Lippincott.

pupil. When the light is withdrawn from one eye, the opposite pupil should dilate simultaneously. Pupillary reaction to light is recorded using descriptive terms or symbols. The descriptive terms used include *brisk, sluggish,* and *nonreactive* or *fixed*. Assessing the size and shape of the pupils and the direct light reaction are ways of gathering data about the presence of brain dysfunction to provide a preanesthetic baseline evaluation (Table 12–7).

Motor Function

The motor assessment is employed in an organized manner, beginning with the neck and proceeding to the upper extremities, trunk, and finally to the lower extremities. The identification of significant changes is important for noting deterioration, improvement, or stabilization in condition. The following should be considered in the basic approach to assessing motor function: muscle size; muscle tone; muscle strength; presence of involuntary movement; and posture and gait. When one muscle or muscle group is assessed, it is always compared with the same muscle or group on the opposite side of the body. Normally, function should be the same on both sides of the body. When assessing muscle size, a tape measure may be used if a difference in size seems to exist. Muscle tone is examined first by palpation at rest and then during passive movement. Muscle strength is assessed by testing active, passive, and active resistive movements. The presence of involuntary movements such as tremors, myoclonus, tics, or spasms are documented.

Sensory Function

The sensory evaluation is usually deferred unless the patient has spinal cord disease (secondary to trauma, neoplasm, infectious processes, or stenosis), intervertebral disk disease, or other conditions that affect the spinal cord or spinal nerves. A sensory assessment is conducted on the patient who is conscious, cooperative, and able to respond appropriately. The sensory modalities assessed include superficial sensation (light touch with cotton-tipped applicator or pain with pinprick) and deep sen-

TABLE 12–6. Nursing Assessment of Pupillary Shape

Descriptive Term	Definition	Findings
Round	Like a circle	• Normal finding
Ovoid	Slightly oval "ovoid"	• Almost always indicates intracranial hypertension and represents an intermediate phase between a normal pupil (round) and a fully dilated fixed pupil; an early sign of transtentorial herniation
Keyhole	Like a keyhole	• Seen in patients who have had an iridectomy (excision of part of the iris). An iridectomy is often part of cataract surgery, a common procedure in the elderly population. (The reaction to light is very slight.)
Irregular	Jagged	• Seen in Argyll–Robertson pupils and with traumatic orbital injuries

From Hickey, J. V. (1997). The clinical practice of neurological and neurosurgical nursing (4th ed., p. 148). Philadelphia: Lippincott.

sation (proprioception) by moving fingers and large toe in various positions.

Vital Signs
The relationship between vital signs and neurologic function is centered on hemodynamics. The hemodynamic concept requires that the brain be supplied with a large and constant volume of O_2-rich blood to support adequate CPP and cell metabolism. Without adequate cerebral perfusion, cerebral ischemia develops, cerebral cell metabolism is affected, and neurologic dysfunction occurs.

Respirations
The respiratory pattern can be correlated with the anatomic level of dysfunction because at certain cerebral

TABLE 12–7. Nursing Assessment of Pupillary Light Responses

Descriptive Term	Symbol	Findings
Brisk	++	Normal finding
Sluggish	+	Found in conditions that cause some compression of the oculomotor (III) nerve; seen in early transtentorial herniation, cerebral edema, and Adie's pupil
Nonreactive or fixed	−	Found in conditions that include compression of the oculomotor nerve; seen with transtentorial herniation syndromes and in severe hypoxia and ischemia (terminal stage just before death)
Swollen closed	c	One or both eyes are tightly closed because of severe periorbital edema; the pupillary light reflex may be difficult to assess.
One other response—the Hippus phenomenon—is included; this does not usually appear on assessment sheets but may be observed in the clinical area and, therefore, needs to be recorded.		
Hippus phenomenon	None	With uniform illumination of the pupil, dilation and contraction are noted. This may be considered normal if pupils are observed under high magnification. The Hippus phenomenon is also observed in patients who are beginning to experience pressure on the third cranial nerve. This is often associated with early transtentorial herniation.

Note: On some pupillary assessment sheets, other symbols are used in place of descriptive terms.
From Hickey, J. V. (1997). The clinical practice of neurological and neurosurgical nursing (4th ed., p. 150). Philadelphia: Lippincott.

levels, specific respiratory patterns are characteristically found. However, the patient may be on a ventilator that is set for a particular rate and rhythm, thus overriding an adequate respiratory pattern. The respiratory centers are located within the pons and medulla. The pons contains the apneustic and pneumotaxic areas. The medulla contains the dorsal respiratory group and ventral respiratory group, which together are referred to as the *rhythmicity center.*

The dorsal respiratory group is located in the dorsal portion of the medulla. This group plays a fundamental role in the control of respirations, mainly by causing inspirations and setting the basic rhythm of respirations. The ventral respiratory group, located in the ventrolateral part of the medulla, can cause either expiration or inspiration, depending on which neurons in the group are stimulated. During normal respirations, the ventral group is almost totally inactive; however, when the respiratory drive for increased pulmonary ventilation exceeds normal limits, some neurons of this group become a back up system to stimulate the dorsal respiratory group, resulting in increased respiratory drive.

The pneumotaxic center is located in the dorsal portion of the upper pons. It continually transmits impulses of varying magnitude for inspirations. The primary function of the center is to limit inspiration; however, by limiting respirations, it exerts a secondary effect on the rate of breathing. Strong pneumotaxic signals can increase the rate of breathing, whereas weak signals will reduce the rate of breathing to only a few breaths per minute. The Hering–Breuer reflex (which will be discussed next) also has an effect on turning. The function of the apneustic center is unclear. Only under special conditions involving transection of the vagus nerve and connections to the pneumotaxic center does the apneustic center function. This center sends signals to the dorsal respiratory group to prevent the *turning off* of inspirations. As a result, the inspiratory phase is long, followed by only occasional, short, expiratory gasps.

The Hering–Breuer reflex is a protective reflex that prevents excessive lung expansion. Stretch receptors located in the bronchi throughout the lungs have stretch receptors that transmit signals through the vagus nerves to the dorsal respiratory group when the lungs are overinflated. This reflex is similar to the pneumotaxic center in that it limits the duration of inspiration through a feedback loop that *turns off* inspiratory effort and reduces the time of inspiration so that the respiratory rate is increased.

The rate, rhythm, and characteristics of the inspiratory and expiratory phases of respirations should be documented. In addition to neurologic causes of respiratory changes, a number of other etiologies should be considered, such as acidosis, alkalosis, electrolyte imbalance, congestive heart failure, anxiety, and various respiratory complications (eg, atelectasis, pneumonia, and pulmo-

nary edema). An acute rise in ICP is reflected by a slowing of respiratory rate. As ICP continues to rise, the rate becomes rapid. The respiratory pattern will also change with a rising ICP.

Pulse
The nuclei in the medulla is responsible for inhibitory and excitatory impulses in the cardiac system. The excitatory or accelerator fibers arise from the spinal nerves T1 to T5. The vagus nerve provides constant inhibitory impulses to slow the heart. Assessment of the rate, rhythm, and quality of the pulse provide significant information related to the CNS. The major changes associated with rate and rhythm are tachycardia, bradycardia, and cardiac arrhythmias. Tachycardia may indicate the end stages of a neurologic disease process. Bradycardia can indicate the late stages of increased ICP. Cardiac arrhythmias are common in the neurosurgical patient and are often associated with subarachnoid hemorrhage, ruptured cerebral aneurysm, and severe head injury. The increased cardiac irritability is most often associated with blood appearing in the CSF. The major changes that occur in pulse quality are characterized by a full-bounding pulse or a thready pulse. A full-bounding pulse is associated with increasing ICP and thready pulse is indicative of catastrophic cerebral sequelae.

Blood Pressure
Blood pressure (BP) regulation is conducted through the vasomotor center of the medulla. Nuclei of the vasomotor center deliver impulses via the spinal cord and spinal nerves to the arteriole walls for constriction or dilation. Measurement of BP usually focuses on comparisons from previous assessment of normotension, hypotension, hypertension, and pulse pressure. Changes in BP during neurosurgery will effect cerebral perfusion and autoregulation (as discussed previously). An elevated BP in the neurologic patient is usually associated with a rising ICP. An elevated systolic BP, widening pulse pressure, and bradycardia are seen in the advanced stages of increased ICP (Cushing's response). Hypotension is rarely attributable to cerebral injury. When it is seen with severe injury, it occurs only as a terminal event and is accompanied by tachycardia. Inadequate cerebral perfusion denies the cerebral tissue an adequate O_2 supply, and the regulatory mechanisms no longer function. During this stage of decompensation, deterioration is rapid and death results. Hypotension and bradycardia may be seen in patients with cervical spinal injury. In these situations, the altered signs would be the result of interruption of the descending sympathetic pathways.

Temperature
The hypothalamus is the center for the regulation of body heat and acts by monitoring the blood tempera-

ture. Regulation of heat is accomplished by afferent impulses to the sweat glands, peripheral vessels, and skeletal muscles for shivering. Through these structures, the body can conserve or divest itself of body heat. An elevated temperature can be caused by a neurologic condition, such as injury to the hypothalamus. The temperature elevation can be high and may occur rapidly. An elevated temperature is treated vigorously in the neurologic patient because it results in an increased cell metabolism that eventually produces increased CO_2 and lactic acid by-products of cell metabolism. As mentioned in the physiology section, CO_2 is a potent cerebral vasodilator and will cause an increase in ICP in a patient who may already have a high ICP. If the O_2 supply to the cerebral tissue is insufficient, cerebral ischemia develops. Therefore, aggressive treatment of hyperthermia to prevent neurologic deterioration is important and necessary. Hypothermia is seen in certain conditions, such as spinal shock when autonomic innervation is lost; metabolic or toxic coma of any origin; drug overdose, especially for depressant drugs (barbiturates); destructive brain stem or hypothalamic lesions; and in terminal stages of certain neurologic disease processes. Hyperthermia can be elevated in conditions such as CNS infection, subarachnoid hemorrhage of the hypothalamus or brain stem, traction on the hypothalamus or brain stem, heat stroke, bacterial endocarditis, pneumonia, overdose of phenothiazines or anticholinergic drugs, and other infections outside the CNS.

Glasgow Coma Score

The Glasgow Coma Scale, which is widely used in the United States, was developed in 1974 at the University of Glasgow in Scotland for the assessment of consciousness in clients with head injuries (Teasdale & Jennett, 1974; Hickey, 1997). The scale (Fig. 12–10) was devised to develop standardized observations for objective and accurate data collection to assess level of consciousness. The scale is especially useful in monitoring changes associated with a recent injury.

The Glasgow Coma Scale is divided into three subscales: eye opening, best verbal response, and best motor response. There are a variety of categories within each subscale. The information collected is plotted on a graph to provide a visual record of improvement, deterioration, or stabilization (Hickey, 1997). In the interpretation of the scale, the numerical values of each subscale may be added for a total score. The range of possible scores is 3 to 15. A score of 15 would indicate a fully alert, oriented client, whereas a score of 3, the lowest possible score, would be indicative of deep coma. Patients with scores of 7 or less are generally considered comatose.

Diagnostic Studies

The latest developments of improved diagnostic and monitoring techniques have positively influenced patient outcomes related to neurosurgical intervention and treatment of neurologic disease states. Computed tomography (CT) and magnetic resonance imaging (MRI) have revolutionized the modalities available in neurologic assessment and evaluation. As a result, the traditional diagnostic procedures, such as the pneumoencephalogram and echoencephalogram, are now obsolete. A CT scan and MRI provide rapid initial identification of pharmacologically or surgically treatable lesions such as tumors, abscesses, hematomas, and edema without significant hazard to the patient because of delayed diagnosis, mechanical complications, or expansion of residual air from pneumoenchalography (Shwiry, 1992).

Electrophysiologic monitoring of the brain via EEG and multimodality evoked potentials (EPs) readily detects abnormal function in the presence of ischemic changes. Consideration of the effects of cardiopulmonary parameters and the pharmacologic influence on intracranial dynamics in conjunction with new diagnostic and monitoring devices has contributed greatly to improved management and outcome of the neurosurgical patient.

Radiographic Studies

Skull films generally include anteroposterior and lateral views. Other angles may be included to provide more detail in specific cases. Skull films provide information about presence of fractures, unusual calcification, the size and shape of skull bones, and bone erosion, particularly of the sella turcica (Hickey, 1997).

Spinal films provide views of various regions of the spine (cervical, thoracic, lumbar, or sacral). The anterior, posterior, and lateral views are most commonly obtained. Abnormal findings from spinal films may include defects in vertebra, such as bone erosion, calcification (spur), narrowing of the vertebral canal, vertebral fractures and dislocations, and spondylosis.

Initially introduced in the early to mid-1970s, CT scans now represent the cornerstone of neurologic diagnostic procedures. The CT scan (with or without contrast medium) is extremely useful in locating and diagnosing various cranial lesions, such as abscesses, cysts, infarctions, hematomas, contusions, hydrocephalus, and primary and metastatic lesions.

Magnetic resonance imaging is noninvasive and painless and carries no known risk to the client. When compared to a CT scan, MRI is technologically different and uses no radiation. The images obtained from MRI are unmatched for sharpness. The cross sections of living tissue provide not only anatomic information, but also in-

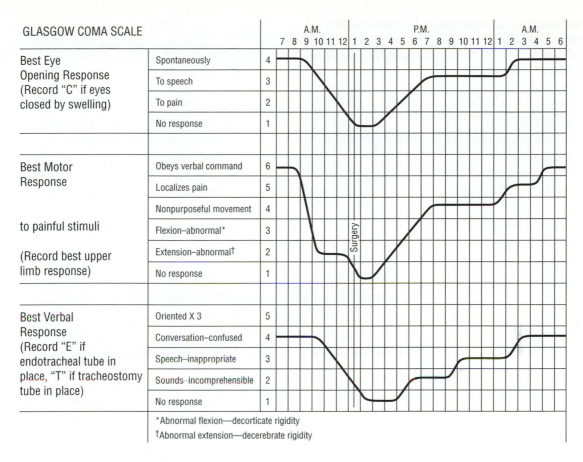

GLASGOW COMA SCALE			A.M.			P.M.			A.M.		
			7 8 9 10 11 12	1 2 3 4 5 6	7 8 9 10 11 12	1 2 3 4 5 6					
Best Eye Opening Response (Record "C" if eyes closed by swelling)	Spontaneously	4									
	To speech	3									
	To pain	2									
	No response	1									
Best Motor Response to painful stimuli (Record best upper limb response)	Obeys verbal command	6									
	Localizes pain	5									
	Nonpurposeful movement	4									
	Flexion–abnormal*	3									
	Extension–abnormal†	2									
	No response	1									
Best Verbal Response (Record "E" if endotracheal tube in place, "T" if tracheostomy tube in place)	Oriented X 3	5									
	Conversation–confused	4									
	Speech–inappropriate	3									
	Sounds–incomprehensible	2									
	No response	1									

*Abnormal flexion—decorticate rigidity
†Abnormal extension—decerebrate rigidity

Scoring of Eye Opening
• 4 Opens eyes spontaneously when the nurse approaches
• 3 Opens eyes in response to speech (normal or shout)
• 2 Opens eyes only to painful stimuli (e.g., squeezing of nail beds)
• 1 Does not open eyes to painful stimuli

Scoring of Best Motor Response
• 6 Can obey a simple command, such as "Lift your left hand off the bed"
• 5 Localizes to painful stimuli and attempts to remove source
• 4 Purposeless movement in response to pain
• 3 Flexes elbows and wrists while extending lower legs to pain
• 2 Extends upper and lower extremities to pain
• 1 No motor response to pain on any limb

Scoring of Best Verbal Response
• 5 Oriented to time, place, and person
• 4 Converses, although confused
• 3 Speaks only in words or phrases that make little or no sense
• 2 Responds with incomprehensible sounds (e.g., groans)
• 1 No verbal response

Figure 12–10. Glasgow Coma Scale (GCS).

formation about the chemical and physiologic components of living tissue. Hickey (1997) reports that with increasing availability of MRI, protocols are being developed to guide clinicians in determining the preferred method (Table 12–8).

Positron emission transaxial tomography (PET) is a noninvasive technique that is useful in studying biochemical and physiologic function in living organisms. Positron emission transaxial tomography is a new, developing technology that is utilized in CNS research focusing on improv-

TABLE 12–8. Comparison of Indications for CT Scans and MRIs

CT Scan	MRI
• Pacemaker in place*	• Allergy to contrast medium
• Metal prosthesis in place*	• Subacute/chronic cerebral trauma
• Uncooperative patient*	• Pituitary tumors
• Acute craniocerebral trauma	• Posterior fossa tumors (eg, acoustic neuroma)
• Acute subdural, acute epidural, or acute intracerebral hemorrhage	• Demyelinating disease (eg, multiple sclerosis)
• Predicting cerebral vasospasm	• Cerebral atrophy
• Aneurysm clipping with metal*	• Seizure disorders when CT scan yields normal results
• Hemorrhagic stroke	• Spinal cord tumors (primary and metastatic)
• Subarachnoid hemorrhage	• Spinal cord trauma
• Ischemic stroke (48 to 72 hours old)	• Intervertebral disk disease when myelographic results are normal
• Supratentorial enhancing tumors	
• Hydrocephalus	

*MRI contraindicated.
From Hickey, J. V. (1997). The clinical practice of neurological and neurosurgical nursing (4th ed., p. 85). Philadelphia: Lippincott.

ing the understanding of epilepsy, dementia, cerebrovascular disease, cerebral trauma, and mental illness. The major drawback is that an on-line cyclotron is necessary for its use and that this equipment is only found in a few major research centers in the United States (Hickey, 1997).

Cerebrospinal Fluid and Spinal Testing

Cerebrospinal fluid and spinal testing techniques include lumbar puncture, cisternal puncture, and myelography. The indications for lumbar puncture can be divided into diagnostic and therapeutic purposes. The diagnostic indications include measuring CSF, examining CSF for presence of blood, collecting CSF for laboratory evaluation, injecting air, O_2, or radiopaque material to visualize parts of the nervous system radiologically, and evaluating the dynamics of CSF flow. A cisternogram is used for diagnosing hydrocephalus, blockage of CSF flow in the vertebral column secondary to spinal compression, blockage by adhesions, and tearing of meninges. A myelogram is a diagnostic procedure that involves injection of a contrast medium into the subarachnoid space to aid in the diagnosis of spinal cord tumor, herniated intervertebral disk, or a ruptured disk.

Noninvasive Carotid Studies

Kistler, MacDonald, Ackerman, and Abbott (1987) identify a battery of complementary noninvasive carotid studies available to assess the presence, location, and severity of artherothrombotic disease at the bifurcation of the common carotid artery. Diagnosis of patients with carotid bruits, transient ischemic attacks (TIAs), or stroke has been greatly facilitated with these mainstay evaluative procedures. These tests have been divided into indirect and direct methods. The indirect method evaluates the indirect effects on pressure and flow in the distal internal carotid artery (ICA) of lesions involving the bifurcation of the common carotid artery (CCA). The direct method directly evaluates the bifurcation of the CCA.

Ocular pneumoplethysmography (OPG) indirectly measures intraocular ophthalmic systolic pressure. The ophthalmic artery is the first major vessel to branch off the ICA. If there is a significant stenosis or partial occlusion of the proximal ICA, it will be reflected by reduced systolic pressure in the ophthalmic artery (Hickey, 1997). Three direct testing procedures are used to examine carotid flow. These include carotid phonoangiography, quantitative phonoangiography, and Doppler flow velocity analysis.

Carotid phonoangiography is a simple, noninvasive technique that uses a transducer to record carotid bruit during systole and diastole. Quantitative phonoangiography is thought to be a highly accurate means of diagnosing bruit-producing stenotic lesions at the origin of the ICA. This test uses the frequency–intensity sound spectrum of the bruit. The examiner notes the point where the intensity begins to decline and can then calculate the residual luminal diameter of the stenotic lesion that is producing the bruit. Finally, the Doppler flow velocity analysis can diagnose carotid artery stenosis or occlusion. These data are amplified and graphic recordings are produced. The test takes only 5 to 10 minutes and is 95% accurate (Kistler, MacDonald, Ackerman, & Abbott, 1987; Hickey, 1997).

Invasive Carotid Studies

Invasive cerebrovascular testing includes digital subtraction angiography (DA), cerebral angiography, and temporal artery biopsy. Digital subtraction angiography is a computer-assisted radiographic procedure for visualizing carotids and other cerebral vessels. The image produced becomes more distinct with the elimination of surrounding and interfering anatomic structures.

A cerebral angiogram consists of injecting a radiopaque contrast medium into an artery for direct visualization of the intracranial and extracranial blood vessels. Cerebral angiography is used to diagnose intracranial lesions and cerebrovascular abnormalities. It is the definitive diagnostic tool for aneurysms and arteriovenous malformation.

Temporal artery biopsy is used for patients who experience facial pain and nonspecific neurologic symptoms. After administration of a local anesthetic, a small piece of temporal artery is removed and is examined for evidence of temporal arteritis.

Electroencephalography

An EEG is a diagnostic tool used to detect abnormal cerebral function. An EEG provides a recording of the electrical activity of the brain. Signals are picked up from surface cerebral cortex neurons and are amplified so that an acceptable recording can be made. The greatest value of the EEG is in evaluating seizure activity. The classification of brain waves is based on the number of cycles per second or hertz (Hz), the amplitude measured in microvolts, and the symmetry of the waveforms. There are four frequency bands identified for EEG interpretation (Johnson, 1996). Delta waves (0 Hz to 4 Hz) are consistent with deep anesthesia, coma, hypoxic ischemia, and deep sleep. Theta waves (4 Hz to 7 Hz) are seen predominantly in premature infants, healthy young children during sleep, during hyperventilation, and with moderate anesthesia. Alpha waves (8 Hz to 13 Hz) are typically seen in the person who is relaxed, alert, with eyes closed and with light anesthesia. Beta waves (14 Hz to 30 Hz) are characterized by low voltage and fast activity seen in the awake, alert (not relaxed) individual.

Evoked Potentials

Evoked potentials are a noninvasive means of applying a specific stimulus and recording the tiny electrical potentials that are subsequently created. As such, normal sensory EPs reflect the integrity of the pathway being observed. These pathways are ascending sensory tracts that usually involve a peripheral or cranial nerve. Evoked potentials are used as a complementary procedure in the battery of testing conducted for problems that are not well defined clinically, or that are readily diagnosed. They are classified into three categories based on the type of stimulus provided and the sensory system stimulated. Each system stimulated produces a characteristic wave formation. The three sensory systems used in EPs are the visual, auditory, and somatosensory pathways. For a more detailed discussion of EEG and EP measurement tools, refer to Chapter 23.

▶ PATHOPHYSIOLOGY OF PATIENTS WITH NEUROLOGIC DISEASES

Seizure Disorders

The incidence of epilepsy is about 0.5% to 2% (Kofke, 1997), with 25% to 30% of epileptics experiencing seizure activity more than once per month. There are about 300 000 people who have medically uncontrolled epilepsy. Of this group, 13% are candidates for epilepsy surgery (Kofke, 1997). Seizures are defined as an excessive discharge of large quantities of neurons that depolarize in a synchronous manner. Poorly controlled epilepsy results in the inability to maintain a normal lifestyle. Intellectual and social deficits may arise from the brain-damaging effects of uncontrolled recurrent seizures, negative attitudes of society, or from the adverse side effects of antiepileptic drug therapies. Seizures are categorized as partial or focal (including simple partial and complex partial); generalized (including absence and myoclonic); and grand mal continuous seizures (status epilepticus).

Perianesthesia Considerations

Preoperative preparation begins by assessing the patient's neuropsychiatric status; determining antiepileptic drug therapy; and determining the impact of drug therapy on organ function, coagulation, and response to anesthetic agents. Sedation produced from antiepileptic drug therapy may have an additive effect with anesthetic agents, whereas drug-induced enzyme induction may alter responses by other agents (including nondepolarizing muscle relaxants, opioids, and barbiturates).

The selection of anesthetic agents for induction, maintenance, and postoperative care should focus on their effects on CNS electrical activity. The more obvious agents (methohexital, ketamine, and enflurane) should be avoided in clients with known seizure disorders. Methohexital may activate epileptic foci and actually has been recommended as a method of delineating these foci in patients undergoing surgical treatment of epilepsy. Ketamine has been known to produce seizure activity in patients at risk. Also, concurrent use of ketamine and theophylline may result in a lower seizure threshold for both drugs. With all of the other sedative/hypnotics available (benzodiazepines, barbiturates, and propofol), the use of ketamine should be avoided.

When selecting muscle relaxants, there is a potential resistance to nondepolarizing agents with clients being treated with carbamazepine and phenytoin. Another concern related to muscle relaxants is the CNS-stimulating effects of laudanosine, a metabolite of atracurium. Avoiding enflurane would seem logical because it has been shown to produce seizure activity in those at risk (Kofke, 1997). Notwithstanding all of the drugs used in anesthesia, it is critical to maintain the preestablished drug therapy throughout the perioperative period.

Intracranial Tumors

Intracranial tumors and masses may be congenital, a benign or malignant neoplasm, an infectious abscess or cyst, or a vascular lesion (hematoma or malformation). Supratentorial tumors arise from portions of the brain superior to tentorium cerebelli. Supratetorial tumors make up the majority of intracranial surgeries. These tumors frequently originate from metastatic lesions in the pulmonary and gastrointestinal systems (Bedford, 1997). Frontal, temporal, and parieto–occipital craniotomies are performed in the supine position. Infratentorial tumors require a posterior fossa exploration. These procedures can be performed in either a modified lateral or prone position; however, the sitting position may be preferred for access to large midline tumors and to enhance CSF and venous drainage (Morgan & Mikhail, 1996). Infratentorial tumors account for about two thirds of intracranial tumors in children (Young, 1997). Prognosis is poor with glioblastoma and infiltrating brain stem glioma. Benign lesions such as meningioma and acoustic neuroma have low morbidity and mortality rates, but may recur if resection is incomplete. The degree of head elevation will influence the incidence and severity of air embolism (sitting > prone > park bench/lateral position).

Perianesthesia Considerations

Preoperative preparation includes assessment of physical status, presence or absence of increased ICP, hydrocephalus, and anxiety level. Avoid narcotic premedication if there is a risk for increased ICP (hypoventilation causes hypercapnia, resulting in increased CBF). Irregular respirations and impaired level of consciousness due to brain stem compression and swelling are common features with infratentorial lesions. Other concerns both with supra- and infratentorial masses include seizure, neurologic deficit, and dementia.

Anesthesia management of supratentorial tumor surgery includes the selection of appropriate anesthetic drugs, intraoperative fluid management, and control of intracranial hypertension (ICH). Determinants of anesthetic drug selection centers on the drugs' effects on CBF, ICP, CMR_{O_2}, CPP, promptness of recovery, potential for brain protection, and compatibility with monitors of neurologic function [somatosensory evoked potentials (SSEPs), EEG, and electromyography (EMG)]. Monitoring considerations include an arterial line for BP control and frequent arterial blood gases; end-tidal CO_2 as a rough guide only, using Pa_{CO_2} to confirm changes; possibe use of ICP measurements; and the use of the nonparetic extremity for neuromuscular monitoring due to increased

cholinergic receptor density. It is critical to avoid both increased BP with intubation/head pins and brain swelling due to venous outflow occlusion (do not permit overflexion or rotation of neck). Because there are no painful structures below the dura, minimal anesthetic requirements with brain manipulation are needed. This can be accomplished with a low-dose inhalation agent and/or a propofol infusion. Although the awake and normocarbic patient allows for early neurologic assessment, the risk of coughing, straining, and possible hematoma formation occurs. The incidence of postoperative hypertension may also develop. With a deep extubation, coughing and hypertension may be avoided; however, early neurologic assessment is difficult.

With infratentorial (posterior fossa) surgery, selection of patient position is an important consideration and choices include prone, lateral, and sitting positions. Use of the sitting position has both advantages and disadvantages. The advantages include better surgical exposure, less tissue retraction and damage, less bleeding, less cranial nerve injury, better access to lesions, and ready access to the airway, chest, and extremities. The disadvantages include venous air embolism, hypotension, and the risk of brain stem ischemia. During the postoperative phase, if hypertension occurs with bradycardia, suspect brain stem compression or hematoma. Avoiding potent narcotic analgesics that may produce hypercarbia and decreased intracranial compliance is recommended.

Occlusive Cerebrovascular Disease

Hampson (1996) describes cerebrovascular disease as abnormalities in both extracranial and intracranial blood vessels that may lead to an inadequate supply of blood, and therefore O_2, to the brain. When the O_2 supply is inadequate to meet the needs of the brain, cerebral ischemia results. The two major groups of symptoms include TIAs and stroke. A TIA develops suddenly, involves neurologic dysfunction for minutes to hours (by definition, never lasting more than 24 hours), clears spontaneously, and is associated with a normal CT scan (Hampson, 1996). Strokes may develop rapidly or in a stepwise fashion over a period of hours, days, or weeks. Strokes usually require a period of months or years to resolve or, more commonly, never resolve completely. Strokes can be classified as minor, with eventual full or nearly full recovery, or major, with severe and permanent disability or death. Strokes are also associated with many other disease states, including but not limited to hypertension, diabetes, coagulopathies, atrial fibrillation, mitral valve disease, substance abuse, and endocarditis.

Perianesthesia Considerations

During the preoperative phase, the focus should be on collecting a neurologic assessment, optimizing control of coexisting hypertension, coronary artery disease, diabetes, chronic obstructive pulmonary disease (COPD), and evaluating normal BP ranges. Although general anesthesia is most often employed for cerebral vascular surgery, repeated neurologic evaluation of conscious clients is cited as the principle reason for choosing regional anesthesia. Monitoring may include arterial line, inferior lead ECG (V_5), and EEG during carotid endarterectomy procedures. Induction and maintenance of anesthesia should include sustaining hemodynamic stability based on BP range and normocapnia reflected by preoperative pH and Pa_{CO_2}. Caution regarding the use of succinylcholine in patients with previous paretic cerebrovascular accident (CVA) should be demonstrated. Patients who are deeply anesthetized and whose systemic vascular resistance (SVR) is supported by an infusion of phenylephrine have more than twice the incidence of myocardial ischemia than those whose BP is maintained by light anesthesia and endogenous vasoconstrictors. Especially during carotid surgery, efforts are made to avoid straining on the endotracheal tube on extubation and emergence. Again, emphasis on awakening the patient immediately following surgery allows early and frequent neurologic evaluation.

Spinal Cord Injury

Patients with spinal cord injuries (SCIs) present a unique challenge for the anesthesia provider. It is essential that these patients be thoroughly evaluated during the perioperative period. Areas that may be highly abnormal include the nervous, cardiovascular, and respiratory systems. The findings of the neurologic assessment are dependent on the level of spinal cord involved in the injury. An injury between T2 and T12 causes paraplegia but leaves the upper extremities and the diaphragm intact. At injury levels between C5 and T1, varying degrees of upper extremity paralysis may be seen. The diaphragm is innervated by cervical roots 3 to 5; thus, involvement at these levels may cause various degrees of diaphragmatic dysfunction and ventilatory inadequacy in addition to quadriplegia. In patients with cervical spine trauma it is critical to avoid neck motion which can produce further cord damage. Flexion is generally more deleterious than extension, but both should be avoided if possible. Sperry (1996) states that in cases of spinal trauma the spinal cord is not usually severed; rather, it is injured by compression from bone, hematoma, edema, and ischemia. Currently, no pharmacologic treatment (steroid, mannitol, naloxone, thyroid-stimulating hormone) or physical measure (local hypothermia) has been clearly shown to be more beneficial than simply maintaining spinal cord perfusion. Spinal cord blood flow is controlled similarly to CBF. Severe hypercapnia should be avoided to prevent increases in intraspinal pressure that may result in ischemia.

Cardiovascular sequlea as a result of SCI include acute spinal shock, which is due to the loss of cardioaccelerator and vasoconstrictor tone at the levels of T1 to L1. The profound systemic hypotension associated with spinal shock may be seen within hours of injury and may persist for weeks, especially with lesions above T6. Loss of sympathetic vascular tone causes blood volume to pool in the periphery. Unopposed parasympathetic tone causes a resultant bradycardia and an inability to increase the chronotropic or inotropic state of the heart. The significance of these cardiovascular derangements is that clients poorly tolerate and compensate for sudden changes in posture, blood loss, or anesthetics with cardiodepressant or vasodilating properties.

Perianesthesia Considerations

Perianesthesia care of SCI patients requires a meticulous focus on appropriate airway management and maintaining hemodynamic stability. The induction of anesthesia in patients with cervical spine injury requires special attention. In some patients, neck immobility must be ensured by placement of a halo device, while others may require assistance to maintain neck alignment during induction and intubation. In general, intubation with careful application of topical anesthetics and sedation is preferred (Devane, 1997). However, a rapid sequence intubation with manual in-line stabilization of the neck is preferred in children and uncooperative adults to avoid further injury. Manual in-line stabilization is used to counter extension or flexion during laryngoscopy and tracheal intubation. Nasal intubation is contraindicated in the presence of a basilar skull fracture and/or in patients with significant coagulopathies. Patients with high cervical lesions have probably been intubated early in the course of treatment, either in the field or in the emergency department. All patients should be presumed to have a cervical spine injury. Elective intubation in the operating room should be performed in an awake patient to allow neurologic evaluation prior to and after intubation. After adequate topical anesthesia to the pharynx, transtracheal and superior laryngeal nerve blocks (contraindicated in patients with a full stomach) may be accomplished in preparation for a fiberoptic oral or nasal tracheal intubation.

Anesthesia must be induced carefully because there may be compromise of the cardiovascular system caused by spinal shock, cardiac trauma, or hypovolemia. The use of an anticholinergic agent may be recommended before intubation to reduce secretions, bronchospasm, and reflex bradycardia. Commonly used induction agents include opioids, etomidate, thiopental, and ketamine. Unlike etomidate and opioids, ketamine acts to increase cerebral blood flow and increase pressure, making its use contraindicated with closed head injuries. Succinylcholine may be used safely within the first 48 hours of an acute SCI. Hypotension on induction should be treated aggressively with fluids, as guided by hemodynamic measures, and with small doses of direct-acting sympathomimetics such as phenylephrine.

One important goal of intraoperative management is maintaining spinal cord perfusion to prevent further damage. Both intravenous and inhalation anesthetics may be used, but inhalation agents have the advantage of providing greater control of intraoperative fluctuations in blood pressure. As mentioned previously, the spinal cord circulation is similar to the cerebral circulation in that severe hypocapnia may lead to vasoconstriction and the potential for ischemia. Attention to positioning is critical in preventing skin breakdown and peripheral nerve injuries. Normothermia is essential and can be maintained via warming blankets, heated humidified gases, increased ambient temperature, and warmed fluids.

Autonomic Hyperreflexia

Autonomic hyperreflexia (AH) is a syndrome of massive reflex sympathetic discharge in response to cutaneous or visceral stimulation below the level of a spinal cord lesion in paraplegic and quadriplegic patients. Autonomic hyperreflexia is seen after the resolution of spinal shock and the return of spinal cord reflexes (about 1 to 3 weeks after injury). According to Liu (1997), those with spinal cord transection at T7 or above have a 65% to 85% risk of developing AH. Normally, sympathetic activity is modulated by inhibitory impulses from supraspinal centers. In AH, the sympathetic nervous system below the level of spinal cord transection is isolated from all inhibitory influences of the brain stem and hypothalamus.

In general, the clinical manifestations of AH are a result of sympathetic nervous system stimulation below the lesion and compensatory parasympathetic nervous system stimulation above the lesion. Severe hypertension and bradycardia with stimulation below the level of cord transection occurs. Below the transection, sympathetically mediated pallor, pilomotor erection, somatic and visceral muscle contraction, and increased spasticity may be seen. Above the lesion, the parasympathetic system evokes vasodilation, resulting in flushing of the face and mucous membranes. In severe cases, arrhythmias, pulmonary edema, cardiovascular collapse, cerebral hemorrhage, seizures, and subsequent death may occur. Bladder distension seems to be a common eliciting factor along with placement of a bladder catheter. Other common triggering causes include gastrointestinal procedures (eg, sigmoidoscopy and enemas), acute appendicitis, temperature extremes, decubitus ulcers, sunburn, and tight-fitting clothing.

Perianesthesia Considerations

During the preoperative phase, assessment should focus on the patient's previous experiences with AH, adequate

cardiovascular and respiratory function, and volume status. The use of an intra-arterial catheter for continuous invasive BP monitoring is essential in these cases. Considerations for central venous pressure and/or pulmonary artery catheters may be necessary when volume changes are expected and when patients present with poor cardiac reserve. Liu (1997) recommends the use of nifedipine 30 minutes prior to procedures most likely to trigger AH.

The use of nondepolarizing muscle relaxants are advocated because succinylcholine can evoke severe hyperkalemia, especially when the SCI occurred less than 6 months before surgery. Considerations for sodium nitroprusside prior to induction may be required. General anesthesia with a volatile agent may be more beneficial than nitrous oxide (N_2O)/narcotic technique in preventing or treating AH. Other treatment options for AH include ganglionic blockers (trimethaphan) and alphaadrenergic blockers (phenoxybenzamine and phentolamine). Subarachnoid blocks are highly effective in preventing AH in procedures involving the lower abdomen, pelvis, and lower extremities. The down side of using spinal anesthetics is the difficulty in assessing height of neuroaxial block because of sensory deficits below transection. Epidural anesthesia may also be effective; however, the most intense stimuli that provoke AH originate from the S2 to S4 segments, an area sometimes missed with epidural bocks.

Autonomic hyperreflexia can occur during the postoperative period. Extubation may be difficult with high transection owing to respiratory impairment. This along with muscle spasticity may require the use of muscle relaxation. Patients with severe hypertension and difficulty in awakening, should be assessed for possible cerebral bleed. Meticulous attention to positioning is necessary to prevent skin breakdown and peripheral nerve injuries. Maintaining normothermia is essential via warming blankets, heated and humidified gases, increased ambient temperature, and warmed intravenous fluids.

Parkinson's Disease (Paralysis Agitans)

Parkinson's disease is described by Sharpe and Zimmermann (1997) as a degenerative disease of the extrapyramidal system characterized by bradykinesia, rigidity, and tremor. It is associated with the loss of dopaminergic fibers and dopamine depletion in the basal ganglia. The results are diminished inhibition of the extrapyramidal motor system and unopposed action of acetylcholine. Fry (1996) explains that patients with Parkinson's disease display increased rigidity of the extremities, facial immobility, shuffling gait, rhythmic resting tremor, dementia, depression, diaphragmatic spasms, and oculogyric crisis. Fry (1996) defines oculogyric crisis as a form of dystonia in which the eyes are deviated in a fixed position for minutes or hours.

The etiology is unknown. There are, according to Sharpe and Zimmermann (1997), some clusters related to the 1927 influenza epidemic. There is no known hereditary component. Secondary causes include post-encephalitis, carbon monoxide poisoning, manganese poisoning, and chronic ingestion of dopamine-inhibiting antipsychotic drugs. These drugs include phenothiazines (eg, chlorpromazine, promthazine, fluphenazine, prochlorperazine); butyrophenones (eg, droperidol), which may antagonize the effects of dopamine in the basal ganglia; and metoclopramide, which inhibits dopamine receptors in the brain (Fry, 1996).

Parkinson's disease is commonly treated with levodopa, which crosses the BBB, and is converted to dopamine. Carbidopa is often combined with levodopa to inhibit the activity of dopa decarboxylase. Patients with mild symptoms may be treated with amantadine or anticholinergic agents such as benztropine and procyclidine. The anticholinergic treatment is limited by the autonomic side effects such as dry mouth and urinary retention. Surgical treatments include the experimental use of fetal tissue transplantation and, in rare cases, stereotaxic procedures.

Perianesthesia Considerations

Levodopa therapy should continue during the perioperative course. Because the half-life of levodopa is short, abrupt withdrawal may lead to skeletal muscle rigidity that interferes with adequate ventilation. Fluctuations in BP and cardiac dysrhythmias may occur. Orthostatic hypotension is a common side effect of levodopa therapy. Increased levels of dopamine may increase myocardial contractility and heart rate. Renal blood flow is likely to increase, causing an increase in glomerular filtration rate and excretion of sodium. Therefore, intravascular fluid volume is decreased and the renin–angiotensin aldosterone system is depressed, leading to orthostatic hypotension (Fry, 1996). Obviously, patients may require aggressive administration of fluids (colloids or crystalloid solutions) especially during induction. Avoidance of phenothiazines and butyrophenones is essential. The use of ketamine in these cases is questionable because of its sympathomimetic effects.

Because autonomic dysfunction is commonly seen in patients with Parkinson's disease, the risk for gastric regurgitation and potential development of aspiration pneumonitis is evident. The autonomic dysfunctions of the gastrointestinal system include excessive salivation, dysphagia, and esophageal dysfunction. During the postoperative phase, patients are more susceptible to confusion and possibly hallucinations.

Myasthenia Gravis

Myasthenia gravis is an autoimmune disease of the neuromuscular junction that is mediated by a reduction in the number of acetylcholine receptors. The disease is mostly a postsynaptic disorder. Characterized by weakness and high fatigability of skeletal muscles, myasthenia gravis primarily affects women of all races and men usually after age 40. Patients are differentiated on the basis of symptoms from a class scale ranging from class 1 to 4. In most cases, the disease has an insidious onset with resulting transient weakness of voluntary muscle groups. This condition is exacerbated by exercise and improves with rest. Some early signs that prompt patients to seek medical attention are diplopia and difficulty swallowing and chewing. Symptoms can be exaggerated by stress, infections, hyperthyroidism, or drugs such as procainamide, quinidine, and aminoglycoside antibiotics. The use of anticholinesterases has been the mainstay for treatment for many years. Pyridostigmine is used effectively because it has fewer side effects than other anticholinesterases and primarily affects the postsynaptic region. In addition, other treatments such as immunosuppressive drugs, intravenous immunoglobulin, plasmapheresis, and surgical thymectomy are also advocated.

Patients with myasthenia gravis may present with symptoms of either undertreatment with anticholinesterase agents (myasthenic crisis) or overtreatment with anticholinesterase agents (cholinergic crisis). An exacerbation of the respiratory-related symptoms occurs in myasthenic crisis and is associated with difficulty in swallowing, increased secretions, muscle weakness, and respiratory infections. Cholinergic crisis is difficult to differentiate from myasthenic crisis in that muscle weakness and increased secretions are also observed. A differential diagnosis is made by a gradual intravenous injection of edrophonium (approximately 10 mg in a 70-kg patient). If improvement is seen, myasthenic crisis is the cause; if the symptoms worsen, cholinergic crisis would be the identifying problem.

Perianesthesia Considerations

The anesthetic problems associated with myasthenia gravis are mainly those related to muscle weakness; thus, whenever possible, the use of muscle relaxants should be avoided. According to Swafford Dahm (1992), these patients may not need muscle relaxants for thymectomies. Class 2 to 4 myasthenic clients need thymectomies (class 1 patients are milder cases, and class 4 are the most severe). The need for postoperative ventilatory assistance is common. The biggest controversy in the anesthetic management of the myasthenic is the use of anticholinesterase agents perioperatively (Swafford Dahm, 1992). The general belief is that anticholinesterase agents should be given throughout the perioperative period to those patients already dependent on them. Complications associated with anticholinesterase agents include vagal response, decrease in the metabolism of local ester anesthetics, and more obviously, difficulty in providing muscle relaxation. Regardless of the cause, patients with muscle weakness tolerate sedation and analgesia very poorly. Perioperative monitoring of the respiratory depressant effects is critical, especially when providing conscious sedation in the spontaneously breathing patient.

Myasthenic syndrome (Eaton–Lambert Syndrome) is associated with carcinoma, and symptoms mimic myasthenia gravis except that they improve with increased physical activity. The bronchus is the most common site of the carcinoma (especially oat cell tumors). Other sites include the prostate, breast, stomach, and rectum. Electromyography reveals a reverse picture to that of myasthenia gravis (Swafford Dahm, 1992). Although there is a reduction in muscle response to single-nerve stimulation, tetanic stimulation shows progressive increase in muscle strength as the frequency in duration of the stimulation is increased. These patients are sensitive to nondepolarizing and depolarizing muscle relaxants, and weakness may last many days after their use. Therefore, most muscle relaxants are to be avoided.

Amyotrophic Lateral Sclerosis

Amyotrophic lateral sclerosis (ALS), also known as Lou Gehrig's disease, is a degenerative process causing upper and lower motor neuron death with denervation and atrophy of corresponding muscle fibers. If the condition is limited to the motor cortex, the disease is termed primary lateral sclerosis with limitations reflecting the brain stem nuclei and spinal cord. Typically, extraocular muscles, bowel/bladder sphincters, sensory system, movement coordination, and intellect remain intact (Cole, 1997). Diagnosis is aided by elevated serum creatinine kinase levels, decreased compound muscle action potential, electromyographic evidence of denervation with reinnervation, and abnormal EP responses. There may be a genetic predisposition in fewer than 5% of cases (autosomal dominant gene) (Swash & Schwartz, 1992). Other etiologic hypotheses include autoimmune factors, exitotoxins, viral factors, exogenous toxins, and other neurotransmitters/neuropeptides. Various patterns of involvement can develop, but the classic pattern begins with a combination of weakness with increased tone, atrophy, and fasiculations of the limbs. Involvement of the upper motor neurons results in spasticity and reduced muscle strength, whereas lower motor neuron involvement results in flaccidity, paralysis, and muscle atrophy.

Perianesthesia Considerations

The major goal of anesthesia care focuses on maximizing respiratory status and ability to communicate effectively with client. Dysfunctions of the pharyngeal muscles and dysphagia contribute to difficulty with speech and diminished gag reflex. This, along with vagal dysfunction, respiratory impairment from muscle weakness, and di-

aphragmatic paralysis, makes these clients susceptible to increased secretions, aspiration, respiratory failure, and infection. Although no technique is shown to be superior, the use of local or regional anesthetics should be considered if possible. If general anesthesia is necessary, avoid succinylcholine (hyperkalemic response) and expect an exaggerated response and increased duration to nondepolarizing muscle relaxants. There is a low risk for postoperative mechanical ventilation requirements if the peak inspiratory pressure is greater than 30 cm H_2O, if the vital capacity is greater than 1.5 L, and if there are no concurrent problems (Cole, 1997). There is a high risk for postoperative mechanical ventilation need when peak inspiratory pressure is less than 20 cm H_2O, if the vital capacity is less than 1.0 L, and if there is hypercarbia and hypoxia, or a concurrent problem.

▶ GENERAL PERIANESTHESIA CONSIDERATIONS

Preoperative Considerations

The patient's overall medical condition must be considered and integrated into the formulation of an anesthetic management plan during the initial preanesthesia evaluation. If the patient is being prepared for a neurosurgical procedure, communication among all of the health care providers is paramount. Neurosurgical procedures tend to require unusual positioning and special techniques such as hyperventilation, cerebral dehydration, and deliberate hypotension. Neurosurgical procedures are usually lengthy, and not all patients can tolerate the position desired by the surgeon. This issue must be addressed and evaluated during the preoperative period. With the routine institution of hyperventilation and osmotic diuretic therapy, organ function may be compromised. Those patients with cardiac dysfunction must be optimized prior to surgery. Except for neurosurgical emergencies (eg, head trauma or impending herniation), most neurosurgical procedures can be delayed to treat medically unstable conditions (Bendo, Kass, Hartung, & Cottrell, 1997).

The preoperative evaluation must include a complete neurologic assessment with focused attention on the patient's level of consciousness, presence or absence of increased ICP, and sensory and motor function. All medications that the patient normally takes should be evaluated, and any history of corticosteroid, diuretic, or anticonvulsant therapies should be clearly identified. In addition to routine laboratory data, evaluation to rule out corticosteroid-induced hyperglycemia, electrolyte disturbances due to diuretics, and abnormalities associated with antidiuretic hormone secretion should be investigated (DeVane, 1997). Also, anticonvulsant drug levels should be evaluated, especially when seizure activities are not clearly defined and/or controlled.

Special attention should be directed to the signs and symptoms frequently associated with intracranial hypertension. These signs and symptoms include headache, nausea, papilledema, unilateral pupillary dilation, and oculomotor or abducens palsy. As the stages of ICH progress, the patient displays a depressed level of consciousness and irregular respiration. The clinical signs do not reliably indicate the level of ICP (Bendo, Kass, Hartung, & Cottrell, 1997). Only a direct CSF pressure measurement can be used to quantify the pressure. However, the level of ICP can be determined by evaluating the MRI or CT scan for a mass lesion accompanied by a midline shift of 0.5 cm or greater and/or encroachment of expanding brain on CSF cisterns.

Premedication should be avoided when level of consciousness is in question, or when ICH is suspected. By all means, those patients who are alert and anxious may receive an anxiolytic prior to arriving in the operating room suite. If there is any doubt about the level of consciousness and the patient is anxious, sedation may be administered as long as an intravenous route is established and proper monitoring and airway equipment are readily available. During the preinduction insertion of invasive monitoring devices in the awake, conversant patient, premedication with small doses of opiates should be considered to alleviate the discomfort from needle punctures (Bendo, Kass, Hartung, & Cottrell, 1997).

Intraoperative Considerations

Monitoring

Routine perianesthesia monitoring applies to neurosurgical patients but should also include indwelling urinary catheterization and intra-arterial BP measurements. Blood pressure fluctuations occur during induction, intubation, hyperventilation, positioning, surgical manipulation, and emergence which requires continuous BP monitoring to ensure adequate cerebral perfusion. The arterial line transducer is zeroed at the level of the external auditory meatus instead of at the level of the right atrium to facilitate the quantitative value for cerebral perfusion pressure (CPP = MAP − ICP or CVP). Also, the use of an arterial line to obtain blood gases is essential to calculate the end-tidal and arterial CO_2 to determine the gradient.

Morgan and Mikhail (1996) emphasize the importance of central venous access and pressure monitoring especially when considering vasoactive agents. The use of the internal jugular vein for access is somewhat controversial because of the risk of carotid puncture and concern that the catheter may interfere with venous drainage from the brain. To avoid this issue, many anesthetists will opt to insert a long-line intravenous catheter centrally through the median basilic vein. Use of the external jugular or subclavian vein may also be a suitable alternative. Monitoring urinary output is necessary because of the frequent use of diuretics and the length of most neurosurgical procedures, and also because it serves as a guide for fluid therapy.

Neuromuscular function must be monitored on the unaffected side of patients with hemiparesis to avoid overdosage. Resistance to nondepolarizing blockade may be falsely assessed by train-of-four when using the paretic extremity. Other monitoring devices such as EEG, EPs, and ICP may be used to monitor CNS function. The EEG is a monitor of cerebral function that provides early evidence of cerebral ischemia during carotid endarterectomy and cardiopulmonary bypass. The EEG has also been advocated to monitor depth of anesthesia. Evoked potentials are the electrophysiologic responses of the CNS to sensory stimulation (somatic, auditory, and visual) that allow assessment of the functional integrity of neural pathways during anesthesia. Intracranial pressure monitoring is advocated in patients with intracranial tumors, to recognize sudden and often unexpected increases in ICP and thus facilitate prompt and aggressive interventions to lower ICP. Although EEG, EPs, and ICP monitoring play an important role in neuroanesthesia, the complexity of interpretation, the variability of unpredictable events (eg, alterations in $Paco_2$ and changes in body temperature), and the effects of anesthetic agents on wave forms and tracings limit its frequent use in practice. Refer to Chapter 23 for a more detailed discussion of monitoring in anesthesia practice.

Positioning

Proper positioning and the physiologic consequences must be clearly understood when providing anesthesia to neurosurgical patients and those with neurologic diseases. Neurosurgical procedures require a variety of positions to enhance CSF and venous drainage facilitating adequate surgical exposure. With the exception of posterior fossa or infratentorial compartment craniotomies, most frontal, temporal, and parieto-occipital procedures are conducted in the supine position. In the supine position, the head is typically elevated from 15° to 30° and possibly turned to one side to accommodate surgical exposure. It is important to keep in mind that excessive twisting of the neck may impede jugular venous drainage and increase ICP. The risk of unrecognized breathing circuit disconnection is increased because many times the operating room table is turned 90° to 180° away from the anesthesia work space, and both the client and breathing circuit are covered with surgical drapes (Morgan & Mikhail, 1996; DeVane, 1997).

Operations in the posterior fossa require unusual positioning (eg, prone, lateral, or sitting), each of which presents with particular problems. The sitting position receives the most attention and poses the greatest anesthesia management issues. Despite the concerns about venous air embolism (VAE), the sitting position is in widespread use and offers many advantages over alternative positions (Todd, Warner, & Maktabi, 1998). These include excellent surgical exposure, particularly of midline structures and those located in or on the high dorsal brain stem or midbrain. Todd, Warner, and Maktabi (1998) also report that there is less pooling of blood and CSF in the surgical field, and blood loss may be less than with nonsitting positions because of lower venous pressures. In the sitting position, the face and airway are accessible, making it easier to monitor facial nerve function. In addition, peak airway pressures may be lowered and ventilation/perfusion matching better than those in the prone position. All of these advantages must be balanced with a few disadvantages, notably VAE and quadriplegia. A VAE can occur whenever the pressure within an open blood vessel is subatmospheric. Because normal right atrial pressure ranges from 2 mmHg to 10 mmHg, this can theoretically occur any time the surgical site is located more than 5 cm above the heart. Quadriplegia can occur due to compression of the cervical spine from excessive neck flexion. Injuries and complications can be prevented with careful positioning. Pressure points such as the forehead, elbows, and ischial spine must be padded well with foam- or jelly-filled pads. Refer to Chapter 24 for further information on positioning in anesthesia practice.

Fluid Management

Fluid and electrolyte *management* during neurosurgery *requires* knowledge of the patient's underlying pathophysiologic disease status. The general principles of fluid management often do not take into account the effects of fluids on cerebral edema, cerebral perfusion, ischemic insults, and water and electrolyte homeostasis. In most neurosurgical clients, fluid that contains sodium in a concentration similar to that of serum (eg, lactated Ringer's solution or 0.9% saline) is administered is a volume that in sufficient for the maintenance of the peripheral perfusion but avoids hypervolemia. Usually, less fluid is given than would be administered for nonneurologic surgery (Prough & Cohen, 1991; DeVane, 1997). Unless hypoglycemia is suspected, solutions containing glucose should be avoided during neurosurgical procedures. Using dextrose in combination with free water (D_5W) is contraindicated because D_5W rapidly equilibrates throughout all intracranial compartments (Spiekermann & Thompson, 1996). The resultant brain edema may interfere with surgical exposure or, if the skull is closed, compromise cerebral perfusion (DeVane, 1997). Prough and Cohen (1991) suggest that the sequestered extracellular fluid can be cautiously replaced with lactated

Ringer's solution or with 0.9% saline. Also, in the absence of diuretic therapy, a urinary output of 0.5 to 1.0 mL/kg/h suggests adequate replacement, as do hemodynamic stability and cardiac filling pressures within the normal range. Refer to Chapter 26 regarding further information on fluid therapy.

Neurophysiologic Effects of Anesthetic Agents

Inhalation Agents. The CNS effects of inhalation anesthetic agents play an integral role in the management of neurosurgical clients. In general, the inhalation agents produce a dose-dependent depression of the CNS with progressive slowing of the EEG. Inhalation agents reduce $CMRo_2$ from 40% to 50% if given in high enough concentrations to produce an isoelectric EEG (Farnsworth & Johnson, 1996).

Inhalation agents uncouple the relationship of CBF and $CMRo_2$. The ratio of CBF and $CMRo_2$ is usually 14 to 18 : 1 in the awake brain. There is an inverse relationship produced by inhalation agents where CBF increases while $CMRo_2$ decreases. The inhalation agents, for the most part produce cerebral vasodilation which increases CBF. With the reduction of $CMRo_2$, blunting of increased CBF can occur. All volatile anesthetics produce an initial increase in CBV of about 10%, which falls to preanesthetic levels after about 3 hours (Farnsworth & Johnson, 1996). This change in CBV occurs early and influences increased ICP. A critical determinant of ICP that is significantly altered by inhalation agents is CSF. The CSF volume depends on its rates of formation and absorption (which is affected by resistance to absorption). All of the anesthetic agents available have an effect on CSF volume. All increase the resistance of CSF absorption except isoflurane. Table 12–9 lists and describes the effects of inhalation agents on cerebral physiology.

NITROUS OXIDE. Although nitrous oxide (N_2O) is mistakenly perceived as being inert physiologically and pharmacologically, it is a cerebral vasodilator that can produce increased ICP. This effect can be clinically significant in neurosurgical patients with decreased intracranial elastance. The effect of N_2O on ICP has been shown to be blocked or blunted by prior administration of narcotics, barbiturates, and hypocapnia. Its effect on $CMRo_2$ in humans is less clear, although most data suggest that it causes an increase. The effects of N_2O on EEG in concentrations of greater than 50% causes most subjects to lose consciousness, and alpha activity is replaced by fast wave activity. It is highly unlikely that N_2O causes seizure activity. Its effects on EPs is minimal, with a slight decrease in amplitude and little effect or no change in the latencies (Bendo, Kass, Hartung, & Cottrell, 1997).

TABLE 12–9. Comparative Effects of Anesthetic Agents on Cerebral Physiology

Halothane	↓↓	↑↑↑	↓	↓	↑↑	↑↑
Enflurane	↓↓	↑↑	↑	↓	↑↑	↑↑
Isoflurane	↓↓↓	↑	±	↑	↑↑	↑
Desflurane	↓↓↓	↑	↑	↓	?	↑↑
Sevoflurane	↓↓	↑	?	?	?	↑↑
Nitrous oxide	↓	↑	±	±	±	↑
Barbiturates	↓↓↓↓	↓↓↓	±	↑	↓↓	↓↓↓
Etomidate	↓↓↓	↓↓	±	↑	↓↓	↓↓
Propofol	↓↓↓	↓↓↓↓	?	?	↓↓	↓↓
Benzodiazepines	↓↓	?	±	↑	↓	↓
Ketamine	±	↑↑	±	↓	↑↑	↑↑
Narcotics	±	±	±	↑	±	±
Lidocaine	↓↓	↓↓	?	?	↓↓	↓↓

Key: ↑, increase; ↓, decrease; ±, little or no change; ?, unknown.
Legend: CMR, cerebral metabolic rate; CBV, cerebral blood volume; CBF, cerebral blood flow; ICP, intracranial pressure; CSF, cerebrospinal fluid.
From Morgan, G. E. & Mikhail, M. S. (1996). Clinical anesthesiology (2nd ed., p. 482). Stamford, CT: Appleton & Lange.

Pneumocephalus can occur during posterior fossa craniotomy or cervical spine procedures while the patient's head is elevated and the CSF spaces are open. In this situation, CSF will continuously drain due to gravity and will be replaced by air. Because N_2O equilibrates with any air-filled space and has a blood solubility 30 times greater than that of nitrogen (N_2), it leads to a transient but significant net increase of gas molecules in the space, and hence an increase in pneumocephalus. This may lead to seizure activity, changes in level of consciousness, and neurologic sequelae. Obviously, N_2O should be discontinued when these conditions exist.

HALOTHANE. Among the five volatile anesthetics in use today, halothane remains the most potent cerebral vasodilator. It produces a dose-related decrease in $CMRO_2$. Critical CBF is defined by Michenfelder (1988) as that flow below which the majority of subjects develop ipsilateral EEG changes indicative of ischemia within 3 minutes following carotid occlusion. Among the critical regional CBFs reported for volatile agents, it is greater for halothane at 18 to 20 mL/100 g/min. As a result of halothane causing an increase in CBF, and hence CBV, it can increase the ICP in patients at risk. However, the establishment of hypocapnia ($PaCO_2 < 30$ mmHg at normothermia) before introducing halothane consistently blocks the effects on ICP. The simultaneous initiation of hyperventilation and halothane administration does not reliably prevent increases in ICP. Halothane also decreases production of CSF but increases the resistance to CSF reabsorption. With regard to EEG, even at clinically relevant concentrations, halothane cannot produce an isoelectric pattern. Halothane effects EP monitoring more or less the same as that of other volatile agents (Farnsworth & Johnson, 1996).

ENFLURANE. Enflurane is a cerebral vasodilator but less so than halothane. Enflurane causes a decrease in $CMRO_2$. However, the production of seizure activity can occur on EEG at high concentrations of enflurane (1.5 to 2 MAC), especially when combined with hypocapnia. Remember that alkalosis with hypocapnia lowers the seizure threshold. With the onset of seizure activity, $CMRO_2$ increases by as much as 50%. Because enflurane is used clinically at much lower concentrations without extreme hypocapnia, its use is not contraindicated in patients with a history of seizure. The critical CBF according to Michenfelder (1988) is 15 mL/100 g/min. Enflurane's potential to increase ICP can be attenuated by prior induction of hypocapnia before its administration, keeping in mind the possibility of seizure activity with combinations of extreme hypocapnia and high concentrations of enflurane. Enflurane increases both CSF production and resistance to reabsorption.

ISOFLURANE. Isoflurane is the least potent cerebral vasodilator of the volatile agents. It depresses $CMRO_2$ more than halothane or enflurane. At 2 MAC, isoflurane causes an isoelectric EEG pattern and up to a 50% decrease in $CMRO_2$. Doubling the isoflurane concentration to 4 MAC has been shown to cause no further decrease in $CMRO_2$ (in contrast to halothane). There is no evidence of neurotoxicity from deep levels of isoflurane. Michenfelder (1988) purports a critical CBF with isoflurane to be the lowest at 10 mL/100 g/min. There is evidence in humans that isoflurane provides a degree of brain protection with incomplete cerebral ischemia but only compared with halothane and enflurane. No comparison was made with the traditional use of barbiturates as the common pharmacologic method of inducing cerebral protection. Increased ICP can be blocked with prior hypocapnia. Isoflurane has no effect on CSF production and actually decreases the resistance to CSF reabsorption. Effects on EP monitoring are the same as with other volatile agents.

DESFLURANE. Desflurane produces cerebrovasodilation and decreases $CMRo_2$. If profound hypotension is induced, CBF decreases but the reduction in $CMRo_2$ maintains the O_2 supply and demand balance. Increasing the concentration of desflurane from 0.5 to 1.5 MAC results in a 28% increase in CBF. Conversely, up to 2.4 MAC of desflurane decreases $CMRo_2$, CPP, and CBF without changing CVR and without evidence of ischemia. In patients with space-occupying lesions who are undergoing craniotomy procedures, desflurane produced a 63% increase in CSF pressure despite previous establishment of hypocapnia, whereas isoflurane had a 20% decrease in CSF pressure (Farnsworth & Johnson, 1996). Therefore, caution is advised when administering desflurane in clients with increased ICP. The EEG effects are similar to those of isoflurane. An isoelectric pattern occurs at about 1.5 MAC. Mental function returns quickly following anesthesia with desflurane as compared to isoflurane.

SEVOFLURANE. The effects of sevoflurane are similar to those of isoflurane (Farnsworth & Johnson, 1996). Sevoflurane has the associated advantages of having a lower solubility than isoflurane, and it is not pungent. Approximately 2% of sevoflurane is metabolized, with the production of two toxic metabolites (inorganic fluoride and hexafluoroisopropanol). Toxic metabolites have not been shown to be of any significant negative clinical effect, although the length of many neurosurgical procedures makes these metabolites of more concern than would be for other types of surgery.

Intravenous Anesthetic and Sedative Agents.
All intravenous anesthetic agents either have little effect or reduce $CMRo_2$ and CBF with the exception of ketamine. For the most part, changes in CBF generally parallel changes in $CMRo_2$. Cerebral autoregulation and CO_2 response are preserved with most agents (Table 12–9).

BARBITURATES. Barbiturates are intravenous agents that are commonly used in neuroanesthesia because of their favorable neurophysiologic features. These clinical features include hypnosis, reduction of CBF due to increased cerebral vascular resistance, depression of $CMRo_2$, and anticonvulsant influence.

Barbiturates produce their pharmacologic effects by enhancing the inhibitory synaptic transmission and blocking the excitatory ones via interaction with the gamma-aminobutyric acid (GABA) receptor complex (Farnsworth & Johnson, 1996). The duration of GABA occupancy is prolonged with barbiturates when compared to benzodiazepines, thus extending the duration of its inhibitory activity. Barbiturates are also potent anticonvulsants. Small doses of these agents increase EEG-recorded beta activity, whereas larger doses lead to burst-suppression and isoelectricity. Larger doses will increase latency and decrease, but not abolish, the amplitude of SSEPs, even when the EEG is *flat.*

Thiopental and thiamylal are the most frequently used barbiturates in neuroanesthesia. They are capable of inducing anesthesia smoothly within one circulation time (about 45 to 60 seconds). Recovery from an induction dose results from redistribution. Thiopental and thiamylal are metabolized hepatically. Dose-dependent cardiac depression can occur.

Methohexital is commonly used during electroconvulsant therapy and other brief procedures for sedation and induction of anesthesia. The metabolism of methohexital is hepatic, but it occurs more rapidly than that of thiopental. The fact that methohexital enhances the epileptogenic activities in patients at risk limits its use in the neurosurgical population. Also, induction with methohexital is not as smooth as with thiopental because of its excitatory phenomena. The one major advantage of methohexital is its effectiveness as a rectally administered induction/sedation agent in the pediatric population.

PROPOFOL. Propofol is an intravenous agent used during the induction and maintenance of anesthesia. Like barbiturates, it offers many favorable properties for the treatment of neurosurgical patients. Propofol lowers CBF, $CMRo_2$, and ICP. Also, propofol causes a dose-dependent cardiovascular and respiratory depression and can decrease CPP. The cardiac depression with propofol is greater than that with thiopental. With a stable BP, propofol is a highly effective agent for maintenance of anesthesia. Recent reports (Farnsworth & Johnson, 1996) indicate that a propofol-based anesthetic for neurosurgical procedures compares favorably to inhalation and N_2O/narcotic techniques in terms of cost, length of intensive care unit stay, and side effects. Propofol blunts the sympathetic response to laryngoscopy and intubation more effectively than thiopental or etomidate. Recovery is rapid and emergence is smooth, with little nausea and vomiting. Obviously, a rapid, smooth recovery is preferred by neurosurgeons in order to assess the patient's neurologic status in the immediate postoperative period.

ETOMIDATE. Etomidate is useful in neurosurgery or with patients who have neurologic disease because of its remarkable hemodynamic stability, especially in cardiac patients at risk. It is a cerebral vasoconstrictor that reduces CBF and ICP without decreasing CPP. The CMR_{O_2} is reduced by 50%, although less globally as with thiopental. Cardiac index, BP, afterload, and preload are minimally changed with etomidate. There is no histamine release with etomidate, and it is metabolized by the liver and renally excreted. It produces an EEG pattern of delta waves that are associated with myoclonic movement. Negative effects of etomidate include the possible precipitation of seizure activity in patients at risk. It also suppresses the adrenocortical axis when administered as a continuous infusion. Nausea, vomiting, and pain on injection are side effects commonly seen with etomidate. The risk/benefit ratio for its use in neurosurgery must be clearly determined.

BENZODIAZEPINES. Benzodiazepines lower CBF and CMR_{O_2}, but to a lesser extent than barbiturates, propofol, and etomidate. They are useful as anticonvulsant agents, especially diazepam (with its longer elimination half-life). Midazolam is the benzodiazepine of choice for anesthesia practice because of its short pharmacokinetic properties. Midazolam induction frequently causes significant decreases in CPP in elderly and unstable clients and may prolong emergence in some instances (Morgan & Mikhail, 1996).

Flumazenil is a specific antagonist for benzodiazepines. Flumazenil is short-acting with an elimination half-life of about 1 hour. Recurrence of the central effects of benzodiazepines (resedation) may occur after a single dose of flumazenil due to residual effects of the more slowly eliminated agonist drug. Obviously, it may be necessary to administer repeated doses or a continuous infusion to sustain antagonism. Reversal of benzodiazepines does not appear to change CBF and CMR_{O_2}. Following midazolam anesthesia for craniotomy, acute increases in ICP have been reported in head-injured patients receiving flumazenil. In addition, seizures may be precipitated by abrupt reversal of benzodiazepines (Chang & Bleck, 1996).

KETAMINE. Ketamine is a dissociative anesthetic agent with limited application in the patient with neurologic disease. It increases CBF (by as much as 50% to 60%), and impedes CSF absorption, therefore increasing ICP. The CMR_{O_2} does not change significantly with ketamine, although it may increase slightly. Seizure activity in the thalamic and limbic areas is also described. In epileptic clients, cortical and subcortical seizures have been reported (Farnsworth & Johnson, 1996). Delirium with hallucinations and agitation may be seen on emergence, although lessened with preadministration of benzodiazepines. A state of dissociation occurs with ketamine because the brain becomes unable to properly analyze sensory information.

OPIOIDS AND NONSTEROIDAL ANTI-INFLAMMATORY AGENTS. Opioids are profound analgesics and produce sedation but do not provide reliable amnesia. They cause dose-dependent slowing of the EEG, with a shift from alpha to delta activity. Opioids do not produce burst-suppression or a flat EEG. The CMR_{O_2} is submaximally reduced, with preservation of decreased CBF. Overall, opioids decrease ICP, although alfentanil, fentanyl, and sufentanil may increase ICP with head injury if hypotension occurs concomitantly (Farnsworth & Johnson, 1996).

Respiratory depression and muscle rigidity are two potential side effects that are of special significance in neurosurgical clients. Opioids cause a dose-dependent depression of CNS respiratory centers, producing a decrease respiratory rate, CO_2 response, and minute volume. If untreated, hypercapnia will result leading to increased CBF and ICP. The incidence of muscle rigidity is related to the dose and speed of intravenous injection of opioids. Truncal rigidity can make ventilation extremely difficult, again leading to hypercapnia and its consequences. In addition, the muscular rigidity can increase CVP and reduce venous drainage from the brain, thereby increasing cerebral blood volume and ICP. Neuromuscular blocking agents should be readily available when large doses of opioids are utilized during induction.

Other common side effects seen with opioids are nausea and vomiting, decreased gastrointestinal motility, increased gastric volume, and urinary retention and urgency. Many of these effects can predispose the patient to aspiration. Therefore, although opioids are excellent anesthetic agents, a thorough knowledge base of their systemic pharmacologic effects is required for safe administration.

The CNS effects of naloxone have been the subject of numerous studies (Todd, Warner, & Maktabi, 1998). When carefully titrated, it normalizes CBF and CMR_{O_2} in narcotized subjects. However, abrupt reversal with excessive doses of naloxone has resulted in hypertension, pulmonary edema, dysrhythmias, and intracranial hemorrhage. Some have suggested that nalbuphine can be used to reverse respiratory depression without reversal of analgesia, and hence without the hemodynamic difficulties (Todd, Warner, & Maktabi, 1998). Clinical trials have shown that when naloxone and nalbuphine are given to equivalent respiratory endpoints, the changes in BP and heart rate are identical.

Nonsteroidal anti-inflammatory agents are an essential component of pain management in many cases. Although ketorolac is used especially for postoperative pain control in nonneurosurgical cases, Farnsworth and Johnson (1996) report that it is avoided after craniotomy because of concern about its inhibitory effect on platelet aggregation.

Neuromuscular Blocking Agents. With the exception of large doses of D-tubocurarine, where histamine release can increase CBV and ICP, many sources (Todd & Warner, 1993; Tarkkanen, Laitenen, & Johanson, 1974), agree that nondepolarizing muscle relaxants have little effect on cerebral physiology. Some argue against atracurium because of the convulsant effects of the metabolite laudanosine. However, no evidence is available to support this, and calculations make it highly unlikely that substantial levels of laudanosine can be achieved except perhaps in anephric individuals (Todd & Warner, 1993).

One practical concern centers on the increased dose requirements for nondepolarizing agents in patients treated with phenytoin (and possibly carbamazepine) for seizure disorders. The mechanism is unknown and the dose–response curves of most relaxants are shifted to the right with the duration of effect markedly reduced (Ornstein, Matteo, & Schwartz, 1987). Another factor that occasionally impacts the use of nondepolarizing relaxants in neurosurgery is the presence of neurologic deficits, particularly hemiplegia. It has long been known that paretic/plegic extremities are relatively resistant to the action of nondepolarizing agents (Moorthy & Hilgenberg, 1980). This poses unique problems, especially in neuroanesthesia when the paretic extremity may be the only one readily available for neuromuscular monitoring. There is potential for overdosage of relaxants. Careful monitoring and titration of nondepolarizing relaxants is clearly evident in these cases.

There is little question that succinylcholine can increase ICP in humans (Todd, Warner, & Maktabi, 1998). Studies report that succinylcholine effects can be clearly differentiated from other events such as laryngoscopy or changes in ventilation. Animal studies indicate that these changes are associated with increased CBF and may be related to muscle spindle afferent activity. In anesthetized patients with brain tumors, succinylcholine increases ICP an average of 4.9 mmHg.

Succinylcholine may also cause hyperkalemia. In normal clients, intubation doses of succinylcholine will increase the serum potassium levels by about 0.5 mEq/L (Farnsworth & Johnson, 1996). In patients with neuromuscular disease, the proliferation of extra junctional acetylcholine receptors will allow a large potassium flux. Pretreatment with a defasiculating dose of a nondepolarizing muscle relaxant will not reliably prevent this hyperkalemic response. Neurosurgical patients with upper motor neuron injury or intracerebral compromise are at risk for the development of hyperkalemia after succinylcholine administration. When considering succinylcholine in rapidly securing the airway, the patient's risks and benefits need to be evaluated carefully, and the appropriate measures and premedication must be used.

Intracranial Hypertension

The etiology of ICH is usually related to a secondary process accompanying other pathology that increases brain, CSF, or cerebral blood volumes (eg, head injuries, hemorrhage, hydrocephalus, abscess, primary and metastatic brain tumors, cerebral infarcts, venous thrombosis, infection, burns, near drowning, and status epilepticus). As mentioned in the neurophysiology section, the intracranial compartment has fixed volumes with three components (brain, CSF, and cerebral blood volume). An increased volume in any one of these components (eg, tumor, hydrocephalus, or hemorrhage) will potentially elevate ICP, causing ICH with an ICP greater than 20 mmHg (Dooley & Gingrich, 1997). Intracranial hypertension reduces cerebral perfusion which increases perioperative risks associated with brain ischemia and herniation leading to brain infarction, disability, coma, and death.

Obviously, the focus is on treatment of the primary disease (eg, surgical removal of tumor, hematoma, or abscess). The anesthetist's major charge is to avoid hypercapnia and hypoxemia and to deliver moderate hyperventilation (maintain $Paco_2$ around 25 mmHg). Other goals for the nurse anesthetist are establishing stable hemodynamics, head elevation (head above the heart) and neutral neck position to promote cerebral venous return; possibly administering osmotic therapy to *shrink* brain tissue; CSF drainage; and maintaining sedation and nondepolarizing muscle relaxants in the responsive, mechanically ventilated client.

Cerebral Protection

Procedures or drugs chosen to protect the brain during an ischemic event should augment, or at least not interfere with, the following mechanisms: maintaining adenosine triphosphate (ATP) levels by reducing the metabolic rate, blocking sodium or calcium influx, scavenging free radicals, blocking receptors for excitatory amino acids, and maintaining blood flow (Bendo, Kass, Hartung, & Cottrell, 1997). When exploring the most effective method for reducing demand when ischemia reduces supply, hypothermia remains the most useful. Estimates in the reduction of $CMRo_2$ range from 50% to 80% as temperature decreases from 37°C to 27°C (Hartung & Cottrell, 1994). Hypothermia lowers $CMRo_2$ by 7% to 13% for each degree centigrade that temperature is reduced. Hartung and Cottrell (1994) stated that "consequently, the brain can withstand complete ischemia for 4 minutes at 38 degrees centigrade, for 8 minutes at 30 degrees centigrade, for 16 minutes at 22 degrees centigrade, and more than 30 minutes at 16 degrees centigrade" (p. 7).

Emergence and Postoperative Considerations

A smooth emergence from anesthesia is the goal, avoiding straining and bucking on the endotracheal tube. Straining and bucking can cause increased ICP and arterial hypertension during the termination of general anesthesia, which can lead to postoperative hemorrhage and cerebral edema. In order to avoid these sequelae, muscle relaxants should not be reversed until the head dressing is applied during intracranial procedures. Intravenous lidocaine (1.5 mg/kg) can be administered 90 seconds before suctioning and extubation to minimize coughing, straining, and hypertension (Bendo, Kass, Hartung, & Cottrell, 1997). Antihypertensive agents such as labatelol, esmolol, and sodium nitroprusside are administered during emergence and postoperatively to control systemic hypertension. Ideally, the patient is extubated when awake and fully reversed from neuromuscular paralysis. If the patient is unresponsive, the endotracheal tube remains in place until the patient is awake and following commands. A brief neurologic examination is performed and compared to the preoperative assessment, and changes are clearly documented and reported. The patient is positioned with a 30° elevation of the head (unless contraindicated by the surgeon) and transferred to the postanesthesia care unit (PACU) with O_2 by mask and O_2-saturation monitoring. Continuous evaluation of the neurologic status is maintained in the PACU.

► CASE STUDY

Perioperative Care of the Patient with Multiple Sclerosis

A 41-year-old female presents to the operating room for vaginal hysterectomy with a recent diagnosis of multiple sclerosis. The patient has been experiencing vague neurologic symptoms that include muscle wasting, emotional lability, pain, and spasticity. These symptoms were exacerbated during the postpartum period of a childbirth experience 2 years ago. The client is currently taking prednisone for steroid supplementation.

1. Describe the pathophysiology, incidence, and assessment of the patient with multiple sclerosis.

Multiple sclerosis (MS) or disseminated sclerosis is a chronic, progressive, degenerative disease that affects the myelin sheath and conduction pathways of the CNS. The classification of MS is based on the clinical course (Hickey, 1997). In relapsing/remitting disease (65% of cases), the relapses develop over 1 to 2 weeks, resolve over 4 to 8 weeks, and then return to their baseline. Relapsing/progressive disease (15% of cases) is similar to the relapsing/remitting form, but with less recovery, so that the client does not return to baseline and is left with significant residual disability. Chronic progressive disease (20% of cases) is characterized by spinal cord and cerebellar dysfunction; symptoms of the spinal cord and the cerebellum are the initial manifestations. The category of stable MS is sometimes used for patients who have had no active disease or any subjective deterioration in their condition in the last year.

The etiology is unknown, although a viral infection has been suggested as the cause. Multiple sclerosis is referred to as the disease of young adults because the highest rate of incidence is between the ages of 20 and 40 years. About 20% experience their first symptoms in their 40s and 50s. Women are slightly more affected than men; the incidence is 15 times greater in first-degree relatives (Hickey, 1997).

Multiple sclerosis affects the white matter of the brain and spinal cord by causing scattered, demyelinated lesions, preventing conduction through the demyelinated zone. On autopsy, MS plaques are found throughout the white matter of the brain and spinal cord. The scattering differs from patient to patient, accounting for the various presenting symptoms.

The signs and symptoms vary from patient to patient and include the following: sensory symptoms (numbness, burning, pricking, tingling pain, and decreased proprioception and sense of temperature); motor symptoms (paresis, paralysis, dragging of foot, spasticity, bladder and bowel dysfunction); cerebellar symptoms (ataxia, loss of balance and coordination, nystagmus, speech disturbances, tremors, and vertigo); and other symptoms such as fatigue, impotence, depression or euphoria, and facial paralysis. In many instances, symptoms of MS may mimic cerebral ischemia, spinal cord compression, and tic douloureux. The diagnosis is made on clinical assessment by exclusion of all other possible neurologic disorders.

There are no known cures for the demyelination process. Corticosteroids have been used to promote remission. The actions of corticosteroids focus on decreasing white matter edema and enhancing neural conduction through partially demyelinated nerve fibers. Treatment for muscle spasticity includes the use of benzodiazipines, dantrolene, and baclofen. The MS patient should avoid excessive fatigue, emotional stress, and hypothermia.

2. Identify the perioperative evaluation and considerations for patients with MS.

Providing anesthesia to the patient with MS presents as a challenge to the clinician because there are numerous factors to be taken into consideration. The current neurologic condition of the patient should be well documented so that any postoperative changes can be interpreted with these findings in mind. Pulmonary function needs to be addressed because kyphoscoliosis may be present, causing restrictive disease. There have been reports of acute respiratory failure and weakness from diaphragmatic paralysis. Lability of the ANS has also been seen in MS patients. With this in mind, efforts should be made to avoid hypotension in the selection of anesthetic agents.

There is no evidence that any particular drugs used to induce general anesthesia, either intravenous or inhaled, cause exacerbations of MS. Succinylcholine may need to be avoided in advanced MS because of the possibility of massive hyperkalemia. Effective management of anesthesia must include temperature control. A rise in temperature may be associated with temporary clinical deterioration. The mechanism is uncertain, but any increase in temperature may inhibit optimal functioning of conduction pathways. Consequently, it may be advisable to avoid agents with anticholinergic properties, such as glycopyrrolate, which may increase the possibility of a temperature rise. Also, antipyretics should be administered when indicated and causes of infection treated promptly.

The issue in this case would be the use of regional anesthesia. Numerous reports exist of exacerbations of MS after spinal anesthesia. The mechanism of this reaction is unclear but may be related to the potential neurotoxic effect of a drug exposed to a spinal cord lacking the protective nerve sheath as a result of demyelination. Successful lumbar epidural anesthesia has been reported in patients with MS, but there remains the possibility of exacerbation of symptoms. Although epidural anesthesia is not absolutely contraindicated in the MS patient, a full discussion of the risks and benefits should be made clear to the patient before proceeding.

▶ SUMMARY

Assessment and perianesthetic management of the patient with neurologic disease is challenging for the nurse anesthetist. A thorough knowledge of anatomy, physiology, and pathophysiology is essential to the perianesthetic plan. Anesthetic agents and pharmacologic adjuncts influence neurophysiology. A variety of advanced nursing assessment skills are required to evaluate these clients, particularly when the level of consciousness is impaired. A thorough integration and knowledge of all parameters of assessment, both subjective and objective, must be incorporated into the perianesthetic care of the patient with neurologic disease in order to execute quality care from the preoperative through the postoperative phase.

▶ ACKNOWLEDGMENTS

The authors would like to acknowledge Julius Migliori, MD, for his dedication and contributions to nurse anesthesia education over the years. Dr. Migliori is the Director, Department of Anesthesia at St. Joseph Hospital in North Providence, Rhode Island.

▶ KEY CONCEPTS

- The constancy of CBF is ensured by maintaining a stable CPP (the difference between MAP and ICP).
- Autoregulation is an active vascular response to maintain a constant CBF in the range of 50 mmHg to 150 mmHg; autoregulation may be affected by hypoxia, hypercapnia, trauma, and some anesthetic agents.
- Alterations in $Paco_2$ and Pao_2 produce distinct variations in CBF.
- Total CBF generally parallels overall $CMRo_2$ and is closely correlated with brain activity.

- Clinical implications associated with the permeability of the BBB focus on those anesthetics with a high solubility coefficient that generally cause unconsciousness more quickly.
- In terms of aids in diagnoses, skull films, spinal films, CT scans, MRI, and PET provide rapid initial identification of pharmacologically or surgically treatable neurologic dysfunction; use of EEG and EPs readily detect abnormal function and the presence of ischemic change.
- Premedication should be avoided when level of

consciousness is in question, or when ICH is suspected.
- Fluid and electrolyte management centers on maintaining peripheral perfusion but avoiding hypervolemia and diuresis.

- With few exceptions, inhalation agents increase CBF, decrease CMR_{O_2}, increase CBF/CMR_{O_2} ratios, and increase CSF resistance to absorption (except isoflurane), while most intravenous agents decrease CBF and CMR_{O_2}.

▶ Study Questions

1. How will knowledge of the anatomy and physiology of the nervous system play a critical role in providing anesthesia to patients with neurologic dysfunction?

2. How will a complete neurologic evaluation influence the nurse anesthetist's ability to provide optimal care?

3. Does knowledge of the pathophysiologic state of specific neurologic diseases have an impact on anesthesia care? If so, how?

4. What are the general perianesthesia considerations for patients with neurologic dysfunction?

5. What are the links among the pharmacologic and physiologic influences in providing anesthesia to patients with neurologic diseases?

KEY REFERENCES

Bendo, A. A., Kass, I. S., Hartung, J., & Cottrell. J. E. (1997). Anesthesia for neurosurgery. In P. G. Barash, B. F. Cullen, & R. K. Stoelting (Eds.), *Clinical anesthesia* (3rd ed., pp. 699–745). Philadelphia: Lippincott-Raven.

DeVane, G. G. (1997). Neurosurgical anesthesia. In J. J. Nagelhout & K. L. Zaglaniczny (Eds.), *Nurse anesthesia* (pp. 795–815). Philadelphia: Saunders.

Hickey, J. V. (1997). *The clinical practice of neurological and neurosurgical nursing* (4th ed.). Philadelphia: Lippincott-Raven.

Morgan, G. E. & Mikhail, M. S. (1996). *Clinical anesthesiology* (2nd ed., pp. 477–504). Stamford, CT: Appleton & Lange.

Newfield, P. & Cottrell, J. E. (Eds.), (1991). *Neuroanesthesia: Handbook of clinical physiologic essentials* (2nd ed.). Boston: Little, Brown & Co.

Stone, D. J., Sperry, R. J., Johnson, J. O., Spiekermann, B. F., & Yemen, T. A. (Eds.), (1996). *The neuroanesthesia handbook.* St. Louis: Mosby.

REFERENCES

Bedford, R. F. (1997). Supratentorial brain tumors. In M. F. Roizen & L. A. Fleisher (Eds.), *Essence of anesthesia practice* (p. 300). Philadelphia: Saunders.

Bendo, A. A., Kass, I. S., Hartung, J., & Cottrell, J. E. (1997). Anesthesia for neurosurgery. In P. G. Barash, B. F. Cullen, & R. K. Stoelting (Eds.), *Clinical anesthesia* (3rd ed., pp. 699–745). Philadelphia: Lippincott-Raven.

Chang, W. J. & Bleck, T. P. (1996). Neuroscience intensive care. In D. J. Stone, R. J. Sperry, J. O. Johnson, B. F. Spiekermann, & T. A. Yemen (Eds.), *The neuroanesthesia handbook* (pp. 437–486). St. Louis: Mosby.

Cole, D. J. (1997). Amyotrophic lateral sclerosis. In M. F. Roizen & L. A. Fleisher (Eds.), *Essence of anesthesia practice* (p. 14). Philadelphia: Saunders.

DeVane, G. G. (1997). Neurosurgical anesthesia. In J. J. Nagelhout & K. L. Zaglaniczny (Eds.), *Nurse anesthesia* (pp. 795–815). Philadelphia: Saunders.

Donegan, J. (1991). Physiology and metabolism of the brain and spinal cord. In P. Newfield & J. E. Cottrell (Eds.), *Neuroanesthesia: Handbook of clinical and physiologic essentials* (2nd ed., pp. 3–29). Boston: Little, Brown & Co.

Dooley, J. & Gingrich, K. J. (1997). Intracranial hypertension. In M. F. Roizen & L. A. Fleisher (Eds.), *Essence of anesthesia practice* (p. 192). Philadelphia: Saunders.

Farnsworth, S. T., Johnson, J. O., & Sperry, R. J. (1996). Neurophysiology. In D. J. Stone, R. J. Sperry, J. O. Johnson, B. F. Spiekermann, & T. A. Yeman (Eds.), *The neuroanesthesia handbook* (p. 37–54). St. Louis: Mosby.

Frost, E. A. M. (1991). Anesthesia for neurosurgical emergencies. *American Society of Anesthesiologists Refresher Course, 19,* 43–54.

Fry, T. (1996). Muscular disorders and neuropathies. In J. Duke & S. G Rosenberg (Eds.), *Anesthesia secrets* (p. 305). Philadelphia: Mosby.

Guy, J. & Gelb, A. W. (1993). Perioperative management of intracranial aneurysms. *American Society of Anesthesiologists Refresher Course, 14,* 1–8.

Haley, E. C., Kassell, N. F., & Torner, J. C. (1992). The International Cooperative Study on the Timing of Aneurysm Surgery: The North American experience. *Stroke, 23,* 205–214.

Hampson, C. (1996). Cerebrovascular insufficiency. In J. Duke & S. G. Rosenberg (Eds.), *Anesthesia secrets* (pp. 251–258). Philadelphia: Mosby.

Harrigan, C. (1997). The central nervous system. In J. J. Nagelhout & K. L. Zaglaniczny (Eds.), *Nurse anesthesia* (pp. 91–115). Philadelphia: Saunders.

Hartung, J. & Cottrell, J. E. (1994). Mild hypothermia and cerebral metabolism. *Journal of Neurosurgical Anesthesia, 6,* 1–14.

Hickey, J. V. (1997). *The clinical practice of neurological and neurosurgical nursing* (4th ed., pp. 81–163). Philadelphia: Lippincott.

Hunt, W. E. & Hess, R. M. (1968). Surgical risk as related to time of intervention in the repair of intracranial aneurysms. *Journal of Neurosurgery, 28,* 14–27.

Johnson, J. O. (1996). Monitoring. In D. J. Stone, R. J. Sperry, J. O. Johnson, B. F. Spiekermann, & T. A. Yemen (Eds.), *The neuroanesthesia handbook* (pp. 87–112). St. Louis: Mosby.

Katz, J. (1997). *Anesthesiology: A comprehensive study guide* (pp. 149–191). New York: McGraw-Hill.

Kistler, J. P., MacDonald, N. R., Ackerman, R. H., & Abbott, W. M. (1987). Carotid invasive studies. *Massachussetts General Hospital Lab Newsletter, 19,* 1–3.

Kofke, W. A. (1997). Seizures—Epilepsy. In M. F. Rozien & L. A. Fleisher (Eds.), *Essence of anesthesia practice* (p. 284). Philadelphia: Saunders.

Liu, M. (1997). Autonomic hyperreflexia. In M. F. Roizen & L. A. Fleisher (Eds.), *Essence of anesthesia practice* (p. 41). Philadelphia: Saunders.

Michenfelder, J. D. (1988). *Anesthesia and the brain* (pp. 23–55, 94–113). New York: Churchill Livingstone.

Moorthy, S. S. & Hilgenberg, J. C. (1980). Resistance to nondepolarizing muscle relaxants in paretic upper extremities of patients with residual hemiplegia. *Anesthesia & Analgesia, 59,* 624–625.

Morgan, G. E. & Mikhail, M. S. (1996). *Clinical anesthesiology* (2nd ed., pp. 477–504). Stamford, CT: Appleton & Lange.

Newfield, P. (1993). Perioperative management of intracranial aneurysms. *American Society of Anesthesiologists Refresher Course, 21,* 13–26.

Ornstein, E., Matteo, R. S., & Schwartz, A. E. (1987). The effects of phenytoin on the magnitude and duration of neuromuscular block following atracurium or vecuronium. *Anesthesiology, 67,* 191–199.

Prough, D. S. & Cohen, N. H. (1991). Fluid management. In P. Newfield & J. E. Cottrell (Eds.), *Neuroanesthesia: Hand-*

book of clinical and physiologic essentials (2nd ed., pp. 161–179). Boston: Little, Brown & Co.

Rando, J. T. (1992). Neurophysiology. In W. R. Waugaman, S. D. Foster, & B. M. Rigor (Eds.), *Principles and practice of nurse anesthesia* (2nd ed., pp. 355–381). Norwalk, CT: Appleton & Lange.

Sharpe, M. D. & Zimmermann, W. (1997). Parkinson's disease. In M. F. Roizen & L. A. Fleisher (Eds.), *Essence of anesthesia practice* (p. 242). Philadelphia: Saunders.

Shwiry, B. (1992). Anesthesia for neurosurgery. In W. R. Waugaman, S. D. Foster, & B. M. Rigor (Eds.), *Principles and practice of nurse anesthesia* (2nd ed., pp. 663–688). Norwalk: Appleton & Lange.

Sieber, F. E. (1997). Cerebral aneurysm clipping. In M. F. Roizen & L. A. Fleisher (Eds.), *Essence of anesthesia practice* (p. 367). Philadelphia: Saunders.

Sperry, R. J. (1996). Anesthesia for spinal cord injury. In D. J. Stone, R. J. Sperry, J. O. Johnson, B. F. Spiekermann, & T. A. Yeman (Eds.), *The neuroanesthesia handbook* (pp. 161–181). St. Louis: Mosby.

Spiekermann, B. F. & Thompson, S. A. (1996). Fluid management. In D. J. Stone, R. J. Sperry, J. O. Johnson, B. F. Spiekermann, & T. A. Yemen (Eds.), *The neuroanesthesia handbook* (pp. 113–126). St. Louis: Mosby.

Stone, D. J. & Bogdonoff, D. L. (1996). Anesthesia for intracranial vascular surgery. In D. J. Stone, R. J. Sperry, J. O. Johnson, B. F. Spiekermann, & T. A. Yemen (Eds.), *The neuroanesthesia handbook* (pp. 313–356). St. Louis: Mosby.

Swafford Dahm, L. I. (1992). Anesthetic management of the patient with neuromuscular or related diseases. In W. R. Waugaman, S. D. Foster, & B. M. Rigor (Eds.), *Principles and practice of nurse anesthesia* (2nd ed., pp. 791–804). Norwalk: Appleton & Lange.

Swash, M. & Schwartz, M. S. (1992). What do we really know about amyotrophic lateral sclerosis? *Journal of Neurological Science, 113,* 4–16.

Tarkkanen, L., Laitenen, L., & Johanson, G. (1974). Effects of D-tubocurarine on intracranial pressure and thalamic electrical impedance. *Anesthesiology, 40,* 247–253.

Teasdale, G. & Jennett, B. (1974). Assessment of coma and impaired consciousness. *Lancet, 2,* 81–88.

Todd, M. M., Warner, D. S., & Maktabi, H. D. (1998). Neuroanesthesia: A critical review. In D. E. Longnecker, J. H. Tinker, & G. E. Morgan, Jr. (Eds.), *Principles and practice of anesthesiology* (2nd ed., pp. 1607–1658). St. Louis: Mosby Year Book.

Young, M. L. (1997). Infratentorial tumors. In M. F. Roizen & L. A. Fleisher (Eds.), *Essence of anesthesia practice* (p. 190). Philadelphia: Saunders.

Assessment of the Renal, Gastrointestinal, and Endocrine Systems of the Adult

John G. Aker, Jane A. Scanlan, and K. Patman Smith

Although the traditional medical work-up, which consists of physical examination and specific laboratory data, provides a general screening of patient health, this approach has been shown to be inefficient for preoperative anesthetic assessment (Carson & Eisenberg, 1982). Preoperative anesthetic assessment conducted via an assessment of individual organ systems enables the anesthetist to identify those systems that may have underlying disease processes and appreciate the functional level of each organ system. Following this assessment, additional medical consultation may be required to further evaluate the specific disease process. To appreciate functional limitations, the anesthetist must have a sound knowledge base of the anatomy and functional physiology of each organ system.

This chapter guides the novice anesthetist in an understanding of the anatomy, physiology, and pathophysiology of the renal, gastrointestinal, and endocrine systems. Relevant anatomy and physiology of each system precedes a discussion of the preoperative assessment. The preoperative evaluation will guide the anesthetist in an assessment of each organ system outlining the essential elements: the patient interview, physical examination, and relevant diagnostic laboratory data. The pathophysiology commonly encountered in the surgical population of each organ system will be reviewed. Integrating the knowledge of functional anatomy, physiology, and pathophysiology, the anesthetist will be guided in the development of an anesthetic plan of care.

▶ RENAL SYSTEM

Anatomy

The kidneys are paired and located retroperitoneally against the posterior abdominal wall extending from L1 to L3 in the upright position, and from T12 to L3 when supine. Each kidney weighs approximately 150 g and receives approximately 1200 mL/min of blood flow or 25% of the total cardiac output. The ureter, renal artery, and renal vein enter through the pelvis of the kidney. In a cross sectional view, the kidney is composed of an outer cortical and an inner medullary area, which is further divided into an inner and outer region.

Each kidney is comprised of approximately 1.2 million nephrons, which are classified as either cortical or juxtamedullary based on location of the glomeruli and length of the loops of Henle. The majority (85%) of nephrons are located in the cortex, receiving 80% to 90%

of the total renal blood flow. Each nephron consists of a glomerulus and a recurrent renal tubule that provides the conduit for glomerular filtrate to be delivered to the renal pelvis as urine (Fig. 13–1). The renal tubule is divided into a proximal convoluted tubule, a descending limb of the loop of Henle, an ascending limb of the loop of Henle, and a distal convoluted tubule that empties into a collecting tubule.

Each kidney is supplied by a single renal artery that branches to form several interlobular arteries, which transverse the medulla at the corticomedullary junction, and undergo further divisions to form afferent arterioles. The afferent arterioles form a capillary tuft—the glomerulus—and supply each Bowman's capsule. Capillaries coalese to form the efferent arteriole which exits the renal corpuscle. This efferent arteriole forms an additional capillary plexus, the peritubular plexus, which surrounds the tubular portion of the nephron. Blood flows progressively through the afferent arteriole (glomerulus), the efferent arteriole, the peritubular capillary, the venules, and ultimately to a single renal vein which drains into the inferior vena cava. The positioning of a capillary bed between two arterioles (between the afferent and efferent arterioles), maintains a high-pressure bed favoring filtration, and the peritubular capillaries, a low-pressure bed favoring reabsorption from the renal tubules.

Innervation of the kidney arises from spinal segments T4 to L1 via the celiac ganglia and renal plexus. Pain from the kidney is conducted through somatic fibers entering the spinal cord at segments T10 to L2. At rest in the supine position, the renal vasculature has little sympathetic tone (Muravchick, 1991). There are alpha, beta, and dopaminergic receptors in the renal vasculature, although sympathetic constrictor fibers that arise from spinal segments T4 to L1 predominate. The re-

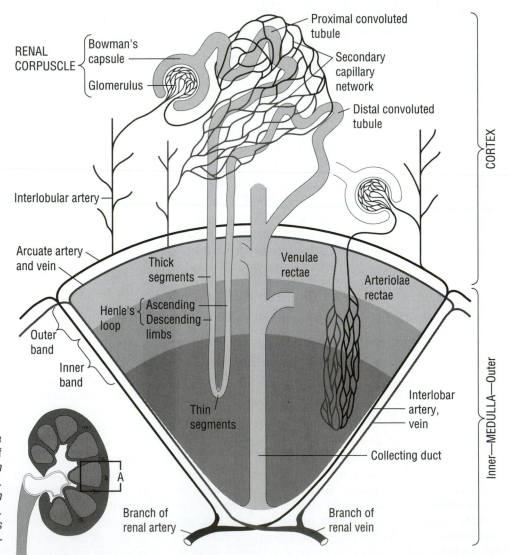

Figure 13–1. Diagram of the nephron. Insert A shows location of the renal tubule in the kidney. *(From King, B. G. & Showers, M. J. [1969]. Human anatomy and physiology [6th ed., p. 325]. Philadelphia: Saunders. Copyright 1969 by W. B. Saunders Company. Reprinted with permission.)*

nal vasculature lacks sympathetic vasodilator or parasympathetic innervation (Mazze, Fujinaga, & Wharton, 1996). Stimulation of dopaminergic receptors results in vasodilation, increased renal blood flow, and glomerular filtration.

Physiology

The kidney functions to eliminate nitrogenous waste products derived from protein catabolism, and maintains fluid and electrolyte balance. This is accomplished through a number of mechanisms involving filtration, the secretion of neurohumoral substances, and the active and passive reabsorption of solutes.

Blood flow through Bowman's capsule produces a glomerular ultrafiltrate at a rate of 125 mL/min or 180 L/day. Only 1.5 L of this tubular ultrafiltrate is excreted as urine, the remainder being reabsorbed into the interstitium and removed by the peritubular capillaries in the renal cortex. The vasa recta or *straight vessels* (Fig. 13–1) formed from the peritubular capillaries, which descend into the medulla of the kidney around the loops of Henle, are responsible for reabsorption of fluid from the renal interstitium in the inner and outer medulla. The vasa recta plays an important role in concentrating the urine via the countercurrent mechanism. Tubular secretion involves the transport of toxins and solutes from the blood, interstitium, and tubular epithelial cells into the tubular lumen. The major functions and unique characteristics of each portion of the nephron are summarized in Table 13–1. Figure 13–2 shows the sites of water and electrolyte exchange in the nephron and relative percentages of glomerular filtrate at each level of the renal tubule.

Glomerular filtration is achieved by a balance of hydrostatic and oncotic forces within the plasma, glomerulus, and Bowman's capsule. Dehydration, hemorrhage, tubular or ureteral obstruction, changes in blood pressure and cardiac output, and alterations in the diameter of the afferent and efferent arterioles will affect the glomerular filtration rate (GFR) and rate of urine production (Patafio, 1996). The GFR parallels the rate of renal blood flow (RBF) (Sladen, 1994).

Renal blood flow, and hence glomerular filtration, are maintained by intrinsic autoregulation and extrinsic neural and humoral influences. Autoregulation refers to the direct and proportional relationship between blood flow and vascular resistance in a particular organ vascular bed. The purpose of renal autoregulation is to maintain a constant GFR which facilitates the control of fluid and solute excretion. Fluctuations in the renal mean arterial pressure (MAP) between 75 mmHg and 160 mmHg produces accompanying changes in afferent arteriolar diameter, maintaining a constant RBF and GFR over this range of arterial pressures. Outside of these limits, RBF and GFR are pressure-dependent. Decreases in MAP below the range of autoregulation will result in decreased RBF, GFR, urine production, and solute excretion. Glomerular filtration ceases when the MAP is less than 40 mmHg (Morgan & Mikhail, 1996). Autoregulation may be overridden by extrinsic neural and humoral influences. Stimulation of alpha-adrenergic receptors in the afferent arterioles produces vasoconstriction, reducing RBF. Sympathetically mediated vasoconstriction induced by high-stress states such as fear, pain, and hemorrhage may produce marked reductions in glomerular filtration. Renal blood flow and glomerular filtration may cease in

TABLE 13–1. Summary of Nephron Functions

Segment	Reabsorption	Secretion	Diuretic Site of Action	Distinctions	Filtrate Remaining (%)
Proximal convoluted tubule	Na^+ (70%), H_2O, Cl^-, K^+, glucose (100%), HCO_3^- (90%), urea, amino acids	H^+	Carbonic anhydrase inhibitors (acetazolamide), mannitol	Na^+/K^+ ATPase pump	33
Descending loop of Henle	H_2O	Na^+, Cl^-		Countercurrent multiplier mechanism	20
Ascending loop of Henle	Na^+ (20%), K^+, Cl^-		Loop diuretics (furosemide, edecrin, bumex)	Thick portion is impermeable to H_2O	15
Distal convoluted tubule	Na^+ (5%), Ca^+, HCO_3^- (10%), H_2O (ADH required)	Renin, K^+, H^+, NH_3	Thiazides	JGA releases renin PTH; vitamin D-mediated Ca^+ reabsorption	15
Collecting duct	Na^+ (5%), H_2O (ADH required)	K^+, H^+, NH_3	K^+ sparing diuretics (aldactazide, spironolactone)	ADH-mediated H_2O reabsorption; Aldosterone-mediated Na^+ reabsorption	5 to 0.5

ADH, antidiuretic hormone; ATPase, adenosine triphosphatase; PTH, parathyroid hormone.

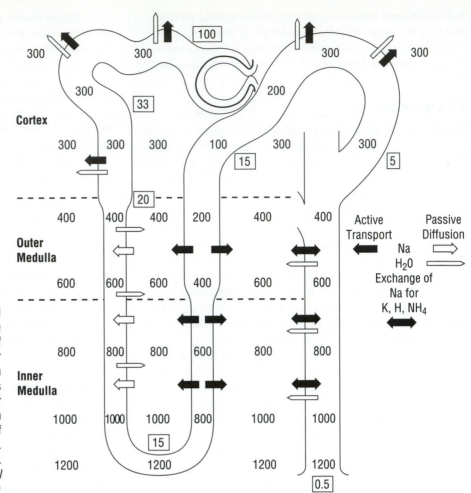

Figure 13–2. Summary of passive and active exchanges of water and ions in the nephron in the course of elaboration of hypertonic urine. Concentrations of tubular urine and peritubular fluid are given in milliosmoles per liter; large boxed numerals are the estimated percentages of glomerular filtrate remaining within the tubule at each level. *(From Pitts, R. F. [1974]. Physiology of the kidney and body fluids [3rd ed., p. 134]. Chicago: Year Book Medical Publishers, Inc. Copyright 1974 by Year Book Medical Publishers, Inc. Reprinted with permission.)*

instances of grave emergency in order to shunt blood to other organs (Pitts, 1974). In disease states such as sepsis, autoregulation may be lost, with periods of hypotension significantly diminishing RBF and GFR (Miller, 1996).

The renal medulla, which receives only 5% to 10% of the total RBF, consumes five times the amount of oxygen (O_2) as the renal cortex (Aronson, 1995a). Accordingly, the renal medulla is more vulnerable to hypoxic cellular injury when O_2 delivery is diminished. Increased solute reabsorption in the medulla may produce additional increases in O_2 consumption which exceeds O_2 delivery. Redistribution of blood flow from the cortex to the medulla serves to protect the medulla from hypoxia by increasing O_2 delivery in the face of increasing O_2 consumption.

Neural control appears to be at least partially responsible for the redistribution of blood flow within the kidney under certain conditions. Hypotension resulting from hemorrhage initiates a redistribution of intrarenal blood flow from the cortical to the medullary nephrons, maximizing sodium, chloride, and water reabsorption to maintain blood volume (Miller, 1996).

Additional factors act to maintain adequate RBF and glomerular filtration. Dopamine, catecholamines, and diuretics can enhance or hinder RBF and GFR. Dopamine promotes diuresis and natriuresis by increasing RBF in a dose-dependent manner. Low-dose dopamine (1 to 2 μg/kg/min) activates dopaminergic receptors (DA_1 and DA_2) in the renal and splanchnic vasculature, producing vasodilation. $Beta_1$-adrenergic stimulation occurs with infusion rates of 3 to 10 μg/kg/min. These doses increase cardiac output and glomerular filtration. At doses exceeding 10 μg/kg/min, alpha-adrenergic stimulation predominates, procuding renal vasoconstriction and diminished RBF and glomerular filtration.

Diuretics increase urine output by decreasing the absorption of sodium and water. Diuretics are generally classified by their site of action in the nephron (Table 13–1). The diuretics most commonly used in anesthesia are the osmotic and loop diuretics. Osmotic diuretics are filtered at the glomerulus but not reabsorbed, remaining in the tubule to influence sodium and water movement into the tubule with subsequent excretion. Mannitol increases RBF and glomerular filtration primarily by volume expansion, and it may block release of renin (Dooley & Mazze, 1996). Rapid intravascular volume expansion may precipitate pulmonary edema in vulnerable patients. Mannitol is frequently used to protect against renal failure when hypoperfusion or sludging is anticipated because the resulting large volumes of dilute urine increase tubular flow and decrease intraluminal tubular obstruction (Morgan & Mikhail, 1996).

Loop diuretics interfere with the ability to form concentrated urine, increasing the excretion of sodium and potassium ions, resulting in large volumes of isosmotic or slightly dilute urine. Loop diuretics also produce renal vasodilation due to increased prostaglandin production, a protective effect that may be inhibited by nonsteroidal anti-inflammatory drugs (NSAIDs) (Hemmings, 1996). However, these diuretics should be used cautiously in hypovolemic patients, as the diuresis may worsen volume depletion, worsen renal ischemia, and concentrate nephrotoxins in the tubules (Dooley & Mazze, 1996). Combinations of diuretics are frequently used. Low-dose dopamine may increase urine output in patients previously unresponsive to fluid boluses or loop diuretics. Dopamine enhances RBF and delivery of the diuretic to the site of action in the tubule (Aronson, 1995a).

Humoral influences play a predominate role in the regulation of water and electrolyte balance. The renin–angiotensin system influences RBF and glomerular filtration. Hypotension, decreased afferent arteriolar wall pressure, $beta_1$-adrenergic stimulation, and plasma volume depletion, as well as decreased plasma and/or decreased extracellular sodium or chloride content, stimulate the release of the enzyme renin from the juxtaglomerular cells (Muravchick, 1991).

The juxtaglomerular cells are modified smooth muscle cells found in the wall of the afferent arteriole that release the proteolytic enzyme renin in response to a decrease in renal afferent arterial pressure, a decrease in filtered tubular sodium presented to the macula densa, the release of circulating catecholamines simulating $beta_1$ receptors, a decrease in right atrial pressure, or a decreased sodium or chloride content (decreased extracellular fluid volume). Figure 13–3 illustrates the physiologic effects of the renin–angiotensin system. The release of renin is inversely related to renal perfusion and may be decreased by atrial natriuretic peptide (ANP), angiotensin II, or vasopressin (Lake, 1992). Atrial cells release ANP in response to distension of atrial stretch receptors. Renin cleaves angiotensinogen formed in the liver producing angiotensin I (an inactive decapeptide). Angiotensin I is rapidly converted by angiotensin-converting enzyme (ACE) in the lungs to form angiotensin II (an octapeptide). It is this important step that is pharmacologically blocked by ACE inhibitors such as captopril. The two most important actions of angiotensin II include constriction of efferent arterioles and a stimu-

latory effect of tubular reabsorption of sodium. Generalized arteriolar vasoconstriction increases peripheral vascular resistance, raising systemic blood pressure. Constriction of efferent arterioles preserves GFR in the face of a decreasing RBF (Sladen, 1987).

Angiotensin II stimulates the release of aldosterone from the zona glomerulosa of the adrenal cortex. This mineralocorticoid influences sodium and water reabsorption in exchange for hydrogen or potassium ions in the distal nephron (distal renal tubule and collecting duct) (Fig. 13–2). Angiotensin II produces vasoconstriction of preglomerular vasculature. The RBF is protected by renin-induced prostaglandin synthesis (Marley, 1993). Prostaglandins produce renal vascular vasodilation that counteracts the vasoconstrictive effects of angiotensin II and decreases ischemia during renin-angiotensin activation. Prostaglandins increase cortical blood flow, resulting in diuresis and increased sodium excretion (Mazze, 1990b). Nonsteroidal anti-inflammatory drugs block prostaglandin synthesis, producing unchecked vasoconstriction and decreased RBF. The inhibition of prostaglandin synthesis when normal states of hydration and sodium balance are present does not affect RBF or glomerular filtration (Miller, 1996). However, during periods of hypotension, hypovolemia, or ischemia, administration of NSAIDs can have deleterious effects on RBF, glomerular filtration, and sodium excretion. Angiotensin II also stimulates the formation and release of erthyropoietin and may explain the finding of mild anemia in patients taking ACE inhibitors (Griffing and Melby, 1982).

Humoral regulation of kidney function extends beyond those factors produced by the kidney itself. Antidiuretic hormone (ADH) is released by the posterior pituitary in response to hypovolemia and increased plasma osmolarity. As shown in Figure 13–2, little water is reabsorbed from the collecting ducts. In the presence of ADH, the distal tubules and collecting ducts are highly permeable to water, increasing water reabsorption and the formation of concentrated urine. Beta-adrenergic drugs and cholinergic agents stimulate ADH release (Mazze, Fujinaga, & Wharton, 1996). Other factors responsible for ADH release include pain, stress, hemorrhage, and hyperthermia. Antidiuretic hormone secretion is inhibited by decreased plasma osmolarity, ethanol, cortisol, and hypothermia. A high-volume dilute urine is produced with ADH inhibition (Stoelting, 1991).

Positive-pressure ventilation may stimulate ADH secretion decreasing urine output (Mazze, Fujinaga, & Wharton, 1996). However, the decreased urine output may be the result of impaired release of ANP (Hemmings, 1996). Atrial natriuretic peptide inhibits sodium reabsorption in the proximal tubule and produces arteriolar vasodilation with increased RBF and GFR, increasing sodium and water excretion. The net effect is an in-

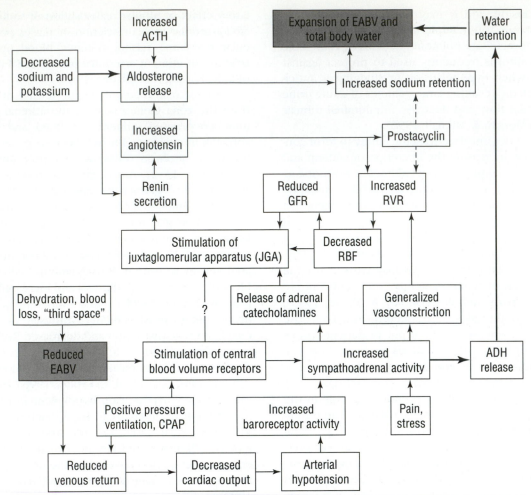

Figure 13–3. Homeostasis of total body water and effective arterial blood volume (EABV). Increases in renovascular resistance (RVR) produce decreased RBF and a reduced GFR. These changes stimulate the juxtaglomerular apparatus (JGA) and activate the renin–angiotensin system. Dashed lines indicate competing vasodilator effects of prostacyclin that reduce the likelihood of renin-induced ischemia during this sequence of events. *(From Muravchick, S. [1991]. The anesthetic plan: From physiologic principles to clinical strategies [pp. 295–296]. St. Louis: Mosby Year Book Co. Copyright 1991 by Mosby Year Book Co. Adapted and reprinted with permission.)*

creased urine output and decreased plasma volume and blood pressure.

The kidney has additional metabolic functions that impact anesthetic management. Acid–base balance is maintained by the kidney's ability to reabsorb bicarbonate from the proximal and distal convoluted tubules, and secrete hydrogen ion into the proximal convoluted tubule and tubular fluid. Under physiologic acid–base conditions, the amount of bicarbonate reabsorbed equals the rate of hydrogen ion excretion, leaving an excess of either to be excreted into the urine. Under abnormal acid–base conditions (metabolic or respiratory acidosis), the kidneys respond by increasing the excretion of hydrogen ion and increasing the reabsorption of bicarbonate. Although the renal response is activated immedi-

ately, the effects are not noticeable for 12 to 24 hours and may not be maximal for 5 days (Morgan & Mikhail, 1996).

The kidneys, although not typically thought of as endocrine organs, play a major role in erythrocyte production via the secretion of erythropoietin. Hypoxia stimulates the kidneys to secrete erythropoietin which activates erythropoiesis, increasing RBC production from stem cells in the bone marrow. The subsequent increase in RBCs increases O_2-carrying capacity, increasing O_2 delivery to the tissues. Although hypoxia increases erythropoietin levels within 24 hours, erythropoiesis and the release of the mature RBC requires 5 to 7 days. Without stem cell stimulation by erythropoietin, severe anemia develops (Guyton & Hall, 1996). The kidneys are also involved in the production of the active form of Vitamin D (1,25-dihydroxy vitamin D_3). Vitamin D is important in the role of phosphate and calcium homeostasis.

History and Preoperative Interview

The assessment of the renal system begins with a complete review of the patient's medical history, including concomitant drug therapy and drug or latex allergies. The general symptoms of renal dysfunction include a history of anorexia, nausea, vomiting, diarrhea, weight loss, pruritus, peripheral edema, and neurologic changes. The anesthetist should remember that clinical evidence of altered renal function may not be evident until renal disease is well advanced (Mazze, 1990a). The assessment should note a family or patient history of previous renal failure or disease, hypertension, diabetes, systemic lupus erythematosis (SLE), peripheral vascular disease, or heart failure (Kaufman & Contreras, 1990). These disease states have a variable effect on renal function. For example, diabetic patients have a tenfold greater risk for renal dysfunction following a period of hypovolemia than nondiabetics (Shusterman, 1987).

A history of calculi, recurrent kidney or bladder infections, abnormal urine character or volume, or change in bladder function should be further investigated. Altered mental status, presence of peripheral neuropathy, and easy bruising may also be findings consistent with abnormalities of the renal system (Larson, 1992). The anesthetist should be suspicious of renal function in patients who take large quantities of NSAIDs or have a recent history of exposure to nephrotoxic drugs (Table 13–2) (Patafio, 1996). It has been estimated that as many as 18% of patients who take NSAIDs may have some renal impairment (Murray, Bater, Tierney, Hui, & McDonald, 1990). Patients at risk of renal impairment who take NSAIDs include the elderly, males, those with intravascular volume depletion, and patients with a history of heart failure, cirrhosis, or preexisting renal disease.

Physical Examination

Many intraoperative factors—including sepsis, hypovolemia, and hypotension as well as cardiac, vascular, and hepatobiliary surgical procedures—predispose patients to renal failure. A thorough assessment of the patient with preexisting renal dysfunction is important to minimize postoperative renal failure. In patients without a previous history of renal dysfunction, clinical evidence of altered renal function may not be evident until more than 75% of the nephrons are nonfunctional (Stoelting & Dierdorf, 1993). However, the presence of certain physical findings should alert the anesthetist to the presence of abnormal renal function that may require further evaluation.

A multitude of signs and symptoms are suggestive of renal dysfunction. Following the acquisition of objective data, the patient should be examined to assess the presence of hypervolemia, peripheral edema, pulmonary congestion, pleural effusions, and congestive heart failure present in the patient with renal dysfunction (Larson, 1992).

Auscultation of the chest and palpation of the peripheral pulses will determine the presence of tachycardia which may be etiologic of hypovolemia or heart failure secondary to activation of the renin–angiotensin system. As previously discussed, patients with renal disease have low levels of erythropoietin and are anemic. Anemia may be clinically evident as fatigue, exercise intolerance, or shortness of breath with normal levels of physical activity. This may be observed during patient ambulation to the examination room. The lung fields should be auscultated to determine the presence of pulmonary edema. Blood pressure determination in both arms quantifies the presence of hypertension, and jugular venous distension provides information relative to intravascular volume. The extremities as well as the sacral area in the bedridden patient should be examined for the presence of edema or sequestered fluid.

Examination of the abdomen may reveal tenderness of the flank or suprapubic region, which is suggestive of the presence of a urinary tract infection. Bladder distension is suggestive of prostatic disease or neurogenic bladder dysfunction. Frequent bladder distension will accompany polyuria of diabetes. Auscultation of the abdomen may reveal a bruit suggestive of renal artery stenosis or abdominal aortic aneurysm. These findings should prompt an immediate medical consultation.

Patients requiring chronic hemodialysis will have a peripheral arteriovenous shunt (AV shunt) in the arm, forearm, ankle, or occasionally in the groin. The patient should be queried as to his or her dialysis schedule and the completion of the most recent dialysis session. The AV shunt should be palpated to determine patency. Intravenous cannulation must be avoided in the extremity containing the shunt to avoid the risk of infection. Noninvasive blood pressure monitoring must also be avoided to prevent clotting of the shunt. In addition, the extremity containing the shunt must be padded and protected during the perioperative period to prevent thrombus formation.

Diagnostic Data

Selective laboratory testing assists in determining the extent of renal disease and guides the development of an anesthetic plan for the preservation of renal function during the perioperative course. If abnormalities of the renal system are suspected by the history and physical, these selective laboratory tests may be indicated to better evaluate renal function. The basic laboratory assessment includes a complete blood count and urinalysis. The complete blood count will provide a measure of serum hematocrit and red blood cell indices. Preoperative hematocrit levels may reflect long-standing anemia. White blood cell count and differential will assist in the determination of ongoing infection.

Urinalysis, a simple and relatively inexpensive test, provides qualitative information of renal function. This test includes the evaluation of urine color, specific gravity, pH, protein, and sediment. Urine color is normally a clear, light yellow, but when substances appear in the urine (casts, red blood cells) the urine appears turbid. The presence of bile pigments can be determined, as the urine becomes tea colored and foams following vigorous shaking. Specific gravity (normal range 1.016 to 1.022) reflects the kidney's ability to concentrate urine and is thus an estimation of the solute concentration of the urine. In states of volume depletion or decreased RBF, the renal tubules reabsorb sodium and water producing a concentrated urine with a specific gravity greater than 1.030. When renal tubular function is lost, specific gravity is fixed at 1.010. The anesthetist should appreciate that specific gravity is influenced by nonrenal factors, including concomitant drug therapy and endocrine abnormalities. Urine osmolarity, electrolytes and fractional excretion of sodium (FE_{Na}) are additional tests that may better evaluate tubular function, and are commonly used to differentiate different types of renal failure (Kellen, Aronson, Roizen, Barnard, & Thisted, 1994). Urine pH, (normal range, 5.5 to 6.5) determined during urinalysis, may reflect tubular function but must be interpreted in relation to the patient's overall acid–base status.

Routine urinalysis may detect pyuria and the presence of leukocyte esterase, suggesting a urinary tract infection. Proteinuria in large amounts (3+ or 4+) suggests glomerular disease, and may be accompanied by systemic hypoproteinemia. The presence of glucosuria is abnormal and may indicate diabetes or proximal tubular damage. The presence of cellular casts in the urine also suggests tubular injury. Hematuria may result from glomerular disease or trauma to any aspect of the genitourinary system.

Coagulation studies should also be evaluated in the patient with known renal dysfunction, particularly if invasive vascular monitoring is planned. Prolonged bleeding time (platelet dysfunction) is the most frequent clotting abnormality found in patients with renal disease. The administration of desmopressin will decrease bleeding time and increase circulating factor VIII and von Willebrand factor, decreasing the risk of operative bleeding.

Blood urea nitrogen (BUN) reflects glomerular filtration and urine-concentrating ability. Urea is filtered at the gomerulus, so increasing serum BUN levels reflect a drop in glomerular filtration. Although BUN (normal range 10 mg/dL to 20 mg/dL) is inversely related to GFR,

abnormalities of BUN can reflect altered production rate or tubular absorption. As an example, BUN may be elevated in spite of a normal GFR as a result of dehydration, degradation of blood following tissue trauma, consumption of a high-protein diet, or following the administration of a loop diuretic. Low tubular flow rates, such as those occuring with volume depletion, decreased renal perfusion, CHF, or tubular obstruction, produce an increased reabsorption of urea into the capillaries and an elevated BUN. Although an abnormal BUN does not always reflect an abnormal GFR, a BUN greater than 50 mg/dL almost invariably reflects a decreased GFR (Stoelting & Dierdorf, 1993).

Creatinine (normal range 0.8 mg/dL to 1.3 mg/dL male; 0.6 mg/dL to 1 mg/dL female) more accurately reflects GFR and is independent of tubular flow. Increased creatinine reflects either increased production, which is directly related to skeletal muscle mass, or decreased filtration. The elderly or chronically ill patient with reduced muscle mass has decreased creatinine production, and normal serum levels may be present despite reduced GFR. Increased levels are clearly indicative of abnormal renal function. Doubling of creatinine reflects a 50% reduction in GFR. Therefore, serial creatinine levels may be a more precise indicator of GFR when renal function is changing (Aronson, 1995b). Creatinine will increase within 8 to 17 hours after an acute change in the GFR (Stoelting & Dierdorf, 1993). However, elevated BUN and creatinine are late signs of renal dysfunction, as levels are not significantly increased until GFR is reduced to 25% of the normal level (Kellen, Aronson, Roizen, Barnard, & Thisted, 1994).

The ratio of BUN to creatinine may reflect decreased RBF and GFR. When tubular flow rates are low, as with dehydration, decreased renal perfusion, or tubular obstruction, there is increased reabsorption of urea, resulting in an elevated BUN. Creatinine filtration is not affected by tubular flow. A BUN to creatinine ratio greater than 20:1 reflects states of renal hypoperfusion, or prerenal azotemia. Kaufman and Contreras (1990) suggest that the ratio should always be calculated as part of the preoperative evaluation to identify states of renal hypoperfusion that could progress to renal failure without treatment.

Creatinine clearance (normal range 100 mL/min to 120 mL/min) is the best estimate of GFR, although it can overestimate GFR in patients with moderate to severe renal dysfunction (Aronson, 1995a). Clearance rates of 60 mL/min to 100 mL/min reflect diminished renal reserve, and rates of 25 mL/min to 50 mL/min are consistent with symptomatic renal insufficiency. Creatinine clearance less than 25 mL/min is consistent with renal failure, and uremia develops with creatinine clearance levels less than 10 mL/min, (Kaufman & Contreras, 1990). The anesthetist should remember that the determination of a creatinine clearance requires an accurate collection of urine for up to 24 hours, and therefore may be impractical to obtain in the immediate preoperative period. However, the creatinine clearance can be estimated via the following formula (Prough & Foreman, 1992):

$$GFR = \frac{(140 - age) \times lean\ body\ weight\ (kg)}{72 \times serum\ creatinine}$$

Patients with renal dysfunction must have their serum electrolytes checked prior to anesthesia. Hyperkalemia is common in patients with renal failure and may develop into a life-threatening problem in the immediate postoperative period. Serum potassium should be determined immediately preoperatively. This value can be compared with the patient's dialysis records to note the degree of hyperkalemia normally tolerated by the patient.

A chest x-ray and electrocardiogram (ECG) should be obtained in the patient with renal dysfunction. The standard anteroposterior chest x-ray will help identify the presence of pleural or pericardial effusion, left ventricular hypertrophy, pneumonia, pulmonary edema, and congestive heart failure. There is a high incidence of ischemic coronary artery disease in patients with chronic renal dysfunction that is attributable to the presence of preexisiting hypertension, hyperlipidemia, and diabetes. It is important to note that ischemic coronary artery disease is the most common cause of death in patients with chronic renal dysfunction (Broyer, 1986). The ECG should be evaluated for evidence of myocardial ischemia, dysrhythmias, or left ventricular hypertrophy. Hyperkalemia may produce peaking of T-waves. Hyperkalemia can be treated with the intravenous administration of calcium. Calcium decreases the threshold potential and myocardial membrane excitability. This treatment must be reserved for the emergency situation as hypercalcemia may result in cardiac arrest.

Pathophysiology

Acute Renal Failure

Acute renal failure (ARF) is defined as an abrupt decline in renal function resulting in accumulation of nitrogenous waste products in the blood (azotemia) without reference to urine volume (Byrick & Rose, 1990). Although oliguria, defined as a urine output below 0.5 mL/kg/h, (or 400 mL/day) implies renal failure, nonoliguric renal failure may be present if waste products accumulate and fluid, electrolyte, or acid–base imbalances develop (Dooley & Mazze, 1996). Table 13–2 lists the etiology of ARF, classified as either prerenal (inadequate perfusion), intrarenal (acute tubular necrosis) or postrenal (obstructive uropathy) (Patafio, 1996). Treatment of prerenal causes of ARF is determined by the specific cause and may include fluid therapy or inotropic agents and di-

TABLE 13–2. Etiology of Acute Renal Failure

Prerenal	Renal	Postrenal
Hypovolemia	Toxins	Surgical trauma
Dehydration	Iodinated intravenous	Prostatism
Hemorrhage	contrast	Calculi
Hypotension	Antibiotics	Pelvic mass
CHF	Aminoglycosides	
Shock due to sepsis	Amphoteracin	
Thromboembolism	Chemotherapy agents	
	Cisplatinum	
	Cyclosporin	
	Fluorinated inhalation agents	
	Sevoflurane	
	Methoxyflurane	
	Enflurane	
	Ischemia due to prolonged	
	renal hypoperfusion	
	Acute glomerulonephritis	
	Free hemoglobin	
	Massive transfusion	
	Transfusion reaction	
	Free myoglobin due to massive	
	muscle necrosis	

CHF, congestive heart failure.

uretics. Treatment of postrenal failure is directed at relief of the obstruction. Both prerenal and postrenal causes are reversible in the early stages, but delayed treatment may result in parenchymal renal failure. The mortality rate for patients with postoperative renal failure is 50% to 100%, and accordingly, identification, prevention, and early treatment are crucial (Novis, Roizen, Aronson, & Thisted, 1994).

Acute tubular necrosis (ATN) accounts for 80% to 90% of the cases of ARF (Patafio, 1996). Sustained ischemia or nephrotoxicity causes necrosis of tubular cells. Damaged tubular cells slough and obstruct the loop of Henle, producing increased tubular pressure and decreased glomerular filtration. Back pressure causes leakage of the ultrafiltrate into the renal interstitium, where waste products are reabsorbed into the circulation. Renal protective therapies, including volume loading, low-dose dopamine infusion, and diuretic administration, are frequently used to lessen the severity of the backleak by flushing the tubules (Byrick & Rose, 1990). The course of acute renal failure is variable. Oliguria persists for 10 to 45 days, and hemodialysis is required during this phase. The diuretic phase signals recovery of renal function and is accompanied by fluid and electrolyte imbalance. Clinical features of ARF are summarized in Table 13–3. Two thirds of those who survive ARF will have a complete return of renal function, and one third will develop chronic renal failure (CRF) (Mazze, 1990a).

TABLE 13–3. Clinical Features of Acute Renal Failure

Progressive increase in blood chemistries (BUN, creatinine, Mg, uric acid)

Daily rise in K^+ (0.3 to 3 mEq/L)

Decreased serum Na^+ and Ca^+

Decreased albumin and serum proteins

Metabolic acidosis

Increased lipids, cholesterol, triglycerides, PO_4

Hyperglycemia

Hypertension due to disorders of aldosterone and renin–angiotensin secretion

Anemia due to decreased erythropoietin production

Congestive heart failure

Coagulation abnormalities

Abnormal liver function

Impaired excretion of drugs and toxins

BUN, blood urea nitrogen.
From Bruton-Maree, N. (1992). Hepatic and Renal Physiology. In W. R. Waugaman, S. D. Foster, & B. M. Rigor (Eds.), Principles and practice of nurse anesthesia (2nd ed., p. 390). Norwalk, CT: Appleton & Lange.

Chronic Renal Failure

Chronic renal failure is progressive and develops with an irreversible loss of functioning nephrons. Decreased GFR results in azotemia. Chronic renal failure results in physiologic changes in all organ systems. Systemic diseases including diabetes, hypertension, polycystic kidney disease, pyelonephritis, glomerulonephritis, and connective tissue disorders may lead to the development of CRF. It is the level to which the GFR has been reduced that determines the perioperative risk for patients with CRF (Kaufman & Contreras, 1990).

Chronic renal insufficiency (GFR 25 mL/min to 50 mL/min) is present when 10% to 40% of the remaining nephrons are functioning. Although hypertension is typically noted in patients with CRF, it is not always present with renal dysfunction; but does occur with damage to particular portions of the kidney. Hypertension usually develops in cases of increased renal vascular resistance, with decreased glomerular capillary filtration, and in cases of excessive tubular reabsorption of sodium. Anemia develops as a consequence of decreased renal secretion of erythropoietin. Elevations in serum potassium, BUN, and creatinine parallel the decrease in functioning nephrons. Polyuria and nocturia develop due to diminished concentrating ability. With the decrease in functioning nephrons, there is little reserve, and excess stress, catabolic loads, or the administration of nephrotoxic agents can lead to a further decrease in functional nephrons (Stoelting & Dierdorf, 1993). Perioperative morbidity should not be increased in patients with chronic renal insufficiency if fluid and electrolyte balance is monitored closely (Kaufman &

Contreras, 1990). The loss of 90% of functioning nephrons (GFR < 10 mL/min) results in uremia and the need for hemodialysis. Dialysis is indicated for severe azotemia, hyperkalemia, fluid overload, and uremic encephalopathy.

Clinical features of CRF are summarized in Table 13–4. Patients with CRF exhibit hyponatremia resulting from an increased intravascular volume. Physiologic compensatory mechanisms for the accompanying chronic anemia (hemoglobin = 5 g/dL to 8 g/dL) include an increased heart rate and cardiac output, a decreased afterload, and an increased production of 2,3-diphosphoglucose (2,3-DPG) which shifts the oxyhemoglobin dissociation curve to the right increasing O_2 delivery to the tissues. Red blood cell transfusion is rarely indicated.

Chronic renal failure produces a metabolic acidosis which also produces a rightward shift of the oxyhemoglobin dissociation curve. Tachypnea accompanies metabolic acidosis. Chronic renal failure also produces changes in cardiovascular function as a direct result of fluid overload. The patient with CRF may develop pericarditis, pericardial effusions, and congestive heart failure. Gastrointestinal abnormalities include nausea, vomiting, increased gastric volumes, and hyperacidity with delayed gastric emptying. These changes increase the risk of regurgitation and aspiration. Decreased vitamin D synthesis results in increased parathormone secretion with calcium ion mobilization from the bone, producing osteodystrophy and increasing the potential of spontaneous fractures.

TABLE 13–4. Clinical Features of Chronic Renal Failure

Altered hydration and electrolyte imbalance
    Fluid overload
    Hyperkalemia, hyponatremia, hypocalcemia, hypophosphatemia

Metabolic acidosis

Systemic hypertension
    LVH
    Atherosclerosis with coronary artery disease

Hematologic abnormalities
    Chronic anemia (Hb 5 to 8 g/100 mL)
    Platelet dysfunction
    Increased incidence of infection

Gastrointestinal abnormalities
    Delayed gastric emptying
    Hyperacidity
    Increased gastric volume

Peripheral and autonomic neuropathies

Osteomalacia

Pruritis

Hypoalbuminemia

LVH, left ventricular hypertrophy.

Nephrotic Syndrome

The nephrotic syndrome is characterized by the excretion of greater than 3.5 g of protein in the urine per day. Renal tubular function is not disturbed. Nephrotic syndrome may develop in patients with toxemia of pregnancy, diabetes, or SLE. Alterations in the glomerular basement membrane increase permeability to proteins, facilitating the loss of albumin and some immunoglobulins. A number of additional clinical findings, including hypoproteinemia, hyperlipidemia, lipiduria, and peripheral edema, accompany the loss of protein. Plasma albumin concentration is reduced to 20% of the normal level, as its loss is greater because of its high plasma concentration and lower molecular weight. Compensatory increases in protein synthesis are not sufficient to maintain plasma oncotic pressure. Hypoalbuminemia and the attendant decrease in plasma oncotic pressure precipitate the development of edema, ascites, pleural effusions, and hypovolemia. Edema is typically the first symptom and presents as soft pitting edema of the lower extremities and periorbital area. Accordingly, these patients have excess total body water and decreased intravascular volume. The estimation of preoperative intravascular volume is essential because the treatment of the nephrotic syndrome typically includes a diuretic as well as corticosteroids. The anesthetist should appreciate that although tubular function is usually preserved in the nephrotic syndrome, chronic hypovolemia may lead to tubular dysfunction.

Vitamin D deficiency may also develop as the hormone 25-hydroxycholecalciferol is bound to plasma globulins that are filtered by the glomerulus. Hypocalcemia occurs as a result of decreased intestinal absorption. The development of hypocalcemia may produce a secondary hyperparathyroidism. Osteomalcia may develop as the required calcium is released from skeletal stores.

Perianesthetic Plan

General Considerations

All anesthetic agents can affect renal function either directly via the release of nephrotoxic metabolites (fluroride secondary to methoxyflurane administration) or indirectly via alterations in the function of the cardiovascular and neuroendocrine systems. A transient, reversible depression of renal function occurs in most surgical patients and is attributed to the effects of anesthesia as well as the type and duration of surgical procedure (Hemmings, 1996). Following general anesthesia GFR, RBF, urine output, and solute excretion decrease. These effects resolve in the early postoperative period and can be attenuated by preoperative hydration. These changes in renal function occur as a result of a decrease in systemic vascular resistance, cardiac output, or anesthetic-induced myocardial depression which reduces RBF. Reductions in systemic blood pressure lead to a loss of renal autoregulation. Recall that the hypertensive patient requires a higher systemic blood pressure to maintain the direct and proportional relationship between blood flow and vascular resistance. Accordingly, a MAP greater than 75 mmHg may be required to maintain GFR in the hypertensive patient.

Additional mechanisms that act to depress renal function following general anesthesia include the redistribution of RBF to the salt-retaining juxtamedullary nephrons, and alterations in neurohormonal regulation. Increased release of angiotensin II, ADH, and plasma catecholamines decrease RBF, GFR, and urine output, although activation of these systems is probably not provoked by anesthetic agents (Sladen, 1987). Surgical stress, pain, anxiety, and hemorrhagic hypovolemia stimulate the sympathetic nervous system, increasing ADH release, the activation of the renin–angiotensin system, and sympathoadrenal systems (Burchardi & Kaczmarczyk, 1994).

Inhaled anesthetic agents decrease cardiac output and systemic blood pressure and reduce GFR, urine output, and sodium excretion. Halothane has been shown to preserve RBF in the face of systemic hypotension (Hemmings, 1996). Using indirect quantification of RBF in humans, enflurane has been demonstrated to decrease RBF (Hemmings, 1996).

Nephrotoxicity of inhalation agents may lead to the development of postoperative renal dysfunction. The contemporary inhalation agents are all suitable for use in the patient with renal failure, as their elimination is renally independent. Biotransformation of the fluorinated inhalation agents may lead to the release of inorganic fluoride (Fi) (specifically methoxyflurane) which may produce direct nephrotoxic effects. Methoxyflurane, an agent no longer available in the United States for clinical use, has been demonstrated to produce fluoride-mediated renal toxicity (Burchardi & Kaczmarczyk, 1994). Dose-dependent elevations in serum Fi levels that reach or exceed a toxic threshold of 50 μm/L are associated with proximal tubular necrosis, polyuria, and progressive azotemia. Serum Fi levels less than 50 μm/L are rarely associated with renal dysfunction (Sladen, 1987). Enflurane and sevoflurane metabolism produces Fi, although peak levels above 30 μm/L are rarely achieved (Conzen, Nuschler, Melotte, Verhaegen, Leupoly, Van Aken, & Peter, 1995). Recent studies (Conzen, Nuschler, Melotte, Verhagen, Leupoly, Van Aken, & Peter, 1995; Tsukamoto, Hirabayashi, Shimuzu, & Mitsuhata, 1996) have revealed that although sevoflurane results in higher Fi levels than enflurane, there is no nephrotoxicity in patients with normal or impaired renal function. Isoflurane and desflurane produce negligible amounts of Fi, which may make them preferred agents in patients with known or suspected renal impairment.

Sevoflurane is readily degraded by carbon dioxide (CO_2) absorbants to produce a vinyl ether (compound A), which has been demonstrated to be nephrotoxic in rats. Several factors including low flow rates, closed-circuit anesthesia, increased ventilation, hyperthermia, high temperatures, the dessication of CO_2 absorbants, and use of baralyme rather than soda lyme CO_2 absorbants increase the production of compound A (Kandel, Laster, Eger, Kerschmann, & Martin, 1996). Renal injury from compound A produces proteinuria and glucosuria, indicating glomerular and proximal tubular damage (Eger, Koblin, Bowland, Ionescu, Laster, Fang, Gong, Sonner, & Weiskopf, 1997). Although renal impairment has not been documented in patients with normal renal function, the effects of compound A in patients with impaired renal function requires further evaluation.

Opioids, benzodiazepines, and barbiturates diminish renal function to a lesser extent, reducing GFR and urine output 10% to15% (Sladen, 1987). Anticholinergics may produce urinary retention and a postrenal pattern of renal failure in susceptible patients via the inhibition of the needed parasympathetic pathways for micturition. Opioids and benzodiazepines are metabolized by the liver and excreted by the kidney. Morphine, meperidine, diazepam, and to a lesser extent midazolam and sufentanil have active metabolites that can accumulate when excretion is reduced in renal failure. Respiratory depression lasting up to 7 days has been documented in patients with renal failure who received morphine (Stoelting, 1991). Fentanyl and alfentanil do not have pharmacologically active metabolites, but may have prolonged depressant effects in patients with renal insufficiency due to decreased protein binding. The pharmacodynamics of remifentanil, which is metabolized by nonspecific esterases in the blood to inactive metabolites, are unaltered in patients with renal failure.

Increased volume of distribution, anemia, hypoalbuminemia, acidemia, and electrolyte balance impact the pharmacokinetics and pharmacodynamics of anesthetic agents. Anemia decreases the blood–gas partition coefficient of volatile agents, resulting in a more rapid induction and emergence (Stoelting, 1991). Decreased protein binding results in increased bioavailability of highly protein-bound intravenous drugs (thiopental, etomidate, propofol, benzodiazepines, opioids) producing an exaggerated pharmacologic response and an increased duration of action. Ketamine is not significantly protein bound and is suitable for use in patients with renal impairment, although accumulation of active metabolites may result in prolonged effects. Acidemia increases the unionized (free) fraction of most sedative/hypnotics and opioids which facilitates penetration of the blood–brain barrier, increasing depressant effects of these agents. As a result of these pharmacokinetic and pharmacodynamic alterations, anesthetic agents should be judiciously

titrated in patients with CRF. Generally, all drug dosages should be reduced by 25% to 50% (Sladen, 1996).

Ionized drugs such as nondepolarizing muscle relaxants, antibiotics, diuretics, cholinesterase inhibitors, and digoxin are water soluble and excreted unchanged by the kidney. Renal dysfunction results in accumulation and prolonged effect of these drugs (Table 13-5) (Morgan & Mikhail, 1992). Atracurium and mivacurium have nonorgan-dependent elimination and may be the muscle relaxant of choice for patients with CRF. Rocuronium and vecuronium are minimally dependent on renal elimination and may be safely used in patients with CRF. Variable clinical duration and increased half-life may result from the increased volume of distribution in patients with renal disease. The effect of all nondepolarizing muscle relaxants may also be enhanced by concurrent electrolyte abnormalities (hypophosphatemia and hypermagnesemia). Succinylcholine administration elevates serum potassium (K^+) 0.5 mEq/L to 1.0 mEq/L. The administration of succinylcholine in the patient with pre-existing hyperkalemia may precipitate fatal dysrhythmias.

Regional anesthesia, including axillary, spinal, and epidural techniques are suitable for patients with renal impairment. Spinal and epidural anesthesias produce sympathetic blockade, protecting against the afferent arteriole vasoconstrictor response induced by the stress of anesthesia and surgery. Spinal blockade to a T1 level produces minimal reductions in RBF and GFR if adequate blood pressure is maintained and epinephrine free solutions are used (Hemmings, 1996). Either spinal or epidural anesthesia may be preferred in patients with renal insufficiency (Sladen, 1987). However, these patients may be more prone to hypotension and may not tolerate the increased fluid load required prior to induction of re-

TABLE 13–5. Drugs with Prolonged Effect in Patients with Renal Insufficiency

---

Muscle relaxants: Pancuronium, doxacurium, pipecuronium, D-tubocurare, metocurine, gallamine

Cholinesterase inhibitors: Neostigmine, physostigmine, pyridostigmine

Anticholinergic agents: Atropine, glycopyrrolate

Antihypertensives: Calcium channel blockers (nifedipine, diltiazem), beta-blockers (atenolol), ACE inhibitors (enalapril, captopril, lisinopril), clonidine, hydralazine, sodium nitroprusside, methyldopa

Cardiovascular agents: Digoxin, isoproterenol, procainamide, amrinone, amphetamines

Diuretics: Furosemide, hydrochlorothiazide, acetazolamide, spironolactone

Antibiotics: Penicillin, caphalosporins, aminoglycosides, vancomycin

Miscellaneous: Metoclopramide, H_2 receptor antagonists, anticonvulsants, phenobarbital

---

ACE, angiotensin converting enzyme.

gional anesthesia to prevent hypotension. The presence of peripheral neuropathy may dissuade the anesthetist from selecting a regional anesthetic technique. Axillary blocks are commonly utilized for the placement of arteriovenous shunts in patients with CRF. Maximal vasodilation provides optimal surgical conditions. However, decreased duration of local anesthetics may be seen in patients with renal failure due to increased cardiac output and uptake of the local anesthetic. Prolonged bleeding time (>15 minutes), despite normal prothrombin time (PT), partial thromboplastin time (PTT) and platelet counts, reflects platelet dysfunction common in patients with CRF and is a contraindication to the use of regional anesthesia. Patients should be evaluated for residual heparinization with a PTT following hemodialysis if a regional anesthetic is anticipated.

Arterial catheters are often placed in the lower extremities to preserve access for future vascular shunt sites in the upper extremities (Stoelting & Dierdorf, 1993). Procedures that involve significant blood loss or fluid shifts may require central venous pressure monitoring, with use of a pulmonary artery catheter if cardiac insufficiency or severe pulmonary disease is present. Monitoring hourly urinary output via an indwelling catheter is indicated, assuming the patient makes urine (Table 13–6). Sepsis is the primary cause of death in patients with CRF (Bastron, 1985); therefore, strict asepsis should be observed during all invasive procedures.

The anesthetist must ensure protection of an arteriovenous fistula from compression by tourniquets, noninvasive blood pressure cuffs, positioning, and encroachment by the surgical team. Patient positioning requires careful and thoughtful preparation because the patient with CRF has an increased potential for fractures from osteodystrophy. Peripheral neuropathy and altered hydration and nutritional status may increase the potential for pressure-related injuries.

Preoperative Considerations

Patients at increased risk of developing perioperative renal failure should be identified in the preoperative evaluation (Table 13–7). Preoperative renal dysfunction, cardiac failure, and advanced age are predictive of postoperative renal failure (Novis, Roizen, Aronson, & Thisted, 1994). Measures to assess and maintain renal perfusion and avoid renal insult should be paramount in the anesthetic plan. In high-risk patients, renal perfusion should be optimized before surgery, including correction of preoperative fluid deficits with intravenous infusions the night before surgery (Byrick & Rose, 1990).

Hyperkalemic cardiac arrest may be the primary cause of perioperative mortality in patients who were poorly prepared for surgery (Kaufman & Contreras, 1990). Acidemia results in increased serum K^+. Therefore, it has been recommended that elective surgery be postponed if serum K^+ is greater than 5.5 mEq/L, and if the pH is less than 7.25 and bicarbonate (HCO_3^-) is below 18 mmol/L (Kaufman & Contreras, 1990).

In patients with documented renal failure, the etiology, duration, and ongoing management should be reviewed. Daily urine output, if any, should be quantified. The type and schedule of dialysis and dialysis access sites (arteriovenous fistula or peritoneal catheter) should be noted. The time of the last dialysis prior to the scheduled surgical procedure, with pre- and postdialysis weight and labs (BUN, creatinine, electrolytes, PTT), should be recorded. Preoperative dialysis can reduce the risk of anesthesia and surgery in the uremic patient by reversing many of the problems associated with uremia, including fluid and electrolyte imbalances, acidemia,

---

TABLE 13–6. Indications for Intraoperative Bladder Catheterization

Renal insufficiency

Electrolyte abnormalities

Lengthy surgical procedures (> 4 hours)

Aortic cross-clamping

Cardiopulmonary bypass

Burns

Anticipation of decreased cardiac output or hypotension

Large fluid shifts

Intraoperative administration of diuretic agents

Surgery that involves or may damage the urogenital system

Extensive trauma

Induced hypotension

From Dooley, J. R. & Mazze, R. I. (1996). Oliguria. In N. Gravenstein & R. R. Kirby (Eds.), Complications in Anesthesiology (2nd ed., pp. 483). Philadelphia: Lippincott-Raven. Copyright by Lippincott-Raven Publishers. Reprinted with permission.

TABLE 13–7. Patients at Risk for Perioperative Renal Failure

Coexisting renal disease

Preoperative hypoperfusion states

Hypovolemia

Cirrhosis

Biliary tract obstruction

Sepsis

Multiple organ system failure

Multiple system trauma

Congestive heart failure

Abdominal aortic aneurysm resection

Cardiopulmonary bypass

Advanced age

From Stoelting, R. K. & Dierdorf, S. F. (1993). Anesthesia and co-existing disease (3rd ed., p. 299). New York: Churchill Livingstone. Copyright by Churchill Livingstone, Inc. Adapted with permission.

platelet dysfunction, gastrointestinal symptoms, and central, peripheral, and autonomic neuropathy (Bastron, 1985). However, hemodialysis creates additional problems, including hypovolemia and residual heparinization, the effects of which may be evident for up to 10 hours after dialysis. Sladen (1996) recommends that hemodialysis be completed the day before but within 48 hours of surgery to allow for the equilibration of fluid and electrolytes. Continuous ambulatory peritoneal dialysis (CAPD) may be continued until the time of surgery.

Preoperative transfusions, although rarely required, are ideally given during hemodialysis to remove excess fluid and K^+ of the stored blood. Anemia with hematocrit (Hct) levels of 15% to 25% are common and generally well tolerated in patients with end-stage renal disease (ESRD). Transfusion criteria are individualized according to the patient's preexisting cardiopulmonary disease but may be indicated if Hct is less than 20%, or significant cardiopulmonary disease exists. In general, transfusions are utilized to maintain Hct above 25% (Kaufman & Contreras, 1990).

Platelet dysfunction as evidenced by bleeding time over 15 minutes should be corrected with cryoprecipitate (10 units) or desmopressin (approximately 0.3 g/kg) 1 hour before major surgery (Sladen, 1996). A serum potassium level should be obtained immediately before surgery. In less urgent situations, exchange resins (Kayexalate 0.5 g/kg) can decrease plasma potassium but cannot be effectively utilized on an emergent basis. Hyperkalemia can be emergently corrected with the intravenous administration of insulin and dextrose or by producing alkalosis via hyperventilation or administration of sodium bicarbonate. Calcium chloride will counteract the cardiac effects of hyperkalemia pending definitive treatment (Sladen, 1996).

Premedication with reduced dosages of midazolam may be safely administered to anxious patients with renal failure who are stable and alert. However, these patients should be closely observed, with the application of a pulse oximeter, as they have increased sensitivity to CNS depressants. Chronic antihypertensive and cardiac medications should be continued until the time of surgery. Aspiration prophylaxis with an H_2 receptor antagonist and metoclopromide is indicated because these patients have delayed gastric emptying.

Intraoperative Considerations

The intraoperative anesthetic goal for patients with impaired renal function is the preservation of existing renal function by maintaining adequate RBF and cardiac output. Increased cardiac output is the primary compensatory mechanism for anemia. Anesthetic agents that minimally alter cardiac output are preferred in these patients. The use of nitrous oxide (N_2O)/opioid technique is acceptable, although Fio_2 should be at least 50% to

maximize O_2-carrying capacity in anemic patients. It is important to recall that O_2-carrying capacity is not only influenced by the inspired O_2 concentration, but the initial hemoglobin and arterial O_2 saturation. All of these factors must be considered in determining the resultant inspired O_2 concentration.

Patients with renal failure frequently experience nausea, vomiting, delayed gastric emptying, and stress ulcer bleeding. Aspiration prophylaxis and rapid sequence induction (RSI) or modified RSI may be indicated. Preoxygenation is important to increase the O_2 content and denitrogenate the functional residual capacity. Hypertension is frequently seen in these patients and should be optimally controlled prior to elective surgical procedures. Hypotension is common with anesthetic induction, particularly if the patient is hypovolemic following a recent dialysis session. Hypotension at induction may be prevented by the judicious administration of a bolus of normal saline in the patient following recent dialysis (Sladen, 1996). Patients with ESRD who are dependent on hemodialysis may safely be given a volume of fluid equivalent to one half of the weight reduced during dialysis (Bready, 1992).

Intraoperative fluid therapy is determined by the degree of renal insufficiency present, but in general should be judicious in patients with any degree of renal dysfunction. Patients with ESRD undergoing minor procedures require only replacement of insensible losses with solutions that are free of K^+ and lactate, such as normal saline. Fluid losses should be replaced with fluids of similar composition: Blood loss may be replaced with packed cells; protein-rich exudates such as ascites should be replaced with plasma substitutes; and third space losses should be replaced with balanced salt solutions that do not contain K^+ (Mazze, Fujinaga, & Wharton, 1996). Careful estimation of intraoperative blood and fluid loss is essential, as there is little margin of safety between insufficient and excessive fluid administration in patients with ESRD.

Patients with insufficient but functioning kidneys challenge the anesthetist to find a balance between renal hypoperfusion and potential fluid overload. When considering fluid therapy in the healthy patient, it should be noted that the consequences of fluid overload, such as pulmonary congestion, are easier to treat than those of ARF (Morgan & Mikhail, 1996). Inadequate renal perfusion resulting from hemorrhage or dehydration are the most frequently recognized insults leading to the development of ARF (Aronson, 1995b). Tests used to assess RBF, such as creatinine clearance, FE_{Na}, urine osmolarity, and electrolytes, are impractical or not readily available during surgery. Therefore, urine output and hemodynamic monitoring remain the best means to ensure adequate RBF. Administration of an isosmotic solution at a rate of 3 to 5 mL/kg/h to maintain a urine output greater than 0.5 mL/kg/h is recommended (Stoelting & Dierdorf, 1993).

Oliguria, defined as a urine output of less than 0.5 mL/kg/h, is a symptom of ARF and is the normal compensatory response to prevent it (Aronson, 1995a). Postrenal causes, such as obstruction of the retention catheter or pooling of urine in the dome of the bladder, should be ruled out first. Initial treatment of oliguria in an adult includes a fluid challenge of 500 mL of crystalloid. Increased urine flow rate indicates that additional fluid should be given, as oliguria does not occur until there is an extracellular fluid deficit of 25% or more (Dooley & Mazze, 1996). If oliguria persists, low-dose dopamine (1 to 2 μg/kg/min) will increase RBF and GFR. When cardiac failure is present, inotropic support with dobutamine, dopamine, or epinephrine should be initiated to increase cardiac output and renal perfusion. To increase tubular flow, mannitol may then be indicated if there is still no response, followed by loop diuretics. It should be noted that the early administration of loop diuretics in hypovolemic patients will worsen renal failure, and they should only be used as the first line of treatment when overt signs of intravascular volume overload are present. The treatment of perioperative oliguria should be prompt and aggressive in high-risk patients, and continue until urinary flow is restored or oliguria persists despite a pulmonary artery wedge pressure of 18 mmHg or more after administration of inotropes, dopamine, and diuretics (Prough & Foreman, 1992).

Although positive-pressure ventilation decreases glomerular filtration, controlled ventilation is frequently chosen to prevent respiratory acidosis. Patients with metabolic acidosis compensate with mild hyperventilation; therefore, minute ventilation should be increased and adjusted to maintain the baseline pH intraoperatively. However, severe hyperventilation with respiratory alkalosis will shift the oxyhemoglobin dissociation curve to the left, inhibiting release of O_2 to the tissues, and should be avoided. Adequate tidal volume with a slow respiratory rate will allow increased venous return and minimize the decreased cardiac output encountered with positive-pressure ventilation.

Intraoperative anesthetic concerns include management of coexisting diseases. Labile blood pressure with intraoperative hypotension and hypertension may be treated by adjusting the depth of anesthesia. Vasodilators, such as hydralazine, droperidol, nitroglycerine, or sodium nitroprusside may be used to treat hypertension. Beta-blockers may also be an acceptable choice.

Emergence from anesthesia may be associated with hypertension, pulmonary edema, prolonged neuromuscular blockade, respiratory depression, and emesis. Anticholinesterases used to reverse muscle relaxants have a prolonged duration of action in patients with renal fail-

ure, with half-lives at least as long as the muscle relaxants. Therefore, recurarization is unlikely to occur. However, prolonged neuromuscular blockade in patients may occur due to acidosis, hypermagnesemia, hypokalemia, hypothermia, or the use of antibiotics and diuretics (Hemmings, 1996). Prolonged neuromuscular blockade due to hypermagnesemia may be partially antagonized by calcium (Sladen, 1996). The continued risk of aspiration should be considered during the period of emergence, and the endotracheal tube should not be removed until neuromuscular blockade is reversed and the patient has a return of protective reflexes.

Postoperative Considerations

Anesthetic concerns in the postoperative period focus on treatment of coexisting diseases, assessing the effect of renal insufficiency on the clearance of drugs, and evaluating renal function. Hemodynamic monitoring is continued during the immediate postoperative period. Signs of fluid overload, including hypertension and pulmonary congestion, may occur if excessive fluid was administered intraoperatively or as systemic vascular resistance increases with resolution of spinal or epidural anesthesia. The treatment of hypertension with vasodilators or beta-blockers should take into account the patient's normal systemic pressure. If hypervolemia exists, patients with ESRD may require hemodialysis. Opioids must be used judiciously in patients with renal failure. Opioid-induced hypoventilation may result in respiratory acidosis, with decreased pH and increased risk of hyperkalemia. Patients with anemia should be discharged from the postanesthesia care unit (PACU) with supplemental O_2.

Postoperative evaluation performed within 24 hours after administering the anesthetic includes assessment of anesthesia-related complications. Physical exam should focus on cardiac and respiratory functions, evaluating for signs of fluid overload, potential cardiac failure, or ischemia. Laboratory evaluation may include Hct, BUN, creatinine, electrolytes, arterial blood gases (ABG), chest x-ray, and 12-lead ECG. Urinalysis revealing proteinuria or glucosuria in the absence of hyperglycemia may represent glomerular and proximal tubular damage from nephrotoxic drugs and anesthetic agents (Eger, Koblin, Bowland, Ionescu, Laster, Fang, Gong, Sonner, & Weiskopf, 1997). Potential complications related to positioning should be evaluated, including neuropathy, pressure sites, and potential fractures due to osteodystrophy. Postoperative oliguria may result from decreased renal perfusion or the administration of nephrotoxic agents intraoperatively. Additional tests, including FE_{Na}, urine and serum creatinine, urea, electrolytes, and osmolarity, may be ordered in the postoperative period to determine if the oliguria is prerenal, intrarenal, or postrenal in origin.

► GASTROINTESTINAL SYSTEM

Although the liver plays a central role in the biodegradation and excretion of ingested or digested drugs and toxic compounds, the anesthetist should appreciate the major physiologic functions of the liver which include the regulation of carbohydrate, protein, fat, lactate, and bilirubin metabolism, as well as bile secretion. Preexisting hepatocellular disease, either acquired (alcoholism) or iatrogenic (viral hepatitis), may interfere with normal physiologic function. Patient mortality may follow general anesthesia in patients with underlying hepatic dysfunction despite the most benign surgical procedures.

Mechanical and physiologic dysfunction of the gastrointestinal system may develop from stress and anxiety, pain, preexisting disease, surgical manipulation of abdominal organs, and concurrent drug therapy. Decreased gastric motility and emptying, increased gastric acid secretion, intestinal obstruction, obesity, or neoplasm of the upper gastrointestinal tract increase patient risk for aspiration pneumonitis. The formulation of an anesthetic care plan requires comprehension of the normal mechanical and physiologic functions of the gastrointestinal system, and the variable impact of anesthetic drugs and adjuvant agents administered in the perioperative period.

Hepatic Anatomy and Physiology

The liver is the largest organ of the body, weighing approximately 1200 g to 1500 g. It has both an exocrine function (the secretion of bile from hepatocytes into the bile duct) and an endocrine function (eg, the secretion of glucose into the blood stream). The liver is divided into right and left lobes that are separated by a fold of peritoneum, the falciform ligament. The liver is covered by a fibroelastic capsule, the capsule of Glisson, which contains vascular and lymphatic channels and sensory nerves. Distension of the capsule of Glisson causes right upper quadrant pain and contributes to the accumulation of ascites via lymphatic leakage.

The right lobe is considerably larger, consisting of the caudate lobe, which occupies the posterior surface, and the quadrate lobe, which occupies the inferior surface (Fig. 13-4). The liver may be further subdivided through a detailed study of the vascular anatomy to delineate eight separate segments; this facilitates surgical resection.

The liver lobule is the basic functional unit formed from cords or plates of hepatocytes (Fig. 13-5). The major physiologic functions of the hepatocytes include the regulation of carbohydrate, protein, fat, bilirubin metabolism, bile secretion, and drug metabolism. The liver lobule is viewed histologically as a hexagonal unit where the portal triads are formed from the angles of the hexagon and the center of the hexagon, is occupied by a cen-

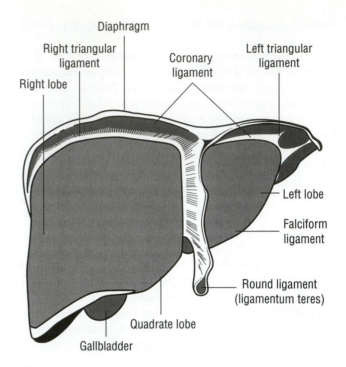

Figure 13–4. Gross structure of the liver. *(From McCance, K. L. & Huether, S. E. (1998). Pathophysiology: The biological basis for disease in adults and children.* Pathophysiology *[3rd ed., p. 1303]. St. Louis: Mosby.)*

tral hepatic vein. However, this histologic description has been refined. The acinus is now defined as the functional unit of the liver and consists of liver parenchyma located between two centrilobar veins. The center of the acinus

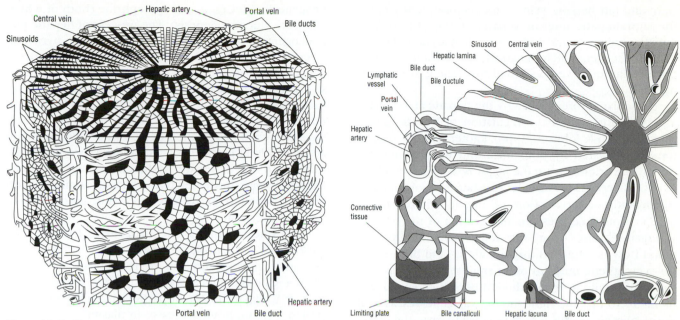

Figure 13–5. Diagram of liver parenchyma detailing blood supply. *(Left: From Leeson, Leeson, & Paparo [1985]. A Brief Atlas of Histology, Philadelphia: Saunders, p. 167; Right: From Ross, Romrell, & Kaye [1995]. Histology: A Text and Atlas [3rd ed]. Baltimore: Williams and Wilkins.)*

is formed by a portal triad that consists of a portal vein, the hepatic arteriole, bile duct, lymphatic ducts, and nerves, whereas the centrilobar vein occupies the peripheral border of the acinus (Fig. 13–6). This description is important because it characterizes the flow of blood from the hepatic arteriole in the sinusoid to the centrilobar vein. Accordingly, hepatocytes adjacent to the portal triad (zone 1 cells) receive oxygenated blood first, whereas those cells farther away (zone 2 cells, and zone 3 cells adjacent to the centrilobar vein) are the last to be perfused. The term *centrilobar necrosis* refers to the death of hepatocytes that lie adjacent to the centrilobar vein.

The liver receives approximately 25% of the cardiac output, or 100 mL of blood flow per 100 g of tissue in order to meet basic metabolic demands, which approximates one fifth of total body O_2 consumption (Strunin, 1977). The liver has a unique dual blood supply that delivers oxygenated blood from the hepatic artery, and partially deoxygenated venous blood from the confluent drainage of the pancreas, spleen, and intestines via the valveless hepatic portal vein. The hepatic artery supplies approximately 25% to 30% of the total hepatic blood flow, and contributes 40% to 50% of the liver O_2 requirement while the portal vein supplies 65% to 75% of the hepatic blood flow and contributes 50% to 60% of the liver's O_2 requirement. The hepatic artery and portal blood intermingle and flow through the hepatic sinusoids. This is a low-resistance circulatory system with sinusoidal pressures of approximately 3 mmHg. The hepatic sinusoids empty into the central veins, which coalesce to form the

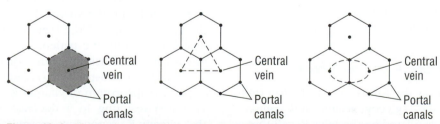

Figure 13–6. Histologic comparison of the liver. The classic liver lobule (far left) has the central vein at the center of the lobule and the portal canals at the periphery. The liver acinus (right) has the distributing vessels at the equator, and the central veins occupy each pole. *(From Weiss, L. [1983]. Histology [5th ed., p. 713]. New York: Elsevier.)*

right and left hepatic veins, which subsequently enter the suprahepatic inferior vena cava. (Fig. 13–6). The hepatic sinusoids are lined with phagocytic cells, the cells of Kupffer, which phagocytize the bacteria transported via portal venous blood from the gastrointestinal tract.

Vascular autoregulation by the hepatic artery plays a very minor role in the regulation of hepatic blood flow (Hansen & Johnson, 1966). Rather, hepatic arterial tone is regulated by both local and intrinsic mechanisms. The arterioles are the major resistance vessels to hepatic arterial flow. Vascular resistance may be altered significantly with reductions of intrahepatic blood volume or sinusoidal pressure. Innervation of the hepatic vasculature arises from the celiac ganglion. Arterial blood flow is regulated through alpha- and beta-receptor sympathetic innervation of smooth muscle, specifically preganglionic sympathetic fibers from spinal segments T7 to T10, the right and left vagus nerves, as well as the phrenic nerves which synapse to form the celiac plexus (Bioulac-Sage, Lafon, Saric, & Balabaud, 1990). Hypotension, hypovolemia, hypoxia, hypercarbia, and insufficient suppression of autonomic reflexes during *light* anesthesia will produce hepatic arterial vasoconstriction.

Spinal and epidural anesthesia will reduce hepatic blood flow via a reduction in portal blood flow (Kennedy, Evereet, & Cogg, 1971). Nitrous oxide does not produce significant alterations in blood pressure or cardiac output, and therefore has no effect on hepatic blood flow. All inhalation agents produce reductions in hepatic blood flow, although halothane produces the most prominent reduction in total hepatic blood flow and hepatic venous O_2 saturation (Goldfarb, Debaene, Ang, Roulot, Jolis, & Lebrec, 1990).

Intravenous anesthetic agents have no direct effects on hepatic blood flow, but alter blood flow through changes in cardiac output and increases in arterial CO_2, which accompanies respiratory depression. A single bolus of propofol has minimal effects on hepatic blood flow; continuous infusions have not been extensively studied. Some general concerns with continuous propofol infusions in patients with hepatic disease surround the issues of propofol metabolism and disposition of the solvent portion of the drug.

Metabolic Functions of the Liver

Metabolic tasks, such as the formation of glucose (gluconeogenesis), storage (glycogenesis), and release (glycogenolysis), are regulated by the liver. Recall that a number of hormones interact in this process, namely insulin (stimulates glycogen synthesis and inhibits gluco: neogenesis), glucagon, and epinephrine (both of which stimulate gluconeogenesis). The process of hepatic gluconeogenesis requires the substrates lactate, pyruvate, glycerol, or amino acids. Glucose enters the hepatocyte and is stored in the form of glycogen (glyconeogenesis). The hepatic capacity for glycogen storage is approximately 75 g, which can be depleted with 24 to 48 hours of fasting. When glycogen reserves are exhausted, active degradation of fat and protein maintain adequate blood glucose concentrations. Accordingly, patients with severe hepatic dysfunction may experience hypoglycemia. Intraoperative glucose administration may be required in patients receiving glucose-based parental nutrition.

Anesthesia inhibits gluconeogenesis. Patients who have fasted for a prolonged period may require intraoperative glucose infusion to reestablish acceptable plasma glucose concentrations (Sieber, Smith, Traystman, & Wollman, 1987). In particular, adult females experience precipitous decreases in plasma glucose with fasting periods in excess of 24 hours (Merimee & Tyson, 1974).

Hepatic protein synthesis is essential for maintaining plasma oncotic pressure, drug binding, and coagulation. All proteins, with the exception of coagulation factor VIII (produced by the vascular endothelium) and gamma globulins, are produced by the rough endoplasmic reticulum of the hepatocyte. Plasma or *pseudocholinesterase* is also synthesized by the hepatocytes. Recall the role of this enzyme in the degradation of both succinylcholine and ester local anesthetic agents.

Albumin, the predominate protein produced by the liver, is the major determinant of plasma oncotic pressure. Daily albumin production approaches 200 mg/kg/day, maintaining a plasma concentration of 3.5 g/dL to 5.5 g dL. The half-life of serum albumin is 14 to 17 days. Albumin production markedly decreases in severe liver disease, while gamma globulins produced in the reticuloendothelial system will be increased in an attempt to compensate for the decreased albumin production. Decreased albumin production increases the pharmacologically active fractions of administered drugs.

Hepatocytes synthesize the clotting factors (fibrinogen, factor I) and the vitamin-K–dependent factors (prothrombin, factor II) VII, IX, and X. Synthetic activity remains intact until the patient is beset with severe liver disease. Impaired gastric absorption of vitamin K may occur with biliary obstruction (recall that bile acids are essential for absorption of vitamin K and other fat-soluble vitamins) resulting in a decrease in the synthesis of the vitamin-K–dependent coagulation factors. Coagulopathies must be suspected in the patient with acute and chronic hepatic dysfunction.

Bile production is essential for the absorption of dietary fat from the gastrointestinal tract. Approximately 1 L of bile is formed by the hepatocytes per day, stored in the gallbladder, and released with the intestinal secretion of cholecystokinin. Absorbed dietary fat is transported via the portal circulatory system as chylomicrons and enters the liver where it is converted to glycerol, and then converted to ketone bodies during periods of fasting, sparing the need for gluconeogenesis. During nonfasting states glycerol is esterified, forming triglycerides, the building blocks for the synthesis of cholesterol. Cholesterol biosynthesis is important in the production of bile salts, the formation of steroid hormones, and the structural components of cell membranes.

It is important to remember that opioids (morphine is the greatest offender) can produce spasm of the sphincter of Oddi with a concomitant rise in pressure in the common bile duct (Radnay, Duncalf, Novakovic, & Lesser, 1984). This biliary spasm can be thwarted with the administration of glucagon, naloxone, atropine, and nitroglycerin (Jones, Fiddian-Green, & Knight, 1978).

Bilirubin is formed from the breakdown of the heme-containing compounds such as myoglobin and hemoglobin. Bilirubin is transported to the liver when it is bound to albumin (unconjugated form). In the liver, bilirubin is conjugated with glucuronic acid, forming a water-soluble compound that can be excreted via the urine. Unconjugated bilirubin is excreted into the bile where it enters the small intestine and is converted by intestinal bacteria into urobilinogen and urobilin. Urobilinogen undergoes hepatic recirculation and is excreted by the kidneys.

Drug Biotransformation

Biotransformation of administered drugs is an essential hepatic function. These enzymatic reactions can be classified as either phase I reactions (oxidation by cytochrome P450, reduction, and hydrolysis) or phase II reactions (conjugation of parent compound into more polar compounds). It should be stated that during biotransformation, metabolically active or potentially toxic compounds can be produced. The microsomal cytochrome P450 enzymes can be *induced* by drugs such as phenobarbital, enhancing their rate of drug metabolism. Lipid-soluble drugs undergo metabolism to water-soluble substances, which can then be excreted by the kidney. Drug availability is dependent on the protein-bound portions and hepatic blood flow. The clearance of drugs (meperidine or lidocaine) which have a high hepatic extraction ratio (the amount of blood removed from the blood during passage through the liver) is de-

pendent on hepatic blood flow. As hepatic blood flow is increased, more drug is available for extraction. On the contrary, drugs that have a low hepatic extraction ratio (thiopental, diazepam, digoxin) are dependent on protein binding and metabolism by the microsomal enzymes.

Chronic liver disease will significantly alter drug metabolism, as hepatocellular damage will decrease hepatic blood flow, decreasing the number of hepatocytes that contain the microsomal enzymes.

Hematologic Function of the Liver

During gestation, the liver is the site of formation of red blood cells with the bone marrow assuming the responsibility of erythropoiesis at approximately 2 months of age. Heme is synthesized in the bone marrow and liver via porphyrin metabolites. The porphyrias represent inherited or acquired disruptions in heme synthesis. These may be classified as to the site of abnormal porphyrin production (liver or bone marrow), presentation (acute or nonacute), and pattern of enzyme deficiency (Jensen, Fiddler, & Striepe, 1995). Acute hepatic porphyrias (acute intermittent, variegate, heriditary coprophyria) can be precipitated with the administration of particular anesthetic agents, most notably thiopental. Table 13–8 lists the safe and unsafe anesthetic agents for patients with acute hepatic porphyrias.

Gastrointestinal Anatomy and Physiology

The gastrointestinal (GI) tract is composed of four basic layers that are modified in different locations of the digestive tube. These four basic layers, from the exterior to the interior are the (1) serosa, a covering of parietal peritoneum; (2) muscularis externa, which consists of an inner circular and an outer longitudinal layer of smooth muscle; (3) connective tissue submucosa; and (4) the mucosa. During embryonic development, a number of glandular structures develop from, and remain connected to, the digestive tube via ducts. These glandular structures—the salivary glands, liver, gallbladder, and pancreas—release their secretory products via specialized ducts that are connected to the digestive tube.

The blood supply to the GI tract is a part of the splanchnic circulation, an extensive parallel circulatory system which includes the spleen, small and large intestine, and liver. The superior mesenteric artery supplies the small intestine and right colon. The inferior mesenteric artery supplies the transverse colon, left colon, and rectum. Venous blood is directed from these structures to the portal vein through the superior mesenteric veins.

TABLE 13–8. Safe and Unsafe Anesthetic Drugs for the Patient with Porphyria

Group	Safe or Likely Safe	Unsafe or Likely Unsafe	Unclear
Intravenous drugs	Midazolam, lorazepam, propofol	Barbiturates, etomidate, chlordiazepoxide, flunitrazepam, nitrazepam	Diazepam, ketamine
Inhaled drugs	Nitrous oxide	Enflurane	Isoflurane, halothane
Neuromuscular blockers	Succinylcholine, vecuronium, D-tubocurarine		Pancuronium, atracurium
Premedicants	Scopolamine, atropine, droperidol, promethazine, chloral hydrate, diphenhydramine, cimetidine		
Opioids	Morphine, fentanyl	Pentazosine	Sufentanil
Anticholinesterases	Neostigmine		
Local anesthetics	Bupivacaine, procaine		Lidocaine
Cardiovascular	Atenolol, labetolol, guanethadine, reserpine, phentolamine	α-methyldopa, hydralazine, phenoxybenzamine	
Other	Glucose-loading anticonvulsants	Oral contraceptive, griseofulvin, endogenous steroids	

From Jensen, N. F., Fiddler, D. S., & Striepe, V. (1995). Anesthetic considerations in porphyrias. Anesthesia and Analgesia, 80, 593.

There are a variety of arterial and venous communications that surround the esophagus. These low-pressure vascular communications become important in pathologic states, namely portal hypertension and cirrhosis of the liver. Cirrhosis produces inflammation with the formation of scar tissue, which encroaches on the hepatic sinusoids, producing a *back-up* of portal blood. As portal pressure rises, these vascular communications become engorged, producing esophageal or rectal varices, forming active bleeding sites. Figure 13–7 provides a pictorial view of this blood supply.

Central nervous system innervation of the GI tract originates from the sympathetic preganglionic fibers of spinal segments T5 to L3. The sympathetic innervation of the esophagus is derived from preganglionic fibers in spinal cord segments T1 to T6; the stomach, small intestine, and ascending and transverse colon T5 to T11, and the descending colon and rectum T12 to L3. Parasympathetic innervation of the GI tract is derived from the dorsal motor nuclei of cranial nerve X (vagus nerve).

Gastrointestinal dysfunction is common in the surgical patient population. The presence of hiatal hernia, gastroesophageal reflux, peptic ulcer disease, and intestinal obstruction increase the risks of regurgitation and aspiration of gastric contents. The esophagus joins the stomach approximately 3 cm below the diaphragm. The distal esophagus contains smooth muscle that receives innervation via preganglionic cholinergic fibers from cranial nerve X. The junction of the stomach and esophagus, the gastroesophageal junction, is controlled by the cardiac or lower esophageal sphincter (LES), which acts to prevent reflux of stomach contents into the esophagus. Lower esophageal function is particularly important in the parturient and the patient with hiatal hernia. The pressure to prevent gastric reflux, referred to as barrier pressure, is determined by the LES pressure minus gastric pressure. Functional LES barrier pressure is generally maintained between 10 mmHg and 20 mmHg. LES function is altered by pain, anxiety, and neural and hormonal influences. Individuals with gastroesophageal reflux have an incompetence of the gastroesophageal junction and experience sour taste and heartburn.

Pharmacologic agents will alter LES tone. Anticholinergic agents (atropine, glycopyrrolate, and scopolamine) decrease LES tone (Brock-Utne, Rubin, McAravey, Dow, Welman, Dimopoulos, & Moshal, 1977; Brocke-Utne, Rubin, Wellman, 1978), whereas metaclopramide increases LES tone (Brock-Utne, Rubin, Wellman, 1978). Pain, anxiety, and the administration of opioids decrease LES tone, increasing the risk of regurgitation. The chronic alcoholic has hypotonia of the LES, and accordingly is at risk for regurgitation and aspiration with the induction of general anesthesia.

Hiatal hernia describes the herniation of the cardiac portion of the stomach through the diaphragm into the thorax. Gastroesophageal reflux, although not uncommon in patients with hiatal hernia, does not typically occur unless the distal esophagus enters the thoracic cavity. Symptoms include fullness after meals, burning retrosternal pain that may mimic angina, dysphagia due to the slow passage of food at the portion of herniation, and postprandial nausea and vomiting.

Gastric Emptying

The time of solid food and liquid ingestion is important to the anesthetist, as these materials empty from the stomach at different rates. Gastric emptying varies between individuals (women empty more slowly than men) and depends on the constituents of the meal in-

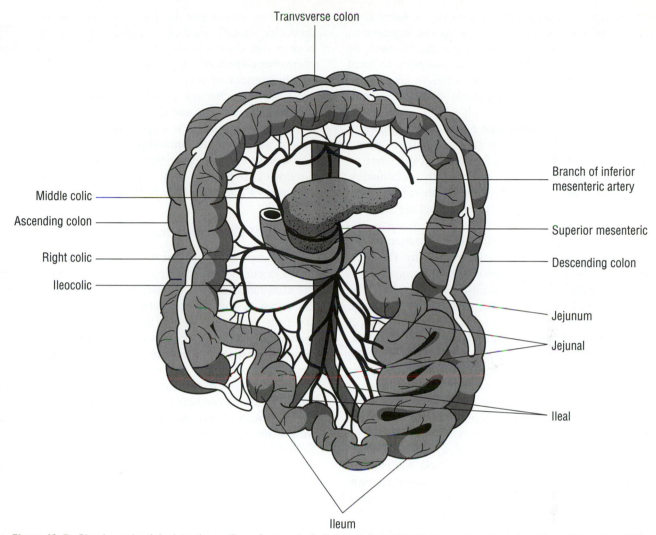

Transvsverse colon

Middle colic

Ascending colon

Right colic

Ileocolic

Branch of inferior
mesenteric artery

Superior mesenteric

Descending colon

Jejunum

Jejunal

Ileal

Ileum

Figure 13–7. Blood supply of the intestines. *(From Guyton, A. C. & Hall, J. E. [1996]. Textbook of medical physiology [9th ed., p. 800]. Philadelphia: Saunders.)*

gested (Notivol, Carrio, Cano, Estorch, Vilaredell, 1984). For example, solid material will pass more slowly than liquids. In addition, a host of factors including preoperative pain and anxiety elicit a neuroendocrine response that decreases gastric motility, gastric emptying, and increases gastric acid secretion. Conditions such as diabetes, peptic ulcer disease, inflammatory intestinal disease, electrolyte disturbances, and pregnancy also decrease gastric emptying and increase the risk of regurgitation and aspiration (Mamel, 1982). Loss of intestinal motility may follow the administration of opioids, producing intestinal atony and increasing gastric volume with resultant abdominal distension. The administration of a preoperative anxiolytic may enhance gastric emptying and reduce gastric acid secretion (Schurizek, Kraguland, Andreasen, Jensen, & Juhl, 1988).

It is impossible to predict gastric emptying time. It may require as long as 2 hours for liquids to empty from

the stomach, and 4 to 6 hours for solids to empty from the stomach. The anesthetist should recall the factors previously discussed that decrease gastric emptying time.

History and Preoperative Interview

The preoperative assessment begins with a complete review of the patient's medical history (preexisting hepatic or GI disease) including concomitant drug therapy and drug or latex allergies. Previous anesthetic records should be reviewed for patient responses to the administered anesthetic agents and techniques. In addition, the previous anesthetic record will provide information regarding airway management, laryngoscopy, and endotracheal intubation, and provides a synopsis of the perioperative period. Pertinent family history must also be elicited.

The chart should be examined for the patient's current prescriptive history and known drug or latex allergies. Patients with a history of atopy may be sensitive to the histamine-releasing pharmacologic agents such as morphine, thiopental, and atracurium. Allergies to local anesthetics, antibiotics, iodine, and adhesive tapes must also be noted, including the patient-specific response when exposed to these agents.

Patients must be questioned regarding the presence of gastric reflux. Symptoms include an acid or a sour taste and substernal or epigastric pain that does not radiate. Gastric reflux generally occurs with recumbancy. The symptoms are generally relieved with antacids and food. Patients at risk for gastric reflux include the parturient, patients with hiatal hernia, obese patients, patients with partial bowel obstruction, and patients with gastroparesis as a result of diabetic neuropathy. The anesthetist should be wary of patients with prolonged bowel obstruction, as the possible aspiration of fecal material is associated with increased mortality. The anesthetist must also inquire as to the NPO status of each and every patient immediately prior to the induction of anesthesia. Anesthesia providers go to great lengths to protect the airway from gastrointestinal secretions. The anesthetist must ask the following questions: (1) Is the stomach empty for the elective or emergency surgical procedure? (2) What food and fluid restrictions should be placed on the patient preoperatively? and (3) What prophylactic treatment is needed to minimize gastric volume and decrease hydrogen ion secretion? Prescribed NPO orders are variable, but in general, the patient is asked to withhold all solid food and drink at midnight when scheduled for an elective surgical procedure the following day. These general guidelines are modified for the neonate and young child.

Patients should also be queried regarding their dietary habits. Any patient who appears unusually thin should be assesed for eating disorders that may manifest in electrolyte imbalance. Adolescent girls and young women may be more vulnerable to disorders such as anorexia nervosa or bulimia. Patients who are suspected of having bulimia may reveal evidence of dental problems such as caries or enamel loss from the acidity of vomitus.

The patient should be questioned to elicit the general symptoms of hepatic or biliary dysfunction, including a history of anorexia, nausea, vomiting, diarrhea, weight loss, abdominal pain, ascites, jaundice, dark urine, pale stools, fever, chills, fatty food intolerance, easy bruising, or repeated epistaxis, and recent behavioral or neurologic changes. The anesthetist should directly question the patient to elicit a previous history of hepatitis or recreational or occupational exposure to hepatotoxins including environmental chemicals, alcohol, and illicit drugs. A history of alcohol consumption should be obtained from all patients. The alcoholic may consume as

many as six drinks per day for a considerable period of time. One shot of whiskey is equivalent to one bottle of beer, or one glass of wine. Alcoholics may also complain of pruritis and anorexia, and appear malnourished.

Incidences of acute abdominal pain accompanied by neurologic changes (confusion, hysteria, peripheral neuropathy), dark-colored urine (red or purple), or a family history of porphyria is suggestive of disease. The parturient with acute abdominal pain needs further evaluation because greater than 50% of parturients who have underlying porphyria will experience a crisis during pregnancy (Jensen, Fiddler, & Striepe, 1995).

Physical Examination

The conduct of the physical examination should focus on all organ systems. During the physical examination, the anesthetist should be attentive to the patient's general physical appearance. Patients with hepatic disease complain of fatigue, weight loss, and general weakness. Spider telangiectasis, gynecomastia, palmar erythema, and Dupuytren's contractures are evident during the physical examination. The extremities should be examined for evidence of bruising. Jaundice and scleral icterus are the hallmarks of hepatic disease. Icterus, a sign of hyperbilirubinemia, can be detected through an examination of the sclera. Patients with Gilbert's disease, an inherited deficiency of the glucuronyltransferase enzyme which is required for the hepatic uptake of unconjugated bilirubin, may have scleral icterus but have no symptoms of liver disease. Scleral icterus accompanying stressors such as fasting, hospitalization or recent illness, exertion, and sleep deprivation, with a lack of physical and laboratory finding of liver disease (other than an increase in unconjugated bilirubin) is suggestive of the disease. These patients do not require a consultant, and no changes in the anesthetic plan is necessitated by the disease.

There are a variety of cardiovascular alterations that accompany hepatic disease. True shunts as evidenced by spider angiomas produce a high cardiac output and a bounding pulse. Despite the increases in cardiac output, these patients have little cardiac reserve. An examination of the extremities and the dilated peripheral vessels (palmar erythema) provides evidence of a decrease in peripheral vascular resistance. A widened pulse pressure is noted with a peripheral blood pressure measurement. It should be noted that alcoholic cirrhotics will have a decrease in cardiac output, and may experience cardiac failure secondary to alcoholic cardiomyopathy. A preoperative ECG is essential to identify underlying ischemia or previous myocardial infarction.

The pulmonary system is generally compromised in patients with hepatic disease. Generally speaking, patients with hepatic disease (the majority of which results from alcoholism) have a long history of tobacco use. Accordingly, underlying chronic obstructive pulmonary disease may also accompany the pulmonary changes of hepatic disease. However, patients with hepatic disease have impaired gas exchange as a result of ventilation/perfusion mismatch, atelectasis as a result of acities, and intrapulmonary arterivenous shunts (Furukawa, Hara, Yasumoto, & Inkuchi, 1984; Rodriguez, Roisen, Roca, Agusti, Mastai, Wagner, & Bosch, 1987). Specific pulmonary abnormalities include pleural effusions, intrapulmonary shunts, restrictive defects due to acities, and ventilation–perfusion mismatch. Physical findings differ markedly from patients with cardiac disease. Arterial O_2 desaturation occurs in the upright position with a decrease in the subjective complaint of dyspnea in the supine position. A preoperative chest radiograph may identify pleural effusions and other pulmonary parenchymal pathology.

An examination of the abdomen may reveal previous scars that may assist the patient in recalling previous anesthetics and surgical procedures. Underlying portal hypertension or vena caval obstruction will produce prominent superficial veins in the abdominal wall. Pressure applied over the liver may result in distension of the ipsilateral jugular vein (hepatic–jugular reflux).

Patients who present with acute right upper quadrant pain, shaking chills, fever, nausea and vomiting, and increases in the white blood count generally have cholecystitis or cholangitis. These patients may present with acute onset of jaundice. The presence of ascites is a clear indication of severe hepatic dysfunction. Patients with acities are generally given the diuretic spironolactone, an aldosterone antagonist. Ascites accumulation increases the patient's body weight and is physically identified by abdominal distension, dilated upper abdominal veins, and an inverted umbilicus. The ascitic fluid may displace the diaphragm cephalad, decreasing lung capacity and resulting in the subjective complaint of dyspnea. This abdominal distension increases the patient's risk for gastroesophageal reflux and aspiration. The hepatologist may initiate elective paracentesis prior to surgery.

Tenderness or increased size of abdominal organs can be determined with abdominal palpation. Pain over the liver margins suggests congestion accompanying congestive heart failure, or the inflammation of hepatitis or gallbladder disease (Frank, 1989). Positive findings suggest a referral for further evaluation. Patients with viral hepatitis are at risk for deterioration in liver function and present a risk to members of the health care team. Hypersplenism may also contribute to abdominal distension. Hypersplenism is probably etiologic in the decrease in circulating platelets.

Renal failure is common in patients with advanced hepatic disease. The etiology of renal failure may be either prerenal azotemia, acute tubular necrosis, or the poorly understood hepatorenal syndrome. Fluid administration must be carefully monitored as the renin-angiotensin system is activated. Cirrhotics will have an underlying metabolic alkalosis, and accordingly, may have dangerously low serum K^+ levels.

Diagnostic Data

Preoperative screening laboratory tests have been used to detect asymptomatic disease, but have been found to be expensive and generally have little impact on patient care. In fact, significant hepatic disease must be present before abnormal laboratory tests are obtained. Routine chemistry panels may detect clearly elevated serum enzyme levels in voluntary hospital surgical admission in 1 out of 700 patients, whereas the incidence of clinical jaundice occurs in 1 out of 2540 patients (Schemel, 1976). Abnormalities in appropriately ordered laboratory tests will assist in the determination between hepatic parenchymal disease and obstruction.

Patients with hepatic disease undergoing major surgical procedures should have the following laboratory indices: serum electrolyte analysis (Na^+, K^+, and Cl^-), complete blood count, creatinine, BUN, blood glucose, albumin, arterial blood gas analysis, and urinalysis. Abnormal clotting and bleeding are also common in patients with hepatic disease. Laboratory evaluation of coagulation should include a prothrombin time (including an international normalized ratio INR value), activated partial thromboplastin time, quantitative platelet count, and bleeding time (to determine platelet function). Recall that patients with hypersplenism may have a decrease in circulating platelets. Hepatic disease decreases production of the vitamin K-dependent clotting factors (II, VII, IX, X) and reduces the plasma concentrations of factors V, XIII, and fibrinogen. In addition, ongoing GI bleeding will decrease the circulating half lives of these factors because they are consumed to arrest bleeding.

Laboratory tests considered *liver function tests,* which are useful for the differentiation of hepatic disease, include the determination of serum albumin, transaminase levels, bilirubin, and alkaline phosphatase levels. Table 13–9 lists the typically ordered liver function tests and the differential diagnosis. As previously discussed, the hepatocytes manufacture albumin, so hepatic

TABLE 13–9. Liver Function Tests and Differential Diagnosis

Hepatic Dysfunction	Bilirubin	Transaminase Enzyme	Alkaline Phosphatase
Prehepatic	Unconjugated	Normal	Normal
Intrahepatic	Conjugated	Elevated	Normal to elevated
Extrahepatic	Conjugated	Normal to elevated	Elevated

From Waugaman, W. R., Foster, S. D., & Rigor, B. M. (Eds.). (1992). Principles and practice of nurse anesthesia (2nd. ed., p. 390). Norwalk, CT: Appleton & Lange.

dysfunction will lead to decreases in production. Levels below 2.5 g/dL are suggestive of chronic hepatocellular disease or malnutrition. Because the half life of albumin is 14 to 17 days, serum albumin is not a sensitive indicator of hepatocellular disease.

Elevations in transaminase levels generally parallel the degree of hepatocellular dysfunction (Greenberger, 1989). In general, transaminases appear in the blood as they are released following heptocellular death. The transaminases most commonly determined are serum alanine aminotransferase (ALT), previously known as serum glutamate pyruvate transaminase (SGOT), and aspartate transaminase (AST), previously known as serum glutamic-oxaloacetic transaminase (SGOT). Alanine aminotransferase is the most sensitive of heptocellular damage because it is contained within the hepatocyte. Aspartate transaminase is present in extrahepatic tissue including the lungs, heart, and skeletal muscle. Accordingly, skeletal trauma or repeated intramuscular injections may produce increases in this transaminase. Serum ALT and AST determinations should be below 35 IU/L. Increases to 300 IU/L are suggestive of cholestasis or carcinomatous disease of the liver.

Bilirubin is the end product of heme metabolism, and is bound to albumin and delivered via the circulation to the liver. When bilirubin levels exceed the normal serum concentrations of 0.3 mg/dL to 1.2 mg/dL and approach levels in excess of 3 mg/dL, clinical jaundice becomes evident. Increases in the unconjugated fractions are suggestive of biliary tract obstruction, Gilbert's disease as previously discussed, and/or hepatocellular disease.

Alkaline phosphatase is present in the bile duct cells and will increase in the presence of bile duct obstruction. Alkaline phosphatase enzyme determination has been used to differentiate between bile duct obstruction and hepatocellular injury; however, the presence of extrahepatic tissue stores of alkaline phosphatase may decrease the specificity.

Transaminase lactic dehydrogenase (LDH) is found in a number of tissues including erythrocytes, skeletal muscles, and the heart and liver. Accordingly, the measurement of plasma LDH is an insensitive indicator of hepatocellular injury. However, the determination of the isoenzyme-5 fraction is thought to be hepatic-specific (Viegas & Stoelting, 1979).

The quantification of a plasma ammonia level may be helpful in the patient with hepatic disease. Deamination of amino acids in the gut results in the formation of ammonia. Intestinal bacteria are also active in the formation of ammonia. Ammonia is transported via the portal blood from the intestine to the liver, where it is converted to urea by the ornithine cycle. The formation of urea from ammonia removes ammonia from the body fluids. With significant hepatic disease, urea is not formed and ammonia accumulates in the blood. Plasma ammonia levels can rise dramatically, producing hepatic coma and death.

Table 13-10 summarizes the differential diagnosis of prehepatic, intrahepatic (hepatocellular), and posthepatic (cholestatic) dysfunction and the accompanying changes in serum protein and transaminase levels.

Mortality Accompanying Hepatic Disease

Mortality from hepatic disease has doubled in the last three decades, primarily as a result of an increase in alcohol consumption (Aranha & Greenlee, 1986; Lebach, 1975; Powell-Jackson, Greenway, & Williams, 1982; Schmidt, 1976). At the conclusion of the preoperative examination and laboratory evaluation, the surgical risk of patients with hepatic disease can be assessed. A number of studies support the conclusion that patients with significant hepatic disease have an increase in perioperative mortality. The incumbent perioperative risks are not necessarily related to the selected anesthetic agents or techniques. This increased mortality is the result of a progression in the underlying hepatic disease, a decrease in hepatic synthetic function (precipitating coagulopathies), a progression of extrahepatic complications (renal failure, encephalopathy), and alterations in the pharmacokinetics and pharmacodynamics of adminis-

TABLE 13–10. Liver Function Tests and Differential Diagnoses

Hepatic Dysfunction	Bilirubin	Transaminase Enzymes	Alkaline Phosphatase	Causes
Prehepatic	Increased unconjugated fraction	Normal	Normal	Hemolysis, hematoma, resorption, bilirubin overload from whole blood
Intrahepatic (hepatocellular)	Increased conjugated fraction	Markedly increased	Normal to slightly increased	Virus, drugs, sepsis, hypoxemia, cirrhosis
Posthepatic (cholestatic)	Increased conjugated fraction	Normal to slightly increased	Markedly increased	Stones, sepsis

From Stoelting, R. K., & Dierdorf, S. F. (1993). Diseases of the liver and biliary tract. In R. K. Stoelting & S. F. Dierdorf (Eds.), Anesthesia and Coexisting Disease (p. 257). New York: Churchill Livingstone.

TABLE 13–11. Modified Child's Classification of Operative Risk

Variable	Group A	Group B	Group C
Bilirubin (mg/dL)	< 2.3	2.3 to 2.9	> 3.0
Albumin (g/dL)	> 3.5	3.0 to 3.5	< 3.0
Ascites	None	Easy control	Poor control
Neurologic disorders	None	Minimal	Advanced
Nutrition	Excellent	Good	Poor
Surgical risk (mortality rate)	Good (10%)	Moderate (10% to 30%)	Poor (> 40%)

tered drugs (Greene, 1981). Progressive hepatic dysfunction following anesthesia and surgery depends on the degree of perioperative hepatic dysfunction, the development of intraoperative and postoperative hypoxia, and intraoperative alterations in hepatic blood flow.

The classification of operative mortality (Pugh, Murray-Lyon, Dawson, Pietroni & Williams, 1973), is a predictive assessment of operative mortality following major abdominal surgical procedures. Table 13–11 describes this classification.

Pathophysiology

Parenchymal Hepatic Disease

Parenchymal hepatic disease produces a global inflammation of the liver (hepatitis) and can be simply classified as either acute or chronic. Table 13–12 lists the major etiologies of parenchymal hepatic disease. Parenchymal hepatic disease may present as acute viral hepatitis, chronic active hepatitis, alcoholic hepatitis, or drug-induced hepatitis. Hepatitis produces progressive alterations in hepatic structure (inflammation and destruction of hepatocytes with fibrosis) and metabolic function. The hepatic metabolic reserve is compromised with the destruction of hepatocytes. The classic features of hepatic disease (malaise, weakness, exhaustion, weight loss, jaundice, dark urine, hypoalbuminemia, portal hypertension, bleeding varices, ascites, and abdominal pain) and alterations in cardiovascular, pulmonary, and renal function then become clinically evident.

Hepatitis A is transmitted through fecal–oral contact (contaminated food and water); however, blood and saliva transmission are also possible. In many cases the infection is subclinical and the affected individual is anicteric. The infection is generally self-limiting and does not progress to chronic hepatitis. The virus is easily trans-

TABLE 13–12. Etiologies of Parenchymal Hepatic Disease

Viral Infection

Chronic active and chronic persistent hepatitis

Viral Etiology	Transmission	Transmission risks	Incubation	Prognosis
Hepatitis A	Fecal–oral saliva	Fecal contact, food contamination	2 to 6 weeks	Self-limited, rarely fatal, no chronic infection
Hepatitis B	Blood, serum, sexual contact	Transfusion, needlesticks, sexual contacts	1 to 6 months	Chronic infection, cirrhosis may develop; 2% mortality
Hepatitis C (non-A, non-B)	Blood, serum, sexual contact, fecal–oral?	As above	1 to 4 months	As above
Hepatitis D	Concurrent hepatitis B infection	As hepatitis B	2 to 9 weeks	Can result in fulminant hepatic failure; 30% mortality
Hepatitis E	Fecal–oral	Food contamination, poor sanitation	2 to 9 weeks	Spontaneous resolution; mortality < 1%

Drugs

Acetaminophen (Tylenol)
Halothane

Chemicals

Ethyl alcohol

Inborn errors of metabolism

Wilson's disease

Miscellaneous

α_1 antitrypsinogen deficiency
Hemochromatosis
Cystic fibrosis

mitted to health care workers who fail to adhere to strict hand-washing techniques and use of universal precautions (eg, glove use) when handling body fluids. It has been estimated that 50% of the US adult population may have serologic evidence of a previous infection (Krugman, Ward, & Giles, 1962). Blood transfusions are rarely responsible for hepatitis A infection. Banked blood is not tested for the presence of hepatitis A virus.

Hepatitis B, unlike hepatitis A, is a progressive and more serious infection; 3% of cases can progress to a chronic hepatitis. Hepatitis B virus is present in the blood and serous fluids of the infected individual. The virus is hardy, surviving up to 1 week in dried blood. The diagnosis is based on the detection of hepatitis B surface antigen in the plasma. Individuals at risk include intravenous (IV) drug users, those with multiple sex partners, patients who require hemodialysis, and health care workers who are exposed to blood and body fluids. The Centers for Disease Control and Prevention (CDC) recommends that all health care providers receive a hepatitis B vaccination (Reingold, Kane, & Hightower, 1988). Transmission to health care workers can occur with exposure to blood of an infected individual through inadvertent needlesticks; blood contact with open cuts or mucosa; or blood that comes into contact with the eyes. Donor-banked blood is routinely screened for hepatitis B surface antigen, although hepatitis B is estimated to account for 5% to 10% of posttransfusion hepatitis.

Hepatitis D (delta hepatitis) is etiologic in patients with hepatitis B and complicates the clinical course of those infected with hepatitis B. The delta virus consists of a ribonucleic acid (RNA) strand that requires concurrent hepatitis B infection for replication. The delta virus and hepatitis B may be contracted together, or the delta virus can develop as a superinfection in individuals with hepatitis B. Intravenous drug abusers and patients who receive multiple transfusions are particularly at risk. Hepatitis D infection resolves as the hepatitis B surface antigen is cleared from the plasma. Mortality may approach 20% in patients who fail to initially recover.

Hepatitis C (formerly known as non-A, non-B hepatitis) has generally been attributed to cases of posttransfusion hepatitis. An enteric form of hepatitis C viral infection is associated with up to 40% of cases in which no blood transfusion was documented (Dienstag, Alaama, Mosley, Redeker, & Purcell, 1977). The hepatitis C viral genome has been successfully cloned, and this has facilitated the development of a sensitive and specific serologic test. Since its development, the number of cases of hepatitis C posttransfusion hepatitis has dropped tenfold, to approximately 6% (Mazze, 1994).

A number of viruses including Epstein–Barr virus, Coxsackie virus, herpes simplex, and cytomegalovirus may produce a hepatitis-like clinical picture. Nonviral etiologies including bacteria, rickettsia, and certain fungi may produce hepatitis with accompanying jaundice.

Cholestasis

Cholestasis, an impairment of bile flow, may develop as a result of intrahepatic obstruction or extrahepatic obstruction (obstructive jaundice) of the biliary tree, or may be precipitated by drugs (phenothiazines, synthetic estrogens, and phenytoin, to name a few). The signs and symptoms of cholestasis include pruritus and jaundice. Extrahepatic biliary obstruction is characterized by progressive jaundice, dark urine, and pale stools. Accompanying fever and chills are suggestive of an accompanying cholangitis. As previously discussed, there is also a failure in the absorption of the fat-soluble vitamins in the absence of bile salts. Extrahepatic cholestasis is readily amenable to surgical treatment (eg, the removal of a common bile duct stone). The clinical features that differentiate cholestasis from parenchymal hepatic disease include the development of hyperbilirubinemia, elevation of bile acids, and an increased alkaline phosphatase with a minimal to moderate elevation in transaminases (Brown, 1988).

Cirrhosis

Parenchymal hepatic disease may progress to the destruction of the hepatic architecture, which is then replaced with collagen. The loss of cellular elements and the disruption of the vascular and bile channels within the liver produce irreversible alterations in hepatic function. The resulting increased resistance to intrahepatic blood flow is etiologic in the development of portal hypertension. The majority of hepatic blood flow is now dependent on the hepatic artery, which transports less O_2 than portal blood, further compromising hepatic oxygenation. Far-reaching systemic and end-organ effects soon develop, such as impaired oxygenation, altered central nervous system function (hepatic encephalopathy), the development of coagulopathies, and altered protein synthesis. The most frequent etiologies of hepatic failure are viral hepatitis (with the exception of hepatitis A) and alcoholic hepatitis.

The development of portal hypertension alters venous portal system collaterals (veins of the esophagus and rectum, stoma of a colostomy, and abdominal adhesions) which dilate with blood. These sites may become active sources of bleeding (particularly esophageal varices), and are extremely difficult to control. Patients with esophageal varices should not electively have esophageal intubations with a stethoscope, temperature probe, or nasal or oral gastric tubes. Table 13–13 lists the diagnostic features of portal hypertension.

TABLE 13–13. Diagnostic Features of Portal Hypertension

Anorexia and loss of skeletal mass, particularly of the head, neck, and arms

Hepatomegaly, splenomegaly, and ascites

Palmar erythema

Subcutaneous bleeding with minor trauma

Hematocrit, 30% to 35%

Hyponatremia

With normal renal function, BUN[a] < 10 mg/dL

With renal insufficiency, BUN > 20

Mild to moderate elevation in alkaline phosphatase, plasma bilirubin, and transaminases

[a] BUN, blood urea nitrogen.

From Waugaman, W. R., Foster, S. D., & Rigor, B. M. (1992). (Eds.). Principles and practice of nurse anesthesia (2nd ed., p. 386). Norwalk, CT: Appleton & Lange.

Perianesthetic Management of Gastrointestinal and Hepatic Dysfunction

General Considerations

Anesthesia management for patients with gastrointestinal dysfunction (eg, hiatal hernia, gastroesophageal reflux, intestinal obstruction) requires the development of an anesthetic care plan that initially is focused on protection of the airway and lungs from gastric secretions. In addition, intravascular volume may be depleted which may contribute to marked changes in cardiovascular stability with the administration of anesthetic induction agents.

Anesthetic induction must be preceded by measures to increase gastric pH (administration of the non-particulate antacid bicitra), decrease gastric acid secretion (H_2 antagonist administration, cimetidine) and enhance gastric emptying (metoclopramide). In addition, the administration of metoclopramide will increase LES tone. Patients with gastric distension may have a nasogastric tube in place for decompression. This tube should be attached to suction, or left open to drain freely during anesthetic induction. The presence of a nasogastric tube may provide a false sense of security; complete emptying of the stomach cannot be guaranteed despite the placement of these tubes. These individuals are still at risk for gastric regurgitation and aspiration.

Following preoxygenation with a tight-fitting face mask, anesthetic induction is facilitated with an IV agent and an appropriate muscle relaxant (either succinylcholine or a suitable alternative such as rocuronium). This anesthetic induction sequence may incorporate titrated doses of fentanyl or another opioid, as well as a benzodiazepine. During the induction sequence, progressive sedation may place the patient at risk of regurgitation and aspiration and decrease LES tone. Cricoid pressure, when properly applied, compresses the lumen of the pharynx between the cricoid and cervical vertebrae. Cricoid pressure is applied by an assistant and maintained until verification of successful endotracheal intubation.

The anesthetist must continue efforts to protect the airway from GI secretions during emergency from anesthesia. Prior to emergence, the anesthetist should document the reversal from neuromuscular blockade via a peripheral nerve stimulator. The patient must be responding appropriately with intact airway reflexes prior to endotracheal extubation. The patient is best placed in the lateral decubitis position for transportation to the recovery room.

Patients with acute or chronic active hepatitis should not undergo elective surgical procedures. Surgical mortality approaches 10% in patients with acute hepatitis, with a subsequent 12% incidence of morbidity in those who survive surgery (Harville & Dummerskill, 1963). Patients with concurrent liver disease who undergo laparotomy have approximately a 30% mortality (Powell-Jackson, Greenway, & Williams, 1982). Mortality was 100% in patients with liver disease secondary to viral or alcoholic etiologies. A 1986 examination of hepatic mortality in the United States found a 91% mortality rate in patients whom the prothrombin time by more than 2.5 seconds (Aranha & Greenlee, 1986).

This poor prognosis is likely due to hepatic blood flow alterations that attend anesthesia and surgery. With compromised hepatic blood flow and O_2 delivery, further reductions precipitate hepatic necrosis in the immediate postoperative period. There is no clear relationship between reductions in hepatic blood flow and administered anesthetic agents, although isoflurane has been shown to have minimal effects on hepatic blood flow in an animal model (Gelman, Fowler, & Smith, 1983). Recall that hypotension, hypovolemia, hypoxia, hypercarbia, and insufficient suppression of autonomic reflexes during *light* anesthesia, as well as positive-pressure ventilation, will produce hepatic arterial vasoconstriction. Hypercarbia elicits splanchnic vasoconstriction, decreasing hepatic blood flow. Accordingly, the intraoperative $Paco_2$ should be maintained in the normal range (35 mmHg to 40 mmHg). The site of operative intervention also influences the alterations in hepatic blood flow. Abdominal surgical procedures interfere with splanchnic blood flow as a result of direct handling of intra-abdominal structures, the placement of retractors, and the placement of abdominal packs. Elevations in transaminase levels will occur following abdominal procedures in patients without hepatic disease and is dependent on the duration of the procedure (Clarke, Hoggart, & Lavery, 1976). Table 13–14 lists a number of factors that alter hepatic blood flow in the surgical patient.

Patients with hepatic disease should be maintained

TABLE 13-14. Factors Altering Hepatic Blood Flow in Surgical Patients

Patient Position

Surgical manipulation of splanchnic vasculature

Placement of retractors, surgical packs

Administration of vasoactive agents
Vasoconstriction (ephedrine, phenylephrine)

Positive-pressure ventilation (including PEEP)

Metabolic factors
$Paco_2$; hypercapnia; release of catecholamines (eg, vasoconstriction); hypocapnia; positive end-expiratory pressure; decreased venous return
Hypoxia; arteriolar vasoconstriction
pH

Blood volume

Preexisting hepatic disease

Inhalation anesthetic agents

---

on their drug regimen throughout the preoperative period. The selection of anesthetic agents must take into account the alterations in pharmacokinetics and pharmacodynamics which accompany hepatic disease. Decreased protein binding (decreased albumin production which increases the active drug fraction) and increases in the volume of distribution require careful, deliberate titration of all IV agents. Of the opioids, alfentanil has been demonstrated to have a decreased plasma clearance, producing a prolonged duration of action in patients with cirrhosis (Ferrier, Marty, Bouffars, Haberer, Levron, & Duvaldestin, 1985). Meperidine clearance is also substantially decreased in patients with hepatic disease. Fentanyl and sufentanil have a predictable duration of action in the cirrhotic, as there is no alteration in pharmacokinetics.

The clearance of benzodiazepines (phase I reaction) is susbtantially decreased and a prolonged duration of action can be expected in patients with hepatic disease. Although midazolam is widely used because of its favorable pharmacokinetic profile (short duration of action, brief hypnotic effects in comparison to diazepam), continued sedation from prolonged elimination can occur in patients with cirrhosis (MacGilchrist, Birnie, Cook, Scobie, Murray, Watkinson, & Brodie, 1986).

Beta-blockers, which may be employed for the control of portal hypertension, have a prolonged duration of action due to decreased clearance in the cirrhotic patient. The clearance of lidocaine is likewise impaired, requiring reduced doses (Thompson, Melmon, Richardson, Cohn, Steinbrum, Cudihee, & Rowland, 1973). The clearance of the H_2 antagonists cimetidine and ranitidine is reduced in patients with ascites and hypoproteinemia (Ziemniak, Bernard, & Schentag, 1983).

In severe hepatic disease, synthetic functions, including the production of plasma cholinesterase may be decreased. The administration of succinylcholine theoretically will lead to an increased and unpredictable duration of action, as succinylcholine hydrolysis depends on adequate concentrations of plasma cholinesterase. Even in cases of fulminant hepatic failure, succinylcholine duration is unlikely to be prolonged (Ward, Knight, Strunin, & Strunin, 1976).

The anesthetist should recall that the nondepolarizing muscle relaxants are water soluble and are excreted in the urine. The long-duration agents D-tubocurarine and pancuronium, both of which have large volumes of distribution in patients with hepatic disease, will have a prolonged duration of action. The steroidal muscle relaxants vecuronium and rocuronium do not have altered pharmacokinetics in patients with cirrhosis (Arden, Lyman, Castagnoli, Cantell, Cannon, & Miller, 1988; Magorian, Wood, Cauldwell, & Miller, 1991). Atracurium, which is not dependent on end organs for elimination, has unchanged pharmacokinetics and pharmacodynamics in patients with hepatic disease. The monitoring of neuromuscular function should always accompany the administration of nondepolarizing muscle relaxants.

General considerations for the patient with hepatic dysfunction undergoing general anesthesia must include consideration of the need for invasive monitoring. Each patient should be assessed on an individual basis to determine the need for aterial and central venous pressure monitoring. The choice is based in part on the planned surgical procedure and the extent of the underlying cardiovascular alterations. Significant bleeding may occur during intra-abdominal procedures in the patient with portal hypertension. Accordingly, one or two large-bore IV lines that are warmed should be established. All IV agents should be carefully titrated to the desired effect. Intraoperative determinations of electrolytes, arterial blood gas, blood glucose, and hemoglobin and hematocrit may be required during lengthy procedures. The anesthetist must maintain the patient's core temperature by raising the operating room temperature, utilizing fluid warmers, warming blankets, or forced air-warming devices.

The choice of regional anesthesia must take into account the potential for underlying coagulation dysfunction. Prior to the use of a regional anesthetic technique, the prothrombin time and activated partial thromboplastin time should be immediately determined.

The selected anesthetic technique must be judiciously administered to minimize the occurrence of hypotension, which will decrease hepatic blood flow. Circulating blood volume, arterial blood pressure, and cardiac output should be optimal. Accordingly, deliberate hypotension should not be considered in an attempt to minimize surgical blood loss.

Renal dysfunction can accompany hepatic disease and must be carefully preserved during the intraoperative period. The placement of a urinary catheter will assist in the assessment of renal perfusion. Furosemide and/or mannitol may be required to maintain urine output (Gelman, 1989).

Postoperative Considerations

Postoperatively, appropriate ventilatory support including O_2, mechanical ventilation, or both to maintain oxygenation is important. Body temperature should be maintained in the postoperative period using adjunctive support such as a Bair Hugger or other body warming system. Gastrointestinal secretions should be evaluated for the presence of blood. Postoperative medications for pain should be administered as needed and the patient's disease state considered when evaluating drug response, uptake, and metabolism. Postoperative laboratory findings should be evaluated and treatment ordered accordingly.

▶ ENDOCRINE SYSTEM

The anesthetic management of the patient with a preexisting endocrine disorder can be extremely challenging. The formulation of an anesthetic plan of care may require consultation with an endocrinologist. Commonly encountered endocrine disorders include diabetes mellitus and hypo- or hyperthyroidism. Occasionally the anesthetist will be confronted with rare and complex disorders (eg, the genetically linked disorders that produce multiple airway abnormalities).

Hormone Structure and Function

The endocrine system synthesizes and secretes mobile chemical messengers to coordinate intracellular communications, which allows multicellular organisms to maintain and adapt to changes in their internal and external environments. The classic definition of a hormone emphasizes that these chemical messengers are synthesized in one organ and transported by the blood to act on a target organ. However, hormones may also act on adjacent cells, or the cell from which they were synthesized.

Structurally, hormones are classified as amino acid derivatives (histamine), protein derivatives (polypeptides like insulin), steroids (androgens, estrogens), or fatty acid derivatives (prostaglandins). Hormones produce their action by combining with a specific cell receptor. These receptor sites vary according to the type of hormone involved. Proteins, peptides, and catecholamines combine with a cell membrane receptor. Steroid hormones bind with receptors located in the cell cytoplasm. Thyroid hormones bind with receptors located in the cell nucleus. The onset and duration of the action of hor-

mones can vary from seconds to days and weeks. The major hormones and their respective secreting glands, major actions, and structures are listed in Table 13-15. Sex hormones and those secreted by the placenta are not included.

Anatomy and Physiology

Hypothalamus and Pituitary

The hypothalamus is located in the middle, basal forebrain, just superior to the pituitary gland. It is intimately associated with the third ventricle and communicates with the limbic system at all levels. The hypothalamus acts to control homeostasis by regulating pituitary gland hormones. The hypothalamus secretes trophic and inhibitory hormones into the hypothalamic–pituitary portal system. These hormones in turn cause the stimulation or inhibition of the hormones of the anterior pituitary. Hormones of the posterior pituitary gland (vasopressin and oxytocin) are synthesized in the hypothalamus and transported down axons arising from either the supraoptic or paraventricular nuclei (Robertson, 1995). These hormones are secreted into the systemic circulation from the posterior pituitary gland. Antidiuretic hormone or vasopressin arises from the supraoptic nuclei, while oxytocin arises from the paraventricular nuclei (Guyton & Hall, 1996; Jeffcoate, 1993).

The pituitary gland lies in the sella turcica below the hypothalamus and is composed of two distinct portions—the anterior and posterior pituitary. The posterior pituitary is derived from neural tissue and is basically an extension of the hypothalamus. The anterior pituitary originates from an invagination of the pharyngeal epithelium, Rathke's pouch. Some of the pituitary gland hormones and their associated physiology and pathophysiology present more commonly and provide more concern, from an anesthetic viewpoint, than others. According to Jeffcoate (1993), adrenocorticotropin (ACTH), or corticotropin, is under the influence of corticotropin-releasing hormone (CRH) from the hypothalamus. Adrenocorticotropin binds with cell membrane receptors in the adrenal cortex to stimulate the release of cortisol. It is also the main pigmentary hormone. Thyroid-stimulating hormone (TSH) is released from the anterior pituitary secondary to stimulation of hypothalamic thyrotropin (TRH). It in turn stimulates the release of thyroid hormones from the thyroid gland. Growth hormone-releasing hormone and somatostatin secreted by the hypothalamus stimulate and inhibit the release of growth hormone. Growth hormone stimulates the formation of insulin-like growth factors (IGFs) in the liver and periphery. Hypothalamic osmoreceptors, baroreceptors, and adrenergic stimulation regulate the release of ADH. Nausea produces ADH secretion 5 to 50 times that of normal levels. Oxytocin is released in response to nipple stimu-

TABLE 13–15. Major Hormones and Their Respective Secreting Glands, Major Actions, and Structures

Hormone	Producing Gland	Actions	Structure
Growth hormone	Anterior pituitary	Growth of cells and tissues	Protein/peptide
Adrenocorticotropin	Anterior pituitary	Stimulates secretion of adrenocortical hormones	Protein/peptide
Thyroid-stimulating hormone	Anterior pituitary	Stimulates secretion of thyroid hormones	Protein/peptide
Follicle-stimulating hormone	Anterior pituitary	Stimulates preovulatory follicle growth; stimulates sperm formation	Protein/peptide
Luteinizing hormone	Anterior pituitary	Helps cause ovulation; stimulates secretion of sex hormones	Protein/peptide
Prolactin	Anterior pituitary	Development of breasts and secretion of milk	Protein/peptide
Antidiuretic hormone	Posterior pituitary	Renal conservation of water; vasoconstriction	Peptide
Oxytocin	Posterior pituitary	Uterine contraction and milk secretion	Peptide
Cortisol	Adrenal cortex	Metabolism of fats, carbohydrates, and proteins	Steroid
Aldosterone	Adrenal cortex	Decreases sodium excretion and increases potassium excretion	Steroid
Epinephrine	Adrenal medulla	Multiple metabolic and pressor effects	Tyrosine derivative
Norepinephrine	Adrenal medulla	Multiple metabolic and pressor effects	Tyrosine derivative
Thyroxine	Thyroid	Cell growth and metabolism	Tyrosine derivative
Triiodothyronine	Thyroid	Cell growth and metabolism	Tyrosine derivative
Calcitonin	Thyroid	Promotes calcium deposition in bones (decreases extracellular calcium)	Peptide
Parathormone	Parathyroid	Regulates extracellular calcium concentration controlling Calcium absorption from the gut Excretion of calcium by the kidneys Release of calcium by the bones	Polypeptide
Insulin	Pancreas	Glucose transport across cell membrane	Polypeptide
Glucagon	Pancreas	Increase release of glucose from liver	Polypeptide

lation and stretching of the lower genital tract (Ferguson's reflex) (Steer, 1990).

Pancreas

The pancreas weighs from 60 g to 140 g and is positioned in the curvature of the duodenum near the spleen and left kidney (Brown, 1991). The endocrine portion of the pancreas is made up of 1 to 2 million islets of Langerhans, each approximately 0.3 mm in diameter. Because these cells secrete insulin and glucagon directly into the bloodstream, they are organized around small capillaries. The islets are further subdivided into alpha, beta, and delta cells. Beta cells constitute approximately 60% of the islet cells and secrete insulin. The pancreas secretes about 0.5 to 1.0 units of insulin per hour. Alpha cells secrete glucagon and make up about 25% of the total. The remaining 10% are delta cells and secrete somatostatin. These hormones are necessary for fat, carbohydrate, and protein metabolism (Jeffcoate, 1993; Guyton & Hall, 1996).

The exocrine portion constitutes about 80% of the gland and is made up of the acinar cells. These cells secrete digestive juices into the duodenum. The pancreas secretes 1.5 L to 3.0 L of an isosmotic alkaline fluid to aid in digestion each day. This fluid consists of various enzymes and proenzymes. The main proteolytic enzymes are trypsin, chymotrypsin, carboxypolypeptidase, ribonuclease, and deoxyribonuclease. The main lipid enzymes are lipase and cholesterol esterase; the main carbohydrate enzyme is amylase (Jeffcoate, 1993; Guyton & Hall, 1996).

Insulin, glucagon, and pancreatic polypeptides are secreted by cholinergic and beta-adrenergic stimuli. Acetylcholine, gastrin, cholecystokinin, and secretin released during digestion stimulate the acinar to secrete enzymes and sodium bicarbonate. The pancreas also contains cells that secrete pancreatic polypeptide which is comprised of 36 amino acids. The exact function and importance of pancreatic polypeptide are unknown (Bonner-Weir, 1995).

Insulin is composed of two peptide chains, 21 and 30 amino acids in length, linked by two sulfhydryl bridges (Halban & Weir, 1995). The pancreas secretes insulin every 13 minutes without stimulation. Secretion of insulin also occurs in response to blood glucose, glucagon, lysine and leucine, growth hormone, vagal stimulation, and other hormones. Hypocalcemia, norepinephrine, and somatostatin inhibit insulin secretion. Because insulin and glucagon produce opposite effects on carbohydrate metabolism, the pancreas secretes these hormones in an integral fashion. Insulin activates glycogen synthesis, inhibition of lipase and lipolysis, prevention of ketone formation, and transport of glucose across cell membranes.

Thyroid and Parathyroids

The thyroid gland lies just below the larynx and anterior and lateral to the trachea. It weighs 20 g to 25 g and is innervated by the superior and recurrent laryngeal nerves (Jeffcoate, 1993). Vascular supply to the thyroid gland is via the superior and inferior thyroid arteries and is 4 to 160 mL/min/100 g, one half the flow to the kidneys. The gland contains closed follicles that are filled with a substance known as colloid. Thyroglobulin is the main constituent of colloid. Cuboidal epithelial cells line and secrete into the follicles. Extracellular iodides are used to form the main thyroid hormones, thyroxin (T4) and triiodothyronine (T3), as components of thyroglobulin (Guyton & Hall, 1996).

Thyroid hormones are released in response to stimulation by the anterior pituitary gland hormone, TSH. Thyroxine and T3 are then cleaved from thyroglobulin and released as free hormone with 90% of the hormones released being T4. Thyroxine and T3 are 99.98% and 99.7%, respectively, bound to plasma proteins—thyroid-binding globulin, albumin, and transthyretin—for transport to the tissues. Thyroxine is deiodinated in the peripheral tissues to become T3 so that most of the action of the thyroid gland is from T3. Equivalent amounts (about 35 µg per day) of T3 and reverse T3 are produced daily; the latter is biologically inactive. Thyroid hormones produce profound effects on the growth, development, and metabolic processes of many different tissues. For example, thyroid hormone is essential for normal brain development in the fetus. In adults, thyroid hormone has a profound effect on basal metabolic, cardiac, and hepatic rates (Usala, 1995).

The thyroid and parathyroid glands share a common blood supply. Parathyroid glands may number from 1 to 12, but there are usually four, one behind each of the upper and lower poles of the thyroid (Livolsi, 1995). Each parathyroid gland measures 2 mm to 7 mm in length, 2 mm to 4 mm wide, and 0.5 mm to 2.0 mm thick, and may appear as dark brown fat when viewed macroscopically (Livolsi, 1995). Each parathyroid gland consists of chief cells that secrete most of the parathyroid hormone and oxyphil cells whose function is unclear (Guyton & Hall, 1996). The major function of parathyroid hormone is the maintenance of a normal level of calcium in the extracellular fluid.

A detected decrease in serum calcium ion concentration stimulates the release of parathyroid hormone. Parathyroid hormone binds with cell membrane receptors on bone and in the renal tubule. Calcium and phosphate are released from bone. At the renal tubule, calcium and H^+ ions are reabsorbed while phosphate and bicarbonate are excreted (Guyton & Hall, 1996).

Adrenal Glands

The adrenal glands each weigh roughly 4 g and lie at the superior poles of the kidneys, at the level of the 11th thoracic to the first lumbar vertebrae (Jeffcoate, 1993). The adrenal gland is composed of a central portion, the medulla, enclosed in the cortex. The adrenal gland produces about 50 different hormones, but only a few have importance. The medulla makes up about 20% of the gland and is the main site of synthesis for the catecholamines epinephrine, norepinephrine, and dopamine (White, Pescovitz, & Cutler, 1995). The cortex secretes mineralocorticoids, glucocorticoids, and androgens. Mineralocorticoids act primarily on electrolyte composition of extracellular fluids whereas glucocorticoids effect carbohydrate, fat, and protein metabolism. The androgens act similarly to sex hormones. The cortex makes up 80% of the adrenal gland and is composed of three distinct layers (White, Pescovitz, & Cutler, 1995). The outer layer, the zona glomerulosa, produces mineralocorticoids, primarily aldosterone. The middle layer, or zona reticularis, makes up about 10% of the cortex and secretes both mineralocorticoids and glucocorticoids. The zona fasciculata makes up 75% of the cortex and secretes glucocorticoids, primarily cortisol. In terms of the type of corticosteroids produced, however, the different zonas are interchangeable under some circumstances.

Cortisol is one of many glucocorticoids secreted by the adrenal gland, yet it is responsible for approximately 95% of glucocorticoid activity (Guyton & Hall, 1996). Cortisol is released from the adrenal gland secondary to ACTH. Adrenocorticotropin is released by the anterior pituitary in response to CRH stimulation from the hypothalamus. This cascade of events occurs in a rhythmic fashion with cortisol levels being high in the morning and in response to stress. Once released, cortisol acts to promote gluconeogenesis, protein and fat metabolism, and multiple anti-inflammatory responses. Cortisol, like most hormones, acts via a negative feedback mechanism to maintain normal plasma levels.

Aldosterone produces 90% of the mineralocorticoid activity. Cortisol produces a comparatively weak mineralocorticoid effect. Because the amount of cortisol secreted is 80 times as much as aldosterone, cortisol contributes a substantial amount to mineralocorticoid activity. Aldosterone is secreted in response to increases in serum K^+ or decreases in serum Na^+ levels, with K^+ concentration being the more important. Activation of the renin–angiotensin system in response to decreased renal blood flow also produces dramatic increases in aldosterone secretion. Aldosterone acts on the renal tubules to produce Na^+ conservation and K^+ excretion.

Serum Na^+ levels usually do not change because of simultaneous reabsorption of water. This increase in extracellular fluid volume increases arterial pressure and acts as a negative feedback mechanism on the renin–angiotensin system (Guyton & Hall, 1996).

Gonads

The gonads, the ovaries and testes, produce hormones necessary for sexual maturation, reproductive function, and the development of secondary sex characteristics. The adrenal glands also contribute to these processes by stimulating the production of androgens (Toto, 1994). Reproductive endocrinolgy does not significantly impact anesthesia practice, and the reader is referred to other literature in this field for more in-depth information. Only those conditions or disorders that specifically impact the perianesthesia process will be discussed.

History of the Endocrine System with Emphasis on Specific Pathophysiology

Diabetes Mellitus

The history of usual glycemic control is determined through patient interview, serial blood glucose records, and glycosylated hemoglobin values, if available. The age of onset compared to the patient's current age provides clues as to the possible presence of preexisting complications. The history should include previous surgical and anesthetic responses. Historical evidence of peripheral and autonomic neuropathies should be pursued and documented. Subjective data concerning distal polyneuropathies include paresthesia, burning and hyperasthesias, and nocturnal discomfort of the lower extremities (Ockert & Hugo, 1992). Complaints of intermittent diarrhea, rectal incontinence, urinary retention and incontinence, impotence, lack of sweating, and early satiety can be indicative of autonomic neuropathy (Ockert & Hugo, 1992; Roizen, 1996).

Pancreatitis—Acute and Chronic

The primary historical markers of pancreatitis are alcohol abuse and biliary disease. These patients may also give a history of hyperlipidemia. Patients with a positive family history of pancreatitis have an increased risk for pancreatitis. Recent blunt abdominal trauma increases the risk for acute pancreatitis. Bacterial and viral infections including mumps, scarlet fever, Coxsackievirus, hepatitis B, campylobacter, and mycoplasma are etiologic factors associated with acute pancreatitis. Less common factors associated with acute pancreatitis include electric shock, pregnancy, lupus erythematosus, polyarteritis nodosa, posttransplantation, exposure to organophosphates, and scorpion venom (Brown, 1991; Krumberger, 1993).

Severe abdominal pain is the chief complaint in these patients. It is characterized as sharp, stabbing, twisting pain in the mid- or periumbilical region, radiating to the costar margins or referred to the lower back. Classically, these patients will assume an upright position with the knees and spine flexed, as a supine position will exacerbate the pain. These patients will give a history of protracted vomiting that is worsened by food or drink (Brown, 1991; Krumberger, 1993).

Chronic pancreatitis occurs chiefly in chronic alcoholics. Other factors for development of chronic pancreatitis include chronic, severe biliary tract disease and a previous history of abdominal trauma. These patients will have long-standing problems that impact anesthetic management but are usually not of the same magnitude as acute pancreatitis (Stoelting & Dierdorf, 1993).

Thyroid and Parathyroid Disorders

Patients with disorders of the thyroid gland present to the operative suite for both thyroid and nonthyroid surgeries. Regardless of the type of surgery, key management of these patients includes assessment of current thyroid state. Elderly patients suffering from thyroid anomalies demonstrate ambiguous findings that warrant an extra measure of vigilance during the perianesthetic course (McMorrow, 1992; Pronovost & Parris, 1995). Hyperthyroid patients complain of nervousness, fatigue, weakness, tremor, heat intolerance, sweating, insomnia, weight loss with concurrent increase in appetite, and palpitations. Elderly hyperthyroid patients may present with a paradoxical anorexia (McMorrow, 1992; Pronovost & Parris, 1995). The hypothyroid patient typically complains of intolerance of cold, dry skin, voice changes (hoarseness), fatigue, hair loss, and weight gain. Patients with severe hypothyroidism may have a history of apathy, neglect, decline in intellect, emotional lability, confusion, or true psychoses (Jordan, 1995). Thyroid masses may cause dysphagia and increasing shortness of breath.

Subjective data in patients with dysfunctions of the parathyroid glands relate to the subsequent hypo- or hypercalcemia produced. The history for patients with hyperparathyroid disease can include renal stones, abdominal pain, nausea and vomiting, peptic ulcer disease, pancreatitis, and, most commonly, skeletal muscle weakness (Stoelting & Dierdorf, 1993). Chronic hypocalcemia, as with hypoparathyroidism, produces muscle cramps, fatigue, and lethargy. The patient with acute hypocalcemia, as with inadvertent parathyroidectomy during thyroid surgery, may complain of perioral paresthesia.

Hypothalamic, Pituitary, and Adrenal Disorders

Disorders associated with the hormones of the adrenal gland may not be localized to the adrenals only but may also involve other parts of the hypothalamic–pituitary–adrenal axis. Regardless of the defect involved, these disorders share similar subjective complaints associated with hormone excess or deficiency. Symptoms associated with glucocorticoid excess (Cushing syndrome) include muscle weakness, back pain, psychologic disorders, headache, polydipsia, polyuria, reports of edema, a rather sudden onset of weight gain, and easy bruising (Orth, 1995). Lee and Gumowski (1992) reported that primary hypoadrenocorticism (adrenal insufficiency) presents acutely as weight loss, abdominal or back pain, weakness, mental status changes, and skin changes. These patients may have symptoms of shock secondary to acute loss of intravascular fluid volume. Patients with secondary hypoadrenocorticism complain mainly of excessive weakness or fatigue. These patients may also have gastrointestinal complaints such as nausea and vomiting, and weight loss with or without anorexia. If the etiology of secondary adrenal insufficiency is panhypopituitarism (total failure of anterior pituitary function), these patients will have complaints involving other hormones as well (Dexter, 1995). Patients with secondary hypoadrenocorticism usually do not present with symptoms of acute hypovolemia (Stoelting & Dierdorf, 1993).

Symptoms of hyper- or hypoaldosteronism are related to the underlying fluid and electrolyte changes produced by the syndrome. Patients with hyperaldosteronism (Conn's syndrome) may report signs consistent with acute hypertension or give a history of acutely elevated diastolic blood pressure. Skeletal muscle weakness, secondary to hypokalemia, is a common complaint. Symptoms of nephrogenic diabetes insipidus are present as well (Stoelting & Dierdorf, 1993). Symptoms of hyperkalemia predominate in patients with hypoaldosteronism. Patients with chronic renal disease, diabetes mellitus, or those taking ACE inhibitors can develop hypoaldosteronism.

Trauma, neoplasm, or other injury to the hypothalamus, posterior pituitary, or kidney can result in disorders of ADH production, secretion, and function. Diabetes insipidus (DI) occurs as a result of decreased ADH production or release, or from failure of the kidney to respond to ADH. Patients will report polyuria with large amounts of dilute urine being produced. These patients ingest voluminous amounts of water and yet continue to complain of thirst. Patients with decreased access to water and those simply unable to keep up with the massive diuresis will report symptoms of hypovolemia (Batcheller, 1992; Blevins & Wand, 1992; Bell, 1994).

Oversecretion of ADH results in the syndrome of inappropriate ADH secretion (SIADH). The symptoms of SIADH are related to hypervolemia and hyponatremia. They include headaches, nausea, vomiting, impaired taste sensation, anorexia, weight gain, and dulled sensorium. As the syndrome progresses, patients will be confused and hostile, and ultimately become comatose (Batcheller, 1992, 1994).

Physical Examination

Pancreas

Diabetes Mellitus. The clinical findings associated with the previously diagnosed diabetic involve delineating and documenting the acute and chronic complications associated with the disease. The acute complications concerning anesthesia providers include hypoglycemia, hyperosmolar coma, and diabetic ketoacidosis (DKA). These complications, especially the latter two, are often included in the admitting factors for the newly diagnosed diabetic (Roizen, 1996).

Siperstein (1992) declares that pure hyperosmolar coma and pure DKA occur rarely; rather, the typical presentation is a mixed hyperosmolar–DKA state even though it may be diagnosed as one or the other. Marked hypovolemia produces thirst, decreased skin turgor, soft eyeballs, hypotension, and orthostasis. Kussmaul breathing occurs as a sign of acidemia in which the pH is less than 7.1. Abdominal pain and vomiting are common, especially toward the DKA portion of the continuum. Stupor, obtundation, seizures, and coma occur later and are signs of a severe hyperosmolar state.

Chronic complications of diabetes mellitus include ocular, peripheral, and autonomic neuropathies, and angiopathies of the peripheral and cardiac vessels. Physical findings consistent with peripheral neuropathy include deficiency of pain and temperature (spinothalamic) sensation, vibration, joint and position sensations (posterior column sensations), and distal extremity muscle weakness (Ockert & Hugo, 1992).

Autonomic neuropathy is one of the most serious diabetic complications. Ishihara, Singh, and Giesecke (1994) performed several bedside tests for autonomic neuropathy. These tests included observing for a decrease in systolic blood pressure of greater than 30 mmHg when compared to lying systolic blood pressure as a positive sign for autonomic neuropathy. Another bedside test involved the measuring of ECG R–R intervals at 15 and 30 beats after standing, followed by calculating the ratio of the R–R interval at the thirtieth beat to that of the fifteenth beat. A ratio of less than 1.0 was considered abnormal.

The primary cardiovascular complications monitored for in the diabetic patient are hypertension and coronary artery disease. One must examine the 12-lead ECG carefully because silent myocardial ischemia is typical in the diabetic patient. Ockbert and Hugo (1992) report that patients with autonomic neuropathy are more likely to have silent myocardial ischemia. Patients with a concurrent diagnosis of hypertension have a 50% incidence of autonomic neuropathy (Roizen, 1996).

A careful physical exam may reveal other potential anesthetic problems related to the diabetic. Patients with nonfamilial short stature and tight, waxy skin may have limited joint mobility. These patients should be assessed for a positive *prayer sign*—an inability to approximate the palmer surfaces of the hands. (Milaskiewicz & Hall, 1992).

Acute and Chronic Pancreatitis. Acute pancreatitis presents as an acute abdomen. Abdominal tenderness, guarding, and distension on palpation are key clinical features. Abdominal rigidity, rebound tenderness, and ascites may be present as well. Hypoactive or absent bowel sounds are common as gastrointestinal motility is altered. These patients usually have a fever of less than 39°C unless peritonitis, cholecystitis, or intra-abdominal abscess is present. Hypotension, tachycardia, respiratory alkalosis, diaphoresis, mottled skin, and weakness are consistent with the marked hypovolemia associated with the disease. Oliguria indicates hypovolemia or acute tubular necrosis secondary to decreased renal perfusion. Accumulation of blood around the flanks or the umbilical area is indicative of hemorrhagic pancreatitis. This produces bluish discoloration known as Grey Turner's sign (for the flanks) and Cullen's sign (for the umbilicus) (Krumberger, 1993).

Chronic pancreatitis develops most commonly in chronic alcoholics. These patients are usually emaciated and about 10% have concurrent jaundice. Fatty liver infiltration and mild diabetes occur commonly. After 80% of the pancreas is destroyed, these patients will have maldigestion of fat and protein (Stoelting & Dierdorf, 1993).

Thyroid and Parathyroid Disorders

Patients diagnosed with myxedema coma, the most serious form of hypothyroidism, present with decreased mental status, hypoventilation, hypothermia, bradycardia, hyponatremia, hypoglycemia, and a precipitating infection (usually pneumonia or a urinary tract infection). These patients have edematous, pale faces with periorbital edema. The skin is cold and dry with sparse body hair. Macroglossia may be present and there is nonpitting edema of the extremities. The classic physical exam reveals distant heart sounds and delayed relaxation of the deep tendon reflexes (Jordan, 1995).

The features of hypothyroidism vary according to the severity of the deficiency. In most cases physical examination reveals a hoarse voice, dry skin, and delayed relaxation of the deep tendon reflexes. All organ systems will be affected; however, it should be noted that the signs and symptoms of this disease are subtle, particularly in the elderly (Pronovost & Parris, 1995).

Hyperthyroidism generally presents as a state of catecholamine excess. Typically the patient is hyperactive, restless, and irritable. These patients may have protruding eyeballs and a neck mass. Cardiovascular signs include palpitations, tachycardia, atrial fibrillation, high-output congestive heart failure, and newly precipitated

or worsened angina. Loss of muscle mass, myopathy of the proximal muscles, and fine tremor may be present (Pronovost & Parris, 1995). Cardiovascular and myopathic signs predominate in the elderly patient (McMorrow, 1992).

Thyroid storm represents an acute and extreme state of hyperthyroidism. Presentation is abrupt with hyperpyrexia and tachydysrhythmias resistant to cardioversion being the hallmarks of the syndrome. Thyroid storm under anesthesia can be confused with malignant hyperthermia; however, it typically lacks muscle rigidity, metabolic acidosis, and malignant arrhythmias (Ambus, Evans, & Smith, 1994). Adrenal insufficiency, leukocytosis, diarrhea, and hyperglycemia also occur during thyroid storm (Pronovost & Parris, 1995).

Manifestations of parathyroid hormone excess or deficiency are due to hyper- or hypocalcemia, respectively. Signs and symptoms of hypercalcemia present primarily as subjective and laboratory findings. Suspected hypocalcemia, secondary to hypoparathyroidism, is verified with laboratory studies but includes classic diagnostic signs as well. Neuromuscular irritability results in facial muscle twitching in response to manual tapping of the facial nerve at the mandibular angle (Chvostek's sign). Trousseau's sign is considered positive if carpopedal spasm is produced secondary to 3 minutes of ischemia produced by a tourniquet. Laryngeal neuromuscular irritability is evidenced by inspiratory stridor.

Hypothalamic, Pituitary, and Adrenal Disorders

Hyperadrenocortic patients present with an atypical physical examination, regardless of the underlying cause. Recent weight gain is usually centralized with thickening of the facial fat and an enlarged dorsocervical hump. These are referred to classically as the *moon face* and the *buffalo hump,* respectively. Fat pads that bulge above the supraclavicular fossae are specific for Cushing's syndrome. Muscle wasting and weakness, a ruddy complexion, and thin fragmented skin that bruises easily are common findings. Osteoporosis, pathologic fractures, and renal calculi occur. Glucose intolerance, hypertension, gastric and peptic ulcers, hirsutism, menstrual irregularities, and various psychologic disturbances are also present in this catastrophic illness. Hyperpigmentation may lead to purple striae on the abdomen, buttocks, and axillae (Gumowski, Proch, & Kessler, 1992; Orth, 1995). This feature is absent in patients with adrenal tumors (Orth, 1995).

Clinically, patients with acute hypoadrenocorticism present with hypovolemic shock unresponsive to volume or vasopressors. Orthostatic hypotension and tachycardia are present secondary to hypovolemia. Hyperpigmentation at pressure points and along the surfaces of the palm are key features of the diagnosis (Lee & Gumowski, 1992). As with subjective findings, clinically observed signs will be less severe in the case of secondary hypoadrenocorticism (Stoelting & Dierdorf, 1993).

The presence of hypertension with a low serum K^+ is indicative of hyperadrenocorticism. Conversely, hyperkalemia with orthostatic hypotension and without concomitant renal insufficiency is suspicious for hypoaldosteronism. Laboratory and subjective findings are the key indicators in these processes (Stoelting & Dierdorf, 1993).

Disorders of the hypothalamus and posterior pituitary involve ADH excess or deficiency. Diabetes insipidus secondary to relative or absolute ADH deficiency produces signs and symptoms consistent with hypovolemia. Orthostatic hypotension, tachycardia, poor skin turgor, and dry mucous membranes, along with subjective complaints, are the primary factors in making the diagnosis. Diagnostic studies confirm the diagnosis (Batcheller, 1992; Blevins & Wand, 1992; Bell, 1994). The SIADH is suspected when there is evidence of water retention and hyponatremia. These patients will gain weight but will not have edema. Classically, progressively worsening neurologic status and laboratory findings confirm the diagnosis (Batcheller, 1992, 1994).

Most disorders of the anterior pituitary present no specific concerns for the anesthesia provider. The defects impacting anesthesia care relate to growth hormone excess or deficiency of panhypopituitarism. Growth hormone excess in the adult produces acromegaly. Excess growth of soft tissue leads to edema and hypertrophy of the face; thick, oily, leathery skin; prominent skin folds; and vocal cord hypertrophy. Bony overgrowth results in prognathism; prominent frontal, nasal, and malar bones; and peripheral entrapment neuropathy. Cardiomegaly and hypertension are also present (Aron, Tyrrell, & Wilson, 1995). Growth hormone deficiency and panhypopituitarism produce dwarfism (Guyton & Iall, 1996).

Gonadal Disorders

Gonadal disorders of particular interest to the anesthetist are Turner syndrome and Noonan syndrome. Both syndromes are genetic disorders. Short stature, primary amenorrhea, and genital immaturity are primary clinical manifestations. Hypertension, possible aortic disease (coarctation or aortic valve stenosis), and pectus excavatum occur as well. These patients tend to have a short neck, high palate, and micrognathia. Noonan syndrome is Turner syndrome with normal chromosomes. The two disorders share short stature and facial characteristics. Differences for Noonan syndrome include mental retardation, right-sided cardiac lesions, and fertility (Campbell & Bousfield, 1992; Schwartz & Eisenkraft, 1992).

Physical findings associated with androgen excess, whether endogenous or exogenous, are of particular concern to the anesthetist. Clinical features include hirsutism, acne, central obesity, male pattern baldness, clitoral hypertrophy, upper torso widening, and an increased waist-to-hip ratio. In addition to these external signs, these women commonly suffer from cardiovascular disease, insulin resistance, and the potential for intravascular thromboses (Derman, 1995).

Diagnostic Data

Pancreas

Diabetes Mellitus. Diabetes is diagnosed based on history, physical examination, and laboratory results. Typically, an abnormal fasting blood sugar and glucose tolerance test confirm the diagnosis. Microalbuminuria, though not routinely performed, may be present. A diabetic with microalbuminuria in excess of 29 mg/dL is at increased risk for the development of renal insufficiency (Roizen, 1996). For the diabetic presenting for surgery, glycemic control is of great importance. Home glucose or in-hospital fingerstick glucose records indicate the level of glycemic control. Glycosylated hemoglobin values, if available, are also indicative of glycemic control. A glycosylated hemoglobin value greater than 10% and a fasting blood glucose value greater than 200 mg/dL suggest poor control (Gavin, 1992). Erratic glycemic control can be an adumbration for perianesthetic hypoglycemia (Roizen, 1996). Furthermore, glycosylated hemoglobin values of 8.5% to 9.0% put the patient at risk for developing retinopathy.

The newly diagnosed diabetic or the diabetic out of glycemic control secondary to infection or injury may present with DKA or hyperosmolar coma. The patient with DKA will usually have a blood glucose less than 300 mg/dL whereas the patient with hyperosmolar coma may have a glucose above 700 mg/dL. The bicarbonate level is less than 15 mEq/L with a pH usually less than 7.2 in DKA. Because a number of compounds that are not osmotically active may give an erroneous serum osmolarity, it is best to calculate osmolarity based on osmotically active molecules using the following equation:

$$\text{Osmolarity} = 2[Na^+] + 2[K^+] + \frac{[glucose]}{20}$$

A normal value is 280 mOsm/L to 295 mOsm/L. Comatose patients will have an osmolarity above 340 mOsm/L. An anion gap can be calculated with this equation:

$$\text{Anion gap} = [Na^+] - ([Cl^-] + [HCO_3^-])$$

Normal is 8 mEq/L to 16 mEq/L with an anion gap of greater than 16 indicating acidosis secondary to organic acids. Potassium may be normal or high and urine ketones confirm the diagnosis of DKA (Siperstein, 1992).

Pancreatitis—Acute and Chronic. Acutely, serum amylase levels are elevated in the patient with pancreatitis. These return to normal after 48 hours. Serum lipase levels are elevated for up to 7 days. The amylase to creatinine ratio is determined by the following equation:

$$\frac{(\text{Serum amylase} \times \text{Urine creatinine})}{(\text{Serum creatinine} \times \text{Urine amylase})} \times 100$$

A normal value is less than 3%; an amylase to creatinine ratio greater than 5% is indicative of pancreatitis (Brown, 1991). Other laboratory results may include an elevated white blood cell count, hyperglycemia, hypocalcemia, hypoalbuminemia, hypomagnesemia, and elevated liver function tests. Potassium can be low or high. Hypoxemia will be present in patients with concomitant respiratory failure (Krumberger, 1993). Computed axial tomography (CAT) scans, magnetic resonance imaging (MRI), ultrasonography, and endoscopic retrograde cholangiography are also used to make the diagnosis.

Thyroid and Parathyroid Disorders

Various thyroid function tests are available to assess for adequate thyroid hormone production and to define the etiology of clinical signs and symptoms. Total serum thyroxine (T4), total serum triiodothyronine (T3), TSH, and resin triiodothyronine uptake (RT3U) are the mainstays of blood tests for thyroid gland function. T4 and T3 levels are increased during hyperthyroidism. An elevated RT3U rules out alterations in T4-binding globulin. In hypothyroidism due to hypothalamic or anterior pituitary dysfunction, all laboratory values are decreased. Primary hypothyroidism presents with an increase in TSH with all other values decreased (Stoelting & Dierdorf, 1993). Routine thyroid function tests are not commonly performed. It should be noted, however, that asymptomatic patients may have abnormal thyroid function tests, indicating subclinical hypo- or hyperfunction (Hart, 1995; Smith, 1995). Patients with subclinical thyroid disease are at the same risk for perianesthetic complications. Thyroid scan, ultrasonography, and thyroid antibody studies may be done to determine the etiology of dysfunction.

Hypercalcemia and renal colic are the key features of hyperparathyroidism. The ECG reveals a prolonged P-R interval and a shortened Q-T interval. Radiographic findings demonstrate subcortical bone resorption in the phalanges and pathologic fractures may be present. Parathyroid hormone assays are elevated in hyperparathyroidism. Conversely, hypocalcemia is the key diagnostic feature in hypoparathyroidism. Significant dysfunction will produce a prolonged Q-T interval on ECG as well as previously mentioned clinical signs. Parathormone levels are obviously decreased (Aurbach, Marx, & Spiegel, 1992).

Hypothalamic, Pituitary, and Adrenal Disorders

Cushing's syndrome due to anterior pituitary tumor or other malignant tumors will demonstrate elevated ACTH levels. Iatrogenic or pure adrenal causes result in elevated cortisol levels only. A dexamethasone suppression test, stimulation test, and 24-hour urine studies establish the diagnosis (Gumowski, Proch, & Kessler, 1992). Contemporaneous findings include hyperglycemia and hypokalemia (Orth, 1995).

Hypoadrenocorticism manifests as decreased ACTH and cortisol levels. In primary hypoadrenocorticism, aldosterone levels are also low. Hyperkalemia, hypoglycemia, hyponatremia, elevated BUN, and evidence of hemoconcentration are present. Electrolyte imbalances produce prolonged Q-T intervals, peaked T-waves, widened QRS with low voltage, and the potential for ventricular dysrhythmias. Chronic adrenal insufficiency has milder forms of the same electrolyte derangements along with anemia. Diagnosis is determined by comparing cortisol levels at baseline and post-ACTH administration (Lee & Gumowski, 1992).

Hyperaldosteronism (Conn syndrome) results in hypokalemia. Plasma aldosterone is increased and urinary K^+ excretion will exceed 30 mEq/L. The patient with hypoaldosteronism has decreased aldosterone levels, hyperkalemia, and hyperchloremic metabolic acidosis. These patients demonstrate ECG changes consistent with the electrolyte imbalance (Stoelting & Dierdorf, 1993).

Excess or deficiency of growth hormone secretion is determined by urinary concentrations of growth hormone. Hyposecretion is usually a diagnosis of exclusion. Hypersecretion is confirmed by urine concentrations determined in conjunction with a glucose tolerance test (growth hormone should be suppressed in response to a glucose load). Serum measurements of IGF may be used in some settings (Jeffcoate, 1993).

Excess ADH secretion, as with SIADH, produces hyponatremia and decreased osmolarity (less than 280 mOsm/kg) secondary to water retention. Urine sodium will be greater than 25 mEq/L and, along with increased urine osmolarity, demonstrates inappropriately concentrated urine (Batcheller, 1992, 1994). Diabetes insipidus manifests as elevated plasma osmolality, decreased urine osmolality, and hypernatremia. Serum ADH levels are decreased with neurogenic DI but are normal or high with nephrogenic DI. Hypokalemia and hypercalcemia are consistent with nephrogenic DI (Blevins & Wand, 1992; Bell, 1994).

Pathophysiology

Pancreas

Diabetes Mellitus. Diabetes is a relative or absolute deficiency of insulin. Diabetes is influenced by genetic predisposition and is believed to be an immunologic disorder (Muir, Schatz, & Maclaren, 1992). Diabetes mellitus can be classified into two types—insulin-dependent

(IDDM) and noninsulin dependent (NIDDM). Historically the insulin-dependent diabetic tends to be young and nonobese, whereas the noninsulin-dependent diabetic tends to be elderly and overweight. Current understanding dictates that age is of little consequence in the diagnosis of the disease. Instead, insulin dependence is determined by the number and functionality of beta islet cells—NIDDM may antedate a stage of insulin dependence in adults. Diabetic stressors (age, obesity, pregnancy) lead to clinical diabetes with varying retention of functioning numbers of beta cells.

Elevated glucose levels lead to diabetic complications. Elevated serum glucose levels disrupt autoregulation, thereby decreasing the protection normally afforded to vital organs. Nonenzymatic glycosylation secondary to hyperglycemia leads to abnormal proteins that can affect joint mobility and wound healing. Hyperglycemia may also lead to multiple alterations in leukocyte function, predisposing the diabetic to infections (Roizen, 1996).

Severe insulin deficiency results in development of the hyperosmolar, ketoacidotic state (Siperstein, 1992). Cell hunger resulting from decreased glucose utilization in the periphery leads to increased gluconeogenesis in the liver. Hydrolysis of adipose tissue results in the release of large amounts of free fatty acids into the plasma. Hepatic metabolism is altered because of the lack of insulin and consequent excess of glucagon, leading to the conversion of fatty acids to ketones—primarily beta-hydroxybutyric acid, acetoacetic acid, and acetone.

The hyperglycemia produces osmotic fluid shifts, severe osmotic diuresis, and loss of electrolytes. Initially, osmotic movement of fluid to the extracellular space from the intracellular space helps to preserve intravascular volume. When the renal hyperglycemic threshold is exceeded, osmotic diuresis of free water and sodium occurs. Continuation of this process results in intra- and extracellular dehydration. As the calculated osmolarity approaches 340 mOsm/L, cellular dehydration produces coma and, potentially, vascular collapse (Siperstein, 1992).

Acidosis is produced by the production of ketones from free fatty acid metabolism. Kussmaul breathing indicates a serum pH of more than 7.2. Acidemia causes K^+ to move out of the intracellular space to the extracellular space. Therefore, serum K^+ measurements can be normal or high, but total body K^+ is always low (Siperstein, 1992).

Pancreatitis—Acute and Chronic. Pancreatitis results from the activation of pancreatic enzymes within the organ to produce autodigestion. Usually, trypsin inhibitor prevents the activation of trypsin within the pancreas. This in turn prevents the activation of other digestive enzymes. Although the precise mechanism is unknown, accumulation of and autodigestion by pancreatic enzymes can result from obstruction of the pancreatic duct system, dysfunction of the secretory cells of the acini, or injury to the pancreas (Brown, 1991; Krumberger, 1993). Because patients with hyperparathyroid hormone excess and other causes of hypercalcemia tend to develop pancreatitis, acinar cell calcium toxicity may be an impetus in the pathogenesis of pancreatitis (Ward, Petersen, Jenkins, & Sutton, 1995).

As the pancreas autodigests, vasoactive compounds and kinins are released. This produces massive third spacing, resulting in hypovolemia. These patients sequester up to 6 L of fluid in the peritoneal space. Protracted nausea and vomiting worsen hypovolemia. Hypocalcemia and hypokalemia occur frequently in these patients and produce dysrhythmias and decreased myocardial contractility. Kinins also decrease myocardial contractility. Phospholipase and free fatty acids damage pulmonary surfactant, predisposing these patients to the development of adult respiratory distress syndrome (ARDS). Pleural effusions secondary to pancreatic exudate are common. Atelectasis develops because of decreased respiratory effort secondary to intense abdominal pain and further complicates the pulmonary status of these patients. Elevated levels of fibrinogen and factor VIII produce a hypercoaguable state and lead to thrombosis or disseminated intravascular coagulation (Krumberger, 1993).

Thyroid and Parathyroid Disorders

Thyrotoxicosis is the overproduction of thyroid hormones. Pronovost and Parris (1995) indicate that, most commonly, thyrotoxicosis occurs as the result of an autoimmune process affecting the thyroid gland (Grave's disease). Postpartum thyroiditis, in which physiologic overproduction of thyroid hormones continues into the postpartum period, and overtreatment with T3 or T4 also occur commonly (Jeffcoate, 1993). Toxic adenoma ("hot nodule"), toxic multinodular goiter, and the toxic phase of Hashimoto's thyroiditis can produce thyrotoxicosis. Less common causes include the toxic phase of subacute (DeQuervain's) thyroiditis and TSH-secreting pituitary tumors (Jeffcoate, 1993; Volpé, 1993). These patients may or may not develop a goiter; if present, the goiter may or may not cause significant pain. Overproduction of thyroid hormones results in an increased metabolic rate, hyperthermia, osteopenia and osteoporosis, increased cardiac output, tachycardia, and extraocular muscle enlargement.

An acute, severe exacerbation of thyrotoxicosis is thyroid storm. This usually occurs when the hyperthyroid patient suffers major physical trauma (eg, surgery, general anesthesia). Hyperpyrexia, tachycardia, congestive heart failure, and hypovolemia should be expected. These patients are at extreme risk for circulatory collapse (Pronovost & Parris, 1995).

Hypothyroidism usually occurs iatrogenically, as the result of treatment for hyperthyroidism. Hashimoto's thyroiditis, autoimmune destruction of the gland, produces hypothyroidism. Subacute (DeQuervain's) thyroiditis and postpartum thyroiditis may be followed by hypothyroidism (Jeffcoate, 1993). Myxedema coma is the most severe state of hypothyroidism (Jordan, 1995).

Lack of adequate levels of thyroid hormone produces changes related to metabolic depression. Bradycardia, decreased stroke volume, decreased blood volume, and altered baroreceptor responses are present. These patients exhibit a decreased response to hypercarbia and hypoxia as well as gastric hypomotility (Pronovost & Parris, 1995).

Hyperparathyroidism occurs secondary to hyperplasia of the parathyroid glands, a benign parathyroid adenoma, or a parathyroid carcinoma. The result is oversecretion of parathyroid hormone resulting in hypercalcemia. Hypercalcemia produces ECG changes, hypertension, renal calculi, polyuria, polydipsia, and the potential for pathologic fractures (Stoelting & Dierdorf, 1993).

Hypoparathyroidism is almost always iatrogenic and results in hypocalcemia. Neuromuscular irritability is the hallmark of hypocalcemia. Of particular concern to the anesthetist is the effect on laryngeal musculature (Stoelting & Dierdorf, 1993).

Hypothalamic, Pituitary, and Adrenal Disorders

Cushing's syndrome will be either corticotropin dependent or corticotropin independent. Corticotropin-dependent hyperadrenocorticism occurs when abnormal levels of corticotropin stimulate the adrenal glands as opposed to excessive production of cortisol by abnormal tissues as in corticotropin-independent Cushing's syndrome. Most commonly, pituitary tumors produce excessive ACTH resulting in Cushing's disease. Small-cell lung carcinoma is the most frequent cause of nonpituitary corticotropin-dependent Cushing's syndrome. Corticotropin-independent Cushing's syndrome is caused by adrenal tumors (adenoma or carcinoma) and rarely by micronodular hyperplasia (Orth, 1995). Iatrogenic Cushing's syndrome results from excessive exogenous steroids and is common (Gumowski, Proch, & Kessler, 1992). In all cases, the result is excessive secretion of cortisol. The physiologic effects of hypercortisolism we described earlier in this chapter.

Hypoadrenocorticism, or adrenal insufficiency, represents a deficiency of cortisol and, in the case of primary adrenal insufficiency, aldosterone. Underlying causes include adrenal cortex destruction by autoimmune disease, bacterial or viral infections, and malignant neoplasms. Prolonged exogenous corticosteroid administration can result in suppression of the hypothalamic–pituitary–adrenal axis (Stoelting & Dierdorf, 1993).

In acute adrenal insufficiency, lack of cortisol and aldosterone results in hyperkalemia, hyponatremia, hypovolemia, decreased cardiac output, tachycardia, and hypotension. Acute adrenal insufficiency is a medical emergency (Lee & Gumowski, 1992). Secondary adrenal insufficiency results from a lack of ACTH. Severe hypovolemia, hyponatremia, and hyperkalemia are not likely in secondary adrenal insufficiency since aldosterone secretion is intact.

Primary hyperaldosteronism is most commonly produced by excess secretion from a functional tumor. Excessive aldosterone leads to hypernatremia and hypervolemia, hypokalemia, and hypertension. Secondary hyperaldosteronism occurs when increased renin results in excess aldosterone production (Gumowski, Proch, & Kessler, 1992).

A defect in the juxtoglomerular apparatus or treatment with ACE inhibitors can produce hypoaldosteronism secondary to hyporeninemia. Indomethacin-induced prostaglandin deficiency can result in decreased renin production that results in hypoaldosteronism. Heparin administration also has the potential to produce hypoaldosteronism (Oster, Singer, & Fishman, 1995). Rarely, aldosterone deficiency occurs as a result of congenital lack of aldosterone synthetase (Stoelting & Dierdorf, 1993).

Growth hormone deficiency is most commonly due to idiopathic growth hormone-releasing hormone deficiency. It may also be secondary to hypothalamic or pituitary tumors. Growth hormone excess is usually secondary to a growth hormone secreting pituitary adenoma (Jeffcoate, 1993).

Severe damage to the hypothalamic–posterior pituitary system results in neurogenic DI. The result is a deficiency of ADH. Nephrogenic DI is caused by failure of the renal tubule to respond to ADH and can be acquired or congenital. Both syndromes result in polyuria and the potential for severe hypovolemia (Blevins and Wand, 1992).

The SIADH can be produced by numerous clinical states and syndromes. A frequent cause is oat cell bronchogenic carcinoma. Excessive ADH secretion results in water intoxication and hyponatremia (Batcheller, 1992, 1994).

Gonadal Disorders

According to Derman (1995), androgen excess can occur concurrently with Cushing's syndrome, polycystic ovary syndrome, congenital adrenal hyperplasia, and ovarian and adrenal tumors. Exogenous androgen excess can result from drug use, including oral contraceptives and anabolic steroids.

Perianesthetic Management

Pancreas

Diabetes Mellitus. The preoperative preparation for anesthesia in the diabetic patient proceeds in a stepwise fashion, focusing broadly and proceeding to the complex. Consultation with an internist or an endocrinologist is a top priority in the management of the diabetic. As with any patient, all aspects of care must be individualized.

The anesthesia provider, through interview or chart review, must determine whether the diabetes is insulin dependent or noninsulin dependent (Gavin, 1992). Preadmission therapeutic regimens, including pharmaceutical, dietary, and exercise regimens, should be noted (Roizen, 1996). Patients with NIDDM on oral hypoglycemics should refrain from taking these medications on the day of surgery (Peters & Kerner, 1995). Patients diagnosed with NIDDM often take insulin for adequate control of glucose levels.

The presence of complications associated with diabetes should be determined and documented preoperatively. The determination of the possible existence of diabetic autonomic neuropathy was outlined earlier in this chapter. Although patients with diabetic autonomic neuropathy may not be at risk because of volume or pH of gastric contents, these patients do have food particles present, even after an 8-hour period of fasting (Ishihara, Singh, & Giesecke, 1994). It may be prudent to consider a rapid sequence induction, especially if other risk factors (obesity, trauma, etc) are present. Nathan (1996) observed that chronic glycemic control is the factor best correlated to complications of diabetes. Patients who demonstrate poor glycemic control should have surgery delayed until tighter glycemic control is achieved.

A plethora of regimens for intraoperative management of the diabetic patient exists in the literature. An improved understanding of the pathophysiology and its impact on the surgical patient renders many of these obsolete. The Diabetes Control and Complications Trial Research Group (1995) has shown that intensive therapy and tight control markedly delay or prevent complications associated with diabetes. Gavin (1992) states that any diabetic patient having major surgery should receive insulin perioperatively and that a major operation is any procedure that requires general anesthesia.

Many providers use half of the patient's usual morning dose of insulin, given subcutaneously, as a method for managing these patients. Because insulin needs may be increased and because of the marked pharmacokinetic variability associated with this route of administration, this technique is not recommended. Intravenous insulin doses, either by bolus or infusion, provide the best method for perioperative glucose control, with infusion being the better of the two.

Estimation of intraoperative insulin needs is based on the history, physical examination, and type of surgery. As recommended by Gavin (1992), any patient (IDDM or NIDDM) using insulin should receive an insulin infusion at 1.5 units per hour (U/h) while patients on oral medications or a controlled diet would be started at 1 U/h. Patients who have a history of poor glycemic control, obesity, or hepatic disease should receive 1.5 times the initial estimated dose. Patients with severe infection, receiving steroid therapy, or having renal transplant surgery should receive 2 times the initially selected dose, whereas coronary artery bypass surgery patients would receive 3 to 5 times that dose. These patients should have an infusion of 5% dextrose at 100 mL/h and have hourly fingerstick glucose monitoring. The insulin drip is adjusted according to fingerstick glucose values. The insulin drip rate, in units per hour, can be determined by dividing the blood glucose value by 100. Although Gavin (1992) reports that patients will rarely experience hypoglycemia, the insulin infusion is discontinued if the blood glucose is less than 80 mg/dL. Blood glucose levels less than 50 mg/dL can be treated with 15 mL of 50% dextrose (Roizen, 1996).

In order for this method to achieve optimum performance, patients should be started on both 5% dextrose and the insulin infusion at least 2 to 3 hours before surgery. There are a variety of methods for mixing an insulin infusion; however, no particular method seems to have any value over the others. An important point with any insulin infusion is to flush the tubing with the mixture before using it in order to fill the insulin binding sites in the plastic tubing.

Postoperatively, the insulin infusion is continued until the patient is tolerating food. At this time, patients can be returned to their preoperative medical regimen or be placed on a regimen using the previous day's total dose as an estimate of insulin need. The patient's internist or endocrinologist should assume management of the patient at this time.

Diabetic patients who present with or develop DKA or hyperosmolar coma are at increased risk perioperatively. As with any diabetic patient, consultation with an endocrinologist should be done early. Elective surgery should be postponed until these patients are stabilized. Correction of hypovolemia is the primary goal. If insulin is administered before beginning fluid replacement, glucose and water move from the vascular compartment to the intracellular space, worsening hypovolemia and hypernatremia and increasing the chance for mortality (Siperstein, 1992). Ockert and Hugo (1992) recommend volume replacement beginning with isotonic saline at 20 mL/kg/h until urine output is 1 mL/kg/h and central venous pressure approaches normal. Volume resuscitation is continued at 5 mL/kg/h. Insulin is given intravenously with a usual loading dose of 0.1 U/kg and an infusion of 0.1 U/kg/h. Potassium should be given at 20 mEq/h to 40 mEq/h. Bicarbonate therapy is not needed unless the pH is less than 7.0, at which time 44 mEq of bicarbonate may be given (Siperstein, 1992).

Pancreatitis—Acute and Chronic. The patient with acute pancreatitis may present for emergency surgery and is likely to be in hypovolemic shock. These patients have severe abdominal pain that may preclude the supine position until the moment of induction. Ileus is common and one should consider a rapid sequence induction. Anesthetic management is geared toward correcting hypovolemia and treating electrolyte imbalances, especially hypocalcemia. Because this disease is commonly associated with chronic alcohol abuse, the patient may have impaired liver function. Pleural effusions and ARDS are common among this population so postoperative ventilatory support may be required.

Chronic pancreatitics generally suffer from malnourishment and concomitant liver disease. Anesthetic management should consider the presence of hypoalbuminemia and altered hepatic metabolism.

Thyroid and Parathyroid Disorders

Patients with hyperthyroid disease may present to the operating room for both thyroid and nonthyroid surgery, whereas patients suffering from hypofunction typically present for nonthyroid surgery. For elective surgery, the goal is to have the patient in a euthyroid state.

Both hypo- and hyperthyroid patients may have neck masses. The presence of hoarseness, dysphagia, or orthopnea should alert the anesthetist to potential airway difficulties. Depending on the size of the mass, preoperative flow–volume loops in addition to x-rays, CAT scans, or MRIs are needed to determine possible airway obstruction. An awake fiberoptic intubation may be required (Todesco, Williams, & Eagle, 1994).

Patients who have hyperthyroidism can receive propythiouracil or methimazole with clinical improvement observed over a period of a few weeks. For rapid treatment, iodine preceded by propylthiouracil inhibits the release of thyroid hormones. If no other contraindications exist, regional anesthesia can be used safely. Lo Gerfo, Ditkoff, Chabot, and Feind (1994) reported almost 40 cases of successful thyroid surgery using deep and superficial cervical plexus blocks and supplemental sedation. The anesthetist should avoid vagolytic drugs such as atropine sulfate and sympathetic stimulants such as ketamine. If exophthalmus exists, the patient may require additional eye protection. Vigilant monitoring of temper-

ature is necessary, and anesthetic requirements will be increased in the hyperthermic patient.

Thyroid storm can develop intraoperatively and up to 18 hours postoperatively. Thyroid storm under anesthesia can be confused with malignant hyperthermia; thyroid storm, however, typically lacks muscle rigidity, metabolic acidosis, and malignant arrhythmias. Treatment of thyroid storm begins at the moment it is considered part of the differential diagnosis (Pronovost & Parris, 1995). Initial treatment begins with propanolol HCl 1 mg/min to 10 mg/min given intravenously and titrated to effect. Patients with coexisting airway disease can be treated with the $beta_1$ selective esmolol HCl, starting at 50 μg/kg/min after an initial loading dose of 250 μg/kg/min. The infusion is increased by 50 μg/kg/min every 5 minutes until achieving the desired effect. Patients with coexisting congestive heart failure should receive digoxin before administration of beta-blockers. Frequent measurement of electrolytes, arterial blood gases, and calcium is required. Pulmonary artery catheterization can assist with fluid management. Antipyretic treatments, such as cooling blankets, should be used but aspirin should be avoided (Pronovost & Parris, 1995).

Patients who are hypothyroid are at increased risk from generalized depressed metabolic activity. Levothyroxine should be prescribed until the patient is euthyroid. It is not necessary for patients to receive levothyroxine on the morning of surgery because it has a half-life of 7 days. The hypothyroid patient can be very sensitive to depressant drugs so premedication with benzodiazepines or opioids is avoided. Induction should be with ketamine or small doses of other hypnotics. Because of perioperative decreases in gastric motility, a rapid sequence induction should be considered, especially if other risk factors are present. Additionally, antiemetics should be administered perioperatively. Although minimum alveolar concentration is not decreased by hypothyroidism, volatile agents should be used minimally because of decreased cardiac output, cardiac reserves, and baroreceptor reflexes. Appropriate measures to prevent hypothermia should be utilized. Because the ventilatory response to hypercarbia and hypoxia is decreased, respiratory depression is common. Intraoperative and postoperative steroids may be used because of decreased adrenal reserves.

The patient with myxedema coma must have aggressive preoperative thyroid replacement—levothyroxine 300 μg to 500 μg intravenously followed by 100 μg daily. Additionally, hydrocortisone 100 mg to 300 mg every 8 hours should be given because of decreased adrenal reserves. Pulmonary artery catheterization along with invasive arterial blood pressure monitoring is necessary. Nitrates should be administered prophylactically in this patient population (Pronovost & Parris, 1995).

Hyperparathyroidism may present as part of multiple endocrine neoplasia (MEN), a classification system of two or more hormone-secreting tumors in the same individual. The first classification, MEN I (Werner's syndrome), consists of tumors of the parathyroid, pancreatic islet cells, and the pituitary. Parathyroid hyperplasia is part of MEN IIa (Sipple's syndrome) in which medullary carcinoma of the thyroid gland and pheochromocytoma are the other tumors (Jeffcoate, 1993). Otherwise, anesthetic management is aimed at avoiding possible complications by maintaining hydration and adequate urine output. Because osteoporosis is a concern, extra care in the positioning of these patients is required. Potentially, muscle relaxation could be prolonged.

The anesthetic management of hypoparathyroidism is aimed at maintaining normal calcium levels. Serial calcium measurements and assessment of neuromuscular signs should be made throughout the perianesthetic period. Because hypoparathyroidism usually occurs iatrogenically, such as during thyroid surgery, postoperative laryngeal muscle involvement is a primary concern and is indicated by the presence of stridor. Hypocalcemia is treated with intravenous calcium and thiazide diuretics.

Hypothalamic, Pituitary, and Adrenal Disorders

Cushing's syndrome, regardless of etiology, produces a patient with hypervolemia and hypokalemia. In the case of elective surgery, these should be corrected preoperatively. These patients may have osteoporosis, so extra care during positioning is warranted. These patients will require steroid supplementation, as their adrenal glands may be unable to respond to stress.

Adrenal insufficiency is managed by adequate steroid replacement during the perioperative period. Concurrent treatment of hypovolemia, hypotension, hyperkalemia, and acidosis may be required in an acute crisis.

Roizen (1996) indicates that perioperative stressors are related directly to the degree of trauma and inversely to the depth of anesthesia. He further adds that only a minority of patients with suppressed adrenal function will have cardiovascular mishaps if they do not receive supplemental steroids. The risk associated with giving supplemental steroids, however, is minimal. Classically, 100 mg of hydrocortisone is administered every 8 hours starting the evening before or the morning of surgery. Alternatively, 25 mg can be given at induction followed by 100 mg given in an infusion over the next 24 hours (Symreng, Karlverg, Kagedal, & Schildt, 1981).

Preoperative correction of hypokalemia and control of hypertension are the mainstays of anesthetic management in the patient with hyperaldosteronism. A normal serum K^+, however, does not guarantee a normal total body K^+. Testing for orthostatic hypotension preoperatively is used to assess volume status. Pulmonary artery catheterization is used to guide volume replacement intraoperatively. Supplemental steroid replacement is indicated in cases where adrenal manipulation is expected (Stoelting & Dierdorf, 1993).

Preoperative preparation is the key to managing patients who present with hypoaldosteronism. An exogenous mineralocorticoid, fludrocortisone, is administered daily in preparation for surgery (Stoelting & Dierdorf, 1993).

Airway evaluation and management are the keys in patients with growth hormone excess or deficiency. Careful airway evaluation and conservative management are in order. Awake fiberoptic intubation may be the first choice in this population. Management also includes careful evaluation of coexisting disease.

Anesthetic management of DI is geared toward correcting the patient's volume status. Volume repletion begins preoperatively. Serum electrolytes and urine output are monitored intraoperatively. Volume replacement intraoperatively is guided by urine output. Preoperative and intraoperative administration of 1-desamino-8-D-arginine vasopressin (DDAVP) may be necessary (Stoelting & Dierdorf, 1993).

Restricted fluid intake is the treatment for SIADH. Demeclocycline and normal saline infusion are used to antagonize the renal tubule effects of ADH. In patients with severe hyponatremia, hypertonic saline administration is required (Stoelting & Dierdorf, 1993).

Turner and Noonan syndrome patients present the challenge of potentially difficult airways and severe cardiac lesions. Regional anesthesia is not contraindicated but may be technically difficult. Careful and conservative airway evaluation and management are required. These patients should have a thorough cardiac evaluation. Cardiac management depends on the type and severity of the lesion.

Gonadal Disorders

Androgen excess in women, whether endogenous or exogenous, should be of particular concern to the anesthetist. These women commonly suffer from cardiovascular disease, insulin resistance, and the potential for intravascular thrombosis (Derman, 1995). Anesthetic management includes thorough preoperative workup and subsequent management based on the underlying disorders.

▶ CASE STUDY

A 42-year-old male, status post-left above the knee amputation (AKA) with an infected left stump, comes to the operating room for incision and drainage, revision left

AKA stump with an estimated surgical time of 1.5 hours. Past medical history includes (1) IDDM poorly controlled with blood sugars ranging from 50 to 350; (2) ESRD, on hemodialysis for 2 years, last hemodialysis via Quinton catheter 36 hours prior to arrival in the operating room; (3) hypertension well controlled on quinapril and diamox; (4) coronary artery disease with history of inferior infarction, 3 years prior to admission, no recent angina; (5) heart failure, with ejection fraction of 30%; and (6) diabetic retinopathy. Regular medications include NPH/regular insulin, diamox, quinapril, epogen, omeprazole, calcium carbonate ($CaCO_3$), and morphine sulfate (MSO_4). Past surgical history includes uneventful general anesthetic for left AKA, axillary blocks for creation of arteriovenous (AV) fistulae, and thrombectomy. Physical examination reveals an alert and oriented thin male in no acute distress. Vital signs were blood pressure (BP), 120/75; heart rate (HR), 75; respiratory rate (RR), 24; and temperature (T), 98.4.

Auscultation of the heart and lungs was normal. Exam revealed no peripheral edema or jugular venous distention but was significant for poor venous access and clotted AV fistulae in both arms. Venous access included a 22-gauge IV and a right femoral Quinton catheter. Diagnostic data obtained before dialysis included complete blood count [hemoglobin (Hb), 9 g/100 mL; Hct, 28%; white blood cells (wbc), 14 000/mm^3; platelet count, 413 000/mm^3), chemistry panel (Na$^+$, 134 mEq/L; K$^+$, 5.2 mEq/L; Cl$^-$, 101 mEq/L; CO_2, 19.3 mEq/L; BUN, 59 mg/100 mL; creatinine, 9.1 g/100 mL; glucose, 64 mg/100 mL; and PT/PTT (14 s/28 s). Chest x-ray revealed cardiomegaly.

The ECG showed left ventricular hypertrophy, Q-waves in leads II, III, and aVF consistent with an old inferior infarct. Postdialysis laboratory data were not available, although the recorded weights had diminished 1.2 kg to 75 kg on a 5'8'' frame.

1. What coexisting conditions and laboratory abnormalities are often found in patients with ESRD?

   Most commonly, patients may exhibit water, electrolyte, and acid–base imbalances; hematologic abnormalities including anemia and coagulopathies; cardiovascular disease such as hypertension, pericarditis, atherosclerosis; infections; hyperparathyroidism; neuropathy; and myopathy. These patients often are on chronic dialysis as the case study illustrates. Some patients with ESRD are treated with steroids and immunosuppressants. This patient exhibited many of these diseases and laboratory disorders including diabetes mellitus, hypertension, heart failure, chronic renal dialysis, and anemia. Laboratory data were reported before dialysis. New data should be obtained prior to surgery as Hct, Hb, BUN, creatinine, and other studies may be different following dialysis.

2. What anesthetic plan should be formulated for this case?

   A rapid sequence induction is indicated because patients with ESRD often experience nausea, vomiting, delayed gastric emptying, and/or stress ulcer. The patient was premedicated with 30 mL of nonparticulate antacid orally, 10 mg of metoclopramide, and 1 mg midazolam via an IV infusion of normal saline. The patient had been NPO for 18 hours, and a preinduction glucose was 120 mg/100 mL. Standard monitors were applied revealing an O_2 saturation of 96% on room air, BP of 150/90 mmHg, and HR of 76, while a preinduction fluid bolus of 300 mL infused. Anesthesia was induced following 100 μg of fentanyl and 100 mg lidocaine with etomidate 20 mg and rocuronium 50 mg via rapid sequence with direct cricoid pressure, followed by uneventful intubation. Anesthesia was maintained with isoflurane 0.5% to 1% and N_2O/O_2 (1:1). Ventilation was controlled throughout the case with a tidal volume of 880 mL and RR of 7. The vital signs remained stable postinduction with a BP of 100/60 mmHg and HR of 76. A tourniquet was applied to the stump, and within 10 minutes of incision there was a 500-mL estimated blood loss (EBL). The BP decreased to 78/54 mmHg.

3. How should hypotension be managed in this case? Should any additional monitoring be implemented? When should transfusion be considered?

   Decreased BP was treated by decreasing anesthetic depth, administering an additional 400 mL of crystalloid and phenylephrine in 100 μg to 200 μg boluses with return of BP to 90 mmHg to 100/60 mmHg. A left external jugular catheter was placed after several unsuccessful attempts to place a central venous catheter. An additional 1 mg of midazolam and 150 μg of fentanyl were administered in 50-μg increments. The EBL was 700 mL, and 1 unit of packed cells was transfused, followed by a second unit when the EBL was 900 mL 10 minutes later.

   At the conclusion of the operation, muscle relaxation was fully reversed with 4 mg of neostigmine and 0.8 mg of glycopyrrolate. The patient was extubated and taken to the recovery room awake, ventilating well, and complaining of pain. Total EBL was 1200 mL; the patient received 500 mL of packed cells and 1 L of crystalloid. Initial vital signs were a BP of 130/84 mmHg, HR of 84, and RR of 28, with O_2 saturation of 90% on O_2 via mask at 8 L/min. The patient was medicated with fentanyl in 2 doses of 50-μg increments with good relief.

4. How could the patient be expected to respond postoperatively and when should dialysis be reinstituted?

Postoperative evaluation should be conducted in the recovery room within the first 24 hours. Dialysis is generally begun within 24 hours postoperatively if the patient is stable. The postoperative evaluation for this patient was conducted 20 hours postoperatively while he was undergoing hemodialysis. Diagnostic data obtained during the first postoperative morning and before dialysis included CBC (Hb, 11.1 g/100 mL; Hct, 33%; wbc, 21 500/mm^3; plt, 345 000/mm^3), chemistry panel (Na$^+$, 130 mEq/L; K$^+$, 5.3 mEq/L; Cl$^-$, 100 mEq/L; CO$_2$, 16.6 mEq/L; BUN, 49 mg/l00 mL; creatinine, 8.4 g/100 mL; glucose, 298 mg/100 mL) and PT/PTT (13.6 s/21.4 s). Postoperative ECG was not obtained, as it was not deemed necessary for this patient. Vital signs were unchanged from preoperative values with BP of 128/66 mmHg, HR of 74, RR of 24, T of 99.4, and O$_2$ saturation of 97% on room air. Auscultation of the heart and lungs was normal, without peripheral edema or jugular venous congestion. The patient had no recall of intraoperative or immediate postoperative events.

► SUMMARY

Patients presenting for surgery require vigilant and complex anesthetic management. A thorough understanding of the pathophysiology and the anesthetic ramifications of each disease entity prepares the anesthetist to provide quality care to these patients.

► KEY CONCEPTS

- The risk factors strongly predictive of postoperative renal failure include perioperative renal dysfunction, cardiac failure, and advanced age.
- Inadequate renal perfusion is the most frequently recognized single insult leading to ARF during surgery, hemorrhage, or dehydration.
- Because of the increased risk of aspiration due to delayed gastric emptying and hyperacidity, rapid sequence induction and aspiration prophylaxis with an H$_2$ receptor antagonist and metoclopramide are indicated for patients with ESRD undergoing surgery.
- Renal dysfunction results in decreased elimination and prolonged effect of ionized drugs including nondepolarizing muscle relaxants, antibiotics, diuretics, cholinesterase inhibitors, and digoxin.
- Anesthetic agents and techniques affect renal function either directly or indirectly, decreasing GFR, urine ouput, and solute excretion; however, these effects are resolved in the early postoperative period and can be attenuated by preoperative hydration.
- Patients with diabetic autonomic neuropathy, which occurs 50% of the time with concurrent hypertension, are more likely to have silent myocardial ischemia.
- Chronic glycemic control is the factor best correlated to complications of diabetes; intensive therapy and tight glycemic control markedly delay or prevent complications associated with diabetes.
- Anesthetic management for patients with gastrointestinal dysfunction require that care be focused on protection of the airway and lungs from gastric secretions and restoring depleted intravascular volume.
- Patients with acute or chronic active hepatitis should not undergo elective surgical procedures, as the mortality approaches 10% with a 12% incidence of morbidity in those who do survive. The poor prognosis is likely due to hepatic blood flow alterations that occur during anesthesia and surgery and may precipitate hepatic necrosis in the immediate postoperative period.
- Anesthetic drug pharmacokinetics and pharmacodynamics are altered significantly in patients with hepatic disease. This includes decreased protein binding, increases in volume of distribution, and decreased drug clearance.
- Anesthetic management of the patient with acute pancreatitis is geared toward correcting hypovolemic shock and treating electrolyte imbalances, especially hypocalcemia. Pleural effusion and ARDS are common among these patients, so postoperative ventilatory support may be required.
- Thyroid storm under anestheisa can be confused with malignant hyperthermia, although thyroid storm typically lacks the muscle rigidity, metabolic acidosis, and malignant arrhythmias associated with malignant hyperthermia. Treatment of thyroid storm should be initiated as soon as the differential diagnosis is made.
- Only a minority of patients with suppressed adrenal function will have cardiovascular mishaps if they do not receive supplemental steroids, and the risk associated with giving supplemental steroids is minimal.

► Study Questions

1. What is the kidney's response to decreased renal blood flow, including neural and humoral mechanisms?

2. What are the anesthetic implications of renal failure?

3. What is autoregulation of the kidney and what conditions and factors affect it?

4. What is the pathophysiology of DKA and hyperosmolar nonketotic syndrome?

5. What are the signs and symptoms of androgen excess and the anesthetic implications?

6. What are the signs, symptoms, and treatment of intraoperative thyroid storm?

7. What is the effect of chronic liver disease on drug metabolism?

8. What cardiovascular and pulmonary alterations accompany hepatic disease?

9. What are the etiologies of parenchymal hepatic disease and the implication for anesthetic mortality and morbidity?

10. What are the symptoms associated with adenopophyseal hormone excess and deficiency and the anesthetic implications of these disorders?

KEY REFERENCES

Aronson, S. (1995). Monitoring renal function in patients with and without transplants. *American Society of Anesthesiologists Refresher Courses in Anesthesiology, 23,* 1–13.

Becker, K. L. (Ed.). (1995). *Principles and practice of endocrinology and metabolism* (2nd ed.). Philadelphia: Lippincott.

Brown, B. R. (1988). Obstructive (cholestatic) jaundice. In B. R. Brown (Ed.), *Anesthesia in hepatic and biliary tract disease* (pp. 253–261). Philadelphia: F. A. Davis.

Dooley, J. R. & Mazze, R. I. (1996). Oliguria. In N. Gravenstein & R. Kirby (Eds.), *Complications in anesthesiology* (2nd ed., pp. 479–491). Philadelphia: Lippincott-Raven.

Gavin, L. A. (1992). Perioperative management of the diabetic patient. *Endocrinology and Metabolism Clinics of North America, 21*(2), 457–475.

Greene, N. M. (1981). Anesthesia risk factors in patients with liver disease. *Contemporary Anesthesia Practice, 4,* 87.

Jeffcoate, W. (1993). *Lecture notes on endocrinology* (5th ed.). Cambridge, MA: Blackwell Scientific Publications.

Kaufman, B. S. & Contreras, J. (1990). Preanesthetic assessment of the patient with renal disease. *Anesthesiology Clinics of North America, 8*(4), 677–695.

Mamel, J. J. (1982). Gastric emptying disorders. In H. J. Nord & P. G. Brady (Eds.), *Critical care gastroenterology* (p. 113). New York: Churchill Livingstone.

Malhotra, V. (Ed.) (1996). *Anesthesia for renal and genito–urologic surgery.* New York: McGraw-Hill.

Pronovost, P. H. & Parris, K. H. (1995). Perioperative management of thyroid disease. *Postgraduate Medicine, 98*(2), 83–98.

Sladen, R. N. (1987). Effect of anesthesia and surgery on renal function. *Critical Care Clinics, 3*(2), 373–393.

Stoelting, R. K. & Dierdorf, S. F. (Eds.). (1993). *Anesthesia and co-existing disease* (3rd ed., pp. 289–312; 339–373). New York: Churchill Livingstone.

Wilson, J. D. & Foster, D. W. (Eds.). (1993). *Williams textbook of endocrine physiology* (8th ed.). Philadelphia: Saunders.

REFERENCES

Ambus, M. D., Evans, S. & Smith, N. T. (1994). Thyrotoxicosis factitia in the anesthetized patient. *Anesthesiology, 81*(1), 254–256.

Arden, J. R., Lyman, D. P., Castagnoli, K. P., Cantell, P. C., Cannon, J. C., & Miller, R. D. (1988). Vecuronium in alcoholic liver disease: A pharmacokinetic and pharmacodynamic analysis. *Anesthesiology, 68*(5), 771–776.

Aranha, G. V. & Greenlee, H. B. (1986). Intraabdominal surgery in patients with advanced cirrhosis. *Archives of Surgery, 121,* 275.

Aron, D. C., Tyrrell, J. B., & Wilson, C. B. (1995). Pituitary tumors: Current concepts in diagnosis and management. *Western Journal of Medicine, 162,* 340–352.

Aronson, S. (1995a). Controversies: Should anesthesiologists worry about the kidney? *Anesthesia & Analgesia, 1995 Review Course Lectures* (suppl.), 68–73.

Aronson, S. (1995b). Monitoring renal function in patients with and without transplants. *American Society of Anesthesiologists Refresher Courses in Anesthesiology, 23,* 1–13.

Aurbach, G. D., Marx, S. J., & Spiegel, A. M. (1992). Parathyroid hormone, calcitonin, and the calciferols. In J. D. Wilson & D. W. Foster (Eds.), *Williams textbook of endocrine physiology* (8th ed., pp. 1397–1476). Philadelphia: Saunders.

Bastron, R. D. (1985). Anesthetic considerations for patients with end stage renal disease. *American Society of Anesthesiologists Refresher Courses in Anesthesiology, 13,* 33–41.

Batcheller, J. (1992). Disorders of antidiuretic hormone secretion. *AACN—Clinical Issues in Critical Care Nursing, 3*(2), 370–378.

Batcheller, J. (1994). Syndrome of inappropriate antidiuretic hormone secretion. *Critical Care Nursing Clinics of North America, 6*(4), 687–692.

Bell, T. N. (1994). Diabetes insipidus. *Critical Care Nursing Clinics of North America, 6*(4), 675–685.

Bioulac-Sage, P., Lafon, M., Saric, J., & Balabaud, C. (1990). Nerves and perisinusoidal cells in human liver. *Journal of Hepatology, 10,* 105.

Blevins L. S. & Wand G. S. (1992). Diabetes insipidus. *Critical Care Medicine 20*(1), 69–79.

Bonner-Weir, S. (1995). Morphology of the endocrine pancreas. In K. L. Becker (Ed.), *Principles and practice of endocrinology and metabolism* (2nd ed., pp. 1187–1191). Philadelphia: Lippincott.

Bready, L. L. (1992). Renal dialysis. In L. Bready & B. Smith (Eds.), *Decision making in anesthesiology* (2nd ed., pp. 150–151). St. Louis: Decker.

Brock-Utne, J. G., Dow, T. G. B., Welman, S., Dimopoulous, G. E., & Moshal, M. G. (1978). The effect of metoclopramide on the lower esophageal sphincter in late pregnancy. *Obstetrics and Gynecology, 51,* 426.

Brock-Utne, J. G., Rubin, J., McAravey, R., Dow, T. G., Welman, S., Dimopoulos, G. E., & Moshal, M. G. (1977). The effect of hyoscine and atropine on the lower esophageal sphincter. *Anaesthesia and Intensive Care, 5,* 223.

Brock-Utne, J. G., Rubin, J., Wellman, S., Dimopoulos, G. E., Moshal, M. G., & Downing, J. W. (1978). The effects of glycopyrrolate (Robinul) on the lower esophageal sphincter. *Canadian Anaesthetists Society Journal, 25,* 144.

Brown, A. (1991). Acute pancreatitis. *AACN Focus on Critical Care, 18*(2), 121–130.

Brown, B. R. (1988). Obstructive (cholestatic) jaundice. In B. R. Brown (Ed.), *Anesthesia in hepatic and biliary tract disease* (pp. 253–261). Philadelphia: F. A. Davis.

Broyer, M. (1986). Demography of dialysis and transplantation in Europe. *Nephrology, Dialysis, and Transplantation, 1,* 1.

Burchardi, H. & Kaczmarczyk, G. (1994). The effect of anesthesia on renal function. *European Journal of Anesthesiology, 11,* 163–168.

Byrick, R. J. & Rose, D. K. (1990). Pathophysiology and prevention of acute renal failure: The role of the anaesthetist. *Canadian Journal of Anaesthetists, 37*(4), 457–467.

Campbell, A. M. & Bousfield, J. D. (1992). Anaesthesia in a patient with Noonan's syndrome and cardiomyopathy. *Anaesthesia, 47*(2), 131–133.

Carson, J. L. & Eisenberg, J. M. (1982). The preoperative screening examination. In D. R. Goldmann (Ed.), *Medical care of the surgical patient* (pp. 16–30). Philadelphia: Lippincott.

Clarke, R. S. J., Hoggart, J. R., & Lavery, J. (1976). Changes in liver function after different types of surgery. *British Journal of Anaesthesia, 48,* 119–128.

Conzen, P. E., Nuschler, M., Melotte, A., Verhaegen, M., Leupoly, P., Van Aken, H., & Peter, K. (1995). Renal function and serum fluoride concentrations in patients with stable renal insufficiency after anesthesia with sevoflurane or enflurane. *Anesthesia & Analgesia, 81,* 569–575.

Derman, R. J. (1995). Effects of sex steroids on women's health: implications for practitioners. *American Journal of Medicine, 98* (suppl 1A), 1A-137S–1A-143S.

Dexter, R. N. (1995). Hypopituitarism. In K. L. Becker (Ed.), *Principles and practice of endocrinology and metabolism,* (2nd ed., pp. 169–180). Philadelphia: Lippincott.

The Diabetes Control and Complications Trial Research Group. (1995). The effect of intensive diabetes therapy on the development and progression of neuropathy. *Annals of Internal Medicine, 122*(8), 561–568.

Dienstag, J. L., Alaama, A., Mosley, J. W., Redeker, A. G., & Purcell, R. H. (1977). Etiology of sporadic hepatitis B surface antigen-negative hepatitis. *Annals of Internal Medicine, 87,* 1.

Dooley, J. R., & Mazze, R. I. (1996). Oliguria. In N. Gravenstein & R. Kirby (Eds.), *Complications in anesthesiology* (2nd ed., pp. 479–491). Philadelphia: Lippincott-Raven.

Eger, E. I., Koblin, D. D., Bowland, T., Ionescu, P., Laster, M. J., Fang, Z., Gong, D., Sonner, J., & Weiskopf, R. B. (1997). Nephrotoxicity of sevoflurane versus desflurane anesthesia in volunteers. *Anesthesia & Analgesia, 84,* 160–168.

Ferrier, C., Marty, J., Bouffars, Y., Haberer, J. P., Levron, J. C., Duvaldeston, P. (1985). Alfentanil pharmacokinetics in patients with cirrhosis. *Anesthesiology 62,* 480.

Frank, B. B. (1989). Clinical evaluation of jaundice. *Journal of the American Medical Association, 262*(21), 3031.

Furukawa, T., Hara, N., Yasumoto, K., & Inkuchi, K. (1984). Arterial hypoxemia in patients with hepatic cirrhosis. *American Journal of Medical Sciences, 287,* 3–10.

Gavin L. A. (1992). Perioperative management of the diabetic patient. *Endocrine and Metabolism Clinics of North America 21*(2), 457–475.

Gelman, S. (1989). Anesthesia and the liver. In P. G. Barash, B. F. Cullen, & R. K. Stoelting (Eds.), *Clinical anesthesia* (pp. 1133–1159). Philadelphia: Lippincott.

Gelman, S., Fowler, F. C., & Smith, K. R. (1983). Liver circulation and function during isoflurane anesthesia in dogs. *Anesthesiology, 59,* A224.

Goldfarb, G., Debaene, B., Ang, E., Roulot, D., Jolis, P., & Lebreu, P. (1990). Hepatic blood flow in humans during isoflurane–N_2O and halothane–N_2O anesthesia. *Anesthesia & Analgesia, 71,* 349–353.

Greenberger, N. J. (1989). *Gastrointestinal disorders: A pathophysiological approach* (4th ed., pp. 95–100). Chicago: Year Book Publishers.

Greene, N. M. (1981). Anesthesia risk factors in patients with liver disease. *Contemporary Anesthesia Practice, 4,* 87.

Griffing, G. T. & Melby, J. C. (1982). Enalapril and white cell count and hematocrit. *Lancet, 1*(82–85), 1361–1363.

Gumowski, J., Proch, M., Kessler, C. A. (1992). Endocrinopathies of hyperfunction: Cushing's syndrome and aldosteronism. *AACN Clinical Issues in Critical Care Nursing 3*(2), 331–347.

Guyton, A. C., & Hall, J. E. (1996). *Textbook of medical physiology* (9th ed., pp. 199–208, 221–238, 297–424, 749–760, 793–854, 883–888, 925–1002). Philadelphia; Saunders.

Halban, P. A., & Weir, G. C. (1995). Islet cell hormones: Production and degradation. In K. L. Becker (Ed.), *Principles and practice of endocrinology and metabolism* (2nd ed., pp. 1191–1198). Philadelphia: Lippincott.

Hansen, K. M., & Johnson, P. C. (1966). Local control of hepatic arterial and portal venous flow in the dog. *American Journal of Physiology, 211,* 712–720.

Hart I. R. (1995, January 15). Management decisions in subclinical thyroid disease. *Hospital Practice,* (Office Edition) *30*(1)43–50.

Harville, D. D., & Dummerskill, W. H. J. (1963). Surgery in acute hepatitis. Causes and effects. *Journal of the American Medical Association, 184,* 257.

Hemmings, H. C., Jr. (1996). Anesthetics, adjuvant drugs, and the kidney. In V. Malhotra (Ed.), *Anesthesia for renal and genito–urologic surgery* (pp. 15–29). New York: McGraw-Hill.

Ishihara, H., Singh, H., & Giesecke, A. H. (1994). Relationship between diabetic autonomic neuropathy and gastric contents. *Anesthesia & Analgesia, 78,* 943–947.

Jeffcoate W. (1993). *Lecture Notes on Endocrinology* (5th ed.). Cambridge, MA: Blackwell Scientific Publications.

Jensen, N. F., Fiddler, D. S., & Striepe, V. (1995). Anesthetic considerations in porphyria. *Anesthesia & Analgesia, 80,* 591–599.

Jones, R. M., Fiddian-Green, R., & Knight, P. R. (1978). Narcotic-induced choledochoduodenal sphincter spasm reversed by glucagon. *Anesthesia & Analgesia, 48,* 437.

Jordan R. M. (1995). Myxedema coma. *Medical Clinics of North America, 79*(1), 185–194.

Kandel, L., Laster, M. J., Eger, E. I., Kerschmann, R. L., & Martin, J. (1995). Nephrotoxicity in rats undergoing a one-hour exposure to compound A. *Anesthesia & Analgesia, 81,* 559–568.

Kaufman, B. S. & Contreras, J. (1990). Preanesthetic assessment of the patient with renal disease. *Anesthesiology Clinics of North America, 8*(4), 677–695.

Kellen, M., Aronson, S., Roizen, M. F., Barnard, J., & Thisted, R. A. (1994). Predictive and diagnostic tests of renal failure: A review. *Anesthesia & Analgesia, 78,* 134–142.

Kennedy, W., Evereet, G., Cogg, L.(1971). Simultaneous systemic and hepatic hemodynamic measurements during epidural anesthesia in normal patients. *Anesthesia & Analgesia, 50,* 1069–1077.

Krugman, S., Ward, R., & Giles, J. P. (1962). The natural history of infectious hepatitis. *American Journal of Medicine, 32,* 717.

Krumberger, J. M. (1993). Acute pancreatitis. *Critical Care Nursing Clinics of North America, 5*(1), 185–202.

Lake, C. L. (1992). Cardiovascular anatomy and physiology. In P. G. Barash (Ed.), *Clinical anesthesia* (2nd ed., pp. 989–1020). Philadelphia: Lippincott.

Larson, C. P. (1992). Evaluation of the patient and preoperative preparation. In P. G. Barash, B. F. Cullen, & R. K. Stoelting (Eds.), *Clinical anesthesia* (2nd ed., pp. 545–562). Philadelphia: Lippincott.

Lebach, W. K. (1975). Cirrhosis in the alcoholic and its relation to the volume of alcohol abuse. *Annals of the New York Academy of Science, 252,* 85.

Lee L. M & Gumowski J. (1992). Adrenocortical insufficiency: A medical emergency. *AACN Clinical Issues in Critical Care Nursing, 3*(2), 319–330.

Livolsi, V. A. (1995). Morphology of the thyroid gland. In K. L. Becker (Ed.), *Principles and practice of endocrinology and metabolism* (2nd ed., pp. 281–284). Philadelphia: Lippincott.

Lo Gerfo, P., Ditkoff, B. A., Chabot, J., & Feind, C. (1994). Thyroid surgery using monitored anesthesia care: An alternative to general anesthesia. *Thyroid, 4*(4), 437–439.

Marley, W. (1993). AANA Journal Course: Update for nurse anesthetists—Essential hypertension, anesthesia and the kidney. *AANA Journal, 61*(6), 597–604.

MacGilchrist, A. J., Birnie, G. G., Cook, A., Scobie, G., Murray, T., Watkinson, G., & Brodie, M. J. (1986). Pharmacokinetics and pharmacodynamics of intravenous midazolam in patients with severe alcoholic cirrhosis. *Gut 27,* 190.

Magorian, T., Wood, P., Cauldwell, J. E., & Miller, R. D. (1991). Pharmacokinetics, onset, and duration of action of rocuronium in humans: Normal vs hepatic dysfunction. *Anesthesiology, 75,* A1069.

Malhotra, V. (1994). Anesthesia and the renal and genitourinary systems. In R. D. Miller (Ed.), *Anesthesia* (4th ed., pp. 1947–1968). New York: Churchill Livingstone.

Mamel, J. J. (1982). Gastric emptying disorders. In H. J. Nord & P. G. Brady (Eds.), *Critical care gastroenterology* (p. 113). New York: Churchill Livingstone.

Mazze, M. (1994). Anesthesia and the liver. In R. D. Miller (Ed.), *Anesthesia* (4th ed., p. 1970). New York: Churchill Livingstone.

Mazze, R. I. (1990a). Anesthesia and the renal and genitourinary systems. In R. D. Miller (Ed.), *Anesthesia* (3rd ed., pp. 1791–1808). New York: Churchill Livingstone.

Mazze, R. I. (1990b). Renal physiology. In R. D. Miller (Ed.), *Anesthesia* (3rd ed., pp. 601–617). New York: Churchill Livingstone.

Mazze, R. I., Fujinaga, M., & Wharton, R. S. (1996). Fluid and electrolyte problems. In N. Gravenstein & R. R. Kirby (Eds.), *Complications in anesthesiology* (2nd ed., pp. 459–478). Philadelphia: Lippincott-Raven.

McMorrow, M. E. (1992). The elderly and thyrotoxicosis. *AACN Clinical Issues in Critical Care Nursing, 3*(1), 114–119.

Merimee, T. J. & Tyson, J. E. (1974). Stabilization of plasma glucose during fasting. *New England Journal of Medicine, 291,* 1275–1278.

Milaskiewicz, R. M. & Hall, G. M. (1992). Diabetes and anesthesia: The past decade. *British Journal of Anaesthesia, 68,* 198–206.

Miller, E. D., Jr. (1996). Understanding renal function and its preoperative evaluation. In V. Malhotra (Ed.), *Anesthesia for renal and genito–urologic surgery* (pp. 1–14). New York: McGraw-Hill.

Morgan, G. E. & Mikhail, M. S. (1996). *Clinical anesthesiology* (2nd ed., pp. 575–649), Stamford, CT: Appleton & Lange.

Muir, A., Schatz, D. A., Maclaren, N. K. (1992). The pathogenesis, prediction, and prevention of insulin-dependent diabetes mellitus. *Endocrine and Metabolic Clinics of North America, 21*(2), 199–219.

Muravchick, S. (1991). Renal function and body fluids compartments. In: *The Anesthetic plan: From physiological principles to clinical strategies* (pp. 286–324). St. Louis: Mosby Year Book.

Murray, M. D., Bater, D. C., Tierney, W. M., Hui, S. L., McDonald, C. J. (1990). Ibuprofen associated renal impairment in a large general internal medicine practice. *American Journal of Medical Sciences, 299*(4), 222–229.

Nathan, D. M. (1996). The pathophysiology of diabetic complications: How much does the glucose hypothesis explain? *Annals of Internal Medicine 124*(1, Pt. 2), 86–89.

Notivol, R. I., Carrio, L., Cano, L., Estorch, M., & Vilaredell, F. (1984). Gastric emptying of solid and liquid meals in healthy young subjects. *Scandanavian Journal of Gastroenterology, 8,* 1107–1113.

Novis, B. K., Roizen, M. F., Aronson, S., & Thisted, R. A. (1994). Association of preoperative risk factors with postoperative renal failure. *Anesthesia & Analgesia, 78,* 143–149.

Ockert, D. B. M. & Hugo, J. M. (1992). Diabetic complications with special anaesthetic risk. *South African Journal of Surgery, 30*(3), 90–94.

Orth, D. N. (1995). Cushing's syndrome. *New England Journal of Medicine, 332*(12), 791–803.

Oster, J. R., Singer, I., & Fishman, L. M. (1995). Heparin-induced aldosterone suppression and hyperkalemia. *American Journal of Medicine, 98,* 575–586.

Patafio, O. (1996). Acute renal failure and perioperative oliguria. In V. Malhotra (Ed.), *Anesthesia for renal and genito–urologic surgery* (pp. 31–43). New York: McGraw-Hill.

Peters, A. & Kerner, W. (1995). Perioperative management of the diabetic patient. *Experimental Clinics in Endocrinology, 103,* 213–218.

Pitts, R. F. (1974). *Physiology of the kidney and body fluids* (3rd ed., p. 134). Chicago: Year Book Medical Publishers.

Powell-Jackson, P., Greenway, B., & Williams, R. (1982). Adverse effects of exploratory laparotomy in patients with suspected liver disease. *British Journal of Surgery, 69,* 449.

Pronovost, P. H. & Parris, K. H. (1995). Perioperative management of thyroid disease. *Postgraduate Medicine, 98*(2), 83–98.

Prough, D. S., & Foreman, A. S. (1992). Anesthesia and the renal system. In P. G. Barash, B. F. Cullen, & R. K. Stoelting (Eds.), *Clinical anesthesia* (2nd ed., pp. 1125–1155). Philadelphia: Lippincott.

Pugh, R. N. H., Murray-Lyon, I. M., Dawson, J. L., Pietroni, M. C., & Williams, R. (1973). Transection of the esophagus for bleeding varices. *British Journal of Surgery, 60,* 646–649.

Radnay, P. A., Duncalf, D., Novakovic, M., & Lesser, M. L., (1984). Common bile duct pressure changes after fentanyl, morphine, meperidine, butorphanol and naloxone. *Anesthesia & Analgesia, 63,* 441–444.

Reingold, A. L, Kane, M. A., & Hightower, A. W. (1988). Failure of gloves and other protective devices to prevent transmission of hepatitis B virus to oral surgeons. *Journal of the American Medical Association, 259,* 2558.

Robertson, G. L. (1995). Physiology of vasopressin and oxytocin, and thirst. In K. L. Becker (Ed.), *Principles and practice of endocrinology and metabolism* (2nd ed., pp. 248–257). Philadelphia: Lippincott.

Rodriguez, R., Roisen, R., Roca, J., Agusti, A. G., Mastai, R., Wagner, P. D., & Bosch, J. (1987). Gas exchange and pulmonary vascular reactivity in patients with liver cirrhosis. *American Review of Respiratory Disease, 135,* 1085–1092.

Roizen M. F. (1996). Endocrine abnormalities and anesthesia: Adrenal dysfunction and diabetes. *Anesthesia & Analgesia* (suppl.), 104–113.

Schemel, W. H. (1976). Unexpected hepatic dysfunction found by multiple laboratory screening. *Anesthesia & Analgesia, 55*(6), 810–812.

Schmidt, W. (1976). The epidemiology of cirrhosis of the liver. In M. M. Fisher & J. G. Rankin (Eds.), *Alcohol and the liver.* New York, Plenum.

Schurizek, B. A., Kraguland, K., Andreasen, F., Jensen, L. V., & Juhl, B. (1988). Gastrointestinal motility and gastric pH and emptying following ingestion of diazepam. *British Journal of Anaesthesia, 61*(6), 712–719.

Schwartz, N. & Eisenkraft, J. B. (1992). Anesthetic management of a child with Noonan's syndrome and idiopathic hypertrophic subaortic stenosis. *Anesthesia & Analgesia, 74,* 464-466.

Shusterman, N. (1987). Risk factors and outcome of hospital-acquired acute renal failure: Clinical epidemiologic study. *American Journal of Medicine, 83,* 65–71.

Sieber, F. E., Smith, D. S., Traystman, R. J., & Wollman, H. (1987). Glucose: A reevaluation of its intraoperative use. *Anesthesiology, 67,* 72–81.

Siperstein, M. D. (1992). Diabetic ketoacidosis and hyperosmolar coma. *Endocrinology and Metabolic Clinics of North America, 21*(2), 415–433.

Sladen, R. N. (1996, October). *Anesthetic concerns for the patient with renal disease.* In 47th annual refresher course lectures and clinical update program, (No. 171). New Orleans: American Society of Anesthesiologists.

Sladen, R. N. (1987). Effect of anesthesia and surgery on renal function. *Critical Care Clinics, 3*(2), 373–393.

Sladen, R. N. (1994). Renal physiology. In R. D. Miller (Ed.), *Anesthesia* (4th ed., pp. 663–688), New York: Churchill Livingstone.

Smith, S. A. (1995). Commonly asked questions about thyroid function. *Mayo Clinic Proceedings, 70,* 573–577.

Steer, P. J. (1990). The endocrinology of parturition in the human. *Balliere's Clinical Endocrinology and Metabolism, 4,* 333–349.

Stoelting, R. K. (1991). *Pharmacology and physiology in anesthesia practice* (2nd ed., pp. 23–25; 737–739; 778–781). Philadelphia: Lippincott.

Stoelting, R. K. & Dierdorf, S. F. (1993). Renal disease. In: *Anesthesia and co-existing disease* (3rd ed., pp. 289–312; 339–373). New York: Churchill Livingstone.

Strunin, L. (1977). The liver in anesthesia. In W. W. Muschin (Ed.), *Problems in anesthesia* (p. 37), Philadelphia: Saunders.

Symreng, T., Karlberg, B. E., Kagedal, B., & Schildt, B. (1981). Physiological cortisol substitution of long-term steroid-treated patients undergoing major surgery. *British Journal of Anaesthesia 53*(9), 945–954.

Thompson, P. D., Melmon, K. L., Richardson, J. A., Cohn, K., Steinbrum, W., Cudihee, R., & Rowland, M. (1973). Lidocaine pharmacokinetics in advanced heart failure, liver disease and renal failure in humans. *Annals of Internal Medicine, 78*(4), 499.

Todesco, J., Williams, R. T, & Eagle, C. J. (1994). Anaesthetic management of a patient with a large neck mass. *Canadian Journal of Anaesthesia, 41*(2), 157–160.

Toto, K. H. (1994). Endocrine physiology: A comprehensive review. *Critical Care Nursing Clinics of North America, 6*(4), 637–653.

Tsukamoto, N., Hirabayashi, Y., Shimuzu, R., & Mitsuhata, H. (1996). The effects of sevoflurane and iosflurane anesthesia on renal tubular function in patients with moderately impaired renal function. *Anesthesia & Analgesia, 82,* 909–913.

Usala, S. J. (1995). Physiology and the thyroid gland II: Receptors, postreceptor events, and hormone resistance syndromes. In K. L. Becker (Ed.), *Principles and practice of endocrinology and metabolism* (2nd ed., pp. 292–299). Philadelphia: Lippincott.

Viegas, O. J. & Stoelting, R. K. (1979). LDH5 changes after cholesystectomy or hysterectomy in patients receiving halothane, enflurane, or fentanyl. *Anesthesiology, 51,* 556–558.

Volpé R. (1993). The management of subacute (DeQuervain's) thyroiditis. *Thyroid, 3*(3), 253–255.

Ward, M. E., Knight, K. M., Strunin, J. M., & Strunin, L. (1976). Serum pseudocholinesterase concentrations in fulminant hepatic failure. *British Journal of Anaesthesia, 48*(8), 818.

Ward, J. B, Petersen, O. H., Jenkins, S. A., & Sutton, R. (1995). Is an elevated concentration of acinar cytosolic free ionized calcium the trigger for acute pancreatitis? *Lancet, 346,* 1016–1019.

White, P. C., Pescovita, O. H., & Cutler, G. B. (1995). Synthesis and metabolism of corticosteroids. In K. L. Becker (Ed.), *Principles and practice of endocrinology and metabolism* (2nd ed., pp. 647–662). Philadelphia: Lippincott.

Ziemniak, J., Bernard, J., & Schentag, J. (1983). Hepatic encephalopathy and altered cimetidine kinetics. *Clinical Pharmacology and Therapeutics, 34,* 375.

The Geriatric Patient

Wynne R. Waugaman and Benjamin M. Rigor, Sr.

Aging is a complex phenomena, partly exogenous and partly endogenous, in which physiologic and pathologic processes are often inextricably mixed. Since World War II, our society has undergone profound changes, including rapid growth and greater sophistication in the delivery and technology of medicine. As a result, we are presented daily with large numbers of patients who have lived longer and survived the physiologic effects of age and disease only to require extensive surgery.

As the elderly population increases, so will the incidence of other associated and chronic diseases such as Alzheimer's disease. The impact of this age factor is significant as demographic trends illustrate that the population susceptible to Alzheimer's disease is increasing rapidly. The risk for developing Alzheimer's disease is more than 10% among adults 80 to 85 years of age and more than 20% among those 85 to 89 years of age (Jenike, 1996). The risk of surgery for many elderly patients is complicated by chronic disease processes. The reported incidence of the most prevalent diseases among the aged are 78% for osteoarthritis, 40% for hypertension, 40% for heart disease, and 4% for diabetes mellitus (Waugaman & Rigor, 1992).

When adequately prepared, elderly people can tolerate many types of operations as well as young people; however, in the case of extensive major operations, the mortality rate for the elderly may be four to eight times higher than that for young patients. Patients older than 70 years have an overall elective surgery mortality less than 5% compared with nearly 10% for emergency surgery, with variations depending on anatomic site and development of complications (Waugaman & Rigor, 1992). At least 2% of this mortality can be attributed to anesthesia. It has been reported that more than 100 000 patients older than 65 years die postoperatively each year (Moritz & Ostfeld, 1990).

The success of anesthesia and surgery with these patients in part depends on the nurse anesthetist's knowledge of physiologic alterations caused by the aging process and of the possible effects of anesthetics and adjuvant and supportive drugs on the elderly. Although age alone does not preclude surgery, it is apparent that the anesthetic management of the elderly is influenced by the frequency and severity of degenerative diseases and chronic illnesses affecting vital organs and organ systems.

▶ AGING AND MORTALITY

There is no consensus as to the true definition of old age, but most authors and experts consider age 65 and older as elderly and the true scope of geriatric medicine. It has been known that chronologic age has no direct relationship with physiologic age, and aging can be characterized as a process in which there are well-documented changes in the chemical composition of the body, a broad spectrum of progressive deteriorative changes, reduced ability to respond and adapt to environmental changes, an increased vulnerability to many diseases, and an increase in mortality. As we approach the twenty-first century, people older than 65 years constitute approximately 13% of the population. This will increase to approximately 20% or 70 million by the year 2030 (U.S. Bureau of Census, 1993). Five million Americans reach the age of 65 every day, and about 1% of the population is 100 years old or older (Treas & Longino, 1997). The average human life span in the United States was 47 in the year 1900 and 76 years in 1993. By 2010, it will be 82.4 years because of improved nutrition, sanitation, and health care, as well as healthier lifestyles, advancements in medical technology, and better drug therapy. This will happen despite the increased incidence of AIDS and "lifestyle" diseases, for example, chemical dependency (alcoholism), domestic violence, abuse of the elderly, and motor vehicle accident (MVA) deaths (Mittlemark, 1994). In fact, MVAs are the leading cause of injury and death among older adults.

As the birth rate decreases, the percentage of geriatric people increases. The biologic limit to the human life span now appears to be around 100 years of age. A person reaching the age of 85 has only 1 in 10 000 chances of reaching the age of 110 (Treas & Longino, 1997). The population of Americans 65 and older is a large and diverse group; however, there is a considerable heterogeneity in the manner in which these people mature, and the elderly population itself is aging. There is also a trend toward higher mortality rates for males compared with females for all age groups. It seems that the elderly of the new era or the coming decades will be better educated and therefore more demanding and sophisticated health care consumers (Mittlemark, 1994).

Eighty percent of Americans older than 65 years have at least one chronic disease, and many have more than one. The most common coexisting conditions in the elderly are congestive heart failure, depression, dementia, chronic renal failure, angina pectoris, ischemic heart disease, osteoarthritis, gait disorders, urinary incontinence, vascular insufficiency, constipation, diabetes, sensory and perceptual deficits, sleep disorders, adverse drug reactions, and anemia. More than 80% of all health care resources in the United States are devoted to care for chronic medical conditions, and 75% of elderly

deaths can be attributed to these causes (Treas & Longino, 1997).

► HEALTH CARE EXPENDITURES FOR THE ELDERLY

The elderly are more likely to have health problems and physical infirmity. The per capita health care cost for persons 65 and older is approximately three times that for the younger person. Whereas older persons represent 11% of the total population, they account for 29% ($41.3 billion) of total personal health care costs. Of these costs, one third is paid by private sources and two thirds by Medicare, Medicaid, and other state and federal programs (Fig. 14–1). More than half of elderly Americans have some chronic medical conditions, and 18% have limited ability to work or care for themselves. The elderly make 40% to 50% more outpatient physician visits and are 2.5 times more likely to be admitted to a hospital where they spend 70% more time per admission than younger patients (Pawlson, 1994). Thus, per capita, the elderly accumulate three times more hospital bed days than do the young, and they constitute over 90% of long-term care patients. These long-term care patients now occupy more beds than all general hospital beds in the United States combined at an annual cost exceeding $15 billion per year. In 1988 alone, the financial risk of an average older adult for long-term care in a nursing home setting was an average of $22 000. The realistic assumption about the current and future cost of health care and personal economic resources of adults are that no more than 30% to 40% of adults will be able to insure long-term care adequately. The other 60% to 70% will depend on public provision for care (Pawlson, 1994). Twelve percent of the elderly had self-pay expenses of more than

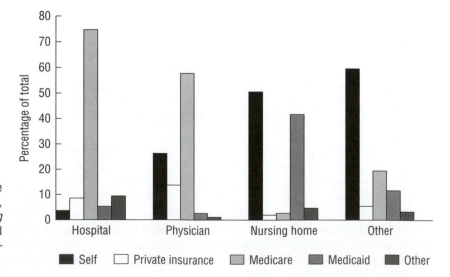

Figure 14–1. Source of payment for health care services for persons 65 and older. *(From Pawlson, L. G. [1994]. Health care implications of an aging population. In* Principles of geriatric medicine and gerontology *[3rd ed., p. 171]. Reprinted with permission of the author.)*

$5000 per year. Those who did average $5000 accounted for nearly 50% of all self-pay expenditures. The 5.9% of Medicare patients who die each year account for nearly 30% of the total program expenditure because of the increase in service volume, intensity of newer technologies, and reimbursement structure of Medicare.

The implications are plain and simple. Aging is here to stay and has many characteristics of a long-term growth industry. The number of individuals aging will increase dramatically as the Baby Boomers turn 65. The elderly are growing older; retirement as currently patterned may no longer be anticipated. The elderly are less homogeneous as a group than the middle-aged, young adults, and children. Statistically, the variability among physiologic and psychologic determinants increases with age: the aged become less alike when compared with other age groups. Aging is a process of change that enhances individual differences in abilities, interests, and background. The elderly have the greatest experience in living. Many have good health, emotional resources, creativity, and a sense of survival that is enviable, and most of the mythology of incapacity is at times unwarranted.

▶ GERIATRICS AND GERONTOLOGY

Gerontology is a field devoted to the study of aging. Care of the aging population requires an interdisciplinary approach. Nurse anesthetists must fully appreciate the lifestyle and health implications of aging beyond the surgical environment. We must emphasize to the practicing nurse anesthetists the "I's" of geriatrics and gerontology, which are as follows:

Impecunity or Income Deficits
Immobility
Incontinence
Isolation
Infections and Immunocompromise
Insomnia
Instability (Falls)
Iatrogenesis

Impecunity. The median income for all elderly households was $16 855 compared with $33 920 for households not headed by an elderly person in 1990. The major source of income for the elderly was Social Security (39%), asset income (25%), earnings (17%), public and private pensions (17%), and other sources (3%). The poverty rate was 10.1% for the elderly Caucasian individual, 22.5% for Hispanic Americans, and 33.8% for African Americans. The poverty rate is higher for those living in nonmetropolitan areas such as those found in the South, those who did not complete high school, and those who were too ill or disabled to work (Tauber, 1992).

Immobility. The most common causes of immobility in the elderly are musculoskeletal, neurologic, and cardiovascular disorders. Degenerative joint diseases, osteoporosis, hip fractures, and podiatric problems such as bunions, calluses, and so on cause pain and reluctance or inability to ambulate. Residual deficit strokes and late stages of Parkinsonism are examples of neurologic conditions. Coronary artery disease with frequent angina, intermittent claudication, and severe chronic obstructive airway disease (COAD) can drastically restrict activity and limit socialization. Some patients restrict their mobility for fear of falling, and the lack of horizontal or upright stability can be due to impaired vision, impaired proprioception, and middle ear pathology. Decreased mobility and increased isolation can also be signs of depression. Excessive medications with sedatives, hypnotics, and antipsychotic drugs impair mobility, and the latter can cause extrapyramidal effects and muscle rigidity (Kane, Ouslander, & Abrass, 1994). The immobile and bedridden surgical patient is usually hypovolemic and in negative nitrogen balance unless proven to the contrary. The anesthetic implications include preoperative orthostatic hypotension, massive hypotension on induction, and hemodynamic cardiovascular instability during the maintenance of anesthesia.

Incontinence. The involuntary loss of urine and/or stools in sufficient amounts or frequency constitutes a social and/or health problem in the elderly. The incidence is about 4% to 6% among community-dwelling older adults, and it is a heterogenous condition that ranges in severity from occasional episodes of dribbling to continuous uncontrolled urination or defecation. It has the potential for severe adverse effects, such as physical (urinary tract infections), psychologic (depression, isolation, and dependency), social (stigmatized by relatives and caregivers as messy and odoriferous), and economic (urologic supplies, caregivers, repeated surgery, etc.) consequences (Kane, Ouslander, & Abrass, 1994).

Isolation. Many elderly patients are isolated and/or insulated from their relatives and family. Of the elderly in community dwellings, 10% to 20% express sadness and 5% have chronic depression (National Institutes of Health, 1991). Loss of memory and other intellectual functions results in depression, and the suicide rate is highest among elderly males older than 80 years (50/100 000 versus 10/100 000 for the general population).

Infections and Immunocompromise. The elderly have a higher incidence of acute and chronic illnesses requiring hospitalization and longer hospital stays, exposing them to nosocomial or hospital-acquired infections. Those who are immunocompromised such as those with malignancies, malnutrition, or chronic debilitating disease are most susceptible to infections. Cell-mediated immunity is also diminished. Many infections are associated with higher morbidity and mortality (Yoshikawa & Norman, 1987). Proper antibiotic therapy must be initiated before surgery, especially in patients who are colonized or immunocompromised, and those with prosthetic devices or parts of the body. The initial dose of the antibiotic must maintain a high blood level after incision of the skin or mucous membrane.

Insomnia. Aging itself is associated with changes in the sleep pattern, such as daytime naps, early bedtime, increased time to onset of sleep, decreased amounts of deeper stages of sleep, and increased periods of wakefulness. Insomnia can be a sign of depression and other psychiatric and medical disorders. It can also be caused by the effects of and/or withdrawal from drugs and alcohol. One third of the elderly population may have specific sleep disorders, including obstructive sleep apnea with associated risks for life-threatening or fatal cardiac dysrhythmias and myocardial and cerebral infarction (Kane, Ouslander, & Abrass, 1994). The anesthetic implications of obstructive sleep apnea are related to sensitivity to agents for premedication and postoperative care, including the possibility of difficult airway management.

Instability (Falls). Nearly one third of those age 65 years and older living at home suffer a fall once a year, and about one in 40 of those are hospitalized; in nursing homes as many as one half suffer a fall each year with 10% to 25% having serious consequences and accounting for two thirds of accidental deaths. Of deaths from falls in the United States, more than 70% occur in the 11% of the population older than 65 (Sattin, Lambert Huber, DeVito, Rodriguez, Ros, Bacchelli, Stevens, & Waxweiler, 1990). Fractures of the hip and lower extremities lead to prolonged disability, hospitalization, and immobility, which can cause deep venous thrombosis (DVT) and the development of hypostatic pneumonia. Instability from various causes, (slower righting reflexes, diminished muscular strength, decreased proprioceptive sense, changes in gait, orthostatic hypotension, and so on) increase susceptibility to falls and other mishaps or accidents, including (MVAs).

Iatrogenesis. Elderly patients are at high risk for iatrogenic complications because they often come from nursing homes and are in poor general/constitutional condition on admission. They also present with a narrower therapeutic window than the younger patient. The hazards of hospitalization include drug and medication errors; environmental hazards; underdiagnosis; dangers of invasive diagnostic procedures, anesthesia, and surgery; falls from hospital beds or in bathrooms, and so on. Among 815 consecutive admissions to a hospital's general medical service, an overall rate of 497 iatrogenic events developed in 36% of patients; 9% resulted in major consequences, and 2% contributed to death (Steel, Gertman, Crescenzi, & Anderson, 1981).

The success of anesthesia and surgery with geriatric patients in part depends on the nurse anesthetist's knowledge of physiologic alterations caused by the aging process and of the possible effects of anesthetics and adjuvant and supportive drugs on the aged. Although age alone does not preclude surgery, it is apparent that the anesthetic management of the elderly is influenced by the frequency and severity of degenerative diseases and chronic illnesses.

▶ ANESTHETIC IMPLICATIONS OF PHYSIOLOGIC ALTERATIONS IN THE ELDERLY

The geriatric patient differs little from the young patient, even when the physiologic aspects of aging are considered because, in general, neither group tolerates prolonged anesthesia or extensive surgery. It can, however, be said that the margin of safety and capacity for compensation are reduced appreciably at the extreme ages of life. The influence of age on the risks of anesthesia and surgery is determined by the type of associated disease and dysfunction; however, separating the effects of aging from those of degenerative disease processes is often difficult.

The aging process is not only a function of chronologic age. Organs and organ systems do not regress at the same rate and speed; thus patients must be assessed individually. Organ function declines 1% per year of the functional capacity present at age 30 (Fig. 14-2). These physiologic changes of aging often interfere with the uptake, distribution, biotransformation, and elimination of anesthetics. The significant physiologic alterations from the aging process and their implications in anesthetic management are discussed in the following sections.

General and Constitutional Changes

The elderly experience a decrease in body fat and adipose tissue, which decreases their ability to retain body heat and, in turn, exposes them to hypothermia in the cool environment of the operating room (OR). Accurate determination of weight and weight changes is profoundly significant. Acute, sudden weight loss is usually due to loss of body water. Chronic weight loss is due to depletion of body stores of protein and fat. As a person ages, his or her body water naturally decreases; however, nutritional deficiencies may also occur in the elderly and are associated with a reduction in intracellular water and total potassium. Hypovolemia, a natural consequence of

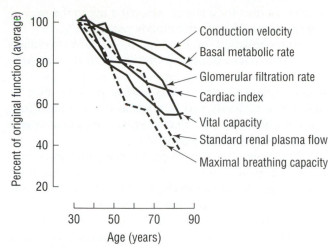

Figure 14–2. Changes in physiologic function with age in humans expressed as percentages of mean values at age 30. *(Reprinted, with permission, from Miller, R. D. [1986]. Anesthesia for the elderly. In R. D. Miller [Ed.], Anesthesia [2nd ed., pp. 1801-1819]. New York: Churchill Livingstone.)*

this decrease in total body water, renders these patients vulnerable to hypotension during induction of anesthesia with potent intravenous agents such as sodium thiopental. Patients who are sedentary, bedridden, or immobilized for long periods are usually hypovolemic and have more difficulty compensating for changes in circulatory physiology caused by altering their posture or position. Their lowered basal metabolic rate (hypothyroid-like state) reduces tolerance to increasing concentrations of premedications, anesthetic agents, postoperative sedatives, hypnotics, and analgesics.

Senile atrophy with collagen loss and decreased elasticity of tissue makes the skin more sensitive to trauma from tape, monitoring electrodes, and surgical tourniquets. When the patient is placed on the operating table, close attention must be paid to bony prominences and other areas sensitive to pressure. Arm boards should be padded properly and the patient's arms positioned comfortably. Care must be taken when a warming blanket is used because burns may occur more frequently in the elderly, particularly in those with peripheral vascular disease or areas of compromised circulation.

The airway of the geriatric patient presents several problems. There is a progressive decrease in reactivity of protective airway reflexes such as coughing and swallowing associated with age. The elderly are often edentulous or have a few loose teeth remaining. These factors make an anesthetic mask fit tenuously and increase the likelihood of regurgitation of stomach contents with aspiration of vomitus into the lungs. Cervical osteoarthritis and laryngeal changes that accompany rheumatoid arthritis, as well as irregular dentition, often increase the difficulty of inserting an endotracheal tube into the tra-

chea to maintain a proper airway and adequately ventilate the lungs.

Cardiovascular System

Arteriosclerotic vascular changes and reduced myocardial reserve decrease cardiac output and stroke volume, prolong circulation time, and decrease perfusion of the vital organs such as the brain, heart, liver, and kidneys. Heart rate also decreases during the aging process. When anesthesia is induced, these cardiac and vascular changes can cause disastrous consequences such as hypotension, myocardial ischemia or infarction, cerebral vascular accidents, and renal failure from decreased renal artery perfusion.

Coronary artery disease is prevalent in younger patients as well as geriatric patients; however, coronary obstructive lesions are seen more frequently in the elderly. It is important to remember that the patient with coronary disease is unable to significantly increase coronary flow. Therefore, preventive measures should be directed against increasing myocardial oxygen demand.

Rapid intravenous induction of potent short-acting barbiturates such as sodium thiopental or methohexital can provoke cardiovascular collapse as a result of poor compensatory hemodynamic response and inadequate cardiac function and blood volume. A prolonged circulation time has profound implications for the intravenous agents. One can anticipate an induction time of up to twice as long as would be expected in a younger patient. This prolonged circulation time not only prolongs the onset of action of succinylcholine, but also decreases the tendency to fasciculate and increases the time during which pseudocholinesterase can act.

The age-related decrease in cardiac index provides a faster induction with volatile inhalation agents of low solubility because of a more rapid rise in alveolar concentration. Hypotension may therefore appear sooner, especially in the patient who is hypovolemic. Bradycardia in the aged is probably best treated with glycopyrrolate, as it does not cross the blood–brain barrier. This drug appears to be more desirable in the elderly than atropine.

The aging myocardium becomes thicker during both systole and diastole. There is a decrease in size and number of individual muscle fibers and an increase in fibrous and adipose tissue. Afterload increases with age. The elastic and muscular tissue in the arterial walls is replaced by fibrous tissue and calcium.

Peripheral vascular resistance increases with age to a greater degree than the decrease in cardiac output, so the blood pressure increases. The most notable increase is generally in the systolic pressure. Hypertension in the elderly, as expected, may be above 160 systolic and 90 diastolic. These numbers may be acceptably increased as age increases. The baroreceptor reflex is diminished during the aging process. There is less tachycardia to warn of hypovolemia and less increase in vascular tone to maintain perfusion pressure.

Respiratory System

Significant respiratory changes that occur with aging include decreased breathing capacity; stiffening and rigidity of air passages as a result of fibrosis; distension of peripheral air sacs; reduction of forced expiratory volume and forced vital capacity; decrease in diffusion properties; and an increase in closing volume. The consequences of these respiratory changes, especially in patients with chronic obstructive airway problems such as emphysema, predispose the elderly to infection and collapse of airways in the early postoperative period. Changes in pulmonary dynamics also decrease or prolong uptake and distribution of less soluble inhalation anesthetics such as sevoflurane.

After age 65, the closing volume becomes greater than the functional residual capacity. There is small airway closure with each breath and relatively decreased ventilation–perfusion, resulting in shunting and a decrease in the Pa_{O_2}. An 80-year-old patient may have normal lungs but have a Pa_{O_2} of 75 torr. This level may be adequate to maintain the oxygen saturation of the blood, but a smaller margin of error exists for periods of hypoxia such as those created by airway obstruction and momentary apnea. This decrease in arterial oxygen tension as a result of age can be predicted by the equation $Pa_{O_2} = 109$ torr $- 0.43 -$ age (in years). Other similar equations exist for the computation of expected Pa_{O_2}.

There is an increased risk of pulmonary embolism in the elderly during the perioperative period, especially for operations conducted in the head-up position or those involving prolonged immobility and bed rest. Miniheparinization, antiembolism stockings, and early ambulation may be helpful in reducing the incidence of pulmonary embolism.

Central and Peripheral Nervous Systems

The decreased requirement for both inhalation and intravenous anesthetics is related not only to circulatory and constitutional changes, but also to decreased neuronal density. Decreased sensitivity to local anesthetic drugs was shown by Bromage (1978) to be caused by changes such as alterations in vascular supply (arteriosclerosis), abnormal neural structures, and differences in the permeability coefficient of the drugs. The peripheral nerve changes that occur with aging are diminution in size and number of motor units.

Brain weight and number of neurons decrease with increased age. This causes the patient to become more sensitive to sedative and hypnotic drugs in terms of a more pronounced initial response and a prolonged recovery. There is also greater sensitivity to the toxic effects of anticholinergic agents such as atropine; doses

that are normal for a young adult (0.4 mg to 0.8 mg) often cause psychosis in the elderly patient.

Autoregulation of cerebral blood flow maintains flow independent of pressure until a critical mean pressure is reached; below this pressure a direct pressure–flow relationship is observed. This critical pressure may be raised in the elderly and in arteriosclerotic individuals. The anesthetist must be alert to avoid even a mild degree of hypotension in these patients.

Reduction in the dopaminergic receptors and postreceptor alterations (cell membrane, ion transport systems, and so on) occur during the aging process. Animal studies have shown that a reduction in total dietary intake of up to 40% causes no change in the number of dopaminergic receptors in the aged versus the young adult (Waugaman & Rigor, 1992). Therefore, one may predict that obesity further contributes to reduction in these receptors.

Hepatorenal System

The decrease in liver enzymes such as plasma pseudocholinesterase reduces the detoxification and elimination of ester-type local anesthetics such as procaine and tetracaine, muscle relaxants such as succinylcholine, and ganglionic blocking agents such as trimethaphan. Therefore, reduced dosages of these drugs are required. Poor or sluggish biotransformation and detoxification prolong and magnify the effects of anesthetics and other adjuvant or supportive drugs.

Changes in renal function as a result of aging influence other body physiology. Degenerative changes in renal circulation begin early. In fact, renal perfusion decreases by 1.5% per year, which means that there is a 40% to 50% decrease from age 25 to age 65. Reduction in plasma albumin and synthesis increases the levels of active drugs, such as barbiturates, local anesthetics, and certain muscle relaxants, that are unbound to plasma proteins. Glomerular filtration rate abruptly decreases after the age of 60, and effective renal plasma flow decreases 10% per decade. Creatinine clearance is the most sensitive indicator of renal function in the elderly. These hepatorenal changes not only reduce drug elimination, but also raise, prolong, or sustain drug levels in blood and tissues.

Other Physiologic Changes Pertinent to Anesthesia

The aged patient has a decreased capacity for thermal regulation, as shown by tests for regional cooling and homeostatic reaction to external temperature. Prolonged and extensive surgery with massive blood loss and exposed body cavities and organs induces hypothermia, which antagonizes the effect of nondepolarizing muscle relaxants such as vecuronium and pancuronium bromide and prolongs the process of awakening from anesthesia.

Although procedures preparing the large bowel for surgery have many advantages from the standpoint of reducing bowel flora, they have the disadvantage of disturbing the fluid and electrolyte balance. Cleansing enemas and cathartics cause significant losses of fluids containing quantities of sodium and potassium. There is also a loss of bicarbonate and chloride. The frequently diminished renal function in the elderly may not permit prompt compensation for these abrupt body fluid and electrolyte shifts. Not only is adequate fluid needed, but additional sodium bicarbonate or sodium lactate is required to correct the hyperchloremic acidosis that may be caused by bowel preparation. Because of a decrease in lean body mass, in the presence of drugs distributed primarily to this compartment, such as diazepam, plasma levels are increased with a calculated dose and the half-life is increased.

Stress accents biologic differences between individuals, and there tends to be a wider variation among the elderly in their responses to stress. The organic and physiologic alterations caused by aging decrease the rate of compensatory responses and recovery from the stress of anesthesia and surgery. This may be compounded by a decrease in adrenocortical secretions, also associated with the aging process.

▶ APPLIED GERIATRIC CLINICAL PHARMACOLOGY

Although only 13% of the American population is age 65 or older, this age group spends about $3 billion per year for prescription and nonprescription drugs, which represents 20% to 25% of the total national expenditure. These numbers are predicted to increase to 35% to 45% over the next four decades. Approximately 25% of all drugs prescribed are consumed by elderly individuals, and an estimated 85% of elderly ambulatory patients and 95% of institutionalized patients receive drugs. About 25% of all drug reactions occur in the elderly, and of the medications prescribed for the elderly, 25% are known to be ineffective or not needed! The average number of drug categories used by patients varies directly with increasing age: 1.64 drug categories for those younger than 70 years and 2.64 categories for those older than 84. The failure rate of the elderly to comply with a physician's treatment plan may be as high as 50%. Three fourths of this noncompliance consists either of omitting necessary medications or taking inappropriate drugs. Fifteen percent of these patients suffered from visual handicaps of a magnitude significant enough to cause problems in reading labels and following instructions accurately. Adverse reactions varied from 10.2% to 24% in a variety of elderly patients. The complexity of these problems relative to multiple drug intake, problems with possible overuse or noncompliance, and gastrointestinal, hepatic, renal, and other significant factors affecting drug absorption, distribution, biotransformation, and rate of excretion presents a challenge to the anesthesia practitioner. Therefore, every professional must be adept and familiar with the pharmacokinetics and pharmacodynamics of drugs used by and for the elderly including their interactions with anesthetics and other adjuvant drugs.

The most commonly used drugs are cardiovascular agents, drugs for hypertension, analgesics and antiarthritic preparations, sedatives and tranquilizers, and gastrointestinal preparations such as laxatives and antacids. About 40% of these medications are over-the-counter drugs, and for all inpatients, the number of drugs prescribed increases linearly with age and the length of stay in the hospital or in a nursing or convalescent home.

The ability of the drug to produce side effects depends on the amount that reaches specific receptors. In the absorption of the drug, the amount administered is very important. In geriatric patients, drugs taken orally can be absorbed slowly or may not be absorbed at all. There are sufficient studies showing that tablets taken orally can appear in the feces of elderly patients unchanged. This poor absorption is related to changes in the gastrointestinal mucosa, a marked reduction in blood supply, alteration in gastric emptying and intestinal motility, and reduction in gastric acidity. Most drugs absorbed by passive facilitation and not involving an active transport process are probably not limited, in contrast to nutrients such as sugar, amino acids, calcium, iron, thiamine, and others that are absorbed by an active transport mechanism. Drugs administered parenterally, either intramuscularly or intravenously, behave differently because with the former there is slower or erratic absorption as a result of poor and slow peripheral and tissue perfusion, and with the latter, slow circulation time and reduced cardiac output together with reduced receptor sensitivity cause a protracted and prolonged onset of effect (eg, sedation with barbiturates during intravenous induction). Systemic availability varies according to the fraction of the drug absorbed and the metabolism of that fraction by the intestine and hepatic enzymes. The amount of drug metabolized during the "first pass" of the absorption phase in the liver decreases with age, increasing the total amount of drug reaching the systemic circulation and necessitating dosage reduction for the elderly. In anesthesia practice, it is prudent and safe to reduce the drug dose, making it one third to one half the adult dose and titrating it to effect after sufficient observation and monitoring for tangible effects or physiologic responses.

There is a 10% to 15% reduction in total body water between ages 20 and 80 years, as well as a reduction in the plasma volume and extracellular fluid. There is a gradual decline in lean body mass and a proportionate increase in body fat, which is about 18% in men and 12% in women. These changes in body composition affect the volumes of distribution of drugs into total body water and fat. The volumes of distribution for some of the lipophilic drugs such as diazepam, chlordiazepoxide, and thiopental will be larger; those of the water-soluble drugs such as cimetidine and digoxin decline with age. The serum albumin concentration can be reduced as much as 15% to 20% with an increase in the globulin fraction and the concentration of alpha$_1$-acid glycoprotein (AGP), which tends to occur with age. Acidic drugs such as diphenylhydantoin and warfarin are bound to plasma albumin, whereas weak bases such as lidocaine and propranolol are bound primarily to AGP. With the decline in albumin and the increase in AGP concentration, there is a reduction in the binding of weakly acidic drugs and an increase in the binding of weak bases. There is a resultant shift in the free drug concentration and an increase in the availability of free drug for metabolism or receptor binding sites. Caution should be exercised when using multiple drug therapy because displacement from receptors and binding sites by drugs competing for the same receptors may liberate other drugs, the pharmacologic effects of which can be toxic and fatal to geriatric patients.

In the elderly there is also a reduction in the activity of the microsomal mixed function oxidase system and microsomal enzyme induction. Hepatic mass and regional blood flow to the liver are reduced as much as 40% to 45%. This is shown by the benzodiazepine class of sedative–hypnotic and analgesic agents. Clearance of midazolam (Fig. 14–3) and of chlordiazepoxide and its metabolite desmethyldiazepam is reduced in older patients, especially men. Many of the other drugs in this class have long elimination half-lives of up to 220 hours, and because of this tendency for accumulation and excessive sedation, doses of these drugs should be reduced in elderly patients. The elimination rates of drugs metabolized by nonmicrosomal enzymes, such as lorazepam, do not seem to be affected by these changes in the liver.

The clearance and excretion of these drugs are heavily influenced by changes in the kidneys, which include reduced or diminished renal function, both glomerular and tubular. There is a decline in the capacity to concentrate urine during water deprivation and renal sodium conservation with an increased sensitivity to hyperosmolarity. It is essential that plasma levels of potentially toxic drugs that accumulate in the body such as digoxin and the newer-generation aminoglycoside antibiotics be measured. Many of the drugs used in anesthesia practice that are eliminated primarily by renal excretion, such as pancuronium and cimetidine, have shown a reduction in excretion with age.

On the basis of our pharmacokinetic knowledge and the recommendation to reduce the dosages and frequency of administration of potent medications for elderly patients, it should be emphasized that older people are more sensitive to the effects of analgesics and sedatives such as the benzodiazepines, but not to the effects of cardiovascular drugs such as propranolol, verapamil, and calcium blockers.

▶ HISTORY

All geriatric patients scheduled for elective surgery must have a preoperative visit from the anesthesiologist or

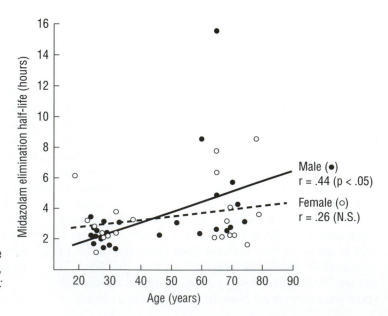

Figure 14–3. Relation of age to midazolam elimination half-life in men and women. *(Reprinted, with permission, from Reves, J. G., Fragen, R. J., Vinik, H. R., et al. [1985]. Midazolam: Pharmacology and uses.* Anesthesiology, 62, *316.)*

anesthetist. Increased fear resulting from a previous unpleasant anesthesia experience may be alleviated by a pleasant preoperative experience and positive reinforcement. These fears and anxieties can provoke sympathetic nervous system responses and cardiac dysrhythmia during induction of anesthesia. Tactful and sympathetic visits allay apprehension and give lasting, genuine reassurance.

It is important to ask specific questions to evaluate how activities of daily living have been affected by normal aging processes, chronic illness, or disability. The general activity level of the older adult must be evaluated, particularly as related to activity and exercise tolerance. Knowledge concerning exercise tolerance gives the anesthetist an indication of cardiopulmonary reserve. The focus should be on the health state during the past 5 years. The nurse anesthetist should assess the quality of the patient's hearing because failure to recognize hearing loss may preclude the taking of an accurate history.

As with adults in general, inquiries should be made concerning other hospitalizations, surgeries, chronic illnesses, and any accidents or injuries. The geriatric patient may provide lengthy responses and not necessarily in chronological order, so the nurse anesthetist may need to guide this discussion carefully.

Elderly patients may take multiple drugs; therefore, a careful history of drug intake will reduce the incidence of undesirable drug interactions (Table 14–1). The nurse anesthetist should request to see the pill bottles if the patient has them. Prolonged intake of steroids in patients with arthritis or allergies indicates the possibility of adrenal insufficiency, necessitating an adjustment in this

medication to compensate for the stress of anesthesia and surgery. Many medications, particularly antihypertensive agents, should be continued up to the time of surgery. The use of clonidine before surgery had been controversial, but recent studies have shown that it can reduce anesthetic requirement, decrease hemodynamic variability during intubation of the trachea, and, in older patients undergoing ophthalmic surgery, decrease anesthetic requirement, improve sedation, and prevent increases in the intraocular pressure (Ghignone, Noe, Calvillo, & Quintin, 1988). At doses higher than 5 μg/kg, hypotension and bradycardia can be a problem, and it also can augment the pressor response to exogenous vasopressors and catecholamines. When used as an adjuvant for controlled hypotension, lower amounts of hypotensive agents are used and hemodynamic stability is maintained. The ability of clonidine to cause sedation and better hemodynamic stability may justify its use as a premedication for patients with ischemic heart disease, and it can have protective effects on the myocardium.

In addition to prescriptive medications, disclosure of any over-the-counter drugs, vitamins, and herbal therapies is necessary to perianesthetic planning. Untoward response to a variety of over-the-counter drugs, such as aspirin and nonsteroidal anti-inflammatory drugs (NSAIDs), can manifest as delirium.

Sleep patterns should be evaluated. What is the usual sleep pattern? Does the patient awaken often at night because of nocturia, shortness of breath, insomnia, or early morning awakenings? Information concerning sleep patterns can be useful in identifying delirium or forms of dementia such as Alzheimer's disease.

TABLE 14–1. Drugs and Adverse Effects After Chronic Intake With Possible Drug–Drug Interactions in the Aged

Drug	Effect/Interaction
Digitalis	Hypokalemia; arrhythmias
Diuretics	Hypokalemia; arrhythmias
Alcohol dependence	Hepatic disease; chronic intake—decreased response to anesthetics
Sedatives, tranquilizers, barbiturates	Liver enzyme induction; need reduced dose of anesthetics following intake
Tricyclic antidepressants	Interference with myocardial conduction; arrhythmias after relaxant reversal; discontinuation 48–72 h preop probably advantageous
Echothiophate eyedrops	Pseudocholinesterase inhibition—avoid or decrease succinylcholine
Monoamine oxidase inhibitors	Discontinue 10–14 d prior to surgery; hypotensive response with most anesthetics; hypertensive crisis with meperidine
Lithium carbonate	Atrial arrhythmias; muscle relaxant interaction
Antibiotics (streptomycin, gentamycin, neomycin)	Muscle relaxant interaction (prolonged response)
Quinidine	Muscle relaxant interaction
Aspirin	Bleeding and ulceration of gastrointestinal tract
Propranolol hydrochloride	Bradycardia and hypotension with potent halogenated anesthetic agents
Calcium channel blockers	Interaction with beta blockers can lead to cardiac decompensation; interaction with halogenated anesthetics at minimum alveolar concentration may enhance drug effects

When assessing the anesthetic and operative risks, potential airway problems should be noted, as described earlier. Individuals with chronic obstructive pulmonary disease or a smoking habit may require respiratory aerosol therapy, bronchial dilators, chest physical therapy, and antibiotic therapy for existing infections for an appropriate length of time preoperatively. Correction or control of other associated medical problems such as diabetes, hypertension, angina, and congestive heart failure is mandatory. Elective surgery should be postponed if the medical conditions cannot be controlled or stabilized in time.

Surgical priorities and criteria for operability should include proper assessment of operative risk, assessment and treatment of functional abnormalities and other associated diseases, and the fine-tuning necessary to optimize conditions for anesthesia and the surgical procedure. It has been shown that surgical mortality rates increase linearly with American Society of Anesthesiologists (ASA) physical status classification (I through V), which can be used to critique operative mortality. Patients can also be classified on the basis of functional cardiorespiratory status derived from physiologic parameters obtained by peripheral, arterial, and central pulmonary artery catheterization (DelGuercio & Cohn, 1980). The proper management of elderly surgical patients requires an understanding of the normal decline in physiologic reserves and the common pathologic conditions associated with the aging process. Assessment of cardiac risk factors (Table 14–2), improvement of pulmonary function including exercise tolerance, and prevention of pulmonary, cardiac, renal, and other vital organ failure are essential to obtaining optimal conditions for the administration of anesthesia and performance of the surgical procedure.

There is consensus that factors associated with increased risks in surgery among elderly patients include age of 75 or older, emergency procedures, anatomic site (eg, chest and upper abdomen), surgical procedure longer than 2 hours, and poor exercise tolerance or low level of activity before procedure. Other significant factors to be considered are the skill of the surgeon and the adequacy of the anesthesia care and management plan. The most common reasons for preoperative medical consultations include chronic medical problems (56%); specific signs and symptoms, for example, angina and fever (18%); electrocardiogram (ECG) and other laboratory anomalies (15%); acute illness or recent change in condition (6%); and specific management and therapeutic issues, for example, antibiotic prophylaxis, steroid coverage, and bleeding and coagulation problems (5%) (Charlson, Cohen, & Sears, 1983). All possible complications, risks, and alternatives must be explained to the patient and family. The type of anesthetic management

TABLE 14–2. Computation of the Cardiac Risk Index

Criterion	Multivariate	"Points"
History		
Age > 70 y	0.191	5
MI[a] in previous 6 mo	0.384	10
Physical examination		
S3 gallop or JVD	0.451	11
Important VAS	0.119	3
Electrocardiogram		
Rhythm other than sinus or PACs	0.283	7
> 5 PVCs/min documented at any time before operation	0.278	7
General status		
$Po_2 < 60$ or $Pco_2 > 50$ mmHg	0.132	3
K < 3.0 or $HCO_3 < 20$ mEq/L		
BUN > 50 or Cr > 3.0 mg/dL		
Abnormal SGOT		
Signs of chronic liver disease or patient bedridden from noncardiac causes		
Operations		
Intraperitoneal, intrathoracic, or aortic operation	0.123	3
Emergency operation	0.167	4
Total possible		53 points

[a]MI, myocardial infarction; JVD, jugular vein distension; VAS, valvular aortic stenosis; PACs, premature atrial contractions; ECG, electrocardiogram; PVCs, premature ventricular contractions; Po_2, partial pressure of oxygen; Pco_2, partial pressure of carbon dioxide; K, potassium; HCO_3, bicarbonate; BUN, blood urea nitrogen; Cr, creatinine; SGOT, serum glutamic–oxaloacetic transaminase.

Reprinted, with permission, from Goldman, L. (1977). Multifactorial index of cardiac risk in non-cardiac surgical patients. New England Journal of Medicine, 297, 848.

planned and the reason for the choice should be discussed with the patient, stressing that the patient's safety and welfare are the foremost considerations in this selection.

The family support network and the persons who will provide care after surgery should also be discussed with the patient. The older adult may have concerns about going home immediately after surgery, particularly if he or she will be cared for by a geriatric spouse. The current health care environment that dictates early discharge after surgical procedures is frightening to the geriatric patient. It is difficult for these patients to understand why they cannot stay in the hospital until they are ready to go home. The anesthesia provider should verify that proper home care support will be provided to the patient on discharge to alleviate his or her fears and reduce stress.

▶ PHYSICAL EXAMINATION

After a review of the patient's chart and results of standard laboratory examinations, a physical examination is conducted with emphasis on the airway and its airway problems, endocrine and metabolic signs of disease, and stability of the hemodynamic components. The patient should be assessed with a simple tilt test. A positive result implies either hypovolemia or an unstable sympathetic nervous system. Neck and jaw mobility should be assessed as part of the airway evaluation. Chronic disease processes such as arthritis may affect the airway. The physical examination should be conducted in a gentle manner as it may be difficult for the older adult to assume certain positions, and he or she may tire easily during the evaluation.

The elderly patient should be assessed for tremors and any difficulty in gait that may suggest Parkinson's disease. The patient's level of consciousness should be evaluated carefully, and family members should assist in identifying any disorientation, memory loss, or uncooperative behavior that differs from typical behavior.

▶ DIAGNOSTIC DATA

Standard laboratory examinations must include a complete blood count, liver and renal function profile, electrolyte analysis, chest x-ray, and ECG. Age-related changes in the ECG occur because of histologic changes in the conduction system. It is not uncommon to see prolonged P–R and Q–T intervals or left axis deviation from mild left ventricular hypertrophy and fibrosis in the left bundle branch (Jarvis, 1996). Other laboratory studies such as arterial blood gases, pulmonary function tests, and blood coagulation profile, as well as highly specialized

studies such as blood volume and urinary steroids should be ordered on an individual basis when indicated.

▶ MANAGEMENT OF PREOPERATIVE MEDICAL PROBLEMS AND PATHOPHYSIOLOGY

Uncontrolled hypertension is a risk for end-organ failures, such as stroke, myocardial infarction, and renal failure, aside from reflecting the inherent hypovolemic state of the patient. In general, patients with uncontrolled hypertension have more hemodynamic instability throughout the perioperative period especially during intubation, conditions causing fluid shifts such as third-space fluid losses, and the emergence period in which there is catecholamine release as a result of pain, stress, hypoxia, and hypercarbia. Elective procedures on patients with diastolic pressures higher than 100 mmHg should be postponed or rescheduled, and the patient's compliance with antihypertensive medication should be monitored for adequate and proper control of blood pressure before surgery. Advances in the pharmacotherapy of hypertension have made blood pressure control easier by adjusting doses of drugs so they are used in a monotherapy mode, preferably once a day, to increase patient compliance, such as angiotensin-converting enzyme (ACE) inhibitor, beta and calcium channel blockers, and the newer generation of antihypertensive medications (Goldman & Caldera, 1979). In a patient with labile hypertension, intraoperative direct arterial line blood pressure monitoring is mandatory with properly prepared and mixed vasopressors and depressor agents to obtain optimal control of blood pressure and prevent extremes (ie, profound hypotension, which can precipitate myocardial infarction, or massive hypertension, which can result in stroke and other cardiac disastrous events such as cardiac arrest).

The classic signs of congestive heart failure in elderly patients include jugular venous distension, dyspnea on exertion, hepatomegaly, dependent pedal edema, and S3 gallop. Depending on the etiology, aggressive treatment with diuretics, inotropes, and vasodilators; close monitoring of hemodynamic parameters with pulmonary artery catheters; and intraoperative transesophageal echocardiographic monitoring of filling pressures, wall motion, and ejection fraction are warranted (Cahalan, Litt, Botvinick, & Schiller, 1987).

There is a greater incidence of ventricular dysrhythmias and conduction abnormalities among elderly patients, probably as a normal progression of heart diseases, but also from a previous myocardial infarction affecting the conduction system. Patients with complete heart block and sick sinus syndrome require preoperative pacemaker placement. Among patients with demand pacemakers, who are undergoing transurethral resection of the prostate, a fixed-rate pacemaker is recommended to decrease the possibility of interference from electrical cautery or other extraneous sources of electricity in the OR. Blood levels of antiarrhythmic agents must be monitored for adequacy of dosage and optimal effect. Conditions that increase arrhythmia perioperatively include anxiety and stress, exogenous catecholamines, adverse hemodynamic extremes, hypoxia, and hypercarbia; these should be prevented and properly monitored.

Changes in the respiratory reserve as a normal part of aging are also magnified in the elderly patient, especially those with a long history of smoking or a history of primary pulmonary lung diseases. The surgical morbidity and mortality resulting from a respiratory complication can be as high as 40%. Anesthetic risk increases because of the obtunded protective airway reflexes such as coughing, gagging, and swallowing, as well as the altered level of consciousness, which increases the probability of aspiration pneumonitis. The decrease in functional cilia of the tracheobronchial tree hampers the clearance of tracheal secretions, which is already aggravated by dry and nonhumidified anesthetic gases. Bedridden and sedentary patients are also more susceptible to venous stasis and pulmonary embolism. High-risk patients should be identified not only by a thorough workup and medical history, but also by pulmonary function tests and evaluation of exercise tolerance. Patients who require pulmonary function tests include those scheduled for thoracic and upper abdominal surgery, those with a prolonged history of heavy smoking and other primary pulmonary diseases, and those 70 years of age and older (Tisi, 1979). Patients with a maximum breathing capacity less than 50% of the predicted value, a forced expiratory volume in 1 second (FEV_1) less than 2 L, and a Pco_2 greater than 45 mmHg are very high pulmonary surgical risks. It is recommended that these patients decrease or stop smoking, submit sputum culture for proper antibiotic therapy, and undergo bronchodilator, aerosol, and humidification therapy as well as postural drainage and chest physiotherapy (Tine & Cassara, 1970). Enteral or parenteral nutrition improves integrity of respiratory muscles. It is important to overemphasize the continuation of a rigorous pulmonary regimen beyond the postoperative period, including well-supervised incentive spirometry, reduction of narcotic and depressant drugs with the use of selected regional anesthesia techniques and epidural opiates, use of effective breathing exercises to prevent splinting during deep breathing, effective coughing, and early ambulation.

The mortality for acute operative–postoperative renal failure is between 40% and 80% in elderly patients. With an awareness of the renal changes in the elderly and the effects of anesthesia and surgery, the goal is to decrease the risk of postoperative renal failure. Factors that compromise renal blood flow during the perioperative period include the decrease in cardiac output caused by halogenated inhalation anesthetics, positive-pressure ventilation, hypovolemia from surgical losses, and retraction and pressure on renal blood vessels by surgical instruments. The patient should be hydrated to ensure a good urinary output of 0.5 to 1 mL/kg/h. As much as possible, the use of potentially nephrotoxic drugs such as aminoglycosides must be avoided. Any patient with terminal renal failure or disease should be dialyzed to treat hypovolemia, hyperkalemia, metabolic acidosis, or uremic encephalopathy (Pompei, 1990). Fluid and electrolyte problems resulting from surgical procedures include water or irrigation fluid absorption during transurethral resection of the prostate, profound hypovolemia and massive fluid replacement in major trauma, vasopressin deficiency in pituitary surgery, gastrointestinal obstruction with continuous vomiting and suction for the decompression of dilated bowels, and any other massive extracellular fluid shifts and translocations must be anticipated.

Many elderly patients with a history of adult- or maturity-onset diabetes (non–insulin-dependent, non–ketoacidosis-prone, type II, or stable diabetes) for many years present as a challenge to the anesthetist because of complications associated with the progress of the disease, such as ketoacidosis, neuropathies, atherosclerosis, microangiopathy, increased incidence of infection, and delayed wound healing. Ketoacidosis is diagnosed in patients with metabolic acidosis and hyperglycemia (more than 300 mg/dL). Glycosuria and osmotic diuresis accent hyperosmolality and loss of electrolytes, resulting in hypovolemia that can lead to circulatory collapse. Patients with severe autonomic neuropathy manifest orthostatic hypotension, resting tachycardia, and reduction of beat-to-beat variability with deep breathing signifying autonomic instability that is resistant to vasopressors, inotropes, and anticholinergic agents. There is an inherent sensitivity to respiratory depressant drugs as well as a higher incidence of silent myocardial infarction and unexplained cardiorespiratory arrest that is resistant to aggressive cardiopulmonary efforts and a greater tendency to aspiration as a result of gastroparesis (Page & Watkins, 1978). Perioperative anesthesia care includes frequent monitoring of blood sugar and ketone bodies in the blood and urine. There is no evidence that tight or close control of blood glucose concentration is beneficial over other methods as long as the blood glucose concentration is maintained between 100 to 250 mg %, with additional glucose or regular insulin as often as necessary. The presence of ketone bodies is a good reason to postpone elective surgery. In the presence of peripheral neuropathy, conduction or regional anesthesia should be used with caution because of a predisposition to nerve injury; this also emphasizes the importance of proper positioning and padding of bony prominences and external nerve distributions to prevent traction, pressure, and ischemia. It is prudent to decrease the dose of local anesthetics, and caution must be exercised in the use of epinephrine and other vasoactive drugs with local anesthetics in patients with diabetes complicated by atherosclerosis. Patients suffering from nonketonic hyperglycemic coma require immediate correction of hypovolemia and hyperosmolarity with intravenous balanced electrolyte solution, potassium supplementation, and small doses of intravenous regular insulin.

The prevalence of hypothyroidism in hospitalized elderly patients is reportedly 9.4% to 13.2% (Livingston, Hershman, Sawin, & Yoshikawa, 1987). The anesthetic implications of hypothyroidism include a marked sensitivity to depressant drugs (eg, drugs for premedication, agents for induction, and medications for pain relief postoperatively); a hypodynamic cardiovascular system with reduced cardiac output, heart rate, and stroke volume; a slower drug metabolism and detoxification (eg, for hypnotics, sedatives, and opiates); unresponsive baroreceptor reflexes; decreased intravascular volume; impaired ventilatory response to arterial hypoxemia, elevated P_{CO_2}, or both; delayed gastric emptying time; impaired clearance of free water resulting in hyponatremia; hypothermia; anemia; hypoglycemia; and primary adrenal insufficiency (Murkin, 1982). There is a reduced requirement for premedication, anesthetic agents, and muscle relaxants because of the previously mentioned effects of the aging process and the fragile general constitution of the patient who is very susceptible to congestive heart failure and hypothermia. Appropriate monitoring modalities are recommended. Conservative use of adjuvant drugs such as vasopressors, inotropes, and other sympathetic amines; maintenance of normal body temperature; optimal ventilatory support; and conservative use of opiate analgesics are essential during the postoperative period.

Bleeding and coagulation problems among elderly patients result from excessive use of aspirin and NSAIDs for degenerative osteoarthritis, vitamin deficiency from poor nutrition and use of broad-spectrum antibiotics, liver disease associated with chronic alcoholism, indiscriminate use of coumadin, and, recently, use of dipyridamole for coronary, cerebral, and other vascular occlusive diseases. Patients with liver disease have complex hemostatic abnormalities and platelet dysfunction. Alcohol or ethanol may interfere with arachidonic metabolism in the platelets. There is now good evidence that aspirin increases operative blood loss in heparinized patients undergoing open heart surgery (Goldman, Copeland, Moritz, Henderson, Zadina, Ovitt, Doherty, Read, Chester, Sako, et al., 1988).

▶ ALZHEIMER'S DISEASE

Alzheimer's disease, or senile dementia of the Alzheimer type (SDAT), is a complex degenerative process involving selective neuronal pathways. At this writing, no risk factors have been confirmed directly with the development of Alzheimer's disease although a familial tendency seems to exist. Advanced chronologic age itself appears to be the only factor directly related to the development of this disorder.

Because people are living longer, more elderly people may be faced with the prospect of elective or emergency surgery. Therefore, the number of patients with Alzheimer's disease undergoing surgery will continue to increase. Significant cognitive impairment is a cardinal sign of the disease and may not be a function of the aging process. Other symptoms of Alzheimer's disease are variable, but the patient may present in a good state of physical health or have a health status compromised by concurrent chronic disease processes. The overall physical condition of the Alzheimer's patient should be a primary factor when considering outpatient, ambulatory, or inpatient surgery.

Cognitive impairment in the patient with Alzheimer's disease may include memory loss and reduced ability to concentrate. These factors make it difficult to take an accurate history from the patient. A close family member or guardian should be queried regarding the patient's past and current medical and surgical history, including drug therapy. Patients with Alzheimer's disease may be taking a cadre of medications to modify behavioral changes such as aggressiveness, anxiety, depression, agitation, insomnia, and paranoia that may have resulted from the disease process. These patients are extremely sensitive to the effects of all medications and generally require reduced dosages to achieve the desired effect. The Alzheimer's patient should be observed carefully for any side effects from medications taken both preoperatively and for concurrent chronic disease processes.

It is very important to rule out treatable and potentially reversible causes of dementia in the elderly patient. A mnemonic has been devised to help in identifying many of the potentially reversible causes of dementia (Lamy, 1980).

D   Drugs
E   Emotional disorders
M   Metabolic and endocrine disorders
E   Eye and ear dysfunctions
N   Nutritional deficiencies
T   Tumor and trauma
I   Infections
A   Arteriosclerotic complications (myocardial infarction, heart failure) and alcohol

Any directions the patient is expected to follow should be written down clearly and concisely. The written word is very helpful to reinforce any preoperative and postoperative instructions for the patient with Alzheimer's disease. In all discussions with the patient regarding the upcoming surgery, the day and time of surgery should be mentioned. This helps the patient to remain oriented to time and place. If the patient will be moved to a new unit or require special care postoperatively, the patient and family should be apprised of this preoperatively if feasible. The family should be involved as much as possible in the plans for postoperative care. In some cases, private duty nurses or family members may plan to stay with the patient. If the quality of care the Alzheimer patient requires can be provided in this manner, this may be optimal. Because of the difficulty with orientation to time and place exhibited by Alzheimer patients, the routines of specialty care units may add to their cognitive difficulties. The continuity of care provided by supportive family members and nurses familiar to the patient reinforces the patient's orientation to time and place. The charge nurse of the patient care unit should make every effort to assign a small number of nurses to care for the patient with Alzheimer's disease. The consistency of caregivers provides stability for the patient during the hospital stay (Waugaman, 1988).

Patients with Alzheimer's disease requiring emergency surgery need special preoperative consideration. Explanations to the family and patient and an accurate accounting of the patient's history, particularly of drug therapy, are crucial. The number of individuals making a preoperative assessment of the patient should be kept to a minimum to reduce the degree of confusion associated with many new faces.

The same physical preparation should be made for Alzheimer's patients as for other elderly patients. A patient in the late stages of Alzheimer's disease may exhibit agitation and combative behavior. Restraint of the patient may be necessary to prevent accidental or self-inflicted injury.

Preoperative medication administered to these patients should be minimal as the patient may exhibit an exaggerated or untoward response to the medication that will make communication with and cooperation by the patient more difficult. Patients with Alzheimer's disease may be very sensitive to the depressant effects of hypnotics and narcotics because they generally are taking tranquilizers of some type. If a narcotic or sedative is administered preoperatively, the patient should be carefully monitored and observed for signs of respiratory depression. Administration of these drugs further depresses airway reflexes, increasing the risk of passive regurgitation and aspiration of gastric contents. Vital signs must be monitored because these patients also may be sensitive to cardiovascular side effects such as hypotension from any narcotic or sedative medications administered preoperatively.

Because the cholinergic system of these individuals has been shown to be impaired, anticholinergics such as atropine and scopolamine should be avoided. The use of these drugs could lead to an exacerbation of behavioral symptoms. The use of preoperative medication should be reserved for those instances in which the patient requires analgesia or treatment of agitation. Patient rapport and understanding often serve as the most effective forms of "preoperative medication."

Most patients with Alzheimer's disease will have their surgery performed under general anesthesia. Because of difficulty with mentation and lack of understanding or cooperation, these patients generally are not good candidates for regional or local anesthesia, except in the very early stages of the disease process when cognitive abilities are well maintained.

Delayed recovery from anesthesia is not uncommon in these patients. Therefore, prolonged observation of the patient will be required in the postanesthesia care unit as well as in the patient care unit. Every effort should be made intraoperatively and postoperatively to keep the patient normothermic. Hypothermia can delay recovery from anesthesia. Confusion in the postoperative phase has been attributed to low body temperature and inadequate hydration.

Preserving optimum body temperature and maintaining adequate hydration help reduce the incidence of confusion postoperatively in patients with Alzheimer's disease. Outpatients should be apprised preoperatively by the surgeon or anesthetist of the prospect of hospital admission overnight after surgery should recovery be delayed. Some patients have shown temporary improvement in their cognitive abilities in response to administration of the anticholinesterase, physostigmine. The long-term effects of using physostigmine as part of the treatment regimen in Alzheimer's disease are still under investigation.

► PERIANESTHESIA MANAGEMENT OF THE GERIATRIC PATIENT

Preoperative Considerations

The basic principle in prescribing and providing preanesthesia medications for geriatric patients include evaluating the need for drug therapy, obtaining a complete history of habits and drug usage, reducing the dose, and titrating the drug dosage on the basis of the patient's response. As much as possible, the patient should be encouraged to comply with a therapeutic regimen that is simple, easy to understand, practical, cost-effective, and characterized by a high margin of safety. The patient's medications should be continuously reviewed, and unnecessary drugs should be discontinued to avoid complex drug interactions and reactions.

Specific medical problems that must be controlled and corrected before elective surgery include hypertension, congestive heart failure, cardiac dysrhythmias, preexisting pulmonary conditions, fluid and electrolyte imbalance, endocrine and metabolic disorders, bleeding and coagulation abnormalities, neuropsychiatric disorders, and possible drug interactions or reactions. The most significant preoperative medical problems encountered during the preoperative period are shown in Table 14–3, and the mortality rates for these conditions are shown in Table 14–4. There is no question that involvement of more than one organ system with organic diseases increases morbidity and mortality from a surgical procedure. The mortality rate is 29% for patients age 95 and older with multiple-organ disease compared with 4.7% among healthy patients of similar age (Denny & Denson, 1972).

For certain patients with specific problems, useful and meaningful laboratory data such as blood volume, electrolytes, renal and hepatic function, chest x-rays, ECG, arterial blood gases, and pulmonary function must be assessed thoroughly and additional tests ordered if necessary. The adequacy of blood volume and compensatory autonomic nervous system reflexes can be as-

TABLE 14–4. Mortality by Selected Preoperative Condition

Condition	Number of Deaths	Number of Operations	Mortality Rate (%)
Cardiac failure	186	1,175	15.8
Impaired renal function	84	779	10.8
Vomiting	154	1,529	10.1
Previous general anesthetic	219	3,014	7.3
Angina, arteriosclerosis, or ischemic heart disease	544	7,776	7.0
Impairment of general health by surgical diagnosis	631	10,681	5.9
Diabetes	82	1,462	5.7
Chronic lower respiratory tract infection	408	8,060	5.1
Obesity	116	5,434	2.1
No preoperative condition	206	43,483	0.5

Reprinted, with permission, from Farrow, S. C., Fowkes, F. G. R., Lunn, J. N., et al. (1982). Epidemiology in anaesthesia. II. Factors affecting mortality in hospital. British Journal of Anaesthesia, 54, 811.

TABLE 14–3. Preanesthetic Complications[a]

Complication	Number of Patients	Percentage
Hypertension	466	46.6
Arteriosclerotic cardiovascular disease	269	26.9
Myocardial infarction	185	18.5
Cardiomegaly	136	13.6
Congestive heart failure	75	7.5
Angina	64	6.4
Cardiovascular accident	58	5.8
Chronic obstructive pulmonary disease	140	14.0
Pulmonary (other)	135	13.5
Diabetes	92	9.2
Renal dysfunction	314	31.4
Liver dysfunction	85	8.5

[a]Preexisting complications by history or examination.
Reprinted, with permission, from Stephen, C. R. (1984). The risk of anesthesia and surgery in the geriatric patient. In S. E. Krechel (Ed.). Anesthesia and the geriatric patient (p. 231). New York: Grune & Stratton.

sessed by blood volume determinations using dye dilution studies. To assess forced expiratory volume and forced vital capacity, simplified pulmonary function tests can be done with a portable respirometer.

Invasive monitoring techniques such as right-sided heart catheterization, balloon-flotation pulmonary artery catheterization (Swan-Ganz), and arterial catheterization for blood pressure measurement and blood sampling may be indicated to assess the physiologic status of the patient undergoing severe or extensive surgery. This invasive preoperative assessment may disclose serious physiologic abnormalities that require a delay in surgery or even cancellation of the procedure. When gross physiologic decompensation is absent, the elderly patient may tolerate and demand effective premedication. Premedication should be prescribed to suit individual situations, but generally consists of a narcotic, a tranquilizer or hypnotic, an anticholinergic, or a combination of these. Doses should be reduced from a "normal adult dose" to one suitable for an elderly patient. Ideally, the patient should be premedicated 1 hour before transport to the OR so the medication can achieve maximum effectiveness. Some controversy exists over the need for a narcotic as part of the preoperative medication routine in a patient who is not in pain. The consequences of producing respiratory depression in these patients must be considered. In addition, anticholinergics should be avoided because they may precipitate delirium in older patients. This may also occur from preoperative use of ophthalmic medications absorbed systemically (Jenike, 1996).

Intraoperative Considerations

No shortcut anesthetic regimen can be used for the elderly because their physiologic condition and the associated risks leave a very narrow margin of safety. The monitoring and surveillance of the elderly must minimally include blood pressure, pulse, respiration, and temperature. In addition to the other standard noninvasive monitoring modes mentioned, monitoring of end-tidal carbon dioxide concentration and oxygen saturation is particularly useful in helping the anesthetist to maintain homeostasis intraoperatively. Invasive monitoring techniques such as measurement of central or peripheral arterial pressure, central venous pressure, and pulmonary artery pressure by catheterization are generally reserved for extensive surgery in which massive blood loss and fluid shifts are anticipated, and for patients with moderate to severe cardiopulmonary disease. Insertion of a urinary catheter for the monitoring of urinary output is helpful but may be contraindicated for patients with histories of multiple genitourinary infections or prostatic obstruction.

Temperature must be carefully monitored intraoperatively. Body temperature may decrease rapidly in the cool OR environment. Preventive measures to maintain body heat include warming or use of a hyperthermia blanket, warmed intravenous and irrigation fluids, a heated nebulizer, and reduction in total gas flows. It is mandatory that the correction of abnormal physiologic parameters be confirmed, including blood volume in patients with chronic or acute hemorrhage, blood pressure stability and control in hypertensive patients taking diuretics and antihypertensive agents, and blood glucose levels in brittle diabetics prone to diabetic ketoacidosis. After prolonged diuretic therapy, the serum potassium level must be measured because electrolyte imbalance can cause fatal arrhythmias during anesthesia. Blood sugar determination by the glucose oxidase method (Dextrostix) is essential for patients who receive their maintenance insulin dose on the day of surgery and may be indicated for other insulin-dependent diabetics as well as for adult-onset diabetics prone to hypoglycemia.

The criteria for operability must take into account the possibility of partial to complete restoration of function, diminution of disability, alleviation of pain, and prolongation of life. Choice of anesthetic is based on the patient's condition, the type of surgery, and the skills of the anesthesia care team and surgeon. The ideal anesthetic is one that can be controlled with very little effect on the patient's already altered physiology. The anesthetic technique should be reversible so if complications arise it can be discontinued abruptly and all vital functions may recover quickly.

General Anesthesia

General anesthesia involves intravenous and inhalation agents. Compared with regional anesthesia, general anesthesia with insertion of an endotracheal tube has the advantages of better airway control and fast, smooth induction of anesthesia with unlimited duration, but it carries the hazard of aspiration of vomitus into the lungs, especially in patients with full stomachs.

Intravenous induction agents should be administered slowly in incremental doses so the drug effect can develop completely and physiologic changes can be analyzed. Hypovolemia is common in the elderly and, coupled with the reduced ability of the circulatory system to compensate for this, tends to make the induction of anesthesia with drugs such as thiopental potentially hazardous by producing poorly controlled swings in blood pressure and pulse. Hypertension and cardiac arrhythmias may occur if laryngoscopy is performed under light anesthesia. This is particularly dangerous in a patient with coronary insufficiency. Rapid, efficient laryngoscopy after intratracheal or intravenous treatment with lidocaine may help control the occurrence of arrhythmias during this procedure.

For many years, a balanced anesthetic technique—nitrous oxide, narcotic, tranquilizer, and muscle relaxant—was considered the safest for the elderly patient. However, this technique has been reexamined and shown to cause myocardial or respiratory depression or both (depending on which narcotic had been used). There is renewed interest in inhalation agents for anesthetic management of the aged, particularly since the introduction of isoflurane, desflurane, and sevoflurane. It has been illustrated that, with age, the minimum alveolar concentration (MAC) of inhaled agents progressively decreases (Table 14–5). Other investigators have made sim-

TABLE 14–5. Minimum Alveolar Concentration for the Frequently Used Agents for Young and Elderly Adults

	Young Adults	Elderly Adults	
	MAC	MAC	Age (y)
Nitrous oxide	104	87.0[a]	80
Halothane	0.77	0.60	80
Enflurane	1.70	1.39[a]	
Isoflurane	1.15	1.05	64
Desflurane	6.0	5.2	70
Sevoflurane	2.6	1.4	80

[a] Calculated.
MAC, minimum alveolar concentration.
From Gloyna, D. F. (1997). Effects of Inhalation Agents. In C. H. McLeskey (Ed.), Geriatric Anesthesiology (p. 290). Copyright 1997 by Williams & Wilkins. Adapted with permission.

ilar findings with different anesthetic agents when comparing MACs of inhalation agents with age (Gloyna, 1997). That is, age decreases the requirements for anesthesia with an inhalation agent.

Some of the effects of halogenated anesthetic agents on organs and organ systems include cerebral vasodilation with an increase in cerebral blood flow, early obtundation of laryngeal and pharyngeal reflexes, respiratory depression, and depression of myocardial and vascular smooth muscles, which causes a decrease in systemic blood pressure, cardiac contractile force, cardiac output, total peripheral resistance, and whole-body oxygen consumption. The anesthetist should recognize the incompatibility of halothane with exogenous and endogenous catecholamines such as epinephrine because, depending on the dose of exogenous catecholamines or blood level of endogenous catecholamines, cardiac arrhythmias may result. The ability of halogenated anesthetic agents to produce hepatorenal toxicity is related to the amount of biotransformation and the final or intermediate products of detoxification. This is possibly not a direct effect but an indirect or autoimmune mechanism.

Inhalation agents have been associated with a higher incidence of intraoperative hypotension and arrhythmias than intravenous agents. The intravenous or balanced anesthetic technique gives a smoother intraoperative course but, reportedly, greater postoperative morbidity and mortality.

Regional Anesthesia

Regional block or conduction anesthesia is ideal for surgery on the extremities and for many types of surgery below the level of the umbilicus. Because geriatric patients may have degenerative and vascular changes, their local anesthetic requirement is low, and incorporating drugs such as epinephrine to prolong nerve blocks is not recommended. The obvious advantages of regional anesthetics are a conscious patient and probably a better, faster recovery with less likelihood of aspiration and other postoperative pulmonary complications.

The disadvantages of spinal or epidural anesthesia are that the sympathetic blockade can result in profound hypotension or cardiovascular collapse, and there may be technical difficulty with inserting the spinal needle into a patient with spinal arthritis or calcified ligaments. Also, some patients refuse this anesthetic technique in spite of its relative safety compared with general anesthesia. Many cling to unscientific, traditional beliefs and fears that spinal anesthesia can cause paralysis, even though this complication is rare today.

▶ SPECIAL ANESTHETIC CONSIDERATIONS

Geriatric Ambulatory Surgery

In many hospitals of the United States today, more than 60% of surgical procedures can be done in outpatient or ambulatory surgery centers. The benefits of outpatient surgery include better psychologic and emotional support from less disruption of daily routines, decreased morbidity and mortality (0.01 to 0.02 deaths per 10 000 procedures), less exposure to hospital-acquired or nosocomial infections, improved utilization of inpatient hospital beds, and greater cost effectiveness. These outweigh the disadvantages of outpatient procedures, such as lack of immediate availability or care should a sudden complication arise. Patient selection is extremely important because of the known physiologic changes of aging and the effects on organ systems, drug action, elimination, and the perioperative and postoperative conduct of anesthesia and surgery. There is always the argument as to whether elderly patients can undergo surgery on an outpatient basis if no responsible adult or guardian will take care of the postoperative needs and requirements (eg, medications, feeding, wound care, and complications). No one refutes the argument that adequate and proper postoperative home care is mandatory for the optimal care of these patients. Many hospital-based ambulatory surgery centers now use the 23-hour postoperative admit unit to handle these concerns, and there is usually no additional charge to the patient or insurance carrier.

The type, anatomic location, and duration of the surgical procedure are also extremely important. Most elderly patients should not require extensive or prolonged medical and nursing postoperative care, which may increase health care costs. In a series of 1553 patients, Meridy (1982) reported that age did not affect the duration of recovery from anesthesia or the complication rate. The selection of anesthesia depends on the surgical procedure, the patient's state of health and psychologic and emotional adequacy, and the skill and experience of the surgeon and anesthesia care team. Local and regional anesthesia when adequate and effective provides patients with a better sense of control and psychologic gratification, and there is evidence to show that there are fewer complications and a more expedient and pleasant recovery. In a series of 65 000 patients and unanticipated postoperative admissions, the overall admission rate was 0.8%, whereas the geriatric admission rate was 1.2%. Perhaps the most significant outcome was an admission rate of 4.6% for geriatric patients who had received inhalation anesthesia (Appelbaum, Kallar, & Wetchler, 1991). The overall ambulatory anesthesia care of these patients must be considerate, sympathetic, understanding, and relaxed; these attitudes are true virtues in addition to the safe conduct of anesthesia and surgery.

▶ POSTOPERATIVE CONSIDERATIONS

Postoperative management includes proper monitoring of all vital signs and parameters, including fluid intake and output, adequacy of ventilation, and cardiac stability. Among the most frequent postoperative complications are those that are pulmonary in nature. Prevention of these problems begins as soon as the operative procedure is completed. Tracheobronchial suctioning before removal of the endotracheal tube and oropharyngeal suctioning are basic methods for ensuring that ventilatory exchange is maintained in the immediate postoperative period. Often it is safer to leave the endotracheal tube in place after the operation until the patient reacts to its presence rather than to remove the endotracheal tube before the patient is conscious, is breathing adequately, and has regained control of all reflexes.

Despite preventive measures, tenacious sputum and atelectasis of the lung still may cause difficulties postoperatively. Forceful coughing must be encouraged and tracheal suctioning must be resorted to if coughing is ineffective. Oxygen should be administered routinely through a high-flow mask; patients with chronic obstructive pulmonary disease who retain carbon dioxide should be provided with a Venturi-type mask for the delivery of low concentrations of oxygen.

If the patient exhibits delirium in the recovery room, hypoxemia should be suspected. If arterial blood gases are normal, 1 to 2 mg of physostigmine may be used to reverse the effect of anticholinergic toxicity when displayed symptoms are related to administration of anticholinergic drugs.

Hypothermia must be prevented in the early postoperative period. Shivering in response to hypothermia increases tissue oxygen demand by as much as 400% to 500%. This can initiate a cycle of increased minute volume and cardiac output. Unless cardiopulmonary compensation occurs, anaerobic cellular metabolism will ensue, leading to severe metabolic acidosis. Postoperative hypothermia is prolonged in the patient who has undergone regional anesthesia rather than general anesthesia.

Narcotics may be used with caution in elderly patients. The usual dosage may produce profound respiratory depression. For the majority of patients, a reduced analgesic dose will control pain and allay restlessness without having an adverse effect on respiratory or circulatory function.

The metabolic response to surgery in elderly patients is similar to that seen in younger patients, but certain important aspects particularly influence postoperative management and are especially important when cardiac or re-nal function is impaired. In the postoperative period, increased output of antidiuretic hormone by the posterior pituitary enhances reabsorption of water by the renal tubules and produces increased water retention. More adrenal hormones, principally aldosterone, are secreted and result in sodium retention. Basic fluid requirements, therefore, are limited to not more than 1000 mL to cover insensible water losses and not more than 1500 mL to provide sufficient water for urine formation to excrete nitrogenous waste products. Not more than 500 mL of this should be isotonic sodium (normal saline solution). As soon as urinary output is ensured, potassium should be added to infused fluids, 40 to 60 mEq daily, to provide for potassium loss. Extrarenal losses of fluid, such as by gastric drainage, should be replaced by volume with appropriate solutions in addition to the quantities outlined.

After an operation, daily weighing is a valuable aid in determining hydration. Patients should be weighed at the same time each morning after voiding. After major surgery, weight loss should be anticipated. If weight loss does not occur by the third day, overhydration should be suspected and administration of fluids curtailed. Overzealous administration of fluids is a common cause of cardiac decompensation in the elderly during the postoperative period.

Early ambulation and mobilization should be encouraged to prevent clot formation in the lower extremities and pelvic vessels. Pulmonary embolism is a complication that frequently occurs in the elderly, particularly if there is no ambulation early in the postoperative period or if patients are not encouraged to wear antiembolism stockings. The goal for these patients is early rehabilitation and return to community activities and functions.

▶ CASE STUDY

A 69-year-old black male, height 6'0", weight 72 kg, is admitted because of progressive urinary frequency, urgency, and nocturia. The patient has a history of hypertension that is being treated with a diuretic and ACE inhibitors. He also takes one baby aspirin daily. For his diabetes, he injects himself with 20 units of NPH insulin daily. He was admitted to the coronary care unit (CCU) of a local hospital 3 years ago for frequent indigestion and chest pains. He has confided to his caregivers that he "passes out" once in a while but has no memory of the events. The results of his cardiology workup while in CCU are not available.

His physical examination reveals an enlarged prostate by rectal examination and a pulsating mass in the midline just below the umbilicus with audible bruit.

Preoperative laboratory studies show hemoglobin, 12.8 g; hematocrit, 36.8%; fasting blood sugar, 175 mg/dL; potassium, 3.2 mEq/L; blood urea nitrogen, 18 mEq/L; creatinine, 1.2 mEq/L; platelet count, 260 000/mm³; prothrombin time, 12 seconds; and partial thromboplastin time, 28.5 seconds. His chest x-ray shows slight hyperinflation and increased bronchovascular markings. His ECG reveals normal sinus rhythm and occasional premature ventricular contractions, borderline left ventricular hypertrophy, and nonspecific ST–T changes.

His preoperative vital signs on admission are blood pressure, 179/92; heart rate 92 beats/min, irregular; respiratory rate, 13 breaths/min; and temperature, 98.7°. The nursing home staff who accompanied the patient claims that he is very nervous about the procedure and would prefer general anesthesia if at all possible.

1. What preoperative considerations are important in planning anesthesia for this patient?

Although the patient does have chronic disease, it appears to be well controlled. Because of his history of hypertension, the anesthetist should have drug therapy appropriate to treat hyper- or hypotensive episodes prepared and immediately available. It is also possible that the patient may be somewhat hypovolemic, and careful fluid hydration should occur. Blood glucose levels should be monitored throughout the perioperative period to ensure that insulin doses are adequate. Because the patient is being transferred from a long-term care facility, he may have no immediate family available. The nurse anesthetist should spend as much time as possible allaying the patient's fears and discussing the perianesthetic process. The patient has already expressed concern to another caregiver that he is apprehensive concerning a regional anesthetic. The nurse anesthestist should discuss these concerns with the patient and particularly discuss the advantages of regional anesthetic for this surgical procedure. The patient should be assured that he will receive medication sufficient to allay his anxiety and produce amnesia. Orientation of the patient to time and place should be continually assessed. The number of different caregivers interfacing with the patient should be kept to a minimum to reduce the probability of the patient developing delirium or confusion in the postoperative period.

2. Is regional or general anesthesia indicated for the transurethral resection of the prostate (TURP) procedure the patient is scheduled to undergo?

Regional Anesthesia would be optimal for this patient undergoing a TURP for a number of reasons, including the patient's chronic hypertension. However, the area of least controversy in the general versus regional anesthesia debate involves the benefits related to perioperative bleeding and coagulation. Regional anesthesia, particularly epidural anesthesia, has been associated with a lower incidence of thromboembolic events than general anesthesia. This includes deep venous thrombosis (DVT) and pulmonary embolism (PE). However, there is still debate as to whether regional anesthesia may produce an increased risk of fibrinolysis during procedures such as prostatectomy due to release of urokinase.

3. What considerations should be addressed in this patient's postoperative care?

The patient should be observed for developing signs and symptoms of TURP syndrome, which can occur as early as during the surgical procedure and up to several hours into the postoperative period. Symptoms that the patient who has undergone regional anesthesia may exhibit include dizziness, headaches, tight feeling in the chest and throat, and shortness of breath. The patient can also act restless or confused. Blood pressure can rise with a concurrent decrease in heart rate that can lead to cardiac arrest if not treated. Some patients present with neurologic symptoms including lethargy leading to unconsciousness. One cause of this syndrome has been circulatory overloading through excessive absorption of irrigation solution through the venous network of the prostate gland. This circulatory overloading can lead to a number of clinical situations including water intoxication, glycine toxicity, ammonia toxicity, and hyponatremia. If TURP syndrome is suspected, immediate intensive therapy should be initiated, including measures to treat pulmonary edema, hyponatremia, or seizures.

The patient should also be observed postoperatively for visual disturbances. Transient blindness has been observed following TURP and is probably due to the toxic effects of glycine absorption on the retina. Vision usually returns to normal as glycine blood levels decrease. Hemolysis and coagulopathies may occur postoperatively following TURP. Some patients develop a systemic coagulopathy, the cause of which remains controversial. However the coagulopathy does seem to be caused by a disseminated intravascular coagulation (DIC). The prognosis for patients who develop DIC is grave.

The patient's blood sugar should be analyzed postoperatively and insulin administered as appropriate. Hypertension should be controlled if necessary with analgesia for pain and other antihypertensive therapy as needed. The psychologic profile should be evaluated including orientation to time and place. Consistency of caregivers and supportive care assist in reducing the incidence of postoperative delirium known to occur in the elderly.

▶ SUMMARY

The field of anesthesia for the elderly or geriatric patient is very broad. This chapter has presented only a brief summary of the major points, issues, and physiologic alterations resulting from the aging process that influence anesthetic management. Information gained through studying our expanding life spans, coupled with increased technology and research in gerontology, will enhance our skill in anesthetic management of the elderly.

▶ KEY CONCEPTS

- Nurse anesthetists must be conversant with the "I's" of geriatrics and gerontology: impecunity, immobility, incontinence, isolation, infections and immunocompromise, insomnia, instability (falls), and iatrogenesis.
- Although age alone does not preclude surgery, it is apparent that the anesthetic management of the elderly is influenced by the frequency and severity of degenerative and associated diseases of the patient.
- The consequences of respiratory changes, especially in patients with chronic obstructive airway disease such as emphysema, predispose the elderly patient to early collapse of the airways and infections in the postoperative period.
- Hepatorenal changes not only reduce drug elimination but also raise, prolong, or sustain drug levels in the blood and tissues.
- It is prudent to reduce the dose of drugs to one third or one half of the adult dose and titrate to effect after sufficient observation and monitoring for physiologic responses.
- Chronologic age has no direct relationship with physiologic age; consequently, no standard anesthetic regimen can be used for the elderly because their physiologic condition and associated risks leave a very narrow margin of safety.
- A mnemonic has been devised to help identify potential reversible causes of dementia: *d*rugs, *e*motional disorders, *m*etabolic and endocrine disorders, *e*ye and ear dysfunctions, *n*utritional deficiencies, *t*umor and trauma, *i*nfections and immunocompromise, and *a*rteriosclerotic complications and alcohol.

▶ STUDY QUESTIONS

1. What are the most prevalent chronic diseases that affect the elderly and how do they influence perianesthetic management?

2. What are the anesthetic implications of a prolonged circulation time in the elderly patient?

3. Because there is a decrease in the synthesis of plasma pseudocholinesterase enzyme in the elderly, what drugs will have a longer duration of action?

4. How does the use of clonidine before surgery affect the elderly patients who take it?

5. What factors increase risks in the surgery of geriatric patients?

6. When should elective or scheduled surgical procedures be postponed?

7. What are the treatable and potentially reversible causes of dementia in the elderly?

8. Why are the elderly at greater risk for aspiration and pneumonia?

KEY REFERENCES

Ferraro, K. F. (Ed.) (1997). *Gerontology perspectives and issues* (2nd ed.). New York: Springer.

Hazzard, W. R., Bierman, E. L., Blass, J. P., Ettinger, Jr., W. H., & Halter, J. B. (Eds.) (1994). *Principles of geriatric medicine and gerontology* (3rd ed.). New York: McGraw-Hill.

Jenike, M. A. (1996). Psychiatric illnesses in the elderly: A review. *Journal of Geriatric Psychiatry and Neurology, 9,* 57–82.

Kane, R. L., Ouslander, J. G., & Abrass, I. B. (1994). *Essentials of clinical geriatrics* (3rd ed.). New York: McGraw-Hill.

McLeskey, C. H. (Ed.) (1997). *Geriatric anesthesiology.* Baltimore: Williams & Wilkins.

Smith, R. B., Gurkowski, M. A., & Bracken, C. A. (1995). *Anesthesia and pain control in the geriatric patient.* New York: McGraw-Hill.

REFERENCES

Appelbaum, J. L., Kallar, S. K., & Wetchler, B. V. (1991). The adult and geriatric patient. In B.V. Wetchler, (Ed.), *Anesthesia for ambulatory surgery* (2nd ed., pp. 197–307). Philadelphia: J. B. Lippincott.

Bromage, P. (1978). *Epidural analgesia.* Philadelphia: W. B. Saunders.

Cahalan, M. K., Litt, L., Botvinick, E. H., & Schiller, N. B. (1987). Advances in noninvasive cardiovascular imaging: Implications for the anesthesiologist. *Anesthesiology, 66,* 356–372.

Charlson, M. E., Cohen, R. P., & Sears, C. L. (1983). General medical consultation: Lessons from a clinical service. *American Journal of Medicine, 75,* 121–128.

DelGuercio, L. R. M. & Cohn, J. D. (1980). Monitoring operative risk in the elderly. *Journal of the American Medical Association, 243,* 1350–1355.

Denny, J. H. & Denson, J. S. (1972). Risk of surgery in patients over 90. *Geriatrics, 27,* 115.

Ghignone, M., Noe, C., Calvillo, O., & Quintin, L. (1988). Anesthesia for ophthalmic surgery in the elderly: The effects of clonidine on introcular pressure, perioperative hemodynamics and anesthetic requirement. *Anesthesiology, 68,* 707–716.

Gloyna, D. F. (1997). Effects of inhalation agents. In C. H. McLeskey (Ed.), *Geriatric anesthesiology* (pp. 283–309). Baltimore: Williams & Wilkins.

Goldman, L. & Caldera, D. L. (1979). Risk of general anesthesia in elective operation in the hypertensive patient. *Anesthesiology, 50,* 285–292.

Goldman, S., Copeland, J., Moritz, T., Henderson, W., Zadina, K., Ovitt, T., Doherty, J., Read, R., Chesler, E., Sako, Y., *et al.* (1988). Improvement in early saphenous vein graft patency after coronary artery bypass surgery with antiplatelet therapy: Results of a Veterans Administration cooperative study. *Circulation, 77,* 1324–1332.

Jarvis, C. (1996). *Physical examination and health assessment* (2nd ed., 70–71, 90–95, 720, 750–751). Philadelphia: W.B. Saunders.

Jenike, M. A. (1996). Psychiatric illnesses in the elderly: A review. *Journal of Geriatric Psychiatry and Neurology, 9,* 57–82.

Kane, R. L., Ouslander, J. G., & Abrass, I. B. (1994). *Essentials of clinical geriatrics* (3rd ed.). New York: McGraw-Hill.

Lamy, P. P. (1980). *Prescribing for the elderly.* Littleton, MA: PSG Publishing.

Livingston, E. H., Hershman, J. M., Sawin, C. T., & Yoshikawa, T. T. (1987). Prevalence of thyroid disease and abnormal thyroid tests in older hospitalized and ambulatory persons. *Journal of the American Geriatrics Society 35,* 109–114.

Meridy, H. W. (1982). Criteria for selection of ambulatory patients and guidelines for anesthesia management: A retrospective study of 1,553 cases. *Anesthesia & Analgesia 61,* 921.

Mittelmark, M. B. (1994). The epidemiology of aging. In W. R. Hazzard, E. L. Bierman, J. P. Blass, W. H. Ettinger, Jr., & J. B. Halter (Eds.), *Principles of geriatric medicine and gerontology* (3rd ed., pp. 135–152). New York: McGraw-Hill.

Moritz, D. J. & Ostfeld, A. M. (1990). The epidemiology and demography of aging. In W. R. Hazzard, R. Andres, E. L. Bierman, & J. P. Blass (Eds.), *Principles of geriatric medicine and gerontology* (2nd ed., pp. 146–156). New York: McGraw-Hill.

Murkin, J. M. (1982). Anesthesia and hypothyroidism: A review of thyroxin, physiology, pharmacology, and anesthetic implications. *Anesthesia & Analgesia, 61,* 371–383.

National Institutes of Health. (1991). Diagnosis and treatment of depression in late life. (November 4–6) NIH consensus statement 9(3):1–27. Available at http://www.mental-health.com/book/p45-dp01.html (2/6/97).

Page, M. M. & Watkins, P. J. (1978). Cardiorespiratory arrest in diabetic autoimmune neuropathy. *Lancet, 1,* 14–16.

Pawlson, L. G. (1994). Health care implications of an aging population. In W. R. Hazzard, E. L. Bierman, J. P. Blass, W. H. Ettinger, Jr., & J. B. Halter (Eds.), *Principles of geriatric medicine and gerontology* (3rd ed., pp 167–176). New York: McGraw-Hill.

Pompei, P. (1990). Preoperative assessment and perioperative care. In C. K. Cassel, D. E. Riesenberg, L. B. Sorensen, & J. R. Walsh (Eds.), *Geriatric medicine* (2nd ed., pp. 111–124). New York: Springer-Verlag.

Sattin, R. W., Lambert Huber, D. A., DeVito, C. A., Rodriguez, J. G., Ros, A., Bacchelli, S., Stevens, J. A., & Waxweiler, R. J. (1990). The incidence of fall injury events among the elderly in a defined population. *American Journal of Epidemiology, 131,* 1028–1037.

Steel, K., Gertman, P. M., Crescenzi, C., & Anderson, J. (1981). Iatrogenic illness on a general medical service at a university hospital. *New England Journal of Medicine, 304,* 638–642.

Tauber, C. (1992). *Income and poverty trends for the elderly.* Bureau of Census Report. Washington, DC: U.S. Department of Commerce.

Tine, M. & Cassara, E. L. (1970). Preoperative pulmonary evaluation and therapy for surgery patients. *Journal of the American Medical Association, 211,* 787–790.

Tisi, G. M. (1979). Preoperative evaluation of pulmonary function: Validity, indications, and benefits. *American Review of Respiratory Diseases, 119,* 293–310.

Treas, J. & Longino Jr., C. F. (1997). Demography of aging in the United States. In K. F. Ferraro (Ed.), *Gerontology perspectives and issues* (2nd ed., pp. 19–50), New York: Springer.

U.S. Bureau of the Census. (1993). Population projections of the United States, by age, sex, race, and Hispanic origin: 1993–2050. In *Current population reports* (P25-1104). Washington, DC: U.S. Government Printing Office.

Waugaman, W. R. (1988). Preoperative and postoperative considerations for patients with Alzheimer's disease. *Geriatric Nursing, 9,* 227–230.

Waugaman, W. R. & Rigor, B. M. (1992). Geriatric anesthesia. In W. Waugaman, S. Foster, & B. Rigor (Eds.), *Principles and practice of nurse anesthesia* (2nd ed., pp. 575–589). Norwalk, CT: Appleton & Lange.

Yoshikawa, T. T., & Norman, D. C. (1987). *Aging and clinical practice: Infectious diseases, diagnosis and treatment.* New York: Igaku-Shoin.

The Neonatal and Pediatric Patient

Susanna K. Cook Lindsey

Trends in the practice of anesthesia have produced changes in the practice of pediatric anesthesia. Enhanced monitoring techniques, increased outpatient surgery, and newer anesthetic techniques have impacted the practice of pediatric anesthesia. Shortened patient stays, morning surgical admissions, and day surgery have necessitated creative approaches to preparation of the child and parent for surgery.

There are multiple unique considerations when administering anesthesia to children. Overall, the risks for untoward events are thought to be greater in the child than in the adult. Children are unable to verbalize as well as adults. The increased incidence of laryngospasm as well as postoperative nausea and vomiting in children is well identified. Neonates and infants have a decreased cardiac reserve coupled with an inability to unload oxygen at the tissue level. Data about autoregulation, although abundant for the adult, has not been well established in infants and children. Cohen and Cameron (1990) reported an overall untoward event rate of 35% in the child, which contrasts with 17% for the adult.

Recognizing sources of perioperative anxiety for the child and family is essential in the preoperative preparation process. There are unique sources of stress for the parents of the child undergoing surgery (Zuckerberg, 1994). These include financial concerns, feelings of guilt, lack of control, separation anxiety, fear of surgical failure, and fear of death. Children, on the other hand, have their own concerns and anxieties. Younger children express fears of the unknown, fears of mutilation and torture, and a universal fear of needles. Older children and teens express concerns over body image, dignity, and modesty.

Although different sources of anxiety emerge at different developmental levels throughout childhood, Zuckerberg (1994) identified separation anxiety as the child's greatest source of anxiety. Thus, in many institutions, parents participate in anesthesia induction by remaining with the child until he or she is obtunded. If parents are prepared properly and present with the child during induction, it seems there are fewer behavioral problems postoperatively in the child. If parental presence is not possible for induction, then the parents or a parent should remain with the child as long as possible during the preoperative period.

▶ PHYSIOLOGIC AND ANATOMIC DIFFERENCES BETWEEN THE PEDIATRIC AND THE ADULT PATIENT

Respiratory System

The respiratory system is of special interest to the anesthetist. It is the route of administration for inhaled anesthetic agents, and its functions may be significantly changed during and after anesthesia. Changes occur continuously from infancy to about age 12 as the system grows to maturity. Developmental changes can be described in four phases from birth to adulthood. The newborn period is considered to be the first 24 hours of life; the neonatal period, the first month; the infancy period, the first year; and the childhood period, from the first year to the teen years.

Steward (1994) described the changes that take place at birth as the newborn moves from a water environment to an air environment. This change occurs within a few breaths. Pulmonary vascular resistance (PVR) decreases as systemic vascular resistance increases with the first breath. This initial decrease in PVR continues slowly over the first 3 months of life. This decrease in PVR parallels the regression in the thickness of the medial muscle layer of the pulmonary arterioles. During the first month of life, the PVR is still relatively high, and muscular pulmonary vessels are highly reactive. Hypoxia, acidosis, and stress caused by endotracheal suctioning may all result in rapid elevation of PVR. This may necessitate a right to left shunt.

Wensley and Sear (1993) described the small radius of the diaphragm curvature that allows the newborn to achieve the high negative pressures necessary to open the lungs. A functional residual capacity (FRC) of approximately 30 mL/kg is soon established. Remaining lung fluid is removed during the first few days of life by the pulmonary lymphatics and blood vessels. Newborns delivered by cesarean section are not subjected to the same thoracic squeeze and may have more residual fluid in the lungs. This may result in transient respiratory distress. In addition to the significant changes at birth in respiratory physiology, certain major anatomic characteristics are important to the anesthetist. The neck of the newborn is relatively short, whereas the tongue and head are large (Berry & Yemen, 1994). The oral airway obstructs easily. The nasal passages are narrow and also easily blocked, which may cause airway obstruction. This is important because newborns are thought to be obligate nose breathers. The larynx is more cephalad and anterior. Its long axis is directed inferiorly and anteriorly. Elevation of the neonate's head will tend to move the larynx anteriorly. The airway is narrowest at the level of the cricoid cartilage just below the vocal cords. The epiglottis is relatively long and stiff. It is U-shaped and projects posteriorly at an angle of 45 degrees above the glottis. The trachea is short; therefore, precise placement and fixation of the endotracheal tube are essential (Fig. 15-1).

Management and assessment of pediatric lung volumes may create challenges for the anesthetist as well. Wensley and Sear (1993) described the lung volumes during the newborn period. It has already been stated that the FRC is established within the first few breaths. When related to body weight, static lung volumes (total lung capacity, functional residual capacity) are close to adult values (Table 15-1). However, neonatal alveolar ventilation is more than twice as high, reflecting an elevated oxygen consumption. Consequently the FRC is a much less effective buffer in the neonate, so changes in

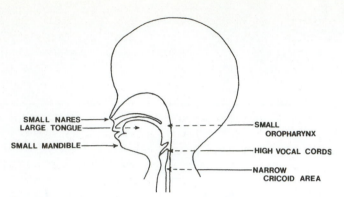

Figure 15–1. The pediatric airway.

the concentration of inspired gases are more rapidly reflected in alveolar and arterial levels. Webster and Lopez (1993) described the elastic properties of the neonatal lung that result in higher closing volumes, which may remain higher well into childhood and may exceed the FRC.

Airway closure during normal ventilation may explain the lower normal values for Pao_2 during infancy and childhood. Normal Pao_2 during the first week of life is 70 mmHg, rising incrementally to 96 by 12 to 16 years. A fall in FRC usually occurs during general anesthesia and persists into the postoperative period (Steward, 1994). This fall in the FRC may be expected to increase the significance of the high closing volume and further increase the alveolar oxygen tension gradient. Higher closing volumes may result in ventilation–perfusion mismatch: the younger the child the larger the decrease in the FRC. This necessitates an increase in the oxygen concentration of inspired gases while anesthesia is administered.

Surfactant decreases the surface tension in the neonatal lung. It stabilizes the alveoli to prevent collapse and decreases the inspiratory force required for expansion of the lungs. Webster and Lopez (1993) briefly described the developmental implications of surfactant development. The quantity of surfactant increases as gestational age increases. Production begins at 22 weeks of

TABLE 15–1. Lung Volumes

	Adult	Child	Neonate
VA (mL/kg/min)	60	80	100–150
Frequency (per min)	10	20	40
TLC[a] (mL/kg)	80	70	60
FRC (mL/kg)	34	32	30
RV (mL/kg)	17	19	20
Vt (mL/kg)	7	7	6

[a] TLC, total lung capacity; FRC, functional residual capacity; RV, residual volume.

gestation and peaks at 36 weeks. After birth, the biochemical pathways for surfactant production can be depressed by hypoxia, hyperoxia, acidosis, and hypothermia. These conditions must be prevented and corrected quickly. Decreased surfactant can result in alveolar collapse, maldistribution of ventilation, impaired gas exchange, decreased compliance, and increased risk of pneumothorax. Pneumothorax is more common in the newborn than at any other age. Inhaled anesthetic gases have little effect on surfactant production.

Respiratory development continues during the first two decades of life. The number of alveoli increases rapidly over the first 6 years, reaching almost adult maturation. Growth of alveoli continues into adolescence.

Laryngospasm occurs more frequently in association with pediatric anesthesia, especially during induction and following extubation. The reason for the increased incidence of laryngospasm in infants and children has not been thoroughly identified. However, it is acknowledged that cough, laryngospasm, apnea, and swallowing are the four protective reflexes of the airway that allow the complex control of the airway required for breathing, swallowing, and phonation (Berry & Yemen, 1994). It was noted by Martin (1994) as well as Tait, Reynolds, and Gutstein (1995) that patients with a recent upper respiratory tract infection tend to have more reactive airways and a higher risk of bronchospasm and laryngospasm. Airway reactivity seems to be increased by endotracheal intubation.

Cardiovascular System

During fetal circulation there are four shunts, which include the placenta, ductus venosus, foramen ovale, and the ductus arteriosis. Newborn adaptation to extrauterine life involves the elimination of these four shunts. Elimination of placental blood flow is accomplished with clamping of the cord. This simultaneously creates an increase in systemic vascular resistance and elimination of blood flow through the ductus venosus and a closure of this shunt. As air enters the lungs there is a decrease in PVR. With this decrease, blood flow increases to the lungs and then via the pulmonary veins into the left atrium. The left atrial pressure is increased above the

right atrial pressure, and the atrial septum is closed over the foramen ovale. The ductus arteriosis anatomically closes during the first 10 to 15 hours of life in response to increases in oxygen saturation and withdrawal of placental prostaglandins. Anatomic closure is accomplished at age 2 to 3 weeks.

According to Steward (1994), there are several hemodynamic considerations when anesthetizing the newborn and child. During the early neonatal period, there are some circumstances that may precipitate persistent fetal circulation. If hypoxia occurs, PVR increases and the ductus arteriosus may reopen, establishing a vicious cycle of hypoxemia, acidosis, impaired blood flow, and hypoxemia. Relative changes in vascular tone caused by the administration of anesthetic agents can alter the effects of intracardiac shunts. A ventricular septal defect (left-to-right shunt) may produce pulmonary vascular overload and subsequent right heart failure.

The limited stroke volume of the newborn is described by Webster and Lopez (1993). Only 30% of fetal cardiac muscle is contractile mass, compared with 60% in the adult. As a result, it is less compliant and less capable of adjusting stroke volume in response to demands for increased cardiac output, which is largely dependent on heart rate. In the newborn the parasympathetic innervation of the heart is complete whereas the sympathetic innervation is still incomplete. Consequently, the newborn is predisposed to bradycardia. During the immediate newborn period, the heart rate is between 100 and 170 beats per minute (BPM) and the rhythm is regular. As the child matures, the heart rate decreases. Sinus arrhythmia is common in children. All other irregular rhythms must be considered abnormal. Neonatal blood pressures increase from a systolic blood pressure of approximately 60 mmHg and diastolic pressure of 35 mmHg to adult levels by about age 16 (Table 15–2).

Hematologic Changes

Hematologic differences must also be evaluated by the anesthetist. Steward (1994) indicated that values for blood volume, hematocrit, and hemoglobin (Hgb) vary from newborn to newborn, depending on the time of umbilical cord clamping. These values tend to be high at

TABLE 15–2. Cardiovascular Data

	Heart Rate	Blood Pressure (mmHg)	Blood Volume (mL/kg)	Hemoglobin (g/100 mL)
Neonate (0–4 wk)	120	60/40	80	16–18
Infant (4 wk–6 mo)	110	90/60	75	10–11
Child (6 mo–6 y)	100	100/70	70	12–14
Adult	80	120/70	60–65	12–14

birth, with the neonatal hematocrit starting about 54% to 60%. After 1 week of life, the hematocrit level starts to fall to a low of 29% to 33% by 3 months of age. Much of the Hgb present at birth is of the fetal type (HbF). The affinity of fetal hbF for oxygen is greater than that of adult Hgb (HbA), but HbF releases O_2 less readily to the tissues than does HbA. Adequate oxygen transport in the newborn requires a higher Hgb concentration. Less than 12 g constitutes anemia in the newborn. By about 3 months of age, Hgb levels have decreased to about 9 g to 11 g (Table 15-2). At this time hbF has largely been replaced by HbA. As a result, oxygen delivery at the tissue level is improved. If development is normal, the Hgb level increases over several weeks to 12 g to 13 g, which is maintained during early childhood.

Thermal Regulation

Thermal regulation in pediatric patients requires attention by the anesthetist. The newborn loses heat through conduction, convection, radiation, and evaporation and thus is unusually susceptible to rapid falls in temperature. Newborns rely primarily on increased metabolic rate to counter any cold stresses. Nonshivering thermogenesis results in metabolic acidosis, increased oxygen consumption, decreased oxygenation of vital tissues, hypoventilation, and decreased cardiac output. Cold stress may also prolong recovery from anesthetic drugs. Frequent and central temperature monitoring is mandatory along with interventions to maintain a neutral thermal environment. Heating lights, elevation of room temperature, blankets, and protective skin covering are all appropriate measures.

Fluid and Electrolyte Status

Fluid and electrolyte status is impacted by maturational level. Glomerulogenesis is complete by about 34 weeks gestation (Siker, 1994). The full-term newborn kidney matures rapidly. Glomerular and proximal tubular function double in the term infant by one month of age. Drugs excreted via the kidneys depend on the glomerular filtration rate (GFR) and tubular secretion capacity, both of which are decreased during the first few weeks of life. The renin–angiotension–aldosterone system is intact at birth. During the first week of life, the infant is an obligate sodium loser because the distal tubule cannot efficiently reabsorb sodium, even while losing sodium.

In the first 48 hours of life, the infant is unable to concentrate or dilute urine. At 1 month of age, renal function is about 70% to 80% of normal adult function. The central osmoreceptors and peripheral volume receptors of infants must act to regulate water and sodium balance. Total body water and extracellular fluid volume of the newborn are larger on a weight basis than those of an adult. In the full-term newborn 73% of total body

Table 15–3. Dehydration Criteria

Physical Sign	Dehydration (%)
Dry mouth and mucous membranes, infrequent voiding	5
Sunken eyes or fontanelle, lethargy, poor capillary filling	10
Tenting of the skin, anuria, hypotension	15

weight is water, whereas only 60% of total body weight is water in the adult. The percentage of extracellular fluid is higher in the neonate than in the adult, whereas the percentage of intracellular fluid is lower. Preoperative assessment of hydration status is necessary for appropriate replacement of water and electrolytes during the preoperative and intraoperative period. Preoperative dehydration can be classified by the size of the deficit as mild, moderate, or severe (Table 15-3). Mild dehydration is characterized by a 5% body weight loss or 50 mL/kg. Moderate dehydration is characterized by a 10% weight loss or 100 mL/kg. Severe dehydration is characterized by a 15% weight loss or 150 mL/kg.

▶ PEDIATRIC PHARMACOLOGY

There are multiple developmental changes that influence the pharmacology of anesthetic drugs in the pediatric patient. In neonates and infants, the total body water is larger than in adults. Because this increase in water is largely extracellular, drugs distributed through this compartment may require a higher dose. The blood volume of the newborn is also larger on a weight basis than that of the adult, which further contributes to the initial larger volume of distribution. Decreased muscle mass and fat stores in the newborn provide less uptake to inactive sites and tend to keep plasma concentrations higher. The smaller amount of fat tissue provides a smaller reservoir for fat-soluble drugs.

The pharmacodynamics and pharmacokinetics of inhalation agents are significantly influenced by the maturational differences in infants and children. Maturational differences in the infant include a higher rate of alveolar ventilation, particularly in relation to the FRC (Chan, 1993). The infant has a higher cardiac output and greater distribution to the vessel-rich organs than does the adult. There is a lower blood solubility related to lower albumin and globulin concentration and a lower tissue solubility as a result of greater water and decreased protein. These differences from the adult accelerate the partial pressure equilibrium in the infant and contribute to the rapid uptake of the inhalation agents. Excretion of inhaled anesthetics is more rapid in infants and small children, provided that ventilation is not depressed. The minimal alveolar concentration for all anesthetic agents is higher in younger children than in older children or adults and is lower in newborns or preterm infants.

▶ HISTORY AND PHYSICAL EXAMINATION

Maxwell, Deshpand, and Wetzel (1994) identified historical areas of particular concern to the anesthetist, which include a history of prematurity as well as history related to neuromuscular, cardiovascular, respiratory, endocrine, hematologic, oncologic, or eating disorders. A history of prematurity may result in apnea or subglottic stenosis. The child should be approached according to the specific needs of the developmental age group. Efforts to maintain modesty of the adolescent are important to establishing rapport. Overall physical growth and development as well as activity level should be assessed. Areas of key interest to the anesthetist in the physical examination include airway anatomy; the presence of stridor, wheezing, or murmurs; and evidence of neurologic deficit.

▶ DIAGNOSTIC DATA

Accurate weight and height is required for every child. Potential emergency drug doses may be calculated in advance to avoid confusion during an emergency. The value of routine urinalysis and hemoglobin screening of healthy children is debatable, but in some regions, this may be a legislated requirement. Many authorities now recommend that these tests be omitted for healthy patients undergoing minor surgery. However, all infants, especially those who were born prematurely, should have a hemoglobin determination to rule out anemia, which is more common in infancy and may increase the risk of complications. Older children with systemic diseases, those with a history of anemia, and those who may lose significant amounts of blood intraoperatively should also have a preoperative Hgb determination. A sickle-cell test is necessary for all patients at risk. If the test is positive, a hemoglobin electrophoresis should be ordered.

Patients receiving anticonvulsant therapy should have blood concentrations measured to ensure therapeutic levels perioperatively. If the child requires theophylline, serum levels should be measured to optimize drug dosing and guide intraoperative bronchodilator therapy. Children with cardiovascular disease on digoxin therapy should have serum sodium, potassium, and digoxin levels measured. An electrocardiogram (ECG) is warranted in a child with obstructive sleep apnea, bronchopulmonary dysplasia, congenital heart disease, or severe scoliosis. Likewise, a chest x-ray is appropriate in a child with chronic aspiration or lower airway disease.

▶ PERIANESTHESIA PLAN FOR THE PEDIATRIC PATIENT

General Considerations of the Pediatric Patient

There are many considerations in the preparation of the pediatric patient, parent, and environment for the provision of a safe and effective anesthetic. One major consideration is proper planning to avoid emergencies, which includes proper equipment for acknowledged potential difficult airway in the child. Standard emergency drugs are also part of planning. Doses for atropine and succinylcholine should be calculated in advance to avoid confusion in case of emergency. Consideration should be given to the appropriateness of an intravenous (IV) versus a mask induction. Multiple sizes of endotracheal tubes and masks should be available (Fig. 15-2).

Appropriate monitoring devices for specific age should be available before induction. Pediatric blood pressure cuffs, pediatric Sao_2 monitors, pediatric size precordial stethoscopes, fluid monitoring devices, and pediatric size angiocaths should be retrieved. Inhalation agents appropriate for child inductions should be available (N_2O, sevoflurane, or halothane). Other inhalation agents are generally avoided because of their pungent odor and ability to irritate the airway during mask inductions. Isoflurane, however, is often used to maintain anesthesia in infants and children.

Preoperative Considerations

The purpose of the preoperative anesthetic visit is fivefold: (1) to identify aspects of the child's history and physical information that may affect the anesthetic management and perioperative course; (2) to obtain information such as height, weight, and appropriate laboratory tests to allow appropriate preparation of drugs and equipment; (3) to alleviate anxiety and provide information regarding the anesthetic plan to the parents and child if appropriate; (4) to premedicate the child and establish NPO parameters; and (5) to ensure that medical issues are addressed to the best extent possible if the case is elective.

Steward (1994) suggested that preoperative fluid replacement take place in three phases: (1) Severe dehydration or impending shock is treated with an initial infusion of the whole blood at 10 mL/kg, or 5% albumin at 20 mL/kg; (2) extracellular water and sodium is replaced over 6 to 8 hours with 0.3 normal saline; and (3) replacement of potassium should be initiated when a good renal output has been established not to exceed

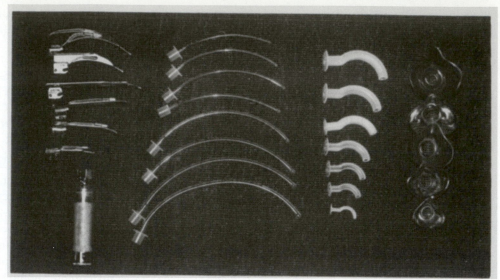

Figure 15–2. Pediatric airway equipment. From left to right, laryngoscope blades—Nos. 0, 1, 2 Miller, No. 1.5 Wis–Hipple, Nos. 2, 3 Macintosh; uncuffed endotracheal tubes—2.5 to 6.0 mm by half sizes; oral airways— 40 to 100 mm; Rendell–Baker–Soucek masks, Nos. 00, 0, 1, 2, 3.

3 mEq/kg in 24 hours. During surgical procedures, sufficient fluid should be given to compensate for preoperative fasting. Hourly infusion rates are based on daily maintenance requirements and adjusted for factors affecting insensible fluid loss or extrarenal losses. Using this maintenance system, the requirements are 4 mL/kg/h for the first 10 kg of weight, 2 mL/kg/h for the second 10 kg, and 1 cc/kg/h for the remaining weight above 20 kg. Maintenance fluids usually consist of 5% dextrose with lactated Ringer's or Plasmalyte for neonates and lactated Ringer's or Plasma-Lyte for older children. The adequacy of fluid losses may be judged by urine output. Adequate urinary output is considered to be 1 mL/kg/h.

The physical status of children is rated using the American Society of Anesthesiologists (ASA) physical status classification just as with adults. In addition to obtaining the history and physical information, the preoperative visit can be used to evaluate and alleviate child and parent anxiety. Perioperative stress is common to all children and their families who undergo anesthesia and surgery. Efforts must be made to make an age-appropriate explanation, provide reassurance, and eliminate disturbing fantasies and misconceptions. Helping the child predict likely postoperative experiences may prevent unexpected and frightening challenges postoperatively.

Premedication should be determined after evaluating and discussing the anesthesia and operative experience with the child (if age-appropriate) and parents. Many practitioners believe that the best premedication is a prepared parent. Some believe that parental presence obviates the need for premedication. This seems clearly related to the quality of the parent–child relationship. The goal is to make the child feel as comfortable and safe as possible when entering the operating suite. Should a premedication be deemed necessary, it should be safe, effective, painless, and capable of rapid anxiolysis. It has already been stated that children have a universal fear of needles; therefore midazolam by mouth (0.3 mg to 0.5 mg/kg) in a clear liquid or dissolved in liquid acetaminophen is often used. Sedative effects are evident within 15 min of administration. Other sedative drugs may be equally appropriate such as rectal brevital, rectal or intramuscular (IM) midazolam, IM or IV ketamine, or intranasal narcotics. The choice the anesthetist makes must be guided by the particular condition of the child.

Preoperative consideration should be given to the blocking of unwanted vagal responses in infants and children. Despite the trend to omit the routine administration of vagal-blocking drugs to adult patients, many authorities such as Steward (1994) believe that they are useful in infants and children. Serious bradycardia resulting from administration of cholinergic drugs such as succinylcholine and halothane is common in young patients. Bradycardia may lead to significant hypotension and serious arrhythmias. If the use of cholinergic drugs or instrumentation of the airway is planned, the prior administration of atropine is suggested. If it is decided not to administer an anticholinergic drug, atropine should still be drawn up and immediately available throughout the anesthetic. Infants younger than 6 months of age should be treated with atropine (0.01 mg/kg) due to their highly vagolytic nature regardless of anesthetic choice.

During the preoperative visit, NPO parameters must be established. Although there has been and continues to be considerable debate regarding the length of the NPO period required for an empty stomach, the vast majority of pediatric anesthetists recommend a 4-hour fast for neonates and infants up to 2 years of age. For children 2 to 6 years of age, a 6-hour fast is recommended, and for those older than 6 years, an 8-hour fast is appropriate. Aspiration is a greater threat in children with feeding and swallowing problems, gastroesophageal reflux, seizures, or other neurologic compromise (such as Guillain–Barré syndrome or myasthenia gravis). The goal of the preoperative evaluation is geared toward minimizing the risks of anesthesia and surgery by having the child in the healthiest possible condition before surgery. Effective communication with parents, child, surgeon, and pediatrician is necessary to ensure that all anesthesia concerns of underlying disease processes are appropriately addressed.

Intraoperative Considerations

Induction

Induction of anesthesia may proceed after careful preparation of the operating room (OR) and anesthesia equipment. The pediatric patient should not be taken to the OR until the room is properly warmed. Warming lights may be used with neonates and young infants. All appropriately sized pediatric monitors, endotracheal tubes, and laryngoscope blades must be available. Straight laryngoscope blades are generally more helpful with infants due to the more cephalad and anterior position of the infant larynx. The Wis–Hippel 1.5 is often an ideal blade for neonates and small infants. Face masks of appropriate size must also be available. Pediatric masks come in different scents to make the inhalation agent more palatable. Endotracheal tubes of appropriate size, one size larger, and one size smaller should be available. A useful equation for determining internal diameter size is age of the child divided by four, plus four. Another equation often used is 16 plus the age of child, divided by four. Uncuffed tubes are appropriate for children younger than 10 years. An IV setup must also be readily available. For children younger than 6 years or those in whom fluids must be closely monitored, a measured infusion chamber (eg, Buretrol® or Soluset®) with a minidrip chamber should be used. The surgeon also must be readily available before the child is introduced to the OR so there is no unnecessary waiting in this stressful environment.

After all necessary preparation, the child may be taken to the OR. All monitors should be placed (ECG, Sao_2 monitor, blood pressure cuff). Depending on the age of the child and the negotiation made with the child, either inhalation or IV induction should proceed. Temperature monitoring should begin soon after induction of anesthesia. Halothane continues to be used frequently for inhalation induction in children; sevoflurane compares very well and is gaining in popularity (Greenspun, Hannallah, Welborn, & Norden, 1994). There seems to be very little laryngospasm, coughing, or breath holding with either halothane or sevoflurane. The other respiratory and circulatory effects of sevoflurane do not appear to be markedly different from those of halothane and isoflurane. Emergence from sevoflurane anesthesia is smooth and rapid; care must be taken to ensure adequate analgesia throughout the procedure.

The inspired concentration of either halothane or sevoflurane should be increased slowly, about 0.2% for each three breaths. Fifty percent to 70% nitrous oxide may be used if the patient's oxygen saturation is satisfactory. If the child begins to cough and hold his or her breath, 100% oxygen must be given until respiration is normal. When respiration is normal and oxygen saturation is satisfactory, the induction pattern may begin again. Added caution is encouraged during the administration of potent inhalation agents in infants and young children because overdose is a leading cause of serious complications. If laryngospasm occurs that does not resolve with 100% oxygen and positive pressure ventilation, treatment should be initiated with either IM or IV succinylcholine (1 to 2 mg/kg) and atropine (0.01 mg/kg).

When the patient is unresponsive to tactile stimuli, IV access should be initiated. In the child who already has IV access, the sequence of induction drugs is similar to that in adults. Methohexital, propofol, midazolam, ketamine, and thiopental all have been used successfully as induction agents in children. In general, neonates are especially sensitive to barbiturates and require only 3 to 4 mg/kg of thiopental for induction. However older infants (1 to 6 months) may require higher than usual doses (6 to 7 mg/kg) to ensure sleep. Children require 5 to 6 mg/kg as a sleep dose.

If succinylcholine is administered, an anticholinergic should be administered first. The use of succinylcholine in infants and children for elective purposes is controversial (Gronert & Brandom, 1994). The Malignant Hyperthermia Hotline in the United States receives about six calls per year reporting cases of intractable, unexpected cardiac arrest after induction of anesthesia with halothane and succinylcholine. Duchenne's muscular dystrophy has subsequently been diagnosed in some of these children. Other, more appropriate nondepolarizing neuromuscular blocking drugs for elective cases include atracurium, rocuronium, vecuronium, mivacurium, or cisatracurium. The use of succinylcholine to produce rapid paralysis allowing endotracheal intubation in patients at risk for hypoxia or aspiration remains acceptable.

After IV access is secured and a muscle relaxant or deep inhalation is administered, the child can be intubated if endotracheal anesthesia is necessary. Depending on the nature and duration of the surgery, the anesthetist may at this point choose a mask general anesthetic or maintain the airway with a laryngeal mask airway instead of endotracheal intubation. Efrat, Kadari, and Katz (1994) reported excellent results with the laryngeal mask airway in children. Because of the large occiput of the infant in relation to body size, a small roll placed under the shoulders can help position the infant for airway management or intubation. If an endotracheal airway is chosen, the endotracheal tube should be placed under direct visualization with laryngoscopy midway between the vocal cords and the carina. The uncuffed tube should allow an air leak at 20 cm H_2O pressure for proper fit. Breath sounds should be bilaterally equal.

Maintenance

In selecting an agent or agents for maintenance of general anesthesia in children several objectives must be considered: (1) Abolish the sensation of pain; (2) prevent awareness; (3) inhibit stress responses; (4) maintain stable cardiopulmonary and metabolic status; and (5) prevent perioperative complications. Many agents are available to help accomplish these objectives. A combination of IV and inhalation agents can be given to successfully maintain general anesthesia. The guiding principle remains "titrate to effect." Only what is needed should be administered, and strict vigilance must be maintained. Muscle relaxation can be maintained with a variety of agents already mentioned. Pancuronium may be beneficial because of its vagolytic effect on the rate-dependent neonate. Neuromuscular blockade must always be monitored. Complete reversal is necessary before emergence.

It should be remembered that there are dose differences related to age. The minimal alveolar concentration (MAC) of anesthetic drugs is higher in infants and children than in neonates or adults. The onset of neuromuscular blocking (NMB) agents is more rapid in the infant than the child. Generally, children require more of all NMB on a mg/kg basis than do infants or adults to achieve the same effect. Children recover from neuromuscular blockade more rapidly than do patients of other ages. Infants may recover more rapidly than any other patients from the effects of drugs such as mivacurium that are metabolized in the plasma.

Emergence

Children are very prone to laryngeal spasm on emergence and extubation, particularly after inhalation anesthesia or if extubated during a light plane of anesthesia. Time required for awakening is dependent on preoperative medication, agents used during the case, age of the child, and length of the case. Extubation should take place when the child is fully awake unless "deep" extubation is beneficial. Examples of cases in which deep extubation is beneficial include neurosurgery and intraocular surgery. Children in whom intubation was difficult or those having emergency surgery must be extubated when fully awake. The oropharynx should be suctioned before extubation. When judging whether the child is "awake" enough for extubation, the anesthetist should wait until the eyes and mouth open sponta-

neously and the child resumes regular spontaneous ventilation after coughing. Only after it is certain that the child is awake, and stable, and that breathing is unlabored should monitors be removed. The child may then be transferred to the postanesthesia care unit while lying in the lateral position. The precordial stethoscope should be left on the chest during transport to monitor heart and respirations.

Postoperative Considerations

The postanesthesia care unit provides an opportunity for the child to recover from the effects of the anesthetic in a closely monitored situation. Although the child is arousable, he or she has not returned to baseline level of consciousness. Each child's cardiorespiratory status is monitored, supplemental oxygen is given, and oxygen saturation is continuously monitored. Minimizing parent–child separation during this time is helpful. In many institutions, once the safe transfer of the child has occurred, parents are encouraged to participate in their child's care. As the recovery proceeds, the child's mental status returns to baseline, and complete protective respiratory and circulatory function returns. Although recovery usually proceeds in an uncomplicated, rapid fashion in children, certain problems may prolong the stay in the postanesthesia care unit. According to Hall (1992) these problems are usually centered around one of the following: (1) emergence delirium; (2) delayed emergence; (3) airway obstruction; (4) hypovolemia; or (5) postintubation croup.

Postintubation croup is treated relative to severity. Mild croup is treated with humidification, oxygen, and hydration. In addition, moderate croup is treated with nebulized racemic epinephrine (0.5 mL of racemic epinephrine 2.25% in 2.5 mL of saline). For more severe croup administration of dexamethasone and reintubation may be considered. These immediate complications must be resolved before discharge from the postanesthesia care unit.

Criteria for discharge tend to differ from unit to unit but usually include the following: (1) stable body temperature; (2) stable, age-appropriate vital signs; (3) recovery of airway reflexes; (4) return to baseline oxygen requirements; and (5) adequacy of analgesia.

Postoperative Pain Management

The philosophy and practice of preemptive pain management has dramatically reduced the need for postoperative pain and analgesic requirements. When the surgical site is appropriate, a caudal epidural injection may be given to the child after induction (Semsroth, Gabriel, Sauberer, & Wuppinger, 1994). This technique dramatically reduces the requirements for general anesthetics and also provides a prolonged postoperative analgesia. The injection of local anesthetic into the surgical site by the surgeon also enhances pain management. Acetaminophen and nonsteroidal anti-inflammatory agents (NSAIDs) such as ibuprofen and ketorolac provide excellent analgesia for many children. Employment of patient-controlled analgesic devices provides the child with a mechanism to assume control as well as prompt and painless analgesia.

Postoperative Nausea and Vomiting

Central effects of the anesthetic as well as the effects of surgical stimulation may produce postoperative nausea and vomiting, which are probably the most common acute complication of pediatric surgery. Risk factors for the child include the type of surgery (particularly strabismus surgery), the anesthetic agent used (N_2O and narcotics), longer procedures, and the age and sex of the child (risk is greater in females between ages 5 and 10 years).

Children undergoing procedures associated with a high incidence of vomiting may benefit from preemptive antiemetic therapy. Various agents have been recommended. Hall (1992) recommended that droperidol (75 μg/kg) be given during surgery or before emergence. This has been shown to decrease the incidence of postoperative nausea and vomiting, but this dosage may be accompanied by prolonged somnolence. Metoclopramide (0.15 mg/kg) may also be used to produce a reduction in vomiting. Other authors recommend small bolus doses of propofol shortly before emergence to reduce the incidence of postoperative nausea and vomiting. Ondansetron (0.15 mg/kg) has also produced a reduction in emesis in the pediatric population. Effective antiemetic and anesthetic drugs continue to be an active area of investigation.

▶ CASE STUDY

A 4-month-old infant was scheduled for surgery to correct a left incarcerated inguinal hernia. The patient was admitted the night before, and NPO status was initiated. An IV of D5.2 normal saline was started at 20 mL/h in the right hand. The parents were interviewed, and attempts were made to alleviate their fears. General endotracheal anesthesia was explained to the parents with a focus on positive outcomes. On examination, the infant was well hydrated, afebrile, well nourished, and without signs or symptoms of URI. There was no recent history of cough, cold, or fever. The term birth infant was well developed. Essentially the anesthesia history and physical was negative. No preoperative sedation was ordered due to the age of the infant. However, because the infant was under

6 months of age, preoperative atropine (0.01 mg/kg IV) was ordered.

The OR was prepared with age-appropriate monitors and airway management equipment. The temperature of the room was increased. Warming lights were provided over the field. The parents were encouraged to stay with the child during the preoperative holding phase. After the infant was carried to the operating room, all monitors were placed. With the IV already in place, a rapid sequence induction was done because of potential for bowel obstruction. Sodium thiopental and succynochline were used for induction. A size 4.0 endotracheal tube was easily passed under direct visualization using a Miller 0 blade. The anesthesia was maintained with a combination of sevoflurane and caudal inserted after the airway was secured.

1. What is the significance of prematurity in the preoperative history?

   Studies have indicated that former premature infants are at greater risk for respiratory complications, especially apnea.

2. What airway option is most appropriate for this patient?

   Because regurgitation is a potential during this procedure, the airway needs to be secured. Endotracheal intubation is the best option.

3. Why is preoperative atropine appropriate for this 4-month-old?

   Infants have a relative predominance of vagal control over cardiovascular function; this vagal predominance is age-related.

4. Why is caudal particularly appropriate for this age group?

   Caudal is appropriate for this age group due to favorable anatomy and effective pain management. Rapid, pain-free recovery without the use of potent analgesics or opioids is especially desirable in this age group.

▶ SUMMARY

The challenges of pediatric anesthesia are numerous. The anesthetist must be prepared with a thorough knowledge of the developmental differences between the newborn, neonate, infant, and child. Special effort is required to appropriately integrate the family into the care of the child. The demand for preparation, vigilance, and planning is more evident in the practice of pediatric anesthesia due to the lack of reserve found in the pediatric patient. Careful attention to detail minimizes complications and enhances recovery.

► **KEY CONCEPTS**

- Parental separation anxiety is the child's greatest source of anxiety.
- Newborns and infants have anatomic characteristics that may make intubation difficult.
- Relative to pediatric pulmonary physiology, laryngospasm occurs more frequently in children than adults, recent URIs increase the potential for bronchospasm and laryngospasm, and the younger the child, the larger the decrease in FRC.
- Relative changes in vascular tone caused by the administration of anesthetic agents can alter the effects of intracardiac shunts.
- The cardiac output of newborns and infants is

largely dependent on heart rate. Newborns and infants are predisposed to bradycardiac episodes.
- Adequate oxygen transport in the newborn requires higher hemoglobin concentrations.
- In neonates and infants, extracellular water and blood volume contribute to an increased volume of distribution.
- Infants and children have a rapid uptake of inhalation anesthetics, and the MAC for all anesthetic agents is higher in younger children than older children, but lower in newborns.
- Preemptive pain management should be regularly employed in infants and young children.

Study Questions

1. What is often the greatest source of anxiety for the child undergoing surgery?

2. What is the relationship between functional residual capacity and the age of the child?

3. Why do neonates and infants have an increased volume of distribution?

4. How does MAC differ according to the age of the child?

5. What anatomic characteristics of the neonate and infant make intubation difficult?

KEY REFERENCES

Berry, F. A. (1990). *Anesthetic management of difficult and routine pediatric patients.* New York: Churchill-Livingstone.

Bloch, E. C. (1992). Update on anesthesia management for infants and children. *Surgical Clinics of North America, 72,* 1207–1221.

Efrat, R., Kadar, A., & Katz, S. (1994). The laryngeal mask airway in pediatric anesthesia: Experience with 120 patients undergoing elective groin surgery. *Journal of Pediatric Surgery, 29,* 206–208.

Lerman, J. (1995). Sevoflurane in pediatric anesthesia. *Anesthesia & Analgesia, 81,* S4–S10.

Littman, R. S. & Keon, T. P. (1991). Postintubation croup in children. *Anesthesiology, 75,* 1122–1123.

Littman, R. S., Perkins, R. M., & Dawson, S. C. (1993). Parental knowledge and attitudes toward discussing the risk of death from anesthesia. *Anesthesia & Analgesia, 77,* 256–260.

Rosen, D. A., Rosen, K. R., & Hannallah, R. S. (1993). Anaesthesia induction in children—Ability to predict outcome. *Paediatric Anaesthesia, 3,* 365–370.

Semsroth, M., Gabriel, A., Sauberer, A., & Wuppinger, G. (1994). Regional anesthetic procedures in pediatric anesthesia. *Anaesthesist, 43,* 55–72.

Steward, D. J. (1991). Screening tests before surgery in children. *Canadian Journal of Anaesthesia, 38,* 693.

Zambricki, C. S. (1992). Pediatric anesthesia: Current thinking. *CRNA-The Clinical Forum for Nurse Anesthetists, 3,* 51–52.

REFERENCES

Berry, F., & Yemen, T. (1994). Pediatric airway in health and disease. *Pediatric Clinics of North America, 41,* 153–171.

Chan, C. Y. (1993). Pediatric Pharmacology. In D. E. Webster (Ed.), *Clinical manual of pediatric anesthesia* (pp. 28–31). New York: McGraw-Hill.

Cohen, M. & Cameron, C. B. (1990). Pediatric anesthesia morbidity and mortality in the perioperative period. *Anesthesia & Analgesia, 70,* 160–167.

Efrat, R., Kadar, A., & Katz, S. (1994). The laryngeal mask airway in pediatric anesthesia: Experience with 120 patients undergoing elective groin surgery. *Journal of Pediatric Surgery, 29,* 206–208.

Greenspun, J., Hannallah, R., Welborn, L., & Norden, J. (1994). Comparison of sevoflurane and halothane in pediatric ENT surgery. *Anesthesia & Analgesia, 78,* 140.

Gronert, B., Brandom, B. W. (1994). Neuromuscular blocking

drugs in infants and children. *Pediatric Clinics of North America, 41,* 73–91.

Hall, S. C. (1992). Perioperative pediatric care. In B. Spiess & J. S. Vendor (Eds.), *Post anesthesia care* (pp. 256–268). Philadelphia: W. B. Saunders.

Martin, L. C. (1994). Anesthetic implications of an upper respiratory infection in children. *Pediatric Clinics of North America, 41,* 121–129.

Maxwell, L. G., Deshpand, J. K., & Wetzel, R. C. (1994). Preoperative evaluation of children. *Pediatric Clinics of North America, 41,* 93–115.

Semsroth, M., Gabriel, A., Sauberer, A., & Wuppinger, G. (1994). Regional anesthetic procedures in pediatric anesthesia. *Anaesthesist, 43,* 55–72.

Siker, C. (1994). Pediatric fluids, electrolytes, and nutrition. In G. A. Gregory (Ed.), *Pediatric anesthesia* (pp. 93–115). New York: Churchill Livingstone.

Steward, D. J. (1994). *Manual of pediatric anesthesia.* New York: Churchill Livingstone.

Tait, A. R., Reynolds, P. E., & Gutstein, H. B. (1995). Factors that influence an anesthesiologist's decision to cancel elective surgery for the child with an upper respiratory infection. *Journal of Clinical Anesthesia, 7,* 491–499.

Webster, D. E. & Lopez, K. (1993). Neonatal and infant anatomy and physiology. In D. K. Rasch & D. E. Webster (Eds.), *Clinical manual of pediatric anesthesia* (pp. 14–30). New York: McGraw-Hill.

Wensley, D. & Seear, M. (1993). Respiratory diseases. In F. A. Berry & D. J. Steward (Eds.), *Pediatrics for the anesthesiologist* (pp. 1–5). New York: Churchill Livingstone.

Zuckerberg, A. (1994). Perioperative approach to children. *Pediatric Clinics of North America, 41,* 15–29.

The Obstetric Patient

Charles H. Moore and Regina Y. Fragneto

The practice of obstetric anesthesia is unlike any other anesthesia specialty. Pregnancy causes major alterations in maternal physiology, and the care of the mother and fetus simultaneously presents unique challenges to the anesthetist. Anesthetists who practice obstetric anesthesia must acquire an understanding of the maternal changes of pregnancy, the uteroplacental unit, and the anesthetic implications of these changes. Labor and delivery are dynamic processes, and emergency situations such as fetal distress or maternal hemorrhage can occur precipitously. For these reasons, vigilant perianesthetic assessment is crucial to providing safe anesthetic care to the mother and fetus.

▶ MATERNAL PHYSIOLOGIC CHANGES OF PREGNANCY

Pregnancy produces profound physiologic changes in all major organ systems (Cohen, 1982). These changes from adult physiology will be highlighted in this section.

Cardiovascular System

The cardiovascular system shows alterations as early as 5 to 8 weeks of gestation. Cardiac output increases 40% to 50% by the end of the second trimester, and this increase is maintained until term (Robson, Hunter, Boyd, & Dunlap, 1989). During labor, cardiac output may increase 50% above prelabor values, and in the immediate postpartum period, cardiac output can increase as much as 80% to 100% above nonpregnant measurements. Cardiac output usually returns to prelabor values by 48 hours postpar-

tum and to normal values within 6 weeks (Robson, Dunlap, & Hunter, 1987).

The cardiovascular system imposes significant demands on the pregnant mother, but these demands are usually well tolerated during gestation. However, the parturient with heart disease or reduced cardiac reserve may not be able to meet the increased requirement during pregnancy or labor.

During pregnancy, red blood cell volume, total blood volume, and total plasma volume all increase. The increase in total blood volume is greater than that in red cell volume; consequently, a physiologic anemia ensues. The total blood volume is usually 40% greater than that of the nonpregnant state, but is ordinarily well tolerated by the gravida.

There is a slight fall in both systolic and diastolic pressure during the second trimester of pregnancy, probably due to a decrease in systemic vascular resistance. A return to the nonpregnant or first trimester level usually occurs in the third trimester. The white blood cell count also increases during pregnancy. The reason for this is not obvious, but the increase may be estrogen induced. In the attempt to evaluate leukocytosis as an indicator of infection, the shift to the left of the white blood cell count is more important than the actual rise in the blood count itself.

Pregnancy produces a hypercoagulable state in the parturient. It is known that there is a change in the coagulation mechanism, with an increase in fibrinogen, prothrombin, and factors VII, VIII, IX, and X, as well as augmentation of the fibrolytic inhibitors. There is a decrease in the concentrations of factors XI and XIII; however, a triggering mechanism is needed to begin the coagulation mechanism (Cohen, 1982).

Respiratory System

The enlarging uterus produces a mechanical change in the configuration of the abdomen and a concomitant rise in the diaphragm of approximately 4 cm. There is an increase in the transverse and anteroposterior diameter of the thoracic cage as well as an outward and upward movement of the ribcage. This produces alterations in lung volume during pregnancy, which usually occur at approximately 4 to 5 months gestation, so that at term, the expiratory reserve capacity is reduced by 20% to 25% from the nonpregnant state. However, respiratory capacity increases, so there is compensation. Minute alveolar ventilation is increased due to a mild increase in the respiratory rate and a greater increase in the depth of the ventilatory tidal volume. Hyperventilation occurs, producing a mild respiratory alkalosis.

A decrease in the functional residual capacity at term is a constant finding. This decrease is exaggerated by the supine or Trendelenburg positions, which are usually assumed by the patient on the delivery or operating table. (This accentuation does not occur in the sitting position.) The decrease in functional residual capacity and the increased alveolar ventilation facilitate washout of anesthetic gases, producing rapid induction of general anesthesia, especially with the more volatile inhalation agents. The reduced functional residual capacity and the low Pa_{CO_2} in the pregnant patient can lead to a rather precipitous decline in Pa_{O_2} during periods of apnea. Denitrogenation before the induction of general anesthesia and intubation is thus essential to minimize the risk of hypoxemia.

Maternal Pa_{O_2} is increased because of the increased alveolar ventilation. Nevertheless, airway closure occurs at normal tidal volume range in many parturients approaching term. This is particularly prevalent among those in the supine position and may lead to ventilation–perfusion abnormalities and reduced Pa_{O_2}. Hyperventilation and mechanical positive-pressure ventilation may reduce uterine blood flow and fetal oxygenation. Similarly, the distraught hyperventilation of uncontrolled labor patients may be detrimental to the fetus, and it is not unusual to see maternal carbon dioxide levels as low as 20 to 25 mmHg and pH levels as high as 7.65 (Cohen, 1982).

Central Nervous System

Increases in intra-abdominal pressure resulting from the enlarged pregnant uterus causes an engorgement of the epidural veins. The swollen epidural veins result in a diminution in the size of the epidural and subarachnoid spaces and a reduction in the amount of local anesthetic required for spinal or epidural block. There is an increase in cerebrospinal fluid pressure, which may contribute to a high dermatome level of local anesthetic spread during pregnancy. Hormonal factors also may make the pregnant woman more sensitive to the effects of local anesthetics. The dosage of local anesthetics used in conduction anesthesia during pregnancy should be 30% to 50% less than that used for nonpregnant patients. There is a reduction in minimal alveolar concentration (MAC) during pregnancy. The cause is not known, but it may be related to the sedative effects of progesterone (Blass, 1979).

Gastrointestinal Tract

As pregnancy progresses, the enlarging uterus pushes the intestines and stomach cephalad. This contributes to the increase in the risk of regurgitation and pulmonary aspiration. There is a rise in intragastric pressure, particularly when the patient is in the lithotomy or modified lithotomy position. There is also a decrease in gastroesophageal sphincter tone. The motility of the stomach is reduced, and there is an increase in gastric contents as well as a reduction in gastric pH. During labor, anxiety and pain tend to reduce the motility of the stomach, delaying emptying time even further and increasing gastric acidity and volume. These changes place the pregnant woman at an increased risk for pulmonary aspiration of gastric contents (Gibbs & Banner, 1984). Measures to reduce the risk of pulmonary aspiration are required when providing anesthesia to a pregnant woman (see section on pulmonary aspiration).

Hepatic, Renal, Endocrine, and Metabolic Changes

The results of many liver function tests are altered during pregnancy. Bromsulfalein excretion is altered, and alkaline phosphate levels are elevated. Serum bilirubin and serum transaminase levels such as alanine aminotransferase (ALT, SGPT) and aspartate aminotransferase (AST, SGOT) may rise to the upper limit of normal (Romalis & Claman, 1962). Total protein and serum albumin concentrations are reduced by 20% to 30% at term. Plasma cholinesterase activity is reduced; however, this is seldom clinically significant and the appropriate dose of drugs such as succinylcholine is safe to use.

Progesterone contributes to the dilation of the smooth muscle of the kidney, pelvis, and ureters starting as early as the third month of gestation. As the pregnant uterus enlarges, it encroaches on the ureters, producing a mechanical cause of kidney dilation. There is a gradual increase in renal blood flow and glomerular filtration, leading to a lowering of blood urea nitrogen (BUN) and creatinine. A patient whose creatinine and BUN are in the normal range for nonpregnant females may have abnormal levels when pregnant, signaling renal dysfunction. As tubular reabsorption of increased amounts of glucose filtered by the glomerulus is relatively fixed, glycosuria during pregnancy is not uncommon.

Pregnancy induces increased activity of the endocrine system. The pituitary gland enlarges during pregnancy, producing more adrenotropic and thyrotropic hormones along with prolactin. The elevated basal metabolic rate during pregnancy has been attributed to pregnancy per se, but studies have shown that this apparent hypermetabolic state is produced by the needs of the fetus for increased oxygen.

There is an increase in thyroxine-binding globulin produced by the excess amount of estrogen in the pregnant state, and there is an increase in the size of the thyroid gland over that of the nonpregnant state. During pregnancy, results of thyroid function tests must be interpreted carefully. The adrenal gland produces more aldosterone, and the parathyroid glands show enlargement. The pancreas is stimulated to increase insulin production in response to the diabetogenic action of pregnancy. Maternal metabolism and oxygen consumption increase steadily throughout gestation, and metabolism of protein, fat, and carbohydrate is altered.

Uteroplacental Circulation

The placenta serves as the point of exchange for maternal and fetal circulation. At term, the maternal uterine arteries deliver nutrient-rich blood to the placenta at a rate of 600 mL/min. Blood flow to the placenta is not autoregulated, and factors that decrease uterine artery blood flow (hypotension from aortocaval compression or sympathetic blockade) or increase uterine vascular resistance (alpha adrenergic stimulation) can severely compromise fetal well-being and should be avoided.

Although the placenta acts as a barrier to the passage of drugs from mother to baby, nonionized, fat-soluble, low-molecular-weight drugs are transferred rapidly. Most muscle relaxants in the usual dosage pass poorly from the mother to fetus, but in doses of high magnitude they readily cross the placenta. Anesthetic gases, narcotics, barbiturates, and most local anesthetics pass readily. Nitrous oxide approaches 80% of the maternal level in about 10 minutes. Pregnancy-induced hypertension (toxemia) and other maternal diseases may interfere with this so-called placental barrier and may allow even more rapid and complete transfer. Whether any drug given to the mother has an adverse effect on the fetus or the mother can be determined only by direct observation. Ideally, maternally administered analgesics should provide maternal pain relief without any adverse effects on the newborn. It is therefore wise to use the minimum amount of anesthetic agents and other drugs to produce any desired effect.

▶ HISTORY TAKING AND THE PREANESTHESIA VISIT

Taking an acceptable preanesthesia history of an anxious, uncomfortable laboring woman can be a challenge. When possible, a preoperative history and physical examination should be performed early in the patient's admission to the labor and delivery suite. This will allow the anesthesia care provider, in many cases, to obtain a more accurate and complete history from a patient who is not yet extremely uncomfortable. In addition, it allows the patient, while in a more comfortable and controlled state, to ask questions about anesthesia procedures and give informed consent. It is imperative that high-risk parturients be evaluated by anesthesia personnel on admission to the labor and delivery unit. In some special situations, including a pregnant cardiac patient or a patient with a history of anesthesia-related complications, a parturient should be evaluated and an anesthetic plan devised before her arrival on the labor and delivery unit. Ideally, all patients on the labor and delivery floor should have at least a brief history and physical examination performed by an anesthesia care provider. Obstetric emergencies can occur in any parturient, including those who have no intention of receiving labor analgesia. Obtaining an adequate history in an emergent situation can be difficult, if not impossible.

Information obtained from the preoperative interview should include the same information that would be obtained from a nonpregnant patient undergoing anesthesia, such as any existing medical problems, current medications, allergies, previous surgical and anesthesia procedures, personal or family history of anesthesia complications, and use of illicit drugs, alcohol, and tobacco. In addition, the parturient should be questioned about any problems associated with her current and previous pregnancies, including the development of pregnancy-induced hypertension, gestational diabetes, and preterm labor. It should also be determined if any difficulties are anticipated with this delivery due to such conditions as placenta previa or a breech or transverse presentation. Information about the status of the fetus, including the presence of conditions such as intrauterine growth retardation (IUGR) or oligohydramnios, which could place the fetus at increased risk of developing distress in utero, should also be obtained. Finally, the parturient should be questioned about the development of any neurologic or orthopedic symptoms during her pregnancy, including the presence of back pain or sciatica. This is especially important when a regional anesthetic technique is being planned.

► PHYSICAL EXAMINATION OF THE PARTURIENT

A preanesthesia physical examination is mandatory in all parturients. The extent of this examination will depend partly on the urgency with which anesthesia must be administered. The most important aspect of the physical exam in a parturient is evaluation of the airway because a difficult airway is more likely to be present in pregnant patients than in nonpregnant patients (Lyons, 1985). When evaluating the airway of a pregnant woman, the neck range of motion, especially the ability to fully extend; the thyromental distance; and the Mallampati airway classification should be determined. The presence of any facial edema, especially in the preeclamptic parturient, which can help predict the presence of laryngeal edema, a factor that contributes to the increased incidence of difficult airway in this patient population, should be noted.

Attention should be paid to the parturient's vital signs, especially to any elevation of blood pressure, which might suggest the presence of preeclampsia. Auscultation of the heart and lungs should be performed in all but the most emergent situations. In the pregnant woman, one might note changes in auscultation of the heart that occur due to the physiologic changes of pregnancy. These changes include accentuation of the first heart sound with exaggerated splitting of the mitral and tricuspid components, presence of a third heart sound, and a grade I or II early to midsystolic ejection murmur. If a patient reports any neurologic symptoms during her pregnancy such as sciatica, or has a history of a neurologic disorder, a complete neurologic examination should be performed and any deficits clearly documented. If neurologic findings are then reported in the postpartum period, the anesthetist will be able to determine if these are pre-existing deficits or new findings that could be associated with positioning or a regional anesthetic procedure.

► DIAGNOSTIC STUDIES

Maternal and Fetal Assessment

Most parturients are healthy and do not require extensive or unusual preanesthesia diagnostic studies. Routine blood analysis will reveal differences in some of the laboratory values when the nonpregnant and pregnant states are compared. These differences reflect maternal adaption to pregnancy rather than a disease process. Table 16–1 compares the results for some of the common laboratory tests between the pregnant and nonpregnant states.

TABLE 16–1. Normal Laboratory Values for the Pregnant and Nonpregnant States

	Nonpregnant	Pregnant
Hemoglobin	12–16 g/dL	10–14 g/dL
Hematocrit	37%–47%	32%–42%
White cell count	4 500–10 000/mm^3	5 000–15 000/mm^3
PT[a]	60–70 seconds	Reduced
PTT	12–14 seconds	Reduced
Platelets	150 000–350 000/mm^3	Reduced
Fibrinogen	250 mg/dL	400 mg/dL
Blood glucose	70–80 mg/dL	60–70 mg/dL
BUN	20–25 mg/dL	8–9 mg/dL
Creatinine	20–22 mg/dL	0.5–0.6 mg/dL

[a] PT, prothrombin time; PTT, partial thromboplastin time; BUN, blood urea nitrogen.

Antepartum Fetal Assessment and Monitoring

Common antepartum tests include the nonstress test (NST), contraction stress test (CST) and the biophysical profile (BPP). Surveillance of the fetus before contemplated delivery is ordinarily not in the province of the anesthesiologist or anesthetist. However, a basic understanding of these antepartum tests of fetal well-being is valuable to the anesthetist practicing obstetrical anesthesia.

Nonstress Test

Because the NST is minimally invasive, it usually is the first test performed when fetal well-being is questioned. The NST involves monitoring of the fetal heart rate and fetal movement. The test is usually interpreted as "reactive" when there are two fetal movements in 20 minutes with fetal heart rate accelerations of at least 15 beats per minute (BPM). An NST is considered "nonreactive" when there is no fetal movement or no accelerations of fetal heart rate with fetal movements. A reactive NST is associated with survival of the fetus for 1 week or more. Further evaluation is indicated when a nonreactive result is obtained.

Contraction Stress Test (Oxytocin Challenge Test)

The CST is indicated following a nonreactive NST. The CST differs from the NST in that intravenous oxytocin is administered in sufficient quantities to stimulate three adequate uterine contractions in a 10-minute period. A CST is positive if persistent late decelerations occur and negative when late decelerations are absent and normal fetal heart rate is present. Further testing or delivery of the infant is indicated when the CST is positive. A CST is contraindicated in the presence of placenta previa, women at risk for premature labor, or women with a previous classical cesarean delivery.

Biophysical Profile

The BPP is a more sophisticated test that is useful for detecting fetal asphyxia. It involves the assessment of five physiologic variables. Ultrasound is used to evaluate (1) fetal movement, (2) fetal tone, (3) fetal breathing movement, and (4) amniotic fluid volume. The fifth variable is the NST. Each variable is scored 0 for an abnormal value and 2 for a normal value. The individual variable scores are summed, and a cumulative score of 10 is possible. Scores of 8 to 10 suggest nonasphyxia, whereas scores of 4 to 6 indicate a suspicion of asphyxia, and delivery should be considered. Scores lower than 4 are strongly indicative of asphyxia, and expedient delivery is usually warranted.

Peripartum Fetal Assessment

The rational use of anesthesia for labor and delivery requires careful surveillance and monitoring of the mother, the uteroplacental unit, and the fetus. Changes in physiology of the obstetric patient may affect the fetus. These changes can increase during the progress of parturition and may be further aggravated by the administration of anesthesia (Fiedler, 1989). The electronic fetal heart rate monitor, developed in the United States by Hon and in Europe by Hammacher, has an advantage over intermittent auscultation of the patient in that it provides a continuous beat-to-beat record of the fetal heart rate and a record of uterine activity. Electronic intrapartum fetal heart rate monitoring is now considered mandatory for high-risk pregnancies, but its value for the low-risk parturient is still undetermined. Electronic monitoring accompanied by an evaluation of the fetal acid–base status has given the obstetrician and anesthetist a more comprehensive understanding of the changes in homeostasis that occur in the fetus and the possible alterations associated with anesthetic administration. Therefore, knowledge of fetal monitoring during labor and in preparation for delivery is essential (Hon, 1968).

Electronic Fetal Heart Rate Monitoring

There are two modes of electronic monitoring: (1) an external mode in which external transducers placed on the maternal abdominal wall are used to determine both fetal heart rate and uterine activity, and (2) an internal mode in which a spiral electrode assists in obtaining the fetal electrocardiogram (ECG) and an intrauterine catheter is used to assess intrauterine pressure.

The technique for obtaining the fetal heart rate by use of the abdominal ECG is associated with problems related to maternal muscle noise and overlapping maternal ECG complexes. Beat-to-beat variability is also more difficult to assess by this method. However, fetal heart rate can be monitored by this method without cervical dilation or rupture of membranes.

Attaching a transcervical bipolar electrode to the fetal presenting part (scalp or buttocks) gives an accurate fetal heart rate, and the beat-to-beat variability can be reliably determined. This direct fetal heart rate determination requires that the fetal membranes be ruptured and that the cervix be dilated at least 1 cm.

Fetal Heart Rate Patterns

Fetal heart rate is considered normal when it is in the range of 100 to 160 BPM. Fetal heart rate faster than 160 BPM is considered tachycardia, and a rate below 100 BPM is bradycardia. Some authorities express the opinion that a rate between 100 and 120 BPM should be termed moderate bradycardia.

When the fetus is stimulated, as with loud sounds or by uterine contractions, the fetal heart rate often changes. These periodic changes may be either decelerations or accelerations. Accelerations, regarded as a sign of an aroused fetus, are generally indicative of an intact internal fetal milieu. In contrast, decelerations may reflect a poor fetal status.

Periodic Decelerations. The three major forms of fetal heart rate decelerations are (1) early, (2) late, and (3) variable. *Early decelerations* (type I) are usually greater than 15 BPM, begin at the onset of a uterine contraction, and return gradually to baseline after the contraction subsides. Early decelerations are generally due to pressure on the fetal skull causing an increase in intracranial pressure or a decrease in cerebral blood flow. This activates the vagus nerve, producing a decrease in the fetal heart rate. Recovery occurs as the pressure is relieved. Head compression may occur from uterine contractions, vaginal examinations, fundal pressure, or occasionally the placement of an internal electronic fetal monitor.

Characteristically, early decelerations have a uniform shape and mirror the contraction phase. They begin early in the contraction phase before the peak of the contraction. The low point of the deceleration occurs at the peak of the contraction. The return to baseline occurs by the end of the contraction. The fetal heart rate rarely drops below 100 BPM, and the depth of the deceleration keeps pace with the intensity of the contraction. These decelerations are usually associated with normal baseline variability and are repetitive with each contraction. Early decelerations are almost always of little clinical significance.

With *late decelerations* (type II), there is a lag between the onset of the uterine contraction and the deceleration, or between the end of the uterine contraction and the return of the fetal heart to its baseline (Fig. 16–1). The deceleration is uniform, and the fetal heart rate seldom drops below 100 BPM. Return of the fetal heart rate to baseline after a contraction most often occurs 15 to 20 seconds after the contraction has ceased. Late decelerations are considered ominous, particularly when they occur with more than 50% of contractions and are associated with the loss of beat-to-beat variability. The smoother the late deceleration and the slower the recovery, the more ominous is the pattern. The etiology is thought to be fetal myocardial hypoxia resulting from uteroplacental insufficiency. Characteristically, uterine hyperactivity or maternal hypotension decreases the intervillous space blood during contractions. This hypoxia and myocardial depression activate a vagal response, producing bradycardia. When accompanied by placental dysfunction, there is anaerobic metabolism and the development of lactic acidosis, which then contributes to the deceleration.

Uteroplacental insufficiency may result from the following: (1) hyperstimulation of the uterus from oxytocin administration; (2) maternal hypotension; (3) toxemia; (4) postmaturity; (5) infection; (6) small-for-gestational-age babies; (7) maternal diabetes; (8) bleeding disorders; and (9) maternal cardiac disease.

Variable decelerations (type III) generally indicate that the fetus is responding to stress. The tracing lacks constancy in its configuration and its time relationship to a uterine contraction. The most common variety of deceleration, it is often preceded or followed by a brief period of acceleration. Variable decelerations are thought to be caused by umbilical cord compression and its consequent cardiovascular reflexes. Administration of oxygen to the mother is without effect; this is not the case with a late deceleration. Fetal acidosis may develop if the compression becomes severe, prolonged, or repetitive.

Variable decelerations that last more than 1 minute or manifest a decrease in heart rate to less than 60 BPM are indicative of acute distress and can indicate impending death in utero. The pathophysiology of this condition is a transitory umbilical cord compression, and accelerations may occur first. The ensuing hemodynamic changes lead to activation of chemoreceptors and baroreceptors that stimulate the vagus nerve, thus producing the deceleration. The etiology is usually umbilical cord compression resulting from maternal position, cord around a fetal part, short cord, knot in the cord, or pro-

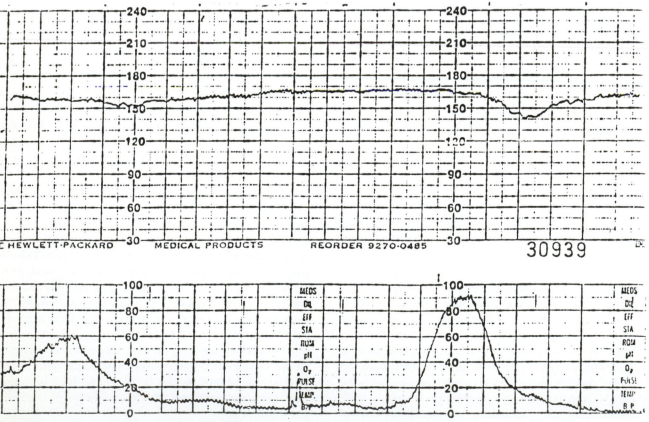

Figure 16–1. Late deceleration. Note that the deceleration occurs after the peak of the contraction.

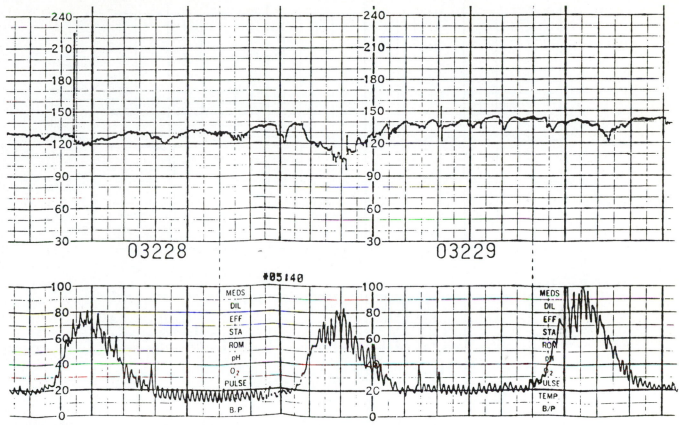

Figure 16–2. Variable deceleration accompanying the middle contraction. Note the acceleration that precedes the deceleration.

lapsed cord. The fetal heart rate usually is slower than 100 BPM and is frequently associated with average baseline variability (Fig. 16–2). It is not necessarily repetitive.

Short-Term Variability (Beat-to-Beat Variability)

The normal fetal heart rate can be described as having a variance of 6 to 10 beats as seen on an electrocardiographic tracing (Fig. 16–3). This is due to the interaction of the sympathetic and parasympathetic divisions of the central nervous system. This beat-to-beat variability of the fetal heart rate, as demonstrated by the fluctuation from the baseline, is an indication of normal neurologic control of the heart rate and a measure of fetal reserve. Increased variability usually is produced by fetal stimulation. This may be caused by uterine contractions, fetal activity, and maternal activity. Decreased variability as seen in Figure 16–4 may be brought about by prematurity, the administration of drugs (narcotics, tranquilizers, anesthetics), hypoxia and acidosis, the physiologic state of fetal sleep, and the suppression of cardiac control mechanisms by heart block in the fetus.

The relationship between reduced fetal heart rate variability and hypoxia was noted by Hon (1962) and has been successfully demonstrated in an animal model.

Normal variability as seen on fetal heart rate tracings can predict a satisfactory neonatal outcome. Clinical studies have demonstrated better acid–base balance and viability in those fetuses with normal variability during labor, regardless of the specific fetal heart rate pattern. There is a greater likelihood of normal neurologic function at one year of age in those infants who displayed normal variability in labor than with infants displaying reduced variability. Shifrin and Dame (1972) showed a significant correlation between normal variability and good Apgar scores. Cetrulo and Schrifin (1976) found that a loss of baseline variability was a consistent feature of fetal heart rate patterns preceding fetal death. Reduced beat-to-beat variability does not always mean that the fetus is hypoxic because several factors can reduce fetal heart rate variability without reducing fetal oxygen tension: fetal sleep, immaturity, fetal tachycardia, congenital anomalies, and drugs such as butorphanol and morphine.

Parasympatholytic agents and local anesthetics have been related to diminished variability. Magnesium sulfate has been reported to decrease variability, but it may actually increase the fetal heart rate because, as a uterine relaxant, it can increase uterine blood flow (Schrifin & Dame, 1972).

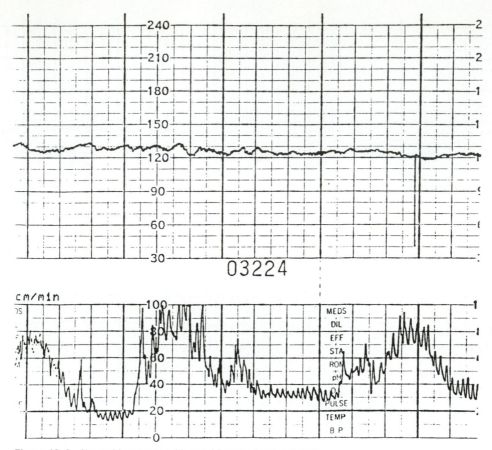

Figure 16–3. Normal heart rate with good beat-to-beat variability.

Prolonged Deceleration

The term *prolonged deceleration* may be applied to a deceleration of the fetal heart rate of more than 30 BPM that persists for more than 2 minutes. It may be caused by hypoxia or may be purely reflex in nature. Even in those cases in which the deceleration is reflex in nature, hypoxemia may occur because, with severe bradycardia, fetal cardiac output is reduced. Prolonged decelerations are frequently observed with compression of the umbilical cord and other hypoxic patterns such as loss of beat-to-beat variability, baseline shifts in fetal heart rate, and late decelerations.

Many factors trigger this reflex or result in sufficient hypoxemia to elicit prolonged decelerations. Hypotension from regional anesthesia, excessive uterine activity, maternal hemorrhage, and supine hypotension can cause fetal bradycardia. Paracervical block in particular has been shown to produce this condition. Management of this pattern requires a coordinated effort in several areas. It occurs frequently in advanced second stage of labor. Delivery can often be accomplished easily by the use of outlet forceps. However, if the patient is not deliverable, more conservative action is indicated and preparations should be made for delivery by cesarean section. Fetal monitoring should be continued even into the delivery room to ascertain if the pattern will spontaneously resolve, thereby averting an operative delivery. Concomitant efforts should be directed to correcting the etiology of the uterine hypertonus, decreased uterine blood flow, or cord compression. Changing maternal position, checking for cord prolapse, and correcting any maternal hypotension should be done quickly.

When the maternal condition is satisfactory, most instances of prolonged bradycardia resolve before fetal acidosis occurs and progression to vaginal delivery may be allowed (Certulo & Schifrin, 1976). If the fetal ECG shows improvement in the fetal heart rate, a fetal scalp blood sample can be obtained to help clarify the condition of the fetus. If the intrauterine environment can be improved to allow fetal recovery, the fetus will correct its hypoxia and acidosis more quickly in utero than if delivered in a hypoxic state. If no trend toward recovery is observed, delivery should be accomplished as soon as possible by an assisted vaginal delivery or cesarean section (Benson, Schubeck, & Deutschberger, 1968).

Baseline Shifts in Fetal Heart Rate

As defined previously, fetal heart rate normally ranges between 120 and 160 BPM. A rate exceeding this range is considered tachycardia, and a rate below, bradycardia. Fe-

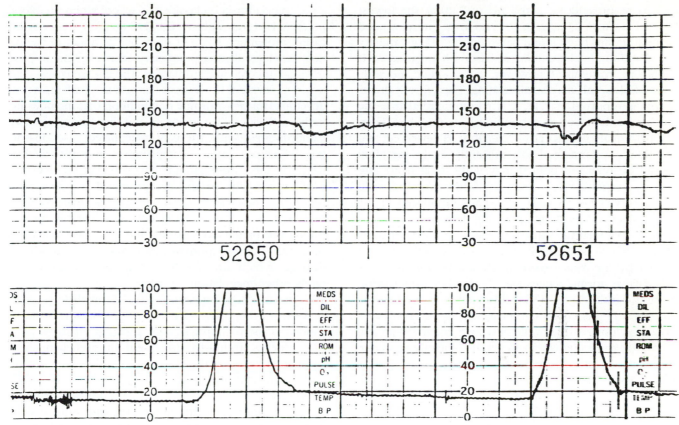

Figure 16–4. Poor beat-to-beat variability with variable decelerations.

tal tachycardia is commonly seen with chorioamnionitis, in which the variability may be reduced and acidosis is also present. Fetal movement, maternal anxiety, and beta-adrenergic stimulation cause fetal tachycardia, but in these situations variability is normal and acidosis is generally absent.

Treatment for Abnormal Fetal Heart Rate Changes

The mother should be turned onto her side, preferably to the left initially, which may relieve compression of the umbilical cord, aorta, and inferior vena cava by the occluding pregnant uterus. Aortocaval compression occurs more frequently when the gravida is supine and if the mother has had major conduction anesthesia. It should be mandatory that gravidas in labor lie on the side or with a left uterine displacement, rather than the supine position. If the mother is receiving oxytocin, this should be discontinued immediately to prevent fetal hypoxia caused by the decreased uterine perfusion produced by the drug. Oxygen should be administered to the mother because maternal hyperoxia may alter the uteroplacental insufficiency as manifested by late decelerations.

Correctable causes of abnormal fetal heart rate patterns (such as hypotension) should be treated with flu-

ids, and ephedrine should be administered as necessary. Fetal scalp biochemical monitoring should be used in these situations.

Biochemical Monitoring

Fetal scalp sampling was introduced initially as an independent means of fetal surveillance during labor. The technique is used when abnormal heart rate patterns occur that cannot be readily abolished or whose significance cannot be determined. The technique consists of analyzing blood drawn from the fetal scalp for determination of pH, Po_2, Pco_2, and base excess (Parer, 1980). This scalp sampling may be accomplished with the patient in the lithotomy or Sim's position, on either the labor bed or delivery table. The cervix must be dilated at least 2 cm to 3 cm, and the presenting part must be in the pelvis. The membranes must be ruptured before the procedure becomes technically feasible. Today most centers determine only the scalp blood pH, and the method is generally reserved for situations in which the fetal heart rate pattern is ominous or confusing.

The reliability of capillary blood in assessing fetal acid–base status has been firmly established. Numerous studies have shown that a fetal capillary blood pH of 7.25 or greater can be classified as normal, a pH of 7.20

to 7.24 as preacidotic, and a pH of 7.20 as the lowest limit of normal (Quilligan, 1979). Furthermore, a good correlation has been found between the pH of capillary blood and the fetal condition as based on Apgar score. It should be recognized, however, that a single measurement of blood pH may be misleading. Therefore, if the fetal pH is reported at 7.18, it is recommended that the mother be delivered as expeditiously as possible. When the pH equals or exceeds 7.25, labor is observed, and samplings are repeated intermittently. Scalp sampling should be repeated immediately if the fetal heart rate pattern becomes more ominous. If, however, the scalp pH is between 7.18 and 7.25, sampling should be repeated every 15 to 20 minutes until delivery.

Normal fetal pH values are found in approximately 10% of infants delivered in a depressed condition as reflected by the Apgar score. Some causes for these so-called false normal values are (1) newborn depression from analgesic drugs or anesthesia administered to the mother; (2) infection; (3) maternal hyperventilation; (4) airway obstruction in the newborn infant; (5) prematurity; (6) congenital anomalies; and (7) asphyxia occurring between the time of sampling and delivery (Chan, Paul, & Toews, 1973).

► MEDICAL CONDITIONS COMPLICATING PREGNANCY

Preexisting medical problems as well as abnormal conditions associated specifically with pregnancy may jeopardize the well-being of the mother, fetus, or both. Women with pregnancy-induced hypertension (preeclampsia), peripartum hemorrhage, and amniotic fluid embolism all fall within this category. A myriad of medical conditions, including diabetes mellitus and cardiac disease may also complicate pregnancy. Such high-risk parturients require special attention, and the anesthetist must understand the anesthetic implications of these diseases.

Preeclampsia/Eclampsia

Preeclampsia is a disease unique to human pregnancy that may involve virtually every organ system including the renal, hepatic, hematologic, and central nervous systems. Certain patients are at increased risk for developing the disease, including young and elderly primigravidae; parturients with diabetes, chronic hypertension, renal and connective tissue diseases, and women with a multiple-gestations pregnancy. The diagnosis of mild preeclampsia is made when a parturient develops hypertension (blood pressure of 140/90 or greater) at 20 weeks gestation or more and also exhibits nondependent edema and/or proteinuria greater than 300 mg/

24 h. Preeclampsia is classified as severe when the blood pressure is elevated above 160/110 on more than one occasion, proteinuria is 5 g or more per 24 hours, or the patient develops oliguria, pulmonary edema, epigastric pain, or visual or cerebral disturbances. The disease is also diagnosed as severe if the patient has seizures (eclampsia) or develops HELLP syndrome (a condition that includes hemolysis, elevated liver enzymes and thrombocytopenia). Pathophysiologically, there is generalized vasoconstriction, which can result in compromised uteroplacental renal perfusion. These patients have a higher incidence of fetal distress due to the compromised uteroplacental perfusion. The majority of patients are also hypovolemic. The central nervous system becomes irritable, predisposing the patient to seizures, and cerebral edema can occur. Another component of the disease is endothelial damage, which can result in thrombocytopenia and, rarely, other coagulation disorders.

The anesthetist must be aware of the obstetric management of this disease as well as the anesthetic implications of the pathophysiology in caring for these high-risk patients. Definitive treatment of preeclampsia is delivery of the fetus and placenta. Therefore, any parturient at term with the diagnosis will be delivered, usually by induction of labor. However, if the fetus is preterm, the obstetrician will attempt to manage mild disease with conservative therapy, such as left-sided bed rest, to allow the fetus more time to mature. However, once the diagnosis of severe preeclampsia is made, delivery must be expedited regardless of gestational age. Magnesium sulfate therapy is instituted to prevent seizures in light of central nervous system irritability. Persistently elevated blood pressure (usually >180/110) requires treatment. The most commonly used antihypertensives in preeclamptic patients are hydralazine and labetolol. Occasionally, hypertension is resistant to these drugs and must be treated with such vasoactive drugs as sodium nitroprusside or nitroglycerin. Titration of these drugs requires the placement of an arterial line.

A minority of patients will develop oliguria that does not respond to a fluid challenge or pulmonary edema. Placement of a pulmonary artery catheter is indicated to guide the management of these patients. The priority in eclamptic patients is the control of seizures. Intravenous (IV) thiopental or diazepam are the preferred drugs for immediate treatment. Generally, a seizing parturient does not require immediate delivery of the fetus. It is usually preferable to stabilize the mother and, provided fetal well-being is documented, subsequent vaginal delivery is acceptable.

Anesthesia providers can help optimize the management of the preeclamptic parturient during the peripartum period. Epidural analgesia is beneficial to the laboring parturient. These women are exquisitely sensitive to vasopressors, including endogenous catecholamines.

Provision of excellent analgesia via an epidural will decrease catecholamine levels. In fact, epidural analgesia in severe preeclamptic patients has been shown to improve uteroplacental perfusion (Joupila, Joupila, Hollmen, & Koivala, 1982). As mentioned previously, the incidence of fetal distress is increased in these patients. If an epidural catheter has been placed for labor analgesia, should an emergent cesarean delivery be required, epidural anesthesia can quickly be established, thus avoiding the risks associated with general anesthesia in these patients.

Before the placement of an epidural catheter, a platelet count should be obtained. If the value is less than 150 000, other coagulation factors including prothrombin time (PT), partial thromboplastin time (PTT), and fibrinogen should be determined to rule out any coagulopathy. The question often arises as to how low a platelet count can reach before it becomes unsafe to place an epidural catheter. Although many anesthetists have used a lower limit of 100 000 in the past, many have now lowered this limit even to 75 000. The risk of epidural hematoma seems to be theoretical in these patients. There is no right answer as to when an epidural catheter should not be placed due to thrombocytopenia. The risk–benefit ratio must be determined for each patient.

Epidural labor analgesia is managed essentially the same in preeclamptic parturients as in normal parturients except for a few caveats. Due to a higher propensity for pulmonary edema, a more conservative fluid bolus should be administered before epidural placement. The further administration of fluid should be based on the patient's blood pressure response to the sympathectomy produced by the epidural. The epidural catheter should be dosed slowly to prevent any significant decreases in blood pressure because uteroplacental perfusion is already compromised. Finally, should hypotension develop, a smaller dose of ephedrine should initially be administered; because these patients have an increased sensitivity to vasopressors.

Should a cesarean delivery be required in a preeclamptic parturient, epidural anesthesia is the technique of choice when possible. Epidural anesthesia allows the anesthetist to raise the sensory level for surgery slowly, making it less likely that hypotension will develop. The use of epidural anesthesia also avoids the risks of general anesthesia in these patients, including aspiration, difficult or failed intubation, and a severe hypertensive response to laryngoscopy. Once intravascular placement of the epidural catheter has been ruled out by a non–epinephrine-containing test dose, any of the commonly used local anesthetics, including 2% lidocaine with epinephrine, may be used to achieve surgical anesthesia. Chloroprocaine should probably be reserved for situations requiring emergent delivery because a major goal generally is to slowly raise the anesthesia level.

In some situations, including the presence of a coagulopathy or fetal distress in the setting of no established epidural, general anesthesia will be required. Many special considerations must be addressed in such a scenario. First, particular attention must be paid to the patient's airway. Because of the nondependent edema characterized by preeclampsia, the glottic opening may be narrowed or distorted. Small endotracheal tubes (as small as 5.0 mm) should be immediately available. If the anesthetist suspects that a difficult intubation may be encountered, an awake intubation will be required. These patients also have a significant risk of developing severe hypertension during laryngoscopy or emergence, which could result in an intracranial hemorrhage. Therefore, if time allows, an arterial line should be placed to better monitor blood pressure. Pretreatment with IV lidocaine and/or labetolol (0.5 to 1.0 mg/kg) should be considered. A rapid-acting, potent antihypertensive agent, such as nitroprusside or nitroglycerin, must be immediately available. Despite the problems associated with general anesthesia in these patients, most anesthesia providers feel this is preferable to spinal anesthesia. Rapid development of a sympathectomy in these patients who are frequently hypovolemic might result in a precipitous drop in blood pressure that could be detrimental to the mother and fetus.

Peripartum Hemorrhage

Peripartum hemorrhage is a leading cause of maternal death in the United States. Placenta previa and abruptio placentae are the most common causes of hemorrhage. Placenta previa results when the placenta implants over or very close to the cervical os. When the fetus attempts to descend, massive hemorrhage will occur. Therefore, in a parturient with placenta previa, the fetus must be delivered via cesarean delivery. Placenta previa occurs in approximately 1 in 200 pregnancies. Risk factors for placenta previa include multiparity, advanced maternal age, previous cesarean delivery, and previous placenta previa. The diagnosis is generally made by ultrasound examination. Occasionally a "double setup" (preparation for both vaginal and cesarean delivery) is required to make the diagnosis. A double setup involves the performance of a vaginal examination in the operating room (OR). If placenta previa exists, this examination could lead to rapid, massive hemorrhage. Therefore, a surgical team must be immediately available to begin an emergency cesarean section. Before the performance of the vaginal examination, the anesthetist should have established IV access with large-bore catheters. Blood must be immediately available in the OR. The patient should be adequately preoxygenated and ready for immediate rapid sequence induction should hemorrhage be precipitated by the examination.

When a cesarean delivery is being performed because of placenta previa, the status of the patient and urgency of delivery will dictate the method of anesthesia. If little or no bleeding is occurring and the woman is hemodynamically stable, regional anesthesia is the preferred method of anesthesia. However, if significant hemorrhage has occurred, maternal instability is present, or the fetus is in a distressed state, general anesthesia is required.

Abruptio placentae occurs when a normally implanted placenta separates prematurely from the uterus, resulting in hemorrhage and interruption of the oxygen supply to the fetus. Unlike placenta previa, which is characterized by painless vaginal bleeding, the bleeding of a placental abruption is frequently accompanied by abdominal pain and a hypertonic uterus. The incidence of maternal and fetal morbidity and mortality is much higher with abruptio placentae than with placenta previa. Risk factors for placental abruption include hypertension, multiparity, advanced age, cocaine use, trauma, and tobacco use. Placental abruption is the most common cause of disseminated intravascular coagulopathy (DIC) in pregnancy and occurs in 10% of cases. The incidence of DIC is highest in situations of severe abruption when fetal distress or demise occurs.

The anesthetic management of women with abruptio placentae is, like that of placenta previa, dictated by maternal and fetal status as well as by the severity of hemorrhage. In some situations of mild or moderate abruption, fetal well-being persists, and the obstetrician opts to deliver vaginally. Once normal coagulation studies have been obtained, it is acceptable to offer that patient epidural analgesia for labor. If an epidural is placed, normal coagulation studies should again be documented before removal of the epidural catheter because DIC could develop later in the patient's course. In the situation of severe abruption requiring emergency cesarean delivery, general anesthesia is usually required. The administration of blood products to replace blood loss and treat coagulopathy is frequently necessary in such a situation.

Amniotic Fluid Embolism

Amniotic fluid embolism is a rare condition that nevertheless accounts for a significant number of maternal deaths because the outcome is frequently catastrophic. The mortality rate is approximately 80%. The syndrome is characterized by sudden peripartum collapse followed by pulmonary edema. The etiology of amniotic fluid embolism remains unclear. Recent work suggests that transient pulmonary vasospasm first occurs with the development of right heart failure, hypoxemia, and hy-

potension. In parturients who survive this first phase, left ventricular failure and pulmonary edema quickly ensue (Clark, 1990). Approximately 40% of these parturients will develop DIC.

Management of amniotic fluid embolism is essentially supportive therapy. Intubation and mechanical ventilation are necessary to support oxygenation. Inotropic support is often needed to support the maternal circulation, and in many situations cardiopulmonary resuscitation must be initiated. Emergency delivery of the fetus is usually required both to salvage the infant and to improve the effectiveness of resuscitative efforts for the mother. Massive fluid resuscitation is necessary, and treatment of DIC requires blood product transfusions.

Diabetes Mellitus

The problems and complications associated with diabetes in pregnancy apply in most cases to women with preexisting disease as well as to those who develop gestational diabetes. An abnormal glucose tolerance test is used to diagnose gestational diabetes. Glucose control can be challenging in the diabetic parturient. Early in pregnancy, when nausea and vomiting may be significant, hypoglycemic episodes frequently occur. As pregnancy progresses, levels of pregnancy hormones that antagonize the effects of insulin increase. As a result, insulin needs during later pregnancy increase and may reach 200% of prepregnancy insulin requirements. Immediately after delivery, insulin requirements markedly decrease and may transiently be less than requirements before pregnancy. Tight glycemic control is the goal during pregnancy because a correlation has been shown between poor glycemic control and an increased incidence of congenital anomalies (Miller, Hare, & Cloherby, 1981). Strict glucose control also is necessary during labor and delivery to avoid a hypoglycemic neonate. Frequently, insulin infusions are used during labor.

Diabetes in pregnancy imposes risks to both the mother and fetus. Diabetic parturients have a higher incidence of preeclampsia and polyhydramnios. Placental abnormalities result in uteroplacental insufficiency, thus increasing the incidence of fetal distress and fetal demise near term. As a result, frequent monitoring of fetal well-being with tests such as the NST are required from approximately 32 weeks gestation until delivery. Macrosomia is another complication of diabetes that increases the incidence of shoulder dystocia and birth trauma. Also, in diabetic mothers fetus lungs mature more slowly, increasing the risk of respiratory distress syndrome.

The anesthetic management of diabetic parturients in labor is similar to that of normal parturients with some special considerations. Because uteroplacental perfusion is compromised, these women can especially benefit from epidural analgesia with the associated decrease in catecholamine levels. The presence of a functioning epidural catheter may also provide the anesthetist with some insurance against the need for general anesthesia should an emergent cesarean delivery be required because of fetal distress. When initiating epidural analgesia, the anesthesia level should be raised slowly to prevent hypotension in a situation of already existing uteroplacental insufficiency. If hypotension does occur, it should be treated aggressively with ephedrine.

If a cesarean delivery is required, regional anesthesia remains the technique of choice. It avoids the risks of general anesthesia, which might be increased in the diabetic patient if gastroparesis exists. Provided that adequate prehydration with lactated Ringer's solution is administered and hypotension is aggressively treated, satisfactory neonatal outcome with no evidence of fetal acidosis has been reported with either epidural or spinal anesthesia. Should general anesthesia be required, the considerations are the same as those for any pregnant woman. Close attention must be paid to glucose control during any delivery. If an insulin infusion has been used, it should be discontinued soon before delivery to avoid hypoglycemia in the immediate postpartum period when the mother's insulin requirements markedly decrease.

Cardiac Disease

The incidence of cardiac disease in the pregnant population is relatively low, but these can prove to be some of the most challenging patients to manage. The types of cardiac disease presenting in pregnant women is changing. In the past, the majority of pregnant cardiac patients had valvular disease associated with rheumatic heart disease. With improved antibiotic therapy, these patients are now significantly fewer. They are being replaced by older parturients with myocardial ischemia and patients with congenital heart disease who are surviving into their childbearing years due to improved surgical techniques.

Regardless of the cardiac disease type, the principles of management include a determination of the patient's clinical status and an understanding of the interaction between the physiologic changes of pregnancy (such as increased blood volume and cardiac output) and the patient's cardiac problem. It is especially important to determine if the patient's status has deteriorated or remained stable with the progression of the pregnancy. Although the prognosis is better for those women who have tolerated pregnancy well, it must be realized that even in those patients the further stresses of labor and delivery could result in cardiac decompensation. In fact, one of the most critical time periods is the immediate postpartum period when the parturient must respond to a large increase in intravascular volume. The anesthetic management, including a determination of the need for invasive monitors, must be determined individually for each patient on the basis of her current clinical status and the predicted effects of labor and delivery on her specific cardiac lesion. Optimal management of these patients requires close communication and collaboration among obstetric, cardiology, and anesthesia personnel. Ideally, this type of patient should be evaluated by an anesthesia provider well before the time she presents in labor to labor and delivery.

▶ PERIANESTHESIA PLAN FOR THE OBSTETRIC PATIENT

Pharmacologic Considerations for the Pregnant Patient

Various physiologic changes of pregnancy will affect the activity of some anesthetic drugs used in both general and regional anesthesia. When halogenated volatile anesthetics are used in a parturient, the MAC has been shown to be reduced by 30% to 40%. Explanations for this decrease in MAC include the elevated level of progesterone in the pregnant woman, which has a sedative effect, and the increased levels of endorphins. In addition to the decreased MAC of the inhalation anesthetics, the rate of rise in the alveolar anesthetic concentration of these agents is more rapid due to the increased minute ventilation and decreased functional residual capacity caused by pregnancy. Probably for the same reasons used to explain decreased MAC in the parturient, the induction dose of thiopental, the most commonly used agent in pregnant patients, is reduced 35%. The elimination half-life of thiopental is prolonged in these women due to a significant increase in the volume of distribution.

Plasma cholinesterase activity is decreased 25% in the parturient. Despite this decrease, the clinical duration of action and elimination half-life are not affected in women who possess normal enzyme. In the postpartum period, a further decrease in plasma cholinesterase activity (40%) as well as a decreased plasma volume does result in a prolonged recovery time. However, this prolongation is small and in most situations is not clinically significant. The pharmacokinetics of some nondepolarizing neuromuscular blocking agents have also been found to be affected by pregnancy. Both vecuronium and pancuronium exhibit an increased clearance and a shortened elimination half-life in pregnant patients. Despite these altered pharmacokinetics, pregnant women actually experience an increased sensitivity to vecuronium with a prolongation of neuromuscular blockade.

The pregnant woman's response to local anesthetics is also altered. Neural susceptibility to local anesthetics has been shown to be increased in these patients. The high level of progesterone is felt to contribute to this increased sensitivity. Spinal dose requirements are decreased 20% to 33% in the parturient. As reported, epidural dose requirements have also been decreased by 30%.

It was once widely believed, on the basis of case reports and previous animal studies, that the cardiotoxicity of bupivacaine is enhanced in pregnancy. It was felt that this increased toxicity resulted from a lesser degree of protein binding of the drug in pregnant women. Decreased protein binding was reported to occur due to a decreased serum concentration of alpha$_1$-acid-glycoprotein, the protein to which bupivacaine preferentially binds. Increased cardiotoxicity of bupivaciane in pregnancy has not been proven.

The chronotropic response to epinephrine is also altered in pregnancy. The increase in heart rate that occurs with its administration occurs to a lesser degree in parturients. Therefore, the use of an epinephrine-containing test dose to detect an intravascular injection during regional anesthesia is less reliable in these women.

Preanesthesia Assessment

It is important to perform a thorough preanesthesia assessment of the mother before administering anesthetic for labor, vaginal delivery, or cesarean section. The preanesthesia assessment is the same whether regional or general anesthesia is planned. Preanesthesia assessment should take into consideration the anatomic and physiologic changes that accompany pregnancy. The airway and cardiorespiratory system need careful assessment. If regional anesthesia is planned, the need for laboratory assessment of coagulation function before preceding is determined by history and physical examination (evidence of easy bruising, diagnosis of pregnancy-induced hypertension, thrombocytopenia, and so on). If serious maternal disease is found, it should be adequately evaluated and the mother should be optimized before proceeding with anesthesia. Fetal status should not be ignored. The fetal heart rate tracing should be examined for evidence of fetal well-being or stress because this can influence anesthesia management.

It is also mandatory that a preanesthesia assessment be performed before anesthesia is induced in emergency situations (such as an emergency cesarean section for fetal distress). The assessment should be efficient and include an evaluation of the airway, health status, previous anesthesia complications, and medication allergies.

Labor Analgesia

Most women experience a great deal of discomfort during labor and delivery. The pain in the first stage of labor is the pain resulting from dilation and effacement of the cervix as well as uterine ischemia because of uterine contractions. This pain is primarily visceral in nature and is transmitted by spinal nerves entering the spinal cord at T10 to T12 and L1. In the second stage of labor, there is the addition of somatic pain resulting from the stretching of the vagina and the distention and tearing of the perineum. These impulses are carried via the pudendal nerves entering S2 to S4. The degree of discomfort that a parturient may experience cannot be accurately predicted and will usually increase as labor progresses. Ideally, analgesia for labor and delivery should alleviate the pain of labor for the mother and not interfere with the mechanics or progress of labor. There should be no undue risk to the mother or to the fetus. Early bonding between the mother and baby should be possible, and adequate working conditions for the obstetrician should not be ignored.

Obstetric analgesia may be provided by such techniques as acupuncture, hypnosis, and natural childbirth, all of which may play a satisfactory role but are beyond the scope of this chapter. Analgesia for labor and delivery can be provided by systemic medications such as narcotics, sedatives, tranquilizers, and inhalation analgesia; local anesthetics and regional anesthesia are increasing in popularity. It is important to remember that all systemic medications used for analgesia or relief of anxiety rapidly cross the placenta.

Nonnarcotic Medications

Tranquilizers, hypnotics, and amnestics may all be given to the mother to alleviate anxiety, but they assist little in the relief of pain and may reduce beat-to-beat variability of the fetal heart rate. Use of these drugs with concomitant narcotics may cause the patient to become disoriented and uncontrollable during painful contractions. Most of these drugs are additive in their depressant effects on both the mother and newborn.

Narcotics

Systemic narcotics are frequently used to lessen the pain in the first stage of labor. Analgesic doses of narcotics cause equal maternal and neonatal depression. The primary difference in the narcotics used is the duration of action in the mother. Thus, longer acting narcotics such as meperidine are indicated early in labor, whereas fentanyl is more appropriate toward the end of labor.

Naloxone is the narcotic antagonist of choice to reverse the maternal and neonatal depressant effects of maternally administered narcotics. It is effective in both the mother and newborn and should not be given to the mother before delivery to reverse anticipated neonatal depression, because it will rapidly antagonize any narcotic analgesia at a time when it is most needed. To antagonize neonatal depression, it is best to administer naloxone directly to the neonate immediately after delivery. The neonatal dose of naloxone is 0.1 to 0.2 mg intramuscularly (IM) or IV. Its duration of action is only about 1 hour, and renarcotization may follow its use. The use of naloxone in patients who are chronic narcotic users or in their newborn children may produce rapid symptoms of narcotic withdrawal.

The opioid agonist–antagonists such as butorphanol and nalbuphine have the advantage of lower incidence of nausea and vomiting and dysphoria as well as a "ceiling effect" on depression of ventilation. Thus, these drugs are to a great extent replacing the pure agonists such as meperidine and morphine. Butorphanol has the disadvantage of producing a high level of maternal sedation, whereas nalbuphine may produce an abstinence syndrome in mothers dependent on morphine-like drugs. Recommended analgesic doses of these agents are 1 mg to 2 mg IM or IV for butorphanol and 10 mg IV or IM for nalbuphine.

Intermittent Inhalation Analgesia

Intermittent inhalation analgesia involves the administration of subanesthetic concentrations of inhalation agents to the mother. Self-administration of volatile inhalation agents during labor and delivery by means of a Duke or Cyprane inhaler, once a popular analgesic technique, has been surpassed by more modern modalities. Nitrous oxide (30% to 50% in oxygen with or without a small added concentration of isofluorane) can give satisfactory analgesia for delivery; however extreme caution must be exercised in administering isofluorane because of the ease of rapid deepening to general anesthesia and loss of protective airway reflexes. When inhalation analgesia is combined with a pudendal block or local infiltration of the perineum, adequate analgesia for episiotomy and outlet forceps delivery can be obtained.

Inhalation analgesia causes little neonatal depression, even when used for long periods. Uterine activity is not depressed, and when inhalation agents are properly administered, the mother remains awake. She maintains the urge to push and can protect her own airways, which minimizes the threat of pulmonary aspiration of stomach contents. However, the depth of analgesia can be rapidly altered, and anesthesia may ensue, increasing the risk of pulmonary aspiration. For this reason inhalation analgesia is only selectively used in modern anesthetic practice. When used, it is essential that inhalation analgesia be carefully and constantly supervised. The mother should be able to answer questions and remain cooperative.

Ketamine

Because of its short duration of action, ketamine is not useful for the first stage of labor and is better suited for use during vaginal delivery. Low-dose ketamine in the range 0.25 to 0.3 mg/kg of maternal body weight provides effective analgesia for vaginal delivery with little or no neonatal depression. There is a minimal amount of hallucinatory response and very little increase in salivation. In moderate to high doses, ketamine produces profound analgesia and amnesia and as such takes away the mother's ability to relate to her newborn and thus could decrease bonding. As far as the fetus is concerned, there is no hypotonia and apparently no thermoregulatory inhibition, nor is there any decrease in the Apgar score. This particular type of analgesia is most satisfactory in those patients who do not want to view the birth because they are giving the baby up for adoption or there is a fetal demise and they do not want to be aware of the delivery. In a normal vaginal delivery, ketamine, except in very low doses, probably does not contribute much because of the amnesia it produces and may even be contraindicated by this fact alone. Ketamine is useful as an adjunct to regional anesthesia.

General Anesthesia

General anesthesia is rarely required for normal vaginal delivery. It abolishes the bearing down reflex and is associated with neonatal depression correlating with the depth of the anesthesia and the elapsed time until delivery. When administered, general anesthesia removes from the mother the awareness of her newborn and definitely increases the risk of pulmonary aspiration. The parturient is particularly prone to aspiration because her stomach usually is not empty even if she has not eaten for a long period, and the enlarged uterus together with the lithotomy position causes a marked rise in intragastric pressure.

When general anesthesia is necessary, it is mandatory that the trachea be intubated with a cuffed endotracheal tube. It may be placed either as an awake intubation or immediately after rapid-sequence induction with correct cricoid pressure (Sellick's maneuver) applied from the time of induction to the time of intubation. General anesthesia for the parturient without intubation is totally unacceptable anesthetic practice.

General anesthesia is indicated when acute fetal distress occurs and prompt vaginal delivery is possible. It may be used in a patient who becomes uncontrollable during delivery or when regional anesthesia is contraindicated or refused and operative obstetrics is required. General anesthesia is often indicated when depression of uterine activity is required. Such uterine relaxation may be necessary to abolish a tetanic uterine contraction or to allow internal uterine manipulation, as in the extraction of a second twin. For uterine relaxation, halothane or isoflurane may be used because they cause rapid relaxation of the uterus; accompanying this relaxation of the uterus, however, is always the danger of hemorrhage. After the baby has been delivered, isoflurane should be discontinued. If it is necessary to maintain general anesthesia, a nitrous oxide–oxygen–narcotic technique is the anesthetic technique of choice.

Regional Anesthesia

Conduction anesthesia is well suited for labor and vaginal delivery, and there are distinct advantages associated with the use of regional anesthesia for both mother and fetus. Maternal airway reflexes usually remain intact provided severe hypotension or reactions to local anesthetics are avoided. The mother remains awake and can react to her newborn early in the postpartum period. There is a decrease in the need for narcotics or sedatives, and regional anesthesia usually eliminates the need for general anesthesia and its potentially depressant effect on the neonate. When properly administered, regional anesthesia is associated with minimal or no neonatal depression.

When regional anesthesia is used, maternal and fetal monitoring are required in both the labor room and the delivery room. A reliable, large-bore IV line must be in place, and it is mandatory that someone be readily available to treat any untoward reaction, whether caused by a high level of anesthetic block, hypotension, or intravascular or accidental intrathecal injection.

Spinal Anesthesia/Analgesia. The profound motor block and finite duration associated with single-dose subarachnoid injection of a local anesthetic makes it unattractive for use during labor. This technique is more suited for use during vaginal or cesarean delivery. Spinal block with a T10 sensory level alleviates all pain of labor and delivery and allows uterine manipulation. Use of 40 mg to 50 mg of lidocaine (5% in 7.5%, dextrose or 1.5% in 7.5% dextrose) provides a satisfactory block for most operative vaginal procedures. For a longer duration block, 5 mg to 7 mg of hyperbaric bupivacaine (0.75% in 8.5% dextrose) gives a satisfactory dermatome level and a block lasting approximately 1.5 to 2 hours.

The major drawbacks of subarachnoid analgesia may include a marked degree of maternal hypotension (James, Greiss, & Kemp, 1970) (particularly if adequate rapid prehydration of IV fluids is not infused prior to initiation), total spinal block, abolishment of the urge to bear down, possible prolongation of the second stage of labor, and postdural puncture headache. Severe and sudden hypotension leading to maternal cardiovascular collapse is a leading cause of maternal mortality. Prophylaxis includes left uterine displacement along with preblock hydration of an IV balanced salt solution. Treatment consists of the preceding dosage plus a primary acting central vasopressor such as ephedrine (10 mg to 20 mg) intravenously and a high Fio_2. Vasoconstrictors such as methoxamine and phenylephrine correct hypotension, but they cause a further decrease in uterine blood flow and compromise the fetus because they are alpha-adrenergic agents.

Total spinal block may lead to apnea, and probably loss of consciousness and cardiovascular collapse. It may be prevented by limiting the dose of local anesthetic to two thirds or even one half that used in a nonpregnant woman and not injecting the medication during a contraction.

Treatment consists of correcting the hypotension and protecting the upper airway with an endotracheal tube and ventilation (ie, intermittent positive-pressure ventilation with 100% oxygen). Even though subarachnoid analgesia abolishes the bearing down reflex, the mother can be coached to push, and forceps delivery is easily performed. Postdural puncture headache occurs very commonly in the parturient, probably because of the increased pressure of cerebrospinal fluid and the venous engorgement discussed earlier. Prophylaxis includes the use of a small-gauge pencil point spinal needle (25 to 27 gauge, Whitacre or Sprotte needle) and adequate hydration.

Caudal Anesthesia. Segmental lumbar epidural anesthesia has replaced caudal anesthesia. The perineal analgesia that caudal anesthesia provides is out of logical sequence, requires more local anesthetic, is less reliable, and technically may be more difficult to perform.

Epidural Analgesia/Anesthesia. Lumbar epidural analgesia has become a very popular anesthetic technique for labor and vaginal delivery. One reason for this is the great versatility epidural analgesia offers. The use of a continuous catheter technique, specifically localized for segmental analgesia and with a T10 to L1 sensory block, is efficacious. This allows a mother to have a relatively pain-free labor and still maintain her motor ability. She can easily push for the vaginal delivery. When the baby is to be delivered, anesthesia of the vagina and perineum (S2 to S4) can be achieved, and if cesarean delivery is necessary, the block can be intensified and extended to the thoracic dermatomes (T4 to T6). Thus, an in situ epidural catheter allows for all necessary obstetric maneuvers. Additionally, continuous epidural analgesia eliminates the necessity for depressant drugs during labor and delivery. The mother remains awake, mostly pain free, and cooperative.

Today, the use of continuous infusions of lower concentration solutions of local anesthetics and opioids are common. This method effectively blunts the pain of labor, even when extremely low concentrations of local anesthetics are used (see Table 16–2 for dosing recommendations). The technique involves administering a standard "test dose" of local anesthetic to detect subarachnoid or intravascular catheter placement. Following a negative response to the test dose, a bolus loading dose is administered to establish patient comfort (T10 sensory

TABLE 16–2. Dosing Recommendations for Labor and Delivery*

Cervical Dilatation At Epidural Administration	Drugs	
	Epidural (plus 3mL test dose 2% lidocaine)	*CSE*
< 6 cm	0.25% bupivacaine (5–8 cc) + 50 μg fentanyl	25–35 μg fentanyl or 10 μg sufentanil
> 7 cm	0.25% bupivacaine (5–12 mL)	Add 2.5 mg of 0.25% bupivacaine to fentanyl 25 μg or sufentanil 35 μg
	+ 50 μg fentanyl or 0.5% bupivacaine (5–8 mL)	
Delivery/forceps[a]	0.25%–0.5% bupivacaine (5–10 mL) 2% lidocaine with epidural (5–10 mL)	Dose epidural if inadequate perinal analgesia

CSE, combined spinal epidural.
*Continuous infusion 1/8th percent bupivacaine with 1–2 μg /mL fentanyl (8–12 mL/hr).
[a] Use higher concentration of local anesthetic if rotational forceps delivery is planned.

level). Once an adequate sensory level is achieved, the continuous infusion can be initiated.

A "top-up" dose before delivery is sometimes necessary and provides superb anesthesia for either forceps delivery or episiotomy repair. An advantage of this technique is that the low concentrations seem to reduce motor block and maintain perineal muscle tone facilitating rotation of the fetal head. In addition, there is no change in the labor pattern or curve. There is no prolongation of labor, and even if, as often occurs with a primigravida, there should be acute pain in the early stages of an extended labor, the possibility of accumulation leading to toxic levels is minimized. The facilitated ease of maintenance does not mean that the patient needs any less observation or monitoring, but safety is certainly enhanced. Furthermore, low-dose continuous infusion provides for a more constant level of analgesia and reduces the magnitude of changes that occur as analgesia wanes.

Hypotension after epidural anesthesia is usually slower in onset than after a subarachnoid block, but its severity can be just as marked. Prevention and treatment are the same as in subarachnoid injection of local anesthetic, and hypotension may be avoided by giving a test dose of 3 mL to 4 mL of local anesthetic, waiting 2 to 3 minutes, and then checking the dermatome level before giving the remainder of the local anesthetic in fractionated or incremental doses. Epidural anesthesia requires 5 to 10 times the amount of local anesthetic to produce the same level of anesthesia as spinal anesthesia. Unrecognized subarachnoid injection usually results in a very high or total block. *To ensure safety, the epidural needle or catheter should always be dosed in a fractionated or incremental fashion with a maximum of 5 mL injected at one time. Signs of intrathecal or intravascular injection should be ruled out before additional fractionated doses are administered.*

Epidural analgesia of the perineum does decrease the urge to bear down and may result in an increased tendency for forceps delivery. There may also be an increase in the incidence of persistent posterior presentations. A disadvantage of lumbar epidural anesthesia as compared with subarachnoid anesthesia is that a larger dose of anesthetic agent is required, resulting in higher local anesthetic blood levels in the mother and fetus.

Combined Spinal Epidural Technique. An exciting development in the field of obstetric anesthesia is the use of a combined spinal epidural (CSE) technique. This technique was first described for use in surgical patients in the early 1980s (Coates, 1982) and is now becoming a popular technique for labor and delivery. A CSE is performed by first placing an epidural needle into the epidural space. Then a spinal needle (long enough to extend beyond the tip of epidural needle) is passed through the epidural needle into the subarachnoid space. A narcotic alone or in combination with a small amount of a local anesthetic is injected into the subarachnoid space. The spinal needle is withdrawn, and an epidural catheter is threaded into the epidural space for use later in labor (Table 16–2). The appeal of this technique is that it combines the dosing advantages offered by spinal administration with the flexibility provided by an indwelling epidural catheter. The major advantage of a CSE is that it provides for a rapid onset of analgesia with small amounts of drugs and produces minimal physiologic alterations. Additionally, if labor is prolonged or cesarean delivery is necessary, the epidural catheter is already in place and can be activated. A CSE can be administered at any time during labor; however, it is probably most useful for relieving pain during very early labor (reducing the total amount of local anesthetic used) and late labor (spinal medication may last through delivery and the epidural may not need to be dosed).

Compared with a "standard epidural," a CSE may be

somewhat more difficult to perform and does require a special spinal or epidural needle. A CSE is also limited somewhat by the high incidence of pruritus caused by the intrathecal injection of narcotics such as fentanyl and sufentanil. Another disadvantage of the CSE technique is that there is usually a delay in dosing the epidural catheter; therefore, it is not known if the epidural will function when needed. Because of this, a CSE should be used cautiously when the mother has a greater than normal chance of having an urgent or emergent cesarean section. This is particularly true for a patient with a difficult airway or some other strong contraindication to general anesthesia. In these situations placing a standard epidural catheter early in labor, one that is known to be functioning, is advisable.

Epidural Analgesia and the Progress of Labor.

Recently, there has been much discussion within the obstetric and anesthesia communities about the effects of epidural analgesia on the progress of labor as well as the mode of delivery. This is a controversial topic because various studies have produced widely differing results. Many obstetricians believe that an epidural placed in early labor will prolong labor. However, in two prospective, randomized studies, no difference in duration of first or second stage labor was found in patients who received an epidural in early versus late labor (Chestnut, Mcgrath, Vincent, & Penning, 1994).

The association between epidural analgesia and the incidence of instrumental and cesarean deliveries is more problematic. Some studies have shown that epidural analgesia is associated with an increased incidence of instrumental deliveries whereas other studies have not. Many of these studies, however, have flaws. Some are retrospective, and in many, the indications for forceps delivery are unclear. Intuitively, one would expect that an obstetrician is more likely to perform an elective instrumental delivery in a patient who already has adequate epidural anesthesia than in a patient with no preexisting anesthesia.

Also, the technique of epidural analgesia differs among studies. The administration of higher concentrations of local anesthesia might, due to pelvic muscle relaxation, interfere with the normal rotation of the fetal head during labor, resulting in a higher incidence of malposition. It is also felt that a dense motor block produced by more concentrated solutions of local anesthesia will result in decreased expulsive efforts by the mother. Both of these factors could contribute to a higher incidence of instrumental deliveries. In fact, the administration of a dilute local anesthetic solution has been shown to decrease the incidence of both malposition and instrumental deliveries (Thorburn & Moir, 1981; Turner, Silk, & Alegesan, 1988). Therefore, the results of one study cannot be extrapolated to other institutions where the technique of epidural analgesia may be very different.

Many of the same problems occur in trying to evaluate the association between epidural analgesia and cesarean delivery rates. The majority of studies that claim an increased incidence of cesarean deliveries associated with epidural analgesia are retrospective, thus introducing selection bias. Even a prospective, randomized study that showed an increased incidence of cesarean deliveries in patients who received epidural analgesia compared with those who received IV meperidine may have introduced bias because the obstetrician who made the decision to perform a cesarean section could not be blinded to the patient's study group (Thorpe, Hu, & Albin, 1993). Of course, there are also retrospective studies that have shown no increase in cesarean delivery rates at various institutions despite marked increases in the use of epidural analgesia. Again, the retrospective nature of these reports make them suspect (Iglesia, Burn, & Saunders, 1991; Socol, Garcia, Peaceman, & Dooley, 1993).

It is clear that the association between epidural analgesia and the progress of labor and delivery requires much more study. As the anesthesia and obstetric communities work to find answers to these questions, it is recommended that anesthetists adopt techniques of epidural analgesia, such as dilute local anesthesia/opioid solutions, that provide adequate analgesia while minimizing marked motor blockade that could contribute to the problems of malposition and inadequate maternal expulsive efforts. However, it must be remembered that there is no well-designed study that proves a cause and effect relationship between epidural analgesia and operative delivery. Therefore, it seems unreasonable to withhold from parturients this superior technique of labor pain management on the basis of current available information.

Spinal Opioids.

The introduction of spinal opioids has greatly influenced the practice of obstetric anesthesia. Opioids, whether by subarachnoid or epidural administration, can be used as sole agent or in combination with local anesthetics. Spinal opioids provide pain relief without producing hypotension or motor blockage and seem to be more effective in relieving visceral pain (first stage of labor) than somatic pain (second stage). When given alone, they may provide complete analgesia in early labor and can be used when the prevention of hypotension is mandatory, such as in a laboring cardiac patient. Epidural opiates such as fentanyl, sufentanil, and alfentanil are also highly effective in reducing the "perineal discomfort" seen during the middle of the first stage of labor. Spinal opioids can also result in bothersome side effects such as pruritus and urinary retention; the frequency of these problems may be dose-related. Pruritus can be treated with diphenhydramine (25 mg to 50 mg) or narcan titrated to effect.

Subarachnoid placement seems to provide more complete analgesia than epidural administration and is also more effective in the latter portion of labor. The subarachnoid injection of an opioid in combination with a small dose of a local anesthetic such as bupivacaine seems to be particularly effective. The more lipid-soluble agents such as fentanyl, alfentanil, and sufentanil are minimally associated with maternal or fetal respiratory depression; however, the hydrophilic opiate morphine has been implicated in producing significant respiratory depression as late as 12 to 16 hours after its administration.

Evaluation and Management of Fetal Distress as Determined by Electronic and Biochemical Measurement

Reassuring signs to both obstetrician and anesthesia personnel would be a normal baseline rate, normal baseline variability, and lack of variable or late decelerations (Quilligan & Paul, 1975). Warning signs would be decreasing variability, increasing baseline rate, variable decelerations with abnormal baseline variability, and meconium staining of amniotic fluid. Ominous signs would be no baseline variability, late decelerations, severe variable decelerations, and bradycardia. With the onset of warning and ominous signs, the position of the patient should be corrected. Uterine activity should be decreased by stopping any oxytocin infusion. If not already being given, oxygen should be administered to the mother with a tight face mask at the rate of 6 to 7 L/min. Preparation should be made for operative delivery. If the ominous fetal heart rate pattern persists 10 minutes after the initiation of these restorative maneuvers, immediate termination of labor should be considered by the most expeditious means: either vaginal delivery or cesarean section.

Anesthesia for Cesarean Section

The type of anesthesia for cesarean section should be determined by the reason for the surgery, any underlying medical problems, and the presence of complicating anatomic abnormalities. The trend, however, in modern obstetric anesthesia is to use regional anesthesia when possible. There are guidelines on which to base the choice of regional or general anesthesia. If the patient has had an uneventful labor and the fetus has shown no signs of depressed heart rate patterns, then the choice between epidural, spinal, or general anesthesia is essentially a decision agreed on by the patient, obstetrician, and anesthetist. An example of this type of situation would be a young mother with cephalopelvic disproportion after a trial of labor without progress. If the fetus has shown signs of hypoxia and has had deleterious changes in fetal heart rate patterns, late decelerations, prolonged tachycardia, or loss of beat-to-beat variability, then general anesthesia may be preferable to either spinal or epidural anesthesia. General anesthesia maintains uterine perfusion more uniformly than regional anesthesia, with less chance of hypotension. In the face of an emergency procedure and a possibly mildly dehydrated acidotic mother with a hypoxic fetus, maternal hypotension is probably an unjustified risk to the fetus. When performed expediently and hypotension is avoided, regional anesthesia (placement of a spinal block or dosing an existing epidural with chloroprocaine) has been used safely in urgent and emergent situations.

For cesarean section for a prolapsed cord or for the patient with hemorrhage, such as a bleeding placenta previa, general anesthesia is preferable (Datta & Alpher, 1980). One of the most important factors in this choice is the longer time required for regional anesthesia to be induced and take effect. This is often noxious to the fetus. The second consideration is the sympathetic blockade produced by regional anesthesia in the face of hemorrhage.

Conduction Anesthesia for Cesarean Section (Spinal or Epidural)

Spinal and epidural block are frequently selected for elective cesarean delivery. To ensure adequate anesthesia, a sensory level of T4 to T6 is necessary. It is important to realize that the subarachnoid or epidural dose of local anesthetic necessary to achieve a T4 to T6 level is approximately two thirds to one half the dose normally used in a nonpregnant patient. Table 16–3 presents dosing recommendations for spinal and epidural anesthesia.

Spinal block offers more rapid and reliable anesthesia and, because anesthesia can be induced with small amounts of local anesthetics, less fetal depression from absorbed local anesthetics occurs. Disadvantages of spinal block include less control of sensory level and duration of action, postdural puncture headache, and a higher incidence of hypotension, nausea, and vomiting. With epidural block the in situ catheter can be used for postoperative analgesia, there is greater control of sensory level, and hypotension is less precipitous; however, the block is less reliable and there is increased absorption of local anesthetics.

Combined spinal and epidural technique can also be used for cesarean delivery. The technique is similar to that described for labor except that a dense surgical level of anesthesia (T4) must be obtained. Anesthetic level can be obtained by injection of a full spinal dose, or, alternatively, by subarachnoid administration of a partial dose, and the remainder can be given through the epidural catheter until a T4 sensory level is achieved. The CSE technique has the advantage of combining the rapid onset and dense block of spinal anesthesia with the versatility of epidural anesthesia. Hypotension can be controlled, and the epidural catheter can be used for postoperative analgesia.

The prevention of hypotension from sympathetic

TABLE 16–3. Dosing Recommendations for Cesarean Section*[‡§]

	Epidural	Spinal	CSE
Elective, no epidural in place	2% lidocaine + (epinephrine 1 : 200 000; 20–25 mL) + fentanyl 50–100 μg)	0.75% bupivacaine with dextrose (9–12 mg) + fentanyl 25 μg or lidocaine (1.5% or 5% with dextrose (60–75 mg) + fentanyl 25 μg	Same as spinal or give 2/3 the amount and use epidural to achieve T4 level
Elective, epidural in place for labor	2% lidocaine + (epinephrine) 1 : 200 000 + fentanyl 50–100 μg (incremental dosing to T4)		

CSE, combined spinal epidural.

* Emergent cesarean section: Use general if epidural is not in place or if there is not enough time to do regional.

‡ Urgent cesarean section: Use 3% 2-chloroprocaine to achieve T4–T6 level if epidural is in place; otherwise perform spinal.

§ To provide surgical anesthesia via epidural only, use high concentration local anesthetics for cesarean section (2% lidocaine, 0.5% bupivacaine, and 3% 2-chloroprocaine).

block during conduction anesthesia for cesarean section is an important consideration. Fluid preload with 1500 to 2000 mL of intravenous fluids (non–glucose-containing crystalloid) before initiating the block is necessary, but this does not pertain to the patient with cardiac compromise (Ramanathan, Masih, & Rock, 1983). The obese patient may require an even greater prehydration volume (25 to 30 mL/kg) (Blass, 1981).

After the block is given and the patient has been placed in the supine position, the operating table should be tilted approximately 10 degrees to the left, and a wedge should be placed under the patient's right hip. After the induction of spinal anesthesia, blood pressure should be checked every 30 seconds to 60 seconds until stable, and thereafter at a minimum of every 5 minutes. Epidural dosing should be fractionated, and dosing should continue until a T4 sensory level is obtained (20 mL to 25 mL of local anesthetic). Heart rate and blood pressure must be taken at a minimum of 5-min intervals after each epidural injection and throughout surgery. Oxygen saturation should be continuously monitored by means of pulse oximetry, and supplemental oxygen may be administered by nasal cannula or face mask.

If the systolic blood pressure begins to fall from its preanesthesia level, it is advisable that the uterus be displaced further to the left and an IV fluid bolus of crystalloid be given. Ephedrine in increments of 10 mg to 12 mg should be given intravenously. No longer is it prudent to wait until the systolic blood pressure drops below 100 mmHg (or 20% less than the preanesthesia block level) before instituting ephedrine as a vasopressor. This is particularly true when spinal anesthesia is performed because blood pressure can decrease rapidly.

The addition of opioids to the spinal or epidural anesthetic helps to reduce intraoperative nausea and vomiting and to blunt the discomfort ("pulling and tugging") associated with peritoneal traction and visceral manipulation. Intraoperative nausea and vomiting is common and can be treated with IV droperidol (0.625 mg) or ondansetron (4 mg to 8 mg). Preoperative

metoclopramide (10 mg) can also be given to facilitate gastric emptying.

General Anesthesia for Cesarean Section

General anesthesia for cesarean section requires the same preliminary maneuvers as for conduction anesthesia. However, capnography and pulse oximetry should be considered mandatory monitoring modalities. Before induction of anesthesia, preoxygenation is necessary for 4 to 5 minutes because of the rapid desaturation that occurs in pregnant patients during periods of apnea. If immediate delivery is necessary and 4 to 5 minutes is not available for preoxygenation, four or five deep breaths of 100% oxygen can be substituted. While the patient is lying on the operating table, the table left lateral displacement should be maintained.

After the patient is completely prepared and draped, rapid sequence induction of anesthesia is performed. To minimize fetal depression, thiopental sodium (3 to 4 mg/kg) is given IV and followed by succinylcholine (80 mg to 100 mg). If succinylcholine cannot be used, rocuronium (0.6 mg/kg) can be substituted. Once successful endotracheal intubation is confirmed, the operation can begin. Muscle relaxation can be maintained throughout the procedure with a succinylcholine drip or an intermediate-duration nondepolarizing muscle relaxant (rocuronium, cisatracurium).

It is accepted practice today for halogenated inhalation agents such as halothane (0.5%), isoflurane (0.75%), and enflurane (1.0%) to be used before abdominal delivery of a fetus to provide supplemental anesthesia and to help in prevention of the mother's recall if the time from skin incision to delivery should be extended. At these concentrations, uterine bleeding is not magnified and can be counteracted by pitocin administration after delivery of the fetus. After clamping and cutting of the cord, the halogenated agents most often are discontinued, and a narcotic agent such as fentanyl and an amnestic such as midazolam are then used to deepen the anesthesia. On termination of the surgery, the patient should be awake and able to maintain her own airway before extubation is performed. Oxygen should be administered, and routine recovery care is appropriate.

When general anesthesia is chosen for cesarean section, it must be anticipated that the anesthetist may be unable to intubate the trachea. It is therefore necessary to have a backup plan to protect the patient from developing hypoxia. Cricoid pressure must be maintained. The patient should be turned head down with her face toward the side, and an airway should be inserted. Oxygenation should be established by face mask while cricoid pressure is maintained. The patient should be ventilated with 100% oxygen, the nitrous oxide turned off, and the anesthetic allowed to wear off. Local or regional anesthesia should be carried out as a safer alternative, or an awake oral intubation or fiberoptic technique should be considered. If the operation is an emergency and there is no time to consider another form of anesthetic technique, the patient should be ventilated using nitrous oxide–oxygen and anesthesia maintained with an agent such as isoflurane to establish surgical anesthesia with spontaneous ventilation after the succinylcholine has worn off. If a nondepolarizing muscle relaxant has been used, ventilation has to be continued by the anesthetist. The operation should be allowed to proceed via the face mask, but cricoid pressure must be maintained. If intubation and mask ventilation are unsuccessful, an emergency cricothyroidotomy should be performed to accomplish transtracheal ventilation.

Intrapartum Complications

Hypotension

Hypotension as a consequence of obstetric anesthesia usually is a sequela of conduction anesthetic techniques (ie, spinal or epidural anesthesia). The development of hypotension may be defined as blood pressure falling 20% below the initial baseline blood pressure, or systolic pressure decreasing below 100 mmHg.

Prevention is preferable to treatment. The patient should not be allowed to labor on her back owing to the consequences of aortocaval compression, which can lead to supine hypotensive syndrome. A mild to moderate drop in blood pressure can usually be corrected by placing the patient in a slight head-down lateral position and giving a rapid infusion of fluids, preferably crystalloid. Oxygen tends to reduce the nausea and vomiting associated with the hypotension and may aid in transplacental oxygenation of the fetus. Ephedrine given in small incremental doses of 10 mg to 12 mg at the initial onset of hypotension usually eliminates the syndrome rather rapidly and helps prevent hypoxia of the fetus. Approximately 1 out of 10 or 12 pregnant women in the last trimester of pregnancy, when placed in the supine position, sustains these significant reductions in blood pres-

sure (Howard, Goodson, & Mengert, 1953). There is definite obstruction of the vena cava and the aorta by the gravid uterus when the patient lies supine. The majority of parturients compensate for this by shunting blood from the lower extremities through the azygos veins and the paravertebral circulation into the superior vena cava and then into the right atrium. There is an accompanying increase in sympathetic tone and peripheral vascular resistance; however, approximately 30% of women who have conduction anesthesia (spinal or epidural) have significant hypotension because the sympathetic blockade produced by the conduction anesthetic tends to eliminate the compensatory mechanisms of the body. Treatment consists of placing the patient on her left side, placing a wedge under her right hip, infusing fluids, and administering oxygen. If she is to be transported to the delivery or operating room, she should always be placed in the lateral position, not on her back.

Pulmonary Aspiration

Several predisposing factors make pulmonary aspiration a great risk in the parturient: (1) General anesthesia may be required with great urgency, for example, in the event of a prolapsed cord, fetal distress, or acute hemorrhage; (2) the patient may have had a meal just before admission or even after the onset of labor; (3) pregnant patients have delayed gastric emptying time, with retention of food and solids, particularly after the onset of labor; sedation, anxiety, and pain also delay gastric emptying; and (4) increased intra-abdominal pressure produced by the pregnant uterus is aggravated by the lithotomy position. Pathophysiologically, particulate matter may cause difficulty. Acid aspiration, particularly if the pH is below 2.5, causes a chemical burn. If the pH is less than 1.2, actual necrosis occurs. When aspiration syndrome occurs, there is intense bronchospasm and an increase in lower airway resistance. There is a rapid fall in arterial blood pressure and an initial rise in pulmonary artery blood pressure followed by a return to normal. This is then followed by a fall in the pulmonary artery pressure. Acute pulmonary edema ensues, with a large loss of plasma into the lungs.

Aspiration may occur during induction, maintenance of, or recovery from anesthesia. Trivial amounts of acid cause severe illness. The syndrome itself may occur immediately after the aspiration or may be delayed several hours. The patient becomes restless, dyspneic, tachypneic, and cyanotic; her blood pressure falls rapidly, and she progresses into shock. Generalized bronchospasm, rales, and rhonchi with sanguineous secretions of frothy sputum from frank pulmonary edema are noted. Chest x-rays show mottled densities, as in pulmonary edema or bronchopneumonia.

The clinical picture of a patient who has aspirated solid particles depends on the size of these particles.

Acute bronchospasm and often massive atelectasis of a lobe or the entire lung may occur. Cyanosis, tachycardia, dyspnea, and mediastinal shift can develop. Prevention is preferable to actual treatment. Although it is not guaranteed that local or regional anesthesia will circumvent pulmonary aspiration, it does lower the incidence. Antacids definitely cause a rise in the pH of gastric contents and help alleviate the potential for acid aspiration. Antacids do not eliminate pulmonary aspiration. Particulate matter antacids may cause pulmonary injury if aspirated. Therefore, the use of a nonparticulate antacid such as sodium bicitrate (Bicitra) is recommended. If general anesthesia is to be used, it is essential that the patient be intubated with a cuffed endotracheal tube and that cricoid pressure be applied and maintained from the moment induction is begun. Awake intubation should not be ignored or neglected in the case of a patient with a difficult airway.

H$_2$ blockers such as cimetidine and ranitidine in conjunction with the gastric emptying drug, metoclopramide, may be of benefit. It should be emphasized that these are useful adjuncts to the armamentarium and they should not be considered a substitute for prevention and vigilance. The management of the actual aspiration, if it should occur, consists of clearing the airway immediately with the head down in a lateral position, the right side being preferred. The pH of the vomitus should be tested, the patient oxygenated, and the airway secured with endotracheal intubation before suction. If solid material is aspirated, immediate bronchoscopy may be required. Artificial ventilation with 100% oxygen, positive end-expiratory pressure, and chest therapy may be necessary. If there is hypovolemia, cardiovascular support based on central venous pressure, arterial blood gases, and the wetness of the lungs should be considered. Antibiotics probably should not be used unless infection supervenes.

Total or High Spinal Anesthesia

Total or high spinal anesthesia can occur after accidental injection of an epidural dose into the subarachnoid space or a miscalculation in the injection of local anesthetic into the subarachnoid space. Epidural anesthesia predisposes to a massive total spinal because the dose of local anesthetics used in epidural anesthesia is 5 to 20 times that used in spinal anesthesia.

Patients with a high spinal characteristically suffer from difficulty in breathing, tingling in the fingers of the hand, difficulty in coughing, nausea, and possibly vomiting. Total spinal anesthesia leads to vascular hypotension, bradycardia cessation of respiration, and unconsciousness. Treatment of a massive subarachnoid injection consists of administration of fluids to support the circulation, immediate intubation with an endotracheal tube, and ventilation with 100% oxygen. Blood pressure, circulation, and respiration should be maintained until the effects of the block are terminated. A vasopressor may be necessary to maintain blood pressure.

Intravenous Injection of Local Anesthetics

A toxic level of local anesthesia may follow from accidental injection of a local anesthetic into a vein or may be the end result of accumulated local anesthetic after prolonged administration. An anesthetist usually encounters the former. This occurs when local anesthetic has been injected into a vein rather than the epidural space. It may occur via the epidural needle or the epidural catheter. The engorged nature of the veins and the fact that there are numerous veins in the epidural space predispose to this situation. There are no valves in the veins of the epidural space, and the local anesthetic therefore easily reaches the brain and heart, producing the symptoms of toxicity. Patients may complain of sleepiness, ringing in the ears (tinnitus), circumoral numbness, or a funny taste in the mouth. Grand mal seizures may rapidly follow. There may be bradycardia and cardiovascular collapse. The drop in blood pressure is due to both the lowering of cardiac output and peripheral vasodilation. Prevention is preferable to treatment. Careful aspiration of the catheter before injection of any local anesthetic and the use of a small test dose help to prevent problems and do decrease their incidence, although they do not guarantee safety. Treatment consists of turning the mother to a lateral position, giving 100% oxygen, and performing tracheal intubation immediately if indicated. Use of a barbiturate such as thiopental (50 mg) or IV midazolam aids in terminating convulsions.

Maintenance of circulation and cardiovascular stability by vasopressors or fluids may be necessary. With a convulsion, there is a tremendous increase in oxygen demand, and oxygenation is mandatory.

Postanesthesia Considerations

Postanesthesia Visit

A thorough postdelivery visit should be scheduled for all patients to whom anesthesia was provided. For regional anesthesia patients, the postanesthesia visit should include an assessment for postdural puncture headache and neurologic complications such as leg weakness or diminished sensation.

Acute Postoperative Pain Relief

Spinal and epidural analgesia for cesarean delivery has enhanced the use of intraspinal narcotics for postoperative pain control. Duramorph (morphine without preservatives) in a dose of 3 mg to 5 mg epidurally or 0.25 mg to 0.5 mg subarachnoid (one time), can provide 12 to 24 hours of satisfactory pain relief. Pruritus, nausea, vomiting, urinary retention, and respiratory depression are the most common complications associated with this technique. Side effects seem to be related, at least in part, to dosage. Factors that may increase the risk of respiratory depression include advanced age, opioid sensitivity, highly water soluble narcotics (morphine), concomitant administration of systemic opioids, and intrathecal versus epidural administration (Rawal & Wattwill, 1984).

Patient-controlled intravenous analgesia (PCIA) and patient-controlled epidural analgesia (PCEA) are newly emerging alternatives to traditional forms of postoperative pain relief. Patient-controlled analgesia (PCA) devices consist of a microprocessor-controlled pump triggered by the patient (pressing a button). When triggered, a preset amount (incremental dose) of narcotic is delivered into the patient's IV line or epidural catheter. A timer in the pump prevents administration of an additional bolus until a specified period has elapsed. This technique has the advantage of allowing for consistent titration of analgesic drugs, which can be tailored to the patient's needs. The PCA techniques have the disadvantage of requiring sophisticated and expensive equipment, but offer the patient a sense of control that may increase patient satisfaction. The use of nonsteroidal anti-inflammatory drugs (NSAIDs) such as ketorolac in non–breast-feeding mothers has also proven to be quite beneficial. The close monitoring of patients receiving postoperative IV and intraspinal narcotics is mandatory because of the variable side effects that may occur in a small percentage of patients.

Postanesthesia Complications

Postdural Puncture Headache. Although not considered dangerous, the postdural puncture headache (often called a postspinal headache) is one of the most annoying and bothersome complications of anesthesia. Postdural puncture headache occurs twice as frequently in postpartum patients as in nonpregnant women of equivalent age. Apparently, the incidence of headache is related to the needle tip design and size. The pencil point design (Sprotte and Whitacre) and the use of small gauge needles (25 to 27 gauge) have helped to dramatically reduce the incidence and severity of these headaches. Presumably leakage of cerebrospinal fluid via the puncture site and a subsequent drop in cerebrospinal fluid pressure cause the headache, which is generally located in the frontal or occipital areas. The headache is relieved when the patient lies flat and aggravated in an upright position. Conservative therapy including bed rest, fluids, and oral analgesics very often eliminate the problem. If severe headache persists, an epidural blood patch usually provides immediate relief. If

there is an accidental dural puncture during lumbar epidural anesthesia, the epidural catheter should be placed either one lumbar space above or one lumbar space below the area of the dural puncture. The catheter is kept in place after the delivery, and a prophylactic epidural blood patch via the in situ epidural catheter can be administered. Prophylactic epidural blood patch has been proven effective as a means of preventing a postdural puncture headache (80%) (Colonna-Romano & Shapiro, 1988) when a volume of no less than 15 mL to 20 mL of autologous blood is injected.

▶ CASE STUDY

A 17-year-old woman, 5´6˝ tall and weighing 186 lbs at 38 weeks gestation, is admitted to the delivery suite with elevated blood pressure for induction of labor. Blood pressure is in the range of 146 /92 mmHg, and there is mild generalized edema and proteinuria. Obstetric examination reveals that the cervix is dilated 2 cm and 40% effaced. Pertinent laboratory data include hematocrit 40% and platelet count 185 000. The woman does not smoke or drink and denies chronic medical problems, allergies, or previous surgeries. The American Society of Anesthesiologists (ASA) classification is IE, and airway evaluation reveals a Mallampati class 2 airway. The patient is started on an IV infusion of oxytocin and magnesium sulfate. After a few hours the membranes are ruptured, and the uterine contractions become painful. The woman is very uncomfortable and would like to have epidural analgesia. Blood pressure and repeat laboratory data including platelet count and coagulation profile are stable. The fetal heart rate tracing shows a rate in the 140s with good variability.

1. What do the laboratory values and physical examination reveal about this patient?

   Physical examination and laboratory data indicate that the patient has mild, stable preeclampsia. Blood pressure and laboratory data including the platelet count are stable, and the fetal heart rate tracing is reassuring.

2. What analgesic/anesthetic technique would be appropriate for this patient?

   The patient is being induced, in pain, and committed to a delivery (receiving pitocin and membranes are ruptured). There is no observable contraindication to regional anesthesia. Epidural or CSE analgesia are appropriate, and both techniques can improve uterine blood flow and obviate the need for general anesthesia. Combined spinal epidural technique is advantageous because it will not cause hypotension, but proper functioning of the epidural catheter is less reliable. Segmental epidural analgesia (T10 to L1) using small doses of dilute bupivacaine and fentanyl can provide satisfactory analgesia with minimal hypotension, and a functioning epidural catheter is already established.

3. How should analgesia be maintained throughout labor?

   A continuous epidural infusion of dilute bupivacaine and fentanyl is maintained throughout labor and, if cesarean section is necessary, the epidural catheter is available for use.

4. How should hypotension be managed?

   Measures to prevent hypotension from occurring should be employed. To prevent hypotension, careful fluid administration of 500 mL to 1000 mL is necessary and ephedrine (5 mg to 10 mg incre-

ments) should be administered to maintain blood pressure at preblock values.

▶ SUMMARY

The practice of obstetric anesthesia requires the anesthesia provider to have a complete understanding of the anatomic and physiologic changes associated with pregnancy that influence anesthetic management. In addition, the anesthetist must be cognizant of fetal physiology and anesthetic implications of perianesthesia care for both the mother and baby. Preexisting medical conditions and those that arise during the pregnancy can complicate not only the pregnancy, but anesthesia management at the time of delivery. Vigilant perianesthesia assessment that incorporates subjective, objective, and diagnostic data is essential in providing safe anesthesia care to mother and baby.

▶ KEY CONCEPTS

- Obstetric anesthesia involves the care of two patients simultaneously, the mother and fetus; consequently the preservation of maternal homeostasis is an important factor in the maintenance of fetal well-being.
- Maternal changes produced by pregnancy increase the risk of anesthesia, including (1) hypotension from aortocaval compression; (2) difficult intubation; (3) rapid development of hypoxia during periods of apnea; and (4) aspiration of gastric contents, as the lower esophageal spinchter tone is reduced and gastric volumes are increased.
- To minimize the risk of hypotension, the parturient should be maintained in the left lateral tilt position, and fluid preload should be administered before conduction anesthesia is attempted.
- When general anesthesia is administered, acid aspiration prophylaxis, rapid sequence intubation preoxygenation, and a backup plan for failed intubation are mandatory.

- Uterine blood flow is not autoregulated and is reduced by factors that decrease uterine arterial pressure (hypotension) or increase uterine vascular resistance (alpha-adrenergic stimulation, hyperventilation).
- In the obstetric patient, ephedrine is the vasopressor of choice for treating most episodes of hypotension.
- The safe administration of regional techniques for labor, vaginal delivery, or cesarean delivery requires a preanesthesia assessment, adequate prehydration and maintenance of blood pressure, incremental dosing of all local anesthetics, the prompt recognition of complications, and the ability to provide immediate resuscitation.
- Medical conditions coexisting with pregnancy can put the mother and fetus at great risk, and parturients with coexisting disease or complications deserve special anesthesia care.

► STUDY QUESTIONS

1. What are the anatomic and physiologic changes that occur in pregnant women, and how do these changes influence anesthesia care?

2. How is the fetus monitored, and how does the fetal monitoring influence anesthesia management?

3. What are the methods of anesthesia/analgesia for labor, vaginal delivery, cesarean section, and postoperative analgesia?

4. How do the presence of a fetus and the maternal changes of pregnancy affect the methods of anesthesia/analgesia for vaginal or cesarean delivery?

5. How does epidural analgesia affect the progress of labor?

6. How does the presence of coexisting medical complications such as (1) preeclampsia/eclampsia, (2) peripartum hemorrhage, (3) amniotic fluid embolus, (4) diabetes mellitus, and (5) cardiac disease influence the anesthesia management of the pregnant woman during labor and delivery?

7. What are some of the acute maternal complications that can occur during the course of administering obstetric anesthesia, and how are these conditions managed?

KEY REFERENCES

Chestnut D. H. (Ed.) (1994). *Obstetric anesthesia principles and practice.* St. Louis: Mosby.

Cruikshank D. P., Wigton T. R., & Hays P. M. (1996). Maternal physiology in pregnancy. In S. G. Gabbe, J. R. Niebyl, & J. L. Simpson (Eds.), *Obstetrics normal and problem pregnancies.* (3rd ed., pp. 91–109). New York: Churchill Livingstone.

Norris M. C. (Ed.) (1993). *Obstetric anesthesia.* Philadelphia: J. B. Lippincott Company.

Norris M. C. & Arkoosh V. A. (1994). Spinal opioid analgesia for labor. *International Anesthesiology Clinics, 32,* 69–81.

Santos A. C. & Pedersen H. (1994). Current controversies in obstetric anesthesia. *Anesthesia & Analgesia, 78,* 753–760.

Vincent R. D. (1994). Anesthesia for the pregnant patient. *Clinical Obstetrics and Gynecology, 37,* 256–273.

REFERENCES

Benson R. C. Schubeck, E., & Deutschberger, J. (1968). Fetal heart rate as a predictor of fetal distress *Obstetrics and Gynecology, 32,* 259–266.

Blass N. H. (1979). Regional anesthesia in the morbidity obese parturient. *Regional Anaesthesia, 4,* 20–22.

Blass N. H. (1981). Anesthesia for the morbidly obese. In J. Katz, J. Benumof, & L. B. Kadis, (Eds.), *Anesthesia and uncommon diseases: Pathophysiology and clinical correlations.* (2nd ed., pp. 450–462). Philadelphia: W. B. Saunders.

Cetrulo C. L., & Schifrin B. S. (1976). Fetal heart rate patterns preceding death in utero. *Obstetrics and Gynecology, 48,* 521–527.

Chan W. H., Paul, R. H., & Toews, J. (1973). Intrapartum fetal monitoring: Maternal and fetal morbidity and perinatal mortality. *Obstetrics and Gynecology, 41,* 7–13.

Chestnut, D. H., McGrath, J. M., Vincent, R. D., & Penning, D. H. (1994). Does early administration of epidural analgesia affect obstetric outcome in nulliparous women who are in spontaneous labor? *Anesthesiology, 80,* 1201–1208.

Clark, S. L. (1990). New concepts of amniotic fluid embolus: A review. *Obstetrics and Gynecology Survey, 45,* 360–365.

Coates, M. (1982). Combined subarachnoid and epidural techniques. *Anaesthesia, 37,* 89–90.

Cohen, S. E. (1982). Why is the pregnant patient different? *Seminars in Anesthesiology, 2,* 73–82.

Colonna-Romano, P. & Shapiro, B. E. (1988). Prophylactic epidural blood patch in obstetrics. *Anesthesiology, 69,* A665.

Conklin, K. A., & Murad, S. (1982). Pharmacology of drugs in obstetric Anesthesia. *Seminars in Anesthesiology, 2,* 83–100.

Crawford, J. S., Burton, O. M., & Davies, P. (1973). Anaesthesia for cesarean section: Further refinements of a technique. *British Journal of Anaesthesia, 45,* 726–731.

Datta, S., Corke, B. C., & Alper, M. H. (1980). Epidural anesthesia for cesarean section: A comparison of bupivacaine, chloroprocaine and etidocaine. *Anesthesiology, 52,* 48–51.

Eckstein, K. L. & Marx, G. F. (1974). Aortocaval compression and uterine displacement. *Anesthesiology, 40,* 92–96.

Fiedler, M. F. (1989). AANA Journal Course: Advanced scientific concepts: Update for nurse anesthetists: An introduction to fetal heart rate monitoring. *AANA Journal, 57,* 257–264.

Gibbs, C. P. & Banner, T. C. (1984). Effectiveness of Bicitra® as a preoperative antacid. *Anesthesiology, 61,* 97–99.

Holmes, F. (1960). The supine hypotensive syndrome: Its importance to the anaesthetist. *Anaesthesia, 15,* 298–306.

Hon, E. H. (1968). The clinical evaluation of fetal heart rate. In E. H. Hon (Ed.), *An atlas of fetal heartrate patterns* (pp. 25–31). New Haven, CT: Harty Press.

Howard, B. K., Goodson, J. H., & Mengert, W. F. (1953). Supine hypotensive syndrome of late pregnancy. *Obstetrics and Gynecology, 1–37.*

Iglesia, S., Burn, R., & Saunders, L. D. (1991). Reducing the cesarean section rate in a rural community hospital. *Canadian Medical Association Journal, 145,* 1459–1464.

James, F. M. III, Crawford, J. S., & Hopkinson, R. (1977). A comparison of general anesthesia and lumbar epidural analgesia for elective cesarean section. *Anesthesia & Analgesia, 56,* 228.

James, F. M. III, Greiss, F. C., & Kemp, R. D. (1970). An evaluation of vasopressor therapy for maternal hypotension during spinal anesthesia. *Anesthesiology, 33,* 25.

Joupila, P., Joupila, R., Hollmen, A., & Koivala, A. (1982). Lumbar epidural analgesia to improve intervillous blood flow during labor in severe preeclampsia. *Obstetrics and Gynecology, 59,* 158–161.

Kotelko, D. M., Dailey, P. A., & Shnider, S. M. (1984). Epidural morphine analgesia after cesarean delivery. *Obstetrics and Gynecology, 63,* 409–413.

Lyons, G. (1985). Failed intubation. Six years' experience in a teaching maternity unit. *Anaesthesia, 40*(8), 759–762.

Miller, E., Hare, J. W., & Cloherby, J. P. (1981). Elevated maternal hemoglobin A in early pregnancy and major congenital anomalies in infants of diabetic mothers. *New England Journal of Medicine, 304,* 1331.

Parer, J. T. (1980). The current role of intrapartum fetal blood sampling. *Clinical Obstetrics and Gynecology, 23,* 565–582.

Quilligan, E. J. (1979). Monitoring the fetus using acid–base studies. *Clinical Obstetrics and Gynecology, 6,* 309.

Quilligan, E. J. & Paul, R. H. (1975). Fetal monitoring: Is it worth it? *Obstetrics and Gynecology, 45,* 96–100.

Ramanathan, S., Masih, A., & Rock, L. I. (1983). Maternal and fetal effects of prophylactic hydration with crystalloids or colloids before epidural anesthesia. *Anesthesia & Analgesia, 62,* 673–678.

Rawal, N. & Wattwil, M. (1984). Respiratory depression after epidural morphine: An experimental and clinical study. *Anesthesia & Analgesia, 63,* 8–14.

Robson, S. C., Dunlop, W., & Hunter, S. (1987). Haemodynamic changes during the early puerperium. *British Medical Journal, 294,* 1065.

Robson, C. S., Hunter, S., Boyd, R. J., & Dunlop, W. (1989). Serial study of factors influencing changes in cardiac output during human pregnancy. *American Journal of Physiology, 256,* H1060–H1065.

Romalis, G., & Claman, A. D. (1962). Serum enzymes in pregnancy. *American Journal of Obstetrics and Gynecology, 84,* 1104–1110.

Schifrin, B. S., & Dame, L. (1972). Fetal heart rate patterns: Prediction of Apgar score. *Journal of the American Medical Association, 219,* 1322–1325.

Socol, M. L., Garcia, P. M., Peaceman, A. M., & Dooley, S. L. (1993). Reducing cesarean births at a primarily private university hospital. *American Journal of Obstetrics and Gynecology, 168,* 1748–1758.

Thorburn, J. & Moir, D. D. (1981). Extradural analgesia: The influence of volume and concentration of bupivacaine on the mode of delivery, analgesic efficacy and motor block. *British Journal of Anaesthesia, 53,* 933–939.

Thorp, J. A., Hu, D. H., & Albin, R. M. (1993). The effect of intrapartum epidural analgesia on nulliparous labor: A randomized controlled prospective trial. *American Journal of Obstetrics and Gynecology, 169,* 851–858.

Turner, M. J., Silk, J. M., & Alegesan, K. (1988). Epidural bupivacaine concentrations and forceps delivery in primaparae. *Journal of Obstetrics and Gynaecology, 9,* 122–125.

IV PART

Applied Pharmacology

Pharmacologic Principles of Anesthesia

Michele E. Gold

To understand the pharmacology of anesthetic agents, the student must build on a solid foundation in chemistry and biochemistry. Both chemical and biochemical principles have an impact on the practice of anesthesia, from the concept of enzyme kinetics to understand in vivo reactions, to the difference in action of a drug based on the structure–activity relationship of the newest anesthetic agent. The science of chemistry and biochemistry has advanced the biomedical field, leading to better treatment and patient prognoses and, in anesthesia, to the development of second-generation pharmaceutical agents that improve anesthesia care and delivery. Once a patient has been assessed, the appropriate anesthetic agents must be selected. A solid and detailed knowledge of the pharmacologic principles of anesthetic agents will facilitate this selection, providing a safe and effective anesthetic course.

► CHEMICAL PRINCIPLES OF DRUG ACTION

Principles of both inorganic and organic chemistry are an integral part of the action of drugs. *Inorganic chemistry* is the study of molecules that serve as the building blocks of structures. *Organic chemistry* explores the chemistry of carbon and related compounds, which constitute fats, sugars, proteins, and amino acids. These compounds are the building blocks of essential life processes. Two examples of inorganic and organic compounds of anesthesia-related pharmacologic agents are

nitrous oxide and halothane. Nitrous oxide is an inorganic gas composed of two molecules of nitrogen and one molecule of oxygen that functions as a weak anesthetic agent. It is insoluble in blood and does not metabolize in vivo, so it enters and leaves the body through inspiration and expiration. It is used as an adjuvant agent because high concentrations of nitrous oxide are necessary to achieve anesthesia. The organic compound halothane is a potent inhalation agent; it is a halogenated hydrocarbon composed of a carbon chain and chemical bonds with fluoride, chlorine, and bromine, and it provides complete anesthesia. Halothane undergoes hepatic metabolism and can result in hepatotoxicity (Gruenke, Konapka, Koop, & Waskell, 1988; Rehder, Forbes, Aller, Hessler, & Stier, 1967; Sipes & Brown, 1976). These two agents are used together often in the delivery of anesthesia.

Chemical Bonding

The chemical bonding of the inorganic compounds occurs because of the distribution of electrons in each element. In the outer shell of elements, a configuration of eight electrons forms a stable compound. Two elements that interact through their electrons in the outer shell will combine to reach a full complement of eight electrons, referred to as an *octet,* and achieve chemical stability. This involves a transfer of electrons, in which one compound has a net gain or loss of electrons. Sodium (Na) will interact with chlorine (Cl) to produce a stable substance, sodium chloride. This results from a transfer of

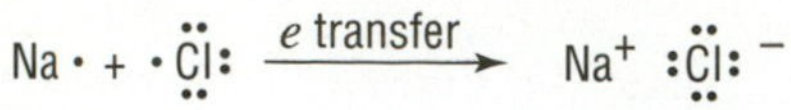

$$Na \cdot + \cdot \ddot{\underset{\cdot\cdot}{Cl}} : \xrightarrow{\;e\;transfer\;} Na^+ \; : \ddot{\underset{\cdot\cdot}{Cl}} : \; ^-$$

Figure 17–1. An example of electron transfer.

an electron from sodium to chlorine. Once combined, the elements form a stable compound (Fig. 17–1).

The air we breathe is formed by two molecules of oxygen to form atmospheric O_2. Oxygen also can combine with carbon to form carbon dioxide (CO_2), a byproduct of respiration, and carbon monoxide (CO), which can result in cellular hypoxemia. The periodic table of the elements provides vertical groupings of similar elements and a listing of each individual element's electron number. This table predicts the chemical reactivity of the elements on the basis of electron number and physical properties, such as metals, nonmetals, and transition elements (Kotz & Purcell, 1991, pp. 363–370; Vollhardt & Schore, 1994, pp. 7–13).

Both inorganic and organic compounds undergo two important types of bonding that form the basis of many biochemical and pharmacologic reactions: covalent bonds and ionic bonds. *Ionic bonds* follow the transfer of one or more electrons from one element to another. The formation of sodium chloride from sodium and chloride is an example of ionic bonding. A *covalent bond* is formed when electrons are shared between two molecules. Ethene (ethylene) is an organic compound and an example of covalent bonding (Fig. 17–2). Covalent bonds can share electrons either equally or not equally. The unequal sharing of electrons in a covalent bond is called a *polar covalent bond* and imparts a polarity (charge) to one element.

Organic covalent bonds can be depicted as straight lines. In addition, these compounds can form two-electron single bonds, four-electron double bonds, and six-electron triple bonds. Each covalent bond will achieve a full complement of eight electrons, a stable octet, and chemical stability. Organic compounds made of single bonds are called *alkanes.* Double- and triple-bonded compounds are called *alkenes* and *alkynes,* respectively. Alkanes are saturated hydrocarbons. Hydrogen atoms have been removed from the alkenes and alkynes, forming unsaturated hydrocarbons.

Examples of alkanes are methane, ethane, and cyclohexane (Fig. 17–3). These compounds are nonpolar

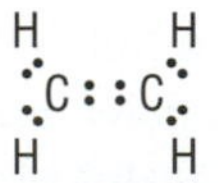

Figure 17–3. Structures of alkanes.

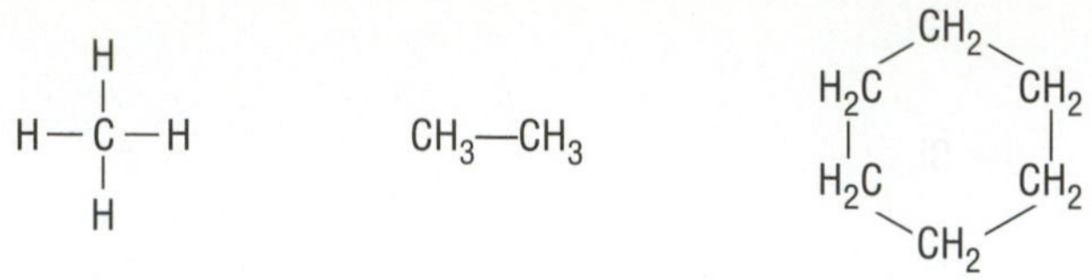

and nonreactive, and all carbon atoms are saturated with hydrogen atoms. Radical groups are formed by removing one hydrogen from a carbon and replacing the -ane stem with a -yl stem. Methane becomes methyl, ethane becomes ethyl, and so on. Alkenes and alkynes have unsaturated double and triple bonds that make these substances more chemically reactive. Organic cyclic compounds can produce saturated hydrocarbons such as the anesthetic cyclopropane, and unsaturated hydrocarbons such as benzene, which is a solvent. The derivatives of benzene made from substitutions on the benzene ring are an integral component of many pharmacologic preparations. Multiple benzene rings can be joined together to form the basic structure of vitamins, steroids, and the nondepolarizing muscle relaxants (Vollhardt & Schore, 1994, pp. 41–45, 421, 467–468).

Isomers

The presence of either single or double bonds in organic compounds will result in the formation of *isomers,* which are compounds that have the same molecular formula but different structures. The inhalation anesthetics isoflurane and enflurane are isomers (Fig. 17–4). These compounds are composed of single bonds, allowing for bond rotation. In compounds with a double bond, such as the alkenes, rotation about the C=C axis is prevented. This results in two possible permanent rotations of functional groups bonded to the carbon molecules. This is called *cis-trans* isomerism. The *trans* have the functional groups on opposite sides of the bond, and the *cis* have the functional groups on the same side of the bond (Fig. 17–5). These compounds are characterized by different structures and different properties. The chemotherapeutic agent cisplatin is active in destroying cancerous cells. The trans isomer has no effect. Other types of isomers present in biologic compounds are stereoisomers, which possess identical structures but different spatial arrange-

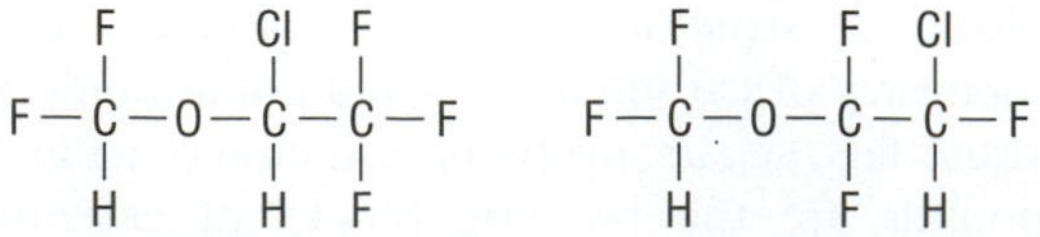

Figure 17–2. An example of covalent bonding.

Figure 17–4. Isoflurane and enflurane are isomers.

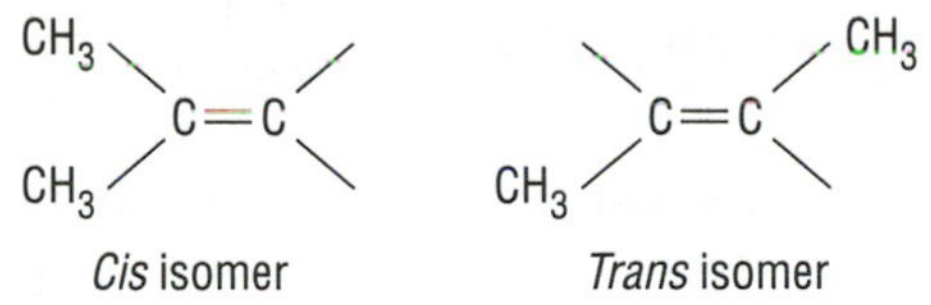

Figure 17–5. *Cis* and *trans* isomers.

ments. They also are called optical isomers because they polarize light in opposite directions. Light polarized to the left is the levorotatory, or *levo (l)*, isomer; light polarized to the right is the dextrorotatory, or *dextro (d)*, isomer. These isomers are mirror images of each other and are also called *enantiomers*. A compound can be a racemic mixture of both *l* and *d* isomers. Ketamine, an intravenous anesthetic, is presently formulated for use as a racemic mixture. When the *d* and *l* isomers of ketamine are separated, Doenicke, Kugler, Mayer, and Hoffmann (1992) found that the *d* isomer of ketamine has less associated adverse effects than the racemic mixture, resulting in improved drug performance and patient outcome.

Class Divisions of Organic Compounds

Organic compounds can be divided into classes based on a functional group. These groups will change the physical properties of the basic compound, altering its lipid solubility and electrical charge.

Halogen Compounds
Substituting hydrogen on a carbon chain for a halogen atom (chlorine, bromine, fluorine, etc.) will form a halogenated compound. The inhalation anesthetic halothane is a halogenated compound comprised of a two-carbon straight chain with chlorine, fluorine, and bromine substitutions. Chloroform, an anesthetic no longer in use today, is a halogenated compound.

Alcohols, Aldehydes, Ketones, and Acids
Alcohols are formed by replacing hydrogen on the carbon chain with the hydroxyl functional group, $R-OH$. For example, replacing a hydrogen of methane with $-OH$ forms methyl alcohol and ethane forms ethyl. Alcohols are further classified as primary, secondary, or tertiary based on the number of carbons attached to the carbon-hydroxyl group.

The functional group of the aldehydes is $R-\overset{\overset{\textstyle O}{\|}}{C}-H$, of which formaldehyde is an example. The aldehydes are formed from the oxidation of a primary alcohol. Ketones are formed by the oxidation of secondary alcohols. Its functional group is $R-\overset{\overset{\textstyle O}{\|}}{C}-R'$ and is called a carbonyl

group. Diabetic ketoacidosis is a metabolic condition defined by an excessive production of ketones. In biologic systems, alcohols are oxidized to aldehydes and ketones. Ethanol is metabolized by the hepatic enzyme alcohol dehydrogenase. The oxidizing agent is nicotinamide adenine dinucleotide (NAD^+).

A carboxyl group ($R-\overset{\overset{\textstyle O}{\|}}{C}-O-H$) will replace a hydrogen to form an organic acid, giving the compound acidic properties. Organic acids have the ability to ionize or react with bases to form neutral salts and water. Carboxylic acid is one part of the basic structure of amino acids (Vollhardt & Schore, 1994, pp. 630-634, 720-723).

Esters and Ethers
Esters are produced by the interaction of an alcohol and an acid (Vollhardt & Schore, 1994, pp. 777-785). Their general formula is $R-\overset{\overset{\textstyle O}{\|}}{C}-O-R'$. The local anesthetics procaine, chloroprocaine, and tetracaine are esters. The hydrolytic metabolism of these compounds takes place at the ester function by cholinesterase in the plasma and to a lesser degree in the liver.

Ethers consist of two carbon chains joined by an oxygen. Their general formula is $R-O-R'$. Isoflurane, enflurane, desflurane, and sevoflurane are all ethers. They are chemically stable and nonexplosive; for this reason they are regarded as safe and effective anesthetics and have replaced diethyl ether and divinyl ether in anesthetic practice today. These compounds undergo minimal hepatic metabolism.

Amines and Amides
Amines have the general formula $R-NH_2$ and can be classified as primary, secondary, tertiary, or quaternary amines (Vollhardt & Schore, 1994, pp. 824-825, 835). The primary, secondary, or tertiary amines are similar to the classification of alcohols. The number of methyl groups attached to a nitrogen atom determines the specific form. Quaternary amines have a positive charge that decreases the hydrophilicity of the compound. The anticholinergic compounds atropine and glycopyrrolate are similar in their vagolytic action. Atropine is a tertiary amine and can cross the blood–brain barrier to produce central nervous system (CNS) stimulation. Glycopyrrolate is a quaternary amine with minimal action on the CNS.

The amide functional group is characterized by $R-\overset{\overset{\textstyle O}{\|}}{C}-NH_2$. The other group of local anesthetics have an amide linkage. These drugs are lidocaine, bupivacaine, mepivacaine, etidocaine, and prilocaine. The amide local anesthetics are metabolized by hepatic microsomal enzymes. The metabolism of amide-linked local anesthetics is slower than that of the ester-linked local anesthetics.

Amino Acids

Amino acids contain both a carboxylic acid group and an amine group. The amino acids are amphoteric and possess both acidic and basic properties because of these two functional groups. Twenty important amino acids are found in humans. Humans can synthesize all but eight amino acids, which are called the *essential amino acids* because they must be taken exogenously. The amino acid tyrosine serves as the precursor to the endogenous synthesis of norepinephrine. In 1988, Palmer, Rees, Ashton, and Moncada suggested that the amino acid arginine was the endogenous precursor for nitric oxide, a reactive molecule that functions as a vasodilator, brain neuromodulator, and neurotoxin. Nitric oxide synthase catalyzes the oxidation of arginine to nitric oxide (Hobbs, Fukuto, & Ignarro, 1994). Nitric oxide also exists as a gas that can be inhaled; it has been studied by Rich, Murphy, Roos, & Johns (1993) in the treatment of pulmonary hypertension due to its local vasodilator effect on the pulmonary vasculature.

The amino acids are the building blocks of protein. Peptides are smaller chains of amino acids. Examples of peptides include the drug insulin, the endorphins that interact on opioid receptors, and hemoglobin. Both proteins and peptides serve essential regulatory biologic functions.

Acid–Base Chemistry

In biologic systems, both acidic and basic compounds are abundant. Physiologically, the body aims to maintain homeostasis and neutralizes acids and bases. An acid is a substance that separates into ions, providing a hydrogen ion (H^+) on dissociation. Basic substances also separate into ions and provide a hydroxide ion (OH^-) as it dissociates. Acids and bases are related by the pH scale. The term *pH* indicates the concentration of hydrogen ion in the body or solution. The pH is determined from the negative logarithm of the hydrogen ion concentration and is measured on a scale of 0 to 14. A pH of 7.00 indicates neutrality, a balance of acids and bases. A pH reading of less than 7.00 indicates an increased acidic or hydrogen ion concentration, and readings from 7 to 14 indicate increasing hydroxide ion concentration or basicity (Kotz & Purcell, 1991, pp. 753–763; Le Bel, 1992a, pp. 71–72).

The relative strength of an acid or base can be expressed quantitatively with the equilibrium constant Ka. Strong acids will dissociate readily and are characterized by a low pKa value. Strong bases also dissociate readily and have a high pKa value. Most biologic acids and bases are weak. The degree of ionization (or the ability of an acid, A^-, and base, *HA,* to dissociate) can be calculated from the Henderson-Hasselbach equation:

$$pH = pKa + \log \frac{[A^-]}{[HA]}$$

This equation expresses the relationship between the pH of the solution and the pKa of a compound. If the pH and pKa are equal, equal distribution of ionized and unionized compound will be present in the solution. The Henderson-Hasselbach equation can be applied to determine the degree of ionization of compounds. A weak acid with a pKa of 4.4 at a physiologic pH of 7.4 will exist only in an ionized form and will be excreted. Pharmacologic agents must be unionized to be effective, and determining the degree of ionization of drugs helps in evaluating their efficacy. Highly charged drugs have limited ability to cross biologic membranes or produce a response. The ideal drug must have a certain concentration of unionized drug at physiologic pH, which results in a therapeutic response (Stryer, 1995, p. 42).

Another application of acid-base chemistry deals with the ability of acids and bases to neutralize and protect the body by maintaining a normal pH. The acid–base balance, and hence the pH of the body, must be tightly regulated to allow for homeostatic mechanisms such as metabolism, tissue oxygenation, and enzymatic functions. Three related mechanisms are responsible for pH balance in the body. They include (1) the chemical buffer systems of the body, most importantly the carbonate-bicarbonate buffer system; (2) the respiratory regulation of CO_2; and (3) the renal excretion of acidic and basic ions.

The carbonate-bicarbonate buffer systems provide for the regulation of the body's pH at about 7.4. The system depends on the CO_2 tension and follows this equation:

$$CO_2 + H_2O \rightleftharpoons H_2CO_3 \rightleftharpoons H^+ + HCO_3^-$$

Carbon dioxide is the end product of cellular metabolism. In the blood it combines with water to form carbonic acid. The dissociation of carbonic acid results in both hydrogen and hydroxide ions. Applying the Henderson-Hasselbach equation to this system at a physiologic pH of 7.4, and using the known pKa value of carbonic acid as 6.1, the ratio of bicarbonate ion to carbonic acid is 20 to 1. This ratio supports the rapid neutralization of both excess hydrogen and hydroxide ions. Increasing acidosis (excess hydrogen ions) will rapidly combine with the hydroxide ions and form carbonic acid and CO_2. Alkalosis following the addition of excess hydroxide ion will be neutralized by carbonic acid. The ability of the carbonate-bicarbonate buffer system to prevent pH changes after alterations in the body's acid and base status serves an important physiologic regulatory function. Other buffering systems include the inorganic buffers phosphate and sulfate, hemoglobin in red blood cells, and plasma proteins (Le Bel, 1992a, p. 72; Marks, Marks, & Smith, 1996, p. 39).

Acid–base status and pH are further regulated by the concentration of CO_2 in the body. The rate and depth of respiration are regulated by the CNS, which is sensitive to pH and the partial pressure of CO_2 (pco_2). When the body pH falls below normal, central stimulation occurs and respiration is increased to lower the pco_2. Elevations in body pH depress the respiratory rate with a rise in pco_2. Once diagnosed, pathophysiologic conditions underlying respiratory acidosis and alkalosis must be treated.

Renal regulation of acid–base status is less rapid than the respiratory regulation. However, over time it appears to be more effective. The kidneys can alter the exchange of hydrogen and bicarbonate ions to maintain the physiologic pH to near-normal values. These physiologic systems will work under normal conditions. Any severe alterations in homeostasis, such as trauma, fluid and blood loss, pulmonary and renal disease, and loss of consciousness, can disrupt their functions. Anesthesia can result in deviations from the normal functioning of these systems, specifically when respiratory abnormalities (ie, hypoxia) and blood loss occur.

▶ BIOCHEMICAL PRINCIPLES OF DRUG ACTION

Proteins, carbohydrates, and lipids provide the basic biochemical structure of the body. Proteins are polymers of amino acids forming long chains that fold and twist. Proteins have important functional roles as enzymes, carriers, receptors, and hormones. They also provide defense mechanisms and structural support to cells. Carbohydrates are organic compounds comprised of carbon, oxygen, and hydrogen that yield simple sugars and starch to provide cellular energy. They can be combined with proteins and lipids to perform structural roles in the body. Lipids have important structural properties and are insoluble in water. The three types of lipids found in cell membranes are phospholipids, cholesterol, and glycolipids.

Biologic cell membranes are comprised of a lipid bilayer. The lipids are amphipathic and contain both a hydrophobic portion and a hydrophilic polar head portion. Proteins are embedded in the bilayer. They can be integral or peripheral proteins or can span the width of the cell membrane. The two most important functions of the cell membrane are to protect the internal cellular environment and to regulate the passage of substances across the membrane. Pharmacologic agents either work at the cellular membrane or need to pass through it to the site of action. Intravenous drugs, such as the neuro-

muscular blockers, interact with nicotinic cholinergic receptors on skeletal muscle. The steroids glucocorticoid and aldosterone interact with intracellular receptors. Both steroids enter the cell by diffusion and combine with a cytoplasmic receptor to form an active steroid-receptor complex. This active complex then can translocate into the cell nucleus and interact with messenger ribonucleic acid (mRNA), resulting in translation to proteins. The inhalation agents possess an even different action at the cell membrane. The lipid-soluble nature of these agents suggest that they readily diffuse into cells within the CNS, which may be responsible for their mechanism of action (Ross, 1996, p. 32).

Enzyme Kinetics

Most important, body processes are catalyzed by enzymes. These include metabolism involving oxidation, reduction, and hydrolytic mechanisms; gastric digestion to aid absorption of food and drugs; substrate formation for cellular energy; and neurotransmitter synthesis and degradation. Enzymes reduce the amount of energy required to initiate or sustain a reaction but are not part of it. Enzymes exhibit a high degree of specificity for substrates. Some enzymes catalyze a reaction by one substrate and are even stereospecific. Other enzymes, such as the family of isozymes of the cytochrome P450 system, are substrate nonspecific (Nebert & Gonzalez, 1987), an important physiologic function. This primary metabolic enzyme system in combination with monooxygenases located in hepatic microsomes is responsible for the degradation of a wide variety of medications possessing diverse chemical structures.

The formation of an enzyme–substrate complex is the first step in an enzymatic reaction. Cofactors may be necessary that function as electron acceptors of donors or as functional groups that can be added or removed from the enzyme. The rate at which an enzymatic reaction occurs depends on the concentration of both enzyme and substrate and the availability of cofactors. The rate of enzyme and substrate combination to form a product proceeds linearly until all functional sites on the enzyme are occupied; the enzyme is saturated with substrate. Further increases in substrate concentration will not increase enzyme–substrate formation or product formation (Stryer, 1995, pp. 190–195). The rate of enzyme-catalyzed reactions can be altered by compounds that compete with the substrate for combination to the active site on the enzyme. This enzyme inhibition could be competitive or noncompetitive, reversible or irreversible. Increased production of enzyme also can occur that depends on a sustained duration of exposure of a particular compound, which acts as an inducing agent of the enzyme. Smoking, excessive alcohol ingestion, and barbiturates are some examples of compounds responsible for enzyme induction of the cytochrome P450-monooxygenase system (Conney, 1967). Enzymes are sensitive to pH and temperature. Extremes of temperature and pH can result in a decline in reaction rates and enzyme denaturation.

Energy Requirements

Physiologic processes require transformation of energy in chemical reactions responsible for movement, growth, and response to stimuli. The metabolic rate is a measure of energy requirements of both body cellular and tissue processes involved in the activity of major organs, such as heart, liver, kidney, brain, as well as muscles, and the mechanical work of respiration, circulation, and peristalsis.

High-energy phosphate compounds are capable of energy storage, transfer, and release. Adenosine tri-phosphate (ATP) is a nucleotide composed of adenine, a ribose sugar, and three phosphate units. Hydrolysis releases a large amount of energy as the terminal bond is split to produce adenosine diphosphate (ADP) and then adenosine monophosphate (AMP). Cellular production of ATP occurs by transfer of electrons within the inner membrane of mitochondria. Protons are transported along an electrochemical gradient to synthesize ATP by oxidative phosphorylation. Another important energy source is the Kreb's cycle, which involves the oxidation of carbohydrates and fatty acids into cellular energy, ATP. The Kreb's cycle is the body's principal metabolic pathway, in which 30 moles of ATP are formed per molecule of glucose (Le Bel, 1992b, pp. 101-102; Stryer, 1995, pp. 551-552).

▶ BASIC PHARMACOLOGIC PRINCIPLES OF DRUG ACTION

The selection and administration of drugs used in anesthesia must encompass a knowledge of the pharmacodynamic and pharmacokinetic principles of these agents. Pharmacodynamics is the study of the actions of chemicals or drugs in producing biologic effects, whereas pharmacokinetic principles identify the factors that determine the time course of drug effects and the amount of drug reaching the site of action to produce a biologic effect. One goal of anesthesia delivery is to administer drugs in the proper dosage range and time interval to ensure appropriate drug concentrations in the organ, tissue, or cellular site of drug action. The determinants of pharmacodynamic and pharmacokinetic principles include (1) drug bioavailability, a consequence of the absorption, distribution, biotransformation, and elimination of drugs; (2) time course of drug effects; and (3) mechanisms of drug action.

Drug Bioavailability

Drugs must be absorbed across biologic membranes to produce a drug effect. The more classic routes of anesthetic delivery are the inhalation, intravenous, topical, and rectal routes. Novel routes of administration include the intranasal (Henderson, Brodsky, Fisher, Brett, & Hertzka, 1988), aerosol (Sinclair et al., 1988), and transmucosal routes (Mock et al., 1986). The bioactive form of a drug is generally the unionized form that is lipid soluble and readily permeates lipid membranes. Ionized drugs are hydrophilic and do not easily permeate lipid membranes. Most therapeutic drugs are weak acids or bases, and the percentage of drug that is unionized can be determined by the Henderson–Hasselbach equation. As noted (see Acid–Base Chemistry), this equation defines the relationship between the pKa of the drug and the pH gradient across a particular membrane. The pKa of a drug is a constant, determined by the pH at which the drug is 50% ionized. This suggests that the local pH surrounding the drug molecule influences the degree of ionization, drug absorption, and bioavailability. Binding of drugs to circulating plasma proteins, such as albumin and globulin, also affects the concentration of the bioactive drug. The degree of protein binding of a particular drug depends on the affinity of the drug for plasma proteins, the pH of the plasma, and temperature. It is the free drug fraction that is responsible for the therapeutic effect. Alterations in protein plasma binding, which might occur in the patient with liver disease, could increase or decrease the amount of free drug available (Winter, 1994; Wood, 1986).

Drug distribution involves the transfer of a drug to its central or peripheral sites of action. Drugs are more rapidly distributed to those organs that are well perfused, such as the brain, heart, liver, and kidney, and less rapidly distributed to muscle, bone, and fat. The concept of redistribution is important and affects certain anesthetic agents. Redistribution involves the removal of a drug from its site of action to muscle and fat. This rapid transfer of drugs away from the site of action is responsible for the short duration of action of sodium thiopental and the fentanyl analogs. After an induction dose of sodium thiopental, the patient recovers within minutes because of the termination of action of sodium thiopental as a result of its removal from active sites in the brain and not as a result of hepatic metabolism. However, a constant infusion of sodium thiopental in the treatment of seizures does depend on hepatic metabolism for termination of drug action.

The absorption of drugs across biologic membranes and their distribution to active sites may be limited by the physical and chemical characteristics of the drug and the cellular barriers. The concentration gradient of the drug and its molecular size determine whether a drug can passively diffuse across membranes. Drugs may be transported by facilitated diffusion, which also depends on the concentration gradient. The active transport of drugs requires energy for passage across membranes, and therefore they are not dependent on the concentration gradient. Specialized membranes, such as the blood–brain barrier and placenta, provide some protection against drug delivery to the CNS and the fetus, respectively; however, because of the high lipophilicity of anesthetic agents, some drugs used in anesthesia (ie, midazolam) can penetrate these protective membranes (Kanto, 1986; Pardridge, 1988). There is a large concentration of gamma amino butyric acid (GABA) receptors in the brain. The benzodiazepine midazolam binds to the GABA receptor, resulting in sedation and relief of anxiety, an important therapeutic action to relieve preoperative anxiety. Wilson, Dundee, Moore, Howard, and Collier (1987) observed that the administration of midazolam to the parturient may result in newborn depression and atony, specifically when given shortly before delivery.

Bioactive lipophilic substances are not readily eliminated by the body and must be metabolized to water-soluble substances. The liver is the predominant metabolic organ, and drug biotransformation occurs here through two distinct metabolic pathways. Phase I processes include oxidative, reductive, and hydrolytic reactions that enzymatically convert the parent compound into more polar metabolites. The cytochrome P450 system, found in the hepatic microsomal fraction, is responsible for enzymatic catalysis of the oxidative and reductive reactions (Fig. 17–6). Due to the lack of substrate specificity, many diverse medications with varying chemical structures are substrates for this microsomal enzyme system (Nebert & Gonzalez, 1987). Conjugation reactions constitute phase II processes and involve the chemical combination of a reactive group on the drug molecule with a variety of endogenous substrates. Glucuronide conjugation is the most common reaction undergone by drugs, but conjugation with sulfate, glycine, and acetate is possible. Certain drugs may need to undergo hepatic metabolism for the enzymatic conversion of a drug into a more pharmacologically active species. The actual drug administered serves as a prodrug, which in itself has little or no biologic activity (Benet, Kroetz, & Sheiner, 1996, pp. 11–16).

Two nondepolarizing muscle relaxant analogs, atracurium and cisatracurium, undergo an organ-independent hydrolytic metabolism (ie, Hofmann elimination) (Fisher et al., 1986; Lien et al., 1996). Hofmann elimination is characterized by spontaneous catalysis of the parent compound at pH 7.4 and normal body temperature. The metabolite is laudanosine, which has insignificant pharmacologic activity and is metabolized by ester hydrolysis.

Hydrolytic enzymes, found in most organs, plasma,

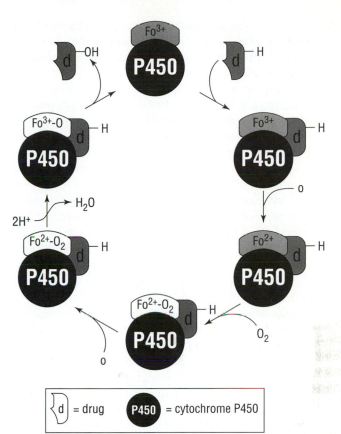

Figure 17–6. Drug biotransformation occurs through the oxidation by the heme-containing protein, cytochrome P450, following NADPH reduction, and the incorporation of oxygen. This increased hydrophilicity of the drug facilitates excretion. *(From Ross, E. M. [1996]. In J. G. Hardman & L. E. Limbird [Eds.], Goodman and Gilman's The pharmacologic basis of therapeutics [9th ed.], Figure 1–3, p. 12. New York: McGraw-Hill. Copyright McGraw-Hill. Reprinted with permission.)*

and tissue, catalyze the metabolism of drugs containing ester or amide linkages. The depolarizing muscle relaxant succinylcholine is rapidly hydrolyzed by plasma esterases to an inactive metabolite, succinylmonocholine. The opioid remifentanil possesses an ester linkage that is susceptible to hydrolysis by nonspecific esterases in blood and tissue resulting in rapid degradation (Egan et al., 1993; Westmoreland, Hoke, Sebel, Hug, & Muir, 1993). These hydrolytic reactions occur rapidly and are responsible for the short duration of action of these drugs. There are certain indications when drugs with a short duration of action are necessary. Succinylcholine is particularly useful in relaxing airway muscles to facilitate intubation when the patient has a full stomach and could aspirate stomach contents or when there is the potential for a difficult airway.

Extensive metabolism of some orally administered drugs (ie, lidocaine) can limit their bioavailability. Following absorption from the stomach, these drugs pass through the liver and undergo hepatic extraction and metabolism. This "first-pass metabolism" results in a subtherapeutic drug concentration and can be prevented by intravenous drug administration.

The rate at which biotransformation of drugs takes place is affected by hepatic blood flow and enzyme induction or inhibition. Alterations in hepatic blood flow by drugs, congestive heart failure, or shock can impair the metabolic rate. The cytochrome P450 enzyme system is subject to enzyme induction, which may increase the amount of metabolic enzyme 25-fold and result in a marked increase in metabolic rate. A variety of drugs, such as phenobarbital and alcohol, are capable of enzyme induction. Enzyme inhibition leads to a decrease in the rate of drug metabolism. Greenblatt et al. (1986) demonstrated that the inhibition of hepatic oxidative enzymes following cimetidine administration led to a decrease in diazepam, but not midazolam, clearance.

Drug elimination most commonly occurs through renal excretion. Most eliminated substances are polar metabolites, but excretion of unchanged drug also can account for the termination of drug action. The renal tubular system depends on the processes of filtration, passive diffusion, and active tubular secretion. Ionized unbound drug molecules of low molecular weight pass through the glomerular filtrate into the renal tubular fluid. Within the renal tubules, the concentration gradient, the molecular size of the ionized drug, and the urinary pH influence passive diffusion. In addition, a number of drugs are substrates for active secretory systems located in the renal tubule cells and are actively transported into the urine. Metabolites formed by conjugation reactions are most likely eliminated by active secretion. Penicillin is one of many compounds that use active secretory processes for elimination (Benet et al., 1996, pp. 16–17).

Other excretory routes include the hepatobiliary system and the lungs. Drugs can pass easily into the liver, but movement into the bile necessitates diffusion mechanisms and active transport systems. Intestinal reabsorption of drugs can occur, and such recycling is referred to as the enterohepatic cycle. The recycled drug ultimately may be further metabolized and excreted in the urine. Inhalation anesthetic agents are eliminated essentially unchanged in the lung. The concentration gradient, solubility, and alveolar ventilation determine the rate of drug elimination.

Time–Response Effects of Drugs

The time course of drug effects can be divided into three phases: (1) time to onset of action; (2) time to peak effect; and (3) duration of action (Levine, 1996, p. 221). The onset of drug action is the length of time from drug administration to the first measurable drug effect; the duration of action is the length of time from drug adminis-

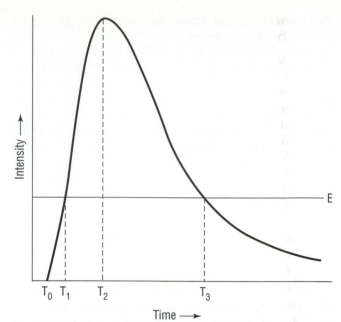

Figure 17–7. Time–response curve illustrates the drug effect over time. The drug is administered at T_0. T_1 is the onset of drug action; T_0 to T_2 is the time to peak effect; and T_1 to T_3 is the duration of drug action. *(From Levine, R. R. [1996].* Pharmacology: Drug actions and reactions *[5th ed., p. 221]. Copyright Parthenon Publishing Group. Reprinted with permission.)*

tration to the cessation of drug effect. Peak effect occurs at the maximal drug concentration (Fig. 17-7). The factors described previously—absorption, distribution, biotransformation, and elimination—influence the time in which a critical concentration of a drug has access to its site of action.

Half-life ($t_{1/2}$), volume of distribution, and clearance can be derived by mathematical principles based on measurements of the drug concentration that occur over time. The *half-life* of a drug is the time required for the plasma concentration of the drug to be reduced by 50% and indicates the time required for drug elimination from the body. The *clearance* of a drug refers to the rate of elimination by the kidneys, liver, or other routes. *Volume of distribution* relates the amount of drug in the body with the same concentration measured in the plasma. Large volumes of distribution indicate the presence of drug in tissues or fluids outside the plasma compartment. Drugs with little protein plasma binding, a high degree of lipophilicity, and tissue binding have a large volume of distribution. Half-life, rate of clearance, and volume of distribution are interrelated. For instance, a decrease in the rate of clearance secondary to renal disease increases the half-life of a drug and possibly intensifies the drug effect. A decrease in plasma protein binding raises the level of free drug in the plasma, increasing the volume of distribution and the rate of drug clearance (Levine, 1996, p. 113; Winter, 1994).

Pharmacologic Principles in Anesthesia Practice

The basic pharmacologic principles provide a framework for understanding the process of anesthesia delivery. Knowledge of the absorption, distribution, biotransformation, excretion, and time course of drugs provides a rationale for the choice, method of administration, and termination of drugs during the course of the anesthesia. Using these principles as the framework, the novice anesthesia provider should be able to incorporate the use of different or new agents. After the evaluation of a patient for a particular operation and after obtaining a history and physical examination, the anesthetist can then choose appropriate anesthetic agents.

The onset and duration of action of anesthetic agents need to be considered when deciding on the choice of drugs. A patient with a diagnosis of hypertension and associated coronary artery disease may have an adverse effect if prolonged hypotension occurred on the induction of anesthesia. Common induction agents, such as sodium thiopenthal, propofol, and etomidate, have a rapid onset of action but can cause hypotension when given in bolus doses and large doses in the debilitated, elderly, or hypovolemic patient. When they are titrated slowly, hypotension is less common. The duration of action of any of these drugs is short, a result of drug redistribution away from its site of action to muscle and fat. The use of a propofol infusion on induction of anesthesia will help to maintain an anesthetic level.

The selection of muscle relaxants also depends on its onset and duration of action. Succinylcholine has the shortest onset and duration of action when compared with other current muscle relaxants in use today. Because of this characteristic, succinylcholine is indicated for rapid sequence induction when the risk of patient aspiration of gastric contents is high. Rocuronium, in increasing doses, has an onset of action of 90 seconds and can be used for rapid sequence induction (Puhringer, Khuenl-Brady, Koller, & Mitterschiffthaler, 1992). If the surgical procedure is lengthy, a muscle relaxant with an intermediate (Fahey et al., 1981) or long (Stanley, Mirajhur, Bell, Sharpe, & Clarke, 1991) duration of action would be appropriate. The duration of action also can be affected by the mechanism of drug metabolism and excretion. Patients with hepatic or renal dysfunction can have an unusually prolonged drug response. Due to their organ-independent metabolic action, the drugs atracurium and cisatracurium are useful in these patients. It is imperative that the patient's history and physical examination be reviewed and that drug management reflect the individual's medical profile.

The ideal anesthetic agent should match the patient's need for onset of anesthesia and duration of surgery. Factors that alter the absorption of drugs such as extensive first-pass metabolism, drug distribution, plasma protein concentration, and hepatic and renal dysfunction will have an impact on the patient's response and an adverse effect. Short-acting agents can be titrated to a predefined end point of sedation or blood pressure control. Because of this, drugs such as midazolam, remifentanil, and esmolol are routinely used in anesthesia. However, this does not preclude the use of longer acting congeners that, when administered according to basic pharmacologic principles, can provide a satisfactory anesthetic course.

Mechanisms of Drug Action

General anesthesia can be induced using either intravenous or inhalation anesthetic agents. The mechanisms of action of these two groups of anesthetics are markedly different. Drug–receptor interactions have been described for most of the intravenous agents used in the administration of anesthesia. Inhalation anesthetics are considered to elicit a drug response following a nonspecific interaction with cellular membranes.

Receptors are protein macromolecules generally bound to the surface of cell membranes. Drug–receptor binding is the initial step in the development of the drug response (see Signal Transduction and Second Messengers). Several subtypes of receptors for the neurotransmitters norepinephrine, epinephrine, acetylcholine, and dopamine have been discovered, isolated, cloned, and sequenced. Receptors can be identified by anatomic localization. For example, $beta_1$- and $beta_2$-receptor subtypes are found in the heart and bronchial smooth muscle, respectively. Activation by epinephrine at the $beta_1$-receptor results in increased inotropy and chronotropy; $beta_2$-receptor activation results in bronchodilation. Acetylcholine is a neurotransmitter used in several different locations, at either the nicotinic or muscarinic receptor subtype. The binding of acetylcholine on nicotinic cholinergic receptors at the neuromuscular junction of skeletal muscle allows for membrane depolarization of muscle; acetylcholine binding to cardiac muscarinic receptors produce bradycardia. The enzyme acetylcholinesterase serves as a "receptor" for acetylcholine.

After site-specific binding to acetylcholinesterase, acetylcholine is broken down to choline and acetate. Competitive inhibition by the anticholinesterases neostigmine, pyridostigmine, and edrophonium prevents acetylcholine breakdown by acetylcholinesterase and is the rationale behind the use of the anticholinesterases to reverse neuromuscular blockade of the nicotinic receptor. The resultant increase in acetylcholine concentration from the competitive inhibition of acetylcholinesterase by these agents competes for receptor occupancy of the nicotinic cholinergic receptor. Steroid receptors differ in that they are localized within the cell cytoplasm. Drugs such as estrogen and progesterone diffuse across cell membranes to cytoplasmic receptors. Local anesthetics bind to voltage-sensitive sodium channels and block sodium conduction and cell membrane depolarization. Intravenous agents used in anesthesia, such as barbiturates, benzodiazepines, neuromuscular blockers, and narcotics, interact reversibly with their specific receptors to elicit a response.

The concept of specific receptors was first introduced by Langley in 1878 to explain the activity of nicotine and curare. The term *receptor* was later coined by Ehrlich in 1913. A review by Ruffolo (1982) summarizes several receptor theories that further expand the role of the receptor. The assumptions included the following: (1) The response of an agonist is proportional to receptor occupancy; (2) the binding of drug is described by the law of mass action; and (3) the quantity of a drug bound to the receptor population is small relative to the total amount of available receptors. Later studies suggested that a maximum effect could be produced when an agonist occupies only some of the receptor population, leaving unbound "spare receptors."

The preceding works led to the discovery of partial agonists, as well as affinity and efficacy of receptor binding. Partial agonists cannot produce a maximal receptor response. Receptor binding affinity describes the rate of drug–receptor complex formation. Efficacy relates to the capacity of a drug to initiate a response dependent on the amount of drug–receptor binding. Receptor desensitization and supersensitivity can occur over time after either the prolonged or diminished exposure, respectively, of a specific drug. Desensitization results in the sequestration of receptor from the surface of the cell membrane (Schwinn, 1993), whereas increase in cell surface receptors can be observed on diminished drug exposure.

The relationship between the concentration of drug and the magnitude of drug effect is important in the administration of either intravenous or inhalation anesthetics. Concentration–response curves evaluate the clinical effects of drugs and provide information about a drug's potency, efficacy, 50% effective concentration (EC_{50}), 50% lethal concentration (LC_{50}), and therapeutic index. Potency refers to the concentration of drug required to produce a maximum response. A relatively potent drug will elicit an effect at a low concentration. Drug efficacy is related to the intrinsic ability of the drug to elicit a response. An agonist has maximum efficacy, whereas an antagonist has zero efficacy. The concentration of drug necessary to elicit a response in 50% of individuals is the EC_{50}, and the LC_{50} is the concentration of drug that results in death in 50% of individuals. The therapeutic index represents the relative safety of a drug and is determined by the ratio between LC_{50} and EC_{50} (Kenakin, 1984). It is relatively easy to determine these drug para-

meters for the intravenous anesthetic agents, most of which produce a response by interacting with specific receptors. The inhalation anesthetics are less amenable to interpretation by these parameters because of the nonspecific nature of their actions and because their receptors are not fully identifiable.

Signal Transduction and Second Messengers

The physicochemical interaction between a drug and a specific receptor triggers a cellular response resulting in a measurable drug effect. This interaction is necessary for cellular communication. Excitable transmembrane proteins (Schwinn, 1993) serve as important means of cell communication to effect cellular and physiologic responses. There are three types of excitable transmembrane proteins: (1) voltage-sensitive ion channels; (2) ligand-gated ion channels; and (3) transmembrane receptors.

Voltage-sensitive ion channels can be considered transport proteins for the translocation of ions through membranes. These transporters are efficient and can transport ions in a very short time, yet they have a large transport capacity that is ion selective between sodium and potassium ions. The function of the voltage-gated sodium channels is to generate the rapid depolarization of the action potential. Local anesthetics block the propagation of action potentials by blocking the voltage-gated sodium channel. The voltage-gated potassium channels will restore the resting membrane potential following the action potential (Wann, 1993).

Nicotinic cholinergic receptors, $GABA_A$, and the serotonin receptors are examples of *ligand-gated ion channels.* These receptors consist of a receptor-binding site that binds the neurotransmitter to a channel formed from several protein subunits (Daniels & Smith, 1993; Schwinn, 1993). Receptor binding causes modulation of the channel to elicit a response. For instance, the site of action of the benzodiazepines is at the $GABA_A$ protein receptor in the CNS (Daniels & Smith, 1993). Binding of a benzodiazepine to the $GABA_A$-receptor increases the affinity of the inhibitory neurotransmitter, GABA, to a specific site on the protein receptor. GABA binding results in an inward flux of chloride ion and a decrease in cellular excitability (Olsen, Stauber, King, Yang, & Dilber, 1986; Richter, 1981).

Activation of *transmembrane receptors* results in a cascade of biochemical changes within the cell to cause signal transduction and amplification by second messengers (Lambert, 1993). The binding of an agonist to its receptor causes a conformational change in the receptor protein that enables the receptor to interact with a second element, a guanine nucleotide protein (G proteins). G protein–coupled receptors include adrenergic, muscarinic, cholinergic, opioid, and dopamine receptors.

Activated G proteins interact with an effector within the cell, either another enzyme system or an ion channel, to produce a physiologic response. Figure 17–8 illustrates the two main enzyme systems that are stimulated by G protein: (1) adenylate cyclase to form cyclic AMP (cAMP); and (2) phospholipase C, resulting in the breakdown of the membrane-bound phospholipid, phosphatidylinositol 4,5-bisphosphate (PIP_2), to yield inositol-1,4,5-triphosphate (IP_3) and diacylglycerol (DAG). Cyclic AMP, IP_3, and DAG serve as second messengers to amplify the initial drug–receptor response.

Furthermore, G proteins can be stimulatory (G_s) or inhibitory (G_i). Beta$_1$-receptor activation interacts with the G_s protein to activate adenylate cyclase, increasing cAMP levels. Stimulation of alpha$_2$ receptors bound to an inhibitory G protein inhibits the activity of adenylate cyclase and decreases cAMP production. Alpha$_1$-adrenoreceptors activate another G protein, G_q (Conklin, Chabre, Wong, Federman, & Bourne, 1992), resulting in IP_3 and DAG production following phospholipase C activation. These second messengers (cAMP, IP_3, and DAG) mediate cellular responses by protein phosphorylation. Cyclic AMP causes phosphorylation and altered cellular responses following stimulation of protein kinase A. Phosphorylation and release of calcium from intracellular stores follow IP_3 and DAG stimulation of protein kinase C (Lambert, 1993).

Drug–Drug Interactions

Current clinical anesthetic practice incorporates the use of many pharmacologic agents that act generally to induce hypnosis, skeletal muscle relaxation, and analgesia and to block reflex responses. Not only do these drugs have specific actions, but a combination of these drugs often produces a variety of different actions and interactions.

A number of pharmacologic principles are relevant to a discussion of drug interactions. *Summation* or an additive dose effect is seen when the combined effect of two or more drugs acting simultaneously is the same as the sum (S) of the effects of the individual drugs ($A + B$) in their selected doses, or $A + B = S$. *Synergism* indicates that the simultaneous total effect of drugs A and B is greater than the effect of either drug A or drug B alone, provided both drugs evoke a similar response ($A + B > A$ or B). *Potentiation,* often considered a special type of synergism, is the augmentation of an effect of drug A by drug B even though drug B may not have any discernible effect on its own ($A + B > A, B = 0$). *Antagonism* is the effect observed when administration of drug A in the presence of drug B decreases the effectiveness of drug B ($A + B < B$). *Agonism* can be seen when an exogenously administered drug mimics the effects observed with endogenous drugs. An exogenously administered drug displays *intrinsic activity* if it can produce an effect usually seen with an endogenous sub-

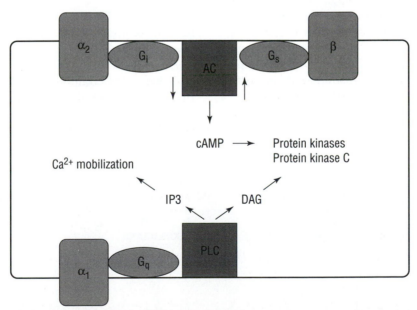

Figure 17–8. Adrenergic receptor subtypes (alpha$_1$ and alpha$_2$; beta) interact with second-messenger systems. Alpha$_1$-receptor interaction with guanine nucleotide proteins (G proteins, G_i, G_s, G_q) results in phospholipase C (PLC) activation and subsequent activation of inositol triphosphate (IP_3) and diacylglycerol (DAG). Alpha$_2$- and beta-receptors activate adenylate cyclase (AC) to produce cyclic AMP (cAMP). *(From Schwinn, D. A. [1993]. Adrenoceptors as models for G protein–coupled receptors: Structure, function and regulation. British Journal of Anaestheia, 71, 80, Figure 5. Copyright 1993 British Journal of Anaesthesia. Reprinted with permission.)*

stance. Drug *allergy* is due to an altered state of reaction to a specific drug or class of drugs produced by a prior sensitization. For example, anaphylaxis is a life-threatening allergic response to a drug that may or may not follow prior drug sensitization. An *idiosyncratic response* is an untoward or abnormal response to a given drug.

Another spectrum of responses includes *tolerance,* which occurs when there is a decreased physiologic response with repeated drug administration of the same or chemically related drug. *Tachyphylaxis* is that special case of tolerance that occurs rapidly with repeated frequent drug administration. *Cumulation* is seen when the body does not completely metabolize one dose of a drug before administration of a second dose. Drug *dependence* may be physical, psychologic, or both. Physical dependence refers to an altered physiologic state that produces profound physiologic symptoms when the drug is suddenly withdrawn. Psychologic dependence denotes emotional reliance on certain drugs. Psychologic dependence often occurs concurrently with physiologic dependence.

Drug interactions may be separated into three categories; however, these categories are strictly a didactic tool. Some drugs, such as the phenothiazines, exhibit interactions that encompass all three categories.

Category 1 includes *pharmacologic interactions* that occur in vitro and in vivo. These drug–drug interactions may be the result of chemical, physical, or physiologic influences. To give several examples, penicillin C and heparin mixed together in a single tube or infusion bag for administration are incompatible; thiopental and opiates cannot be combined together in the same syringe because precipitation will occur; agents that alter gastric pH influence the absorption of acetylsalicylic acid by the gut; and opiate administration alters gastric motility and slows the drug absorption processes.

Category 2 includes *pharmacokinetic factors* that may be attributed to the physiologic state of the patient or the influence of other drugs. As examples, the presence of lipids slows the absorption of alcohol from the gut; alcohol and phenylbutazone alter the plasma protein binding of warfarin; kidney disease prolongs the duration of action of those drugs requiring the kidney as the primary route for elimination; the interaction between succinylcholine and atypical pseudocholinesterase is well documented; propranolol administration produces bronchoconstriction and increases airway resistance, thereby decreasing the ventilation–perfusion ratio in patients; and sulfonamides inhibit and barbiturates stimulate the hepatic microsomal drug-metabolizing enzyme system.

Category 3 includes *pharmacodynamic interactions* resulting from the ongoing effects of endogenous and exogenous drugs as associated with active or silent receptors. For example, halothane produces cardiac arrhythmias when endogenous catecholamine levels are elevated or when exogenous catecholamines are administered simultaneously; administration of a therapeutic concentration of potassium modifies the influence of digitalis on cardiac muscle; and neostigmine alters the effects of succinylcholine.

As drug effects can be strictly quantified only in a mathematical sense, the clinician is constrained to deal with mean distributions for normal and abnormal responses. In the clinical setting, however, this information may not be readily available, and the anesthetist must be aware of and prepared to treat any possible untoward drug interaction response.

Molecular Theories of Anesthetic Action

Several theories of molecular mechanisms of action have been proposed for the inhalation anesthetics. The inhalation anesthetics used in clinical practice (Fig. 17–9) are all halogenated compounds with diverse structures, but the suggestion of a discrete general inhalation anesthetic site needs further investigation. However, a molecular site of action that offers anesthetic specificity and com-

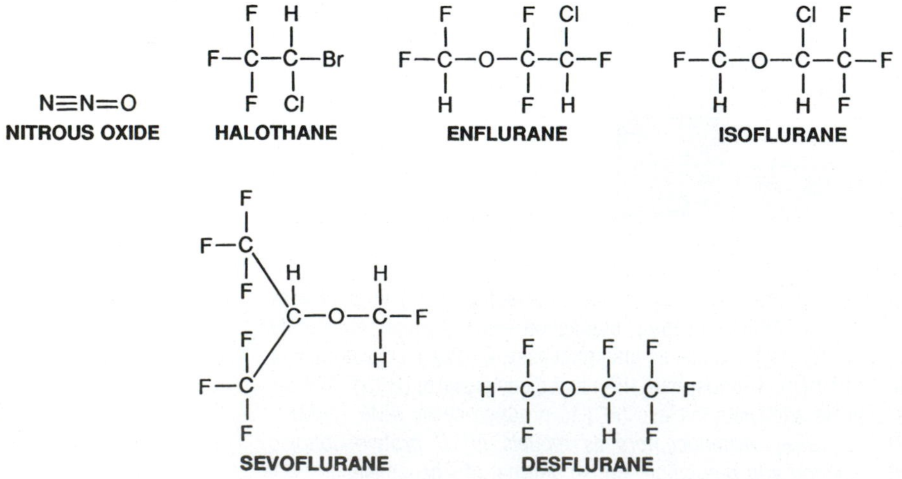

Figure 17–9. Molecular structures of inhalation anesthetics.

bines several different actions most accurately characterize the molecular anesthetic action (Kissin, 1993). This mechanism of action may be unique in current receptor theory. Theories of anesthetic mechanisms include (1) the lipid theory; (2) the physicochemical theory; and (3) the molecular mechanism theory.

The *lipid theory,* described in 1901, is based on the affinity of an anesthetic molecule for lipid, specifically nerve cell membranes composed of a lipid matrix. The potency of an anesthetic correlates with its degree of lipid solubility. Oil : gas coefficients for the inhalation anesthetics are a measure of the lipid solubility of these agents. Miller, Paton, Smith, and Smith (1973) studied the *physicochemical theory,* which explains that the lipid component of the nerve cell membrane expands and thereby increases fluidity or perturbs the membrane, which can lead to an alteration in the membrane channels and result in an anesthetic action. This expansion in the physicochemical properties of the nerve cells can be reversed at high hydrostatic pressures.

Advances in molecular pharmacology have led to investigations into *molecular mechanisms* of anesthetic action. Research since the mid-1980s has focused on the inhibitory neurotransmitter GABA as a molecular mechanism of action for inhalation anesthetics: benzodiazepines, barbiturates, propofol, and etomidate (Cheng & Brunner, 1975, 1984, 1985; Franks & Lieb, 1994; Pocock & Richards, 1993). GABA is the primary inhibitory neurotransmitter in the CNS. Two GABA-receptors have been identified: $GABA_A$- and $GABA_B$-receptors. These receptors are functionally distinct; the $GABA_A$-receptor is a ligand-gated ion channel, and the $GABA_B$-receptor is a G protein coupled receptor. The $GABA_A$-receptor is composed of five membrane-spanning subunits forming the receptor channel, GABA activation of this receptor results in a fast inhibitory postsynaptic potential; activation of the $GABA_B$-receptor causes a slow protracted inhibitory signal (McCormick, 1989).

The mechanism of action of both benzodiazepines and barbiturates is linked to GABA transmission. The intravenous anesthetic propofol also activates the $GABA_A$-receptor channel (Hara, Kai, & Ikemoto, 1994). At clinical concentrations, two or more molecules of propofol activate the channel, leading to an increase in chloride conduction and synaptic inhibition. Furthermore, the binding site of propofol is distinct from the binding sites of benzodiazepines, barbiturates, and steroids.

Early studies demonstrated that clinical concentrations of halothane, enflurane, and isoflurane enhanced the GABA-induced ionic current, resulting in postsynaptic membrane hyperpolarization (Nakahiro, Yeh, Brunner, & Narahashi, 1989). Cheng and Brunner (1985) found that the GABA analog 4,5,6,7-tetrahydroisoxazolo[5,4-*c*] pyridin-3-ol (THIP) is capable of inducing general anesthesia. In a separate study (Fontenot, Wilson, Norris, & Ho,

1984), the use of GABA agonists and antagonists caused an increase or decrease, respectively, in the amount of sleep induced by halothane anesthesia. These "receptor-specific" actions suggested that general anesthetic action may occur directly on a specific target site. To substantiate the receptor specificity further, Harris, Moody, and Skolnick (1992) demonstrated the stereoselectivity of isoflurane binding. In 1996 Mason, Owens, and Hammond identified the $GABA_A$-receptor subtype in the spinal cord of rats as the site of the nocifensive action of halothane. Rengasamy, Pajewski, and Johns (1997) investigated the effect of isoflurane on the N-methyl-D-aspartate (NMDA) receptor, an excitatory neurotransmitter receptor in the brain. In addition, NMDA increases nitric oxide and cyclic guanine monophosphate (cGMP) levels in the brain; after isoflurane administration, NMDA stimulated nitric oxide synthase activity and decreased cGMP levels. It was also found that NMDA receptor antagonists decrease minimum alveolar concentration values of inhalation anesthetics (Scheller, Zornow, Fleischer, Shearman, & Gerber, 1989), which might suggest that the NMDA receptor is involved in an inhalation anesthetic site of action. The potential variety of sites of action for the chemically and behaviorally diverse inhalation agents supports the idea that there is a "multisite agent-specific theory of anesthesia" where the anesthetics can act at specific sites, yet undergo unique mechanisms to produce CNS depression (Tanelian, Kosek, Mody, & McIver, 1993). This may begin to explain the behavioral diversity seen among inhalation anesthetics.

Significant advances have been made in explaining the mechanism of action of general anesthetics. Such advances will improve current drug delivery and allow for the discovery of new drugs that have safe and effective anesthetic action.

▶ CASE STUDY

A 58-year-old male arrives in the emergency room after a motor vehicle accident. He has sustained a right leg fracture necessitating emergency surgery for an open reduction and internal fixation of his right tibia.

His past medical history is remarkable for chronic active hepatitis. The patient had a hernia repair under spinal anesthesia 15 years ago without complications. He does not take any medications, over-the-counter drugs, or drugs of abuse. Smoking history reveals a 25-pack-year history. Laboratory values are normal except for elevated liver function tests. His serum glutamic oxaloacetic (SGOT) and serum glutamic pyruvic transaminase (SGPT) levels are twice the normal levels.

1. Describe the pharmacologic agents that can be used to induce anesthesia.

Propofol or sodium thiopental can be used to induce anesthesia. To secure the airway, a rapid sequence induction and endotracheal intubation are necessary as it must be assumed this patient has a full stomach and is at risk for pulmonary aspiration and airway compromise. Succinylcholine, a depolarizing muscle relaxant, is the agent of choice to cause muscle relaxation within seconds.

A second agent of choice would be rocuronium. In high doses (1 to 1.2 mg/kg) this nondepolarizing muscle relaxant provides adequate muscle relaxation to facilitate endotracheal intubation in less than 90 seconds.

2. What type of general anesthetic agent is appropriate for anesthesia maintenance?

The inhalation anesthetic isoflurane has minimal hepatic metabolism and would be appropriate for anesthesia maintenance. A second type of anesthetic technique could be total intravenous anesthesia using narcotics. Fentanyl is an appropriate narcotic agent. It does have a rapid onset of action (30 to 60 seconds), and its short duration of activity following single doses reflects its redistribution to inactive tissue sites. It does have a prolonged elimination half-life (approximately 200 minutes), which suggests that during prolonged cases with continuous dosing the clinical activity of fentanyl would be prolonged. Remifentanil, due to its rapid hydrolysis by plasma esterases, has a very short clinical duration. Postoperative analgesia must be considered.

► SUMMARY

Successful use of pharmacologic agents in anesthesia depends on a strong foundation of knowledge of the basic principles of pharmacology. Understanding chemical principles of structure and bonding, acid–base chemistry, biochemical principles of cell membrane structure, energy requirements, and enzyme kinetics are essential to understanding drug action. The action of a drug in vivo depends on its pharmacodynamic and pharmacokinetic properties. Following delivery of the drug to its site of action, drug–receptor interaction allows for signal transduction and second-messenger amplification that result in drug effect. As the molecular theories of anesthetic action become more fully identified and understood, the pharmacologic foundation of knowledge for a wide range of anesthetics, such as propofol, barbiturates, and inhalation anesthetics, will expand.

► KEY CONCEPTS

- In the outer shell of elements, a configuration of eight electrons forms a stable compound. Two elements that interact through their electrons in the outer shell will combine to reach a full complement of eight electrons.
- Organic compounds can be divided into classes based on functional groups that change the physical properties of the basic compound, altering its lipid solubility and electrical charge.
- The Henderson–Hasselbach equation expresses the relationship between the pH and the pKa of a solution and calculates the degree of ionization.
- The absorption of drugs across biologic membranes and the distribution to active sites may be limited by the physical and chemical characteristics of the drug and by the cellular barriers.
- Bioactive, lipophilic substances are not readily eliminated by the body and must be metabolized to water-soluble substances.
- The half-life of a drug is the time required for the plasma concentration of the drug to be reduced by 50% and indicates the time required for drug elimination from the body.
- The physicochemical interaction between a drug and a specific receptor triggers a cellular response via excitable transmembrane proteins: voltage-sensitive ion channels, ligand-gated ion channels, and transmembrane receptors.
- The inhibitory neurotransmitter gamma amino butyric acid (GABA) may function as a site for the molecular mechanism of action of inhalation anesthetics, barbiturates, benzodiazepines, propofol, and etomidate.

► STUDY QUESTIONS

1. The inhalation anesthetics differ in structure. Describe the differences in their structure by identifying the chemical bonds and the functional groups.

2. What is the relationship between tissue solubility, protein binding, and ionization on the volume of distribution of the muscle relaxant vecuronium?

3. How does carbon dioxide, the end product of cellular metabolism, function to regulate the body's pH?

4. Drug–receptor binding stimulates a series of steps resulting in a cellular response. How are G proteins and second messengers (ie, cAMP and diacylglycerol) important in the development of cellular response?

5. Many molecular theories of action for inhalation and intravenous anesthetics involve GABA function. What is the proposed mechanism of action for isoflurane, midazolam, sodium pentothal, and propofol?

KEY REFERENCES

Franks, N. P. & Leb, W. R. (1994). Molecular and cellular mechanisms of general anaesthesia. *Nature, 367,* 607–613.

Kissin, I. (1993). General anesthetic action: An obsolete notion? *Anesthesia & Analgesia, 76,* 215–218.

Lambert, D. G. (1993). Signal transduction: G proteins and second messengers. *British Journal of Anaesthesia, 71,* 86–95.

Pocock, G. & Richards, C. D. (1993). Excitatory and inhibitory synaptic mechanisms in anaesthesia. *British Journal of Anaesthesia, 71,* 134–147.

Ruffolo, R. R., (1982). Review: Important concepts of receptor theory. *Journal of Autonomic Pharmacology, 2,* 277–295.

REFERENCES

Benet, L. Z., Kroetz, D. L., & Sheiner, L. B. (1996). Pharmacokinetics: The dynamics of drug absorption, distribution, and elimination. In J. G. Hardman & L. E. Limbird (Eds.), *Goodman & Gilman's The pharmacologic basis of therapeutics* (9th ed.) (pp. 3–28). New York: McGraw-Hill.

Cheng, S. C. & Brunner, E. A. (1975). A neurochemical hypothesis for halothane anesthesia. *Anesthesia & Analgesia, 54,* 242–246.

Cheng, S. C. & Brunner, E. A. (1984). Anesthetic effects on GABA binding. *Anesthesiology, 61,* A326. Abstract.

Cheng, S. C. & Brunner, E. A. (1985). Inducing anesthesia with a GABA analog, THIP. *Anesthesiology, 63,* 147–151.

Conklin, B. R., Chabre, O., Wong, Y. H., Federman, A. D., & Bourne, H. R. (1992). Recombinant Gq alpha. *Journal of Biological Chemistry, 267,* 31–34.

Conney, A. H. (1967). Pharmacological implications of microsomal enzyme induction. *Pharmacologic Reviews, 19,* 317–320.

Daniels, S. & Smith, E. B. (1993). Effects of general anaesthetics on ligand-gated ion channels. *British Journal of Anaesthesia, 71,* 59–64.

Doenicke, A., Kugler, J., Mayer, M., & Hoffmann, P. (1992). Ketamine racemate or S-(+)-ketamine and midazolam. The effect on vigilance, efficacy and subjective findings. *Anaesthetist, 41,* 610–618.

Egan, T. D., Lemmens, H. J. M., Fiset, P., Hermann, D. J., Muir, K. T., Stanski, D. R., & Shafer, S. L. (1993). The pharmacokinetics of the new short-acting opioid remifentanil (GI87084B) in healthy adult male volunteers. *Anesthesiology, 79,* 881–892.

Fahey, M. R., Morris, R. B., Miller, R. D., Sohn, Y. J., Cronnelly, R., & Gencarelli, P. (1981). Clinical pharmacology of ORG NC45 (Norcuron). *Anesthesiology, 55,* 6–11.

Fisher, D. M., Canfell, P. C., Fahey, M. R., Rosen, J. I., Rupp, S. M., Sheiner, L. B., & Miller, R. D. (1986). Elimination of atracurium in humans: Contributions of Hofmann elimination and ester hydrolysis versus organ-based elimination. *Anesthesiology, 65,* 6–12.

Fontenot, H. J., Wilson, R. D., Norris, J. C., & Ho, I. K. (1984). The GABA system: New evidence of neurotransmitter involvement in the mechanism of anesthesia. *Anesthesiology, 61,* A327.

Franks, N. P. & Lieb, W. R. (1994). Molecular and cellular mechanisms of general anaesthesia. *Nature, 367,* 607–613.

Greenblatt, D. J., Locniskar, A., Scavone, J. M., Blyden, G. T., Ochs, H. R., Harmatz, J. S., & Shader, R. I. (1986). Absence of interaction of cimetidine and ranitidine with intravenous and oral midazolam. *Anesthesia & Analgesia, 65,* 176–180.

Gruenke, L. D., Konapka, K., Koop, D. R., & Waskell, L. D. (1988). Characterization of halothane oxidation by hepatic microsomes and purified cytochrome P450 using a gas chromatographic mass spectrometric assay. *Journal of Experimental Pharmacotherapeutics, 246,* 345–350.

Hara, M., Kai, Y., & Ikemoto, Y. (1994). Enhancement by propofol of the gamma-aminobutyric acid$_A$ response in dissociated hippocampal pyramidal neurons of the rat. *Anesthesiology, 81,* 988–994.

Harris, B., Moody, E., & Skolnick P. (1992). Isoflurane anesthesia is stereoselective. *European Journal of Pharmacology, 217,* 215–216.

Henderson, J. M., Brodsky, D. A., Fisher, D. M., Brett, C. M., & Hertzka, R. E. (1988). Pre-induction of anesthesia in pediatric patients with nasally administered sufentanil. *Anesthesiology, 68,* 671–675.

Hobbs, A. J., Fukuto, J. M., & Ignarro, L. J. (1994). Formation of free nitric oxide from L-arginine by nitric oxide synthase: Direct enhancement of generation by superoxide dismutase. *Proceedings of the National Academy of Science, 91,* 10992–10996.

Kanto, J. (1986). Obstetric analgesia: Clinical pharmacokinetic considerations. *Clinical Pharmacokinetics, 11,* 283–298.

Kenakin, T. P. (1984). The classification of drugs and drug receptors in isolated tissues. *Pharmacological Reviews, 36,* 165–222.

Kissin, I. (1993). General anesthetic action: An obsolete notion? *Anesthesia & Analgesia, 76,* 215–218.

Kotz, J. C., & Purcell, K. F. (1991). *Chemistry and chemical reactivity* (2nd ed.). Philadelphia: W. B. Saunders.

Lambert, D. G. (1993). Signal transduction: G proteins and second messengers. *British Journal of Anaesthesia, 71,* 86–95.

Le Bel, L. A. (1992a). Principles of chemistry and physics in anesthesia. In W. R. Waugaman, S. D. Foster, & B. M. Rigor (Eds.), *Principles and practice of nurse anesthesia* (2nd ed., pp. 57–84). Norwalk, CT: Appleton & Lange.

Le Bel, L. A. (1992b). Principles of organic chemistry and biochemistry in anesthesia. In W. R. Waugaman, S. D. Foster, & B. M. Rigor (Eds.), *Principles and practice of nurse anesthesia* (2nd ed., pp. 85–104). Norwalk, CT: Appleton & Lange.

Levine, R. R. (1996). *Pharmacology: Drug actions and reactions* (5th ed.). New York: Parthenon.

Lien, C. A., Schmith, V. D., Belmont, M. R., Abalos, A., Kisor, D. F., & Savarese, J. J. (1996). Pharmacokinetics of cisatracurium in patients receiving nitrous oxide/opioid/barbiturate anesthesia. *Anesthesiology, 84,* 300–308.

Marks, D. B., Marks, A. D., & Smith, C. M. (1996). *Basic medical biochemistry: A clinical approach.* Baltimore: Williams & Wilkins.

Mason, P., Owen, C. A., & Hammond, D. L. (1996). Antagonism of the antinocifensive action of halothane by intrathecal administration of GABA$_A$ receptor antagonists. *Anesthesiology, 84,* 1204–1214.

McCormick, D. A. (1989). GABA as an inhibitory neurotransmitter in human cerebral cortex. *Journal of Neurophysiology, 62,* 1018–1027.

Miller, K. W., Paton, W. D., Smith, R. A., & Smith, E. B. (1973). The pressure reversal of general anesthesia and the critical volume hypothesis. *Molecular Pharmacology, 9,* 131–143.

Mock, D. L., Streisand, J. B., Hague, B., Dzelzkalns, R. R., Bailey, P. L. Pace, N. L., & Stanley, T. H. (1986). Transmucosal narcotic delivery: An evaluation of fentanyl (lollipop) premedication in man. *Anesthesia & Analgesia, 6,* S102.

Nakahiro, M., Yeh, J. Z., Brunner, E., & Narahashi, T. (1989). General anesthetics modulate GABA receptor channel complex in rat dorsal root ganglion neurons. *FASEB Journal, 3,* 1850–1854.

Nebert, D. W. & Gonzalez, F. J. (1987). P450 genes: Structure, evolution and regulation. *Annual Review of Biochemistry 56,* 945–993.

Olsen, R. W., Stauber, G. B., King, R. G., Yang, J., & Dilber, A. (1986). Structure and function of the barbiturate-modulated benzodiazepine/GABA receptor protein complex. In G. Biggio & E. Costa, (Eds.), *GABAergic transmission and anxiety* (pp. 21–49). New York: Raven.

Palmer, R. M. J., Rees, D. D., Ashton, D. S., & Moncada, S. (1988). L-arginine is the physiological precursor for the formation of nitric oxide in endothelium-dependent relaxation. *Biochemical and Biophysical Research Communications, 153,* 1251–1256.

Pardridge, W. M. (1988). Recent advances in blood–brain barrier transport. *Annual Review Pharmacology and Toxicology, 28,* 25–39.

Pocock, G., & Richards, C. D. (1993). Excitatory and inhibitory synaptic mechanisms in anaesthesia. *British Journal of Anaesthesia, 71,* 134–147.

Puhringer, F. K., Khuenl-Brady, K. S., Koller, J., & Mitter-schiffthaler, G. (1992). Evaluation of the endotracheal intubating conditions of rocuronium (ORG 9426) and succinylcholine in outpatient surgery. *Anesthesia & Analgesia, 75,* 37–40.

Rehder, K., Forbes J., Aller H., Hessler, O., & Stier, A. (1967). Halothane biotransformation in man, a quantitative study. *Anesthesiology, 45,* 622–625.

Rengasamy, A., Pajewski, T. N., & Johns, R. A. (1997). Inhalational anesthetic effects on rat cerebellar nitric oxide and cyclic guanosine monophosphate production. *Anesthesiology, 86,* 689–698.

Rich, G. F., Murphy, G. D., Roos, C. M., & Johns, R. A. (1993). Inhaled nitric oxide: Selective pulmonary vasodilation in cardiac surgical patients. *Anesthesiology, 78,* 1028–1035.

Richter, J. J. (1981). Current theories about the mechanisms of benzodiazepines and neuroleptic drugs. *Anesthesiology, 54,* 66–72.

Ross, E. M. (1996). Pharmacodynamics: Mechanisms of drug action and the relationship between drug concentration and effect. In J. G. Hardman & L. E. Limbird (Eds.), *Goodman & Gilman's The pharmacologic basis of therapeutics* (9th ed., pp. 29–42). New York: McGraw-Hill.

Ruffolo, R. R. (1982). Review: Important concepts of receptor theory. *Journal of Autonomic Pharmacology, 2,* 277–295.

Scheller, M. S., Zornow, M. H., Fleischer, J. E., Shearman, G. T., & Greber, T. F. (1989). The noncompetitive N-methyl-D-aspartate receptor antagonist, MK-801 profoundly reduces volatile anesthetic requirements in rabbits. *Neuropharmacology, 28,* 677–681.

Schwinn, D. A. (1993). Adrenoceptors as models for G protein–coupled receptors: Structure, function and regulation. *British Journal of Anaesthesia, 71,* 77–85.

Sinclair, R., Cassuto, J., Hogstrom, S., Linden, I., Faxen, A., Hedner, T., & Ekman, R. (1988). Topical anesthesia with lidocaine aerosol in the control of postoperative pain. *Anesthesiology, 68,* 895–90l.

Sipes, I. G. & Brown, B. R., Jr. (1976). An animal model of hepatotoxicity associated with halothane anesthesia. *Anesthesiology, 45,* 622–628.

Stanley, J. C., Mirajhur, R. K., Bell, P. F., Sharpe, D. E., & Clarke, R. S. J. (1991). Neuromuscular effects of pipecuronium bromide. *European Journal of Anaesthesiology, 8,* 151–156.

Stryer, L. (1995). *Biochemistry* (4th ed.). New York: Freeman.

Tanelian, D. L, Kosek, P., Mody, I., & MacIver, M. B. (1993). The role of the $GABA_A$ receptor/chloride channel complex in anesthesia. *Anesthesiology, 78,* 757–776.

Vollhardt, K. P. C. & Schore, N. E. (1994). *Organic chemistry* (2nd ed.). New York: Freeman.

Wann, K. T. (1993). Neuronal sodium and potassium channels: Structure and function. *British Journal of Anaesthesia, 71,* 2–14.

Westmoreland, C. L., Hoke, J. F., Sebel, P. S., Hug, C. C., & Muir, K. T. (1993). Pharmacokinetics of remifentanil (GI87084B) in patients undergoing elective inpatient surgery. *Anesthesiology, 79,* 893–903.

Wilson, C. M., Dundee, J. W., Moore, J., Howard, P. J., & Collier, P. S. (1987). A comparison of the early pharmacokinetics of midazolam in pregnant and nonpregnant women. *Anaesthesia, 42,* 1057–1062.

Winter, M. (1994). *Basic clinical pharmacokinetics* (3rd ed.). Vancouver, WA: Applied Therapeutics.

Wood, M. (1986). Plasma drug binding: Implications for anesthesiologists. *Anesthesia & Analgesia, 65,* 786–804.

Inhaled Anesthetics

Michele E. Gold and Linda S. Finander

The physical principles of states of matter, solubility, vapor pressures, and therapeutic gases are presented to provide a foundation for understanding the uptake and distribution of inhaled anesthetics. The uptake and distribution of inhaled anesthetics differ with each agent, and a comparative analysis of the inhaled anesthetics is presented in this chapter. The minimum alveolar concentrations (MAC) of anesthetics is defined, along with the impact of drug solubility, physiologic circulation, tissue uptake, and ventilation–perfusion abnormalities on delivery of the inhaled agents.

The inhaled agents halothane, enflurane, isoflurane, desflurane, sevoflurane, and nitrous oxide have important clinical effects. The anesthetist must know the effects of these agents on the cardiac, renal, pulmonary, and central nervous systems. This chapter provides the anesthetist with information necessary to make a rational choice of inhaled agent for any surgical procedure.

▶ PHYSICAL PRINCIPLES OF DRUG ACTION

The inhalation agents used in anesthesia are defined by physical laws and concepts that differ from the pharmacologic principles of intravenous agents. Inhalation agents are vaporized. The ability of the inhalation agents to function as effective and safe anesthetics is determined by the physical principles of solubility, vapor pressure, and gas laws.

States of Matter

The three states of matter (gases, liquids, and solids) are differentiated by the activity of the molecules that make up the substance. Water is the most familiar example of a compound that can exist in all three states of matter. The activity exerted on water, that is, temperature, can alter its state. Liquid water can be cooled to a solid form that has definite shape and cannot be compressed by the molecular forces drawing together. Alternatively, heat can be applied to water to accelerate molecular activity and create a gas. The same principle applies to liquid anesthetics (halothane, enflurane, isoflurane, desflurane, and sevoflurane), which are vaporized (Le Bel, 1992).

Oxygen and nitrous oxide are gases administered during anesthesia. Vapor is the gaseous phase of a substance that at ambient temperature and pressure can exist as a liquid. Gas is a substance that does not exist as a liquid at ordinary temperature and pressure. Vaporizers on anesthesia machines function to enrich the gas (oxygen) being delivered to the patient with the vapor of a liquid anesthetic agent. Inside the vaporizer, the surface area of the liquid anesthetic is exposed to a moving stream of oxygen gas. A portion of the liquid molecules can overcome the cohesive forces of the liquid to escape into the surrounding atmosphere. This vapor is then carried by the oxygen, which is mixed and diluted with nitrous oxide and additional oxygen. The final concentration of anesthetic vapor depends on the flow of carrier gas and the total flow delivered to the patient. In a closed container the molecules that escape the liquid phase to enter the gaseous phase reach an equilibrium, at which time a vapor pressure is exerted by the gas over the liquid. Vapor pressure can be increased by high temperatures that allow more molecules to escape from the liquid. Anesthesia vaporizers are temperature regulated to prevent this occurrence.

The Gas Laws

The actions of gases and vapors follow the ideal gas laws that exist in a specialized environment where no inter-molecular forces are exerted. In anesthesia, the gases and vapors deviate from ideal gases because they are subject to specific forces: Van der Waal's forces. The net effect of these forces is not generally significant, and it can be assumed that the anesthetic gases approximate the ideal gas laws (Davis, Parbrook, & Kenny, 1995). The first gas law is Boyle's law. Boyle's law states that at constant temperature the volume of a given mass of gas varies inversely with the absolute pressure. Boyle's law explains the increase in pressure when the volume occupied by a vapor is decreased and the temperature remains constant. When the volume of a gas decreases by one half, the pressure is doubled. The second gas law is Charles' or Gay-Lussac's law. Charles' law states that at constant pressure, the volume of a gas varies directly with the temperature. This law explains that a gas will expand or increase in volume when heated, and will become less dense. The third ideal gas law states that at constant volume, the pressure of a gas varies directly with temperature. This third gas law explains the increase in pressure seen when heat is exerted on a gas in a closed container. As the temperature of the gas increases, the pressure increases proportionately.

Calculation of volume of the ideal gases must be done on the basis of standard temperature (0°C) and standard pressure (STP, 760 mmHg). A general gas law combines all three gas laws and is calculated at STP to determine the relationship of all variables that affect the behavior of an ideal gas.

Dalton's law of partial pressure of gases also explains how gases behave. This law states that the total pressure exerted by a mixture of gases is equal to the sum of the partial pressures exerted by the individual gases. A cylinder of ambient air containing approximately 21% oxygen mixed with 79% nitrogen can be used as an example of Dalton's law. Atmospheric pressure is 760 mmHg. The partial pressures exerted by oxygen and nitrogen, respectively, are 159 mmHg and 593 mmHg. Dalton's law also applies to the delivery of an inhalation anesthetic. When liquid volatile anesthetics are vaporized, they become a constituent of the combined gas mixture and exert a partial pressure. When delivering a 50:50 gas mixture of nitrous oxide and oxygen at a 5-L flow (2500 mL of nitrous oxide and 2500 mL of oxygen) combined with 100 mL of carrier gas and 50 mL of anesthetic vapor, the final anesthetic concentration is approximately 1%.

Solubility Coefficients

The solubility of gases in liquids can be explained by Henry's law (Davis et al., 1995), which states that, when temperature is constant, the amount of gas dissolved in a liquid is directly proportional to the partial pressure of the gas in equilibrium with the liquid. The diffusion of anesthetic molecules from the alveoli to the blood and between blood and other body tissues flows in accordance with Henry's law. The gas tensions that develop between the two interphases determine the amount of anesthetic agent transfer and influence the time for induction and emergence from anesthesia.

The volume of gas dissolved in a liquid can be described by the Bunsen solubility coefficient or the Ostwald solubility coefficient. The Ostwald solubility coefficient has preferred applicability in anesthesia practice and is closely related to another parameter, the partition coefficient. The Ostwald solubility coefficient is a measure of the volume of gas that dissolves in a unit volume of liquid at ambient temperature. The partition coefficient is defined as the ratio of the volume of gas that can dissolve in the same volume of a liquid phase, such as blood or tissue.

The concepts of Ostwald solubility coefficient and partition coefficient have clinical applications to the uptake of anesthetics and can provide information regarding how rapidly an anesthetic agent acts. The inhalation agent ether has an Ostwald solubility of 12, which suggests that ether is very soluble in blood (12 molecules of ether can partition into the liquid phase, blood). As ether solubilizes into blood, its alveolar concentration is low, which mimics low blood and brain concentrations of ether. Sevoflurane and desflurane are less soluble and have Ostwald solubility coefficients of 0.65 and 0.42, respectively (Table 18–1). The low solubility is responsible for the development of an alveolar concentration approximating the inspired concentration in 10 to 15 minutes resulting in a rapid onset of anesthesia.

The Therapeutic Gases

The gaseous agents oxygen, nitrous oxide, nitrogen, carbon dioxide, and helium have medical applications in anesthesia and respiratory therapy. Oxygen is the most widely used. It is stored as a compressed gas in green or green and white cylinders of various sizes at pressures of approximately 2000 psi. Oxygen can be delivered in various concentrations by mask, nasal catheter, or endotracheal tube. It comprises one fifth of the atmosphere and is essential for delivery in anesthesia. Nitrous oxide is stored as a liquid in blue cylinders at 750 psi and is given as a mixture with either air or oxygen. Nitrous oxide is relatively insoluble in blood, which accounts for its rapid action on induction and emergence from anesthesia. Because of its rapid diffusibility, nitrous oxide enters closed body compartments and may be cause for concern in patients with a bowel obstruction or during surgery. Carbon dioxide is the biochemical end product of the body's respiration. In the past, inhalation of 5% carbon dioxide was used as a respiratory stimulant. This is no

TABLE 18–1. Physical Properties of Inhalation Anesthetics

	Halothane	Enflurane	Isoflurane	Desflurane	Sevoflurane	Nitrous Oxide
Molecular weight (g)	197.4	184.5	184.0	168.0	200	44.0
Boiling point (°C)	50.2	56.5	48.5		58.5	−88.0
Vapor pressure at 20°C	243.0	175.0	250.0	664.0	157.0	39 000
Partition coefficient at 37°C						
Blood : gas	2.3	1.9	1.4	0.42	0.65	0.47
Oil : gas	224.0	98.5	97.8	18.7	53.4	1.4
Water : gas	0.7	0.8	0.61			0.47
Brain : blood	2.0	1.4	1.6	1.3	1.7	1.1
Fat : blood	62.0	36.0	52.0	30.0	55.0	2.3
Minimum alveolar concentration (%)	0.75	1.7	1.3	6.0	2.1	110
Metabolites (%, approximate)	15–20	2.4–9	0.2	0.02–0.2	2–5	

Sources: Wallin, W. F., Regan, B. M., Napoli, M. D., & Stern, I. J. (1975). Sevofluorane: A new inhalational anesthetic agent. Anesthesia & Analgesia, 54, 758; Wade, J. G. & Stevens, W. C. (1981). Isoflurane: An Anesthetic for the eighties? Anesthesia & Analgesia, 60, 667–682; Koblin, O. D., Weiskopf, R. B., Holmes, M. A., Konopka, K., Rampil, I. J., Eger, E. I., & Waskell, L. (1989). Metabolism of I-653 and isoflurane in swine. Anesthesia & Analgesia, 68, 147; Eger, E. I. (1994). New inhaled anesthetics. Anesthesiology, 80, 907.

longer an acceptable technique due to the potential disadvantages of inhaled carbon dioxide. End-tidal carbon dioxide monitors are standard for measuring exhaled carbon dioxide levels in anesthetized patients. Nitrogen and helium have limited medical use in anesthesia. Both are used as diluents with oxygen. Helium–oxygen mixtures are used in patients with severe respiratory obstruction. Nitrogen has been used as a cooling agent in cryosurgery and to freeze tissue samples (Le Bel, 1992).

▶ UPTAKE AND DISTRIBUTION OF INHALATION AGENTS

The pharmacologic properties of the inhalation agents used in anesthesia differ significantly from those of the intravenous agents. The most striking difference is the unique mechanism of action of the inhalation agents. Because the inhalation agents are gaseous molecules that can interact with particular nerve cell membranes to cause an alteration in synaptic transmission, distinct pharmacodynamic and pharmacokinetic properties, including uptake and distribution, metabolism and recovery, apply to these anesthetics.

Minimum Alveolar Concentration

The minimum alveolar concentration (MAC) of an inhaled anesthetic relates the inhalation anesthetic concentration to the observed effect and is a measure of anesthetic potency. The MAC is defined by the concentration of anesthetic that produces immobility in 50% of those patients or animals exposed to a noxious stimulus (Eger, 1974). Therefore, the MAC indicates the relative concentration of anesthetic necessary to achieve surgical anesthesia. The MAC is measured as the alveolar partial pressure of anesthetic, which reflects the partial pressure of

anesthetic at the active site, the brain, at equilibrium. Clinical measurements of intraoperative anesthetic concentrations have been made easy by the advent of mass spectrometry. The MAC values of the inhalation anesthetics are noted in Table 18-1. The MAC values of the various anesthetic agents are used as the basis for comparison among agents: 1-MAC levels of these agents produce equivalent anesthetic states. In addition, MAC values of the anesthetics are additive: A combination of 0.5 MAC of nitrous oxide with 0.5 MAC of halothane produces the same anesthetic effect as each agent used separately. In addition, Drasner, Bernards, and Ozanne (1988) and Valverde, Dyson, and McDonnell (1989) demonstrated that the simultaneous use of other anesthetic agents such as intrathecal morphine with inhalation anesthetics has been shown to cause a reduction in the anesthetic requirements of the inhalation anesthetics.

Many factors are known to alter anesthetic requirements, necessitating an increase or decrease in MAC. For example, hyperthermia, chronic alcohol abuse, and young age (ie, neonates) may increase the anesthetic requirement, whereas hypothermia, pregnancy, preoperative medication, hypotension, and advancing age may decrease MAC (Antognini, 1993; Eger, 1974).

Partial Pressure of Inhaled Anesthetics

The principal objective of inhalation anesthesia is to deliver an optimal concentration of drug to the site of anesthetic action, the brain. Administration of an inhalation anesthetic results in a partial pressure gradient of anesthetic at the alveolar–arterial membrane. The desired anesthetic effect occurs when the partial pressure at the alveolar–arterial membrane is equal to the partial pressure in the brain. The partial pressure at the alveolar membrane is an indirect measure of concentration of anesthetic in the brain. The partial pressure of a gas is described by Dalton's law, which states that the tension (pressure) of an individual gas in a mixture of gases is proportional to its concentration (Dale & Brown, 1987). Development of the alveolar partial pressure depends on the concentration of the inspired anesthetic (concentration effect), the presence of a second gas (second-gas effect), the ventilatory rate, and the solubility of the gas in blood. An increase in these parameters affects the speed of induction of anesthesia.

The concentration effect describes the impact of the inspired concentration of anesthetic on the rate at which the alveolar partial pressure can equilibrate with the inspired concentration. A high inspired concentration of anesthetic will accelerate the rate at which the alveolar partial pressure rises. This principle is demonstrated during the induction of an anesthetic because the initial concentration of anesthetic delivered to the patient is higher than the MAC of that anesthetic. The use of nitrous oxide during the induction of anesthesia also influences the rate at which alveolar partial pressure reaches equilibrium with the inspired partial pressure. Figure 18-1 illustrates the effect of high inspired concentrations of nitrous oxide on a second, more potent anesthetic agent such as halothane, which is delivered at a higher concentration because its inspiratory inflow is augmented (Epstein, Rackow, Salanitre, & Wolf, 1964). It is important to recognize, however, that the effect of delivering a high initial concentration of an anesthetic or concurrent administration of a high nitrous oxide concentration on the rate of anesthetic equilibration in the lung depends on ventilation. The inhalation anesthetics are respiratory depressants that impair the inflow of anesthesia and slow induction. This can be overcome by mechanical ventilation of the patient to provide an adequate anesthetic depth.

Uptake and Distribution

The inspired concentration of an inhalation anesthetic influences the rate at which the anesthetic reaches equilibrium and therefore influences the induction of anesthesia. The inspired concentration of anesthetic is offset by the uptake of inhalation agent from the alveolus into the bloodstream. Anesthetic uptake depends on (1) the solubility of the anesthetic in blood; (2) the circulatory system (ie, cardiac output); and (3) tissue uptake of anesthesia.

Anesthetic solubility is a physical property of the individual drug and is measured as the degree to which the drug can partition itself between a gaseous phase and a liquid phase at equilibrium. Blood:gas partition coefficients have been determined for the inhalation anesthetics in clinical use (Table 18-1) and are used as a relative index of solubility: The more insoluble an anesthetic agent (ie, nitrous oxide, desflurane, and sevoflurane), the sooner equilibrium of the alveolar partial pressure gradi-

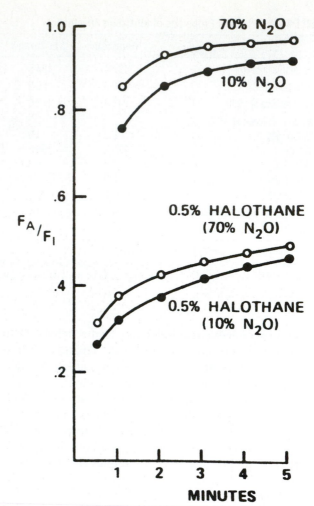

Figure 18–1. Uptake of nitrous oxide (N_2O) and halothane is plotted as the ratio of the alveolar anesthetic concentration (F_A) to inspired concentration (F_I) for each agent. High inspired concentrations of nitrous oxide can augment the inspiratory inflow of halothane. *(From Epstein, R. M., Rackow, H., Salanitre, E., & Wolf, G. L. [1964]. Influence of the concentration effect on the uptake of anesthetic mixtures: The second gas effect.* Anesthesiology, 25, *367. Copyright 1964 by the American Society of Anesthesiologists. Reprinted with permission.)*

ent is reached. The more potent inhalation anesthetics (ie, halothane, enflurane, and isoflurane) are moderately soluble, indicating that a larger amount of anesthetic needs to be dissolved in the blood before a state of equilibrium is reached and an anesthetic effect observed (Fig. 18-2). Again, the use of high inspired initial concentrations of these anesthetics (greater than the MAC) will overcome the solubility factor and speed induction.

Cardiac output carries blood away from the lung and increases the uptake of anesthetic into the blood from the alveolus. This produces a decrease in the alveolar concentration of the anesthetic. An increase in cardiac output slows the rate of induction of anesthesia because the larger blood volume perfusing the lung

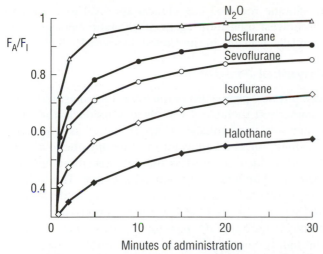

Figure 18–2. The rise in alveolar (F_A) anesthetic concentration toward the inspired (F_I) concentration is most rapid with the least soluble anesthetic agents: nitrous oxide (N_2O), desflurane, and sevoflurane. The moderately soluble anesthetic agents halothane and isoflurane have a slower rate of F_A to F_I ratio rise. *(From Eger E. I. [1993]. Desflurane (Suprane): A compendium and reference [p. 16]. NJ: Healthpress Publishing Group, Inc. Reprinted with permission.)*

TABLE 18–2. Tissue Group Characteristics

	Vessel-Rich	**Muscle**	**Fat**	**Vessel Poor**
Body mass (%)	9	50	19	22
Perfusion (% of cardiac output)	75	18.1	5.4	1.5

Source: Eger, E. I. (1974). Anesthetic uptake and action (p. 88). Baltimore: Williams & Wilkins. Adapted with permission.

effectively dilutes the concentration of anesthetic in the arterial blood. Although the anesthetic agent is taken up more rapidly and may be delivered to the blood circulation faster, a lower arterial blood concentration limits the onset of an anesthetic state. Conversely, a decrease in cardiac output may result in an excessive anesthetic depth. As a lowered cardiac output may be present in the elderly, debilitated, or trauma patient, slow, cautious induction of anesthesia is necessary.

Tissue uptake of the inhalation anesthetics influences the uptake of anesthetic at the alveolus by creating an alveolar-to-venous anesthetic partial pressure difference (Eger, 1994). The amount of anesthetic removed from the bloodstream to the tissues depends on the tissue solubility of the anesthetic agent, the tissue blood flow, and the partial pressure difference between the arterial blood and the tissue. Tissue solubility is influenced by the amount of blood flow to a particular tissue.

Four tissue groups have been identified (Table 18–2) on the basis of their solubility and perfusion characteristics. The vessel-rich group includes the brain, heart, liver, and kidney, which receive 75% of the cardiac output. Tissue solubility of these organs is high, resulting in rapid equilibration of anesthetic. Tissues in the muscle group (muscle and skin) and fat group are poorly perfused. Anesthetic partial pressure in the muscle group equilibrates slowly with the blood, but, because fat has a very high affinity for the inhalation anesthetics, equilibration usually does not occur in the fat. The fat group can continue to take up the anesthetic for several hours.

The vessel-poor group includes ligaments, tendons, cartilage, and bone. Blood perfusion to this group is insignificant and does not influence tissue uptake.

Anesthetic uptake can be limited by ventilation–perfusion abnormalities that may occur in the healthy patient or in patients with problems such as emphysema, atelectasis, and cardiac anomalies. Ventilation–perfusion abnormalities produce an increase in the alveolar partial pressure of anesthetic and a decrease in the arterial partial pressure of anesthetic. A partial pressure difference develops between the alveolus and arterial blood that influences the induction of anesthesia. Perfusion of an unventilated alveolus prevents the uptake of anesthetic. The blood leaving this area mixes with blood from ventilated areas and lowers the arterial partial pressure. In a well-ventilated alveolus with poor perfusion, the arterial partial pressure in the blood may increase and compensate for the diminished arterial partial pressure emerging from a poorly ventilated area (Eger & Severinghaus, 1964).

Recovery from Inhalation Anesthetics

Recovery from anesthesia occurs after the elimination of anesthetic from its site of action, the brain. The concentration, duration, and solubility of the inhalation anesthetic affect the time to recovery from anesthesia (Eger & Johnson, 1987). On termination of the inspired anesthetic, the inspired partial pressure is zero, creating a partial pressure gradient between the tissue and the blood. The anesthetic is rapidly eliminated from vessel-rich tissues, but depending on the duration of anesthesia, the muscle and fat tissues most likely have not reached equilibrium. Anesthetic elimination from these tissues is thereby prolonged, although the continued uptake of anesthetic into fat may contribute to recovery. Recovery from anesthesia is longer with the more soluble anesthetics, that is, halothane, enflurane, and isoflurane. Use of the insoluble anesthetics nitrous oxide, sevoflurane, and desflurane, which have significantly lower blood-gas solubility coefficients (Table 18–1), results in more rapid recovery.

Diffusion hypoxia can occur during recovery from anesthesia secondary to the discontinuation of nitrous oxide. The rapid elimination of nitrous oxide from the tissues and blood into the lung causes a dilution of the other gases present and a relative hypoxemia. Oxygen saturation decreases but can be prevented by the administration of 100% oxygen (Brodsky, McKlveen, Zelcer, & Margary, 1988).

Hepatic metabolism of the anesthetics is not a contributing factor during the maintenance of anesthesia. The high concentrations of drug present during anesthesia appear to saturate the hepatic microsomal enzymes responsible for metabolism, preventing metabolic breakdown. As the anesthetic concentration falls, metabolic breakdown can contribute to the recovery from anesthesia (Sawyer, Eger, Bahlman, Cullen, & Impelman, 1971). The impact of metabolism on recovery may be significant only with the anesthetic halothane because this agent is more highly subject to hepatic metabolism than other inhalation agents (Table 18-1).

Nitrous Oxide Special Considerations

The low solubility of nitrous oxide is advantageous in the delivery, maintenance, and emergence from anesthesia. However, its low solubility also is responsible for the diffusion of nitrous oxide into hollow body cavities such as closed bowel loops and emphysematous bullae. The rapid diffusion of nitrous oxide can interfere with certain surgical procedures. Therefore, nitrous oxide should be discontinued in prolonged gastrointestinal surgery, during placement of a tympanic membrane graft, or in ophthalmologic procedures involving air–fluid exchanges in enclosed spaces. Nitrous oxide also must be discontinued when sudden air emboli occur, as in neurosurgery, and when pneumothorax is present or suspected. Diffusion of nitrous oxide into endotracheal tube cuffs can exert pressure on tracheal mucosa, resulting in local ischemia. Endotracheal tube cuff pressures should be routinely monitored during anesthesia.

▶ PHARMACOLOGY OF INHALATION AGENTS

History

Because the older inhalation anesthetics had many disagreeable properties, including nausea and vomiting, flammability, slow induction, and toxic metabolism, the search for the ideal inhalation agent has continued for many years. The discovery that the addition of a halogenated atom decreased flammability and increased potency led to the exploration of many chemical compounds for possible use in anesthesia. Isoflurane, desflurane, and sevoflurane are in widespread use today, whereas halothane and enflurane, two of the initially employed inhalation agents, have been experiencing a dramatic decline. Halothane was released in the United States in 1957, enflurane in 1972, and isoflurane in 1981.

Desflurane received U.S. clinical approval in 1994, and the newest inhalation agent, sevoflurane, became commercially available in the United States in 1995.

Physical Properties

The physical properties of the inhalation anesthetics are summarized in Table 18-1. Nitrous oxide is the most commonly used inhalation agent, either as a primary anesthetic or as an adjuvant to other anesthetic agents. Nitrous oxide is a colorless, odorless gas stored in liquid form in cylinders at 50 atm of pressure. The volatile anesthetics halothane, enflurane, isoflurane, desflurane, and sevoflurane are liquids at room temperature and are readily vaporized by passing a carrier gas, oxygen, through the liquid. These agents are nonflammable and nonexplosive. Halothane is a halogenated hydrocarbon that differs from enflurane, isoflurane, desflurane, and sevoflurane. Enflurane and isoflurane are isomers and possess an ether linkage, as do desflurane and sevoflurane. Because its vapor pressure is close to atmospheric pressure, desflurane requires the use of a larger, specially developed vaporizer that uses electrical power and converts desflurane to a gas by heating and then blending this gas with diluent fresh gas flow. The molecular structures of these inhalation anesthetics are shown in Figure 18-3.

Nitrous Oxide

Respiratory Effects

The respiratory effects of 50% to 67% and even 1 MAC (110%) of nitrous oxide include a decrease in tidal volume with an increase in respiratory rate and minute ventilation, keeping $Paco_2$ normal (Eger, II, 1985). Although nitrous oxide causes minimal respiratory depression (Fig. 18-4), it does predispose the patient to atelectasis in isolated alveoli because of how easily it is absorbed. Indeed, postoperative Pao_2 levels are lower when nitrous oxide has been used (Gawley & Dundee, 1981). Nitrous oxide is commonly used as an adjuvant anesthetic with the other inhalation agents to reduce their respiratory depressant effects.

Cardiovascular Effects

Nitrous oxide is a direct myocardial depressant. This cardiovascular depression is counterbalanced by the ability of nitrous oxide to increase sympathetic outflow from the brain and to inhibit the removal of norepinephrine by the lung. These actions together usually result in comparatively little cardiovascular depression at 1 MAC (Figs. 18-5 and 18-6). However, adding nitrous oxide to a narcotic anesthetic may depress cardiovascular function more than with nitrous oxide or the narcotic alone. The probable mechanism of action is the ability of narcotics to block sympathetic stimulation. The overall cardiovas-

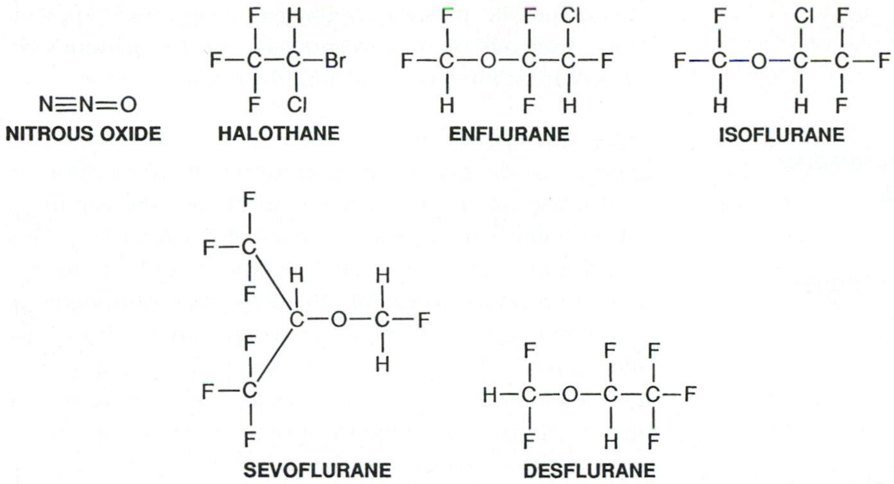

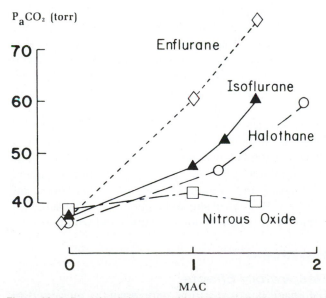

Figure 18–3. Molecular structures of inhalation anesthetics.

cular depressant effects of nitrous oxide must be evaluated in terms of resting sympathetic tone, presence of cardiopulmonary disease, and use of other analgesic and anesthetic drugs.

The use of nitrous oxide with a potent inhaled anesthetic may decrease the necessary concentration of the inhalation agent and diminish the cardiovascular depressant effect of that agent. Nitrous oxide causes a slight increase in pulmonary vascular resistance that may be detrimental in patients with increased pulmonary blood flow and may increase ventilation–perfusion abnormalities and impair oxygenation.

Central Nervous System Effects

Changes in the central nervous system (CNS) when nitrous oxide is administered often are inconsistent and probably reflect its limited potency and the need to combine it with other anesthetic agents. Fifty percent to 75% of nitrous oxide appears to dilate cerebral blood vessels, which causes an increase in intracranial pres-

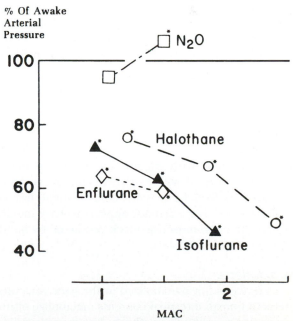

Figure 18–4. $P_a CO_2$ levels increase with all the anesthetic agents, but enflurane is the most potent respiratory depressant. Nitrous oxide causes minimal respiratory depression with a normal $P_a CO_2$. *(From Eger, E. I. [1981]. Isoflurane: A review. Anesthesiology, 55, 559. Copyright 1981 by the American Society of Anesthesiologists. Reprinted with permission.)*

Figure 18–5. The anesthetic agents are cardiovascular depressants and thus cause a decrease in mean arterial blood pressure in anesthetized, normocapnic volunteers. *(From Eger, E. I. [1981]. Isoflurane: A review. Anesthesiology, 55, 559. Copyright 1981 by the American Society of Anesthesiologists. Reprinted with permission.)*

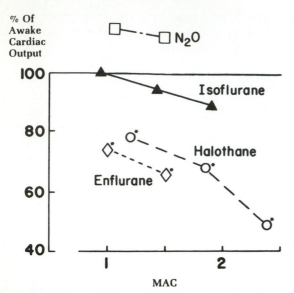

Figure 18–6. The anesthetic agents produce a decrease in cardiac output in anesthetized, normocapnic volunteers. *(From Eger, E. I. [1981]. Isoflurane: A review.* Anesthesiology, 55, 559. *Copyright 1981 by the American Society of Anesthesiologists. Reprinted with permission.)*

sure. These changes may be decreased or prevented by hyperventilation and administration of barbiturates (Frost, 1985). Unlike the other inhalation anesthetics, nitrous oxide does not protect the brain by decreasing cerebral oxygen consumption.

Nitrous oxide also has variable effects on the electroencephalogram (EEG). At 30% nitrous oxide, there is an increase in EEG frequency with lower voltage, and at higher nitrous oxide concentrations an increase in voltage is observed. Somatosensory evoked potentials remain essentially unchanged with nitrous oxide. Nitrous oxide can be used in patients undergoing surgery in which evoked potentials are to be monitored.

Neuromuscular Effects

Nitrous oxide may increase skeletal muscle activity and can be associated with rigidity and increased muscle tone when combined with narcotics. The precise mechanism for this skeletal activity enhancement has not been established. Nitrous oxide appears to have minimal effect on the neuromuscular block produced by nondepolarizing muscle relaxants.

Metabolism

Nitrous oxide is not metabolized in the liver. Anaerobic bacteria in human intestinal contents metabolize nitrous oxide through a reductive pathway, forming free radicals that can produce toxic intermediates, even though the end metabolite is inert (Hong, Trudell, O'Neil, & Cohen, 1980). Only 0.004% ± 0.005% of the nitrous oxide may be metabolized, and this amount is reduced when antibiotics are given. Presently, the clinical importance of

this metabolic pathway is unclear. Respiratory elimination of nitrous oxide is responsible for the patient's recovery from nitrous oxide administration.

Special Considerations

Nitrous oxide inactivates a component of methionine synthetase, an enzyme involved in the metabolism of folate (Koblin, Waskell, Watson, Stokstad, & Eger, 1982). This inactivation can impair DNA synthesis and produce a condition similar to vitamin B_{12} deficiency. Although this condition occurs after prolonged exposure to nitrous oxide inhalation (>24 hours in normal patients and shorter periods in ill patients), (Skacel et al., 1983), more recent investigations have failed to show a clinically relevant effect of nitrous oxide on folate and vitamin B_{12} metabolism (Koblin et al., 1990).

No teratogenic, carcinogenic, or mutagenic effects of nitrous oxide have been consistently reported in the scientific literature. The most contested finding is the increased incidence of spontaneous abortion among women exposed to waste anesthetic gases, specifically nitrous oxide (Cohen, Bellville, & Brown, 1971). More recently, a 10-year prospective study on occupational risks in the operating room determined that exposure to trace anesthetic gases did not cause increased rates of spontaneous abortion or congenital anomalies (Spence, 1995).

Conflicting reports also exist concerning the relationship between nitrous oxide and postoperative nausea and vomiting. Nitrous oxide administered alone induces nausea and vomiting, but adding nitrous oxide to other anesthetic regimens also may increase the incidence. Recently published analyses of large, randomized, controlled studies that compare the incidence of postoperative nausea and vomiting after anesthesia with or without nitrous oxide have concluded that nitrous oxide causes significant postoperative emesis (Divatia, Vaidya, Badwe, & Hawaldar, 1996; Hartung, 1996). Omitting nitrous oxide may reduce the risk of nausea and vomiting to the greatest extent in female patients, perhaps because of hormonal changes during the menstrual cycle (Beattie, Lindblad, Buckley, & Forrest, 1993). Many other factors, including patient age, history of prior postoperative nausea and vomiting, perioperative narcotics, and variations in surgical site and technique may obscure the influence of nitrous oxide on nausea and vomiting.

Halothane

Respiratory Effects

Halothane is a respiratory depressant, as measured by the arterial $Paco_2$ response during spontaneous ventilation in unstimulated volunteers (Fig. 18–4). Tidal volume and minute ventilation are lower at 1 MAC, although respiratory rate is higher. The tachypnea observed with halothane may be due to an increase in the discharge of pulmonary stretch receptors (Eger, II,

1985). Halothane does not stimulate secretions, but it does depress mucociliary flow in a dose-related fashion. Halothane relaxes constricted airways and is the most potent bronchial smooth-muscle dilator of all of the inhalation agents. It often is the agent of choice for patients with asthma or chronic obstructive pulmonary disease.

Cardiovascular Effects

Halothane is a direct myocardial depressant. It decreases all cardiovascular variables including cardiac output, stroke volume, and myocardial contractility by at least 20% at 1 MAC (Figs. 18-5 and 18-6). This cardiovascular depression parallels the decrease in mean arterial pressure and is dose related. The elevation in mean right atrial pressure seen with halothane administration is due to a decrease in stroke volume.

Halothane is unique in its sensitization of the myocardium to catecholamines, producing premature ventricular contractions. The amount of epinephrine that can be administered to a patient anesthetized with halothane is limited to 1 to 3 μg/kg over 10 minutes, and this may be repeated up to three times in 1 hour (Katz & Bigger, 1970). Halothane depresses sympathetic nervous system outflow and may decrease conduction time in atrioventricular nodal pathways.

Central Nervous System Effects

Halothane is the most potent cerebral vasodilator of all the inhalation agents. Cerebral blood flow increases dramatically with 0.6 to 1.6 MAC of halothane and increases almost 200% at 2 MAC (Fig. 18-7). This drastic increase in cerebral blood flow and, hence, in intracranial pressure can be prevented or greatly attenuated by hyperventilation and the establishment of hypocapnia before halothane administration.

Neuromuscular Effects

Halothane potentiates the neuromuscular block produced by nondepolarizing muscle relaxants. The probable mechanisms of action for this augmentation are a decrease in the responsiveness of the motor endplate to acetylcholine and a rise in the threshold for depolarization (Viby-Mogensen, 1985). Blockade is minimally altered when halothane is used with the depolarizing muscle relaxant succinylcholine.

Renal Effects

Halothane is a renal depressant because of its effects on the renal circulation. Renal blood flow is decreased by 38% and glomerular filtration rate is reduced by 20% at 2 MAC. Urine output also is lower during halothane administration, but the urine formation rate returns to normal after halothane is discontinued. Halothane does not cause the release of antidiuretic hormone (ADH). Radioimmunoassay techniques for ADH measurement show that an increase in ADH and, ultimately, a decrease in urine output are due to a secondary stress response that can be attenuated with deeper levels of anesthesia and positive pressure ventilation (Philbin & Coggins, 1980). There is no histologic evidence of renal injury in animals after prolonged administration of halothane.

Hepatic Effects

Because halothane reduces cardiac output, it produces a decrease in total hepatic blood flow. Halothane is distinct from the other inhalation agents in that it actually may decrease hepatic flow to a greater extent by increasing hepatic arterial resistance (Therlin, Andreen, & Irestedt, 1975). Halothane-associated hepatic dysfunction has an incidence of 1 in 35 000 and may be caused by hypoxic liver injury from reduced blood flow or may reflect a genetic predisposition, an allergic reaction to initial damage, or an immunologically mediated injury. Clinical recommendations include avoidance of halothane in patients with preexisting liver dysfunction, patients undergoing liver or biliary surgeries, and adult patients in whom halothane has been used within the preceding 6 months.

Metabolism

Fifteen percent to 20% of inhaled halothane may be metabolized by oxidative and reductive metabolism to trifluoroacetic acid (TFA), Cl^-, F^-, Br^-, and other volatile metabolites detectable in urine or exhaled air (Sharp, Trudell, & Cohen, 1979). Patients taking drugs known to induce cytochrome P450 activity of liver microsomes (ie, phenobarbital) tend to metabolize halothane at a higher than normal rate.

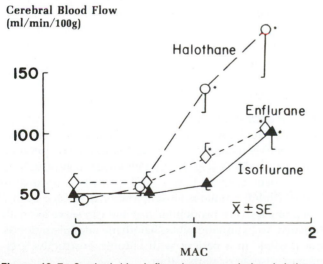

Figure 18-7. Cerebral blood flow increases during halothane, enflurane, and isoflurane anesthesia. Systemic blood pressure and Paco₂ were held at normal levels. SE, standard error. *(From Eger, E. [1985]. Isoflurane [Forane]: A compendium and reference [2nd ed., p. 84]. WI: Anaquest. Reprinted with permission.)*

Special Considerations

Halothane is a dose-dependent uterine smooth-muscle relaxant, decreasing uterine tone and contractility and reducing uterine responsiveness to oxytocic agents. It should be used cautiously in patients undergoing therapeutic abortion and dilation and curretage.

Halothane is the only inhalation anesthetic that contains a preservative. Adding 0.01% of thymol helps to stabilize halothane and prevents its decomposition on exposure to light. A high concentration of thymol may coat the rotary valves on anesthesia vaporizers, causing stickiness, which may affect the accuracy of the halothane vaporizer.

Enflurane

Respiratory Effects

Enflurane is the most potent respiratory depressant of all the inhalation agents (Fig. 18-4). Unstimulated volunteers have a $Paco_2$ of 61 at 1 MAC and become apneic at 2 MAC. Both minute ventilation and respiratory rate are decreased during enflurane administration. Enflurane's pungent odor may stimulate secretions, which limits the inspired concentration that can be given without eliciting coughing or laryngospasm. Enflurane also is a bronchodilator, although its pungency limits its use in relaxing constricted airways. Patients allowed to breathe spontaneously during enflurane anesthesia may occasionally sigh. The mechanism for this reaction is unknown.

Cardiovascular Effects

Enflurane is the most potent myocardial depressant of the inhalation agents (Figs. 18-5 and 18-6). The depression of cardiovascular variables, stroke volume, cardiac output, mean arterial pressure, and myocardial contractility is proportional to the anesthetic concentration of enflurane. The mechanism of action for the direct myocardial depressant effects of enflurane may be a reduction in free calcium ion concentration or an alteration in the sensitivity of contractile proteins to available calcium (Pavlin & Su, 1990).

Enflurane decreases systemic vascular resistance to a greater extent than halothane. Enflurane does not sensitize the myocardium to catecholamines, thus providing a stable heart rhythm and allowing administration of more than twice the dose of injectable epinephrine as halothane to be administered.

Central Nervous System Effects

Enflurane causes cerebral vasodilation, which is equivalent to less than 50% of the amount produced by halothane (Fig. 18-7). Cerebral blood flow is increased, and cerebral metabolic rate is decreased. Enflurane is unique in its ability to promote epileptogenic activity in the anesthetized patient. An increase in the depth of anesthesia with more than 1.5 MAC of enflurane is ac-companied by the appearance of slow EEG waves with increased voltage, progressing to burst suppression at 3%. These EEG effects are more pronounced in the presence of hypocapnia. As seizure activity can greatly increase cerebral metabolism, the use of enflurane in high doses and in combination with a decreased $Paco_2$ should be avoided in patients with seizure disorders or occlusive cerebrovascular disease.

Neuromuscular Effects

Enflurane potentiates the neuromuscular block produced by nondepolarizing muscle relaxants three times more than halothane. Increased concentrations of enflurane will increase the degree of neuromuscular depression.

Renal Effects

Like halothane, enflurane produces a 20% to 25% reduction in the glomerular filtration rate because it decreases cardiac output and renal blood flow. Enflurane does not cause the release of ADH and generally is not nephrotoxic, although prolonged enflurane exposure (>9.0 MAC hours) has been shown to diminish renal concentrating ability (Frink et al., 1994). Enflurane administration is not advised in patients with preexisting renal dysfunction.

Hepatic Effects

Hepatic dysfunction and histologic changes following the administration of enflurane are rare, although there is a reduction in total hepatic blood flow secondary to the reduction in cardiac output from enflurane.

Metabolism

Enflurane is metabolized by the liver, and the metabolites (8% of absorbed enflurane) are excreted in the urine. Equal amounts of organic and inorganic fluoride ions are excreted. Peak serum fluoride levels depend on the number of MAC hours and the concentration of enflurane administered. Peak levels occur 4 to 12 hours after anesthesia.

Isoflurane

Respiratory Effects

Isoflurane depresses ventilation in a dose-related fashion. It falls between enflurane and halothane in its respiratory depressant effects (Fig. 18-4). Pulmonary compliance is slightly decreased at 1 MAC and returns to normal at 2 MAC (Rehder, Mallow, Fibach, Krabill, & Sessler, 1974). Isoflurane also is a bronchodilator and can serve as an alternative to halothane when halothane administration is not possible in a patient with chronic obstructive pulmonary disease or with asthma.

Cardiovascular Effects

Isoflurane produces minimal direct myocardial depression. A decrease in the contractility of isolated cardiac muscle occurs, although this depression is significantly less in vivo. In volunteers, myocardial contractility and cardiac output are only mildly affected by 1 to 1.8 MAC of isoflurane (Figs. 18-5 and 18-6) (Eger, 1981). Isoflurane produces a large decrease in systemic vascular resistance and has a tendency to cause an increase in heart rate, which may be the result of a greater depression in vagal activity than in beta sympathetic activity (Eger, 1984). Isoflurane provides a stable cardiac rhythm and does not sensitize the heart to catecholamines. Administration of 7 to 10 μg/kg epinephrine will not result in cardiac arrhythmias.

Isoflurane can dilate small coronary resistance vessels in the dog. In patients with multivessel coronary artery disease, this action may potentially divert blood flow away from collateral dependent areas of borderline perfusion toward areas that are already adequately perfused. This coronary steal phenomenon has been extensively investigated since Reiz et al. (1983) reported that almost one half of their study patients exhibited evidence of inadequate coronary perfusion (ischemic electrocardiographic changes) when anesthetized with isoflurane and nitrous oxide. Subsequent researchers have been unable to duplicate Reiz's results. Contrasting reports of minimal or no vasodilation (Lunden, Manohar, & Parks, 1983; Sahlman, Henriksson, Martner, & Ricksten, 1988), mild and dose-related vasodilation (Hickey, Sybert, Verrier, & Cason, 1988; Sill et al., 1987), or even near-maximal coronary vasodilation (Crystal et al., 1991) make it difficult to assess the extent and importance of isoflurane's effect on coronary steal. Multiple factors determine collateral blood flow. Inhaled anesthetics have many effects on resistance and pressure in the coronary circulation. The safest clinical course is to maintain normal coronary artery perfusion pressure by maintaining preanesthesia cardiovascular indices. Isoflurane should be avoided in patients with critical coronary artery stenosis. In other patients with documented coronary artery disease, isoflurane should be combined with narcotics to reduce the possibility of coronary steal.

Central Nervous System Effects

Isoflurane produces less cerebral vasodilation than halothane or enflurane (Fig. 18-7). The MAC of isoflurane produces only small increases in cerebral blood flow. Isoflurane can cause EEG spiking but is not associated with the epileptogenic activity produced by enflurane. It is currently the inhalation agent of choice for neurosurgical procedures.

Neuromuscular Effects

Potentiation of nondepolarizing muscle relaxants is greater with isoflurane than with enflurane or halothane, and the same mechanisms of action were proposed for this augmentation: a decrease in the responsiveness of the motor endplate to acetylcholine and a rise in the threshold for depolarization (Viby-Mogensen, 1985).

Renal Effects

As with the other inhalation agents, renal blood flow, glomerular filtration rate, and urinary flow rate are decreased during isoflurane anesthesia. Antidiuretic hormone is not released by isoflurane. Tissue changes indicative of renal ischemia or injury are not present after prolonged anesthesia or after chronic exposure to subanesthetic concentrations of isoflurane (Eger, 1984).

Hepatic Effects

Isoflurane does not produce liver injury. In fact, it has been shown to increase hepatic artery blood flow at 1 and 2 MAC (Gelman, Fowler, & Smith, 1984).

Metabolism

Minimal oxidative metabolism of isoflurane results in the formation of TFA and F^-. Less than 0.2% of isoflurane is metabolized, and this amount is insufficient to cause any effects on renal function and other organ systems of the body (Holaday, Fiserova-Bergerova, Latto, & Zumbiel, 1975).

Desflurane

Respiratory Effects

Desflurane depresses ventilation in a dose-dependent manner and produces apnea at 1.5 to 2 MAC. At higher MAC levels, desflurane causes respiratory depression comparable to that observed with enflurane (Lockhart, Rampil, Yasuda, Eger, & Weiskopf, 1991). Desflurane has a pungent odor (similar to enflurane) and causes increased salivation, breath holding, coughing, and laryngospasm when used for inhalation inductions at concentrations exceeding 1 MAC, or 6% (Eger, 1994). These airway reactions are significant in the pediatric population, causing oxygen hemoglobin desaturation below 90% during induction. Desflurane is *not* recommended for inhalation indications in children, although anesthesia can be safely maintained with desflurane if induced with a different anesthetic (Zwass et al., 1992).

Cardiovascular Effects

Desflurane closely resembles isoflurane in its overall cardiovascular profile. Desflurane decreases mean arterial pressure in a dose-dependent manner through peripheral vasodilatation (Fig. 18-8), but it will maintain cardiac output at clinical concentrations. At end-tidal concentrations of more than 1.2 MAC, depression of myocardial contractility and of cardiac output occurs, similar to that with isoflurane. At more than 1.5 MAC, cardiovascular depression is more profound (Warltier & Pagel, 1992).

Increases in heart rate are minimal at 1 MAC or less, but the heart rate may increase dramatically with higher concentrations of desflurane (Fig. 18-9). Rapid increases in desflurane concentrations from 0.5 MAC to 1.5 MAC

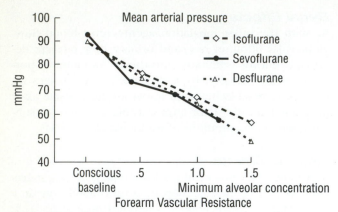

Figure 18–8. Alteration in mean arterial pressure with administration of isoflurane, desflurane, and sevoflurane in healthy volunteers. Increases in MAC levels decreased blood pressure similarly for each anesthetic agent. *(From Ebert, T. J., Harkin, C. P., & Muzi, M. [1995]. Cardiovascular responses to sevoflurane: A review. Anesthesia & Analgesia, 81, S14. Copyright 1995 by the International Anesthesia Research Society. Reprinted with permission.)*

cause significant, transient increases in heart rate, mean arterial pressure, and plasma epinephrine concentrations during induction or steady-state periods of anesthesia (Ebert & Muzi, 1993). To decrease this sympathetic stimulation, Moore et al. (1994) advised 1% increases in end-tidal desflurane concentrations in 30-second intervals when attempting to increase the anesthetic concentration.

Desflurane does not sensitize the myocardium to

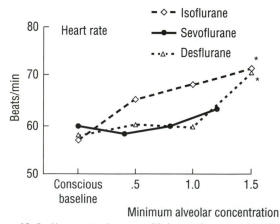

Figure 18–9. Heart rate changes with increasing concentrations of inhalation agents in healthy volunteers. Isoflurane causes an initial increase in heart rate. Sevoflurane maintains a near-resting heart rate, whereas desflurane is associated with a significant increase at 1.5 MAC. *p < .05 vs. sevoflurane. *(From Ebert, T. J., Harkin, C. P., & Muzi, M. [1995]. Cardiovascular responses to sevoflurane: A review. Anesthesia & Analgesia, 81, S12. Copyright 1995 by the International Anesthesia Research Society. Reprinted with permission.)*

catecholamines, and recommended injectable epinephrine limits are similar to those of isoflurane. Coronary steal phenomenon has not been elicited with desflurane and, compared with other inhalation or opioid anesthetics, the risk of untoward postoperative outcomes is the same in patients with coronary artery disease (Eisenkraft et al., 1992; Helman et al., 1992).

Central Nervous System Effects

Desflurane parallels isoflurane in its ability to decrease cerebral vascular resistance and cerebral metabolic rate (Lutz, Milde, & Milde, 1990). Intracranial pressure is minimally affected by desflurane concentrations up to 0.8 MAC, but higher concentrations increase intracranial pressure (ICP) in a dose-related fashion. Cerebrovascular responses to increases in CO_2 are present during desflurane anesthesia (Ornstein, Young, Fleischer, & Ostapkovich, 1993).

Neuromuscular Effects

Like isoflurane, desflurane enhances the action of nondepolarizing muscle relaxants. Like all the other inhalation agents, desflurane can trigger malignant hyperthermia.

Renal Effects

Due to its minimal degradation to inorganic fluoride, desflurane is not associated with any untoward renal effects and does not cause release of ADH. Administration of desflurane does not worsen chronic renal disease, even after repeated or prolonged use (Zaleski, Abello, & Gold, 1993).

Hepatic Effects

Desflurane is not associated with any known adverse hepatic function effects. Reductions in portal blood flow occur at 0.5 MAC, and hepatic arterial blood flow is not decreased until 1.0 MAC, leading to an overall dose-dependent decrease in hepatic blood flow consistent with decreased cardiac output (Armbruster et al., 1997). One case of hepatic injury has been reported after anesthesia with desflurane (Martin et al., 1995).

Metabolism

Even more than isoflurane, desflurane strongly resists degradation by strong acids and bases (Fig. 18–10). Less than 0.02% to 0.2% of inhaled desflurane is recovered as urinary metabolites of inorganic fluoride and trifluoroacetate (Sutton et al., 1991).

Special Considerations

Because it causes a transient increase in heart rate, blood pressure, and catecholamines, desflurane should not be used as the only induction agent in patients with coro-

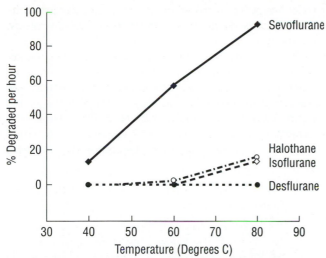

Figure 18–10. Degradation of inhalation agents placed in a sealed flask with 100 g of soda lime at temperatures ranging from 40°C to 80°C. The lower temperature equals that found in soda lime with low-flow circuits. *(From Eger E. I. [1993]. Desflurane [Suprane]: A compendium and reference [p. 7]. NJ: Healthpress Publishing Group, Inc. Reprinted with permission.)*

nary artery disease or in patients for whom increases in blood pressure are undesirable.

Sevoflurane

Respiratory Effects

Sevoflurane is a respiratory depressant that dose-dependently decreases minute ventilation and the ventilatory response to increases in CO_2, as observed with desflurane (Doi & Ikeda, 1987). The degree of respiratory depression also parallels that of halothane up to a MAC equivalent of 1.1, but at a MAC of 1.4 sevoflurane produces more respiratory depression. Its bronchodilating actions are similar to those of isoflurane and are believed to be caused by an inhibition of vagal reflexes (Mitsuhata, Saitoh, & Shimizu, 1994).

Sevoflurane is readily accepted by pediatric and adult patients for inhalation inductions. Its pleasant odor makes it amenable to the vital capacity rapid inhaled induction technique (Yurino & Kimura, 1993). Anesthetic inductions in pediatric patients are smoother with sevoflurane than with halothane because its induction time is faster and it causes less respiratory irritation (Naito, Tamai, Shingu, Fujimori, & Mori, 1991).

Cardiovascular Effects

Both sevoflurane and isoflurane have similar basic cardiovascular profiles, although some key differences do exist. With sevoflurane, systemic vascular resistance is decreased in a dose-dependent fashion, leading to a reduction in mean arterial pressure (Fig. 18–8). Sevoflurane reduces cardiac output at 1.0 and 1.5 MAC levels, but at

2.0 MAC cardiac output recovers almost to preanesthesia values (Calahan, 1996). Heart rate increases with sevoflurane are seen only at deep levels of anesthesia (>1.5 MAC) and are lower than at MAC equivalent concentrations of isoflurane (Fig. 18–9). The neurocirculatory excitation seen with rapid increases in desflurane does not occur with sevoflurane (Ebert, Muzi, & Lopatka, 1995).

Like isoflurane and desflurane, sevoflurane decreases myocardial contractility. Potentiation of epinephrine-induced cardiac arrhythmias is not observed, and epinephrine injection limits are the same. Sevoflurane does not reduce or abnormally redistribute myocardial blood flow derived from coronary collateral vessels and is not associated with coronary steal (Kersten, Brayer, Pagel, Tessmer, & Warltier, 1994). In fact, in cardiac patients undergoing noncardiac surgery, sevoflurane and isoflurane were comparable in incidence and severity of intra- and postoperative myocardial ischemia and in the frequency of adverse cardiac outcomes (Ebert et al., 1997).

Central Nervous System Effects

The effects of sevoflurane on the CNS are similar to those of isoflurane. CO_2 response and cerebral autoregulation are well maintained with 0.88 MAC sevoflurane (Kitaguchi, Uhsumi, Kuro, Nakajima, & Hayashi, 1993). Sevoflurane does not cause convulsive activity at either deep levels of anesthesia or in the presence of decreased CO_2.

Neuromuscular Effects

Like isoflurane and desflurane, sevoflurane enhances the neuromuscular block produced by nondepolarizing muscle relaxants.

Renal Effects

The potential renal toxicity of sevoflurane is related to its metabolism to inorganic fluoride, the proposed etiologic agent responsible for anesthetic nephrotoxicity and sevoflurane's degradation by carbon dioxide absorbents to Compound A (see Special Considerations for further discussion on Compound A). In some patients, peak fluoride concentrations after sevoflurane anesthesia exceed 50 μM, the long-held renal "toxic threshold" (Frink et al., 1994), although key indices of renal function have indicated no postoperative renal changes in patients with no preexisting renal disease (Higuchi et al., 1995). Sevoflurane does not cause release of ADH.

Hepatic Effects

Like isoflurane, sevoflurane increases hepatic arterial blood flow while reducing portal blood flow. The potential for hepatotoxicity from cytochrome P-450 enzyme metabolism is low, and no detrimental effects on overall hepatic function have been observed (Eger,

1994). In Japan, where over 5 million sevoflurane anesthetics have been administered, there have been isolated reports of hepatic injury after sevoflurane anesthesia in adults and children. No causal relationship could be established (Ogawa, Doi, Mitsufuji, Satoh, & Takatori, 1991; Shichinohe et al., 1992; Watanabe et al., 1993).

Metabolism

Approximately 2% to 5% of sevoflurane is metabolized to equal parts of inorganic fluoride and organic hexafluoroisopropanol.

Special Considerations

Sevoflurane reacts to the strong base in carbon dioxide absorbents (Fig. 18–10); baralyme slightly more than sodalime and decomposes to a vinyl ether olefin known as Compound A. This breakdown occurs during clinical anesthesia in low-flow (<2 L/min) or closed circuits, with increased concentrations of sevoflurane, higher absorbent temperatures from rebreathing, and fresh absorbent. Compound A is nephrotoxic in rats, causing proximal tubule lesions and necrosis at 50 ppm (Gonsowski, Laster, Eger, Ferrell, & Kerschmann, 1994). Extrapolation of such findings to humans is very controversial at present, and a publication "miniwar" is raging between the company that markets desflurane, the company that sells sevoflurane, and their paid research consultants.

Although usual renal measurements of blood urea nitrogen, creatinine, and urine concentrating ability are unchanged in humans after sevoflurane administration, more sensitive indicators of renal tubular function and glomerular filtration have recently shown transient renal injury in healthy human volunteers when Compound A levels were 50 ± 4 ppm, obtained after 8 hours of 1.25 MAC sevoflurane concentration at 2 L/min of fresh gas flow (Eger et al., 1997). However, Kharasch et al. (1997) have not demonstrated any evidence of renal impairment in 73 patients using low-flow (<1 L/min) rates of sevoflurane. Although the controversy continues, avoiding factors that increase the concentration of Compound A may prevent potential harmful renal effects when sevoflurane is administered.

▶ CASE STUDY

Mr. Jones is a 66-year-old, 75-kg gentleman with a history of coronary artery disease and hypertension. Mr. Jones is on isosorbide dinitrate, enalapril, and amlodipine. He presents in the emergency room with abdominal pain, elevated blood pressure (210/116), and tachycardia (118). A diagnosis of abdominal aortic aneurysm is made. Mr. Jones is transferred to the surgical intensive care unit for blood pressure control and invasive cardiac monitoring.

The next day, Mr. Jones is your patient in the operating room. He is on a nitroglycerin drip, his blood pressure is 140/88, and his heart rate is 80. For induction, Mr. Jones receives propofol (100 mg), fentanyl (100 μg), and cisatracurium (7 mg). Desflurane (3% to 6% in titrated increments) is used for anesthesia maintenance. Ten minutes after induction, Mr. Jones becomes hypertensive and tachycardic.

1. Describe the possible etiologies of Mr. Jones' hypertension and tachycardia.

   The possible causes of hypertension and tachycardia could be the inadequate depth of anesthesia, the underlying disease process (abdominal aneurysm), or the desflurane anesthetic. Induction of anesthesia can cause initial hypotension, especially with inhalation anesthetics because of the myocardial depressant activity of these agents and the lack of surgical stimulation. Hypertension and tachycardia can follow when surgical stimulation occurs and the concentration of the inhalation anesthetic is inadequate. Mr. Jones has a history of hypertension and coronary artery disease and has been diagnosed with an abdominal aneurysm. His blood pressure is being controlled with the vasodilator, nitroglycerin, which may need to be increased to control the acute episode of hypertension. Desflurane can cause transient rapid increases in heart rate and mean arterial pressure.

2. How can desflurane increase heart rate and mean arterial pressure?

   Rapid increases in desflurane concentrations from 0.5 to 1.5 MAC can transiently increase heart rate and mean arterial pressure as a result of catecholamine release. To decrease this response, end-tidal desflurane concentrations should be increased slowly by 1% increments over 30-second intervals.

3. What is the "coronary steal" phenomenon, and is this happening to Mr. Jones?

   Coronary steal occurs when blood flow is diverted away from collateral dependent areas of borderline perfusion toward areas that are already adequately perfused, causing ischemia in areas of the myocardium in which perfusion is compromised. This can occur in patients with multivessel coronary artery disease and has been observed in patients receiving the inhalation anesthetic, isoflurane. Desflurane has not been associated with coronary steal. It is important to maintain coronary artery perfusion by controlling the heart rate and mean arterial pressure. In this case, controlling the rate of desflurane administration, increasing the nitroglycerin concentration, or adding narcotics will help to prevent hypertension, tachycardia, and poor myocardial perfusion.

► SUMMARY

Nitrous oxide, halothane, enflurane, isoflurane, desflurane, and sevoflurane all provide optimal anesthesia. Sometimes one agent is preferred or is the drug of choice when a certain agent is contraindicated. For instance, halothane is a potent bronchodilator and can be used in the asthmatic patient. If this patient has hepatic dysfunction and presents with elevated liver enzymes, isoflurane or sevoflurane can be given because both agents also cause bronchodilation. Enflurane and sevoflurane should not be used in the patient with renal dysfunction. The tachycardia seen with isoflurane and the potential for coronary steal may preclude the use of isoflurane in the patient with serious coronary artery stenosis. Ventilation–perfusion abnormalities or altered circulatory states, possibly as a result of trauma, can affect anesthesia induction with all of these agents. All inhalation agents potentiate neuromuscular blockade. The relative ease of mask induction with sevoflurane makes this drug unique. Because desflurane and sevoflurane are insoluble, they provide for a rapid induction and emergence from anesthesia. Inhalation agents are commonly used in conjunction with intravenous narcotics. This can lead to a decrease in the concentration of the inhalation agent, and the narcotic has the additional action of providing postoperative analgesia. The choice of an inhalation agent for general anesthesia can be made only after a critical analysis of the cardiac, respiratory, renal, CNS, and metabolic effects of each agent and the physical properties of the drugs that will influence the uptake and distribution of the drug throughout the body.

► KEY CONCEPTS

- A vapor is the gaseous phase of a substance that at ambient temperature and pressure can exist as a liquid.
- The minimum alveolar concentration (MAC) of an inhaled anesthetic relates the concentration of an inhalation anesthetic to the observed effect and is a measure of anesthetic potency.
- The desired anesthetic effect of an inhalation anesthetic occurs when the partial pressure at the alveolar-arterial membrane is equal to the partial pressure in the brain.
- Anesthetic solubility is a physical property of an individual drug and is measured as the degree to which the drug can partition itself between a gaseous phase and a liquid phase: the more insoluble an agent, the sooner equilibrium of the alveolar partial pressure gradient is reached.
- Anesthetic uptake can be limited by ventilation–perfusion abnormalities that may occur in the healthy patient or in patients with problems such as emphysema, atelectasis, and cardiac anomalies.
- Ventilation–perfusion abnormalities produce an increase in the alveolar partial pressure of anesthetics and a decrease in the arterial partial pressure of anesthetics.
- Recovery from anesthesia occurs after the elimination of anesthetic from its site of action, the brain. The concentration duration and solubility of the inhalation anesthetic affect the time to recovery from anesthesia.

► STUDY QUESTIONS

1. Desflurane is formulated as a liquid. However, it functions as an inhalation anesthetic after vaporization. Describe the difference between a vapor and a gas. How does Henry's law apply to the vaporization of desflurane?

2. What is the impact of cardiac output on the anesthesia uptake and induction time with an inhalation anesthetic?

3. What types of patients would benefit from induction with sevoflurane? How may a desflurane induction be detrimental for some patients?

4. Controversies surround all the inhalation agents in use today. What factors should you consider to help you determine the best inhalation agent for your patient?

5. How do desflurane and sevoflurane come closer to being "ideal anesthetic agents" than halothane, enflurane, and isoflurane?

KEY REFERENCES

Dale, O. & Brown, B. R. (1987). Clinical pharmacokinetics of the inhalational anesthetics. *Clinical Pharmacokinetics, 12,* 145–167.

Davis, P. D., Parbrook, G. D., & Kenny, G. N. C. (1995). *Basic physics and measurement in anesthesia* (4th ed). Oxford: Butterworth-Heinemann.

Eger, E. I., II. (1984). The pharmacology of isoflurane (review). *British Journal of Anaesthesia, 56* (suppl. 1), 71S–99S.

Eger, E. I., II. (1994). New inhaled anesthetics. *Anesthesiology, 80,* 906–922.

REFERENCES

Antognini, J. F. (1993). Hypothermia eliminates isoflurane requirements at 20°C. *Anesthesiology, 78,* 1152–1156.

Armbruster, K., Noldge-Schomburg, G., Dressler, I., Fittkau, A., Haberstroh, J., & Geiger, K. (1997). The effects of desflurane on splanchnic hemodynamics and oxygen in the anesthetized pig. *Anesthesia & Analgesia, 84,* 271–277.

Beattie, W. S., Lindblad, T., Buckley, D. N., & Forrest, J. B. (1993). Menstruation increases the risk of nausea and vomiting after laparoscopy: A prospective, randomized study. *Anesthesiology, 78,* 272–276.

Brodsky, J. B., McKlveen, R. E., Zelcer, J., & Margary, J. J. (1988). Diffusion hypoxia: A reappraisal using pulse oximetry. *Journal of Clinical Monitoring, 4,* 244–246.

Calahan, M. K. (1996). Hemodynamic effects of inhaled anesthetics. *Anesthesia & Analgesia, 82* (suppl. 1), 14–18.

Cohen, E. N., Bellville, J. W., & Brown, B. W. (1971). Anesthesia, pregnancy and miscarriage: A study of operating room nurses and anesthetists. *Anesthesiology, 34,* 343–347.

Crystal, G. J., Kim, S. J., Czinn, E. A., Salem, M. R., Mason, W. R., & Abdel-Latif, M. (1991). Intracoronary isoflurane causes marked vasodilation in canine hearts. *Anesthesiology, 74,* 757–765.

Dale, O. & Brown, B. R. (1987). Clinical pharmacokinetics of the inhalational anesthetics. *Clinical Pharmacokinetics, 12,* 145–167.

Davis, P. D., Parbrook, G. D., & Kenny, G. N. C. (1995). *Basic physics and measurement in anesthesia* (4th ed., pp. 44–60, 77–88). Oxford: Butterworth-Heinemann.

Divatia, J. V., Vaidya, J. S., Badwe, R. A., & Hawaldar, R. W. (1996). Omission of nitrous oxide during anesthesia reduces the incidence of postoperative nausea and vomiting. *Anesthesiology, 85,* 1055–1062.

Doi, M. & Ikeda, K. (1987). Respiratory effects of sevoflurane. *Anesthesia & Analgesia, 66,* 241–244.

Drasner, K., Bernards, C., & Ozanne, G. M. (1988). Intrathecal morphine reduces the minimal alveolar concentration of halothane in man. *Anesthesia & Analgesia, 67,* S52.

Ebert, T. J. & Muzi, M. (1993). Sympathetic hyperactivity during desflurane anesthesia in healthy volunteers: A comparison with isoflurane. *Anesthesiology, 79,* 444–453.

Ebert, T. J., Muzi, M., & Lopatka, C. W. (1995). Neurocirculatory responses to sevoflurane in humans: A comparison to desflurane. *Anesthesiology, 83,* 88–95.

Ebert, T. J., Kharasch, E. D., Rooke, G. A., Shroff, A., Muzi, M., & The Sevoflurane Ischemia Study Group. (1997). *Anesthesia & Analgesia, 85,* 993–999.

Eger, E. I. (1974). *Anesthetic uptake and action.* Baltimore: Williams & Wilkins.

Eger, E. I. (1994). Uptake and distribution. In R. D. Miller (Ed.), *Anesthesia* (4th ed., pp. 101–123). New York: Churchill Livingstone.

Eger, E. I. & Johnson B. H. (1987). Rates of awakening from anesthesia with I-653, halothane, isoflurane, and sevoflurane. *Anesthesia & Analgesia, 66,* 977–982.

Eger, E. I., Koblin, D. D., Bowland, T., Ionescu, P., Laster, M., Fang, Z., Gong, D., Sonner, J., & Weiskopf, R. (1997). Nephrotoxicity of sevoflurane vs. desflurane in volunteers. *Anesthesia & Analgesia, 84,* 160–168.

Eger, E. I. & Severinghaus, J. W. (1964). Effect of uneven pulmonary distribution of blood and gas on induction with inhalation anesthetics. *Anesthesiology, 25,* 620–626.

Eger, E. I., II. (1981). *Isoflurane (forane): A compendium and reference.* Madison, WI: Ohio Medical Products.

Eger, E. I., II. (1985). Respiratory effects of nitrous oxide. In E. I. Eger, II (Ed.), *Nitrous oxide* (p. 111). New York: Elsevier.

Eisenkraft, J., Abel, M., Bradford, C., Whitten, C., Elmore, J., & Wiley, J. (1992). Safety and efficacy of desflurane in peripheral vascular surgery (abstract). *Anesthesia & Analgesia, 74,* S84.

Epstein, R. M., Rackow, H., Salanitre, E., & Wolf, G. L. (1964). Influence of the concentration effect on the uptake of anesthetic mixtures: The second gas effect. *Anesthesiology, 25,* 364–371.

Frink, E. J., Malan, T. P., Isner, J., Brown, E. A., Morgan, S. E., & Brown, B. R. (1994). Renal concentrating function with prolonged sevoflurane or enflurane anesthesia in volunteers. *Anesthesiology, 80,* 1019–1025.

Frost, E. A. M. (1985). Central nervous system effects of nitrous oxide. In E. I. Eger, II (Ed.), *Nitrous oxide* (pp. 157–176). New York: Elsevier.

Gawley, T. F. & Dundee, J. W. (1981). Attempts to reduce respiratory complications following upper abdominal operations. *British Journal of Anaesthesia, 53,* 1073–1078.

Gelman, S., Fowler, K. C., & Smith, L. R. (1984). Liver circulation and function during isoflurane and halothane anesthesia. *Anesthesiology, 61,* 726–730.

Gonsowski, C. T., Laster, D. V. M., Eger, E. I., Ferrell, L. D., & Kerschmann, R. L. (1994). Toxicity of compound A in rats. *Anesthesiology, 80,* 556–565.

Hartung, J. (1996). Twenty-four of twenty-seven studies show a greater incidence of emesis associated with nitrous oxide than with alternative anesthetics. *Anesthesia & Analgesia, 83,* 114–116.

Helman, J., Leung, J., Bellows, W., Pineda, N., Mangano, D., & SPI Research Group. (1992). The risk of myocardial ischemia in patients receiving desflurane vs. sufentanil anesthesia for CABG surgery. *Anesthesiology, 77,* 47–62.

Hickey, R. F., Sybert, P. E., Verrier, E. D., & Cason, B. A. (1988). Effects of halothane, enflurane and isoflurane on coronary blood flow autoregulation and coronary reserve in the canine heart. *Anesthesiology, 68,* 21–30.

Higuchi, H., Sumikura, H., Sumita, S., Arimura, S., Takamatsu, F., Kanno, M., & Satoh, T. (1995). Renal function in patients with high serum fluoride concentrations after prolonged sevoflurane anesthesia. *Anesthesiology, 83,* 449–458.

Holaday, D. A., Fiserova-Bergerova, V., Latto, I. P., & Zumbiel, M. A. (1975). Resistance of isoflurane to biotransformation in man. *Anesthesiology, 43,* 325–332.

Hong, K., Trudell, J. R., O'Neil, J. R., & Cohen, E. N. (1980). Metabolism of nitrous oxide by human and rat intestinal contents. *Anesthesiology, 52,* 16–19.

Katz, R. L. & Bigger, J. T. (1970). Cardiac arrhythmias during anesthesia and operation. *Anesthesiology, 33,* 193–213.

Kersten, J. R., Brayer, A. P., Pagel, P. S., Tessmer, J. P., & Warltier, D. C. (1994). Perfusion of ischemic myocardium during anesthesia with sevoflurane. *Anesthesiology, 81,* 995–1004.

Kharasch, E. D., Frink, E. J., Zanger, R., Bowdle, T. A., Artru, A., & Nogami, W. M. (1997). Assessment of low flow sevoflurane and isoflurane effects on renal function using sensitive markers of tubular toxicity. *Anesthesiology, 86,* 1238–1253.

Kitaguchi, K., Uhsumi, H., Kuro, M., Nakajima, T., & Hayashi, Y. (1993). Effects of sevoflurane on cerebral circulation and metabolism in patients with ischemic cerebrovascular disease. *Anesthesiology, 79,* 704–709.

Koblin, D. D., Tomerson, M. S., Waldman, F. M., Lampe, G. H., Wauk, L. Z., & Eger, E. I. (1990). Effect of nitrous oxide on folate and vitamin B_{12} metabolism in patients. *Anesthesia & Analgesia, 71,* 610–617.

Koblin, D. D., Waskell, L., Watson, J. E., Stokstad, E. L., & Eger, E. I. (1982). Nitrous oxide inactivates methionine synthetase in human liver. *Anesthesia & Analgesia, 61,* 75–78.

Le Bel, L. A. (1992). Principles of chemistry and physics in anesthesia. In W. R. Waugaman, S. D. Foster, & B. M. Rigor (Eds.), *Principles and practice of nurse anesthesia* (2nd ed., pp. 57–84). Norwalk, CT: Appleton & Lange.

Lockhart, S., Rampil, I., Yasuda, N., Eger, E. I., II., & Weiskopf, R. (1991). Depression of ventilation by desflurane in humans. *Anesthesiology, 74,* 484–488.

Lunden, G., Manohar, M., & Parks, C. (1983). Systemic distribution of blood flow in swine while awake and during 1.0 and 1.5 MAC isoflurane anesthesia with or without 50% nitrous oxide. *Anesthesia & Analgesia, 62,* 499–512.

Lutz, L., Milde, J., & Milde, L. (1990). The cerebral, functional,

metabolic and hemodynamic effects of desflurane in dogs. *Anesthesiology, 73,* 125–131.

Martin, J. L., Plevak, D. J., Flannery, K. D., Charlton, M., Poterucha, J. J., Humphreys, C. E., Derfus, G., & Pohl, L. R. (1995). Hepatotoxicity after desflurane anesthesia. *Anesthesiology, 83,* 1125–1129.

Mitsuhata, H., Saitoh, J., & Shimizu, R. (1994). Sevoflurane and isoflurane protect against bronchospasm. *Anesthesiology, 81,* 1230–1234.

Moore, M. A., Weiskopf, R. B., Eger, E. I., II, Noorani, M., McKay, L., & Damask, M. (1994). Rapid 1% increases of end-tidal desflurane concentration to >5% increases heart rate and blood pressure in humans. *Anesthesiology, 81,* 94–98.

Naito, Y., Tamai, S., Shingu, K., Fujimori, R., & Mori, K. (1991). Comparison between sevoflurane and halothane for paediatric ambulatory anaesthesia. *British Journal of Anaesthesia, 67,* 387–389.

Ogawa, M., Doi, K., Mitsufuji, T., Satoh, K., & Takatori, T. (1991). Drug induced hepatitis following sevoflurane anesthesia in a child. *Masui, 40,* 1542–1545.

Ornstein, E., Young, W. L., Fleischer, L. H., & Ostapkovich, N. (1993). Desflurane and isoflurane have similar effects on cerebral blood flow in patients with intracranial mass lesions. *Anesthesiology, 79,* 498–503.

Pavlin, E. G. & Su, J. Y. (1990). Cardiopulmonary pharmacology. In R. D. Miller (Ed.), *Anesthesia* (4th ed., p. 125). New York: Churchill Livingstone.

Philbin, D. M. & Coggins, C. H. (1980). The effects of anesthesia on antidiuretic hormone. *Contemporary Anesthesia Practice, 3,* 29–38.

Rehder, K., Mallow, J. E., Fibach, E. E., Krabill, D. R., & Sessler, A. D. (1974). Effects of isoflurane anesthesia and muscle paralysis on respiratory mechanics in normal man. *Anesthesiology, 41,* 477–482.

Reiz, S., Balfors, E., Sorensen, M. B., Ariola, S., Friedman, A., & Truedsson, H. (1983). Isoflurane: A powerful coronary vasodilator in patients with coronary artery disease. *Anesthesiology, 59,* 91–97.

Sahlman, L., Henriksson, B. A., Martner, J., & Ricksten, S. E. (1988). Effects of halothane, enflurane and isoflurane on coronary vascular tone, myocardial performance, and oxygen consumption during controlled changes in aortic and left atrial pressure. *Anesthesiology, 69,* 1–10.

Sawyer, D. C., Eger, E. I., Bahlman, S. H., Cullen, B. F., & Impelman, D. (1971). Concentration dependence of hepatic halothane metabolism. *Anesthesiology, 34,* 230–234.

Sharp, T. H., Trudell, J. R., & Cohen, E. N. (1979). Volatile metabolites and decomposition products of halothane in man. *Anesthesiology, 50,* 2–8.

Shichinohe, M. Y., Masuday, T. H., Kotaki, M., Omote, T., & Shichino, M. (1992). A case of hepatic injury after sevoflurane anesthesia. *Masui, 41,* 1802–1805.

Sill, J. C., Bove, A. A., Nugent, M., Blaise, G. A., Dewey, J. D., & Grabau, C. (1987). Effects of isoflurane on coronary arteries and coronary arterioles in the intact dog. *Anesthesiology, 66,* 273–279.

Skacel, P. O., Hewlett, A. M., Lewis, J. D., Lumb, M., Nunn, J. F., & Chanarin, I. (1983). Studies on the haemopoietic toxicity of nitrous oxide in man. *British Journal of Haematology, 53,* 189–200.

Spence, A. (1995). Occupational risks of the operating room? Data from the UK ten year prospective study. *Bulletin New York State Postgraduate, December,* 140.

Sutton, T. S., Koblin, D. D., Gruenke, L. D., Weiskopf, R. B., Rampil, I. J., Waskell, L., & Eger, E. I., II. (1991). Fluoride metabolites following prolonged exposure of volunteers and patients to desflurane. *Anesthesia & Analgesia, 73,* 180–185.

Therlin, L., Andreen, M., & Irestedt, L. (1975). Effect of controlled halothane anesthesia on splanchnic blood flow and cardiac output in the dog. *Acta Anaesthesiologica Scandinavica, 19,* 146–153.

Valverde, A., Dyson, D. H., & McDonnell, W. N. (1989). Epidural morphine reduces halothane MAC in the dog. *Canadian Journal of Anaesthesia, 36,* 629–633.

Viby-Mogensen, J. (1985). Interaction of other drugs with muscle relaxants. In R. L. Katz (Ed.), *Muscle relaxants: Basic and clinical aspects* (p. 249). Orlando, FL: Grune & Stratton.

Warltier, D. C. & Pagel, P. S. (1992). Cardiovascular and respiratory actions of desflurane: Is desflurane different from isoflurane? *Anesthesia & Analgesia, 75,* 17–31.

Watanabe, K., Hatakenaka, S., Ikemune, K., Chigyo, Y., Kubozono, T., & Arai, T. (1993). A case of suspected liver dysfunction induced by sevoflurane anesthesia. *Masui, 42,* 902–905.

Yurino, M. & Kimura, H. (1993). Vital capacity rapid inhaled induction technique: Comparison of sevoflurane and halothane. *Canadian Journal of Anaesthesia, 40,* 440–443.

Zaleski, L., Abello, D., & Gold, M. (1993). Desflurane vs. isoflurane in patients with chronic hepatic and renal disease. *Anesthesia & Analgesia, 76,* 353–356.

Zwass, M., Fisher, D., Welborn, L., Cote, C., Davis, P., & Dinner, M. (1992). Induction and maintenance characteristics of anesthesia with desflurane and nitrous oxide in infants and children. *Anesthesiology, 76,* 373–378.

Pharmacology of Intravenous Anesthetics

Ilze Ducis

A number of agents that exhibit significant lipid solubility are presently utilized as intravenous anesthetics to induce general anesthesia. Compared to most other routes of drug administration, the intravenous (IV) route is one of the fastest and most precise routes of drug administration, resulting in a rapid onset of drug action. Agents that are commonly utilized as IV anesthetics often are subdivided into two major categories, the opioid and the nonopioid anesthetics. Examples of commonly administered nonopioid IV anesthetics are thiopental, methohexital, thiamylal, midazolam, propofol, etomidate, and ketamine. The opioid IV anesthetics include fentanyl, sufentanil, alfentanil, morphine, and remifentanil.

▶ PHARMACOKINETICS OF INTRAVENOUSLY ADMINISTERED DRUGS

Pharmacokinetics is the subdivision of pharmacology that deals with the absorption, distribution, and clearance of drugs from the body as described in Chapter 17. Pharmacokinetics of particular interest to the study of IV anesthetics are described in this chapter.

Absorption

Bioavailability

Bioavailability is the speed and completeness of the absorption of a drug. It refers to the fraction of unchanged drug that reaches the systemic circulation following administration by any route. If all of the administered drug molecules reach the systemic circulation without chemical modification, the bioavailability of the agent is equivalent to 1, or 100%. The bioavailability of intravenously administered drugs, however, is equivalent to 1 or approaches 1 because these drugs bypass the absorption phase.

First-Pass Phenomena

Some parenterally administered drugs may be extensively metabolized before reaching the systemic circulation. The first-pass phenomenon (also called presystemic elimination) involves metabolism by gut enzymes and bacteria together with liver uptake and metabolism. It involves the hepatic portal circulation, which delivers drugs that have passed through the intestinal wall to the liver. Because many drugs are metabolized in the liver, it is sometimes important not to administer a drug orally, especially if it exhibits a significant first-pass effect.

Intravenously administered drugs bypass the liver, but do pass through the lungs. The lungs also exhibit a first-pass effect before the blood is delivered to the arteries. The drugs that are metabolized in the lungs, however, are mainly weak bases. Only intra-arterial injections bypass both the liver and the lungs. If given orally, many of the intravenously administered anesthetics exhibit a significant hepatic first-pass effect. Unlike intravenously administered drugs, enteral preparations, as well as most other routes of drug administration, exhibit a latency period between administration and onset of drug action. Usually, the intensity and time of onset of the drug effect also are less predictable when drugs are administered by a non-IV route.

Distribution

Factors that Determine the Rate of Tissue Uptake

Once a drug has been absorbed into the blood, it may be distributed to other body compartments (Fig. 19–1) that are separated from one another by semipermeable membranes. An intravenously injected drug is distributed throughout the blood volume in approximately 1 minute. From the blood, the agent may be distributed into interstitial space, and ultimately within tissue cells. The rate at which the anesthetic leaves the systemic circulation, passes through the walls of the systemic capillaries, and reaches the active sites in the central nervous system (CNS) is determined partly by the physicochemical characteristics of the drug's molecules. The rate of tissue uptake of the intravenously administered drugs depends on the following factors: (1) rate of drug delivery to the tissue (fraction of the cardiac output or blood flow to the tissue); (2) molecular size of the drug; (3) fraction or degree of ionization of drug molecules; (4) lipid solubility (lipophilicity) of the drug, particularly of the unchanged form of the drug; (5) degree of plasma protein binding of the drug; and (6) the difference in concentration of free drug molecules between blood and the target tissue. If blood flow to a tissue remains constant and the rate of uptake of two drugs at a given dose is compared, the lipid solubility and degree of ionization of the drug are the most important properties that will determine the rate of distribution of the drug to various tissues. With an increase in lipid solubility of a drug, a faster rate of uptake by a tissue occurs.

Ionization of a Drug

Simple Diffusion. The most common process by which drugs pass through membrane barriers and the walls of systemic capillaries is by the passive process of diffusion. Compounds that cross plasma membranes by simple diffusion always are taken up independently of

each other. With a simple diffusion process, a constant fraction, not amount, of drug moves from one body compartment to another over a unit time period.

Volume of Distribution

Body compartments can be considered to be real volumes of distribution (V_d) for drugs that do not bind extensively to plasma proteins and that do not bind or sequester extensively in extravascular sites (eg, bone, muscle, fat). Large hydrophilic molecules would be expected to exhibit V_d values approximating the volume of plasma or extracellular fluid (ECF). Highly lipid-soluble substances, however, will often exhibit V_d values that are very large and do not represent the volume of a real body compartment. In theory, the V_d of a substance is the fluid volume in which the free drug or unbound drug is dissolved. Finding the V_d of a drug is analogous to finding the volume of fluid in a container by adding a known amount of a substance to the container, mixing, and then determining the resulting concentration of the added substance after equilibrium has occurred. The following equation is used to determine the volume of distribution:

$$V_d = \frac{X}{C'}$$

where X is the amount of substance added and C is the concentration of the substance at equilibrium. Specific substances have been utilized in this manner to determine ECF volume, plasma and blood volumes, and the volume of total body water (Table 19–1).

Compartment Models

A two-compartment model describes the distribution of many drugs used in anesthesia and illustrates the basic concepts of pharmacokinetics that also apply to more complex models (Stanski & Watkins, 1982). In a two-compartment model, a drug is introduced by IV injection or by the inhalation route directly into the central compartment that is comprised of plasma. An initial rapid phase, the alpha (α) phase, reflects the distribution of the drug from the central compartment to the peripheral compartment. The latter compartment is comprised of various organs and tissues. When the kinetics of drug distribution are plotted using a two-compartment model, a biphasic curve is generated. The first phase is the distribution phase of a drug. This phase also is called the α phase. The second, slower process is referred to as the beta (β) phase and reflects elimination of the drug from the body. For some highly lipid-soluble agents used in anesthesia, a two-compartment model may not be sufficient to describe the distribution of the agent, so a triphasic curve is generated. This triphasic curve represents three distinct processes that are oc-

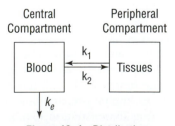

Figure 19–1. Distribution.

TABLE 19–1. Body Compartments

Compartments	Volume	Measurement of Body Fluids
Total body water (0.6 L/kg)	41 L	Small, water-soluble molecules (ethanol, urea, D_2O)
Extracellular fluid (0.2 L/kg)	12 L	Larger, water-soluble molecules (mannitol, insulin, sucrose, Na^+, Cl^-, Br^-)
Plasma (0.04 L/kg)	3 L	Binds strongly to plasma protein and very large molecules (Evan's blue dye, heparin, radiolabeled plasma proteins)
Whole blood (0.08 L/kg)	6 L	Calculated from plasma volume (assume 50% hematocrit) or directly measured by using radiolabeled red blood cells (^{51}Cr)

curring, each with a progressively slower rate. The first phase reflects distribution into systemic blood and highly perfused organs such as the brain, liver, heart, and lungs. The second phase reflects distribution of the agent into less perfused tissues and organs (peripheral compartment). This latter phenomenon of drug transfer from richly perfused tissues to less perfused tissues is called redistribution. The third phase represents a second conceptual peripheral compartment. In a three-compartment model, the drug would go through another phase of decline in plasma concentration in this second peripheral compartment (Schwinn, Watkins, & Leslie, 1994). The rate of drug transfer (rate constant k) between the central and peripheral compartments may decrease with age, because of decreased perfusion of peripheral sites and loss of muscle mass, resulting in high plasma concentrations of drugs such as thiopental. Any residual drug present in the peripheral compartment at the time of another IV injection also will result in an exaggerated drug response because depot sites in the peripheral compartment are saturated or partially saturated with the drug.

Some of the other concepts important in first-order kinetics that apply to compartment models, such as absorption, distribution, and clearance, are discussed in Chapter 17. The reader also should refer to that chapter for information concerning plasma protein binding, the blood–brain barrier, and drug metabolism, which apply to IV anesthetics as well as other pharmacologic agents used in anesthesia practice.

▶ NONOPIOID INTRAVENOUS ANESTHETICS

Barbiturates

Classification of a particular compound as a hypnotic, such as a barbiturate, indicates that its major therapeutic use is to induce sleep or unconsciousness. Several drugs that are hypnotics also are classified as IV anesthetics and are used to induce anesthesia. Induction of general anesthesia by IV barbiturates incorporates both rapid onset of effect and patient satisfaction and acceptability. Induction often is produced by barbiturates classified as ultrashort-acting barbiturates, such as thiopental (Pentothal®), thiamylal (Surital®), and methohexital (Brevital®). Although IV agents usually are used to induce anesthesia, inhalation anesthetics, nonbarbiturate IV anesthetics, and opioid anesthetics may be combined with barbiturate anesthetics to maintain anesthesia.

Chemistry

Structure–Activity Relationships. Barbiturates are derived chemically from barbituric acid (2,4,6-trioxohexahydropyrimidine), a compound that lacks CNS depressant hypnotic activity. Barbituric acid, a cyclic ureide, is derived from the condensation of urea and ethyl malonate, an ester (Fig. 19–2). Barbiturates are synthesized by making substitutions on the carbon 2 (C2)

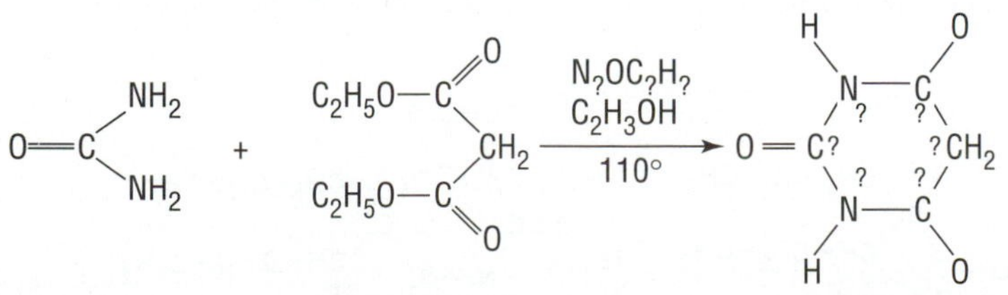

Urea   Ethyl malonate   Barbituric acid (Malonylurea)

Figure 19–2. Barbituric acid, a cyclic ureide, is synthesized by the condensation of urea and ethyl malonate, an ester.

and carbon 5 (C5) atoms of the cyclic ureide ring (Fig. 19-3). Substitutions of phenyl groups or alkyl groups, especially if the latter are branched on C5, result in centrally active compounds that exhibit hypnotic activity. Both hydrogen atoms associated with C5 must be substituted to produce sedation and hypnosis. The length of the alkyl group, which is covalently bonded to C5, also influences the potency and duration of action of the barbiturate. Substituting a sulfur atom for an oxygen atom on C2 of barbituric acid influences an agent's lipophilicity, onset of action, and the duration of action.

The two classes of barbiturates important in anesthesia practice are the oxybarbiturates and thiobarbiturates. The oxybarbiturates have an oxygen atom on the C5, whereas substituting the oxygen atom with a sulfur atom produces a thiobarbiturate. Thiobarbiturates are more lipophilic than oxybarbiturates. The thiobarbiturates thiopental and thiamylal exhibit a greater potency, a more rapid onset of action, and a shorter duration of action than the analogous oxybarbiturates pentobarbital and secobarbital. Substituting an alkyl group on the nitrogen at position number 1 in the ring not only increases the lipid solubility of the agent, accelerates the rate of onset of action, and decreases the duration of action, but also increases the frequency of excitatory side effects, which include tremor and spontaneous involuntary movements (Dundee, 1971, 1979). The thiobarbiturates, as well as pentobarbital and secobarbital, contain a tetrahedral stereocenter, or chiral carbon, on the longest side chain associated with C5. These barbiturates have two stereoisomers and are sold as racemic mixtures. Methohexital contains two different tetrahedral stereocenters, one of which is associated with the longest side chain bonded to C5 and the second asymmetric carbon is ring C5. Methohexital has four stereoisomers, as it has two chiral carbons in its structure. Although the potency of the *l* isomers of pentobarbital, secobarbital, thiopental, and thiamylal is twice as great as that of the *d* isomers, these barbiturates are produced and sold as racemic drug mixtures. The most potent stereoisomer of methohexital that produces hypnosis is the β*l* isomer, which also stimulates motor activity. Therefore, methohexital is produced and sold as a racemic mixture of αD and αL isomers.

Commercial Preparation of Barbiturates. Barbiturates are weak acids and are poorly soluble in water in their acidic form (conjugate acid form). They are prepared commercially for clinical use as water-soluble sodium salts (conjugate base form) in the presence of sodium carbonate. Keto-enol or lactam–lactim tautomerism occurs with the barbiturates in solution. The acidic (enol or lactim) form of a barbiturate, whether it is an oxybarbiturate or a thiobarbiturate, is favored in an alkaline environment. The enol form (conjugate acid form) permits the formation of water-soluble sodium salts.

The purpose of adding sodium carbonate to the barbiturate solution is to maintain the barbiturate in its con-

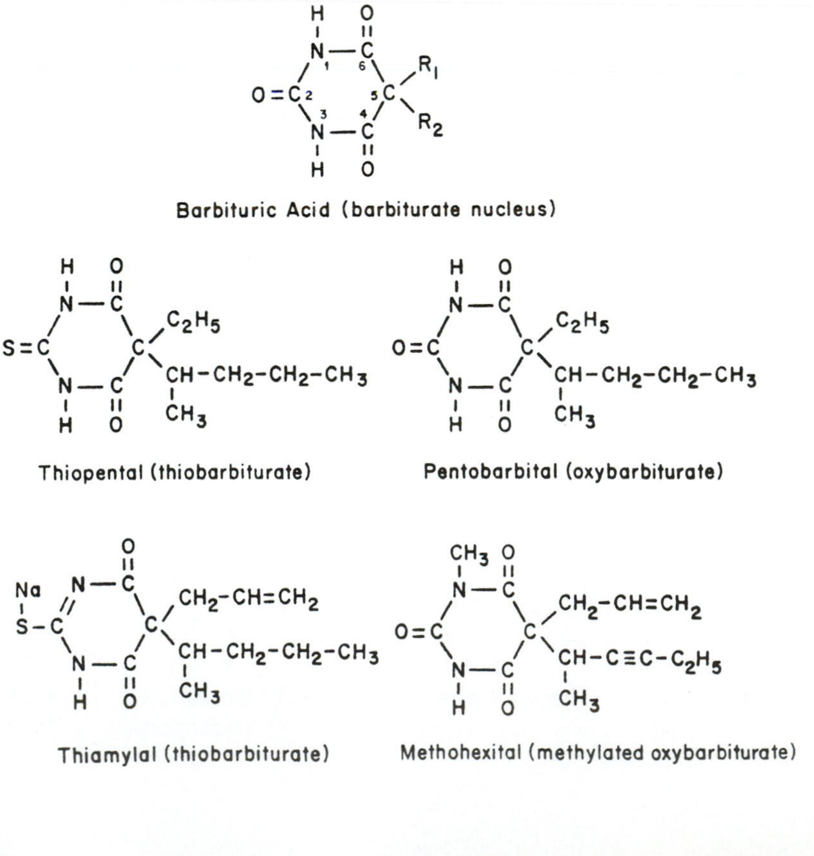

Figure 19–3. Barbituric acid and four different barbiturates resulting from specific substitutions on the barbiturate nucleus.

jugate base form by maintaining an alkaline pH of 10.0 to 11.0 that prevents precipitation of the conjugate acid form of the barbiturate in the presence of atmospheric carbon dioxide. Although the alkalinity of these solutions makes them bacteriostatic, these solutions may result in severe tissue damage if injected inadvertently into extravascular sites or intra-arterially. Intra-arterial injection of thiobarbiturates, but not methohexital, can produce severe arterial spasm and thrombosis, resulting in gangrene of the extremity. Precipitation of weakly basic drugs, such as catecholamines, neuromuscular blocking agents, opioid analgesics, and local anesthetics, also may occur. Therefore, barbiturates should not be administered simultaneously with basic drugs that are soluble in acidic solutions, as precipitation of the barbiturate, as well as the weakly basic drug, can occur in the IV infusion line. The barbiturates utilized for induction of anesthesia are thiopental, thiamylal, and methohexital.

Reconstitution of the sodium salts of the barbiturates should be carried out with sterile water or a 0.9% sodium chloride solution to produce approximately a 2.5%, 2.0%, or 1% solution of thiopental, thiamylal, and methohexital, respectively. A decrease in the alkalinity of the barbiturate solutions can result in their precipitation as free acids. For this reason, barbiturate solutions should not be reconstituted with lactated Ringer's solution, nor should the reconstituted barbiturate solutions be mixed with any acidic solutions. Once the barbiturate is delivered to the circulation, the alkaline solution becomes neutralized and the ratio of percent ionized to nonionized molecules of the barbiturate changes because of the change in pH. A greater portion of the drug particles is now in the acidic or nonionized form in plasma. A high percentage (75% to 85%) of the thiobarbiturate (thiopental, thiamylal) molecules are bound to the inert binding sites of albumin at therapeutic drug concentrations.

Pharmacokinetics

A single IV injection of the ultrashort-acting barbiturates (thiopental, thiamylal, methohexital) produces a rapid onset of CNS depression resulting in a state of anesthesia that lasts for a brief period, followed by a rapid and complete recovery. Depending on the cardiac output, maximal uptake of these ultrashort-acting barbiturates into the brain occurs between 30 to 60 seconds, which accounts for their rapid induction of anesthesia within one arm-to-brain circulation time.

The short duration of action of these agents is due to their pharmacokinetic properties, which can be represented by a three-compartment model of drug distribution (Price, Kovnat, & Safer, 1960). The rate of redistribution to other tissues and organs and the elimination of these IV anesthetic agents from the body are represented by the half-life, $t_{1/2\alpha}$ and $t_{1/2\beta}$, respectively, and depend on the clearance (Cl) and volume (V_d) of distribution. The

V_d is determined by factors such as the pK_a of the drug, percentage of the drug that is protein bound, the fat–blood partition coefficient, age, gender, and percentage of body fat of an individual. Many lipophilic agents, including the ultrashort-acting thiobarbiturates, are extensively bound to plasma proteins and exhibit large apparent volumes of distribution at equilibrium (steady state) because of ultimate sequestration in adipose tissue. Following a rapid bolus IV injection, the ultrashort-acting barbiturates distribute quickly throughout the central compartment, which consists of blood (intravascular space) and the vessel-rich group (VRG) of organs (Table 19–2). These organs, which include the brain, contribute only a small percentage of the body mass (10%) but receive a large percentage of the cardiac output (75%). The rate of distribution of an IV anesthetic to the brain is influenced by the agent's lipophilicity, the rate of blood flow to the brain, the extent of binding to plasma proteins, the unit capacity and total capacity of the brain for the agent, and the percentage of ionization of the drug molecules, the latter of which is determined by the pK_a of the drug and the local pH. Because of its high perfusion rate, the VRG is exposed to and takes up IV anesthetic agents almost immediately. The ultrashort-acting barbiturates readily cross the blood–brain barrier and rapidly equilibrate between brain tissue and arterial blood because of their high lipid solubility, their rapid diffusion rate, and the low drug-binding capacity of the brain. A low capacity implies that the depot sites available in brain tissue are readily and quickly filled, thus permitting the free drug concentration rapidly to rise and equilibrate with the free drug concentration in arterial blood. After a brief period (5 minutes), the concentration of the ultrashort-acting barbiturate in plasma and in the

TABLE 19–2. Distribution of Blood Flow to Various Organs and Tissues

Organs/Tissues	Body Weight (%)	Cardiac Output (%)
Vessel-rich group (70% to 75% of cardiac output)		
Brain	2.0	14
Heart	0.5	5
Liver	4.0	28
Kidney	0.5	23
Total	7.0	70
Intermediate group		
Skeletal muscle	49	15
Skin	6	8
Total	55	23
Fat group	18	6
Vessel-poor group (ligaments, tendons, bone)	19	1

VRG significantly decreases because of the redistribution (α phase) of the agents to skeletal muscle [muscle group (MG)]. Although the short-acting barbiturates are highly lipid soluble and favor the very high-capacity fat group (FG) over other groups, equilibration with the FG is a slow process resulting in a slow delivery of the drug to this site. Therefore, after an IV bolus administration, adipose tissue is the only tissue in which the barbiturate concentration is still increasing after approximately 30 minutes.

Maximal uptake of the short-acting barbiturates by adipose tissue occurs in about 2.5 hours. Importantly, adipose tissue may act as a reservoir or depot site for anesthetic agents. Following prolonged administration of such highly lipophilic drugs, the fat depots may accumulate a large (lipophilic) amount of drug that will be slowly released to the central compartment as blood plasma levels decrease due to metabolism (β phase) of the drug. When this occurs, the usual rapid awakening will not occur. Excess storage of barbiturates in fat depots accounts for the small, but measurable, concentration of anesthetics found in blood for days after anesthesia. These low levels of anesthetic can produce prolonged impairment of cognitive or mental functions after surgery and result in delayed recovery. For these reasons, the optimal administered dose of the ultrashort-acting anesthetics should be calculated using lean body mass, not total body mass.

The redistribution of the ultrashort-acting barbiturates into adipose tissue does not significantly influence the time it takes to return to consciousness after a single IV dose of an ultrashort-acting barbiturate, as the most significant redistribution into skeletal muscle occurs earlier. Ultimately, however, elimination of the agents from the body depends on metabolic enzymes because the barbiturates are too lipid soluble to be filtered at the glomerulus and excreted in urine without chemical modification. Less than 1% of these IV anesthetic agents are recovered unchanged in the urine (Stoelting, 1991).

Thiopental is the most commonly used IV anesthetic to induce anesthesia (Ghoneim, Pandya, Kelly, Fisher & Corry, 1976). Thiopental is approximately 80% bound to albumin. Displacement of thiopental from albumin by drugs, such as aspirin and phenylbutazone, or endogenous compounds such as uric acid, has been reported to enhance the effects of thiopental (Chaplin, Roszkowski, & Richard, 1973). Decreased plasma protein binding of thiopental occurs in conditions such as uremia and cirrhosis of the liver and results in increased drug sensitivity in these patients (Ghoneim & Pandya, 1975).

Clearance

Renal. All barbiturates are filtered, to some degree, at the glomerulus. However, with the more lipophilic agents (thiobarbiturates) that are extensively bound to plasma proteins, the rate of filtration is significantly lower than that for barbiturates that exhibit less protein binding. These highly lipophilic agents also can be readily reabsorbed across the wall of the nephron and returned to the circulatory system after filtration.

Hepatic. Thiopental exhibits a capacity-dependent elimination by the liver that is reflected in its low extraction ratio (ER < 0.3). The clearance of thiopental, unlike that of methohexital, does not depend on the rate of blood flow to the liver. Methohexital is cleared by the liver and is perfusion dependent. A decrease in blood flow to the liver, as is observed in heart failure, will decrease the rate of clearance of methohexital from blood.

Metabolism. Barbiturates are metabolized by the liver mixed–function oxidases (phase I reactions) to more water-soluble compounds that are excreted in urine. Some metabolites that are produced during the first major phase of drug metabolism may also be conjugated (phase II reactions). Biotransformation accounts for the complete removal of the ultrashort-acting barbiturates from the body. Metabolism of the ultrashort-acting thiobarbiturates, however, does not contribute to the termination of an induction dose that produces a short-term hypnosis. The metabolism of these agents (~12% to 15% per hour) is very slow compared to the uptake of drug by the skeletal muscles during redistribution. To efficiently excrete the ultrashort-acting barbiturates, biotransformation of the parent compound to a more water-soluble metabolite must occur. The liver is the primary site of metabolism of both the thiobarbiturates and oxybarbiturates. The metabolites of the ultrashort-acting agents lack pharmacologic activity.

Aliphatic hydroxylation, or side-chain oxidation, of the substituents on the C5 atom is one of the most important metabolic steps that terminates the biologic activity of the ultrashort-acting barbiturates. Furthermore, the thiobarbiturates undergo desulfuration, which results in replacing the more lipophilic sulfur atom with a more polar oxygen atom or hydroxyl group on the C2 atom and hydrolytic opening of the ureide ring. The metabolites that are produced after the phase I reactions are generally conjugated to glucuronic acid to further increase the polarity of the metabolite. Ninety-nine percent of a dose of thiopental is metabolized, but this degradation occurs at a slow rate, with 10% to 15% of a single dose of the drug being transformed by the liver each hour (Breimer, 1977).

Aliphatic hydroxylation of methohexital produces hydroxymethohexital, which is an inactive compound. A significantly greater fraction of methohexital is metabolized per unit time period than that of thiopental. Although volumes of distribution are similar for thiopental and methohexital, the rates of clearance of these agents differ significantly (Hudson, Stanski, & Burch, 1983). The hepatic clearance of methohexital is approximately three times greater than that of thiopental. Methohexital also has a significantly shorter elimination half-life (3 to 5 hours) than thiopental (8 to 10 hours), which again reflects its greater rate of metabolism by the liver.

When a series of doses of methohexital or thiopental are administered to a patient, recovery from methohexital anesthesia occurs more readily than with thiopental. The patient returns to consciousness more rapidly with methohexital, and cognitive functions return more quickly after administration of methohexital than with thiopental (Korttila, Linnoila, Ertama, & Hakkinen, 1975). For these reasons, methohexital is useful for outpatient procedures. If larger or repeated doses of the thiobarbiturates, or methohexital, are administered, the rate of metabolism may be modified. For example, alterations in the rate of drug metabolism could occur because of age, chronic liver disease (cirrhosis), induction of the microsomal enzymes due to previous exposure to an inducing agent such as phenobarbital, or inhibition of metabolism due to the presence of an inhibiting agent (drug–drug interactions). In older patients or patients with a severe liver dysfunction, the elimination half-life of the barbiturate anesthetics may be increased. However, the ability of the liver to metabolize (oxidize) barbiturates is significant; therefore, any hepatic disease that is present has to be severe before an increased duration of action is observed with these anesthetic agents.

Children have a faster rate of metabolism, so elimination half-times of thiopental are significantly shorter than for adults (Sorbo, Hudson, & Loomis, 1984). Recovery after large or repeated doses of thiopental may be more rapid in pediatric patients than in adults. The V_d and plasma protein binding of thiopental are not different in children and adults.

Redistribution. Induction of the cytochrome P450 isoenzymes (mixed-function oxidases) or their inhibition does not appear to modify significantly the duration of the hypnotic effect produced by a single dose of thiopental. Although clearance of thiopental by the liver is classified as capacity dependent, Pandele, Chaux, Salvadori, Farinotti, and Duvaldestin (1983) observed that, in patients with cirrhosis of the liver, clearance of a single dose of thiopental from plasma after redistribution had occurred was not different from control values. Most of a dose of thiopental after redistribution is located in lean tissues and fat depots. Sequestration of thiopental in body tissues results in a very rapid decline of blood plasma levels from redistribution. Very low concentrations of thiopental (15%) remain in blood after 1 minute. Because of this phenomenon and because thiopental is slowly metabolized, even individuals with hepatic dys-

function (cirrhosis) can readily metabolize the amount of drug presented to the liver per unit time period. If, however, increased or multiple doses were administered to the patient with cirrhosis, thiopental may saturate or approach near saturation of tissue depot sites, resulting in higher thiopental blood concentrations and prolonged elimination.

The elimination half-time of thiopental is higher in obese individuals than in individuals with normal weight (Jung, Mayerson, Perrier, Calkins, & Saunders, 1982) when drug dose is calculated using total body mass and not lean body mass. In the elderly, a smaller V_d and smaller lean tissue mass may result in higher plasma concentrations of thiopental for a longer time. The elimination half-time for thiopental may be increased in pregnancy because of an increase in the V_d and plasma protein binding.

Mechanism of Action

The barbiturates appear to have many sites of action in the CNS. They exert a strong inhibitory effect on the reticular activating system (RAS), which is important in maintaining alertness and wakefulness. Barbiturates appear to produce their depressant effects by increasing inhibition in the CNS and by decreasing excitation. They stimulate the central gamma-aminobutyric acid (GABA) receptors, producing increased inhibition of the CNS. They produce decreased excitation of the CNS by inhibiting the actions of glutamic acid, an excitatory neurotransmitter, at selective sites.

Barbiturates interact selectively with the GABA_A-receptor and, thus, are able to modify chloride ion fluxes either indirectly or directly, resulting in an increased inhibition of excitatory signals postsynaptically by either prolonging GABA responses or by mimicking the actions of GABA directly (Olsen, 1988).

Pharmacologic Effects

Central Nervous System. The CNS is the most sensitive to the depressant effects of the barbiturate anesthetics. The barbiturates can produce various levels of CNS inhibition, from mild sedation to unconsciousness. Even at anesthetic doses leading to unconsciousness, peripheral effects may be minor or insignificant. Selective CNS effects cannot usually be observed with the barbiturates without producing generalized CNS depression, with the exception of the anticonvulsant effects of phenobarbital and mephobarbital (metharbital). The CNS sensitivity to the depressant effects of the ultra-short-acting thiobarbiturates does not change with age (Homer & Stanski, 1985). In the presence of pain, small doses of barbiturates may increase the perception and reaction to nociceptor stimulation. Perception of pain generally occurs until unconsciousness is reached. In some individuals, or if pain is present, a paradoxical response can occur, which may include restlessness, excitation, and delirium rather than sedation after administration of a sedative-hypnotic. Therefore, in the presence of noxious stimuli, the behavioral and physical consequences of barbiturate administration cannot always be predicted. However, the elderly have a greater tendency than younger individuals to exhibit confusion and agitation after administration of barbiturates. Excitation occurs more commonly with phenobarbital and N-methylbarbiturates, such as methohexital.

Physical tolerance, referring to a decrease in responsiveness to the effects of a drug after chronic exposure to the agent, is commonly observed with sedative-hypnotics. Tolerance usually results in a need to increase the dose of a drug to produce the desirable drug effects and to prevent the development of a withdrawal syndrome. Withdrawal effects may include increased excitability that may lead to convulsions. Tolerance to the barbiturates is both a pharmacokinetic and pharmacodynamic phenomenon.

The barbiturates generally exhibit a narrow margin of safety (therapeutic index). A dose that is 10 times the therapeutic dose may be lethal (Clarke, Brater, & Johnson, 1992). The margin of safety becomes narrower as physical tolerance develops. Pharmacodynamic tolerance to barbiturates results in cross-tolerance to all drugs that cause CNS depression, including other IV anesthetics, benzodiazepines, volatile anesthetics, and ethanol. When barbiturates are administered in combination with other CNS inhibitors, such as ethanol, benzodiazepines, antihistamines, monoamine oxidase inhibitors, and volatile anesthetics, severe CNS depression can occur.

Cardiovascular System. A transient fall in blood pressure (10 mmHg to 20 mmHg) occurs when the IV barbiturates (thiopental, thiamylal, and methohexital) are administered to normovolemic adult patients during anesthesia induction. The fall in blood pressure usually is accompanied by an increase in heart rate (15 to 20 beats/minute), which returns the blood pressure back to normal. Anesthetic concentrations of the barbiturates result in selective inhibition of specific ion channels (sodium and potassium) in cardiac muscle cells (Nattel, Wang, & Matthews, 1990; Pancrazio, Frazer, & Lynch, 1993) that results in a slightly decreased cardiac output. The peripheral vascular resistance, however, is either increased or unchanged. With the exception of the skin and brain, blood flow to most organs and tissues of the body remains unchanged. Blood flow to the brain and skin, however, is reduced. Cardiac arrhythmias are rarely observed during anesthesia induction with barbiturates, but may result when hypercapnia or hypoxemia develops.

In the presence of circulatory shock (hypovolemic,

cardiogenic, septic, neurogenic), an induction dose of a barbiturate may result in hypotension, leading to circulatory collapse and cardiac arrest because of the partial inhibition of sympathetic ganglia and the blunting of cardiovascular reflexes by the barbiturate anesthetics. If blunting of sympathetic reflexes occurs in the hypovolemic patient, a significant fall in blood pressure could take place.

Cerebral Metabolism and Blood Flow. Cerebral blood flow and cerebral oxygen consumption are decreased in individuals receiving thiopental or other barbiturates. The degree of depression of cerebral metabolism is in direct proportion to the amount of the barbiturate administered. A decrease in cerebral blood flow also accompanies a decrease in cerebral metabolism, but the former effect occurs to a lesser degree than the latter. Decreased cerebral blood flow also will reduce the intracranial pressure. This decrease in intracranial pressure after barbiturate administration is useful in patients with cerebral edema or those undergoing specific neurosurgical procedures that require a reduction in increased intracranial pressure (Shapiro, 1985).

Respiration. During induction, thiopental produces a dose-related depression of the dorsal respiratory group (DRG) of neurons in the medulla, as well as a dose-related depression of the chemoreceptor drive. The compensatory reflex mechanisms initiated by the stimulation of chemoreceptors, when elevated blood levels of carbon dioxide are present or when decreased concentrations of oxygen occur, are reduced or even abolished (Hirshman, McCullough, Cohen, & Weil, 1975). Barbiturate-induced respiratory depression can inhibit or abolish protective airway reflexes, such as coughing, hiccupping, laryngospasm, and bronchospasm. Although thiopental is not considered to be irritating to the tissues of the respiratory tract, airway hyperreactivity is frequently observed. The presence of an irritant such as saliva or the insertion of an endotracheal tube may activate airway reflexes. The activity of these reflexes becomes progressively more inhibited as a deeper plane of anesthesia is reached. Following a dose of thiopental that causes hypnosis, tidal volume and minute volume are decreased and the functional residual capacity may also be reduced (Marshall, Hanson, & Marshall, 1995). Central nervous system stimulants such as doxapram can be given to reverse respiratory depression from clinical doses of thiobarbiturates. The patient must be observed continually following administration of doxapram to ensure maintenance of adequate ventilation.

Barbiturate intoxication or overdose can result in hypotension from hypoxia and/or may result from inhibition of the medullary vasomotor center and sympathetic ganglia. If intoxication occurs with the ultrashort-acting barbiturates, or any other barbiturates, hemodialysis and hemoperfusion can be used to increase drug clearance from the body. Alkalinization of the urine, together with a forced diuresis with the use of an osmotic diuretic, is more effective for long-acting barbiturates. Whether the intoxicating agent is an ultrashort-acting or long-acting barbiturate, oxygen should be administered and a patent airway and adequate ventilation maintained.

Liver and Kidney. Chronic use of barbiturates, particularly of the long-acting phenobarbital, is known to cause a significant increase in liver microsomal enzymes that are responsible for the biotransformation of many endogenous compounds and xenobiotics. Inhalation anesthetics, barbiturate IV anesthetics, and ethanol are metabolized and can induce the mixed-function oxidases that are cytochrome P450 dependent. Induction of cytochrome P450 enzymes by the ultrashort-acting barbiturates would not be expected to occur in patients who are not chronically taking barbiturates.

Thiopental may reduce the glomerular filtration rate because of decreases in the mean systemic blood pressure. If excessive doses of thiopental are administered, however, oliguria or anuria may occur as a result of the development of a significant hypotension.

Pregnancy (Placenta). The barbiturates, particularly the highly lipid-soluble ultrashort-acting agents, readily cross the placenta and can depress the fetus.

Skeletal Muscle. At the neuromuscular junction (NMJ), induction doses of the ultrashort-acting barbiturates inhibit depolarization of the motor end plate by acetylcholine, causing a transient relaxation of skeletal muscles at the onset of anesthesia. Thus, the inhibitory effects of nondepolarizing neuromuscular blocking agents, such as pancuronium, at the NMJ are enhanced during barbiturate anesthesia (Roth, Forman, Brasswell, & Miller, 1989).

Gastrointestinal Tract. The oxybarbiturates cause relaxation of the smooth muscle associated with the wall of the gastrointestinal (GI) tract, and they also tend to decrease the amplitude of intestinal contractions. The effects are caused by both central and peripheral mechanisms.

Porphyria. The presence of variegate or acute intermittent porphyria is a contraindication to the use of barbiturates. In these inherited disorders, barbiturates may cause acute and even fatal attacks of porphyria, resulting in demyelination of central and peripheral nerves, leading to weakness, paralysis, abdominal pains, psychiatric disturbances, and even death.

Propofol

Propofol (Diprivan®) is one of the more recent additions to the IV anesthetic group of drugs. Propofol is classified as a sedative-hypnotic but is unrelated chemically to any of the other agents in this class. Propofol is used as an induction agent and also to maintain anesthesia during surgery. It also can be used as a sedative during regional anesthesia, conscious sedation, and in intubated, mechanically ventilated patients in the intensive care unit.

Chemical and Physical Properties

Chemically, propofol (2,6-diisopropylphenol) is a substituted phenol with a molecular mass of 178.27 and a molecular formula of $C_{12}H_{18}O$. The structure of propofol is shown in Figure 19–4. Because propofol is an alkylated phenol, it is an oil at room temperature and is only slightly soluble in water. It is a weakly acidic drug with a pK_a of 11.03. The octanol-to-water partition coefficient for propofol is 5012 to 1 at physiologic pH.

Because of its high lipophilicity, propofol is formulated in an oil-in-water emulsion that appears as a slightly viscous milky substance. The sterile, nonpyrogenic emulsion is isotonic to body cells and contains 10 mg/mL of propofol, 100 mg/mL of soybean oil, 22.5 mg/mL of glycerol, 12 mg/mL of egg lecithin, and sodium hydroxide for pH adjustment. The emulsion has a pH range of 7.0 to 8.5 and is marketed in 20-mL or 50-mL glass ampules. Propofol should be stored away from direct light, at temperatures between 40°F and 72°F (4°C to 22°C), because it contains no preservatives and would be an excellent medium for microbe growth.

Pharmacokinetics

Although propofol is extensively bound to plasma proteins, an induction dose (2.0 mg/kg to 2.5 mg/kg) produces unconsciousness as rapidly as thiopental, within one arm-to-brain circulation time, about 40 seconds (Waugaman & Foster, 1991). The high perfusion rate of the brain, combined with the high lipid solubility of propofol, contributes to propofol's rapid uptake into the brain and its rapid equilibration with it. Undesirable effects are rare but include pain at the site of injection, coughing and hiccupping, and involuntary skeletal muscle movements. Injection of propofol is rarely associated with the release of histamine or nausea and vomiting.

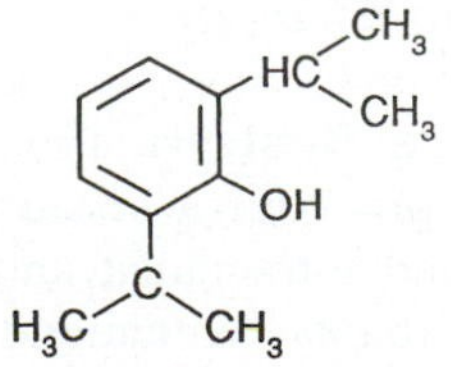

Figure 19–4. Chemical structure of propofol.

Pain at the site of injection of propofol can be decreased by using larger veins and by administering lidocaine before or with propofol.

Usually, hypnosis is produced pleasantly with minimal excitation and adverse effects. Following a bolus IV injection, blood concentrations of propofol decline quickly because of the rapid redistribution of propofol into less highly perfused tissues and from metabolism by the liver. Redistribution accounts for approximately 50% of the decline in plasma concentration after a bolus IV dose of propofol. As with thiopental, the pharmacokinetics of propofol can be described by a three-compartment model of drug distribution (Hull, 1989), which includes a rapid equilibration with plasma and the VRG ($t_{1/2}$ of 2 minutes), redistribution into peripheral tissues (intermediate $t_{1/2}$ of 50 minutes), and a slower elimination phase (terminal $t_{1/2}$ of 4.8 hours).

After a bolus injection of propofol, the patient returns to consciousness in approximately 4 to 8 minutes, with less CNS depression than observed with barbiturates. A continuous infusion of propofol alone or with other agents, such as alfentanil, sufentanil, or inhalation agents, also may be used to maintain anesthesia during surgery. Induction doses should be reduced in elderly and premedicated patients. Recovery from anesthesia after a bolus dose of prolonged infusion with propofol is more rapid than from the ultrashort-acting thiobarbiturates and is associated with less depression of the CNS postoperatively. This feature has made propofol a popular choice for short procedures and outpatient surgery.

Propofol clearance is blood flow dependent. Virtually all propofol delivered to the liver is extracted and metabolized to inactive compounds by phase I reactions (oxidation) and phase II reactions (conjugation to glucuronic acid and sulfate) (Simons, Cockshott, & Douglas, 1985). The inactive metabolites are subsequently excreted in the urine. The clearance of propofol is not lower in patients with chronic hepatic cirrhosis or chronic renal impairment than it is in normal adults.

Mechanism of Action

The mechanism of action of propofol is not completely understood. Propofol inhibits synaptic transmission by increasing the inhibition of the CNS by binding to $GABA_A$-receptors. Propofol also exhibits antiemetic, anticonvulsant, antipruritic, and anxiolytic effects.

Pharmacologic Effects

Central Nervous System. Propofol is useful during neurosurgical procedures because it reduces cerebral blood flow and intracranial and intraocular pressures. It also exhibits antiemetic, anxiolytic, and anticonvulsant properties. Unlike thiopental and other barbiturates, propofol does not promote hyperalgesia and may even provide analgesia.

Cardiovascular System. During induction of anesthesia, a significant drop (25% to 40%) in the mean, diastolic, and systolic blood pressures occurs (Blouin, Seifert, & Conard, 1992; Coates, Monk, Prys-Roberts, & Turtle, 1987; Conti, G., Dell' Utri, D., Vilardi, V., DeBlasi, R. A., Pelaia, P., Antonelli, M., Bufi, M., Rosa, G., & Gasparetto, A., 1993; Mehr, Hirshman, & Lindeman, 1992; Vermeyen, Erpels, & Janssen, 1987). Decreases in blood pressure usually are more marked with propofol than with thiopental. The observed decrease in blood pressure with propofol is due to vasodilation resulting from a decrease in peripheral vascular resistance and reduction in cardiac output from direct myocardial depression. Both the decrease in peripheral vascular resistance and the decrease in cardiac output are dose-dependent effects (Rouby, Andrew, Leger, Arthaud, Landault, Vicaut, Maistre, Eurin, Gandjbakch, & Viars, 1991).

Blood pressure also has been reported to decrease significantly (by 20% to 30%) during maintenance of anesthesia with propofol (Claeys, Gepts, & Camu, 1983; Coates, Monk, Pry-Roberts, Turtle, 1987). Propofol results in blood pressure decreases that are greater than those seen with the thiobarbiturates when equivalent doses are administered. Administration of an opioid analgesic simultaneously with propofol could result in an exaggerated hypotensive effect. Hypotension may be exaggerated in individuals who are hypovolemic, who have compromised left ventricular function, and who are elderly.

Propofol infusion can result in a significant decrease in the metabolic rate and perfusion rate of the heart (Fragen & Caldwell, 1979). Although there is a decrease in the mean blood pressure after an induction dose of propofol, the heart rate does not change significantly. Cullen et al. (1987) have suggested that the baroreceptor reflex mechanism is either reset or inhibited by propofol, resulting in an attenuated response in heart rate during hypotension.

An increase in blood pressure due to the increase in sympathetic activity during endotracheal intubation is less significant with propofol than with the ultrashort-acting barbiturates (Ebert et al., 1992). Propofol does not directly cause cardiac arrhythmias or ischemia or appear to sensitize the heart to catecholamines.

Respiratory System. Propofol is a significant respiratory depressant and may produce apnea in both adults and children for 30 to 60 seconds following an induction dose. Tidal volume, minute volume, functional residual capacity, and the respiratory response to carbon dioxide and a low partial pressure of oxygen are all reduced (Blouin, Seifert, Babenco, Conard, & Gross, 1993). Concurrently, there is an increase in the arterial partial pressure of carbon dioxide. These previous effects are exaggerated by opioid analgesics that are given concomitantly with propofol (Gold, Abraham, & Herrington, 1987). If the patient is being mechanically ventilated (positive-pressure ventilation), the degree of inhibition of the myocardium is increased, resulting in a further decrease in cardiac output. Because depression of respiration and the heart can occur at higher plasma levels of propofol, a 3- to 5-minute time interval should be allowed between each adjusted dosage.

Undesirable responses, such as hiccough, cough, and laryngospasm, occur less often with propofol than the barbiturates. Although not as effective as halothane, propofol has been observed to induce bronchodilation in individuals with chronic obstructive pulmonary disease (Conti et al., 1993).

Liver and Kidney. The clearance of propofol by the liver is perfusion dependent, which is reflected in its high extraction ratio (ER = 1). Because the rate of metabolism of propofol is greater than its rate of delivery to the liver, it has been implied that it is metabolized partly at extrahepatic sites. Propofol has no significant direct effects on renal function.

Skeletal Muscle. Propofol has no direct effect on the NMJ. Propofol does not interfere with administered nondepolarizing and depolarizing neuromuscular blocking agents at the NMJ (De Grood et al., 1985; Nightingale et al., 1985). Propofol administration has not been associated with precipitating malignant hyperthermia in patients (Hopkinson & Denborough, 1988; Richardson, 1987).

Porphyria. Unlike the barbiturates, propofol has not been associated with precipitating acute or fatal attacks of porphyria in susceptible individuals.

Etomidate

Etomidate (Amidate®) is a potent ultrashort-acting sedative-hypnotic that lacks analgesic activity. Etomidate is a nonbarbiturate that is chemically unrelated to other general anesthetics. It is used to induce general anesthesia by IV injection and to supplement less potent anesthetic agents, such as nitrous oxide, for specific and brief surgical procedures.

Chemical and Physical Properties

The isomer of etomidate that exhibits hypnotic activity is a carboxylated imizadole that is chemically designated as R (+) ethyl-1-(1-phenylethyl)–1H–imidazole–5-carboxylate. The molecular mass of etomidate is 342.36. Etomidate is a weakly basic drug with a pK_a of 4.2. The chemical structure of etomidate is represented in Figure 19–5.

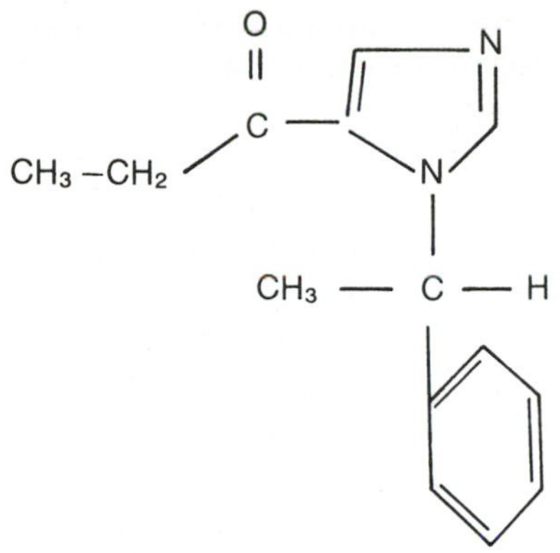

Figure 19–5. Chemical structure of etomidate.

Commercial Preparation of Etomidate

Etomidate is supplied as a sterile, nonpyrogenic solution, containing 2 mg/mL of propylene glycol at pH 6.9. Etomidate is water soluble at an acidic pH and only slightly water soluble at pH 7.38.

Pharmacokinetics

An induction dose (0.3 mg/kg) of etomidate produces unconsciousness as rapidly as thiopental and methohexital, within one arm-to-brain circulation time (approximately in 30 seconds) (Nauta et al., 1983; Nimmo & Miller, 1983). The hypnotic state lasts for approximately 3 to 5 minutes. The high perfusion rate of the brain, combined with the high lipid solubility of etomidate, contribute to its rapid uptake into the brain and its rapid equilibration with it. The duration of unconsciousness of a patient is directly proportional to the magnitude of the single dose of etomidate administered. The duration of anesthesia is usually 3 to 5 minutes when the dose injected is 0.3 mg/kg. As with the other ultrashort-acting anesthetics, multiple doses of etomidate will prolong the duration of anesthesia.

The undesirable effects of etomidate include pain on injection, hiccups, muscle spasms, thrombophlebitis of the veins, nausea, and vomiting (Craip et al., 1982; Doenicke, 1974; Famewo and Adugbesan, 1978; Fragen & Caldwell, 1979; Giese et al., 1985; Nimmo & Miller, 1983; Wells, 1985). A high incidence (30% to 40%) of nausea and vomiting occurs with etomidate. When etomidate administration is accompanied by an opioid analgesic, the incidence of nausea and vomiting is even higher. The frequency of nausea and vomiting can be reduced by the prophylactic administration of IV droperidol. As with propofol, pain at the site of injection of etomidate can be decreased by using larger veins and by administering lidocaine before etomidate administration or simultaneously with etomidate (Canessa et al., 1991; Doenicke, 1974; Famewo & Adugbesan, 1978; Galloway, Nicoll, & Leiman, 1982). Involuntary muscle movement frequency can be decreased by administering either an opioid analgesic or a benzodiazepine (Zacharias et al., 1979).

Thrombophlebitis of a vein used for etomidate injection can occur 2 to 3 days after drug administration; particularly if the dose of etomidate was delivered via a small-gauge IV needle (Kortilla & Aromaa, 1980). A single average induction dose of etomidate inhibits the metabolic functions of the adrenal cortex for up to 8 hours. During this time, the adrenal cortex does not respond to adrenocorticotrophic hormone (ACTH) stimulation. The lack of response to ACTH prevents the secretion of glucocorticoids that mediate the protective responses against stresses (Anonymous, Lancet, 1983; Longneck, 1984). Increased mortality has been observed when bolus etomidate injection has been used for chronic sedation of critically ill patients. Induction doses of etomidate range between 0.2 mg/kg and 0.6 mg/kg. The distribution of a single bolus dose of etomidate is best described by a three-compartment model of drug distribution, which includes a rapid equilibration with the VRG group ($t_{1/2}$ of 27 minutes), redistribution ($t_{1/2}$ of 29 minutes) into less perfused tissues (skeletal muscle and adipose tissue), and an elimination phase (terminal $t_{1/2}$ varies between 2.9 to 5.3 hours (De Ruiter et al., 1981; Hebron, Edbrooke, Newby, & Mather, 1983; Van Hamme, Ghoneim, & Amber, 1978).

Rapid awakening after a single dose of etomidate, which occurs even more quickly than with the ultrashort-acting barbiturates, reflects redistribution and the extensive hydrolysis of etomidate. Because of the rapid rate of return to consciousness during emergence, etomidate is very useful in outpatient procedures where a quick return to consciousness with little impairment of cognitive function is highly desirable. At steady state, the V_d of etomidate is approximately 2.5 L/kg to 4.5 L/kg (De Ruiter et al., 1981; Fragen, Avram, & Henthorn, 1983; Hebron et al., 1983; Schuttler, Schwilden, & Stoeckel, 1985; Van Hamme, Ghoneim, & Amber, 1978).

Etomidate exhibits significant protein binding (75%). Kidney or liver diseases that modify plasma protein concentrations may produce an exaggerated pharmacologic response to the increase in free drug etomidate molecules after loss of excess plasma proteins in urine or due to inhibition of synthesis of these proteins in the liver (Meuldermans & Heykants, 1976).

Etomidate can be administered both to induce and maintain anesthesia. Induction or maintenance doses of etomidate should be reduced in patients that have liver dysfunction or in the elderly. In individuals with hepatic cirrhosis the elimination half-life of etomidate is significantly longer because of an increase in the V_d (Van Beem, Manger, & Van Boxtel, 1983). In the elderly a decreased initial volume of distribution and a decreased clearance rate of etomidate are observed (Carden et al., 1986).

Metabolism

The rapid clearance of etomidate allows it to be administered in a single dose, multiple doses, or as a continuous infusion. Etomidate is rapidly converted to an inactive carboxylic acid derivative after hydrolysis of the ester linkage of the ethyl ester side chain, resulting in an inactive metabolite. Less than 3% of an administered dose of etomidate is excreted via the kidney as unchanged drug. The clearance rate of etomidate (18 to 24 mL/min/kg) is significantly greater than that of thiopental. Etomidate is mainly metabolized in the liver by ester hydrolysis (Corssen, Reves, & Stanley, 1988a).

Mechanism of Action

Evidence suggests that the biologically active isomer of etomidate promotes CNS depression via its interactions with the central $GABA_A$-receptor (Evans & Hill, 1977). The $GABA_A$-receptor also may play an important role in the central actions of propofol.

Pharmacologic Effects

Central Nervous System. Etomidate induction is associated with a transient 20% to 30% decrease in cerebral blood flow and intracranial pressure with no alteration of mean blood pressure (Renou, Viemhet, & Macrez, 1978). As with other IV induction agents, reduction in cerebral metabolic rate, reflected as the rate of oxygen utilization, is approximately proportional to the reduction in cerebral blood flow. A dose of 0.3 mg/kg rapidly reduces intraocular pressure by 30% to 60% (Thomsen et al., 1982).

Cardiovascular Effects. The maintenance of hemodynamic stability in patients after administration of etomidate is unusual among the potent and ultrashort-acting sedative-hypnotics (Gooding & Corssen, 1977; Lamalle, 1976). The use of etomidate is most beneficial to patients with cardiovascular disease, reactive airway disease, and intracranial hypertension. Etomidate imposes few effects on the cardiovascular system in normal patients or individuals with mild cardiovascular disease. In these individuals, etomidate does not produce any significant effects on heart rate, stroke volume, cardiac output, and ventricular filling pressures. Reductions in arterial blood pressure are generally minor and mainly reflect decreases in peripheral vascular resistance. It appears that the maintenance of hemodynamic stability in the presence of etomidate may be from lack of effect on the autonomic nervous system and autonomic reflexes. Etomidate does not promote the release of histamine (Guldager, Sodergaard, Jensen, & Cold, 1985).

Respiratory System. Less respiratory depression occurs with etomidate than with barbiturates. In most patients tidal volume is decreased and the ventilatory rate is increased after etomidate administration. Although etomidate decreases the sensitivity of the central respiratory center in the medulla to carbon dioxide, it may stimulate respiration independently of the medullary center (Choi et al., 1985). Therefore, etomidate may be useful when maintaining spontaneous ventilation is desirable. Inhibition of ventilation, however, may be increased when etomidate is administered as a continuous infusion in combination with inhaled anesthetics or opioid analgesics. Other effects, observed during induction with etomidate, are apnea of short duration (5 to 90 seconds with spontaneous recovery), laryngospasm, hiccupping, and snoring.

Endocrine System. Etomidate, when administered as a bolus injection or as a continuous infusion, inhibits the production of both glucocorticoids (eg, cortisol) and mineralocorticoids (eg, aldosterone) in the adrenal cortex. Direct inhibition of cytochrome P450 by etomidate results in blocking vitamin C resynthesis. Prolonged sedation of patients with etomidate in the intensive care unit is now contraindicated because of enzyme inhibition resulting in decreased levels of corticosteroids and mineralocorticoids with subsequent increase in morbidity.

Liver and Kidney. Etomidate has no significant effects on hepatic and renal function. In contrast to the actions of other anesthetics, both IV and volatile, there is no reduction in renal blood flow.

Skeletal Muscle. Etomidate is an inhibitor of the enzyme that hydrolyzes succinylcholine, plasma cholinesterase. It may prolong the action of succinylcholine in patients who are slow metabolizers of succinylcholine. Etomidate also may increase the degree of inhibition of nondepolarizing neuromuscular blockers at the NMJ (Booij & Crul, 1979). Etomidate administration has not been associated with precipitating malignant hyperthermia in patients. It is potentially porphyrinogenic and should be avoided in patients with porphyria.

Ketamine

Ketamine (Ketalar®) hydrochloride is an ultrashort-acting nonbarbiturate anesthetic that is a potent analgesic. Ketamine produces dissociative anesthesia. The term *dissociative anesthesia* refers to the strong feeling of dissociation of the subject from the surroundings. This latter state is characterized by amnesia, analgesia, catatonia, and nystagmus. Although the patient appears to be awake, the individual is noncommunicative and appears to be in a trance-like state. Ketamine produces dissociation between the thalamus and the limbic system. Keta-

mine is a nonbarbiturate anesthetic that is a powerful analgesic. It is used rarely today in general surgery because of its frequent (approximately 30%) associated emergence phenomena, which include undesirable effects such as disorientation, vivid dreams, unpleasant visual and auditory illusions, and delirium. Ketamine is useful in anesthesia for trauma and emergency surgical procedures as well as for patients who are elderly or in shock because of its ability to maintain the patient's hemodynamic status. It also is used in some types of outpatient surgeries, obstetrics, and in children that have sustained burns that require repeated changes of dressing. Administering benzodiazepines before or after induction of anesthesia with ketamine decreases the incidence of emergence reactions.

Chemical and Physical Properties

Ketamine [D,L-2-(o-chlorophenyl)-2-(methylamino)cyclohexanone hydrochloride] is a phencyclidine derivative that is partially water soluble and has a molecular mass of 238. The ketamine molecule contains one tetrahedral stereocenter, and therefore can exist as two stereoisomers or a pair of entantiomers. The structure of ketamine is shown in Figure 19–6. The pK_a of ketamine is 7.5.

Commercial Preparation

Ketamine is prepared as an acidic (pH 3.5 to 5.5) sterile solution for IV or intramuscular injection. Ketamine, a racemic mixture, is formulated in doses equivalent to 10 mg/mL, 50 mg/mL, and 100 mg/mL. The 10 mg/mL solution has been adjusted with sodium chloride to produce an isotonic solution. The commercial preparation is a racemic mixture of the two optical isomers, $S(+)$ and $R(-)$. The $S(+)$ isomer, however, is a more potent analgesic of the two isomers and also is less likely to cause undesirable emergence effects.

Pharmacokinetics

A calm, quiet environment is necessary to produce optimal results during induction of dissociative anesthesia with ketamine. An IV induction dose (1 mg/kg to 2 mg/kg) of ketamine produces surgical anesthesia in one arm-to-brain circulation time that occurs less than 60 seconds after administration and lasts 5 to 10 minutes.

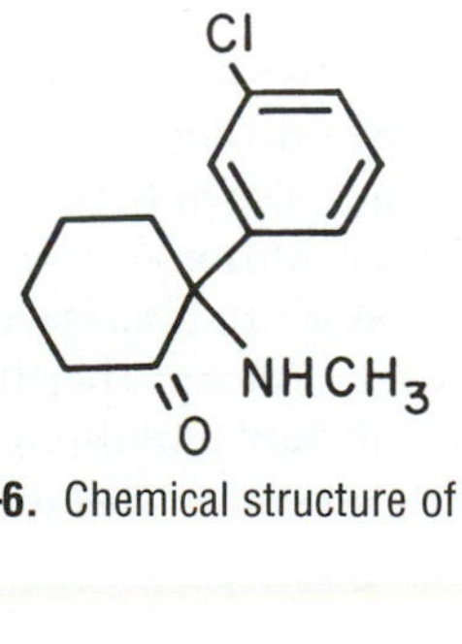

Figure 19–6. Chemical structure of ketamine.

Unconsciousness occurs only 2 to 4 minutes after an intramuscular injection (5 mg/kg to 10 mg/kg) of the 10-mg/mL formulation and lasts approximately 15 to 30 minutes. Ketamine is 5 to 10 times more lipophilic than thiopental. Although it is highly lipid soluble, it is not significantly bound to plasma proteins. The high perfusion rate of the brain, combined with the very high lipid solubility of ketamine, contributes to its rapid uptake into the brain, its rapid equilibration with the brain, and its fast onset of action. During and after the induction of dissociative anesthesia, muscle tone may be increased and purposeless body movements can occur. Occasionally, violent responses to stimuli are produced. Following a bolus IV induction dose of ketamine, the distribution of ketamine is analogous to the distribution of other ultrashort-acting anesthetics. Distribution includes a rapid equilibration with the VRG organs, including the brain, redistribution into less perfused tissues (skeletal muscle and adipose tissue), and an elimination phase, the latter of which includes metabolism and both urinary and biliary–fecal excretion of drug metabolites. Like the other ultrashort-acting drugs, redistribution from the VRG tissues to skeletal muscles and adipose tissues is responsible for the short duration of action of ketamine, which is not significantly affected by hepatic or renal disease following a single dose. With repeated doses of ketamine, cumulative drug effects can occur, as ketamine ultimately depends on hepatic metabolism for clearance. The V_d of ketamine is approximately 3 L/kg. Using a two-compartment model of drug distribution, the $t_{1/2\alpha}$ is approximately 16 minutes and the $t_{1/2\beta}$ is approximately 3 hours.

Metabolism

The clearance (19 mL/kg/min) of ketamine is approximately equal to the perfusion rate of the liver. Ketamine is a rapidly metabolized drug that exhibits a high extraction ratio and perfusion-dependent metabolism. Reductions in cardiac output will decrease the rate of ketamine metabolism. Ketamine undergoes *N*-demethylation and oxidation of the cyclohexane ring (phase I reactions). The metabolites derived from the first phase of drug metabolism are further conjugated to highly polar endogenous compounds (phase II reactions) and are subsequently excreted in the urine and feces. Approximately 93% of the metabolites are excreted in the urine, and approximately 3% are excreted via the biliary–fecal route. It has been suggested that the major effect of ketamine is to interact with specific receptors in the cortex and limbic system, but not the reticular activating system (Reich & Silvay, 1989). Although the mechanism of action of ketamine is not completely understood, much evidence supports the concept that the primary site of action of ketamine is the inhibition of the *N*-methyl-D-aspartate (NMDA) receptor. The inhibitory effects of ketamine are due to its antagonistic actions on the NMDA receptor, a ligand-gated ion channel resulting in blockage of excitatory signals that are normally initiated by the binding of glutamic acid to the receptor. Ketamine also may exert some of its pharmacologic effects by interacting with the GABA$_A$-receptor and increasing the inhibitory signals of this system. The analgesic effects of ketamine, which occur at lower doses, may be due to the actions of the $S(+)$ isomer at specific opioid receptors (μ-receptor).

Pharmacologic Effects

Central Nervous System. Ketamine greatly increases cerebral blood flow, oxygen consumption, and intracranial pressure because of its significant vasodilator actions. Therefore, ketamine is contraindicated in individuals with intracranial hypertension. Intracranial pressure, however, can be reduced by administering barbiturates or benzodiazepines, or by decreasing arterial blood partial pressure of carbon dioxide. Ketamine causes excitation of the CNS, which is reflected in the development of theta (θ) activity on the electroencephalogram. Recovery from ketamine anesthesia often involves unpleasant psychologic events. Emergence reactions occur most frequently during the first hour of recovery from anesthesia. These reactions include confusion, euphoria, vivid dreams, hallucinations, fear, and excitement. The frequency of these reactions occurs most often in adults and is observed less in children and the elderly. The frequency of emergence phenomena can be reduced by administering a benzodiazepine, accompanied by a lower induction dose of ketamine. Ketamine also produces mydriasis and nystagmus in patients.

Cardiovascular System. Unlike the other ultrashort-acting anesthetic agents, which produce no change or cause depression of the heart and blood pressure, ketamine increases the heart rate, systemic and pulmonary arterial blood pressure, myocardial oxygen consumption, coronary blood flow, and cardiac output by stimulating the sympathetic nervous system. The greatest increase in these hemodynamic parameters during administration of ketamine occurs 2 to 4 minutes after IV injection of the drug; values return to normal after 10 to 20 minutes. These cardiovascular stimulatory effects can be blocked by a number of pharmacologic agents, including α- and β-receptor antagonists, clonidine, benzodiazepines, and volatile anesthetics. Ketamine is contraindicated in patients with coronary artery disease and pulmonary hypertension. Ketamine has a direct depressant effect on the contractility of the heart, which is usually masked by the sympathetic responses that are elicited under normal circumstances. If depletion of adrenergic agents occurs, however, the direct effects of ketamine on the heart can be more readily observed. These direct effects may become apparent in patients who are critically ill or in shock. When ketamine is used to induce anesthesia in hypovolemic or critically ill patients who have depleted stores of catecholamines, cardiac output may decrease and hypotension may result.

Respiratory Effects. During anesthesia induction, ketamine transiently decreases the ventilatory rate for 2 to 3 minutes. Apnea may occur after rapid administration of an induction dose of ketamine. Although upper airway reflexes usually are functional and the muscle tone of airways is maintained, ketamine administration stimulates salivary and tracheobronchial secretions that can lead to airway obstruction, laryngospasm, and coughing. For this reason, anticholinergics, such as glycopyrrolate, should be administered preoperatively. Ketamine decreases airway resistance and bronchospasm via its sympathomimetic effect and by a direct smooth-muscle relaxant effect. Ketamine does not significantly decrease the ventilatory response to excess carbon dioxide or to a decrease in the partial pressure of oxygen in arterial blood. Pulmonary vascular resistance also is not altered and ketamine does not inhibit hypoxic pulmonary vasoconstriction.

Liver and Kidney. Ketamine is metabolized by the hepatic microsomal enzymes by *N*-demethylation and hydroxylation. Glucuronidated ion metabolites are mainly excreted in the urine. The metabolites of ketamine have significantly less pharmacologic activity than the parent compound and are not clinically significant. Chronic administration of ketamine, however, can result in induction of the hepatic enzymes involved in its metabolism. Ketamine does not impair hepatic or renal functions.

Skeletal Muscle. Ketamine enhances the action of nondepolarizing neuromuscular blockers but does not markedly prolong the action of succinylcholine.

▶ BENZODIAZEPINES

Diazepam

A number of benzodiazepines are presently available and are primarily used as antianxiety agents and central-acting muscle relaxants. Diazepam is considered the prototype drug for the benzodiazepines (Fig. 19–7) and will be discussed first as a generic model for their classification. Of the benzodiazepines, diazepam was at one time the most widely used and accepted. More recently, midazolam has gained popularity in anesthesia as an IV sedative.

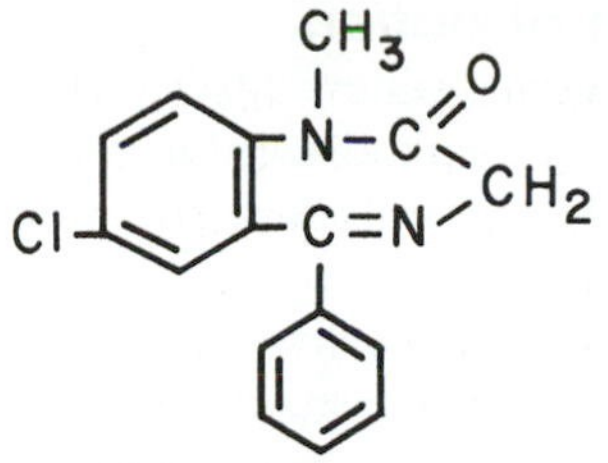

Diazepam
Figure 19–7. Chemical structure of diazepam.

Chemistry and Physical Properties

Diazepam is a benzodiazepine derivative; it is a colorless crystalline compound that is insoluble in water. It contains propylene glycol, ethyl alcohol, 5% sodium benzoate, benzoic acid as a buffer, and benzyl alcohol as a preservative. Each milliliter contains 5 mg of diazepam. The pH of the solution ranges from 6.4 to 6.9. A transient cloudiness occurs when diazepam is diluted with water or saline, but this does not affect the potency. The manufacturer does not recommend dilution because it produces an emulsion of small, particulate matter. Diazepam should not be mixed with other drugs.

Metabolism and Excretion

After IV administration, redistribution is rapid and follows kinetics similar to those of highly lipid-soluble agents. Diazepam is 80% to 90% bound to plasma proteins. After distribution is complete, elimination proceeds at a slow rate because of a relatively long half-life (20 to 40 hours).

The major metabolic pathway involves *N*-demethylation by hepatic microsomal enzymes. This process yields a pharmacologically active product, *N*-desmethyldiazepam, which is only slightly less potent than the parent compound. There is a constant rise in *N*-desmethyldiazepam levels over the first 24 hours, which is mirrored by the steady decline in diazepam levels (Rall, 1990). After 24 hours, levels of both the metabolite and diazepam decline at approximately the same rate. There is an increase in plasma diazepam levels 6 to 8 hours after administration and then a second smaller rise at approximately 10 to 12 hours (Dundee, 1979; Dundee & Wyatt, 1974; Rall, 1990). This is believed to result from enterohepatic recirculation, but this has not been substantiated. The rise in plasma levels at 6 to 8 hours is of clinical significance because patients may become sedate and sleepy again at this time. Oxazepam, an active metabolite of diazepam, reaches a peak plasma concentration in 4 hours and is excreted as the glucuronic acid conjugate in the urine (Benet, Mitchell, & Sheiner, 1990). Approximately 70% of the drug is excreted in the urine as glucuronide and other inactive metabolites.

Mechanism of Action

Benzodiazepines are believed to exert their CNS effects by occupying the benzodiazepine receptor that modulates GABA neurotransmission. The binding of benzodiazepines at these receptor sites causes inhibition of synaptic transmission by hyperpolarizing postsynaptic neurons. The effects of benzodiazepines can vary from tranquility to sedation and, with larger doses, sleep. Diazepam also produces relaxation of striated muscles by a central action. Intravenous administration produces anterograde, but not retrograde, amnesia (Dundee, 1979; Dundee & Wyatt, 1974; Heisterkamp & Cohen, 1975).

Pharmacokinetics and Pharmacodynamics

Gastrointestinal absorption of diazepam is rapid and complete, with plasma levels peaking shortly after administration. Intramuscular injections of diazepam are not as reliable in terms of absorption and distribution. When diazepam is administered intravenously, there is a delay of approximately 60 to 90 seconds before maximum depression occurs; however, there is a great deal of individual variation in response to diazepam. The amnesic action is rare after oral or intramuscular administration, but after IV injection of 10 mg of diazepam, the peak effect occurs in approximately 2 minutes and persists about 5 minutes, declining over the next 30 to 40 minutes. The amnesic actions of benzodiazepines are most marked when sedation is produced. Patients may respond appropriately to questions or commands, but recall for these events is suppressed.

Diazepam is infrequently used in anesthesia for sedation in IV doses and is primarily administered before the procedure in an oral form (5 mg to 10 mg PO) to reduce anxiety. Benzodiazepines are not analgesic and do not enhance the action of narcotics. The antianxiety effect combined with the narcotic action may sometimes appear to produce analgesia. Diazepam possesses anticonvulsant properties that can promptly control seizure activity by abolishing seizure discharge within a few seconds of injection. It often is used as the drug of choice in status epilepticus. The anticonvulsant properties and the elevation of the seizure threshold by diazepam may be of clinical importance in patients who are to receive large doses of local anesthetics. Diazepam can be administered intramuscularly or intravenously for seizure control.

Benzodiazepines have a centrally mediated muscle-relaxant property that is effective in treating muscle spasms of varying etiology. This effect is believed to result from the action of these drugs on the polysynaptic pathways within the spinal cord or on supraspinal structures (Dundee & Wyatt, 1974). Diazepam has been used successfully to control rigidity and muscle spasms caused by tetanus. Although diazepam produces a significant amount of relaxation of muscle rigidity and spasm, it does not produce adequate muscle relaxation for abdominal surgical procedures.

Pharmacologic Effects

Central Nervous System. Diazepam and all benzodiazepines have potent anticonvulsant properties and can be used to prevent propagation and generalization of seizure activity. Although diazepam does not reduce intracranial pressure significantly, reduction in intraocular pressure has been observed.

Cardiovascular System. The cardiovascular changes occurring with diazepam injection appear to be minimal. There is little change in ventricular contractility, heart rate, or pressures even with large doses (0.5 mg/kg to 1.0 mg/kg) (Dundee & Wyatt, 1974; Rao et al., 1973). Although the cardiovascular depressant effects of diazepam appear to be minimal in most patients, the drug must be used cautiously with patients in hypovolemic shock, of advanced age, or in a debilitated state of health. Wide variations in the response to diazepam should always be kept in mind.

Diazepam has been used for cardioversions in poor-risk and emergency situations. With this procedure diazepam produces a significantly lower incidence of ventricular arrhythmias and hypotension than with thiopental.

Respiratory System. Clinical doses of diazepam cause a slight degree of respiratory depression. The hypoventilation is due primarily to a decrease in tidal volume, resulting in a slight reduction in P_{O_2} and a slight rise in P_{CO_2} (Dundee & Wyatt, 1974). Even small doses of diazepam administered intravenously have been reported to cause a transient period of apnea, especially if given with a narcotic. Large doses of diazepam should be given with caution in patients with respiratory impairment, those receiving other CNS depressants such as barbiturates, and those who may have recently ingested alcohol. All these factors can lead to respiratory compromise or an exaggerated response.

Clinical Considerations

Diazepam is an excellent premedicant because of its efficacy in relieving anxiety and simultaneous production of sedation and amnesia. Intravenous diazepam can be administered in doses of 2.5 mg to 10 mg with or without a narcotic. If both narcotic and benzodiazepines are to be given, the doses should be adjusted accordingly. Oral diazepam also is very effective as a premedicant in doses of 5 mg to 10 mg. The oral and intramuscular routes do not produce amnesia. If amnesia is to be a desired effect of premedication, diazepam must be injected intravenously.

Intravenous diazepam in doses of 0.2 mg/kg to 0.6 mg/kg (in 5- to 10-mg increments at 1- to 2-minute intervals) may be required to induce general anesthesia. The dose may vary according to the degree of preoperative sedation. The onset of sleep occurs 1 to 2 minutes after diazepam injection. Intravenous diazepam had been used extensively for sedation for endoscopic procedures under local anesthesia and other minor surgical procedures carried out with local anesthesia, such as dental procedures and plastic surgery. However, use of midazolam has exceeded that of diazepam in these outpatient settings.

When administered intravenously, diazepam must be injected slowly to reduce the possibility of venous thrombosis, phlebitis, local irritation, and swelling. Breimer (1976) found that there is a significantly higher incidence of venous sequelae after IV diazepam than after lorazepam. Both thrombosis and phlebitis were found on the second and third days after injection, with an incidence of 23% for diazepam and 8% for lorazepam. Painless thrombosis that extended to the upper arm and axilla was noted at 7 to 10 days. Very long thrombosed segments of vein were found more often after diazepam administration; the incidence was 39% with diazepam and 15% with lorazepam at 7 to 10 days (Hegarty & Dundee, 1977). The complications occur most frequently when smaller vessels are selected for use. Venous thrombosis after diazepam anesthesia is related to age (Dundee, 1979). The incidence increases with age and increases sharply after age 60. Patients who are 70 years or older have almost a 100% chance of venous thrombosis sequelae.

Hypotension and apnea always are possible complications of intravenously administered CNS depressants. Resuscitative equipment should be available when moderate to large doses are administered. Diazepam must be administered with caution to patients in shock; patients taking barbiturates, phenothiazines, narcotics, monoamine oxidase inhibitors, or alcohol; and elderly or debilitated patients.

Midazolam

Midazolam is the benzodiazepine most commonly used in anesthesia practice today and has properties similar to those of diazepam. The principal differences between the two drugs are (1) the shorter duration of action; (2) the rapid metabolism; and (3) the water solubility. Midazolam is approximately three times more potent than diazepam.

Chemistry and Physical Properties

Midazolam, imidazole-1,4-benzodiazepine (Fig. 19–8), is water soluble in an acidic aqueous medium (pH < 4.0).

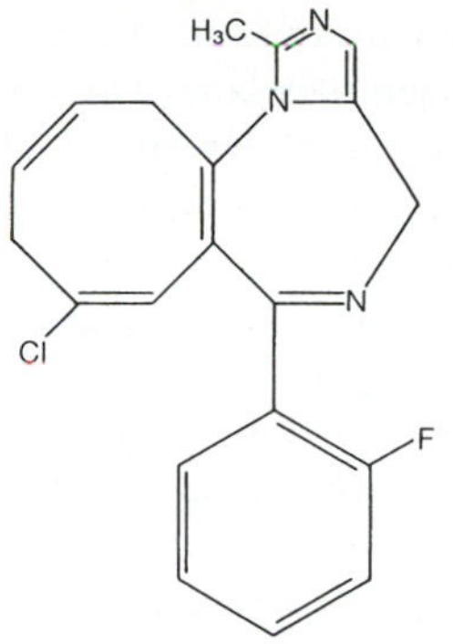

Figure 19–8. Chemical structure of midazolam.

At physiologic pH, midazolam becomes highly lipid soluble and is one of the most lipid-soluble benzodiazepines. The high lipid solubility promotes rapid entry of the drug into brain tissue. Studies have indicated that in an acid medium, the benzodiazepine ring opens and creates the desired water-soluble solution. At a pK_a close to 7.4 the ring closes and the drug becomes lipid soluble and readily crosses the blood–brain barrier (Aldrete & Stanley, 1980). Each milliliter contains midazolam hydrochloride equivalent to 1 or 5 mg. The compound contains sodium chloride and disodium edetate, and benzyl alcohol as a preservative.

Pharmacokinetics, Metabolism, and Excretion

Intravenous administration of midazolam at physiologic pH produces a rapid onset of activity. Entry into brain tissue and clinical activity occurs within 30 to 90 seconds. Midazolam's high lipid solubility and rapid distribution and metabolism contribute to the drug's short duration of action. Midazolam is the shortest-acting benzodiazepine available. The initial phase of drug disappearance is a result of drug distribution. This phase is followed by the less rapid phase, which is attributed mainly to biotransformation. After distribution and equilibration, midazolam is rapidly eliminated. The half-life ranges from 1 to 4 hours.

Oral midazolam is rapidly absorbed from the gastrointestinal tract. Peak plasma concentrations and clinical effects are noted within 1 hour. After oral administration, only 40% to 50% of the dose is available in the systematic circulation in the intact form (Allonen, Ziegler, & Klotz, 1981). This is due to extensive first-pass hepatic extraction and necessitates oral doses approximately twice the IV dose to achieve the same effect. The elimination half-lives of oral and IV midazolam are similar and are independent of the route of administration.

Midazolam is approximately 96% to 97% protein bound. The biotransformation involves hydroxylation by hepatic microsomal enzymes. The major metabolite is 1-hydroxymethyl-midazolam. Two other metabolites formed in very small amounts are 4-hydroxymidazolam and 1,4-dehydroxymidazolam. The metabolites are excreted in the urine in the form of glucuronide conjugates. Both the 1-hydroxy and 4-hydroxy metabolites possess less pharmacologic activity than the parent compound; this is not believed to be a significant factor in the overall clinical effects.

Pharmacologic Effects

Central Nervous System. Once midazolam has crossed the blood–brain barrier, it works at the level of the CNS benzodiazepine receptors. Midazolam appears to have three to four times the affinity for these receptors as has diazepam; thus it is estimated that it has approximately three to four times the potency of diazepam (Reves & Glass, 1990). Midazolam has clinical effects similar to those of diazepam. Premedicated patients usually lose consciousness after an IV dose of 0.2 mg/kg. Unpremedicated patients may require 0.3 mg/kg or higher doses. Such doses sufficient to cause loss of consciousness are recommended to induce anesthesia. Midazolam is an excellent hypnotic, anxiolytic, and amnesic. Anterograde amnesia can be obtained by both the IV and intramuscular routes of administration; the duration of amnesia is dose related. Sedation and reduction in the level of anxiety are easily achieved with IV doses of approximately 1.0 mg to 2.5 mg. Intramuscular doses for adequate sedation range from 0.07 mg/kg to 0.08 mg/kg.

Midazolam possesses anticonvulsant actions similar to those of diazepam. The electroencephalographic changes produced by midazolam also are similar to those observed with diazepam. Cerebral blood flow and cerebral oxygen consumption are reduced much more effectively by midazolam than by diazepam. Intraocular pressures are reduced to a degree similar to that achieved with diazepam.

Cardiovascular System. Midazolam's cardiovascular actions are very similar to those of diazepam. The decrease in blood pressure occurs by two mechanisms: (1) systemic vascular resistance is reduced, and (2) venous return is therefore reduced. When pulmonary artery occlusion pressures are initially high, midazolam has been shown to reduce them. Midazolam appears to maintain hemodynamic values in patients with ischemic heart disease (Reeves, Samuelson, & Linnan, 1980). Samuelson, Reves, Kouchoukos, Smith, and Dole (1981) reported a small increase in heart rate; small decreases in blood pressure, pulmonary artery pressure, and pulmonary artery occlusion pressure; and no change in cardiac output after induction with 0.5 mg/kg of midazolam. Cardiac arrhythmias have not been reported to be a problem.

Elderly patients and other poor-risk patients are more sensitive to the effects of midazolam. Volume-depleted patients may respond to midazolam with serious decreases in blood pressure; it is therefore wise to reduce the dose and to use caution with such patients. Although midazolam appears to produce only minimal cardiovascular depression, it has not been proven to be a safe induction agent in hemodynamically unstable patients.

Respiratory System. Intravenous induction doses of midazolam cause a transient respiratory depression (tidal volume reduction), apnea, or both. Ventilatory depression peaks at about 3 minutes and can last up to 15 minutes after doses of 0.2 mg/kg (Gross et al., 1983). The respiratory depression and apnea appear to occur most frequently in patients premedicated with narcotics. Recovery from this depression and from unconsciousness occur at the same time.

In patients with chronic obstructive pulmonary disease there is a more profound and persistent depression of ventilation (Gross & Smith, 1981). This is also probably true for elderly and poor-risk patients, who are more sensitive to drugs. Sedation and respiratory depression can be reversed with physostigmine (Caldwell & Gross, 1982). Coughing, breath holding, and laryngospasms occur less frequently with midazolam than with thiopental. Sedative doses of midazolam given intravenously may in some patients cause transient respiratory depression; therefore, patients should be observed closely whenever IV midazolam is used.

Kidneys. Midazolam induction reduces renal blood flow and glomerular filtration rate (GFR) and increases renal vascular resistance. These results are comparable to those observed with thiopental, with the exception of GFR reduction: A smaller reduction occurred in patients who received midazolam (Lebowitz, Cote, Daniels, & Bonventine, 1982). Patients with chronic renal failure had shorter induction times and longer recovery times. These findings can be related to the lower degree of binding of midazolam to albumin and the greater availability of the active, unbound drug in these patients, who also exhibited a lower free drug clearance than normal subjects (Vinik, Reves, Greenblatt, & Abernethy, 1983).

Clinical Considerations

Intravenous midazolam can be used for many of the same indications as diazepam: (1) induction agent; (2) maintenance agent; (3) sedation for local anesthesia or regional techniques; and (4) premedication. Induction doses for midazolam range from 0.2 mg/kg to 0.34 mg/kg. The dose is influenced by premedication, age, physical status, speed of injection, and serum albumin concentration. Opioid premedication appears to decrease the dose of midazolam required and shortens induction time. Sedatives and hypnotic premedications do not have the same ability to reduce dosage or induction times.

Induction times vary from 30 seconds to almost 5 minutes depending on the speed of injection. Compared with thiopental, midazolam induction and emergence are considerably slower. Patients regained consciousness after midazolam administration in approximately 15 minutes. Although this is longer than with thiopental, patients were considered street fit 3 to 4 hours after induction with either midazolam or thiopental induction. Induction and emergence times may be abnormal in patients with chronic renal failure.

Midazolam offers no advantage over thiopental for speed of induction and is not more effective in maintaining cardiovascular dynamics than etomidate. The advantages of midazolam as an induction agent are that it has higher reliability, speed of induction, and duration of action than diazepam. Midazolam can be used during anesthetic maintenance in the same manner as diazepam. Midazolam lacks analgesic properties, so it must be used in combination with opioids in a balanced technique or as an adjunct to an inhalation anesthetic. For short procedures, midazolam may be used similarly to thiopental by infusion after induction, supplemented by nitrous oxide and a narcotic premedication.

To supplement a regional or local anesthetic, small doses of IV midazolam in combination with small doses of narcotics will produce hypnosis, sedation, and amnesia. Both midazolam and narcotic should be carefully titrated to obtain the desired effect. Close observation of blood pressure and respirations is crucial when any IV agent is administered for sedation.

Premedication with midazolam can be accomplished intravenously, intramuscularly, or orally. Intravenous premedication may supplement previously administered oral or intramuscular drugs or may be used for acute sedation in an unpremedicated patient. When used for sedation, IV midazolam should be titrated to obtain the desired effect. Intramuscular premedication with midazolam produces much of the same effects obtained by the IV route, namely hypnosis, amnesia, and anxiolysis. The recommended intramuscular dose is 0.07 mg/kg to 0.08 mg/kg approximately 1 hour before surgery.

Advantages over Diazepam

Midazolam causes minimal local irritation and pain after IV or intramuscular administration. Intravenous midazolam has not been associated with the venous sequelae common with diazepam. Other advantages are the rapid onset of action, metabolism, and half-life. Midazolam is superior to diazepam for outpatient and short surgical or diagnostic procedures that require sedation and amnesia.

Lorazepam

Chemistry and Physical Properties

Lorazepam is a benzodiazepine derivative with actions very similar to those of diazepam (Fig. 19–9). It is a white powder that is insoluble in water. Each milliliter contains polyethylene glycol in propylene glycol with benzyl alcohol as a preservative. Each milliliter of sterile injection contains 2 mg or 4 mg of lorazepam. Lorazepam can be diluted with sterile water, sodium chloride, or D5W for injection. The drug should be administered slowly. The incidence of venous sequelae is much lower than with diazepam, probably because of the lower concentration of propylene glycol in lorazepam.

Absorption, Metabolism, and Excretion

Lorazepam is rapidly and virtually completely absorbed by the intramuscular route. Peak plasma concentrations are reached in 60 to 90 minutes. Maximum depressant effects after IV administration of lorazepam do not occur for 10 to 20 minutes. After oral administration, peak plasma levels are reached within 2 hours. Absorption from the gastrointestinal tract is essentially complete. The mean half-life for IV or intramuscular lorazepam is approximately 16 hours. It is 85% bound to plasma proteins. Lorazepam is conjugated in the liver into its major metabolite, lorazepam glucuronide. The metabolite is inactive and is excreted in the urine. The extent of drug accumulation with multiple-dose therapy is considerably less than that seen with diazepam. Dilution of lorazepam with an equal volume of compatible solution is recommended before IV use.

Pharmacologic Effects

Lorazepam and diazepam basically have very similar effects on the central nervous, cardiovascular, and respiratory systems. Lorazepam has a much slower onset of action and a longer amnesic action (Blitt et al., 1976). If lorazepam is to be given for sedation or to relieve preoperative anxiety, it must be given earlier than most preoperative medications (Dundee, 1979). The effects of a clinical dose of lorazepam usually last 6 to 8 hours. The

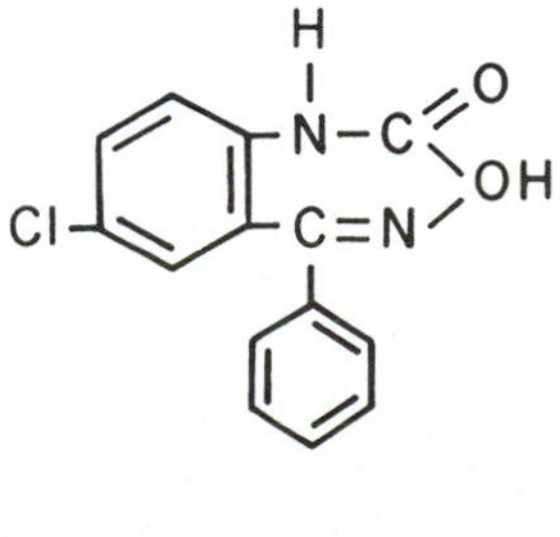

Lorazepam

Figure 19–9. Chemical structure of lorazepam.

amnesic action peaks at 15 to 20 minutes intravenously and 2 hours intramuscularly and can continue for 4 to 8 hours. The degree of sedative and anxiety-relieving effects is similar for both diazepam and lorazepam. The amnesic effects occur more rapidly and also subside more rapidly with diazepam. Lorazepam is indicated when longer sedation and amnesia are desired.

Clinical Considerations

Premedication and sedation for local or regional procedures can be accomplished readily with lorazepam; however, induction of anesthesia with lorazepam is not recommended because of the slow onset of action. Other situations indicating benzodiazepines and requiring rapid onset of action would best be handled with diazepam or midazolam. On the other hand, sedation and amnesia for intensive care patients on a respirator may best be accomplished with lorazepam. The suggested dose for intramuscular premedication with lorazepam is 0.05 mg/kg up to 4 mg. For optimum amnesic effects, intramuscular lorazepam should be administered 2 hours before the anticipated procedure. For IV sedation and relief of anxiety, 0.04 mg/kg up to a total dose of 2 mg may be given. If optimum amnesic effects are required and would be beneficial, 0.05 mg/kg up to 4 mg may be administered intravenously. The manufacturer does not recommend using lorazepam for patients under 18 years of age.

Other Sedatives: Butyrophenones

Droperidol

Droperidol is a potent butyrophenone, a fluorinated derivative of phenothiazine (Fig. 19–10). Each milliliter of drug contains 2.5 mg of droperidol. The pH of the clear, colorless solution is adjusted to 3.5. The 10-mL vial contains methylparaben and propylparaben as preservatives. The onset of action after IV injection is 3 to 5 minutes. The full effect may not be apparent for 30 minutes. The duration of action is generally 2 to 4 hours, but the effects of the drug may be noted for up to 12 hours.

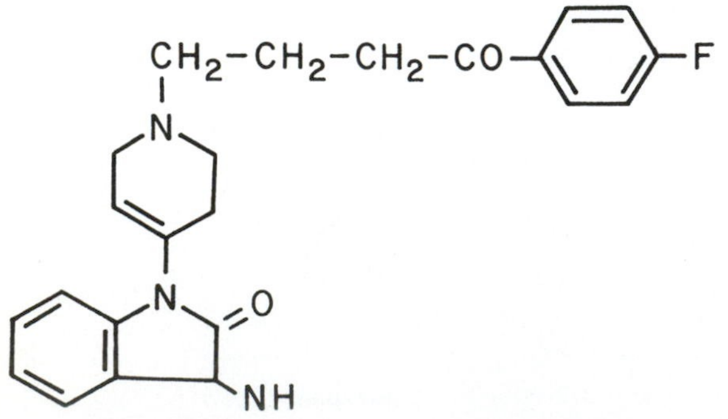

Figure 19–10. Chemical structure of droperidol.

Metabolism and Excretion. Droperidol is metabolized in the liver. Drug is excreted in the urine and feces, and the majority of the metabolites are excreted within 24 hours. Approximately 10% of the drug is excreted intact through the kidneys. No untoward effects on the liver or kidneys have been noted.

Pharmacologic Effects

CENTRAL NERVOUS SYSTEM. Droperidol produces marked tranquilization and inhibits operant (learned) behavior. The butyrophenones are able to induce cataleptic immobility, in which patients appear tranquil and dissociated from the environment but responsive when addressed. These drugs also inhibit symptoms of delusions, hallucinations, paranoia, and mania. This inhibition effect results in the ability to competitively antagonize the norepinephrine-, serotonin-, and dopamine-mediated synapses in the brain. The action is on the postsynaptic neuron, where dopamine is the neurotransmitter. At certain synapses, GABA is the inhibitory transmitter and dopamine the stimulatory transmitter. It is believed that butyrophenones compete for the dopaminergic receptors to decrease transmission (Corssen et al., 1988b).

Droperidol and other butyrophenones have a predilection for areas in the brain that are high in dopaminergic receptors, including the chemoreceptor trigger zone (CTZ) and the nigrostriatum. The marked antiemetic activity of droperidol is due to its action on the CTZ in the medulla. Droperidol does not antagonize motion sickness originating in the labyrinth. Extrapyramidal symptoms sometimes occur in a small percentage of patients as a result of dopamine blockade at the extrapyramidal nigrostriatum, and pseudoparkinsonian effects can be noted, though they may sometimes be delayed up to 24 hours. Such effects usually are associated with high doses but also have been reported with low doses administered intramuscularly. These effects respond to anticholinergics or antiparkinson therapy.

Droperidol can potentiate the effects of other CNS depressants such as thiopental, other tranquilizers, narcotics, and general anesthetics. Dosage adjustments should be made accordingly.

CARDIOVASCULAR SYSTEM. Droperidol has little or no effect on the myocardium, heart rate, or cardiac output. The systemic blood pressure falls slightly (in a normovolemic patient) because of the alpha-adrenergic blocking activity (Yelnosky, Ketz, & Dietrich, 1964). This action is usually very mild, but marked hypotension can occur in a hypovolemic patient. There also is a small decrease in pulmonary vascular pressures caused by decreased resistance. In general, the cardiovascular hemodynamics are well maintained. There has been some evidence that droperidol may reduce the incidence of epinephrine-induced arrhythmias, but it does not appear to prevent other cardiac arrhythmias (Yelnosky et al., 1964).

RESPIRATORY SYSTEM. Droperidol has not been found to produce any significant degree of respiratory depression. The respiratory depression occurring with the administration of Innovar®, a combination of droperidol and fentanyl, is due to the narcotic component, fentanyl.

▶ OPIOID INTRAVENOUS ANESTHESIA

Neuroleptanalgesia

Neurolepsis is a term coined by Delay and his colleagues in 1959 to describe a drug-induced behavioral syndrome consisting of diminished aggression, indifference to surroundings, and somnolence with easy arousability to full rational attention. Neuroleptic is the term used to describe drugs that produce neurolepsis or a neuroleptic state and is synonymous with the term *major tranquilizer.*

In the same year that Delay defined neurolepsis, DeCastro and Mundeleer introduced neuroleptanalgesia at the French Anesthesia Congress in Lyon. Neuroleptanalgesia has since become an extremely popular and useful anesthetic technique. As the name suggests, it is a state produced by combining a potent neuroleptic drug with a potent narcotic. DeCastro and Mundeleer emphasized the uniqueness of this technique with respect to "balanced anesthesia" techniques in that the patients were neither asleep nor awake but in a state of profound analgesia and psychomotor sedation. DeCastro and Mundeleer originally used haloperidol with a narcotic, muscle relaxant, and oxygen. With the introduction of the potent narcotic fentanyl and the neuroleptic droperidol in 1963, use of the previously mentioned drugs was discontinued and Innovar®, a mixture of these two drugs, came into frequent use. The effects produced by Innovar are the result of each component exerting its own pharmacologic effect independently of the other. The combination contains fentanyl and droperidol in a fixed ratio of 1 to 50; each milliliter of Innovar® contains 0.05 mg fentanyl and 2.5 mg droperidol. The use of Innovar® has declined as most anesthesia providers prefer to give the drugs individually to have a more controlled effect of the analgesic and sedative effects. Much less droperidol is generally needed intraoperatively to achieve desired effects than is found in the fixed ratio of Innovar®.

Neuroleptanalgesia has been described as a state of tranquilization and intense analgesia with little or no hypnosis. The technique affects the subcortical areas of the brain, the thalamus, hypothalamus, and reticular system to provide analgesia and sedation, leaving cortical functions intact. The CNS characteristics of this state include somnolence without loss of consciousness, psychologic detachment from the environment, inhibition of learned behavioral activity and reflexes, and analgesia (Reves & Glass, 1990).

From an anesthetic viewpoint, neuroleptanalgesia offers several advantages: (1) mental withdrawal from the immediate situation with an ability to respond and cooperate when the need arises; (2) a disinclination to move; (3) potent antiemetic effects; (4) analgesia; and (5) cardiovascular stability. When undisturbed, the patient remains in a state of calm detachment. The technique has been especially useful for diagnostic or surgical procedures that require consciousness and cooperation of the patient. If an anesthetic agent is added to produce unconsciousness and amnesia, the technique is termed *neuroleptanesthesia.* If required, a muscle relaxant can be added, and this technique then becomes a balanced anesthesia technique.

Opioid Intravenous Anesthetics

Opium is derived from the poppy plant, *Papaver somniferum.* Opium is not one compound, but consists of approximately 25 different plant alkaloids. These plant alkaloids have been identified and separated into a number of groups, including the phenanthrene and the phenylpiperidine groups. Alkaloids in both the phenanthrene group and the phenylpiperidine group include most of the narcotics used in anesthesia practice today. The benzoisoquinoline group yields drugs such as papaverine and noscapine that lack narcotic activity but are used as antitussives and smooth-muscle relaxants.

Chemical and Physical Properties

Morphine constitutes approximately 10% of the opium powder and is the oldest opioid in use. It also is the standard against which all other opioids are compared. The opioids described in this chapter are morphine, meperidine, fentanyl, sufentanil, alfentanil, and remifentanil (Fig. 19–11). Morphine and the other naturally occurring analgesic alkaloids are phenanthrene derivatives. Meperidine, fentanyl, sufentanil, alfentanil, and remifentanil are

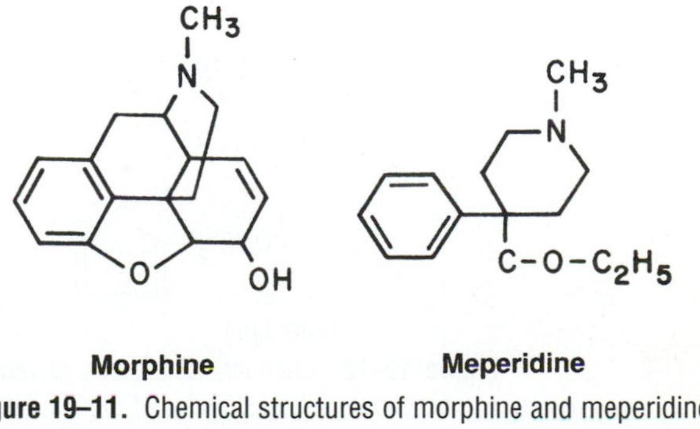

Figure 19–11. Chemical structures of morphine and meperidine.

chemically dissimilar to morphine and are phenylpiperidine derivatives (Fig. 19–12).

The analgesic activity of the opiates is highly stereospecific in that the levoisomer produces the analgesic effects (Beckett & Casey, 1954; Thorpe, 1984). A tertiary nitrogen, a quaternary carbon separated from the nitrogen by an ethane chain, and an electrophilic carbon that attaches to a phenylic or ketone group appear to be common structural characteristics (Beckett & Casey, 1954). Meperidine is a totally synthetic opiate. It was originally studied because of its atropine-like effect and the similarity of its chemical structure to that of atropine. Initial tests demonstrated a narcotic analgesic property and subsequent studies verified this effect. Like meperidine, fentanyl, sufentanil, alfentanil, and remifentanil are synthetic piperidine derivatives. The newest of the available synthetic opioids used in anesthesia are chemical analogs of fentanyl with very similar effects. Remifentanil is unique among the currently utilized agents in anesthesia because of its alkyl ester substituting for the aryl group on the piperidine nitrogen (Bowdle, 1996).

Absorption and Distribution

The opioids are absorbed completely from all routes of administration. Those used for anesthesia are usually administered by IV injection. Regarding distribution with respect to tissue uptake and distribution, opioids follow the same pharmacokinetic principles as other drugs injected intravenously (Table 19–3). Plasma levels of narcotics fall rapidly after injection, and only a small percentage of the injected drug actually reaches CNS tissues. The uptake of opioids by various organs and tissues is a function of both physiologic and chemical factors. Alfentanil possesses a high nonionized fraction at physiologic pH, and it has a small volume of distribution. This increases the amount of alfentanil available for binding in the brain (Morgan & Mikhail, 1996). Although all opioids bind to plasma proteins with varying degrees of affinity after absorption, the compounds rapidly leave the blood and localize in highest concentrations in tissues such as the lungs, liver, kidneys, and spleen. Although drug concentrations in skeletal muscle may be much lower, this tissue serves as the main reservoir of the drugs because of its greater bulk. Accumulation in adipose tissue also can become important, particularly after frequent high-dose administration of highly lipophilic opioids that are slowly metabolized (eg, fentanyl).

Concentrations of opioids are usually relatively lower in the brain than in other organs. An intact blood–brain barrier, however, is not present in infants. Because the opioid analgesics also cross the placenta, their use for obstetric analgesia can result in the delivery

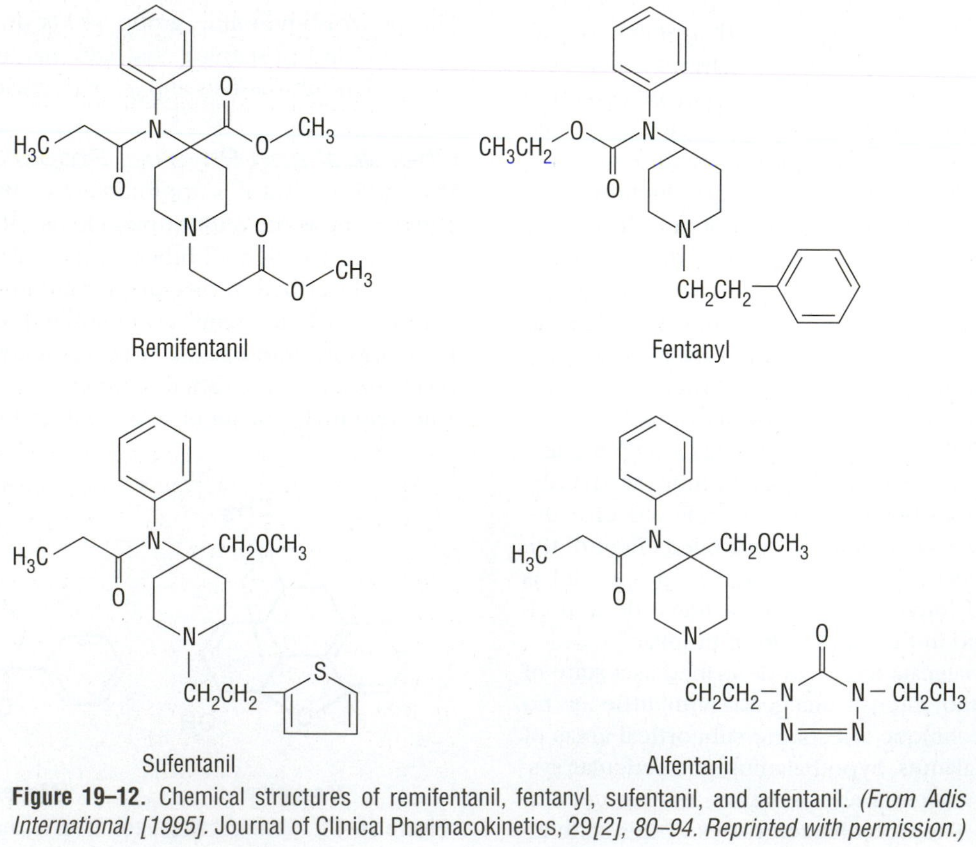

Figure 19–12. Chemical structures of remifentanil, fentanyl, sufentanil, and alfentanil. *(From Adis International. [1995]. Journal of Clinical Pharmacokinetics, 29[2], 80–94. Reprinted with permission.)*

TABLE 19–3. Comparison of Fentanyl, Sufentanil, Alfentanil, Remifentanil, and Morphine

	Fentanyl	**Sufentanil**	**Alfentanil**	**Remifentanil**	**Morphine**
Potency	130	1250	30	65	1
Therapeutic index	277	26 000	1080		70
Elimination half-life (min)	219	164	94	10	180
Volume of distribution (L/kg)	4	3	1	0.39	3
Clearance (L/kg/min)	13.0	12.7	5.0	2.8	14.7

of an infant with depressed respiration. Plasma concentrations of opioids have been noted to be higher in older individuals (Berkowitz et al., 1975). The elderly also are more sensitive to the respiratory depressant effects of opioids.

Metabolism and Excretion

Opioids are metabolized in the liver, and their primary route of excretion is the kidneys. Approximately 5% of morphine is N-demethylated, and almost all of this is excreted as normorphine in the urine. Only about 5% to 10% of free morphine or any of its metabolites can be detected in the feces. Respiratory depression after morphine anesthesia has been found to be inversely related to urinary flow rate and excretion of morphine. Patients with low urine outputs have been shown to have a longer period of respiratory depression after high-dose morphine anesthesia (Stanley & Lathrup, 1977).

Meperidine is N-demethylated to normeperidine and hydrolyzed to meperidinic acid. N-demethylation of the meperidinic acid occurs, forming normeperidinic acid in the liver. After conjugation of the phase I metabolites to glucuronic acid, they are excreted in the urine (Jaffe & Martin, 1990).

Fentanyl (80% to 90%) is hydrolyzed in the liver, producing 4-n-(N-proprionylanilino)piperidine and proprionic acid as metabolites. An oxidative reaction also occurs, but to a much smaller extent. Only about 10% of fentanyl is excreted unchanged. Approximately 70% of the administered drug is excreted in 4 days, with the greatest concentration detected between 8 and 24 hours after administration. The brevity of action of fentanyl is due primarily to rapid redistribution rather than to rapid metabolism and excretion.

Sufentanil is metabolized both in the liver and small bowel. Approximately 80% of the drug is excreted in the urine and feces within 24 hours; 20% of the drug is excreted unchanged. Alfentanil has a shorter duration of action than either fentanyl or sufentanil. The duration of action is approximately one third that of fentanyl. The shorter duration of action of alfentanil reflects its kinetic profile. Alfentanil is less lipid soluble than sufentanil and fentanyl. Its volume of distribution and clearance are lower, and its elimination half-life is much shorter. The

smaller volume of distribution results in greater access of the drug to clearing organs and a shorter elimination half-life despite the low clearance. In contrast to fentanyl, the clinical duration may depend more on metabolism than on redistribution. There is less of a cumulative effect than with fentanyl. The liver is the major site of biotransformation of alfentanil. Approximately 81% of the administered dose is excreted within 24 hours; 0.2% of the dose is eliminated unchanged. Excretion is primarily by the renal route (Hull, 1983).

Remifentanil is a novel ultrashort-acting opioid agonist. Remifentanil undergoes metabolism in extrahepatic sites by plasma and tissue esterases resulting in an extremely rapid clearance of approximately 3 L/min. The metabolism of remifentanil by ester hydrolysis is its distinguishing feature and accounts for its ultrashort duration of action (Bowdle, 1996). Unlike fentanyl and related opioids, termination depends mainly on metabolism (clearance), and not on redistribution. The primary metabolite produced after hydrolysis of the ester linkage of remifentanil is a carboxylic acid metabolite. Most of the drug (90%) is recovered unchanged in the urine in the form of an acid metabolite (Glass et al., 1993).

Pharmacologic Effects

Central Nervous System. Opioid effects on the CNS include analgesia, drowsiness, mood changes, mental clouding, euphoria, sedation respiratory depletion, and cough suppression. The site and mechanism of analgesic action are in the CNS. Receptors in the brain are concentrated in the periaqueductal gray matter, corpus striatum, and hypothalamus. One receptor primarily located in the brain is responsible for supraspinal analgesia. Two subpopulations of this receptor exist. The mu$_1$-receptor mediates supraspinal analgesia, whereas the mu$_2$-receptor mediates unwanted effects, such as hypoventilation, bradycardia, euphoria, and physical dependence. The mu-receptors and mu-antagonists include morphine, fentanyl, alfentanil, sufentanil, and remifentanil. Naloxone is a specific mu-receptor antagonist that reverses the effects of the mu-agonists. K-receptors also mediate analgesia, but are located primarily in the spinal cord. The receptors are excited by endorphins, encephalins, and electrical stimulation. Stimulation of this system is believed to cause descending inhibition of transmission of nociceptive information through the spinal cord. Opioids also induce an alteration in the limbic system response to painful stimuli without significantly altering sensory pathways. Opioids do not alter the threshold or responsiveness of the nerve endings to painful stimuli, nor do they affect peripheral nerve conduction.

Clinically, pain threshold is raised and the perception of response to pain is blunted. The painful stimulus may be noted but not perceived as painful. Patients often report that the pain is present but tolerable. Dull, continuous pain can be relieved more effectively than sharp intermittent pain, but most types of pain can be relieved by narcotics if sufficient doses are administered. Analgesia usually occurs without loss of consciousness, but sedation, drowsiness, and mental clouding become more prominent as the dose is increased. Therapeutic doses usually produce minimal sedative effects, but increasingly larger doses produce effects that range from sedation to coma.

When an appropriate amount of opioid is administered to a patient who experiences pain, discomfort, fear, anxiety, or tension, the patient reports that he or she is less distressed. Drowsiness, euphoria, or sleep may ensue. The onset of sedation is slower than that of the analgesic effect, but its duration is greater. Opioids given to patients who do not experience pain may cause dysphoria rather than euphoria and unnecessary anxiety or fear. Although narcotics provide excellent analgesia, they do not always provide amnesia when used alone. Amnesia may be associated with loss of consciousness after large doses of narcotics. Opioids combined with nitrous oxide will produce amnesia during general anesthesia but narcotic-with-oxygen techniques should not be relied on to produce amnesia.

Nausea and vomiting are due primarily to the ability of opioids directly to stimulate the CTZ located in the medulla (Benet et al., 1990). A vestibular component also may be involved because there appears to be a greater incidence of emesis in ambulatory patients. Other causes of nausea and vomiting after opioid administration include delayed emptying of gastrointestinal contents, increased tone of smooth muscle and sphincters, and increased volume of pancreatic and biliary secretions. Hypotension and inadequate cerebral perfusion also may stimulate the CTZ. Very large doses of opioids may depress it. The emetic effect is counteracted by opioid antagonists, phenothiazines, droperidol, and drugs used for motion sickness.

Cardiovascular System. Fentanyl derivatives, including remifentanil, cause a dose-dependent decrease in heart rate, arterial blood pressure, and cardiac output that is produced by a central stimulation of vagal activity

(James et al., 1992). Morphine and fentanyl derivatives have a positive inotropic effect that depends on the release of endogenous catecholamines (Vasko et al., 1966); this effect can be blocked by beta-blockers. Plasma and urine catecholamine levels usually are elevated after meperidine or morphine administration as in plasma histamine (Flacke et al., 1987). Meperidine has been found to cause significant depression (Sugioka, Boniface, & Davis, 1957).

With the exception of meperidine, all opioids can cause a vagal-induced bradycardia. The decrease in heart rate may be related to the dose, the rate of injection, or both. Bradycardia is less likely to occur with alfentanil than with other fentanyl analogs. Hypotension following opioid injections may be caused by a number of factors. Hypotension after morphine administration usually is attributed to increased plasma histamine, resulting in lower vascular resistance or contributing to a direct effect of morphine on vascular smooth muscle. Meperidine releases histamine and may produce hypotension. Administration of fentanyl, sufentanil, or remifentanil may cause hypotension because of an accompanying bradycardia. Sufentanil also may have a direct effect on vascular smooth muscle that contributes to hypotension (Starck et al., 1989). Hypotension can occur with any opioid and usually is related to the rate of injection and the volume status of the patient. Fluid administration and a slight Trendelenburg position usually correct the hypotensive episode.

Intravenous opioids combined with nitrous oxide produce cardiovascular effects quite different from the effects of the opioid alone. Often, a decrease in arterial pressure and cardiac output occurs with a concurrent increase in peripheral vascular resistance.

Cerebral blood flow is not directly affected by narcotics. Respiratory depression and carbon dioxide retention caused by large doses of narcotics will produce cerebral vasodilation and an increase in intracranial and cerebrospinal fluid pressure. Artificial ventilation that maintains $Paco_2$ at normal levels will maintain a normal cerebral blood flow despite large doses of narcotics.

Respiratory System. Therapeutic doses of opioids produce respiratory depression that can be detected without other apparent signs of CNS depression. The respiratory depression is dose related and can proceed to apnea with large doses. The mechanism of respiratory depression involves direct depression of the medullary centers active in ventilatory control (Tabatabai, Kitahara, & Collins, 1989). The response of the central chemoreceptors to carbon dioxide levels and of the carotid and aortic chemoreceptors to hypoxia also is lower. The carbon dioxide threshold is elevated, and the Pco_2's alveolar ventilation curve is shifted to the right. The pontine and medullary centers involved in ventilatory rhythmicity also are depressed, which may result in irregular and periodic breathing. Often, the inspiratory phase is pro-longed and the expiratory phase is delayed.

Respiratory rate, minute volume, and tidal volume are all depressed. Small doses of opioids decrease the respiratory rate without significantly affecting tidal exchange, whereas anesthetic doses may terminate involuntary respirations. Voluntary mechanisms for ventilation remain intact and the patients are able to respond to commands to breathe. The respiratory rate is greatly depressed, but at this stage the tidal volume is markedly increased to compensate. Opioid overdoses and deaths usually result from profound respiratory depression and respiratory arrest. Other effects of narcotics on respiration include depression of ciliary action within the bronchial tree, inhibition of the cough reflex caused by action on the cough center located in the medulla, and increased bronchial tone. It is not clear whether the last effect is mainly a direct effect on smooth muscle or an indirect action caused by histamine liberation or elevation of Pa_{CO_2} levels.

Kidneys. It was previously thought that the antidiuretic effect of morphine was due to the release of ADH. The decrease in urine output noted with the use of morphine anesthesia is now believed to be related to renal hemodynamics (Deutsch, Bastron, Pierce, & Vandam, 1969). Rapid administration of the drug and the addition of nitrous oxide may decrease hemodynamic function enough that the GFR and urine output are markedly diminished. Fentanyl, sufentanil, alfentanil, and remifentanil are believed to cause only minimal changes in renal function.

Uncatheterized patients may have decreased urine output caused by the increased detrusor tone and contraction of muscles and urethral sphincters, which makes urination difficult (Jaffe & Martin, 1990). The central effects of the drugs may render the patient inattentive to the stimuli arising in the bladder.

Miscellaneous Effects. Opioids decrease gastric and intestinal secretions and motility and decrease lower esophageal sphincter tone (Dowlatshahi, Evander, Walther, & Skinner, 1985). There is a delay in gastric emptying and the passage of bowel contents. Because of the delay, water is more completely absorbed. This is believed to contribute to the constipating effects of narcotics. Propulsive contractions of the bowel are virtually abolished, and the tone may be increased to the point of spasm. Atropine partially antagonizes the spasmogenic action but has little effect on the decreased propulsive activity.

Opioids tend to stimulate smooth muscle of the gastrointestinal and genitourinary tracts, and the resulting spasms can create increased pressure within these tracts, producing pain or rupturing smooth muscle that has been weakened by surgery or disease. Biliary colic

and spasm are intensified by morphine. Meperidine and fentanyl also can precipitate biliary colic but to a lesser degree than morphine. It has been noted that patients who are already suffering from colic can be relieved of their pain from opioids even though these do increase the intensity of the spasm.

The opioids cause pupillary constriction, which occurs even in total darkness. The exact mechanism by which narcotics induce miosis is uncertain but is believed to be a central effect via the Edinger–Westphal nucleus of the oculomotor nerve rather than an effect on the pupillary sphincter. Anticholinergics can counteract the opioid-induced miosis. Tolerance to the miotic effect is not usually seen, and miosis can be detected even in heroin addicts.

Clinical Considerations

In anesthesia opioids often are used (1) for premedication; (2) as adjuncts to regional or local anesthesia; (3) for postoperative analgesia; and (4) as anesthetic agents. Table 19–4 depicts the uses and doses of common opioids used in anesthesia practice.

Premedication. Opioid premedications should not be used routinely but usually are reserved for patients who experience pain or who may require some analgesia before anesthesia induction. There also are those who believe that opioid premedications lower the anesthetic requirements during general anesthesia and that certain opioids in themselves provide tranquilizing effects. Most anesthetists ordering an opioid premedication will order a combination with a benzodiazepine, phenothiazine, barbiturate, or other major tranquilizer. This combination often is used for patients about to undergo surgery with regional or local anesthesia or narcotic–nitrous oxide general anesthesia. Opioid premedication may provide some postoperative analgesia after inhalation anesthesia for a short surgical procedure.

Opioid premedication should be avoided in patients who cannot tolerate even mild respiratory depression (eg, those at risk of increasing intracranial pressure or with severe pulmonary compromise). Although histamine release from premedicant doses rarely is a problem, this should be kept in mind when ordering morphine or meperidine for asthmatics. Administration of morphine to patients with biliary colic or some history of significant biliary tract disease is contraindicated.

Adjunct to Regional or Local Anesthesia. Intravenous opioids are used in conjunction with tranquilizers such as midazolam, diazepam, lorazepam, and droperidol to provide sedation and analgesia. Some patients receiving a regional or local anesthetic are very anxious and will require sedation, amnesia, or both. The narcotic and tranquilizer must be titrated to achieve the desired effect. The desired effect usually is a calm, sedate, but responsive and

TABLE 19–4. Uses and Doses of Common Opioids

Agent	Use	Route	Dose*
Morphine	Premedication	IM	0.05 to 0.2 mg/kg
	Intraoperative anesthesia	IV	0.1 to 1.0 mg/kg
	Postoperative analgesia	IM	0.05 to 0.2 mg/kg
		IV	0.03 to 0.15 mg/kg
Meperidine	Premedication	IM	0.5 to 1 mg/kg
	Intraoperative anesthesia	IV	2.5 to 5 mg/kg
	Postoperative analgesia	IM	0.5 to 1 mg/kg
		IV	0.2 to 0.5 mg/kg
Fentanyl	Intraoperative anesthesia	IV	2 to 150 µg/kg
	Postoperative analgesia	IV	0.5 to 1.5 µg/kg
Sufentanil	Intraoperative anesthesia	IV	0.25 to 30 µg/kg
Alfentanil	Intraoperative anesthesia		
	Analgesia	IV	3 to 7 µg/kg
	Loading dose	IV	8 to 100 µg/kg
	Maintenance infusion	IV	0.5 to 3 µg/kg
Remifentanil	Intraoperative anesthesia		
	Loading dose	IV	1 to 5 µg/kg
	Maintenance infusion	IV	0.1 to 0.8 µg/kg
	Conscious sedation infusion	IV	0.025 to 0.1 µg/kg

*The wide range of opioid doses reflects a large therapeutic index and depends on which other anesthetics are simultaneously administered.
Modified with permission from Morgan, G. E. & Mikhail, M. S. (1996). Clinical anesthesiology (2nd ed., p. 141). Stamford, CT: Appleton & Lange.

cooperative patient. Care should be taken not to oversedate and render the patient apneic or unresponsive.

Immediate Postoperative Analgesia. Nurse anesthetists often administer analgesics in the recovery room for postoperative pain. The IV route is the route of choice because the effects are immediate and the uncertainty of the rate of absorption is not a problem. The drug must be titrated, starting with small doses. It must be remembered that the postoperative patient is frequently still depressed from the anesthetic agents received during the surgery. These patients usually require very small doses of narcotics to obtain analgesia. The respiratory rate should be monitored closely in patients receiving IV analgesics in the recovery room.

"Balanced Anesthesia" Technique. Opioids often are used with nitrous oxide, oxygen, and a muscle relaxant for a technique known as balanced anesthesia, or with oxygen and muscle relaxants without nitrous oxide. The opioid provides analgesia; the nitrous oxide supplements the analgesic effect and provides amnesia. Muscle relaxation is achieved by any nondepolarizing relaxant. The aim of balanced anesthesia is to maintain a consistent level of narcosis during the anesthetic. This can be accomplished by titrating the opioid by intermittent doses or by continuous infusion. The advantages of the opioid–nitrous oxide technique are that it (1) produces very little alteration in cardiovascular dynamics;

(2) decreases laryngeal, tracheal, and cough reflexes; (3) does not cause myocardial sensitization to catecholamines; (4) permits a smooth emergence; (5) provides postoperative analgesia; and (6) decreases metabolic rate. The technique does, however, have disadvantages, including (1) possible cardiovascular depression in the susceptible patient, especially if nitrous oxide is added; (2) chest wall rigidity with rapid administration; (3) no muscle relaxation; (4) requirement of at least 50% nitrous oxide (thus it may not be a wise choice for middle-ear surgery or bowel obstruction); (5) possible renarcotization after reversal; and (6) decreased cough reflex postoperatively.

▶ BENZODIAZEPINE AND OPIOID ANTAGONISM

Benzodiazepine and opioid effects can be antagonized by competitive antagonism. Flumazenil is an imidazobenzodiazepine and is a specific and competitive antagonist of benzodiazepines at the benzodiazepine receptor (Morgan & Mikhail, 1996). It promptly reverses the sedative effects of benzodiazepines, and amnesia is more likely to occur. Tidal volume and minute ventilation return to normal following reversal, although the slope of the carbon dioxide curve may remain depressed (Morgan & Mikhail, 1996). Flumazenil antagonism usually is accomplished in doses of 0.2 mg each minute until the desired level is reached (total dose 0.6 mg to 1 mg). The nurse anesthetist is cautioned that rapid administration of the antagonist may promote anxiety reactions in previously sedated patients. Patients who have chronically ingested benzodiazepines may be prone to symptoms of withdrawal when given flumazenil.

Naloxone is a popular opioid antagonist in anesthesia practice. It is a competitive antagonist at opioid receptors. It reverses the agonist activity associated with endogenous or exogenous opioid compounds. Abrupt reversal of analgesia can result in sympathetic stimulation (tachycardia, ventricular irritability, hypertension, pulmonary edema) caused by a variety of factors. The recommended dose for postoperative patients experiencing respiratory depression from opioids is 0.5 µg/kg to 1 µg/kg every 3 to 5 minutes until adequate ventilation and alertness are achieved. Intravenous doses of more than 0.2 mg seldom are indicated (Morgan & Mikhail, 1996). Naloxone has a brief duration of action (30 to 45 minutes) because of its rapid redistribution.

▶ CASE STUDY

A 55-year-old, 65-kg female patient is scheduled for a lung biopsy under conscious sedation in the radiology department. After evaluating the patient preprocedure, the CRNA starts an IV infusion. The patient has an unremarkable history, except for sinus bradycardia (rate of 50 to 55) without other symptoms, and a lesion was noted on the right upper lobe during a recent physical exam that included a chest x-ray. The patient is quite apprehensive about the procedure. The CRNA administers 1 mg of midazolam and 250 µg of alfentanil immediately prior to local anesthetic infiltration of the needle biopsy site by the radiologist. The blood pressure, pulse, respirations, and pulse oximetry remain at preprocedure levels of 120/80, 55, 14, and 99%, respectively. An additional 0.5 mg of midazolam and 250 µg of alfentanil are given 5 minutes later. The patient's blood pressure transiently decreases to 80/60 with no change in pulse, but within 1 minute it returns to 120/80. Pulse oximetry measurements read 99%. The patient is complaining of discomfort from the needle and is apprehensive about being in the scanner. An additional 0.5 mg of midazolam and 250 µg of alfentanil are administered 5 minutes after the last dose with no change in vital signs. The procedure ends within a few minutes and the patient assists in moving herself back to the guerney. For the 20-minute procedure, the patient received a total of 750 µg of alfentanil and 2 mg of midazolam.

1. Was the dose of midazolam appropriate for this procedure, and what should the CRNA consider when administering this drug for conscious sedation with alfentanil?

The sedative dose range for midazolam is 0.01 mg/kg to 0.1 mg/kg. Based on this patient's weight, the dose range is 0.65 mg to 6.5 mg, and she received a total of 2 mg in divided doses. This dose seemed to be appropriate in providing sedation for the procedure, particularly given the length of the diagnostic procedure. Because midazolam was administered with alfentanil, a synergistic effect can occur that may produce a decease in blood pressure and reduce peripheral vascular resistance. After the second dose of midazolam and alfentanil, the patient's blood pressure decreased transiently, but no signs of respiratory depression were observed. Redistribution is fairly rapid for benzodiazepines, especially midazolam, and the sedative effects generally last between 3 and 10 minutes.

2. Was the dose of alfentanil appropriate for this patient?

The sedative bolus dose for alfentanil is approximately 3 µg/kg to 7 µg/kg and can be repeated as clinically indicated. The bolus dose range for this patient based on her weight is 195 µg to 455 µg. The patient received an initial bolus of 250 µg, which was repeated twice during the 20-minute procedure. Based on the fact that the patient did not demonstrate any symptoms of respiratory depression and was able to move herself from the x-ray table to the guerney, it seems that the dose was appropriate.

3. Is alfentanil a good choice for conscious sedation? What are the pros and cons of using this drug for diagnostic procedures?

Alfentanil has a rapid onset of action, and its peak drug effect occurs in under 2 minutes. Alfentanil is less potent than fentanyl, but it has a higher nonionized fraction than fentanyl, making more drug available for binding in the brain. Although respiratory depression after alfentanil administration is shorter than with comparable doses of fentanyl, it may appear to be more intense because the onset of action of the drug is so rapid. The CRNA should observe the patient closely for any signs of respiratory depression or apnea, particularly when giving this drug concurrently with midazolam. Chest wall rigidity has been reported with all of the fentanyl analogs but occurs most often after large drug doses. Alfentanil must be monitored carefully by the provider, but it does appear to provide more intense analgesia and euphoria than fentanyl even when administered without benzodiazepines.

► SUMMARY

A variety of drugs can be used to achieve anesthesia intravenously. This chapter has provided an overview of the use of barbiturates, particularly thiobarbiturates and oxybarbiturates, propofol, etomidate, ketamine, and benzodiazepines, opioids, opioid antagonists. The focus of this chapter has been on the pharmacology and clinical applications of these drugs in anesthetic practice.

ACKNOWLEDGMENT

The author acknowledges Doris J. Tanaka for her original contribution to this chapter.

► KEY CONCEPTS

- A two-compartment model describes the distribution of many drugs used in anesthesia and illustrates the basic concepts of pharmacokinetics that also apply to more complex models.
- Thiobarbiturates occur when a sulfur atom is substituted for an oxygen on the C2 of barbituric acid, which influences the agent's lipophilicity, onset, and duration of action.
- Thiopental remains the most widely used IV anesthetic, even though it is unstable in solution, produces cardiac and respiratory depression, and often is associated with a postoperative drowsiness and sedation uncharacteristic of other agents such as propofol.
- Recovery from anesthesia following a bolus dose or a prolonged infusion with propofol is more rapid than with an ultrashort-acting thiobarbiturate and is associated with less CNS depression postoperatively.
- Etomidate is a potent ultrashort-acting sedative hypnotic that lacks analgesic activity but promotes hemodynamic stability.
- Ketamine is a nonopioid anesthetic with analgesic properties that produces dissociative anesthesia, causing the patient to "dissociate" from the environment.
- Benzodiazepines exert their central effects by binding to selective sites associated with the GABA-receptor, causing inhibition of synaptic transmission by hyperpolarizing postsynaptic neurons.
- Intravenous anesthetics, with the exception of ketamine and etomidate, depress the cardiovascular and respiratory systems.
- The concurrent administration of opioids and sedatives, including benzodiazepines, creates a synergistic drug effect and may potentiate untoward effects such as respiratory depression.
- The most commonly administered opioids in anesthesia practice are the fentanyl analogs, including fentanyl, sufentanil, alfentanil, and remifentanil.

► STUDY QUESTIONS

1. How does the two-compartment model explain the kinetics of drug distribution for IV anesthetics?

2. What barbiturates are used in anesthesia practice, and how do they differ chemically and in distribution and clearance from other barbiturates?

3. What properties make propofol a highly desirable IV anesthetic?

4. How are benzodiazepines employed in anesthesia practice, and how do the drugs in this classification differ?

5. What are the pharmacologic actions of opioid anesthetics and the distinguishing features of the various fentanyl analogs?

KEY REFERENCES

Bowdle, T. A. (1996). Remifentanil: The first ultrashort-acting opioid. *Current Reviews in Clinical Anesthesia, 16,* 217–224.

Estanfanow, F. G. (Ed.). (1990). *Opioids in anesthesia,* (Vol. II). Boston: Butterworth-Heinemann.

Haefely, W. E. (1988). Benzodiazepines. *International Anesthesiology Clinics, 26,* 262.

Hull, C. J. (1991). *Pharmacokinetics for anesthesia.* Boston: Butterworth-Heinemann.

Olsen, R. W. (1988). Barbiturates. *International Anesthesiology Clinics, 26,* 254–261.

Reich, D. L., & Silvay, G. (1989). Ketamine: An update on the first twenty-five years of clinical experience. *Canadian Journal of Anaesthesia, 36,* 186–197.

Smith, I., White, P. F., Nathanson, M., & Gouldson, R. (1994). Propofol: An update on its use. *Anesthesiology, 81,* 1005–1043.

REFERENCES

Aldrete, J. A., & Stanley, T. H. (Eds.). (1980). *Trends in intravenous anesthesia.* Chicago: Year Book Medical.

Allonen, H., Ziegler, G., & Klotz, U. (1981). Midazolam kinetics. *Clinical Pharmacology and Therapeutics, 30,* 653.

Anonymous. (1983). Etomidate (Editorial). *Lancet, 2,* 24.

Beckett, A. H., & Casey, A. P. (1984). Synthetic analgesics, stereochemical considerations. *Journal of Pharmacy and Pharmacology, 6,* 986.

Benet, L. Z., Mitchell, J. R., & Sheiner, L. B. (1990). Pharmacokinetics: The dynamics of drug absorption, distribution and elimination. In G. A. Goodman, T. W. Rall, A. S. Nies, & Taylor P. (Eds.), *The pharmacological basis of therapeutics* (p. 3). New York: Pergamon Press.

Berkowitz, B. A., Ngai, S. H., Yang, J. C., Hempstead, J., & Spector, S. (1975). The disposition of morphine in surgical patients. *Clinical Pharmacology and Therapeutics, 17,* 629.

Bischoff, K. B., & Dedrick, R. L. (1968). Thiopental pharmacokinetics. *Journal of Pharmacological Science, 57,* 1346.

Blitt, C. D., Petty, W. C., Wright, W. A., & Wright, B. (1976). Clinical evaluation of injectable lorazepam as a premedicant: The effect on recall. *Anesthesia & Analgesia, 55,* 522–525.

Blouin, R. T., Seifert, H. A., Conard, P. F., & Gross, J. B. (1992). Propofol significantly depresses hypoxic ventilatory drive during conscious sedation. *Anesthesiology, 77,* A1215.

Blouin, R. T., Seifert, H. A., Babenco, H. D., Conard, P. F., & Gross, J. B. (1993). Propofol depresses the hypoxic ventilatory response during conscious sedation and isohypercapnia. *Anesthesiology, 79,* 1177–1182.

Booij, L. H., & Crul, J. F. (1979). The comparative influence of gamma-hydroxy butyric acid, althesin and etomidate on the neuromuscular blocking potency of pancuronium in man. *Acta Anaesthesiologica Belgica, 30,* 219.

Bowdle, T. A. (1996). Remifentanil: The first ultrashort-acting opioid. *Current Reviews in Clinical Anesthesia, 16,* 217–224.

Breimer, D. D. (1976). Pharmacokinetics of methohexitone following intravenous infusion in humans. *British Journal of Anaesthesia, 48,* 643–648.

Breimer, D. D. (1977). Clinical pharmacokinetics of hypnotics. *Clinical Pharmacokinetics, 2,* 93–109.

Caldwell, C. B., & Gross, J. D. (1982). Physostigmine reversal of midazolam induced sedation. *Anesthesiology, 57,* 125.

Canessa, R., Lema, G., Urzua, J., Dagnino, J., & Concha, M. (1991). Anesthesia for elective cardioversion: A comparison of four anesthetic agents. *Journal of Cardiothoracic and Vascular Anesthesia, 5,* 566.

Choi, S. D., Spaulding, B. C., Gross, J. B., & Apfelbaum, J. L. (1985). Comparison of the ventilatory effects of etomidate and methohexital. *Anesthesiology, 62,* 442.

Chaplin, M. D., Roszkowski, A. P., & Richard, R. K. (1973). Displacement of thiopental from plasma proteins by nonsteroidal anti-inflammatory agents. *Proceedings of the Society for Experimental Biopsy and Medicine, 143,* 667–671.

Claeys, M. A., Gepts, E., & Camu, F. (1983). Haemodynamic changes during anaesthesia induced and maintained with propofol. *British Journal of Anaesthesia, 60,* 3.

Clark, W. G., Brater, D. C., & Johnson, A. R. (1992). *Goth's medical pharmacology* (13th ed., p. 273). St. Louis: Mosby Year Book.

Conti, G., Dell'Utri, D., Vilardi, V., De Blasi, R. A., Pelaia, P., Antonelli, M., Bufi, M., Rosa, G., & Gasparetto, A. (1993). Propofol induces bronchodilation in mechanically ventilated chronic obstructive pulmonary disease (COPD) patients. *Anaesthesiologica Scandinavica, 37,* 105.

Coates, D. P., Monk, C. R., Prys-Roberts, C., & Turtle, M. (1987). Hemodynamic effects of infusions of the emulsion formulation of propofol during nitrous oxide anesthesia in humans. *Anesthesia & Analgesia, 66,* 64.

Corssen, G., Reves, J. G., & Stanley, T. H. (1988a). Etomidate. In *Intravenous anesthesia and analgesia* (p. 285). Philadelphia: Lea & Febiger.

Corssen, G., Reves, J. G., & Stanley, T. H. (1988b). Neuroleptanalgesia and neuroleptanesthesia. In G. Corssen, J. G. Reves, & T. H. Stanley (Eds.), *Intravenous anesthesia and analgesia.* Philadelphia: Lea & Febiger.

Craig, J., Cooper, G. M., & Sear, J. W. (1982). Recovery from daycase anesthesia. Comparison between methohexitone, althesin and etomidate. *British Journal of Anaesthesia, 54,* 477.

Cullen, P. M., Turtle, M., Prys-Roberts, C., Way, W. L., & Dye, J. (1987). Effect of propofol anesthesia on baroreflex activity in humans. *Anesthesia & Analgesia, 66,* 1115.

Doenicke, A. (1974). Etomidate, a new intravenous hypnotic. *Acta Anaesthesiologica Belgica, 25,* 307.

Doenicke, A., Lorenz, W., Stanworth, D., Duka, T., & Glen, J. B.

(1985). Effects of propofol (Diprivan) on histamine release, immunoglobulin levels and activation of complement in healthy volunteers. *Postgraduate Medical Journal, 61,* 15.

De Grood, P. M., Van Egmond, J., Van De Wetering, M., Van Beem, H. B., Booij, L. H., & Crul, J. F. (1985). Lack of effects of emulsified propofol (Diprivan) on vecuronium pharmacodynamics—Preliminary results in man. *Postgraduate Medical Journal, 61,* 28.

de Ruiter, G., Popescu, D. T., de Boer, A. G., Smeekens, J. B. & Breimer, D. D. (1981). Pharmacokinetics of etomidate in surgical patients. *Archives Internationales de Pharmacodynamie et de Thérapie, 249,* 180.

Deutsch, S., Bastron, R. D., Pierce, E. C., & Vandam, L. D., (1969). The effects of anaesthesia with thiopentone, nitrous oxide, narcotics and neuromuscular blocking drugs on renal function in normal man. *British Journal of Anaesthesia, 4,* 807.

Dowlatshahi, K., Evander, A., Walther, B., & Skinner, D. B. (1985). Influence of morphine on the distal oesophagus and the lower oesophageal sphincter—A manometric study. *Gut, 26,* 802.

Dundee, J. W. (1971). Comparative analysis of intravenous anesthetics. *Anesthesiology, 35,* 137–148.

Dundee, J. W. (1979). Intravenous anesthetic agents. In H. S. Feldman, Q. E. Scurr (Eds.), *Current topics in anesthesia.* Chicago: Year Book Medical.

Dundee, J. W. & Wyatt, G. M. (1974). *Intravenous anesthesia* (pp. 64–127). Edinburgh: Churchill Livingstone.

Ebert, T. J., Muzi, M., Berens, R., Goff, D., & Kampine, J. P. (1992). Sympathetic responses to induction of anesthesia in humans with propofol or etomidate. *Anesthesiology, 76,* 725.

Evans, R. H. & Hill, R. G. (1977). GABA—Mimetic action of etomidate. *British Journal of Pharmacology, 61,* 484.

Famewo, C. E. & Adugbesan, C. O. (1978). Further experience with etomidate. *Canadian Journal of Anaesthesia, 25,* 131.

Flacke, J. W., Flacke, W. E., Bloor, B. C., Van Etten, A. P., & Kripke, B. J. (1987). Histamine release by four narcotics: A double blind study in humans. *Anesthesia & Analgesia, 66,* 723.

Fragen, R. J. & Caldwell, N. (1977). Comparison of a new formulation of etomidate with thiopental side effects and awakening times. *Anesthesiology, 50,* 242.

Fragen, R. J., Avram, M. J., Henthorn, T. K., & Caldwell, N. J. (1983). Pharmacokinetics designed etomidate infusion regimen for hypnosis. *Anesthesia & Analgesia, 62,* 654.

Galloway, P. A., Nicoll, J. M., & Leiman, B. C. (1982). Pain reduction with etomidate injection (Letter). *Anaesthesia, 37,* 352.

Ghoneim, M. M., Pandya, H. B., Kelly, S. E., Fisher, L. J., & Corry, R. J. (1976). Binding of thiopental to plasma proteins. Effects of distribution in the brain and heart. *Anesthesiology, 45,* 635–639.

Ghoneim, M. M., & Pandya, H. (1975). Plasma protein binding of thiopental in patients with impaired renal or hepatic function. *Anesthesiology, 42,* 545–549.

Glass, P. S., Hardman, D., Kamiyama, Y., Quill, T. J., Marton, G., Donn, K. A., Grosse, C. M., & Hermann, D. (1993). Preliminary pharmacokinetics and pharmacodynamics of an ultra-short acting opioid: Remifentanil (GI87084B). *Anesthesia & Analgesia, 77,* 1031–1040.

Gold, M. I., Abraham, E. C., & Herrington, C. (1987). A controlled investigation of propofol, thiopentone and methohexitone. *Canadian Journal of Anaesthesia, 34,* 478–483.

Gooding, J., & Corssen, G. (1977). Effect of etomidate on the cardiovascular system. *Anesthesia & Analgesia, 56,* 717.

Guldager, H., Sodergaard, I., Jensen, F. M., & Cold, G. (1985). Basophil histamine release in asthma patients after in vitro provocation with althesin and etomidate. *Acta Anaesthesiologica Scandinavica, 29,* 352.

Gross, J. B., & Smith, T. C. (1981). Ventilation after midazolam and thiopental in subjects with COPD. *Anesthesiology, 55,* A384.

Gross, J. B., Zebrowski, M. E., Carel, W. D., Gardner, S. & Smith, T. C. (1983). Time course of ventilatory depression after thiopental and midazolam in normal subjects and in patients with chronic obstructive pulmonary disease. *Anesthesiology, 58,* 540–544.

Hebron, B. S., Edbrooke, D. L., Newby, D. M., & Mather, S. J. (1983). Pharmacokinetics of etomidate associated with prolonged IV infusion. *British Journal of Anaesthesia, 58,* 281.

Hegarty, J. E., & Dundee, J. W. (1977). Sequelae after the intravenous injection of three benzodiazepines—Diazepam, lorazepam and flunitrazepam. *British Medical Journal, 2,* 1384–1385.

Heisterkamp, D. V., & Cohen, P. J. (1975). The effect of intravenous premedication with lorazepam (Ativan), pentobarbitone or diazepam on recall. *British Journal of Anaesthesia, 47,* 79–81.

Hirshman, C. A., McCullough, R. E., Cohen, P. J., & Weil, J. V. (1975). Hypoxic ventilatory drive in dogs during thiopental, ketamine, or pentobarbital anesthesia. *Anesthesiology, 43,* 628–634.

Homer, T. D. & Stanski, D. R. (1985). The effect of increasing age on thiopental disposition and anesthetic requirement. *Anesthesiology, 62,* 714–724.

Hopkinson, K. C. & Denborough, M. (1988). Propofol and malignant hyperpyrexia. (Letter). *Lancet, 1,* 191.

Hudson, R. J., Stanski, D. R., & Burch, P. G. (1983). Pharmacokinetics of methohexital and thiopental in surgical patients. *Anesthesiology, 59,* 215–219.

Hull, C. J. (1983). The pharmcokinetics of alfentanil in man. *British Journal of Anaesthesiology, 55,* 1575–1645.

Hull, C. J. (1989). Pharmacokinetics and pharmacodynamics, with particular reference to intravenous anesthetic agents. In J. F. Nunn, J. E. Ulting, & B. R. Brown, Jr. (Eds.), *General anaesthesia,* (5th ed., pp. 96–114). London: Butterworth.

Jaffe, J. H. & Martin, W. R. (1990). Opioid analgesics and antagonists. In G. A. Goodman, T. W. Rall, A. S. Nies, & P. Taylor (Eds.), *The pharmacological basis of therapeutics* (p. 485). New York: Pergamon Press.

James, M. K., Yuong, A., Grizzle, M. K., Schuster, S. V. & Shaffer, J. E. (1992). Hemodynamic effects of GI 87084B, an ultra-short acting mu-opioid analgesic, in anesthetized dogs. *Journal of Pharmacology and Experimental Therapeutics, 263*(1), 84–91.

James, R. & Glen, J. B. (1980). Synthesis, biological evaluation, and preliminary structure-activity considerations of a series of alkylphenols as intravenous anesthetic agents. *Journal of Medical Chemistry, 23,* 1350.

Jung, D., Mayersohn, M., Perrier, D., Calkins, J., & Saunders,

R. (1982). Thiopental disposition in lean and obese patients undergoing surgery. *Anesthesiology, 56,* 269.

Korttila, K. & Aromaa, U. (1990). Venous complications after intravenous injection of diazepam, thiopentone and etomidate. *Acta Anaesthesiologica Scandinavica, 24,* 227.

Korttila, K., Linnoila, M., Ertama, P., & Hakkinen, S. (1975). Recovery and stimulated driving after intravenous anesthesia with thiopental, methohexital, propanidid, or alphadione. *Anesthesiology, 43,* 291–299.

Lamalle, D. (1976). Cardiovascular effects of various anesthetics in man. Four short-acting intravenous anesthetics: Althesin, etomidate, methohexital, and propanidid. *Acta Anaesthesiologica Belgica, 27,* 208–224.

Longnecker, D. (1984). Stress free: To be or not to be? (editorial). *Anesthesiology, 61,* 643.

Marshall, B. E., Hanson, C. W., & Marshall, C. (1995). Clinical physiology and pathophysiology of the respiratory system. In D. Healy & P. J. Cohen (Eds.), *A practice of anaesthesia* (pp. 119–145). London: Edward Arnold.

Mehr, E. H., Hirshman, C. A., & Lindeman, R. S. (1992). The effect of halothane, propofol and thiopental on peripheral airway reactivity. *Anesthesiology, 77,* A1212.

Meuldermans, W. E. G., & Heykants, J. J. P. (1976). The plasma protein binding and distribution of etomidate in dog, rat and human blood. *Archives Internationales de Pharmacodynamie et de Thérapie, 221,* 150.

Morgan, G. E. & Gikhail, M. S. (1996). *Clinical Anesthesiology* (2nd ed., pp. 128–148). Stamford, CT: Appleton & Lange.

Nattel, S., Wang, Z. G., & Matthews, C. (1990). Direct electrophysiological actions of pentobarbital at concentrations achieved during general anesthesia. *American Journal of Physiology, 259,* H1743–H1751.

Nauta, J., Stanley, T. H., de Lange, S., (1983). Anaesthetic induction with alfentanil: Comparison with thiopental, midazolam and etomidate. *Canadian Journal of Anaesthesia, 30,* 53.

Nightingale, P., Petts, N. V., Healy, T. E. J., (1988). Induction of anaesthesia with propofol (Diprivan) or thiopentone and interactions with suxamethonium, atracurium and vecuronium. *Postgraduate Medical Journal, 61,* 31.

Nimmo, W. S. & Miller, M. (1983). Pharmacology of etomidate. *Contemporary Anesthesia Practice, 7,* 83.

Olson, R. W. (1988). Barbiturates. *International Anesthesiology Clinics, 26,* 254.

Pancrazio, J. J., Frazer, M. J., & Lynch, C., III. (1993). Barbiturate anesthetics depress the resting K^+ conductance of myocardium. *Journal of Pharmacology and Experimental Therapeutics, 265,* 358–365.

Pandele, G., Chaux, F., Salvadori, C., Farinotti, M., & Duvaldestin, P. (1983). Thiopental pharmacokinetics in patients with cirrhosis. *Anesthesiology, 59,* 123–126.

Price, H. L., Kovnat, P. J., & Safer, J. N., (1960). The uptake of thiopental by body tissues and its relation to the duration of narcosis. *Clinical Pharmacology and Therapeutics, 1,* 16.

Rall, T. W. (1990). Hypnotics and sedatives: Ethanol. In G. A. Goodman, T. W. Rall, A. S. Nies, & P. Taylor (Eds.), *The pharmacological basis of therapeutics* (p. 345). New York: Pergamon Press.

Rao, S., Sherbaniuk, R. W., Prasad, K., Lee, S. J., & Sproule,

B. J. (1973). Cardiopulmonary effects of diazepam. *Clinical Pharmacology and Therapeutics, 14,* 482.

Renou, A. M., Vemhiet, J., & Macrez, P. (1978). Cerebral blood flow and metabolism during etomidate anesthesia in man. *British Journal of Anaesthesia, 50,* 1047.

Reich, D. L., & Silvay, G. (1989). Ketamine: An update on the first twenty-five years of clinical experience. *Canadian Journal of Anaesthesia, 36,* 186–197.

Roth, S. H., Forman, S. A., Braswell, L. M., & Miller, K. W. (1989). Actions of pentobarbital enantiomers on nicotinic cholinergic receptors. *Molecular Pharmacology, 36,* 874–880.

Reves, J. G., Glass, P. S., & Lubarsky, D. A. (1994). Nonbarbiturate intravenous anesthetics. In R. D. Miller (Ed.), *Anesthesia* (4th ed., pp. 247–289). New York: Churchill Livingstone.

Reves, J. G., Samuelson, P. N., & Linnan, M. (1980). Effects of midazolam maleate in patients with elevated pulmonary artery occluded pressure. In J. A. Aldrete and T. H. Stanley (Eds.), *Trends in intravenous anesthesia* (pp. 253–257). Chicago: Year Book Medical.

Richardson, J. (1987). Propofol infusion for coronary artery bypass surgery in a patient with suspected malignant hyperpyrexia (Letter). *Anaesthesia, 42,* 1125.

Rouby, J. J., Andreev, A., Leger, P., Arthaud, M., Landault, C., Vicaut, E., Maistre, G., Eurin, J., Gandjbakch, I., & Viars, P. (1991). Peripheral vascular effects of thiopental and propofol in humans with artificial hearts. *Anesthesiology 75,* 32–42.

Samuelson, P. N., Reves, J. G., Kouchoukos, N. T., Smith, L. R. & Dole, K. M. (1981). Hemodynamic responses to anesthetic induction with midazolam or diazepam in patients with ischemic heart disease. *Anesthesia & Analgesia, 60,* 802.

Schuttler, J., Schwilden, H., & Stoeckel, H. (1985). Infusion strategies to investigate the pharmacokinetics and pharmacodynamics of hypnotic drugs: Etomidate as an example. *European Journal of Anaesthesiology, 2,* 133.

Shapiro, H. M. (1985). Barbiturates in brain ischaemia. *British Journal of Anaesthesia, 57,* 82–89.

Schwinn, D. A., Watkins, W. D., & Leslie, J. B. (1994). Basic principles of pharmacology related to anesthetics. In R. D. Miller (Ed.), *Anesthesia* (4th ed., pp. 43–65).

Simons, P. J., Cockshott, I. D., Douglas, E. J., Gordon, E. A., Knott, S., & Ruane, R. J. (1985). Blood concentrations, metabolism and elimination after a subanesthetic intravenous dose of ^{14}C-propofol (Diprivan) to male volunteers (Abstract). *Postgraduate Medical Journal, 61,* 64.

Sorbo, S., Hudson, R. J., & Loomis, J. C. (1984). The pharmacokinetics of thiopental in pediatric surgical patients. *Anesthesiology, 61,* 666–670.

Sugioka, K., Boniface, K. J., & Davis, D. A. (1957). The influence of meperidine on myocardial contractility in the intact dog. *Anesthesiology, 18,* 623.

Stanley, T. H., & Lathrup, G. D. (1977). Urinary excretion of morphine during and after valvular and coronary-artery surgery. *Anesthesiology, 46,* 166.

Stanley, T. H. & Webester, L. R. (1978). Anesthetic requirements and cardiac vascular effects of fentanyl–oxygen and fentanyl–diazepam–oxygen anesthesia in man. *Anesthesia & Analgesia, 57,* 411.

Stanski, D. R. & Watkins, W. D. (1982). *Drug disposition in anesthesia.* Orlando, FL: Grune & Stratton.

Starck, T., Hall, D., Freas, W., *et al.* (1989). Peripheral vascular depression with sufentanil in the dog. *Anesthesia & Analgesia, 68,* S277.

Stoelting, Robert K. (1991). Pharmacology and physiology in anesthetic practice. (2nd ed., pp. 102–115). Philadelphia: Lippincott.

Tabatabai, M., Kitahata, L. M., & Collins, J. G. (1989). Disruption of the rhythmic activity of the medullary respiratory neurons and phrenic nerve by fentanyl and reversal with nalbuphine. *Anesthesiology, 70,* 489.

Thomson, M. F., Brock-Utne, J. G., Bean, P., Welsh, N., & Downing, J. W. (1982). Anesthesia and intraocular pressure: A comparative of total intravenous anesthesia using etomidate with conventional inhalational anaesthesia. *Anaesthesia, 37,* 758.

Thorpe, A. H. (1984). Opiate structure and activity: A guide to understanding the receptor. *Anesthesia & Analgesia, 63,* 143.

Van Beem, H., Manger, F. W., Van Boxtel, C., & Van Benten, N. (1983). Etomidate anaesthesia in patients with cirrhosis of the liver: Pharmacokinetic data. *Anaesthesia, 38,* 61.

Van Hamme, M. J., Ghoneim, M. M., & Amber, J. J. (1978). Pharmacokinetics of etomidate, a new intravenous anesthetic. *Anesthesiology, 49,* 274.

Vasko, J. S., Henney, R. P., Brawley, R. K., Oldham, H. N., & Morrow, A. G. (1966). Effects of morphine on ventricular function and myocardial contractile force. *American Journal of Physiology, 210,* 329.

Vermeyen, K. M., Erpels, F. A., Janssen, L. A., Beeckman, C. P., & Hanegreefs, G. H. (1987). Propofol-fentanyl anaesthesia for coronary bypass surgery in patients with good left ventricular function. *British Journal of Anaesthesia, 59,* 1115.

Vinik, H. R., Reves, J. G., Greenblatt, D. J., & Abernethy, D. R. (1983). Pharmacokinetics of midazolam in chronic renal failure patients. *Anesthesiology, 59,* 390–394.

Waugaman, W. R., & Foster, S. D. (1991). New advances in anesthesia. *Nursing Clinics of North America, 26,* 451–461.

Wells, J. K. G. (1985). Comparison of IC135868, etomidate and methohexitone for day-case anesthetic. *British Journal of Anaesthesia, 57,* 732.

Yelnosky, J., Katz, R., & Dietrich, E. V. (1964). A study of some pharmacologic actions of droperidol. *Toxicology and Applied Pharmacology, 6,* 37.

Zacharas, M., Dundee, J. W., Clark, R. S., & Hegarty, J. E. (1979). Effect of preanesthetic medication on etomidate. *British Journal of Anaesthesia, 51,* 127.

Pharmacology of Local Anesthetics

John G. Aker

The flow of information between the peripheral and central nervous system (CNS) occurs from the production of electrical and chemical potentials relayed between neurons and conducted along 43 pairs of nerve fibers. The functional cell of the peripheral nervous system is the neuron, whose cell body resides within the CNS. The axon of these neurons projects to the periphery to form the peripheral nervous system. Local anesthetic agents produce a reversible cessation of the electrical and chemical potentials at the axonal membrane. A number of local anesthetic agents are available for clinical use. The selection of a suitable local anesthetic is based on the inherent potency, onset, and expected duration of action. The basic pharmacologic action of local anesthetics involves the inhibition of excitation and conduction in peripheral nerve fibers and nerve endings. Although the normal sensory and motor functions of peripheral nerves can be reversibly altered by local anesthetics, some substances, such as absolute alcohol or phenol, can also interrupt nerve conduction permanently. This chapter reviews the history of local anesthesia, the basic mechanisms of action of local anesthetics, and the structure–activity relationships of contemporary local anesthetics.

▶ HISTORY OF LOCAL ANESTHESIA

Regional anesthesia was first used when a pharmacologic agent that would temporarily interrupt nerve transmission was discovered: Cocaine, the first available local anesthetic, was isolated by Niemann in 1860 from *Erythroxylon coca,* a plant indigenous to Peru. The Austrian ophthalmologist Koller discovered the application of cocaine to produce local anesthesia of the cornea. This fact was publicized by a colleague at the Congress of Ophthalmology in Heidelberg on September 15, 1884 (Faulconer & Keyes, 1993). Following this report, a number of medical journals began publishing accounts of the various uses of cocaine. Burke (1884) chronicled the use of cocaine in the *New York Medical Journal* for conduction anesthesia in the debridement of a gunshot wound to the hand. The patient described his sensations of the hand following ulnar nerve blockade as "being numb or asleep." Later in the same journal, both Richard Hall and William Halstead reported the successful application of cocaine for minor surgical operations (Halstead, 1885). Cocaine was employed for spinal anesthesia in Germany by Bier and by Halstead for brachial plexus block. Because of the widespread uses of cocaine, a variety of the unwanted characteristics of the drug were discovered, including a propensity to elicit allergic reactions and tissue irritation and its insolubility in aqueous solution. Because of its unique quality in producing local vasoconstriction, cocaine has a limited, but specific, application as a topical anesthetic for the mucous membranes.

The synthesis of additional local anesthetic agents used the chemical structure of cocaine, an ester of benzoic acid. Benzocaine, the first of these agents, was less toxic than cocaine, exhibited good anesthetizing properties, yet was poorly soluble in water. Procaine, another derivative of *para*-aminobenzoic acid, synthesized by

Einhorn and Braun in 1905, proved to be sufficiently water soluble and to have a satisfactory margin of safety so that its clinical application as an injectable agent was assured. Although the duration of action of procaine was relatively short, Braun (1903) discovered that the addition of epinephrine prolonged the duration of action. Local anesthetic drugs have intrinsic vasodilator properties that potentiate the removal of the local anesthetic from the site of action. The addition of epinephrine reduces local blood flow and prolongs the presence of local anesthetic at the nerve.

Many additional ester local anesthetics were synthesized between 1880 and the 1950s. Tetracaine, synthesized in 1931, and chloroprocaine, following in 1952, are the remaining clinically important ester anesthetics. The synthesis of additional ester local anesthetics was probably abandoned because esters of *para*-aminobenzoic acid are associated with hypersensitivity.

The synthesis of a new class of compounds derived from amino amides began with the synthesis of dibucaine in the 1930s. Lidocaine was synthesized by Lofgren in 1943. Lidocaine, which is devoid of the ester linkage, was the first compound in the series of amino amides. Lidocaine is more potent than procaine, has a short onset of action, a minimal degree of toxicity, and is a superior and more reliable local anesthetic agent than procaine.

▶ STRUCTURAL CHARACTERISTICS OF NERVE TISSUE

Neurons transmit impulses because of the structural nature of the nerve membrane or *axolemma*. The physiologic mechanism involves changes in the permeability that permit the flow of ions through the axolemma. As discussed later, the physiochemical properties of local anesthetics (ie, water solubility, lipid solubility, ionization at physiological pH, and protein binding) determine the degree of interaction with the nerve cell membrane and the resulting clinical characteristics of the block. The following brief review of neuronal anatomy will assist the reader in understanding the principles of local anesthetic pharmacology.

The nerve cell membrane consists of a bilaminar lipoprotein matrix derived from phospholipid molecules arranged with their attached fatty acid chains facing one another, producing an inner hydrophobic membrane (Fig. 20–1). The membrane surface, which is in contact with the extracellular fluid, is formed from polar hydrophilic groups of the phospholipid molecules. Globular structural proteins, some of which penetrate the entire thickness of the membrane, form ionic channels that provide a pathway for the transport of ions across the cell membrane. In addition to serving as structural components of the membrane and forming ion channels,

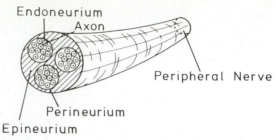

Figure 20–1. Principal structures of a peripheral nerve fiber.

these integral globular proteins may also serve as enzymes (eg, adenylate cyclase), membrane pumps, and cell receptors (eg, the Y-shaped immunoglobulin receptors).

Peripheral nerves are "mixed" nerves that contain both afferent (sensory) and efferent (motor) fibers. Accordingly, peripheral nerves contain both myelinated and unmyelinated fibers. The dorsal nerve root contains the cell bodies of afferent nerve fibers that enter the spinal cord. Ventral nerve roots contain the cell bodies of efferent fibers whose axons leave the spinal cord. It is important to appreciate that some afferent or autonomic nerve fibers are without a myelin sheath, although these fibers receive structural support from Schwann cells.

Local anesthetics must penetrate a number of membranes to reach their sites of action. As illustrated in Figures 20–2 and 20–3, a peripheral nerve or axon contains many fascicles or nerve bundles. The entire nerve is surrounded by the *epineurim*, a connective tissue sheath. This sheath extends into the interior of the nerve and subdivides the nerve into fascicles of nerve fibers. The connective tissue that delineates these nerve fascicles is referred to as the *perineurim*. It is the perineurim that serves as the main diffusion barrier to local anesthetics. The perineurim continues and surrounds each individual nerve fiber as the *endoneurim*. The blood supply of the nerve is distributed within the epineurim and perineurim and divides to form the capillary network which resides inside the endoneurim.

The conduction of a nerve impulse in an unmyelinated nerve fiber increases with the square root of the diameter of the fiber. To double the rate of impulse con-

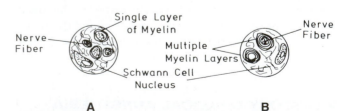

A   **B**

Figure 20–2. Cross sections of a peripheral nerve showing the basic differences between **(A)** unmyelinated and **(B)** myelinated nerves. Schwann cell nuclei, from which myelin is produced, can also be seen.

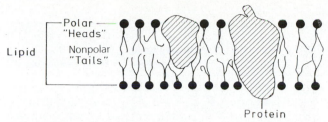

Figure 20–3. Nerve cell membrane as a bilaminar lipoprotein matrix. Note that the protein molecules can "bridge" the entire membrane thickness in places.

duction requires a quadrupling in fiber size. In contrast, the impulse conduction in a myelinated nerve fiber varies directly with the diameter of the fiber; doubling the size of the fiber doubles the rate of impulse conduction. Imagine if you will, the required diameter of the spinal cord provided it contained only unmyelinated fibers! The speed of impulse conduction in small unmyelinated fibers (eg, C fibers) is between 1 and 2 m/s.

Myelin in the peripheral nervous system is produced by the differentiation of the Schwann cell plasma membrane. During the process of myelin formation, the Schwann cell wraps itself concentrically around the nerve fiber to produce successive layers of plasma membrane. Junctions form between successive Schwann cells and myelin along the axon, forming regions called the *nodes of Ranvier*. The axolemma is exposed to tissue fluids at the nodes of Ranvier, facilitating the exchange of ions between the interior and exterior of the axon. In myelinated nerve fibers, excitation of the nerve membrane occurs along the length of the axon from one

node of Ranvier to another in a process called *saltatory conduction* (Fig. 20-4). The speed of impulse conduction in large myelinated A fibers approaches 120 m/s. The categorization and physiologic function of peripheral nerves are provided in Table 20-1.

► ELECTROPHYSIOLOGY

The physiologic basis for the propagation of a nerve impulse lies in the structural nature of the axolemma and depends on the differential concentration of electrolytes within the axolemma and the extracellular space and the semipermeability of the axolemma to these ions. The resting nerve cell has a potential difference, or voltage, that is created by the asymmetric distribution of sodium and potassium ions. The extracellular medium is approximately 10-fold richer in sodium ions than the interior, and the interior of the cell is approximately 10-fold richer in potassium ions. The excess of positive charges on the extracellular surface and the excess of negative charges on the interior of the cell membrane creates a *resting membrane potential*. During this "resting" state the nerve is said to be *polarized* (Fig. 20-5).

In the resting state, the permeability of the axolemma to sodium ions is so low that there is little transfer of sodium ions from the exterior to the interior of the cell despite the large concentration difference. Although larger than sodium ions, potassium ions are freely permeable through the axolemma creating a net deficit of positive ions in the interior of the axolemma. This ionic asymmetry is maintained by the sodium–potassium

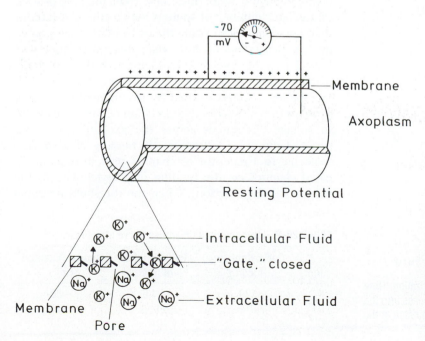

Figure 20–4. Unmyelinated nerve fiber at rest. Note the resting potential of −70 mV, the inside of the cell being negative with respect to the outside. The magnified section of the nerve membrane illustrates the ionic relationships during the resting phase. Note that ionic passage through the pores is controlled by "gates" that, when closed, allow free passage to potassium ions (K^+) but prevent ingress of sodium ions (Na^+).

TABLE 20-1. Categorization and Physiologic Function of Peripheral Nerves

	A-Alpha (Motor)	A-Beta (Touch Pressure)	A-Gamma (Proprioception)	A-Delta (Pain Temperature)	B (Preganglionic Autonomic)	C (Pain Temperature)
Myelin	+++	++	++	++	+	−
Diameter (mm)	12–20	5–12	5–12	1–4	1–3	0.5–1
Conduction Speed (m/s)	70–120	30–70	30–70	12–30	14.8	1.2

adenosine-triphosphate pump (sodium pump, ATP). With the hydrolysis of one molecule of ATP, three sodium ions are transported to the exterior of the cell, with two potassium ions being transported into the interior of the cell. The distribution of sodium ions outside the cell produces a negative resting membrane potential of approximately −60 to −90 mV. The electrical potential that results from the distribution of univalent ions both inside and outside the cell at normal body temperature (37°C) can be calculated by the Nernst equation (Guyton and Hall, 1996):

$$EMF\ (mV) = \pm 61 \log \frac{Concentration\ inside}{Concentration\ outside},$$

where EMF is the Nernst potential in millivolts on the cell interior. The potential is negative for a positive ion and positive for a negative ion. Table 20-2 lists the ionic distribution of electrolytes in mammalian nerve fibers and the corresponding Nernst potentials. As explained, the nerve fiber is essentially a potassium electrode whose resulting resting membrane potential is altered by changes in extracellular and intracellular potassium concentrations. The axolemma is highly permeable to potassium (50-100 times greater) but relatively impermeable to sodium ions; therefore, it is the diffusion of potassium ions that contributes to the development of a membrane potential. For example, an increase in extracellular potassium produces a decrease in the resting membrane potential. The cell is now in a state of hyperpolarization, as the inside of the cell is now less negative or partially depolarized and can reach the threshold potential relatively easily. In contrast, alterations in sodium concentration have little, if any, effect on the resting membrane potential.

Nerve impulses are transmitted through *action potentials* that are generated with alterations in membrane permeability of the axolemma to sodium and potassium ions. *Depolarization* occurs when a stimulus of sufficient intensity (threshold potential) produces an increase in membrane permeability, facilitating the passage of a greater number of sodium ions to the cell interior than potassium ions exiting the cell and producing a cell interior that is less negative than the cell exterior. The lowering of the voltage difference across the axolemma occurs as a result of "gating," or opening and closing, of membrane channels formed by the integral membrane proteins previously discussed. Gating occurs in response to voltage differences across the axolemma (voltage-gated channel) or following the binding of a specific molecule to a receptor or channel protein (chemically gated channel, eg, the binding of acetylcholine to the neuromuscular junction). When the threshold potential

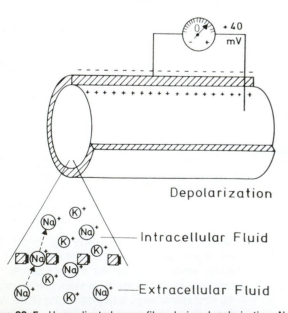

Figure 20–5. Unmyelinated nerve fiber during depolarization. Note that the "gates" are now open, allowing sodium ions to pass into the cell. The electrical potential is momentarily 40 mV, the outside of the cell now being negative with respect to the inside.

TABLE 20–2. Ionic Distribution across Nerve Membrane

Ion	Cell Cytoplasm (mEq/L)	Extracellular Fluid (mEq/L)	Nernst Potential (mV)
K$^+$	120	4.5	−86
Na$^+$	14	142	+61
Cl$^-$	8	107	−70

is reached, sodium channels open, facilitating a rapid influx of sodium into the interior of the axolemma and producing depolarization. The flow of sodium ions is self-perpetuating, as initial sodium ion flow opens additional sodium channels. The action potential develops as the cell interior undergoes a transition from negative to positive (Fig. 20–6). At the peak of depolarization, the electrical potential is approximately 40 mV higher than the cell exterior, and sodium channels become inactivated, which decreases sodium permeability. The action potential develops as a result of the change from the resting potential of −60 to −90 mV to a peak of +40 to +50 mV at the completion of depolarization (for a total change of 110 mV). For an action potential to occur, a critical threshold potential or stimulus must be achieved. For myelinated mammalian nerves, the threshold potential is 20 to 30 mV less than the resting potential (−40 to −70 mV). The threshold potential can be modified by local factors, including pH, P_{O_2}, and P_{CO_2}, as well as the strength of the preceding action potentials. Alkalosis increases, but hypoxemia and acidosis depress neuronal excitability.

Following the completion of depolarization, cell *repolarization* is initiated with the closing of sodium channels, preventing the inward flux of sodium ions, and potassium channels open, allowing the flow of potassium ions out of the axon to return the axon to the resting potential of −60 to −90 mV. The sodium pump is actively involved in reestablishing this ionic asymmetry. During the period of repolarization, the axolemma is refractory or unable to respond to an additional stimulus, no matter how strong (it will not respond to an action potential). In the later phase of repolarization, the axolemma is said to be in a state of relative refractoriness, that is, depolarization can be initiated only by a stimulus whose intensity is greater than that which produced the original depolarization. The refractory period is necessary to limit the impulses that can be conducted by the nerve fiber per unit of time. The relative refractory period can be altered by a number of pharmacologic agents (recall the effect of lidocaine on cardiac conduction), as well as by the frequency of stimulation.

► CHEMISTRY OF LOCAL ANESTHETICS

Commercially available local anesthetics belong to one of two chemical groups: amino esters or amino amides. Amino ester local anesthetics are characterized by an ester linkage (COO−) between the aromatic end of the molecule and the middle intermediate chain, whereas amino amides are characterized by an amide (NH) linkage between the aromatic end of the molecule and the middle intermediate chain. Both molecules terminate with a hydrophilic end formed by a tertiary amine. There are additional local anesthetics that do not fit into either of these categories and may be classified as "miscellaneous" local anesthetics. Dibucaine, a quinoline derivative; dyclone, a ketone derivative; and benzocaine, an ester topical anesthetic devoid of the amino group common to other esters, are examples of "miscellaneous" local anesthetics. Table 20–3 characterizes the commercially available local anesthetics. Table 20–4 provides the chemical structure and physicochemical properties of the commercially available local anesthetics.

Lipid solubility may be altered with changes in either the aromatic or tertiary amine structures of the drug. Lipid solubility and protein binding are increased with the addition of side chains to the aromatic ring. For example, the addition of a butyl group to the aromatic ring of procaine results in the chemical structure tetracaine, which is more potent and has a longer duration of action. Both the potency and the toxicity of the agent can be increased with a corresponding increase in the length of both the intermediate chain and the terminal groups attached to the tertiary amine. The addition of a butyl group to the tertiary amine group of mepivacaine results in the chemical structure of bupivacaine, which is more lipid soluble and highly protein bound. There is a limit to the increase in length of the intermediate chain; when a critical length is reached, anesthetic potency will decrease (Wood, 1990). Optimum binding of local anesthetic to the sodium channel is facilitated with an intermediate chain length of 4 to 5 atoms. The intermediate chain is also important in determining the route of biotransformation of the drug. Agents with ester intermediate chains are hydrolyzed by plasma esterases, and agents with amide intermediate chains are metabolized more slowly by the liver (Wood, 1990).

Physicochemical properties are important in determining local anesthetic action. Molecular weight is an important determinant of the diffusion coefficient of the agent. Diffusion is inversely proportional to the square

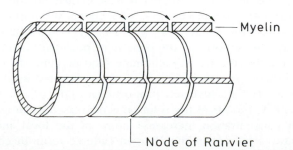

Figure 20–6. Depolarization in a myelinated nerve fiber showing propagation of the electrical impulse from node to node. Voltage changes similar to those described for unmyelinated nerve fibers occur.

TABLE 20–3. Local Anesthetics, Clinical Dosages, and Clinical Application

| Agent | Maximum Single Dose (mg)[a] | | Clinical Use |
	Without Epinephrine	With Epinephrine	
Ester-linked			
Cocaine	150		Topical
Benzocaine	Unknown		Topical
Procaine	800	1000	Infiltration, spinal
Tetracaine	100		Topical, spinal
Chloroprocaine	800	1000	Infiltration, peripheral nerve blocks, obstetric epidural anesthesia
Amide-linked			
Lidocaine	400	500	Topical, infiltration, intravenous regional, peripheral nerve blocks, epidural, spinal
Prilocaine	500	600	Infiltration, intravenous regional, surgical epidural anesthesia
Mepivacaine	300	500	Infiltration, peripheral nerve blocks, epidural
Bupivacaine	175	250	Infiltration, peripheral nerve blocks, epidural, spinal
Ropivacaine	250		Peripheral nerve blocks, surgical epidural anesthesia
Etidocaine	300	400	Infiltration, peripheral nerve blocks, surgical epidural anesthesia
Miscellaneous			
Dibucaine	50		Spinal
Articaine			Infiltration, epidural

[a] Recommended safe dose is influenced by many factors (see text) and should be adjusted for each site of injection. The total dose of epinephrine should not exceed 0.25 mg.
From Brown, D. L. (1996). Regional Anesthesia and Analgesia. (p. 189). Philadelphia: W.B. Saunders.

root of the molecular weight. Molecular weight may play a role in the diffusion of the local anesthetic in the sodium channel (Courtney, 1980).

Lipid solubility determines the intrinsic anesthetic potency of a specific agent. Local anesthetics that are highly lipid soluble readily penetrate the cell membrane and have an increased duration of action (or clinical effect). The amino esters procaine and chloroprocaine have very low lipid solubility, and accordingly they require higher concentrations (2%–3%) to produce an effective neural blockade. In contrast, the amino amides bupivacaine and etidocaine have a high lipid solubility and produce effective neural blockade with relatively low concentrations (0.25%–0.5%). The amino amides lidocaine and mepivacaine and the amino ester prilocaine are intermediate in solubility and anesthetic potency, and require concentrations ranging from 1% to 3%.

▶ MECHANISM OF ACTION OF LOCAL ANESTHETICS

Local anesthetics decrease the excitability of peripheral nerves but do not affect the resting membrane potential. Recall that the resting membrane potential is a function of potassium ion distribution, which is not affected by local anesthetic agents. As discussed, the action potential is generated by increased permeability of the axolemma to sodium ions. Local anesthetic agents interfere with axolemma sodium permeability, increasing the threshold

potential of the cell. Minimal concentrations of local anesthetics can also decrease conduction velocity and increase the refractory period of the nerve, decreasing the ability of the nerve to react to additional repetitive stimuli (eg, lidocaine).

The commercially available local anesthetics are prepared as the hydrochloric (acid) salt of a basic amine. The cation, which is positively charged, is in dissociation equilibrium with the uncharged local anesthetic base according to the Henderson–Hasselbalch equation:

$$pH = pK_a - \log [(B)/(BH^+)],$$

where pH = the hydrogen ion concentration, pK_a is a dissociation constant, $[B]$ is the concentration of the uncharged base, and $[BH^+]$ is the concentration of the positively charged cation.

The pK_a defines the pH at which equal amounts of ionized and unionized forms of a chemical compound exist. The pK_a influences the onset of action as the uncharged base form of the drug is responsible for diffusion across the nerve membrane. The percent of local anesthetic present in base form when injected into tissue at pH 7.4 is inversely proportional to the pK_a of the agent. As the pH of the solution is decreased (hydrogen ion concentration increases), more of the local anesthetic is present in the charged cationic form. In contrast, when the pH increases (a decrease in hydrogen ion concentration), the free-base form of the local anesthetic predominates. This relationship can be expressed by the following equation:

TABLE 20–4. Properties of Local Anaesthetics

Agent	Chemical Configuration			Physiochemical Properties			Pharmacological Properties		
	Aromatic Lipophilic	Intermediate Chain	Amine Hydrophilic	Molecular Weight (Base)	pK$_a$ (25°C)	Protein Binding (%)	Onset	Relative Potency	Duration
Procaine	H—N(H)—⟨benzene⟩	—COOCH$_2$CH$_2$—N	C$_2$H$_5$ / C$_2$H$_5$	236	8.9	6	Slow	1	Short
Tetracaine	H$_9$C$_4$N(H)—⟨benzene⟩	—COOCH$_2$CH$_2$—N	CH$_3$ / CH$_3$	264	8.5	76	Slow	8	Long
Chloroprocaine	H$_2$N—⟨benzene, Cl⟩	—COOCH$_2$CH$_2$—N	C$_2$H$_5$ / C$_2$H$_5$	271	9.3	—	Fast	1	Short
Amides Prilocaine	⟨CH$_3$ benzene⟩—NHCOCH(CH$_3$)—	—N	H / C$_3$H$_7$	220	8.0	55	Fast	2	Moderate
Lignocaine	⟨CH$_3$, CH$_3$ benzene⟩—NHCOCH$_2$—	—N	C$_2$H$_5$ / C$_2$H$_5$	234	8.2	64	Fast	2	Moderate
Mepivacaine	⟨CH$_3$, CH$_3$ benzene⟩—NHCO—	⟨piperidine N—CH$_3$⟩		246	7.9	78	Fast	2	Moderate
Bupivacaine	⟨CH$_3$, CH$_3$ benzene⟩—NHCO—	⟨piperidine N—C$_4$H$_9$⟩		288	8.2	96	Moderate	8	Long

(Continued)

TABLE 20–4. Properties of Local Anaesthetics *(Continued)*

| Agent | Chemical Configuration | | | Physiochemical Properties | | | Pharmacological Properties | | |
	Aromatic Lipophilic	Intermediate Chain	Amine Hydrophilic	Molecular Weight (Base)	pK_a (25°C)	Protein Binding (%)	Onset	Relative Potency	Duration
Ropivacaine		—NHCO		274	8.1	94	Moderate	—	Long (shorter motor block)
Etidocaine		—NHCOCH		276	8.1	94	Fast	6	Long

Source: Adapted from Strichartz, G. R. (1993). Local anesthetics. In S. A. Feidman, W. Patun, & C. Scurr (Eds.), Mechanisms of drugs in anesthesia (Table 18–2, p. 325). Hodder and Stoughton Publishers.

$$pK_a = pH + \log \frac{Base}{Cation}$$

The cationic moiety is responsible for producing neural blockade. After the local anesthetic penetrates the base form through the nerve sheath and axolemma, the cationic species diffuses to the receptor sites on the sodium channels (Fig. 20–7) (Covino & Strichartz, 1993). The binding of the cationic species with the sodium receptor inhibits sodium conductance, producing conduction blockade. However, the penetration of the local anesthetic through the charged axolemma requires a specific concentration of the base form of the drug. In an experiment evaluating the effects of pH on local anesthetic activity of lidocaine in intact isolated nerves, Ritchie, Ritchie, and Greengard (1965a, 1965b) found that raising the pH of the bathing solution markedly reduced the height of the generated action potential. Clinically speaking, the pH of tissues and nerve membranes may vary greatly. In tissues with a high pH, the rate and amount of the absorption of a local anesthetic are greater. However, in tissues of lower pH (infected or inflamed tissue), the rate and amount of local anesthetic absorbed is lower. The discovery that alkaline solutions containing a greater relative proportion of uncharged base act more quickly to produce neural blockade in intact nerves forms the basis for the addition of sodium bicarbonate to local anesthetic solutions to hasten their onset of action. Carbonated local anesthetics, which are not currently available in the United States, are thought to improve anesthetic activity by increasing the CO_2 content around the nerve, producing a decrease in the pH in the interior of the nerve, resulting in an increase in the cationic moiety of local anesthetic within the nerve.

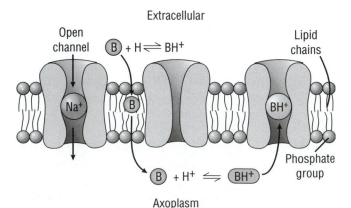

Figure 20–7. The penetration of local anesthetic base (B) and equilibration in axoplasm with the cationic species (BH^+) with subsequent blockade of the sodium channel. *(From Brown, D. L. [1996]. Regional Anesthesia and Analgesia [Figure 14–2, p. 233]. Philadelphia: W. B. Saunders. Modified from de Jong, R. H. (1994) Local anesthetics [p. 49]. St. Louis: Mosby-Yearbook.)*

▶ LOCAL ANESTHETIC ACTION

The specific site (receptor) where local anesthetics produce their effects is thought to be at the internal end of the sodium channel. The displacement of calcium ions from their lipoprotein receptors by the cationic species of the local anesthetic blocks the sodium channel, decreasing sodium conductance across the axolemma and inhibiting depolarization. Following deposition, the local anesthetic moves by diffusion along a concentration gradient through the tissue into the nerve. The concentration of local anesthetic continually decreases as a result of diffusion and absorption through lymphatic and vascular channels. Much of the deposited local anesthetic is also lost to the nerve through binding to protein and lipid structures.

▶ THE ADDITION OF VASOCONSTRICTORS

With the exception of cocaine, all local anesthetics produce concentration-dependent vasoconstriction and vasodilation of vascular smooth muscle. Vasoconstriction is produced with dilute concentrations, whereas concentrations employed for regional anesthesia produce vasodilation at the site of administration (Blair, 1975). Combining a local anesthetic with a vasoconstrictor inhibits the systemic absorption of the local anesthetic and prolongs its duration of action. Adding a vasoconstrictor decreases local anesthetic absorption into vascular channels and maintains a higher concentration of local anesthetic available to the nerve.

Epinephrine is the most popular and widely used vasoconstrictor. The alpha-adrenergic effects are the predominant reason for incorporating epinephrine with local anesthetics. Epinephrine is rapidly oxidized with sterilization, and so it is better to add the desired amount to the local anesthetic immediately prior to use. Local anesthetics commercially prepared with epinephrine contain concentrations of 1:200 000 (5 µg/mL) and the antioxidant metabisulfite. This antioxidant allows a single heat sterilization without loss of potency. The toxic effects of epinephrine manifest clinically as beta-adrenergic stimulatory effects (tachycardia, bradycardia, tachydysrhythmias). However, high doses can produce alpha-adrenergic stimulation that results in hypertension. When epinephrine-containing solutions are used for epidural anesthesia, there may be an increased tendency for hypotension to develop, even in normovolemic subjects, because of the widespread beta-adrenergic effects that oppose compensatory vasoconstriction in the arms and torso (Bonica, Akamatsu, Berges, Morikawa, & Kennedy, 1971). The total dose of epinephrine should not exceed 200 µg. Epinephrine should be used with caution in patients with hypertension and avoided in patients with pheochromocytoma and thyrotoxicosis.

Phenylephrine is the only additional vasoconstrictor that has been combined with local anesthetics. Unlike epinephrine, phenylephrine is a pure alpha-adrenergic agonist. Phenylephrine has been a popular adjunct in spinal anesthesia in concentrations of 1:20 000 (20 µg/mL), and its use is limited as widespread systemic effects may occur when used for other regional anesthetic procedures.

Epinephrine and phenylephrine have a varied ability to prolong the effects of a local anesthetic. The ability to prolong the clinical effects of local anesthetics may be limited due to the inherent vasodilator property of the local anesthetic, its lipid solubility, and the blood flow of the area where the local anesthetic is deposited. For example, adding epinephrine to prilocaine is less effective in prolonging the duration of block because prilocaine is a weak vasodilator. The high lipid solubility of bupivacaine decreases the effectiveness of epinephrine to prolong the duration of block. However, epinephrine substantially increases the duration of action of a tetracaine subarachnoid block (Conception et al., 1984). Epinephrine also prolongs the effects of lidocaine, mepivacaine, or procaine when administered for epidural block or infiltrative block of a peripheral nerve (Buckley, Littlewood, Covino, & Scott, 1978; Bromage, 1965; Gramling, Ellis, & Volpitto, 1964; Kier, 1974).

▶ DIFFERENTIAL AND FREQUENCY-DEPENDENT NERVE BLOCK

Historically, the ability of a local anesthetic to produce neural blockade was thought to depend in part on the size of the nerve fiber to be blocked. The nerve action potential can skip over one, two, or three blocked nodes of Ranvier. In larger nerve fibers there is a greater distance between each node of Ranvier. Each nerve has a critical blocking length, which is proportional to the diameter of the nerve. Three nodes of Ranvier must interact with a local anesthetic to ensure complete blockade of the action potential. Perhaps more nodes of Ranvier need to be blocked to cease conduction of the action potential in smaller unmyelinated fibers.

A mixed peripheral nerve is composed of A, B, and C nerve fibers. Fibers that innervate proximal structures are arranged concentrically on the peripheral aspect, or mantle, of the nerve, and fibers that innervate more distal structures lie in the innermost portion, or core, of the nerve. Clinically, the onset of neural blockade starts with motor and sensory anesthesia of proximal structures, followed by blockade of distal structures as the local anesthetic diffuses into the center of the nerve bundle and blocks the core fibers.

Because the small C fibers appear to be more easily blocked than large fibers, one might expect that it would be possible to block structures innervated by these fibers by a given concentration of local anesthetic, sparing the function of the myelinated A fibers. This phenomenon does occur clinically and is referred to as *differential block*. Experimental evidence demonstrates that what appears to be a greater sensitivity to local anesthetic action by small C fibers is caused by diffusion barriers and is not a function of fiber size (Bromage, Burfoot, Crowell, & Truant, 1967; Gissen, Covino, & Gregus, 1980). To produce blockade of myelinated A fibers the local anesthetic must be administered in sufficient concentrations to overcome the barriers to diffusion. The minimum blocking concentration (C_M) of a local anesthetic was defined by de Jong (1970) as the lowest concentration of a local anesthetic required to produce blockade of all fibers of the nerve in vitro and is analogous to the minimum alveolar concentration (MAC) of an inhalation anesthetic. As with MAC, the administration of an initially higher drug concentration is needed to produce an effective drug concentration at the site of action. Accordingly, local anesthetic concentrations greater than C_M must be administered to produce neural blockade reliably.

An additional factor that may affect local anesthetic action is the frequency with which nerve impulses travel along nerve fibers. An isolated nerve is more sensitive to a particular local anesthetic when the frequency of impulse conduction along the nerve is increased (Courtney, Kendig, & Cohen, 1978). The cationic moiety of local anesthetics preferentially binds to open sodium channels producing neural blockade. An increase in the frequency of nerve impulses increases the number of open sodium channels for binding of local anesthetic. Partial neural blockade in a given axon may be produced with a weak anesthetic solution under low-frequency conduction, but the same axon is completely blocked when subjected to higher frequencies of nerve stimulation. This *frequency-dependent conduction blockade* occurs with all the clinically available local anesthetics, particularly the highly lipid-soluble agents tetracaine, bupivacaine, and etidocaine.

► PHARMACOKINETICS OF LOCAL ANESTHETICS

The duration of neural blockade and clinical recovery depend on the pharmacokinetics of the local anesthetic, governed by absorption, diffusion of the local anesthetic against concentration gradients, affinity of the local anesthetic for lipoprotein structures, metabolism, and excretion.

Absorption of a local anesthetic depends on the vascularity at the site of injection. The more vascular the area, the faster the absorption and the higher the plasma concentrations. The highest blood concentrations, in decreasing order, are obtained after intercostal administration, caudal administration, epidural administration, brachial plexus, sciatic–femoral, and subcutaneous infiltration, provided that equal volumes and concentrations of local anesthetic are administered. In the case of intercostal deposition of local anesthetic, greater uptake occurs as a result of increased vascularity, greater surface area, and lower proportion of adipose tissue. The simultaneous administration of a vasoconstrictor prolongs the duration of the neural blockade and reduces the potential toxicity that may occur from the vascular uptake of the anesthetic. Epinephrine is commonly employed in concentrations of 1 : 200 000 (5 mg/mL). Higher concentrations of epinephrine (except perhaps in oral mucous membranes where solutions may be used in concentrations of 1 : 80 000) may attain durations that are only marginally longer. Although epinephrine combined with the long-acting agents bupivacaine and etidocaine reduces peak plasma concentrations, the increase in duration of action is negligible. This might be explained in part because of the higher lipid solubility of these agents. The local absorption of the agent by protein in the surrounding tissue and the nerve provides a depot and a concentration gradient in favor of the nerves that result in a longer duration of action. This effect offsets the high lipid solubility and favors vascular uptake. The process of absorption of a local anesthetic from its site of administration is reflected in the blood, producing a profile that rises and falls at rates that depend on the rate of distribution from the vascular compartment to other tissue compartments and the elimination by metabolism and excretion. The circulatory concentration of local anesthetics may be expressed either as whole-blood or plasma concentrations, and these values may differ because of different rates of uptake in blood.

Local anesthetics must reach their target site by diffusing through the tissue barriers (the perineurim for the peripheral nerve, the arachnoid mater in the CNS) (Bernards & Hill, 1991). During clinical recovery the diffusion gradient is reversed, as the outer concentric layer of the nerve is exposed to a decreasing concentration of local anesthetic that is lost to the extracellular fluid. The concentration of the local anesthetic in the core of the nerve is maintained for a longer period. The clinical implication of this reversed diffusion sequence can be demonstrated by examining recovery from spinal anesthesia. During recovery, the proximal portion of the legs recover more quickly from neural blockade than does the distal portion of the legs. This mechanism of recovery from neural blockade may be important in the genesis of tourniquet pain.

Local anesthetic agents with a high protein-binding capacity also have an increased duration of action, as there is thought to be a relationship between protein binding and the binding of the agent to the proteins in the axolemma. Bupivacaine and etidocaine are 90% to 97% protein bound and exhibit a long duration of action. Procaine, which is weakly protein bound, has a relatively short duration of action. Prilocaine, mepivacaine, and lidocaine are intermediate in terms of protein binding (55%–75%) and have an intermediate duration of action.

Biotransformation is determined by the chemical structure of the intermediate chain of the local anesthetic. Agents with ester intermediate chains are hydrolyzed to derivatives of *para*-aminobenzoic acid by pseudocholinesterase as well as red cell esterases. The *para*-aminobenzoic acid derivatives may serve as haptens (molecules capable of stimulating the production of antibodies), contributing to the development of allergic reactions. The metabolism of these compounds is faster than the metabolism of the amino amide local anesthetics. For example, chloroprocaine undergoes rapid hydrolysis, whereas procaine is hydrolyzed four times more slowly and tetracaine 16 times more slowly. The clinical significance of this rapid metabolism of amino esters is that any toxic reactions that may occur are usually short-lived.

The amino amide local anesthetics undergo one or more primary degradation steps in the liver. The clearance of the amino amide agents occurs as follows: bupivacaine, then ropivacaive, mepivacaine, lidocaine, etidocaine, and prilocaine. The resultant metabolites, which may have inherent pharmacologic action, differ with each drug. These metabolites are generally inconsequential, but, with concurrent renal or cardiac failure, may accumulate and interact with the parent compound to produce toxic side effects.

Severe liver dysfunction can also precipitate the clinical presentation of toxic side effects with the accumulation of the parent compound in the circulation. The selection and administration of local anesthetics for regional anesthesia in these patients must take this factor into consideration, particularly if large doses of local anesthetics are necessary.

Impaired metabolism alters the clearance of local anesthetics from the body. Generally, more than 90% of all local anesthetics are excreted as metabolites of their parent compound. In humans, the kidney is the primary excretory organ. Significant renal dysfunction also directly affects the clearance and excretion of the local anesthetic metabolites. Renal disease may also contribute to the genesis of toxic side effects from systemically absorbed local anesthetic agents when the local anesthetic is displaced from plasma protein by uremia.

► LOCAL ANESTHETIC POTENCY

The C_M of a local anesthetic is determined by observing a 50% reduction in the action potential spike height in a sheathed frog sciatic nerve within 5 minutes, when the nerve is stimulated at a frequency of 30 impulses per second, in a solution with a pH of 7.2 to 7.4. Using this standard, the potency of local anesthetics can be determined. As illustrated in Table 20–4, there is a strong correlation between anesthetic potency and lipid solubility. Procaine (the least lipid-soluble local anesthetic) has a relative potency of 1, whereas etidocaine (the most lipid-soluble local anesthetic) has a relative potency of 16. Local anesthetics with a high potency are effective at concentrations lower than those for agents of intermediate or low potency. In addition, high-potency agents are more likely to block all the components of the nerve (eg, types A, B, and C fibers), provided sufficient concentrations are used. Clinically, latency of onset of anesthesia and duration of neural blockade are the two most important characteristics. In a manner similar to the standard determination of C_M in the frog sciatic nerve, latency is determined by the concentration of a local anesthetic that depresses the action potential by 50% in 10 minutes. Latency has no relation to potency, pK_a, or lipid solubility but depends on the site of injection. Doubling the anesthetic concentration reduces the latency by approximately one third. Etidocaine, which is highly lipid soluble and has the lowest pK_a, has the shortest latency of all the commercially available local anesthetics (Table 20–4). The duration of neural blockade also depends on lipid and protein affinities. Accordingly, local anesthetics can be separated into three distinct groups: (1) agents of low potency and short duration (procaine, chloroprocaine); (2) agents of intermediate potency and duration of action (lidocaine, mepivacaine, and prilocaine); and (3) agents with high potency and long duration of action (tetracaine, bupivacaine, etidocaine, and ropivacaine). Although in vitro modeling is important for pharmacologic comparisons of local anesthetics, the reader should appreciate that differences do exist between in vitro and in vivo applications. Factors that may account for these differences include the administration within different tissue sites with varying vascularity as well as the inherent vascular tone. The most useful elements clinically are potency, on-set or latency, and duration of action.

► CLINICAL PHARMACOLOGY

Table 20–3 lists the primary uses of the commercially available local anesthetics with the accompanying maximum dosages. Each of these agents has specific properties that are properly suited for a specific use.

Amino Ester Local Anesthetics

The family of amino ester local anesthetics includes co-caine, benzocaine, procaine, chloroprocaine, and tetra-caine.

Cocaine

Cocaine is the historic prototype of the amino esters. It is supplied in a 1% to 20% solution and has a pK_a of 8.6. Cocaine is the only local anesthetic that produces vaso-constriction in clinically useful dosages. Accordingly, so-lutions from 5% to 10% are used in otolaryngology for topical anesthesia of the mucous membranes of the nose and pharynx. The expected duration of anesthesia is ap-proximately 60 minutes.

The maximum safe clinical dose is 150 mg to 200 mg. Cocaine produces stimulatory effects on the sympathetic nervous and cardiovascular systems by in-hibiting the uptake of catecholamines at the nerve ter-minal. Drug toxicity is manifest clinically with excite-ment, tachycardia, hypertension, and seizures, all of which precede the development of depressant effects. Because of its inherent addictive properties and in-creased potential to produce systemic toxicity, cocaine is used only as a topical agent.

Benzocaine

Benzocaine is an ethyl-ester of *para*-aminobenzoic acid. The pK_a of 3.5 indicates that the compound exists al-most entirely in the free-base species at physiologic pH. It is insoluble in water and produces tissue irritation if in-jected. Benzocaine is used as a topical anesthetic agent and is an essential component of topical aerosol agents, such as Hurricaine® and Cetacaine®. The maximum safe clinical dose is unknown.

Procaine (Novacain®)

Procaine is a derivative of *para*-aminobenzoic acid and is formulated as the hydrochloride with a pK_a of 9.0. Pro-caine is a weak local anesthetic that has a long latency and short duration of action and is rarely used today. A 0.5% solution of procaine used to be administered for skin incision, and it was also used in combination with D5W for spinal anesthesia. Because of its low potency and rapid plasma hydrolysis, procaine infrequently pro-duces systemic toxicity. The maximum safe clinical dose is 800 mg, and increases to 1000 mg with the addition of epinephrine. *Para*-aminobenzoic acid is a product of procaine hydrolysis and may be responsible for the rare allergic reactions that follow repeated use.

Chloroprocaine (Nesacaine®)

Chloroprocaine is a 2-chloro derivative of procaine and is available in 1%, 2%, or 3% solutions. Its pK_a is 8.7, and it has a rapid onset of action and a short duration of ac-tion. Chloroprocaine undergoes hydrolysis more rapidly than procaine and is believed to have a low potential for toxicity. The 1% solution is reserved for infiltrative tech-niques. The expected duration of action approaches 45 minutes, but it may be extended to 90 minutes by adding epinephrine. A 3% solution decreases the latency and improves neural blockade. The maximum safe clini-cal dose is 800 mg and increases to 1000 mg with the ad-dition of epinephrine. As with procaine, chloroprocaine is hydrolyzed by pseudocholinesterase and excreted by the kidneys.

Chloroprocaine has been popular for obstetric epidural anesthesia. The rapid onset, incomplete motor blockade, low toxicity, and ability of the fetus to metabo-lize the drug (at one-half the rate as in maternal plasma) contribute to its popularity. However, popularity has de-creased since the publication of reports about its poten-tial for myelotoxicity and neurotoxicity (de Jong, 1981; Gissen, Datta, & Lambert, 1984; Raymond & Strichartz, 1990; Ready, Plumer, Haschke, Austin, & Sumi, 1985; Stevens, Urmey, Urquhart, & Kao, 1993). The original for-mulation of chloroprocaine contained the acid stabilizer sodium metabisulfite in a concentration of 0.2% to pre-vent oxidation during storage. Sodium metabisulfite, when hydrolyzed from sodium bisulfite, leads to the for-mation of sulfurous acid, a neurotoxic agent (Raymond, & Strichartz, 1990). In vivo experiments demonstrated neurotoxicity with 2-chloroprocaine, whereas lidocaine and bupivacaine did not exhibit this effect (Gissen et al., 1984). The neurotoxicity was attributed to the stabiliz-ing agent. Reformulation was accomplished with the substitution of ethylenediaminetetraacetic acid (EDTA) for sodium metabisulfite. Subsequent reports with the use of this product have reported severe lumbar mus-cle spasm as a result of the calcium-chelating action of EDTA (Fibuch & Opper, 1989; Rigler et al., 1991). A new, preservative-free formulation is now available in 2% to 3% Nesacaine-MPF® or chloroprocaine hydrochloride (HCL), U.S.P.

Tetracaine (Pontacaine®)

Tetracaine, an ester of *para*-aminobenzoic acid, is 10 times as potent and is hydrolyzed three to four times more slowly than procaine, providing a longer duration of action and a more intense degree of neural blockade. The pK_a is 8.5. Tetracaine is more lipid soluble than is chloroprocaine and is readily bound to protein. The drug is associated with a long latency when used for peripheral nerve blocks. Complete neural blockade re-quires up to 30 minutes. The maximum safe clinical dose is 100 mg.

Tetracaine is commercially available as a solution or crystals, the latter being more stable to heat sterilization. By virtue of its potency, tetracaine is used in very low concentrations (0.1% or 0.2%) for peripheral nerve block. The drug has found great use for spinal anesthesia, as the administration of 10 mg to 15 mg of a 1% solution provides anesthesia to a midthoracic dermatome for up to 3 hours. The onset of anesthesia is rapid (5 to 10 minutes) following subarachnoid administration. The addition of 0. 2 mg of epinephrine (0.2 mL of a 1:1000 solution) prolongs the duration of action by 50% to 60%. Prolongation of the duration of action by up to 100% can be accomplished by adding 5 mg of phenylephrine (0.5 mL of 1% solution).

Amino Amide Local Anesthetics

The family of amino amide local anesthetics includes lidocaine, prilocaine, etidocaine, mepivacaine, bupivacaine, and ropivacaine. Most of the amides are anilides; however, dibucaine is a quinoline derivative. Mepivacaine, bupivacaine, and ropivacaine are derivatives of the pipecolyl xylidides family.

Lidocaine (Xylocaine®)

Lidocaine is the most frequently used local anesthetic agent as it has a rapid onset of action, inherent potency, and intermediate duration of action. It has a pK_a of 7.9, is moderately lipid soluble, and is 65% plasma-protein bound. Carbonated lidocaine marketed outside the United States is buffered to a pH of 6.5, facilitating the penetration of the axolemma by the uncharged free-base moiety.

Lidocaine is commercially available in 0.5% 1%, 2%, 4%, and 5% solutions, with or without epinephrine. The 0.5% solution should be used for infiltrative anesthesia when large volumes are required. The duration of action of the 0.5% solution can be increased up from 75 to 240 minutes with the addition of 1:200 000 epinephrine. A 1% solution provides 120 minutes of anesthesia and up to 400 minutes with the addition of epinephrine. Because of the encountered vascularity, a 2% solution with 1:80 000 epinephrine is used for dental anesthesia with an expected duration of 150 minutes.

A 0.5% preservative-free solution is used for intravenous regional anesthesia. Higher concentrations unnecessarily increase the risk of toxicity. A 0.5% solution provides satisfactory digital anesthesia, and plexus and peripheral nerve blocks require a 1% solution.

Latency is short with lidocaine, ranging from 5 minutes for peripheral infiltration to 20 minutes following plexus infiltration. A 1% solution is acceptable for epidural or caudal anesthesia; however, the 2% solution produces a greater degree of motor blockade. The addition of epinephrine 1:200 000 shortens latency, improves the degree of motor blockade, increases duration, and may reduce the potential for toxicity when large volumes are used. The duration of anesthesia is increased by up to 100 minutes with the addition of epinephrine.

A 5% solution of lidocaine combined with 7.5% dextrose for spinal anesthesia has enjoyed a remarkable safety record. The customary dosages range from 15 mg to 100 mg. Yet, in 1991, Rigler and colleagues reported three cases of cauda equina syndrome that occurred following continuous spinal anesthesia with this solution and one case following the use of 0.5% tetracaine in 7.5% dextrose. An additional eight cases were reported in 1992, prompting a withdrawal of small-bore catheters for continuous spinal anesthesia (Lambert & Hurley, 1991). The etiology of neurologic injury is thought to result from a direct effect of the local anesthetic administered in a relatively high concentration and a restricted distribution of the anesthetic within the subarachnoid space (Benson, 1992; Rigler & Drasner, 1991). Studies are ongoing to evaluate and understand the mechanisms of transient or permanent neurologic injury following central neural axis blockade.

A 4% solution of lidocaine is reserved for topical anesthesia. A 10% spray is also marketed for this purpose. The maximum safe clinical dose is 400 mg, or 500 mg with the addition of epinephrine. Lidocaine is metabolized by the liver, and less than 4% is excreted by the kidneys as parent drug.

Prilocaine (Citanest®)

Prilocaine is a secondary amine derived from a toulidine and a teritary amine. The clinical features are similar to those of lidocaine with a short onset of action, intermediate duration of action, providing profound neural blockade. The pK_a is 7.9. Prilocaine is less lipid soluble than lidocaine and has less protein binding (55%).

Prilocaine is commercially available in concentrations of 0. 5%, 1%, 2%, and 3% with or without epinephrine. Solutions of 0.5% and 1% are sufficient for infiltrative anesthesia and provide a duration of action from 75 to 280 minutes with the addition of epinephrine. A 0.5% solution has been used for intravenous regional anesthesia as prilocaine is the least toxic of the amide local anesthetics and, therefore, the least likely to produce systemic toxicity in the event of a tourniquet failure. Peripheral nerve block can be accomplished with either the 0.5% or 1% solution.

A 2% or 3% solution is used for caudal or epidural anesthesia, although its selection in these situations is infrequent. The quality of anesthesia is not different from that obtained from lidocaine. A 2% solution without a vasoconstrictor provides minimum motor blockade, low potential for toxicity, and is an excellent choice for ambulatory surgical procedures.

The maximum safe clinical dose is 500 mg, and it increases to 600 mg with the addition of epinephrine. Dosages in excess of 600 mg may lead to the development of methemoglobinemia, a state where hemoglobin is oxidized to the ferric state and is unable to carry oxygen. Prilocaine is partially metabolized by the liver to o-toludine. Under normal physiologic conditions, less than 1% of hemoglobin exists in the ferric state. The clinical manifestations include cyanosis, which is not corrected by the administration of oxygen. Methylene blue, 1 to 2 mg/kg, reduces hemoglobin from the ferric to the ferrous state. Although prilocaine is the safest of the amide local anesthetics (less cardiotoxicity and neurotoxicity), its propensity to produce methemoglobin has led to its abandonment for obstetric anesthesia.

Mepivacaine (Carbocaine®)

Mepivacaine is structurally related to lidocaine and has a similar lipid solubility but a greater protein-binding capacity (up to 84%). Its pK_a is 7.6. The potential for systemic toxicity is similar to that of lidocaine. As with lidocaine, it has a rapid onset of action; however, its duration of action is longer. When administered with epinephrine, the duration of action can be increased by 75%.

Mepivacaine is equipotent to lidocaine and is commercially available in similar concentrations. Clinical applications also parallel those of lidocaine with the exception of obstetric anesthesia, because neonatal metabolism is slower than lidocaine and placental transfer is greater.

The maximum safe clinical dose is 300 mg and increases to 500 mg with the addition of epinephrine. However, epinephrine has a limited effect in decreasing plasma concentration and prolonging the duration of block when combined with mepivacaine. As with lidocaine, mepivacaine is metabolized by the liver, with renal excretion of the metabolites.

Bupivacaine (Marcaine®)

Bupivacaine, a derivative of mepivacaine, has a more rapid onset of action and a prolonged duration of action than mepivacaine. A butyl group replaces the methyl group in the piperidine ring, which confers a greater lipid solubility than mepivacaine. The increased lipid solubility accounts for its increased potency and greater toxicity (greater cardiotoxicity than lidocaine). Bupivacaine is 95% plasma-protein bound. Its pK_a is 8.1.

A 0.25%, 0.5%, or 0.75% solution is commercially available, although the 0.75% solution has limited use and is not recommended for obstetric anesthesia. There are no commercially available topical preparations.

Bupivacaine is an ideal choice when a long duration of anesthesia is desirable. A 0.25% or 0.5% solution is used for infiltration anesthesia; however, more dilute solutions should be used when the administration of large volumes of anesthetic is anticipated. When applied for peripheral nerve block, latency is long, particularly for

plexus anesthesia that may require 30 minutes for complete neural blockade. The 0.5% solution provides superior motor blockade as compared to the 0.25% solution. The duration of anesthesia is variable and may range from 400 minutes to as long as 24 hours. The addition of epinephrine produces an unreliable effect on the duration of action but decreases the toxicity by reducing plasma–drug concentrations.

Bupivacaine is unique in that it produces a concentration-dependent differential block of sensory and motor fibers. Bupivacaine has great utility in obstetric anesthesia as it is used to provide sensory analgesia without significant motor blockade during labor and the postoperative period.

A 0.5% solution is most commonly employed for caudal and epidural anesthesia. Bupivacaine is also available as a 0.5% isobaric or hyperbaric solution for spinal anesthesia. A customary total dose ranges from 15 mg to 20 mg. The duration of action is similar to that of tetracaine, although bupivacaine provides a superior sensory block but a less profound motor block. The maximum safe clinical dose is 175 mg (1–2 mg/kg) and increases to 200 mg when combined with epinephrine. As with lidocaine and mepivacaine, bupivacaine is metabolized by the liver, with renal excretion of the metabolites.

In 1979, Albright detailed the occurrence of six cases of sudden cardiac arrest, resistant to resuscitation, that followed the administration of bupivacaine and etidocaine for brachial plexus, caudal, and epidural anesthesia. Additional cases of maternal mortality were reported and presumed to have resulted from the accidental intravascular injection of 0.75% bupivacaine during epidural anesthesia (Marx, 1984). Data was presented to the U. S. Food and Drug Administration (FDA), which issued an urgent statement indicating that 0.75% bupivacaine was no longer recommended for obstetric anesthesia. Bupivacaine is more cardiotoxic than lidocaine and when administered intravenously can produce cardiac dysrhythmias (supraventricular tachycardia, atrioventricular conduction blocks, multifocal premature ventricular contractions, ventricular tachycardia, and ventricular fibrillation). Bupivacaine is formulated as a racemic mixture, that is, it contains equal portions of the $R (+)$ and $S (-)$ enantiomers. The cardiac sodium channel and the medullary respiratory neurons have a greater affinity for the $R (+)$ enantiomer, which may be the mechanism responsible for the greater cardiorespiratory toxicity.

The high lipid solubility of bupivacaine reduces the absorption from the intended site of action. However, if the drug is administered intravascularly, the drug is transported to the vessel-rich group organs (heart, brain, liver, kidneys), and the high concentration of unbound drug is free to cross the lipid membranes of the heart and brain. Although the FDA attempted to limit the concentration of the drug, it was bupivacaine itself, and not the concentration, that was responsible for the cardiac toxicity. Slow, fractionated dosing of bupivacaine during regional anesthesia reduces the risk of sudden high intravascular drug concentrations and aids the detection of systemic toxicity.

Etidocaine (Duranest®)

Etidocaine is related structurally to lidocaine and has the highest lipid solubility of the commercially available local anesthetics, but it is less toxic than bupivacaine. Its pK_a is 7.74, and the plasma-protein binding is 94%. Etidocaine is not equipotent with bupivacaine, has a shorter latency, provides similar durations of action, and has a more profound degree of motor blockade. The profound blockade of motor fibers and less intense blockade of sensory fibers can be disturbing to patients as they experience motor weakness and inadequate analgesia. Accordingly, etidocaine is not used for obstetric anesthesia.

Epidural and caudal anesthesia can be accomplished with a 1% or 1.5% solution, and a greater degree of motor blockade occurs with the latter solution. A 1% etidocaine solution provides a superior motor block than that provided by 0.5% bupivacaine. Epinephrine has no effect on the expected duration of action but may intensify the degree of motor blockade.

The maximum safe clinical dose is 300 mg, and it increases to 400 mg with the addition of epinephrine. The drug is metabolized by the liver, and less than 1% is excreted unchanged by the kidneys.

Dibucaine (Nupercainal®)

Dibucaine, a quinoline derivative with an amide link in the intermediate chain, has a pK_a of 8.5. The clinical application of dibucaine is limited to spinal and topical anesthesia. The duration of action is slightly longer than with tetracaine. The latency is greater than that of tetracaine (expected duration—3 hours). The duration may be increased up to 4 hours with the addition of 0.2 mg of epinephrine. The drug undergoes hepatic metabolism. Dibucaine is not available commercially in the United States.

Ropivacaine (Naropin®)

Ropivacaine is a new long-acting amide local anesthetic chemically related to mepivacaine and bupivacaine. These three agents differ chemically as mepivacaine has a methyl group, bupivacaine a butyl group, and ropivacaine a propyl group attached to the piperdine nitrogen atom.

The local anesthetics previously discussed are racemic mixtures—that is, they contain equal portions of R (+) and S (−) enantiomers. Ropivacaine is distinctly different as the drug is formulated from the single "S" enantiomer. The S (−) enantiomer is less cardiotoxic but

is clinically equivalent to bupivacaine in its ability to produce neural blockade. The physiochemical properties of ropivacaine are similar to those of bupivacaine; their pK_a is the same (8.1), and the plasma-protein binding is slightly lower (94%) in ropivacaine.

Clinical studies demonstrate that ropivacaine has a similar onset of action and produces a sensory block similar to that of bupivacaine when equipotent doses are administered for epidural and peripheral nerve block. The resultant motor blockade produced by ropivacaine is slower in onset, less intense, and shorter in duration than that produced by equipotent doses of bupivacaine. Increasing concentrations and increasing doses produce a greater degree of motor blockade.

The current clinical applications of ropivacaine are limited to epidural and local infiltrative anesthestic techniques. The drug is available in 0.5% (epidural anesthesia), 0.75%, and 1% concentrations (infiltrative, brachial plexus block). A formulation for spinal anesthesia is not available commercially. Studies evaluating the efficacy of ropivaciane for retrobulbar block and use in pediatric patients (younger than age 12) have not been completed.

The maximum safe clinical dose is 250 mg. Ropivacaine produces vasoconstriction when injected subcutaneously. Epidural blood flow also decreases following epidural administration. As with mepivacaine and bupivacaine, ropivacaine is metabolized by the liver, with renal excretion of the metabolites.

Local Anesthetic Mixtures (Compounding)

Clinicians have combined mixtures of local anesthetics to obtain both a rapid onset of action and a long duration of action. A popular combination for epidural administration was 2-chloroprocaine and bupivacaine. However, 2-chloroprocaine shortened the duration of action of bupivacaine, perhaps by a metabolite of 2-chloroprocaine, which inhibits membrane binding of bupivacaine (Corke, Carlson, & Dettbarn, 1984). Combining local anesthetics does not appear to offer any real clinical advantages. The use of intermittent or continuous dosing of a local anesthetic with a rapid onset of action through an anatomically placed catheter can provide a regional technique with an indefinite duration of action.

Preservatives

A variety of preservatives are added to local anesthetic solutions, including the *para*-aminobenzoic acid derivatives, methyparaben, ethylparaben, and propylparaben, or sodium bisulfite (metabisulfite) and EDTA.

The *para*-aminobenzoic acid derivatives are added to multidose vials to inhibit bacterial growth. As discussed, *para*-aminobenzoic acid derivatives are allergenic and may be the causative agents in allergic reactions following local anesthetic administration. Recall that the ester amino local anesthetics (procaine, 2-chloroprocaine, and tetracaine) are *para*-aminobenzoic acid derivatives. In contrast, allergic reactions are rare with amino amide local anesthetics. Current commercially supplied local anesthetics for spinal and epidural anesthesia are prepared as paraben-free single-dose vials.

The concerns regarding the formulation of chloroprocaine with the preservative metabisulfite was discussed. Because this preservative is neurotoxic, all local anesthetics formulated for spinal or epidural anesthesia should contain a low (0.1%) concentration of bisulfite.

Toxic Effects of Local Anesthetics

A variety of reactions may follow the administration of a local anesthetic. Allergic reactions (*para*-aminobenzoic acid derivatives), skeletal muscle irritation (sodium metabisulfite preservative in 2-chloroprocaine), methemoglobinemia (prilocaine), and addiction (cocaine) are a few of the reactions that have been discussed. However, local anesthetics have far-reaching effects on excitable membranes, producing toxic reactions that manifest clinically as alterations in the CNS and cardiovascular system function. These symptoms develop with increasing plasma concentrations of the specific drug.

The majority of local anesthetic toxic reactions involve the CNS. Initial toxicity is evident clinically as CNS excitation, as there is a selective blockade of the cerebral cortex inhibitory pathways (de Jong, Robles, & Corwin, 1969; Tanaka & Yamasaki, 1966). Subjective excitatory symptoms include lightheadedness, dizziness, tinnitus, and dyplopia. Objective excitatory symptoms include slurred speech, shivering, muscle rigidity, and tremors. Seizures develop with increasing plasma concentrations. With continued rising plasma concentrations, generalized CNS depression and respiratory arrest develop as both inhibitory and facilitatory neural pathways are depressed. Local anesthetic toxicity is enhanced (a decrease in the convulsive threshold) with elevations in P_{CO_2} and hydrogen ion concentration (decreased pH). The clinical care of a patient during regional anesthesia serves as a case illustration. The administration of intravenous sedation during a regional anesthetic may produce respiratory depression and an increase in P_{CO_2}, increasing cerebral blood flow. A decrease in the plasma protein binding of the local anesthetic will also follow, making more free drug available to the CNS. Increases in hydrogen ion concentration change the dissociation equilibrium of the local anesthetic according to the Henderson–Hasselbalch equation, with enhanced conversion of the uncharged base form to the charged cationic species, which is responsible for neural blockade. Acidosis decreases the convulsive threshold by as much as 50%. More local anesthetic is delivered to the CNS as local anesthetic plasma concentrations increase. The development of seizure activity requires attention to airway management, the delivery of supplemental oxygen to thwart the development of hypoxia, and the intravenous administration of thiopental 4 mg/kg or diazepam 0.1 mg/kg to stop seizure activity. de Jong (1970) has suggested that diazepam can be administered prophylactically to prevent the development of seizure activity, although studies do exist that challenge this suggestion. Although the administration of a neuromuscular relaxant such as succinylcholine stops the skeletal manifestations of seizures, the electrical seizure activity of the brain continues. However, neuromuscular blockade may be required to establish a patent airway and provide ventilatory support. It is not generally appreciated that all local anesthetics have anticonvulsant activity; however, the plasma concentrations responsible for these effects are considerably lower than those that elicit seizure activity.

Local anesthetics also produce biphasic effects on cardiac and peripheral vascular smooth muscles. Low concentrations produce stimulatory effects, and depressant effects develop with high plasma concentrations. These cardiovascular reactions have been of intense interest and have been studied extensively. The margin of safety from cardiovascular toxicity with local anesthetics is quite large. Blood concentrations must be ten times greater for short-acting local anesthetics and four times greater for long-acting agents than those necessary to produce toxic CNS effects. The reader must remember that excessive plasma concentrations of any local anesthetic produce depression of both the myocardium and peripheral vascular smooth muscle.

Predictable changes in myocardial function occur with rising plasma concentrations of local anesthetic. These physiologic effects include a prolongation of myocardial conduction as noted by increased P–R interval, increasing QRS duration, bradycardia, and cardiac arrest.

Vasoconstriction of peripheral vascular smooth muscle is produced at low plasma concentrations and progresses to vasodilation with increasing concentrations. The predominant effect depends on the particular vascular bed and the underlying vascular tone. For example, the intra-arterial administration of mepivacaine to human volunteers produces a decrease in forearm blood flow; however, with increasing concentrations, peripheral vascular resistance falls. As discussed, the only local anesthetic that exclusively produces vasoconstriction is cocaine. Accordingly, the toxic peripheral vascular effect is widespread peripheral vasoconstriction with resultant hypertension.

Myocardial depression and cardiovascular collapse originating from peripheral vasodilation follow high plasma concentrations of all other local anesthetics (Reiz & Nath, 1986). In contrast to the peripheral vasculature, the pulmonary vasculature vasoconstricts in response to high concentrations of most local anesthetics.

► CASE STUDY

A 55-year-old auto mechanic was brought to the hospital for emergency repair of lacerated tendons and nerves in his left hand caused by a crush injury at work. He was given morphine 10 mg IM on admission. He had no significant medical history but was taking verapamil daily for migraine prevention. His last meal was 2 hours before the injury. He denied any use of tobacco or recreational drugs. He drinks approximately one to three beers per week. He weighed approximately 70 kg. Following the preoperative evaluation, the patient consented to a brachial plexus block. He was premedicated with 2 mg of midazolam and 100 μg of fentanyl prior to initiation of the regional anesthetic. The anticipated length of the surgery is 3 to 4 hours.

1. What local anesthetics might be considered for this brachial plexus block?

   One percent mepivacaine with epinephrine or 1% prilocaine or a mixture of mepivacaine and tetracaine with epinephrine should provide anesthesia for 3 to 4 hours. Bupivacaine 0.25% to 0.5% would provide excellent blockade, which may range from 6 to 24 hours. Bupivacaine 0.5% provides superior motor blockade. Use of bupivacaine would provide analgesia into the postoperative period. Tetracaine 0.15% to 0.2% with epinephrine can provide regional anesthesia for approximately 5 to 6 hours.

2. What is the maximum safe dose of the local anesthetic if either tetracaine or bupivacaine is selected?

   The maximum safe dose of tetracaine without epinephrine would be approximately 100 mg and with epinephrine would be 150 mg to 200 mg. The maximum safe dose of bupivacaine is 175 mg. If epinephrine is employed, the maximum safe dose is approximately 250 mg or 3 mg/kg.

3. Local anesthetic toxicity may manifest itself in cardiovascular or CNS symptoms. What symptoms should alert the anesthetist to the potential development of this toxic side effect, and what concurrent conditions may facilitate the development of local anesthetic toxicity?

   Toxic symptoms develop with increasing plasma concentrations of the local anesthetic. The majority of local anesthetic toxic reactions involve the CNS. Subjective excitatory symptoms include lightheadedness, dizziness, tinnitus, and dyplopia. Objective excitatory symptoms include slurred speech, shivering, muscle rigidity, and tremors. Seizures develop with increasing plasma concentrations. A continued rise in plasma concentrations produces generalized CNS depression and respiratory arrest from depression of both inhibitory and facilitatory neural pathways. Local anesthetic toxicity is enhanced with elevations in P_{CO_2} and a decreased pH. Intravenous sedation during a regional anesthetic may produce respiratory depression and increase P_{CO_2}, thereby increasing cerebral blood flow. Decreased plasma protein binding of the local anesthetic then occurs and more free drug is available to the CNS. Increases in hydrogen ion concentration change the dissociation of equilibrium of the local anesthetic according to the Henderson–Hasselbach equation and enhance the conversion of the uncharged base form to the charged cation responsible for neural blockade. Acidosis increases the convulsive threshold by as much as 50%.

   Local anesthetics also produce biphasic effects on cardiac and peripheral vascular smooth muscle. At low concentrations, stimulatory effects are produced, and depressant effects develop with high plasma concentrations, which depress both the myocardium and peripheral vascular smooth muscle. The margin of safety from cardiovascular toxicity with local anesthetics is wide. The blood concentration of short-acting local anesthetics must be ten times greater and long-acting agents four times greater than those necessary to produce toxic CNS effects.

► SUMMARY

The majority of clinically applied local anesthetics can be classified according to their chemical structure as amino esters or amino amides. The pharmacologic properties of local anesthetics are important to determine the potential toxicity, onset and duration of action, and the degree of neural blockade of motor and sensory fibers. The anesthetist should appreciate the pharmacology and toxicity of each local anesthetic to make informed choices for each specific clinical situation.

ACKNOWLEDGMENT

The author acknowledges Michael D. Stanton-Hicks for his original contribution to this chapter.

► KEY CONCEPTS

- Local anesthetics act by binding to a protein receptor in the sodium channel, preventing depolarization.
- Physiochemical properties, such as water solubility, lipid solubility, ionization at physiologic pH, and protein binding, determine the degree of interaction with the nerve cell membrane.
- The administration of increasing concentrations of local anesthetic decreases the latency (shortens the onset) and produces a denser and longer-lasting block.
- Epinephrine is added to local anesthetics to decrease the vascular absorption from the deposited site of action and improves the density of the block as well as the duration of action.
- Local anesthetics produce dose-dependent depression of the CNS and the cardiovascular system, eliciting initial toxicity symptoms of lightheadedness, dizziness, vertigo, tinnitus, and visual disturbances.
- Amino ester local anesthetics are metabolized by pseudocholinesterase, whereas amino amide local anesthetics are metabolized by the liver.
- Bupivacaine has the highest protein binding and is the most cardiotoxic of all local anesthetics.

► STUDY QUESTIONS

1. What physiologic property is responsible for the potential difference or voltage across the cell membrane?

2. Name the physiochemical properties that determine the degree of local anesthetic interaction with the nerve cell membrane.

3. What clinical effect results from the addition of sodium bicarbonate to a local anesthetic?

4. Why is epinephrine added to local anesthetics?

5. What is the specific mechanism for the metabolism of amino ester local anesthetics?

6. Which local anesthetic has been identified as etiologic in the development of cauda equina syndrome?

7. Which local anesthetic has the highest degree of protein binding and cardiotoxicity?

KEY REFERENCES

Blair, M. R. (1975). Cardiovascular pharmacology of local anesthetics. *British Journal of Anaesthesia, 47,* (Suppl.), 247–252.

Courtney, K. R. (1980). Structure–activity relations for frequency-dependent sodium channel block in nerve by local anesthetics. *Journal of Pharmacology and Experimental Therapeutics, 213,* 114–119.

Covino, B. G. & Strichartz, G. R. (1993). Local anesthetics. In S. A. Feldman, W. Paton, & C. Scurr (Eds.), *Mechanisms of drugs in anesthesia* (2nd ed., p. 322). London: Hodder & Stroughton Publishers.

de Jong, R. H. (Ed.)(1970). *Physiology and pharmacology of local anesthesia* (p. 32). Springfield, IL: Charles C Thomas.

de Jong, R. H. (1981). The chloroprocaine controversy. *American Journal of Obstetrics & Gynecology, 140,* 237–239.

Halstead, W. S. (1885). Practical comments on the use and abuse of cocaine; suggested by its invariable successful employment in more than a thousand minor surgical operations. *New York Medical Journal, 42,* 292–295.

Lambert, D. H. & Hurley, R. J. (1991). Cauda equina syndrome and continuous spinal anesthesia. *Anesthesia & Analgesia, 72,* 817–819.

Reiz, S. & Nath, S. (1986). Cardiotoxicity of local anesthetic agents. *British Journal of Anaesthesia, 56,* 736–746.

Wood, M. (1990). Local anesthetic agents. In M. Wood & A. J. J. Wood (Eds.), *Drugs in anesthesia: Pharmacology for anesthesiologists* (2nd ed., p. 324). Baltimore: Williams & Wilkins.

REFERENCES

Albright, G. A. (1979). Cardiac arrest following regional anesthesia with etidocaine or bupivacaine. *Anesthesiology, 51,* 285–287.

Benson, J. S. (1992, May). *FDA Safety Alert: Cauda Equina Syndrome Associated with the Use of Small-Bore Catheters in Continuous Spinal Anesthesia.* Rockville, MD: Food and Drug Administration.

Bernards, C. M. & Hill, H. F. (1991). The spinal root sleeve is not preferred route of redistribution of drugs from the epidural space to the spinal cord. *Anesthesiology, 75,* 827–832.

Blair, M. R. (1975). Cardiovascular pharmacology of local anesthetics. *British Journal of Anaesthesia, 47* (suppl), 247–252.

Bonica, J. J., Akamatsu, T. J., Berges, P. U., Morikawa, K., & Kennedy, W. F., Jr. (1971). Circulatory effects of peridural block. II. Effects of epinephrine. *Anesthesiology, 34,* 514–522.

Braun, H. (1903). Ueber den Einfluss der Vitalität der Gewebe auf die Örtlichen und Allgemeinen Giftwirkungen Localkanäthesirender Mittel und über die Bedeutung des Adenalins für die Localanästhesis. *Archiv für Klinische Chirurgie, XIX,* 541–591.

Bromage, P. R. (1965). A comparison of the hydrochloride salts of lignocaine and prilocaine for epidural analgesia. *British Journal of Anaesthesia, 37,* 753–761.

Bromage, P. R., Burfoot, M. F., Crowell, D. E., & Truant, A. P. (1967). Quality of epidural blockade. 3. Carbonated local anaesthetic solutions. *British Journal of Anaesthesia, 39,* 197–209.

Buckley, F. P., Littlewood, D. G., Covino, B. G., & Scott, D. B. (1978). Effects of adrenaline and the concentration of solution on extradural block with etidocaine. *British Journal of Anaesthesia, 50,* 171–175.

Burke, W., Jr. (1884). Hydrochlorate of cocaine in minor surgery. *New York Medical Journal, 40,* 616–617.

Concepcion, M., Maddi, R., Francis, D., Rocco, A. G., Murray, E., & Covino, B. G. (1984). Vasoconstrictors in spinal anesthesia with tetracaine—A comparison of epinephrine and phenylephrine. *Anesthesia & Analgesia, 63,* 134–138.

Corke, B. C., Carlson, C. G., & Dettbarn, W. D. (1984). The influence of 2-chloroprocaine on the subsequent analgesic potency of bupivacaine. *Anesthesiology, 60,* 25–27.

Courtney, K. R. (1980). Structure–activity relations for frequency-dependent sodium channel block in nerve by local anesthetics. *Journal of Pharmacology and Experimental Therapeutics, 213,* 114–119.

Courtney, K. R., Kendig, J. J., & Cohen, E. N. (1978). Frequency-dependent conduction block: The role of nerve impulse pattern in local anesthetic potency. *Anesthesiology, 48,* 111–117.

Covino, B. G. & Strichartz, G. R. (1993). Local anesthetics. In S. A. Feldman, W. Paton, & C. Scurr (Eds.), *Mechanisms of drugs in anesthesia* (2nd ed., p. 322). London: Hodder & Stroughton Publishers.

de Jong, R. H. (Ed.). (1970). *Physiology and pharmacology of local anesthesia* (p. 32). Springfield, IL: Charles C Thomas.

de Jong, R. H. (1981). The chloroprocaine controversy. *American Journal of Obstetrics & Gynecology, 140,* 237–239.

de Jong, R. H., Robles, R. A., & Corwin, R. W. (1969). Central actions of lidocaine–synaptic transmission. *Anesthesiology 30,* 19–23.

Faulconer, A. & Keys, T. E. (Eds.). (1993). Conduction anesthesia. In *Foundations of anesthesiology* (p. 769). Park Ridge, IL: Wood Library—Museum of Anesthesiology.

Fibuch, E. E. & Opper, S. E. (1989). Back pain following epidurally administered Nesacaine-MPF. *Anesthesia & Analgesia 69,* 113–115.

Gissen, A. J., Covino, B. G., & Gregus, J. (1980). Differential sensitivity of mammalian nerve fibers to local anesthetic agents. *Anesthesiology, 53,* 467–474.

Gissen, A. J., Datta, S., & Lambert, D. (1984). The chloroprocaine controversy. II. Is chloroprocaine neurotoxic? *Regional Anesthesia, 9,* 134–135.

Gramling, Z. W., Ellis, R. G., & Volpitto, P. P. (1964). Clinical experience with mepivacaine (Carbocaine). *Journal of the Medical Association of Georgia, 53,* 16–18.

Guyton, A. C. & Hall, J. E. (Eds.). (1996). Organization of the nervous system: Basic functions of synapses and transmitter substances. In *Textbook of medical physiology* (9th ed., pp. 575–581). Philadelphia: W. B. Saunders.

Halstead, W. S. (1885). Practical comments on the use and abuse of cocaine; suggested by its invariable successful employment in more than a thousand minor surgical operations. *New York Medical Journal, 42,* 292–295.

Kier, L. (1974). Continuous epidural analgesia in prostatectomy: Comparison of bupivacaine with and without adrenaline. *Acta Anaesthesiologica Scandinavica, 18,* 1–4.

Lambert, D. H. & Hurley, R. J. (1991). Cauda equina syndrome and continuous spinal anesthesia. *Anesthesia & Analgesia, 72,* 817–819.

Marx, G. F. (1984). Cardiotoxicity of local anesthetics—The plot thickens. *Anesthesiology, 60,* 3–5.

Raymond, S. A., & Strichartz, G. R. (1990). Further comments on the failure of impulse propagation in nerves marginally blocked by local anesthetic. (Letter to the Editor.) *Anesthesia & Analgesia, 70,* 121–122.

Ready, L. B., Plumer, M. H., Haschke, R. H., Austin, E., & Sumi, S. M. (1985). Neurotoxicity of intrathecal local anesthetics in rabbits. *Anesthesiology, 63,* 364–370.

Reiz, S. & Nath, S. (1986). Cardiotoxicity of local anesthetic agents. *British Journal of Anaesthesia, 56,* 736–746.

Rigler, M. L., & Drasner, K. (1991). Distribution of catheter-injected local anesthetic in a model of the subarachnoid space. *Anesthesiology, 75,* 684–692.

Rigler, M. L., Drasner, K., Krejcie, T. C., Yelich, S. T., Scholnick, F. T., DeFontes, J., & Bohner, D. (1991). Cauda equina syndrome after continuous spinal anesthesia. *Anesthesia & Analgesia, 72,* 275–281.

Ritchie, J. M., Ritchie, B., & Greengard, P. (1965a). The active structure of local anesthetics. *Journal of Pharmacology and Experimental Therapeutics, 150,* 152–159.

Ritchie, J. M., Ritchie, B., & Greengard, P. (1965b). The effect of the nerve sheath on the action of local anesthetics. *Journal of Pharmacology and Experimental Therapeutics, 150,* 160–164.

Stevens, R. A., Urmey, W. F., Urquhart, B. L., & Kao, T. C. (1993). Back pain after epidural anesthesia with chloroprocaine. *Anesthesiology, 78,* 492–497.

Tanaka, K. & Yamasaki, M. (1966). Blocking of cortical inhibitory synapses by intravenous lidocaine. *Nature, 209,* 207–208.

Wood, M. (1990). Local anesthetic agents. In M. Wood & A. J. J. Wood (Eds.), *Drugs in anesthesia: pharmacology for anesthesiologists,* (2nd ed., p. 324). Baltimore: Williams & Wilkins.

Pharmacology of Neuromuscular Blockade and Antagonism

Gary D. Zarr

The history of muscle relaxants can be divided into two phases: the early investigational research and the initial medical and anesthetic uses of muscle relaxants. The group of drugs referred to as muscle relaxants have the pharmacologic action of blocking neuromuscular transmission, resulting in muscle paralysis. The muscle relaxants discussed in this chapter have no central muscle relaxant capabilities, such as does diazepam. Skeletal muscle relaxants have no sedative, analgesic, or amnestic properties; their primary contribution to the anesthetic process is to provide a quiet relaxed surgical field. The early history of muscle relaxants is actually a discussion of the history of curare, the first muscle relaxant to be studied. The use of curare as arrow poison by various South American Indian tribes is well known. Work by Brody in 1811 demonstrated that death in curare-treated animals could be prevented with artificial ventilation. Additional investigation by Claude Bernard demonstrated that the site of action of curare was the neuromuscular junction. His work showed that a muscle paralyzed by curare could still contract if stimulated directly. The absence of the equipment and expertise necessary to perform oral endotracheal intubation delayed the safe introduction of curare into clinical use. Initial clinical uses by Chisholm in the American Civil War in 1862 and Lawen in 1912 were attempts to reduce the dose of ether necessary to produce muscle relaxation. Because a spontaneous ventilatory pattern was an essential component of

the open-drop ether technique, these early trials were regarded as unsatisfactory.

The successful clinical use of muscle relaxants is noted in the use of curare to control skeletal muscle spasms in patients with tetanus (West, 1932). Curare was also used as an adjunct in electroconvulsive therapy (Bennett, 1940). The first use of curare in modern clinical anesthesia was reported in 1942 (Griffith & Johnson, 1942). Reports of higher complication rates in surgical patients who received muscle relaxants caused many anesthetists to avoid the use of muscle relaxants (Beecher & Todd, 1940). As the halogenated anesthetics were introduced into clinical practice, it became apparent that the use of a muscle relaxant would be necessary to achieve adequate relaxation for intraabdominal procedures if potentially toxic concentrations of these agents was to be avoided. With increased clinical experience and the use of anticholinesterase–antimuscarinic combinations to reverse residual muscle relaxation, the incidence of postoperative respiratory complications decreased. The transition from diethyl ether to halogenated anesthetics to opiate and nitrous oxide anesthesia resulted in the continued and increasing use of muscle relaxants in clinical practice.

Neuromuscular blockade monitoring was introduced into clinical practice in the latter part of the 1960s and the early portion of the 1970s (Gissen & Katz, 1969) and has resulted in better titration of muscle relaxant to maintain the desired levels of muscle relaxation. In addition, neuromuscular blockade monitoring can aid in deciding when the muscle relaxant is ready to be reversed, completely reversed, or if reversal is required at all.

The research efforts to develop nondepolarizing muscle relaxants with intermediate duration of action, such as rocuronium and *cis*-atracurium, have helped to improve patient safety when muscle relaxants are used as adjuncts to anesthesia. These agents have fewer complications and a shorter duration of action, giving the clinician better control over the depth and duration of muscle relaxation, which is useful in reducing the amount of anticholinesterase drug necessary for reversal and the potential for recurization to occur in the postoperative phase. Because of the introduction of a long-acting nondepolarizing neuromuscular blocking agent such as pipecuronium and doxacurium, along with the intermediate-acting drugs such as rocuronium, vecuronium, and *cis*–atracurium, it would appear that the remaining challenge to improve patient safety related to muscle relaxant drugs would be the introduction of a nondepolarizing agent with a rapid onset and short duration of action, such as that associated with succinylcholine. Introduction of this type of rapid-onset, short-acting, nondepolarizing agent would provide the anesthetist with a selection of muscle relaxants that have minimal side effects and a wide spectrum of duration of action from which to choose.

▶ NEUROMUSCULAR FUNCTION AND CONDUCTION

Physiology of Nerve Conduction

The transduction of an electrical impulse from a nerve to a chemical impulse that stimulates the end-plate of a muscle fiber and produces muscular contraction at the neuromuscular junction. Upper motor neurons that have their origin in the cerebral motor cortex synapse with group A, fast-conducting, somatic, efferent, lower motor neurons that have their cell bodies originating in the gray matter of the anterior horns of the spinal cord. Collections of these lower motor neurons form the efferent spinal motor nerves. When a motor nerve approaches a muscle, it loses its myelin sheath and branches to multiple nerve fibers. A single nerve fiber and the muscle fibers that it supplies constitute a functional motor unit. Muscle function determines how many muscle fibers are supplied by a single nerve fiber. Muscles that perform fine movements are supplied by nerve fibers that supply relatively few muscle fibers, whereas muscles that are responsible for course-sustained contraction are supplied by nerve fibers that supply many muscle fibers. This variability in the size of motor units and the potential for re-

cruitment of additional motor units allows for a high degree of control over the precision and strength of motor movement. The space between the nerve fiber and the muscle fiber it supplies constitutes the neuromuscular junction. The prejunctional nerve fiber axonal ending contains mitochondria, endoplasmic reticulum, and synaptic vesicles, all of which are necessary for the synthesis and storage of the neurotransmitter acetylcholine (ACh). The postjunctional surface is separated from the prejunctional surface by a synaptic cleft 20 to 30 nm wide and is continuous with the extracellular fluid space (Drachman, 1978). The postjunctional surface, or the motor end-plate, is a highly specialized region that is invaginated to increase the surface area of the synapse. Nicotinic cholinergic receptors, the receptors for the neurotransmitter ACh, are located on both the presynaptic axonal terminal and postsynaptic end-plate surface. Acetylcholinesterase (true or tissue cholinesterase), the enzyme necessary to hydrolyze ACh and allow for end-plate repolarization, is located in the synaptic cleft.

The resting membrane potential of both large nerve and skeletal muscle fibers is about -90 mV, and the reference area inside the cell is 90 mV more negative than the extracellular fluid space outside the cell. This negative resting membrane potential is maintained by a combination of selective membrane permeability to sodium and potassium ions and an energy-dependent electrogenic sodium potassium pump. In the resting state, the membrane is much more permeable to potassium than it is to sodium; in fact, the resting membrane potential is closest to the Nernst potential for potassium, which is -94 mV. By using the Goldman equation and the diffusion potentials for sodium and potassium, -86 mV would be the predicted resting membrane potential. The energy-dependent sodium potassium electrogenic pump, which pumps more sodium out of the cell than it pumps potassium into the cell, contributes an additional -4 mV to the resting potential. Electrophysiologic measurements have confirmed the calculated resting membrane potential in large nerve and muscle fiber cells (Guyton, 1996).

When a nerve is stimulated, the resting membrane potential of -90 mV becomes less negative because of the opening ion channels that allow sodium to enter the nerve. If the membrane potential is reduced to about -65 mV, the threshold potential for an action potential will be reached. When the threshold potential is reached, voltage-sensitive ion channels open and allow sodium to rush into the nerve, causing propagation of an action potential along the course of the nerve. As the wave of depolarization moves along the nerve, a wave of repolarization follows. The depolarization that is due to sodium entry into the nerve causes the membrane potential to approach 0 mV, which triggers the opening of voltage-sensitive ion channels and the movement of potassium ions out of the neuron, causing repolarization to −90 mV. Ultimately the restoration of potassium ion concentration inside the nerve and sodium outside the nerve is due to electrogenic sodium–potassium adenosine-triphosphate (ATP)–dependent pump. When the action potential wave of depolarization reaches the nerve fiber axonal terminal, it causes voltage-sensitive calcium channels to open and calcium rushes into the axonal ending. The entry of calcium into the axonal terminal is essential for the exocytotic release of ACh and low calcium levels, or high magnesium levels will inhibit the release of ACh (Hubbard, Jones, & Landau, 1968; Katz, 1966). The released ACh diffuses across the synaptic cleft and binds to the two alpha subunits of the postsynaptic nicotinic cholinergic receptor as well as the presynaptic cholinergic receptors (Taylor, 1985). The postsynaptic nicotinic cholinergic ACh receptor is composed of five protein subunits that form an ion pore that opens when the two 40 000-dalton alpha-subunits bind the neurotransmitter ACh (Fig. 21–1) (Guy, 1984). For the ion pore of the ACh receptor to open each of the alpha-subunits must bind with a molecule of ACh. Binding of a single antagonist molecule or a molecule of alpha-toxin from venoms of the krait or cobra snake to either one of the alpha-subunits prevents ion channel opening (Taylor, Brown, & Johnson, 1983). The ACh-induced opening of this channel enables the movement of sodium into the end-plate region, the depolarization of the region, and the generation of an end-plate potential (EPP). An EPP is unlike a nerve action potential, which is governed by the all-or-none phenomenon. In a nerve, if threshold is reached, an action potential is propagated. The EPPs due to ACh activation of multiple receptors can be summated to produce an end-plate voltage change from −90 mV to about −50 mV, which then results in a propagated action potential in the muscle fiber. As the action potential spreads throughout the muscle, it results in the release of calcium from the sarcoplasmic reticulum and a rise in the free calcium concentration within the muscle fiber. It is believed that the rise in calcium within the muscle fiber results in troponin–tropomyosin interaction with actin, which then allows the active sites on actin to interact with myosin and slide together, producing muscle contraction. Muscle contraction is terminated when calcium is pumped back into the sarcoplasmic reticulum of the muscle fiber, where it is stored until another action potential causes it to be released.

The sustained depolarization of the end-plate region is prevented by the action of the enzyme acetylcholinesterase (AChE), which rapidly hydrolyzes ACh to acetate and choline. As AChE rapidly lowers the concentration of ACh present at the receptor, the equilibrium of binding of ACh to the nicotinic receptor alpha-subunits reverses. The removal of ACh from the nicotinic receptor allows the channel pore to close and the end-plate region to repolarize. The process of diffusion of ACh away from the synaptic region may play a role in terminating its effect as well. However, the fact that the end-plate region is repolarized over a time course of milliseconds would seem to indicate that the rapid action of AChE is the primary mechanism for the termination of the effects of ACh at the synapse.

Acetylcholine Synthesis, Storage, and Release

Synthesis of ACh, a quaternary ammonium ester, takes place within cholinergic nerve terminals. Acetylcholine is synthesized from acetylcoenzyme A derived from glucose metabolism and choline. Choline is present in the extracellular fluid surrounding the nerve terminal. The supply of choline is derived from dietary intake as well as from the enzymatic breakdown of ACh. It has been estimated that as much as 50% of the choline used in the synthesis of ACh is derived from this transmitter's breakdown (Plotter, 1970). Uptake of choline into cholinergic nerve terminals is an active process. It is of pharmacologic interest that hemicholinium can block the uptake of choline and block nerve transmission (Elmqvist & Quastel, 1965). However, the nonspecific blockage of choline uptake in all cholinergic nerves demonstrates the lack of any clinical use for hemicholinium.

In the nerve terminal, choline is combined with the acetyl group from the acetylcoenzyme A under the influence of choline-O-acetyltransferase to yield ACh and free coenzyme A (Fig. 21–2). After ACh is synthesized in the nerve terminal cytosol, it is stored in vesicles. Estimates of the number of ACh molecules in each vesicle range from 1000 to 10 000, a phenomenon known as the *quantal content of each vesicle* (Del Castillo & Katz, 1954). Under physiologic conditions the production of ACh is able to keep pace with release due to action potentials generated in motor nerves. However, if a motor nerve is stimulated with a tetanic impulse of 200 Hz × 5 seconds, the rate of ACh release is diminished (Riker, 1975). This fact would explain why newer clinical blockade monitors have a limitation of 50 Hz to 100 Hz for tetanic stimulation.

When an action potential in a nerve reaches the nerve terminal, it is proposed that adenylate cyclase is activated and causes the conversion of ATP to cyclic AMP, allowing calcium channels to open and calcium to enter the nerve terminal. Entry of calcium into the nerve terminal facilitates the fusion of ACh-containing vesicles with the nerve terminal membrane, resulting in the exocytotic release of ACh into the synaptic cleft (Fig. 21–3) (Standaert & Dretchen, 1981). The number of vesicles or quanta released into the synaptic cleft by a single nerve terminal has been estimated to be 200 to 400 (Hubbard

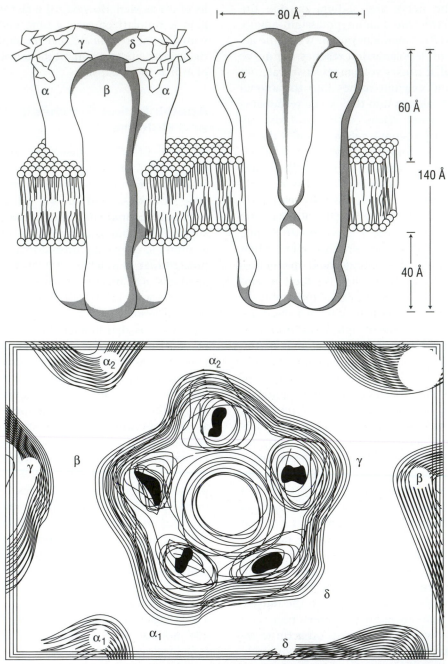

Figure 21–1. Molecular structure of the nicotinic cholinergic receptor. The structure of the nicotinic ACh receptor is described in the text. The top of the figure shows a side view of the receptor. The five subunits are arranged to form an ion channel that extends through the lipid bilayer of the cell membrane. The two alpha-subunits are the binding site for the neurotransmitter ACh or neuromuscular blocking drugs and toxins. The bottom portion of the figure shows a cross-sectional view of an electron density map of the receptor. The five subunits are visible and the mouth of the ion channel can be seen at the center of the subunits. Electron densities of portions of other receptors can be seen as well.

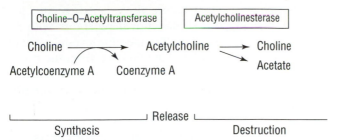

Figure 21–2. Enzymatic synthesis of ACh in the nerve terminal and degradation of ACh at the synaptic cleft.

& Wilson, 1973). The importance of cyclic AMP generation and of calcium entry into the nerve terminal to allow ACh release has been demonstrated by numerous experimental and clinical observations. Aminophylline has been shown to facilitate the formation of cyclic AMP and to promote neuromuscular transmission. Calcium channel-blocking drugs such as verapamil and aminoglycoside antibiotics inhibit calcium entry, which inhibits neurotransmitter release and decreases neuromuscular transmission. Botulinum toxin and tetanus toxin alter calcium entry into the neuron terminal and inhibit ACh re-

lease. Magnesium, a divalent cation, can enter the nerve terminal and replace or decrease the amount of calcium that enters, thereby reducing the release of ACh. Magnesium therapy, such as may be used in obstetrics for preeclamptic and eclamptic patients, has been shown to cause muscular weakness in high doses. In addition, magnesium therapy in obstetric patients has been demonstrated to potentiate both depolarizing and nondepolarizing muscle relaxants (Ghoneim & Long, 1970).

Neuromuscular Margin of Safety

It should be apparent to the reader that under normal conditions the safety margin to maintain neuromuscular function is high. A single action potential at a nerve terminal results in the release of hundreds of vesicles, each with a quantal content of thousands of molecules of ACh capable of binding with an excessive quantity of postsynaptic nicotinic cholinergic receptors to ensure the generation of an EPP and muscular contraction. It has been demonstrated that a 0.1-Hz supramaximal stimulus causes a stable twitch response over a long period of time. For the twitch height response to a 0.1-Hz stimulus to begin to decrease, it has been estimated that 75% of

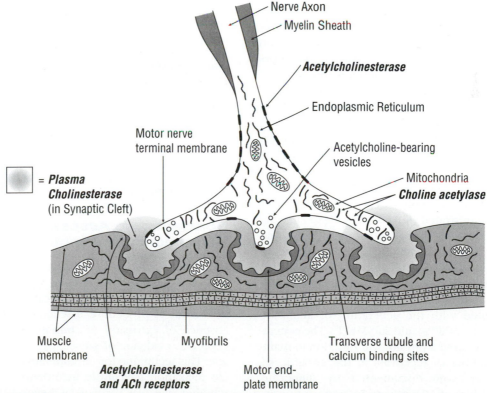

Figure 21–3. Motor nerve terminal and the specialized surface of the muscle that constitutes the neuromuscular junction. Vesicles of ACh can be seen in the motor nerve terminal and are released to bind with ACh receptors located at the top of the folds of the postsynaptic surface of the end-plate region of the muscle. *(From Ali, H. H. & Savarese, J. J. [1976]. Monitoring of neuromuscular function. Anesthesiology, 45, 216–249. Reprinted with permission.)*

the postsynaptic receptors need to be blocked by a non-depolarizing neuromuscular blocking agent before any reduction in motor response occurs (Ali & Savarese, 1976). Fade with train-of-four (TOF) stimulation occurs when 70% to 75% of receptors are blocked (Waud & Waud, 1972). In addition, fade with tetanic stimulation at 100 Hz occurs when 50% of the receptors are blocked at the synapse (Waud & Waud, 1971). The implications of these observations have significant clinical importance. The fact is that a patient may have normal neuromuscular function documented by blockade monitoring and motor responses such as sustained head lift for 5 seconds or longer and still have a large number of nicotinc cholinergic receptors blocked, reducing their margin of safety for neuromuscular transmission. The inability to evaluate residual receptor blockade totally by a competitive nondepolarizing agent would make it a reasonable practice to use an appropriate reversal agent if there is any question of neuromuscular function. The anesthetist's decision regarding the presence of adequate paralysis or the need for reversal of paralysis from neuromuscular blocking agents is probably based on the evaluation of as little as 25% to 50% of the postsynaptic receptors in skeletal muscle, depending on the type of blockade-monitoring criteria used. The remaining 50% to 75% of the receptors is similar to an iceberg in that the largest part cannot be seen. In patients receiving neuromuscular blocking agents, loss of muscle strength is not noted until 75% of available receptors are occupied by muscle relaxant, and normal function returns when 25% of available receptors are available to interact with ACh. Therefore, the status of up to 50% to 75% of postsynaptic receptors at the neuromuscular junction is essentially unknown early in the postanesthesia recovery phase.

Although much of ACh is stored in vesicles, the action potential–dependent all-or-none discharge of ACh vesicle contents to the synaptic cleft does not allow for other forms of storage and release of ACh. Evidence for nonvesicle, nonaction potential–dependent release of ACh has been demonstrated (Katz & Miledi, 1977). In addition, vesicle release of quantal amounts of ACh that are not calcium dependent has been shown to occur (Thesleff & Molgo, 1983). These alternate forms of ACh storage and release do not generate sufficient EPPs to produce muscle contraction. These alternate forms of release are associated with the generation of miniature end-plate potentials (MEPPs) and sub-MEPPs. The generation of MEPPs may serve a physiologic function to maintain a normal number of receptors in the synaptic region. It has been well documented by numerous experiments that loss of ACh release by denervation injuries or disease states results in an extrajunctional overgrowth of nicotinic cholinergic receptors (Carter & Sokoll, 1981). When denervated muscle is exposed to a nicotinic cholinergic agonist or a depolarizing muscle re-

laxant such as succinylcholine, there is exaggerated ion channel opening of extrajunctional receptors with resulting hyperkalemia. Tonic leakage of nonvesicle ACh or isolated vesicle quantal amounts of ACh from the presynaptic nerve terminal may play a role in maintaining normal densities and the type of cholinergic receptors present in the synaptic region.

Presynaptic Effects of Acetylcholine

Postsynaptic effects of released ACh binding to the nicotinic cholinergic receptor in the end-plate region of the muscle has been well understood for some time. The possibility that ACh released from the motor nerve terminal could have presynaptic effects that would result in a positive feedback mechanism to increase mobilization and release of ACh has been recognized more recently. Evidence for this presynaptic action of ACh at presynaptic nicotinic cholinergic receptors has been supported by experimental data using cholinergic agonists and depolarizing muscle relaxants as well as nondepolarizing muscle relaxants. Depolarizing muscle relaxants have been shown to increase the mobilization of ACh in motor nerve terminals, a fact that may further explain the reason for fasciculations commonly seen after depolarizing muscle relaxant administration. The fade seen with tetanic and TOF nerve stimulation after administration of a nondepolarizing muscle relaxant is thought to be associated with decreased mobilization of ACh in the nerve terminal due to presynaptic receptor blockade (Bowman, Marshall, & Gibb, 1984). The nondepolarizing muscle relaxant competitively blocking the presynaptic ACh receptor prevents the binding of ACh and the activation of the positive feedback loop to maintain adequate mobilization of ACh for release.

▶ MONITORING NEUROMUSCULAR FUNCTION

Nonelectronic Assessment of Neuromuscular Function

Early intraoperative assessment of satisfactory neuromuscular blockade required a visual evaluation of reduced muscle tone. If the surgical procedure was an intraabdominal procedure, a relaxed abdominal wall and absence of extrusion of abdominal contents were accepted as evidence of satisfactory neuromuscular blockade. This technique for intraoperative assessment of muscle relaxation gave little quantitative knowledge as to whether one was near or far beyond the ideal level of neuromuscular blockade. Evaluation of adequate reversal of neuromuscular blockade relied on clinical assessment of the ability to sustain head lift, adequate vital capacity, negative inspiratory force, handgrasp, or the capability to keep the arms in an extended position. These valuable criteria for adequate reversal of neuromuscular blockade are still used today. However, these reversal criteria are unreliable in the presence of postoperative pain, or if the patient is uncooperative, or is still under the influence of sedatives or narcotics. Poor performance on clinical evaluations that require voluntary skeletal muscle movement may be due to several causes not associated with residual muscle paralysis secondary to neuromuscular blocking agents.

Electronic Assessment of Neuromuscular Function

The need for a reliable mechanism to evaluate residual muscle paralysis that did not require a cooperative patient led to the use of an electrical impulse to stimulate an action potential in a motor nerve and to the measurement of the evoked response of the muscle supplied by the nerve (Gissen & Katz, 1969). Early quantitative evaluation of neuromuscular blockade with electrical stimulation of motor nerves used three types of electronic stimulation. Single twitch or single stimulus at intervals of 0.1 Hz to 1.0 Hz (1 stimulus/10 seconds to 1 stimulus/second, respectively), tetanic stimulation at a frequency of 30 Hz to 200 Hz (30–200 stimuli/second), and posttetanic potentiation. The single twitch at a frequency of 0.1 Hz was discovered to be of the greatest clinical relevance (Ali & Savarese, 1980). However, there are problems with the use of single-twitch stimuli, even at 0.1 Hz. For single-twitch stimuli to be of value, a control height prior to the administration of a neuromuscular blocking agent must be established to estimate the percentage of reduction in control height after the neuromuscular blocking agent is given. In addition, it has been demonstrated that, when muscle response to single-twitch stimuli and sustained contraction in response to 50-Hz tetanic stimuli have returned to control height, there may be a significant fade to the fourth stimulus of the more sensitive TOF test (Lebowitz, Ramsey, Savarese, & Ali, 1980). In current routine clinical practice, single-twitch stimuli are useful for monitoring the degree of neuromuscular blockade during succinylcholine drip administration.

The appropriate stimulus setting to be used for tetanic stimulation of a nerve during blockade monitoring has varied between authors over time. Gissen and Katz in 1969 recommended the use of high-frequency tetanic stimulation at 100 Hz to 200 Hz to test for fade in muscle contraction that would be associated with residual nondepolarizing blockade. In 1975, Riker demonstrated that high-frequency tetanic stimulation at 200 Hz for 5 seconds or longer could produce fade in normal muscle in the absence of neuromuscular blocking agents. In 1954, Merton showed that the maximal voluntary muscle contraction was equal to the contraction response to tetanus at 50 Hz. In view of these findings, tetanic stimulation for 5 seconds at 50 Hz seems to be the most relevant physiologic and clinically useful frequency to use. Sustained response to tetanic stimulation has been used as partial evidence for absence of neuromuscular blockade. However, as mentioned earlier, in spite of sustained tetanic contraction without fade, significant fade to the fourth stimulus in the more sensitive TOF test has been demonstrated. Monitoring tetanic stimulation has been useful during continuous infusion of succinylcholine. After establishing a baseline response to 50-Hz tetanic stimulation, repeat evaluation of the tetanic response should show a dose-dependent suppression of tetanic contraction without fade. The appearance of fade to tetanic contraction during succinylcholine administration is accepted as evidence of conversion from a phase I block to a phase II block. In addition, tetanic stimulation can be used to differentiate between depolarizing and nondepolarizing neuromuscular blockade, the latter being associated with fade in the tetanic contraction. Evaluation of neuromuscular blockade with tetanic stimulation is not well accepted by conscious patients because it is painful.

Posttetanic twitch stimulation involves the administration of a single-twitch stimulus 5 to 10 seconds after a tetanic stimulus at the same intensity as for single-twitch stimuli prior to the tetanic stimulation. In the presence of a nondepolarizing neuromuscular block or residual nondepolarizing block, posttetanic potentiation or posttetanic facilitation (posttetanic single-twitch greater than pretetanic twitch response) is seen. The increased single-twitch response is due to increased ACh mobilization for release during the tetanic stimulus. Monitoring for the presence of posttetanic potentiation during continuous succinylcholine administration has been valuable in detecting conversion from a phase I depolarizing block to a phase II block, as posttetanic potentiation is not present during a normal depolarizing phase I block.

Train-of-four monitoring of neuromuscular blockade that involves the administration of four single-twitch stimuli at a frequency of 2 Hz (1 stimulus/0.5 seconds) has numerous advantages over the previously discussed types of nerve stimulation. Train-of-four monitoring can provide a quantitative assessment of the degree of nondepolarizing neuromuscular blockade that is present without the need for establishing a baseline control (Waud & Waud, 1972). As described earlier, TOF is the most sensitive measure of neuromuscular function and is much less painful than tetanic stimulation (Ali & Savarese, 1981). The ratio between the amplitude of the fourth twitch to the amplitude of the first twitch has been used to determine the degree of nondepolarizing neuromuscular blockade. A ratio of T_4 to T_1 amplitude of 0.5 to 0.7 generally indicates satisfactory return of muscle function after administration of nondepolarizing neuromuscular blocking agents (Jones, Pearce, & Williams,

"Train of four" suppression		% Neuromuscular block
All 4 responses equal	0	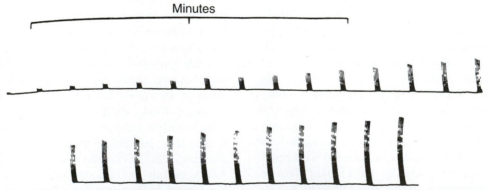
4th response abolished	75	
3rd response abolished	80	
2nd response abolished	90	
1st response abolished	100	

Figure 21–4.   Train-of-four (TOF) suppression correlated with percent of neuromuscular block that is associated with increasing loss of responses to peripheral nerve stimulation.

1984). Although the electromyographic or mechanomyographic equipment necessary to establish T_4-to-T_1 ratios is valuable in a research or teaching environment, it is expensive and time-consuming in daily clinical practice. A simpler clinical evaluation of the degree of nondepolarizing neuromuscular paralysis using TOF involves observing the number of responses to TOF stimulation that are abolished and correlating this with a percentage of paralysis. As shown in Fig. 21–4, when all four responses are present without fade, no neuromuscular blockade exists; when the fourth response in TOF is abolished, 75% neuromuscular block exists; 80% neuromuscular block is present with the loss of the third response; 90% neuromuscular block is present with the loss of the second response; and 100% neuromuscular block is present when the first response is abolished (Jones, 1980). Adequate muscle relaxation for laryngoscopy and abdominal procedures generally is noted with 90% to 95% neuromuscular blockade as measured by TOF monitoring. When using TOF to evaluate neuromuscular blockade during single-dose or continuous infusion of succinylcholine, a dose-dependent reduction of all four responses should be noted during a normal phase I depolarizing block. If fade in response from the first to the fourth response is noted or if part of the responses in the TOF are abolished, this is evidence for early onset of phase II block. Figures 21–5 and 21–6 illustrate depolarizing block TOF monitoring; Figure 21–7 shows TOF monitoring in the presence of nondepolarizing neuromuscular blocking agents.

Stimulus Strength of Blockade Monitor

When any form of electrically evoked potential blockade monitoring is used, it is assumed that the intensity of all stimuli is supramaximal. The use of supramaximal stimuli

Minutes

Figure 21–5.   Both panels show spontaneous recovery from depolarizing neuromuscular blockade after 1 mg/kg succinylcholine under nitrous oxide–oxygen–narcotic anesthesia. Tracing represents thumb adduction in response to TOF stimulation repeated once every 10 seconds. Note the dose-dependent reduction in twitch height, which is equal in all four stimuli of TOF stimulation and the lack of evidence of fade during spontaneous recovery.

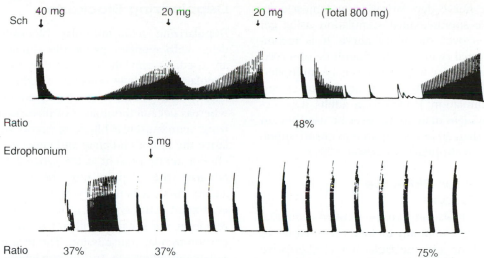

Figure 21–6. Both panels are from the same patient from Figure 21–5, where muscle relaxation was maintained with a succinylcholine infusion of 10 mg/kg given over 2 hours. The upper panel shows response to three bolus doses of succinylcholine after the infusion was discontinued (recorder speed is 10 mm/min). Note the marked development of fade in response to TOF stimulation after the third bolus dose. The bottom panel is a continuation of the upper panel at the same recorder speed. A T_4-to-T_1 ratio of 0.37 is present at the start of the lower tracing. In spite of good recovery of single twitch height and recovery of the height of TOF response after 2 minutes, a T_4-to-T_1 ratio of 0.37 is still present. The potential for reversal of phase II block after succinylcholine administration is demonstrated by the administration of 5.0 mg of edrophonium at the arrow marks. The T_4-to-T_1 ratio improved from 0.37 to 0.75 over 2 minutes.

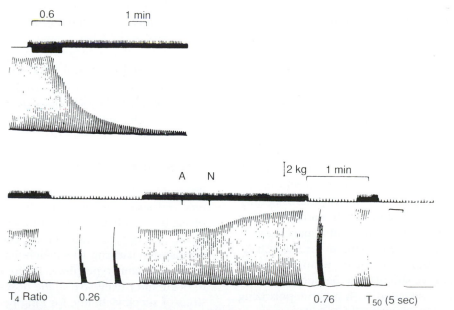

Figure 21–7. The upper panel shows a tracing of loss of twitch height measured by thumb adduction in response to ulnar nerve stimulation at 0.15 Hz after D-tubocurarine, 0.6 mg/kg. The lower panel shows evidence of fade in response to TOF stimulation with a T_4-to-T_1 ratio of 0.26 150 minutes after injection of the 0.6-mg/kg bolus dose of D-tubocurarine, even though single-twitch height has recovered to 75% of control height. Four minutes after administration of atropine and neostigmine, single-twitch height has recovered to control height, and within another minute the T_4-to-T_1 ratio has recovered to 0.76, with no evidence of fade in response to tetanus at 50 Hz for 5 seconds.

ensures adequate nerve depolarization and muscle response. To ensure supramaximal stimulation using gel surface electrodes over the ulnar nerve, it is recommended that maximal twitch in the thumb be observed and the current necessary to produce this be multiplied by 2.75, using the resultant current setting to ensure supramaximal stimulation. However, in adults it is recommended that no less than 20 mA ever be used and, in most cases, more than 20 mA is required to ensure supramaximal stimulation (Kopman & Lawson, 1984).

Anatomic Sites for Blockade Monitor Stimulation

Sites for nerve stimulation during evoked potential blockade monitoring commonly include the ulnar nerve at the wrist or elbow and the facial nerve. Alternative nerve sites for stimulation have included the radial nerve at the wrist and the peroneal nerve at the ankle. When stimulating the facial nerve, the leads should be placed near the tragus of the ear and not over the orbital rima thereby preventing potential for direct stimulation of the orbicularis oculi muscle, which would lead to inaccurate assessment of the lack of neuromuscular blockade (Moore & Williams, 1984). In the presence of 100% neuromuscular blockade, direct electrical stimulation of muscle results in muscle depolarization and contraction.

▶ CHARACTERISTICS OF NONDEPOLARIZING, DEPOLARIZING, AND PHASE II NEUROMUSCULAR BLOCKADE

Nondepolarizing Blockade

Nondepolarizing neuromuscular blockade can also be referred to as a *competitive block*. The nondepolarizing muscle relaxants, of which curare is the classic prototype, are ACh antagonists. They bind competitively to the two alpha-subunits of the ACh receptor, blocking the effects of ACh and preventing depolarization and neuromuscular transmission. Binding of nondepolarizing muscle relaxants is reversible, and when enough of the nondepolarizing agent is excreted or "pharmacologically reversed," ACh can successfully compete for the ACh receptor and neurotransmission can be restored. A summary of peripheral nerve stimulation measurements and clinical observations associated with a nondepolarizing neuromuscular blocking agent would include:

- Fade with TOF and tetanic nerve stimulation
- Posttetanic facilitation or potentiation
- Dose-dependent reduction in single-twitch height
- Dose requirement reduced by prior depolarizing agent administration
- Reversible by administration of ACh agents
- No fasciculations of muscle noted

Depolarizing Blockade

Depolarizing neuromuscular blockade results when drugs with agonistic properties similar to those of ACh are used. Succinylcholine and decamethonium are two depolarizing muscle relaxants. Of these two drugs, succinylcholine continues to be in common clinical use, whereas decamethonium is of historic interest. Depolarizing neuromuscular blocking agents such as ACh depolarize the motor end-plate and generate an EPP. The true cholinesterase present at the synapse is not able to metabolize the depolarizing neuromuscular blocking agents. As long as drug levels maintain an effective concentration at the synapse, repolarization of the end-plate region at the synapse will not occur, thereby blocking neuromuscular transmission. The termination of this depolarizing blockade by succinylcholine primarily depends on plasmacholinesterase or pseudocholinesterase hydrolysis of succinylcholine to succinylmonocholine in the plasma. The rapid hydrolysis of succinylcholine in plasma rapidly lowers the effective concentration in plasma, resulting in lower effective concentrations present at the synapse. Termination of depolarizing blockade by decamethonium primarily depends on renal excretion, as plasma cholinesterase is unable to hydrolyze decamethonium. Peripheral nerve stimulation and clinical findings associated with depolarizing blockade or phase I block include:

- Dose-dependent reduction in single-twitch, TOF, and tetanic stimulation response without fade in any of the tests
- No evidence of posttetanic potentiation
- Fasciculations in skeletal muscle commonly noted
- Anticholinesterase drugs given during depolarizing phase I block showing either no effect on the peripheral nerve stimulator or intensifying the degree of neuromuscular block

Phase II Blockade

Phase II block has been reported in individuals who have received succinylcholine. In the past, other names for phase II block have included desensitization block, dual block, and open-channel block. The conversion from a normal depolarizing succinylcholine phase I block to a nondepolarizing-type phase II block has been reported to occur after excessive single doses or continuous infusions of succinylcholine for long periods in normal individuals. In patients with atypical pseudocholinesterase, inhibition of pseudocholinesterase (organophosphate exposure), or decreased levels of pseudocholinesterase due to disease processes, prolonged paralysis followed by phase II block with 1-mg/kg intubation doses of succinylcholine has been reported. It has been established that the occurrence of phase II block with succinylcholine administration occurs at lower doses 4 to

5 mg/kg if halothane is used, whereas doses of 7 to 8 mg/kg may be required in N_2O/O_2 narcotic anesthesia techniques (Futter, 1983). The cause for occurrence of phase II block is not well defined. The most accepted theory is that the prolonged exposure of the ACh receptor to depolarizing agents such as succinylcholine results in a conformational change of the receptor and the inability to depolarize and repolarize normally in response to cholinergic-type agonists (Bowman, 1980). The pre- and postjunctional ACh receptor conformational change or "desensitization" results in a block with the following peripheral nerve stimulator and clinical observations:

- Fade with TOF and tetanic nerve stimulation
- Posttetanic facilitation or potentiation
- Reduction in single-twitch height
- May be reversed by administration of anti-cholinesterase agents

The capability to reverse a succinylcholine phase II block has been demonstrated (Donati & Bevan, 1985). However, because of the predictability of the quality or safety margin associated with reversal of a phase II block, the conservative clinician may choose to support ventilation and let the passage of time reverse a phase II block.

▶ PHARMACOLOGY AND STRUCTURE-ACTIVITY RELATIONSHIPS OF NEUROMUSCULAR BLOCKING AGENTS

All neuromuscular blocking agents have at least one, and in most cases two, quaternary nitrogen groups on each molecule (positively charged at physiologic pH) that interact or bind to a negatively charged region on the two 40 000-dalton alpha-subunits on the ACh receptors. The charged quaternary nitrogen moiety of the muscle relaxants results in poor absorption from the gastrointestinal (GI) tract and poor transfer across the placenta and the blood–brain barrier. The depolarizing neuromuscular blocking agents are long slender molecules that have structural similarities to the neurotransmitter ACh (Fig. 21–8). In fact, succinylcholine is a dimer of two acetylcholine molecules, and decamethonium is composed of two quaternary ammonium nitrogen groups separated by 10 carbon atoms. The structural similarity of succinylcholine and decamethonium to ACh accounts for the depolarizing agonistic properties at the ACh receptor. The primary action of succinylcholine and decamethonium is to bind to nicotinic ACh receptors in skeletal muscle, producing a depolarizing neuromuscular blockade. Many of the complications associated with the administration of depolarizing muscle relaxants are associated with their capability to bind to muscarinic and nicotinic cholinergic receptors at sites not related to skeletal muscle. Some of the significant sites include nicotinic ACh re-

ceptors in the autonomic ganglia and muscarinic parasympathetic ACh receptors in the heart, GI tract, bladder, and bronchi. In contrast to the depolarizing muscle relaxants, the nondepolarizing muscle relaxants have a large, rigid, bulky structure with at least one, and in most cases two, quaternary nitrogen groups that can bind to the ACh receptor and prevent the binding of ACh to its receptor in a competitive reversible fashion. Other than a quaternary nitrogen group, the nondepolarizing muscle relaxants bear little resemblance to ACh (Fig. 21–8). The nondepolarizing muscle relaxants have no agonistic properties of their own and in sufficient concentration by mass action are able to compete for the ACh receptor-binding site preventing depolarization of the end-plate region by ACh. The primarily monoquaternary structure of D-tubocurarine is thought to be associated with its potential for autonomic ganglionic blockade and histamine-releasing properties. The additional methylation of D-tubocurarine results in the *bis*-quaternary compound dimethyltubocurarine, which is associated with less autonomic ganglionic blockade and histamine-releasing properties. The triquaternary structure of gallamine is thought to be associated with its capability for strong blockade of muscarinic cholinergic receptors, whereas the muscarinic blocking properties of pancuronium are primarily limited to the muscarinic ACh receptors in the heart and M_2 receptors in the autonomic nervous system. The minor modification of removing one methyl group from the steroid structure of pancuronium results in the production of vecuronium, a nondepolarizing muscle relaxant devoid of cardiovascular side effects and that has a shorter duration of action than pancuronium. If there are less than eight CH_2 groups between the quaternary nitrogen groups, significant autonomic ganglionic blocking increases and the potency to block nicotinic ACh receptors in skeletal muscle decreases. Hexamethonium, a *bis*-quaternary compound with six methylene groups between the quaternary nitrogen groups, is associated with significant autonomic ganglionic blocking properties, whereas decamethonium, a compound with 10 methylene groups between the quaternary nitrogen groups, shows significant neuromuscular blocking properties with minimal autonomic ganglionic blocking properties (Paton & Zaimis, 1954). This finding demonstrated significant differences in the binding affinities for ligands and presumably differences in structure between nicotinic ACh receptors in skeletal muscle and autonomic ganglia.

Depolarizing Muscle Relaxants

Types of Depolarizing Drugs

Two drugs, decamethonium and succinylcholine, are depolarizing muscle relaxants that have been used clinically. Decamethonium is not in common clinical usage today; it has most of the side effects of succinylcholine

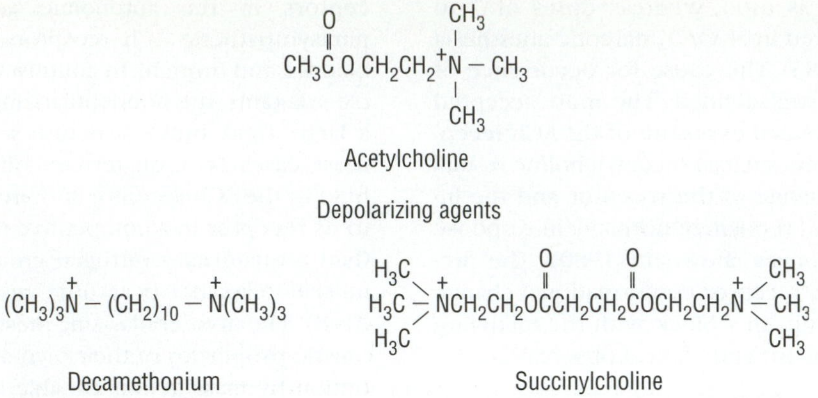

$$CH_3C\overset{O}{\overset{||}{}}O\ CH_2CH_2\overset{+}{N}\overset{CH_3}{\underset{CH_3}{|}}CH_3$$

Acetylcholine

Depolarizing agents

$$(CH_3)_3\overset{+}{N}-(CH_2)_{10}-\overset{+}{N}(CH_3)_3$$

$$\overset{H_3C}{\underset{H_3C}{\overset{|}{H_3C-}}}\overset{+}{N}CH_2CH_2O\overset{O}{\overset{||}{C}}CH_2CH_2\overset{O}{\overset{||}{C}}OCH_2CH_2\overset{+}{N}\overset{CH_3}{\underset{CH_3}{|}}CH_3$$

Decamethonium   Succinylcholine

Figure 21–8. The chemical structure of ACh and of the depolarizing muscle relaxants decamethonium and succinylcholine.

and its usual duration of action after a single bolus dose is about 20 to 30 minutes. Decamethonium is not broken down by pseudocholinesterase and its termination of action is primarily by renal excretion of unchanged drug. The introduction of intermediate duration of action non-depolarizing muscle relaxants such as vecuronium and atracurium have negated any rational choice that would allow the clinical use of decamethonium. The remaining discussion of depolarizing muscle relaxants is limited to the pharmacology and clinical use of succinylcholine.

Succinylcholine

History. Hunt and de Taveau (1906) became aware of the cardiovascular effects of succinylcholine while studying a variety of ACh congeners. Evidently their experiments were performed on curarized animals and the neuromuscular blocking effects of succinylcholine was not noted by these investigators. The neuromuscular blocking effects of succinylcholine were not noted until 1949 (Dorkins, 1982). By 1952, Foldes, McNall, and Borrengo-Hinojosa had introduced succinylcholine into clinical use in the United States.

Drug Action. Succinylcholine was rapidly accepted into clinical practice due to its capability to produce satisfactory paralysis for intubation or short surgical procedures within 1 minute. The effective dose required for paralysis ranges from 0.3 to 1.1 mg/kg, and most clinicians choose a dose of 0.5 to 1 mg/kg, which produces satisfactory intubation conditions in 30 to 60 seconds, maximal paralysis for 3 to 5 minutes, and full spontaneous recovery within 10 minutes in normal patients. Succinylcholine infusions at a rate of 0.5 to 5 mg/min monitored by a peripheral nerve stimulator can be used to maintain paralysis for extended periods of time. The possibility of developing a phase II block with increasing

doses of succinylcholine over extended periods has resulted in the recommendation to avoid the use of succinylcholine infusions for longer than 1 hour. The introduction of vecuronium and atracurium and a continued trend to avoid the use of depolarizing agents has resulted in a decline in the use of succinylcholine for long surgical procedures. However, succinylcholine bolus and continuous infusion are useful for short procedures requiring muscle relaxation, such as Cesarean sections, closed reduction of fractures, and endoscopic procedures. If a succinylcholine in-fusion is to be used, methylene blue added to color the infusion provides an additional safety factor to avoid confusion with other infusions.

Physical and Chemical Properties. Succinylcholine is a dimer of two ACh molecules bonded together resulting in a *bis*-quaternary compound that has two positively charged regions to interact with the 40 000-dalton alpha-subunits of the ACh receptor. Succinylcholine powder is a white crystalline substance that is stable over a wide range of conditions in its unreconstituted state. The water solubility of succinylcholine is high, and it easily goes into solution with most common intravenous solutions. Once succinylcholine has been placed in solution, it is best to keep the solution refrigerated to avoid hydrolysis and loss of potency. Infusions of succinylcholine should only be used for 24 hours after being mixed to avoid the potential for bacterial contamination.

Pharmacokinetics and Pharmacodynamics. Succinylcholine can bind to the ACh receptor and produce persistent depolarization of the skeletal muscle end-plate region because true AChE present at the synapse and in red blood cells cannot hydrolyze succinylcholine. Unlike true AChE, pseudocholinesterase or plasma cholinesterase is synthesized in the liver and high concentrations are present in the plasma but not at the synaptic region. The rapid termination of succinylcholine's effect is due to the capability of pseudocholinesterase to hydrolyze succinylcholine in the plasma rapidly to succinylmonocholine and choline, relatively inactive metabolites of succinylcholine. The elimination half-time ($t_{1/2}$) for succinylcholine is 1 to 2 minutes. The short $t_{1/2}$ of succinylcholine indicates that only a small portion of the total dose administered reaches the synaptic region and that within 5 $t_{1/2}$'s (5–10 minutes) breakdown of succinylcholine to succinylmonocholine and choline is nearly 100% complete. Pseudocholinesterase also is responsible for the slower hydrolysis of succinylmonocholine to succinic acid and choline, which is usually complete after 3 hours. The termination of succinylcholine's effect is due to its rapid hydrolysis in the plasma allowing residual succinylcholine to diffuse out of the synapse to the extracellular fluid, which then allows repolarization of the end-plate.

If there are abnormally low levels of pseudocholinesterase, the reduction of the pseudocholinesterase activity will be directly related to the increased duration of paralysis (Viby-Mogensen, 1980). In individuals with atypical pseudocholinesterase, succinylcholine hydrolysis is lower and renal excretion of this polar drug becomes significant in terminating succinylcholine's effect. When the capability for succinylcholine hydrolysis is significantly altered, the prolongation of paralysis requires sedation and positive pressure ventilation of the patient until complete spontaneous reversal of paralysis occurs. The use of a peripheral nerve stimulator to document sustained presence of a depolarizing block and the duration of its presence enables the clinician to decide rationally when it is safe to extubate the patient. Whenever succinylcholine is administered, a peripheral nerve stimulator should be used to demonstrate complete reversal of succinylcholine before additional succinylcholine or a nondepolarizing muscle relaxant is given.

Pseudocholinesterase. Problems with pseudocholinesterase enzyme are either qualitative (the ability to metabolize succinylcholine) or quantitative (the amount of enzyme available to metabolize succinylcholine). Some of the earliest complications that were associated with succinylcholine administration were related to reductions in quality or the quantity of pseudocholinesterase present to metabolize succinylcholine, resulting in unexpected prolongation of paralysis after apparently normal doses of the drug. Liver dysfunction, pregnancy, and starvation have been shown to produce reductions in the amount of pseudocholinesterase produced. Due to the rapid capability of pseudocholinesterase to metabolize succinylcholine, severe disease or drug inhibition is necessary before a prolongation of succinylcholine paralysis is noted. Foldes, Rendell-Baker, and Birch (1956) demonstrated that liver

disease must be severe before there is an increase in the duration of paralysis from succinylcholine. Term pregnancy has been shown to produce a 40% reduction in pseudocholinesterase activity without a significant increase in the duration of paralysis after succinylcholine administration (Leighton et al., 1986). The remaining 60% functional enzyme capability and the increase in the volume of distribution of succinylcholine are sufficient to prevent any increase in duration of paralysis. The AChE-inhibiting agents that are used in insecticides or the organophosphate AChE-inhibiting agents present in military nerve toxins, such as Saran® and Soman®, would inhibit both true and pseudocholinesterase and potentiate the effects of endogenous ACh and exogenous succinylcholine. In addition, the AChE-inhibiting drugs used to treat glaucoma (ecothiopate), myasthenia gravis (mestanon), and the chemotherapeutic agents (nitrogen mustard and cyclophosphamide) have been associated with a reduction of pseudocholinesterase activity and increased duration of paralysis after succinylcholine administration.

In 1957, Kalow and Genest were able to demonstrate three phenotypes of pseudocholinesterase expressed by use of an in vitro assay using the amide local anesthetic dibucaine. Normal or typical pseudocholinesterase hydrolyzes succinylcholine and benzylcholine. When typical pseudocholinesterase is exposed to benzylcholine in the presence of dibucaine, the hydrolysis of benzylcholine is inhibited to 80% of normal. Therefore, the "dibucaine number" is an expression of the percentage of pseudocholinesterase inhibition of hydrolysis of benzylcholine in the presence of dibucaine. Individuals with normal or typical pseudocholinesterase show 80% dibucaine inhibition, comprise 96.25% of the population (Canadian population data), and react normally to succinylcholine. Individuals who are heterozygotes (one normal and one abnormal allele for pseudocholinesterase) have dibucaine numbers of 70% to 30% inhibition, comprise 3.7% of the population, and may show a modest prolongation of paralysis after normal doses of succinylcholine. Individuals that are homozygotes for atypical pseudocholinesterase (two abnormal alleles for pseudocholinesterase) have dibucaine numbers showing less than 30% inhibition, comprise 0.05% of the population, and may require 2 to 4 hours or more to recover from a single 1-mg/kg dose of succinylcholine.

In about 20% of the homozygote atypical pseudocholinesterase individuals, a third type of allele is thought to exist and has been referred to as the silent allele. The genotype of one atypical allele and one silent allele results in the phenotype of an atypical homozygote. The genotype of two silent alleles results in the phenotypical expression of an individual with no pseudocholinesterase activity at all and would therefore have a dibucaine number of 0% inhibition because there is no enzyme to inhibit. An individual who is a homozygote for the silent allele would demonstrate severe sensitivity to succinylcholine since the only mechanism for termination would be by renal excretion.

A fourth allele is thought to exist based on the observation that rare forms of serum cholinesterase are not resistant to inhibition by dibucaine but are resistant to inhibition by fluoride. If an individual is heterogeneous or a homozygote for the "fluoride-resistant" allele, there is some degree of increased sensitivity to the paralytic effects of succinylcholine.

A fifth isoenzyme of pseudocholinesterase has been identified. The existence of this fifth isoenzyme for pseudocholinesterase would suggest the existence of a fifth allele governing the production of pseudocholinesterase. It is of interest that, unlike the other forms of atypical pseudocholinesterase that show increased sensitivity to succinylcholine, this fifth isoenzyme of pseudocholinesterase is associated with a shorter than normal duration of paralysis and presumably an increased rate of hydrolysis of succinylcholine (Sugimori, 1986).

If a patient is known or suspected of having a form of atypical pseudocholinesterase, it would be reasonable to choose a nondepolarizing muscle relaxant that would have a predictable duration of action. In many cases it would be acceptable to use the priming principle with a nondepolarizing agent in conjunction with ventilation through cricoid pressure to achieve intubating conditions in a slightly longer time than would be noted with succinylcholine. In a patient with atypical pseudocholinesterase, the short duration of action of succinylcholine could not be relied on even if the dose were significantly lower.

Adverse Effects of Succinylcholine

Hyperkalemia. In normal patients succinylcholine produces an increase in serum potassium of about 0.5 to 1 mEq/L (Lowenstein, 1966). Reports of severe hyperkalemic episodes after succinylcholine administration to burn patients were made initially by Lowenstein in 1966 (Mazze, Escue, & Houston, 1969). Since this report was published, conditions associated with hyperkalemia that result in ventricular fibrillation and cardiovascular collapse after succinylcholine administration have expanded to include massive trauma, severe intraabdominal infections, denervation with muscle atrophy, upper motor neuron lesions, tetanus, muscular dystrophy, and multiple sclerosis. The mechanism for hyperkalemia in massive trauma is thought to be related to muscle membrane dysfunction and an inability to move potassium back to the intracellular space after depolarization by succinylcholine. The mechanism for hyperkalemia in patients with upper motor neuron disease or denervation

injuries is better understood. The loss of presynaptic neurotransmitter release results in the excessive growth of extrajunctional cholinergic receptors on the muscle surface, and when succinylcholine binds to these extrajunctional receptors and depolarizes the muscle there is a large release of intracellular potassium to the extracellular space. The duration after injury when the patient is at risk for a hyperkalemic response after succinylcholine administration varies. In burn patients, serum potassium may begin to rise within days after the burn and peak 3 weeks after burn injury. The burn patient remains at risk for hyperkalemia following succinylcholine administration until all burns are healed. In patients with upper motor neuron denervation injuries, patients are at risk for 6 to 12 months after the initial injury if disease has not continued to progress. Succinylcholine has not been associated with hyperkalemia when given less than 24 hours after a burn injury or within the first 1 to 2 hours after injury in trauma patients. It is reasonable to avoid the use of succinylcholine more than 24 hours after initial burn injury or 1 to 2 hours after a traumatic injury until all wounds or burns are healed or infection has been cleared. In the case of denervation injuries and upper motor neuron injuries, it may be safest to avoid succinylcholine for 6 to 12 months after neurologic loss has stabilized.

In the case of a patient with a potassium of 5.5 or greater, the slight increase in potassium of 1 to 0.5 mEq seen in all patients who are given succinylcholine may be sufficient to cause the patient to have an acute onset of arrhythmias. In chronic renal failure patients with potassium elevations who are dialysis dependent and present for emergency surgery, the use of succinylcholine may be contraindicated. Pretreatment or defasciculation with a nondepolarizing neuromuscular blocking agent (10% of a normal paralyzing dose) has been shown to attenuate the hyperkalemic response. However, defasciculation has not been shown reliably to provide full protection against hyperkalemia.

Cardiac Dysrhythmias. The development of dysrhythmias without associated hyperkalemia is associated with the capability of succinylcholine to stimulate cholinergic receptors at autonomic ganglia in both the sympathetic and the parasympathetic nervous system, as well as muscarinic receptors for ACh in parasympathetic effector organs such as the conduction system of the heart. The supraventricular dysrhythmias most commonly reported after the use of succinylcholine have included sinus bradycardia, junctional rhythms, and, more rarely, sinus arrest. Sinus bradycardia after an initial dose of succinylcholine is more common in nonatropinized children who normally have a higher resting sympathetic tone. When the sympathetic nervous system is very active, as it is in many children, additional equal stimulation of both limbs of the autonomic nervous system results in what appears to be greater effect in the parasympathetic nervous system, because there is greater potential for change in activity in the limb of the autonomic nervous system that was less active (the parasympathetic nervous system). As noted, this parasympathetic nervous system activation is due to succinylcholine stimulating the autonomic nervous system at nicotinic cholinergic receptors at the autonomic ganglia as well as cholinergic muscarinic receptors in the cardiac conduction system. Stoelting (1977) has noted that gallamine 0.3 mg/kg is more effective than atropine 0.006 mg/kg in preventing bradycardia after the initial dose of succinylcholine.

The occurrence of junctional bradycardia is most commonly reported in adults who have received a second dose of succinylcholine 5 minutes after the initial dose. The occurrence of this dysrhythmia is most likely due to greater stimulation of muscarinic receptors in the sinus node than in the atrioventricular node, resulting in the atrioventricular node becoming the predominant pacemaker. The time course of 5 minutes between doses suggests that hydrolysis of succinylcholine and generation of succinylmonocholine play a role in potentiating the bradycardic effects of succinylcholine. Mathias, Evans-Prosser, and Churchill-Davidson (1970) demonstrated that the occurrence of junctional bradycardia is increased after a second dose of succinylcholine, but it can be prevented by prior administration of D-tubocurarine, which can reduce the incidence of junctional bradycardia.

Increases in heart rate and blood pressure also have been reported after succinylcholine administration. The magnitude of the heart rate increase would be potentiated by a preexisting high parasympathetic nervous system tone (the opposite effect that is seen with high sympathetic tone in children). In addition, the prior administration of small doses of atropine increases the heart rate because the effects of succinylcholine on the parasympathetic system are blocked by atropine at the muscarinic receptors, thus leaving the effects of succinylcholine in the sympathetic ganglia unopposed (Perez, 1970). The increased blood pressure is due to succinylcholine stimulating nicotinic cholinergic receptors at the autonomic ganglia, resulting in an increased release of norepinephrine and epinephrine from the adrenal medulla. The potential for increased blood pressure and heart rate can be significant in patients who have coronary insufficiency, cerebral aneurysms, or other vascular conditions in which sudden changes in blood pressure could be damaging.

INTRAGASTRIC PRESSURE INCREASES. Succinylcholine is often the muscle relaxant of choice when it is necessary to intubate a patient who presents with a full stomach.

The thought that the drug that can establish intubating conditions the fastest could put the patient at increased risk for regurgitation and aspiration is disturbing. There are conflicting reports in the literature as to succinylcholine's effects on intragastric pressure. Miller and Way (1971) have suggested that the fasciculations associated with succinylcholine can increase intragastric pressure significantly to produce regurgitation of gastric contents. Salem, Wong, and Lin (1972) found that succinylcholine did not significantly alter intragastric pressure in infants and children. Miller and Way (1971) suggested that D-tubocurarine 3 mg, gallamine 20 mg, or lidocaine 6 mg/kg may prevent succinylcholine-mediated increases in intragastric pressure. A study by Smith, Dalling, and Williams (1978) demonstrated that the difference between the intragastric pressure and the high pressure zone of the lower esophageal sphincter was the critical element that prevented gastric regurgitation. As long as the pressure in the high-pressure zone of the lower esophageal sphincter is higher than the intragastric pressure, regurgitation will not take place. In addition, Smith, Dalling, and Williams (1978) found that during succinylcholine administration increases in intragastric pressure were always associated with increases in high-pressure zone esophageal sphincter pressures, preventing any increased risk of regurgitation with succinylcholine administration. Marchand (1957) demonstrated that intragastric pressures greater than 28 cm H_2O resulted in incompetence of the cardioesophageal junction in cadavers. However, the assumption that if intragastric pressure is always below 28 cm H_2O regurgitation will not occur is not always accurate. Intragastric pressures of 15 cm H_2O are sufficient to produce gastroesophageal incompetence in patients who have increased intraabdominal content (pregnancy, bowel obstruction, obesity, ascites, or hiatal hernia) and conditions that alter the normal oblique angle of entry of the esophagus into the stomach.

In current practice, if succinylcholine is to be used for a patient at risk for vomiting or regurgitation and aspiration, it would be reasonable to pretreat the patient with a dose of a nondepolarizing relaxant. In addition, if time and patient condition permit, pharmacologic pretreatment with metoclopramide, an H_2-receptor blocker (ranitidine), and a nonparticulate antacid can be beneficial. Finally, whenever the induction agent and succinylcholine are administered, Sellick's maneuver is maintained until the airway is secured. Should arterial desaturation become evident during a rapid-sequence induction on a patient with a full stomach, mask ventilation with Sellick's maneuver in place is more acceptable than the effects of persistent hypoxemia. If the patient's condition permits, light sedation and awake intubation can overcome many of the concerns of regurgitation in the patient with a "full stomach."

INTRAOCULAR PRESSURE INCREASES. The patient with an open-eye injury poses a dilemma to the anesthetist. In most cases patients with open-eye injuries present emergently and have a "full stomach." Succinylcholine muscle relaxation allows the most rapid intubation and control of the airway. However, it is well known that succinylcholine produces an increase in intraocular pressure that peaks within 2 to 4 minutes and lasts for 5 to 10 minutes (Pandey, Badola, & Kumar, 1972), presumably because of succinylcholine's ability to produce contracture or fasciculations of extraocular and orbital muscles (Katz & Eakins, 1968). It was suggested that a small dose or defasciculatory dose of a nondepolarizing muscle relaxant (3-6 mg of D-tubocurarine) would reduce or prevent succinylcholine-induced increases in intraocular pressure. Cook (1981) has since demonstrated that no pretreatment regimen can reduce succinylcholine-induced intraocular pressure increases consistently. The recommendation that succinylcholine not be given to patients with open-eye injuries remains valid clinically. Common practice techniques to intubate the patient with an open-eye injury generally involve using a priming dose followed by an intubation dose of a nondepolarizing muscle relaxant and mask ventilation with Sellick's maneuver until intubating conditions exist. However, a case that could possibly justify the use of succinylcholine with an open-eye injury would be a patient who also has a difficult airway and visualization to intubate may be a problem. In this case, defasciculation prior to succinylcholine and the possibility for a slight rise in intraocular pressure may be more tolerable than inability to intubate a patient who will be paralyzed for an extended time.

INTRACRANIAL PRESSURE INCREASES. Succinylcholine in doses of 1 mg/kg has been shown to increase intracranial pressure in animals and, more important, in humans. Minton, Grosslight, Stirt, and Bedford (1986) demonstrated that in anesthetized patients with brain tumors succinylcholine produced average intracranial pressure increases of 4.9 mmHg and maximal increases of 9 mmHg in some patients. The rise in intracranial pressure can be prevented by defasciculation with a nondepolarizing muscle relaxant (Stirt, Grosslight, & Bedford, 1987). In cases where immediate control of the airway is not necessary, induction of adequate depth of anesthesia, maintenance of ventilation and hypocarbia, and slower production of muscle paralysis with nondepolarizing nonhistamine-releasing muscle relaxants avoids increases in intracranial pressure. If the need for more rapid intubating conditions exists, succinylcholine can be safely used if the patient is defasciculated, has adequate anesthetic depth, and is under controlled ventilation with hypocarbia.

MYOGLOBINEMIA AND MYOGLOBINURIA. Myoglobinemia after succinylcholine administration has been reported in pediatric patients (Ryan, Kagen, & Hyman, 1971). Significant elevations of plasma creatine phosphokinase (CPK) have also been demonstrated following the administration of succinylcholine. These findings would indicate some degree of muscle damage in children who receive succinylcholine. However, the occurrence of actual myoglobinuria in conjunction with the myoglobinemia is rare. The mechanism responsible for myoglobinemia after succinylcholine administration in children is poorly understood and rarely seen in normal adult patients who have received succinylcholine. There is no correlation between the occurrence of fasciculations, the use of defasciculatory doses of nondepolarizing muscle relaxants, or the total dose of succinylcholine administered and the degree of myoglobinemia seen in children (Harrington, Ford, & Striker, 1983). Based on the long history of clinical use of succinylcholine in normal children, it would appear that myoglobinemia after succinylcholine administration is an interesting biochemical finding that has minimal clinical significance.

MYALGIA. Muscle pain in the shoulders, back, neck, abdomen, chest, and extremities after succinylcholine administration has been reported. The incidence is highest in young adults undergoing minor surgical procedures that are associated with minimal postoperative pain and allow for early ambulation. The onset of pain usually is noted less than 1 day after succinylcholine administration and generally lasts a couple of days. The type of pain is described as that which usually is associated with extended physical exertion. Initially, the myalgia after succinylcholine was thought to be due to fasciculation of skeletal muscle, which is most likely due to presynaptic ACh receptor depolarization by succinylcholine (Riker, 1975). Drugs with the strongest presynaptic ACh receptor blocking capability, such as D-tubocurarine, have been found to be the most reliable defasciculatory agents. The use of defasciculatory doses of nondepolarizing muscle relaxants clearly reduces the incidence of fasciculations as well as the incidence and severity of postoperative myalgia (Stoelting & Peterson, 1975). However, a study by Manchikanti, Grow, Colliver, Canella, and Hadley (1985) showed little correlation between the incidence of fasciculation and postoperative myalgia. Other pharmacologic agents that have been used to prevent fasciculations or reduce myalgias include lidocaine (Chatterji, Thind, & Daga, 1983), fentanyl (Lindgren & Saarnivaara, 1983), calcium gluconate (Shrivasta, Chatterji, Kachhawas, & Daga, 1983), and diazepam (Davies, 1983). The incidence of succinylcholine-induced myalgia in the absence of fasciculations leaves the exact mechanism of action open to question.

ABNORMAL MUSCLE RESPONSES. Rare conditions exist where succinylcholine produces muscle contraction rather than relaxation. Patients with myotonia congenita or myotonia dystrophica who are given succinylcholine develop jaw as well as generalized body rigidity that can make intubation and ventilation difficult. The rigidity that is observed in patients with myotonias given succinylcholine is rarely related to the malignant hyperthermia syndrome, and symptoms of a hypermetabolic state are not noted.

The syndrome of malignant hyperthermia was first described by Denborough, Forster, Lovell, Maplestone, and Villiers in 1962. There are a wide variety of stimuli that can precipitate the onset of malignant hyperthermia in genetically sensitive individuals; in fact, in genetically sensitive pigs, the stress of transport to market was sufficient to trigger fatal episodes of malignant hyperthermia. Rare reports of hyperthermia and death associated with ether anesthesia had been reported in the early 1900s prior to the report by Denborough et al. (1962). Halogenated anesthetics (most commonly halothane) by themselves can be triggering agents for sustained muscle contraction and a malignant hyperthermic episode. However, halogenated anesthetics in conjunction with succinylcholine constitute an especially potent pharmaceutical trigger that can start this hypermetabolic state. Any muscular rigidity that occurs in association with unexplained tachycardia after succinylcholine administration must be evaluated as a potential case of malignant hyperthermia until proved otherwise. For a detailed discussion of malignant hyperthermia, the reader is referred to a review by Gronert (1980).

ALLERGIC RESPONSES AND HISTAMINE RELEASE. Succinylcholine has a low potency for producing clinically significant histamine release and is stated to have 1/100 of the histamine-releasing potency of D-tubocurarine. The possibility for anaphylaxis exists for nearly every pharmacologic compound that has ever been introduced into clinical practice. Rare, true anaphylaxis related to succinylcholine administration has been reported with signs and symptoms of tachycardia, hypotension, bronchospasm, and pharyngeal and facial edema. As with any anaphylatic reaction, maintaining effective circulation and oxygenation are paramount in patient survival.

USE IN PREGNANCY. Succinylcholine has been used safely in obstetric patients for years without adverse effects on the fetus. The quaternary ammonium structure of succinylcholine results in a substance that is highly charged and poorly transferred across the placental barrier in normal clinical doses. Succinylcholine has not been shown to reduce the rate or force of uterine contraction.

SUMMARY OF DEPOLARIZING RELAXANTS. Succinylcholine has enjoyed a unique role in clinical anesthesia. Its primary advantages are its rapid onset and short duration of action. In spite of its many potential complications and drug interactions, it remains in clinical use until a nondepolarizing muscle relaxant with rapid onset and duration of action profile similar to those of succinylcholine is introduced. The introduction of mivacurium is the beginning of the rewards of research and development that is directed at isolating nondepolarizing muscle relaxants that may one day replace succinylcholine (Goldhill et al., 1991).

Nondepolarizing Muscle Relaxants

Common Factors of Nondepolarizing Relaxants

The mechanism of action of all nondepolarizing muscle relaxants is their capability to function as competitive antagonists at the ACh receptor. These agents have no cholinergic agonist activity and by binding to the ACh receptor block the action of ACh. The inhibition of neuromuscular transmission and the development of EPPs depend on a greater concentration of nondepolarizing muscle relaxant than ACh being present at the synapse to compete effectively for ACh binding sites at the alpha-subunits of the ACh receptor. The competitive reversible binding of the nondepolarizing relaxants to the ACh receptor is the basis for reversal of paralysis. When the concentration of nondepolarizing agent decreases or the concentration of ACh is increased by an anticholinesterase drug, the binding of ACh to the ACh receptor is favored and neuromuscular transmission is restored. Activation and channel opening of the ACh receptor requires occupation of both alpha-subunits, and competitive blockade of the ACh receptor channel can be accomplished when only one alpha-subunit of the ACh receptor is occupied.

The available nondepolarizing agents available for clinical use would include D-tubocurarine, metocurine, gallamine, pancuronium, pipecuronium, and doxacurium, all of which have moderately long durations of action. Nondepolarizing agents with intermediate durations of action include atracurium and vecuronium. Mivacurium is a short-acting nondepolarizing relaxant with a duration of roughly half that of atracurium or vecuronium.

Long-Acting Nondepolarizing Muscle Relaxants

D-Tubocurarine

HISTORY AND PHARMACOLOGIC ACTION. D-Tubocurarine (Fig. 21–9) was the first muscle relaxant used clinically and is often the prototype muscle relaxant with which

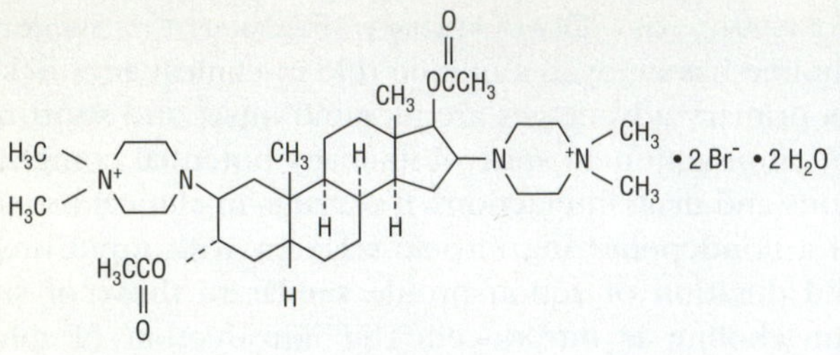

(Pipecuronium Bromide)

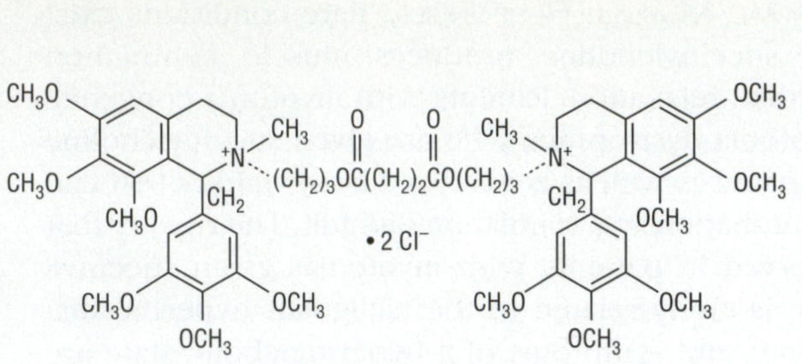

(Doxacurium Chloride)

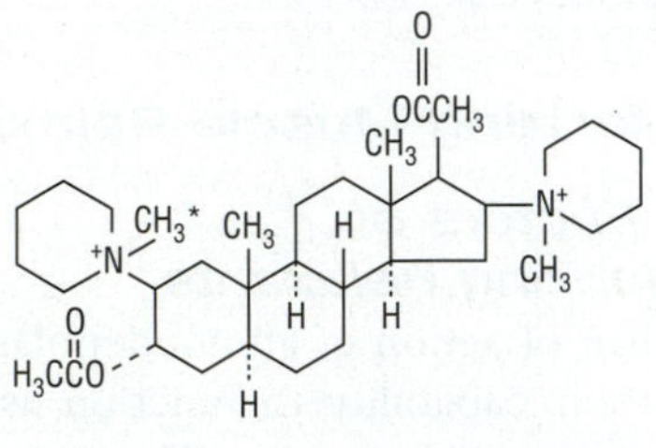

Pancuronium

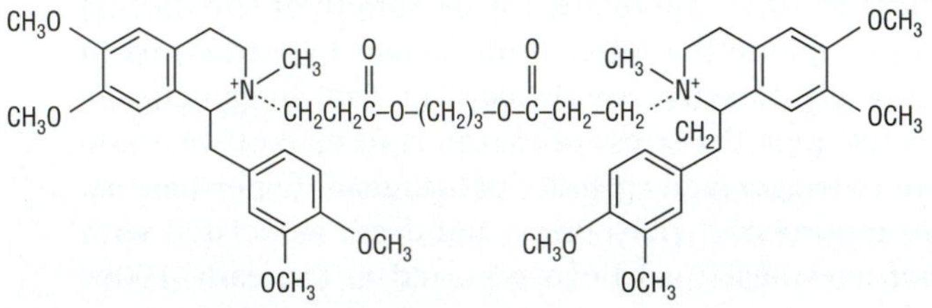

Atracurium

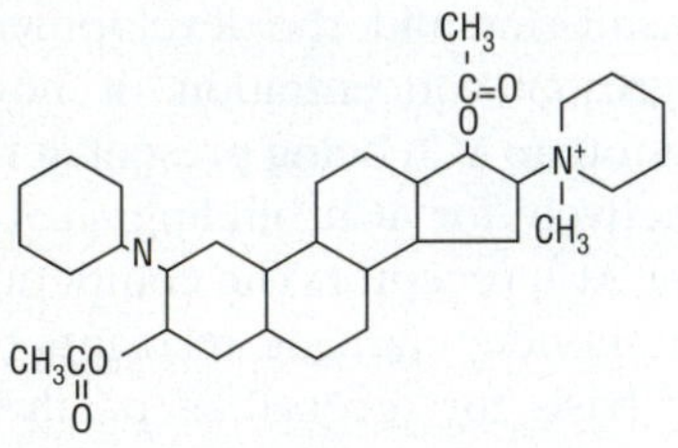

Vecuronium

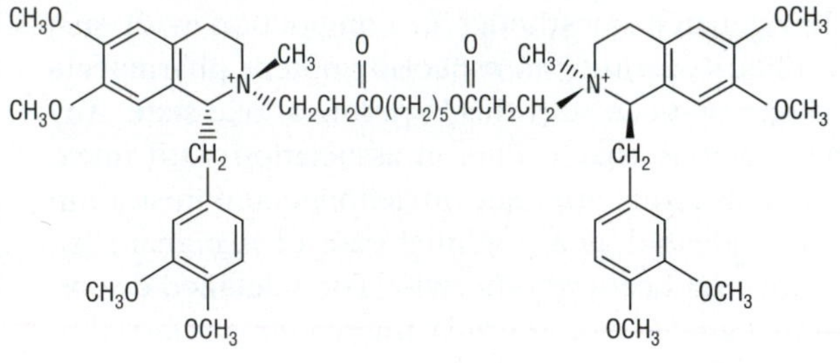

Cisatracurium

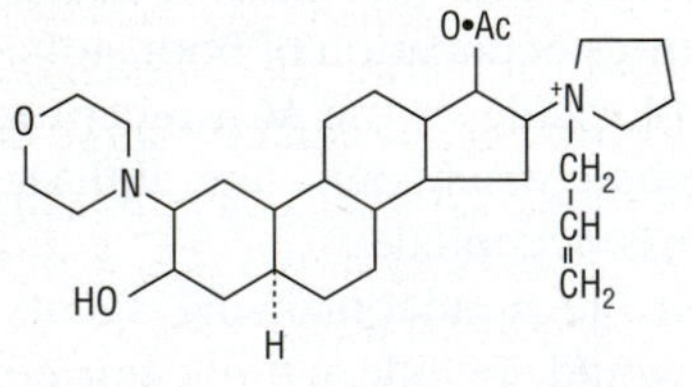

Rocuronium

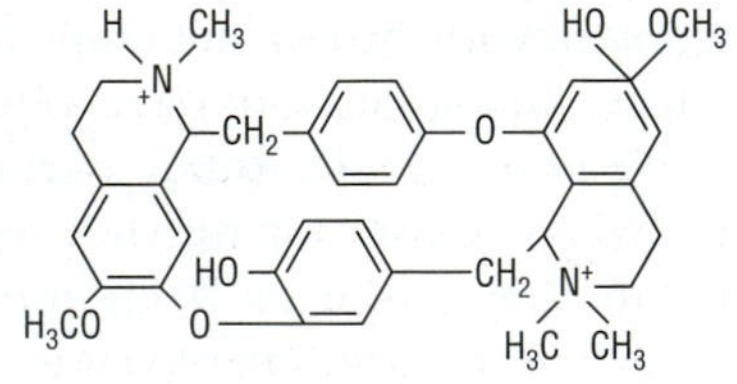

D–Tubocurarine

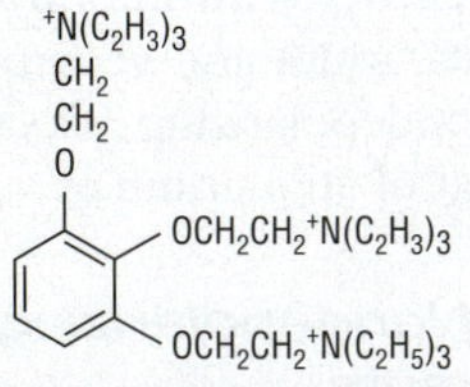

Gallamine

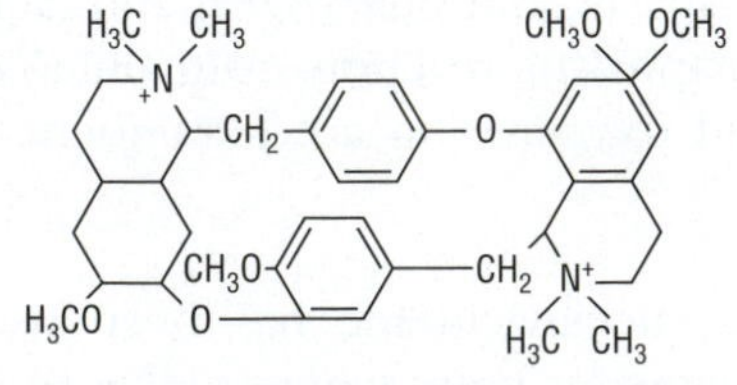

Dimethyltubocurarine

Figure 21–9. The chemical structure of some common nondepolarizing neuromuscular blocking agents.

all new nondepolarizing muscle relaxants are compared as far as potency, side effect profile, and duration of action. Therefore, an understanding of the pharmacology of D-tubocurarine is essential to the understanding of other nondepolarizing agents. The history and clinical pharmacology of D-tubocurarine have been discussed. All nondepolarizing neuromuscular blocking agents produce paralysis by competing with ACh for binding to nicotinic cholinergic receptors at the motor end-plate. Neuromuscular blocking agents are highly ionized at physiologic pH and cross the lipid barriers of cell membranes poorly. Measurable amounts of D-tubocurarine have been detected in cerebrospinal fluid (Matteo, Pua, Khambatta, & Spector, 1977). No alteration in cognitive function or analgesic properties has been shown to be associated with any nondepolarizing muscle relaxant in clinical use. Characteristics of nondepolarizing neuromuscular blockade can be summarized by (1) dose-dependent reduction in single-twitch height, (2) fade with TOF and tetanic stimulation, (3) posttetanic potentiation, (4) absence of fasciculations, (5) reversible with anti-AChE agents, and (6) augmentation of nondepolarizing agent effect by prior administration of a depolarizing agent. Paralysis of skeletal muscle is first noticed in the small muscle groups of the eyes, which explains the frequency of diplopia after defasciculatory doses of nondepolarizing agents. As the plasma concentration of nondepolarizing increases, larger muscle groups are paralyzed, with the diaphragm being the most resistant to paralysis by nondepolarizing muscle relaxants.

PHYSICAL AND CHEMICAL PROPERTIES. D-Tubocurarine (Fig. 21-9) is a monoquaternary compound with one stable quaternary ammonium group (Everett, Cowe, & Wilkinson, 1970). The monoquaternary structure is thought to be related to the potential for histamine release and autonomic ganglia–blocking properties. Methylation of the tertiary amine group of D-tubocurarine to yield dimethyltubocurarine or metocurine (Fig. 21-9) results in a muscle relaxant with three times less autonomic ganglia–blocking properties and histamine-releasing properties than the parent compound (Hughes & Chapple, 1976). D-Tubocurarine, unlike succinylcholine, is not subject to hydrolysis and has a stable shelf life in solution without refrigeration.

PHARMACOKINETICS AND PHARMACODYNAMICS. The ED_{95} for D-tubocurarine is 0.51 mg/kg, and the bolus loading dose for intubation is 0.6 mg/kg and has a duration of action of 60 to 90 minutes. Subsequent maintenance doses under N_2O/O_2–narcotic anesthesia are approximately 0.1 mg/kg, or one fifth the original dose because the initial loading dose continues to occupy the receptor. The maintenance dose during concurrent halogenated agent anesthesia is recommended to be

0.05 mg/kg due to the potentiation of nondepolarizing muscle relaxants by all halogenated anesthetics. Halothane at 1.25 a minimum alveolar concentration (MAC) reduces the requirement of D-tubocurarine by 50% when compared to an equipotent dose required to produce a similar degree of muscle relaxation during N_2O/O_2–opiate anesthesia. Isoflurane and enflurane under similar conditions reduce the dose of D-tubocurarine by 70% (Ali & Savarese, 1976). It should be noted that maximal potentiation of nondepolarizing muscle relaxants is achieved once a stable MAC is reached. During the initial induction or during emergence, when inspired concentrations of inhaled anesthetic are low, the magnitude of potentiation will be lower.

D-tubocurarine is not highly bound to plasma proteins (40% to 50%). Cohen, Corbasci, and Fleischli (1965) demonstrated that in dogs D-tubocurarine is not highly metabolized and that 75% of the dose administered is recovered unchanged in the urine, whereas 10% to 15% of the dose is recovered in the bile within the first 24 hours after administration. This group also demonstrated that in nephrectomized animals hepatic elimination of D-tubocurarine increased three to fourfold (Cohen, Corbascio, & Fleischli, 1965). Elderly patients require similar doses as younger patients to achieve effective plasma concentrations for paralysis. However, the $t_{1/2}$ for terminal elimination in elderly patients is longer than that seen in younger patients (Matteo et al., 1985). Presumably the reduction in glomerular filtration is primarily responsible for the increased time required for terminal elimination of D-tubocurarine and the resulting increased duration of action in the elderly.

CARDIOVASCULAR EFFECTS. It is well known that rapid administration of intubating doses of D-tubocurarine is associated with significant hemodynamic changes. Rapid administration of D-tubocurarine 0.4 mg/kg is associated with reductions in mean arterial pressure (MAP) of 20% or more, which in turn is associated with reductions in systemic vascular resistance (SVR), cardiac output (CO), central venous pressure (CVP), stroke volume (SV), and increases in heart rate (HR) (Stoelting, 1972). The hemodynamic changes associated with D-tubocurarine are due primarily to its histamine-releasing properties and to a lesser extent to the potential for blockade of nicotinic cholinergic receptors in autonomic ganglia. D-Tubocurarine reductions in MAP are associated with a parallel dose-dependent increase in plasma histamine concentrations (Moss, Rosow, Savarese, Philbin, & Kniffen, 1981). The extent of MAP reduction with D-tubocurarine use is related to the total dose administered and the depth of anesthesia (Munger, Miller, & Stevens, 1974). The magnitude of histamine release and the reduction in MAP are also related to the rate of D-tubocurarine administration. The administration of an intubating dose of

D-tubocurarine over 90 seconds rather than a single rapid bolus reduces the magnitude of MAP reduction (Stoelting, McCammon, & Hilgenberg, 1980). The rate of histamine release and reduction in MAP can be further reduced by slow administration of the paralyzing dose of D-tubocurarine over a period of 5 to 10 minutes. In view of the relationship between plasma histamine increases and hemodynamic changes associated with D-tubocurarine, it appears that autonomic ganglionic blockade is minimal in clinically relevant dosages. In the past the hypotensive effects of D-tubocurarine have been exploited when controlling hypotension was part of the anesthetic plan. With the current availability of hypotensive agents that are more predictable and titratable, this practice has decreased. The hemodynamic effects of D-tubocurarine are of greatest concern in patients with compromised cardiovascular systems or individuals who are extremely sensitive to the effects of histamine.

USE IN PREGNANCY. D-Tubocurarine is a quaternary ammonium compound, and because of its highly ionized nature crosses the placental barrier poorly. No reports of significant fetal blood levels or effects on the fetus have been reported. Current clinical use in obstetrics is generally limited to defasciculatory doses prior to succinylcholine administration, which further limits the potential for fetal effects. The duration of action of succinylcholine is generally too long for many obstetric procedures.

Metocurine

HISTORY AND PHARMACOLOGIC ACTION. Metocurine is a synthetic derivative of D-tubocurarine that has three additional methyl groups added to its structure. It is a long-acting, nondepolarizing muscle relaxant with the same mechanism of action as the parent compound that was introduced into clinical practice in 1950.

PHYSICAL AND CHEMICAL PROPERTIES. Adding an additional methyl group to D-tubocurarine results in the production of metocurine, which has two stable quaternary nitrogen groups. This structural modification results in a muscle relaxant that is twice as potent as D-tubocurarine and exhibits markedly histamine-releasing properties or autonomic ganglia–blocking properties.

PHARMACOKINETICS AND PHARMACODYNAMICS. The ED_{95} dose of metocurine of 0.28 mg/kg produces a 95% reduction in twitch height in 3 to 5 minutes and a duration of 60 to 90 minutes. As with D-tubocurarine, metocurine is potentiated by halogenated anesthetics, and it is recommended that the normal incremental dose of 0.07 mg/kg be reduced to 0.04 mg/kg in the presence of halogenated anesthetics. The recommended intubation dose is 0.4 mg/kg. Metocurine does not undergo significant metabolism and primarily depends on unchanged excretion in the urine (Brotherton & Matteo, 1981). The availability of atracurium provides a reasonable alternative to metocurine use in renal failure that is not associated with elimination that is dependent upon renal function.

CARDIOVASCULAR EFFECTS. Metocurine is not associated with any of the vagal blocking properties that are seen with pancuronium or gallamine. Large bolus doses of metocurine 0.4 mg/kg, given rapidly, are associated with slight increases in heart rate and a 7% reduction in MAP (Savarese, Ali, & Antonio, 1977). As with D-tubocurarine, the hypotensive effect is thought to be due primarily to histamine release (Savarese et al., 1977) and can be eliminated when the dose is administered more slowly (Hughes, Ingram, & Payne, 1976). Combinations of pancuronium 0.025 mg/kg and metocurine 0.1 mg/kg have been recommended to exploit the synergistic combinations of these two nondepolarizing muscle relaxants. Synergistic combinations of metocurine and pancuronium potentiate neuromuscular blockade and significantly reduce the increase in heart rate that is seen with pancuronium administration alone (Lebowitz, Ramsey, Savarese, & Ali, 1980). The sympathomimetic and vagolytic properties of intubating doses of pancuronium promote the potential for myocardial ischemia that can be reduced by administration of metocurine pancuronium combinations (Thompson & Putnins, 1985). Introduction of agents such as doxacurium, pipecuronium, vecuronium, rocuronium, cis-atracurium, and atracurium have resulted in a decreased need for metocurine or metocurine combined with pancuronium in many practice settings. With the continued passage of time, metocurine will most likely become a drug of historic pharmacologic interest.

Pancuronium Bromide

HISTORY AND PHARMACOLOGIC ACTION. Pancuronium bromide (hereafter referred to as pancuronium) is a bis-quaternary ammonium steroid without steroid activity that was synthesized in 1964 and introduced into clinical practice in 1977 by Baird and Reed (Fig. 21-9). It is considered to be a long-acting nondepolarizing relaxant that is not associated with significant histamine release or autonomic ganglionic blockade, which was a major advantage when it was introduced. Pancuronium is a highly ionized compound and lacks the structural modifications that would allow it to cross lipid barriers to bind to intracellular steroid receptors or produce receptor–steroid complexes that would translocate to the nucleus. Pancuronium is the precursor of the more modern steroid nondepolarizing muscle relaxants vecuronium and pipicuronium. Pancuronium has the capability to inhibit plasma cholinesterase, which can prolong the action of succinylcholine. When pancuronium is used for defasciculation, the normal nondepolarizing muscle relaxant inhibition of succinylcholine is offset by decreased pseudocholinesterase breakdown of succinylcholine, which results in higher effective succinylcholine concentrations. Defasciculation with nondepolarizing agents other than pancuronium increases the dose of succinylcholine needed for effective blockade.

PHARMACOKINETICS AND PHARMACODYNAMICS. The ED_{95} required for a 95% suppression of twitch height is 0.07 mg/kg and produces satisfactory muscle relaxation for 60 to 90 minutes. Maintenance doses of pancuronium are 0.015 mg/kg without halogenated agents and 0.007 mg/kg with halogenated agents. Initial doses of 0.03 to 0.04 mg/kg after recovery from succinylcholine for intubation have provided adequate muscle relaxation for abdominal surgery. Attempts to shorten the time to onset of paralysis with pancuronium by increasing the dose from $1 \times ED_{95}$ to $2 \times ED_{95}$ given as a single rapid bolus have been successful. The time of satisfactory blockade is shortened from 4.2 to 1.8 minutes, with an increase in the intensity of blockade and time to 5% spontaneous recovery of twitch height increasing from 43 to 129 minutes (Lebowitz, Ramsey, & Savarese, 1981). Should this increased duration of blockade be undesirable when attempting to avoid succinylcholine for intubation, vecuronium can be substituted for pancuronium. At low doses of 0.02 mg/kg, pancuronium is approximately five times as potent as D-tubocurarine, and at higher doses of 0.08 mg/kg, pancuronium is approximately eight times more potent than D-tubocurarine.

As with other highly ionized compounds, pancuronium is eliminated unchanged by the kidneys. The liver has a limited capability to deacetylate pancuronium to less active metabolites, which can be excreted in the bile. When anephric patients are given pancuronium, the $t_{1/2}$ for elimination is increased to five times the normal and prolonged paralysis is noted (McLeod, Watson, & Rawlins, 1976).

CARDIOVASCULAR EFFECTS. The classic hemodynamic effect of pancuronium is to produce a dose-dependent 10% to 15% increase in heart rate, cardiac output, and mean arterial pressure (Stoelting, 1972). The hemodynamic effects of pancuronium are due primarily to increases in heart rate as little change in systemic vascular resistance is noted (Scott & Savarese, 1985). Pancuronium's capability to increase heart rate is principally due to its capability to block muscarinic ACh receptors (M_2 subtype) in the sinoatrial node. Heart rate increases associated with pancuronium can be blocked by prior administration of atropine, which blocks muscarinic ACh receptors.

The clinical significance of the sympathomimetic effects of pancuronium in the autonomic nervous system are difficult to interpret because of the potential for species variation differences in some studies. However, the drug interactions between pancuronium and other sympathomimetic drugs may be explained by the potential for activation of the sympathetic nervous system with pancuronium administration. Experimental evidence indicates that vagal cholinergic nerve terminals synapse with the sympathetic nerve terminals and decrease the release of norepinephrine (Loffelholz & Muscholl, 1970). Pancuronium and gallamine possibly block the muscarinic receptors (M_2 subtype) on the sympathetic nerve terminals and block the inhibitory effects of vagal cholinergic nerve terminal transmitter release, resulting in increased release of norepinephrine (Vercruysse, Bossuyt, Hanegreefs, Verbeuren, & Vanhoutte, 1979). In addition, pancuronium and gallamine have the capability to increase the release of norepinephrine in a noncholinergic muscarinic receptor–blocking mechanism (Brown & Crout, 1970). In addition to increasing the release of norepinephrine from nerve terminals, it is proposed that pancuronium inhibits the reuptake of norepinephrine into the postganglionic sympathetic neurons (Ivankovich, Miletich, Albrecht & Zahed, 1975; Salt, Barnes, & Conway, 1980; Vercruysse et al., 1979).

A final mechanism for sympathomimetic effects of pancuronium at the autonomic ganglionic level is related to its capability to block muscarinic receptors (M_2 subtype) for ACh on dopaminergic interneurons that synapse with postganglionic norepinephrine neurons. Normally, the release and binding of ACh to the muscarinic receptors on the dopamine interneurons increase the release of dopamine, an inhibitory transmitter, which hyperpolarizes the postganglionic norepinephrine neuron, decreasing the release of norepinephrine (Greengard & Kebabian, 1974). The capability of pancuronium and gallamine to block the muscarinic receptors on dopaminergic interneurons inhibits this negative effect on norepinephrine release, and the net effect is an increase in the release of norepinephrine from postganglionic sympathetic neurons (Gardier, Tsevdos, Jackson, & Delaunois, 1978).

The hemodynamic effects of pancuronium are probably of greatest concern in patients with compromised cardiovascular systems due to coronary artery disease or patients on tricyclic antidepressants. Patients with coronary artery disease require slow heart rates to decrease myocardial oxygen demand and to increase myocardial oxygen supply during diastolic time. Many patients with coronary artery disease are treated with calcium channel–blocking agents and beta-adrenergic receptor–blocking compounds to maintain slow heart rates. The greatest increases in heart rate with pancuronium have been reported to occur in patients who had low resting heart rates. Increases in heart rate can be especially detrimental in this population of patients because of increases in myocardial oxygen consumption and corresponding decreases in oxygen supply (Thompson & Putnins, 1985). Dogs pretreated with imipramine, a first-generation tricyclic antidepressant, and given pancuronium during halothane anesthesia develop a high incidence of severe premature ventricular contractions that rapidly progress to ventricular tachycardia and ventricular fibrillation (Edwards, Miller, & Roizen, 1979). This finding has resulted in the recommendation to avoid the triad of pancuronium, halothane, and tricyclic antidepressants.

Gallamine

HISTORY AND PHARMACOLOGIC ACTION. Gallamine is a synthetic triquaternary ammonium compound (Fig. 21–9) with nondepolarizing muscle relaxant properties that has one sixth to one seventh the potency of D-tubocurarine. It was first prepared by the Frenchman Bovet in 1947, and first used in clinical anesthesia in France by Huguenard and Boue in 1948. Gallamine has two outstanding pharmacologic features: Its capability to increase heart rate reliably by its potent vagal blocking properties and its near total dependence on renal function for elimination. Since the advent of newer drugs, gallamine is seldom used in current anesthesia practice.

PHARMACOKINETICS AND PHARMACODYNAMICS. Gallamine 2 mg/kg produces good intubating conditions that are equivalent to a 0.4- to 0.5-mg/kg dose of D-tubocurarine, and the duration of neuromuscular blockade is equal or greater than for D-tubocurarine. The duration of action is prolonged and is best avoided in renal disease because gallamine is almost totally eliminated unchanged by the kidneys (Agoston, Vermeer, Kersten, & Scaf, 1978). In the event of renal failure, the liver is a poor alternative organ for excretion since minimal amounts of gallamine are excreted in bile by the liver and the remaining mechanism of elimination would be dialysis.

CARDIOVASCULAR EFFECTS. Gallamine causes dose-dependent increases in heart rate, with an average of 30% to 40% noted within 1 to 2 minutes after drug administration, which is maximized at a dose of 1 mg/kg (Stoelting, 1973). Like pancuronium, gallamine is associated primarily with blockade of muscarinic ACh receptors (M_2 subtype) in the sinoatrial node. Heart rate increases of nearly 100% have been noted when the resting heart rate is slow prior to administration of gallamine (Stoelting, 1973). The potent vagal blocking properties of gallamine are comparable to those of IV atropine administration when as little as a 20-mg defasciculatory dose is given prior to succinylcholine ad-

ministration (Stoelting, 1977). The vagolytic effects of gallamine administration persist even after the neuromuscular blocking effect is wearing off (Longnecker, Stoelting & Morrow, 1973). Heart rate increases with gallamine 0.5 to 2 mg/kg result in MAP increases of 10 to 20 mmHg and cardiac output increases of 25% to 50% (Stoelting, 1973).

The primary hemodynamic effects of gallamine are most likely due to the vagolytic block and the resulting increase in heart rate. However, experimental evidence shows that gallamine has the potential for sympathomimetic effects at the autonomic ganglia and at postganglionic nerve endings. As seen with pancuronium, gallamine can increase the release of norepinephrine from postganglionic adrenergic nerve terminals (Loffelholz & Muscholl, 1970; Vercruysse et al., 1979), prevent dopaminergic interneuron hyperpolarization of postganglionic adrenergic neurons (Gardier, Tsevdos, Jackson, & Delaunois, 1978; Greengard & Kebabian, 1974), and increase norepinephrine release by a mechanism not related to muscarinic receptor blockade (Brown & Crout, 1970). If the patient's compromised cardiovascular status causes concern about the use of pancuronium, then gallamine certainly is a neuromuscular blocking agent to be eliminated from the anesthetic plan.

Doxacurium Chloride

CHEMICAL PROPERTIES. Doxacurium is a competitive nondepolarizing muscle relaxant with a *bis*-quaternary structure (Fig. 21–9) that is compatible with commonly used intravenous solutions and requires no refrigeration. As a dose of 0.025 mg/kg (1 ED_{95}) has a volume of distribution of 0.15 L/kg, the indication is that the drug is poorly lipid soluble and not widely distributed in body tissues. Doxacurium is associated with a low plasma protein binding of approximately 30% and is 2.5 to 3 times more potent than pancuronium. Its duration of action is dose dependent; doses of 0.025 mg/kg (1 ED_{95}), 0.05 mg/kg (2 $\times$ ED_{95}), or 0.075 mg/kg (3 $\times$ ED_{95}) are associated with mean clinically effective blockade times to 25% recovery of 60 minutes, 100 minutes, and 160 minutes, respectively. Satisfactory intubating conditions in 90% of patients after a dose of 0.05 mg/kg are achieved in 5 minutes, and increasing the dose to 0.08 mg/kg decreases the time to satisfactory intubating conditions by only 1 minute (Scott & Norman, 1989). Doxacurium is not associated with significant drug accumulation after repeated doses, and plasma clearance remains stable over a wide range of dosages in normal patients (Basta, Savarese, & Ali, 1988). Incremental doses after 25% recovery of blockade are usually one fifth the initial dose (0.005 mg/kg after a bolus of 1 ED_{95} or 0.01 mg/kg after a bolus of 2 $\times$ ED_{95}) and are associated with additional clinical relaxation for 30 to 45 minutes. As with other nondepolarizing relaxants, doxacurium is potentiated by inhalation anesthetics up to approximately 25%.

CARDIOVASCULAR EFFECTS. Doxacurium is a nondepolarizing muscle relaxant with a duration of action similar to that of pancuronium and a cardiovascular profile similar to that of vecuronium. In doses up to 0.075 mg/kg ($3 \times ED_{95}$), no significant changes in MAP were noted (Emmott, Bracey, Goldhill, Yate, & Flynn, 1990). A slight reduction in heart rate was observed; however, it was not as great a reduction as was noted with comparable doses of vecuronium. After high-dose doxacurium no increase in plasma histamine levels was noted (Basta et al., 1988). Doxacurium is an agent with a high margin of safety and provides a reasonable alternative when a muscle relaxant with a longer duration than atracurium or vecuronium is desired and the vagolytic effects of pancuronium are not desired.

METABOLISM. Doxacurium is not metabolized in the body. It is excreted unchanged in the urine and the bile. It is reasonable to expect that there will be an increased duration of action if renal or hepatic failure is evident. In addition, higher patient response variability is noted in elderly patients due to varying degrees of reduced renal and hepatic function.

REVERSAL. As with all other long-acting nondepolarizing muscle relaxants, it is not recommended that reversal be attempted until some signs of spontaneous reversal are evident on blockade monitoring. Prostigmine is recommended for reversal, and edrophonium has not been recommended for reversal of doxacurium muscle relaxation (Scott & Norman, 1989).

Pipecuronium Bromide

HISTORY AND CHEMICAL PROPERTIES. Pipecuronium bromide (hereafter referred to as pipecuronium) has been studied extensively in 1980 by Ka'rpa'ti and Bir'o. Its initial clinical use in 1980 was reported by Boros, Szenohradsky, Marosi, and Toth, and it was introduced into common clinical practice in the United States in 1991.

Pipecuronium is a competitive nondepolarizing neuromuscular blocking agent that is structurally similar to the other steroid-based muscle relaxants vecuronium and pancuronium. Both pipecuronium and pancuronium have *bis*-quaternary ammonium structures, but pipecuronium has piperazine rings attached to the steroid nucleus, whereas pancuronium has piperadine rings (Fig. 21-9). The structural modifications of pipecuronium result in a muscle relaxant that lacks cholinergic muscarinic receptor–blocking properties in the sinoatrial node and remarkable hemodynamic sta-

bility. It is supplied as a sterile lypoophilized white crystalline cake that requires reconstitution prior to IV use. Pipecuronium is approximately 30% more potent than pancuronium (Tassonyi, Neidhart, Pittet, Morel, & Gemperle, 1988).

PHARMACOKINETICS AND PHARMACODYNAMICS. Estimates of the ED_{95} range from a high of 0.05 mg/kg (Tassonyi, et al., 1988; Wierda, Richardson, & Agoston, 1989) down to 0.035 mg/kg for pipecuronium during IV-balanced anesthesia (Larijani et al., 1989; Caldwell et al., 1988). The rate of onset of blockade with pipecuronium does not seem to be dose dependent. A 90% suppression of T_1 twitch height in TOF testing was noted at 2.6, 2, and 2.1 minutes following doses of 0.07, 0.085, and 0.1 mg/kg, respectively (Larijani et al., 1989). Good intubation conditions are generally achieved within 2 to 3 minutes after administration of pipecuronium 0.07 mg/kg, and maximum paralysis is achieved 5 minutes after administration. Mean time to 25% recovery of initial twitch height is dose dependent: showing 69.9, 98.3, 94.6 minutes after doses of 0.07, 0.085, and 0.1 mg/kg, respectively, under nitrous oxide–narcotic anesthesia (Larijani et al., 1989). The duration of action for pipecuronium 0.07 mg/kg and pancuronium 0.1 mg/kg showed similar prolongation by halothane anesthesia in normal patients, with mean duration to 25% recovery of initial twitch height 98 minutes and 117 minutes, respectively (Caldwell et al., 1988).

Data from Caldwell et al. (1989) confirm the potentiation of pipecuronium (0.07 mg/kg) by concurrent halothane administration with the time to recovery to 25% of initial twitch height, showing a mean time of 98 minutes in normal patients and 103 minutes for patients with end-stage renal disease. The similar mean recovery times for pipecuronium in normal patients and those with end-stage renal disease may seem confusing on the surface since pipecuronium is heavily dependent on renal elimination. It has been demonstrated that up to 56% of the administered dose is recovered in the urine within 24 hours and 25% of the recovered drug is the metabolite 3-desacetyl pipecuronium (Wierda et al., 1990). However, further evaluation of data from Caldwell et al. (1989) demonstrates a greater degree of variability of recovery in normal patients and patients with end-stage renal disease of 55 to 198 minutes and 30 to 267 minutes, respectively. In addition, the mean clearance and $t_{1/2}$ for elimination (normal vs renal failure) were 2.4 vs 1.6 mL/kg/min[-1] and 118 minutes vs 247 minutes, respectively (Caldwell et al., 1989). The increased variability in time to 25% recovery of twitch height, decreased clearance, and increased time for terminal elimination of pipecuronium indicate a high possibility for increased duration of action of pipecuronium in patients with renal disease.

If succinylcholine is used prior to pipecuronium, it is recommended that the initial dose of pipecuronium be reduced to 0.05 mg/kg to avoid excessive increases in duration of action.

CARDIOVASCULAR EFFECTS. In numerous studies pipecuronium in doses as high as 0.15 mg/kg has not been associated with any significant hemodynamic changes (Foldes, Nagashima, Nguyen, Duncalf, & Goldiner, 1990; Larijani et al., 1989; Tassonyi et al., 1988). Pipecuronium has not been associated with any significant histamine release or autonomic ganglia–blocking properties. This remarkable cardiovascular stability has allowed the bradycardic effects of high-dose narcotic to be more evident in some cases. Pipecuronium is a reasonable choice when a muscle relaxant with cardiovascular stability is desired for procedures that will last 90 minutes or longer.

USE IN PREGNANCY. Current studies on placental transfer and fetal accumulation of pipecuronium are not available. Should experience with other highly ionized *bis*-quaternary ammonium compounds hold true for pipecuronium, significant placental transfer that could produce effects in the fetus would not be expected. The duration of action of pipecuronium is longer than that of many obstetric procedures, and, in most cases, would be a poor choice for use even if studies showed that it was safe to use in pregnancy.

REVERSAL. Patients with spontaneous mean recovery of T_1 to 28.7% and a T_4-to-T_1 ratio of 9.2% demonstrated adequate reversal with T_1 greater than 90% and a T_4-to-T_1 ratios greater than 75% within 10 minutes of 2.5 mg neostigmine with appropriate antimuscarinic agent. Those with spontaneous mean recovery of T_1 to 13.2% showed mean T_1 recovery of 67.9% and a T_4-to-T_1 ratio of 51.4% 10 minutes after reversal with 2.5 mg neostigmine and required additional time for adequate reversal or additional neostigmine administration (Larijani et al., 1989).

Edrophonium 0.5 mg/kg, given to patients with spontaneous recovery of 25% TOF, produced adequate reversal of pipecuronium (>70% recovery of TOF) within 10 minutes in patients who received pipecuronium with nitrous oxide–oxygen–narcotic anesthesia. In patients who received isoflurane 10 minutes after the initial 0.5-mg/kg dose of edrophonium, an additional 0.25-mg/kg dose of edrophonium was required to achieve marginally acceptable reversal at slightly more than 70% recovery of TOF (Wierda et al., 1989). Edrophonium has been judged to be a less than safe antagonist for pipecuronium, as are most of the other long-acting nondepolarizing agents at 0.5- to 0.75-mg/kg doses.

Intermediate-Duration Nondepolarizing Muscle Relaxants

Vecuronium

CHEMICAL PROPERTIES. Vecuronium, a competitive nondepolarizing muscle relaxant, is a structural analog of pancuronium that has had the methyl group removed from the A ring of the steroid nucleus of pancuronium (Fig. 21-9). This minor structural modification results in major clinical differences between vecuronium and pancuronium. Vecuronium has not been associated with muscarinic receptor-blocking properties in clinically relevant doses. The absence of muscarinic receptor-blocking capability results in loss of the vagolytic effects and potential sympathomimetic effects that were associated with pancuronium. The monoquaternary structure of vecuronium is still ionized and hydrophillic, but the loss of one quaternary nitrogen results in a slight increase in lipid solubility and a higher dependence on hepatic function for elimination. When equipotent doses are compared, vecuronium duration of action of clinically effective muscle relaxation is approximately 30% that of pancuronium. Because of its lack of stability in solution, vecuronium is supplied as a lypophilized cake that is reconstituted with sterile water prior to use.

PHARMACOKINETICS AND PHARMACODYNAMICS. If given at $1 \times ED_{95}$ (0.05 mg/kg), vecuronium has an onset time of 4 minutes (Kreig, Crul, & Booij, 1980). Attempts to increase the rate of onset time with vecuronium have employed the priming principle, giving larger doses ($3-5 \times ED_{95}$) or a combination of both. The rate of onset of vecuronium is dose dependent: onset times with doses of $3 \times ED_{95}$ and $5 \times ED_{95}$ are 2.8 minutes and 1.1 minutes, respectively. Recovery from vecuronium is also dose dependent at $5 \times ED_{95}$; 83 minutes are required to recover the second twitch in TOF monitoring (Lennon, Olson, & Gronert, 1986). Incremental doses of 0.01 to 0.02 mg/kg, given when the initial twitch returns to 10% of control or when the fourth twitch in TOF monitoring becomes prominent, maintain satisfactory abdominal muscle relaxation.

Use of the priming principle with vecuronium is an attempt to increase the rate of onset and to enhance the ability to reverse residual paralysis earlier than is allowed with vecuronium at $5 \times ED_{95}$. One technique of priming involves giving one tenth the calculated $2 \times ED_{95}$ dose of vecuronium (0.01 mg/kg) and after 4 minutes, giving the full calculated $2 \times ED_{95}$ dose of vecuronium (0.1 mg/kg) (Taboada, Rupp, & Miller, 1986). Using vecuronium and the priming principle, time to intubation can be reduced to less than 1.5 minutes. After $2 \times ED_{95}$ bolus doses of ve-curonium can be reversed successfully within 20 to 30 minutes. When recovery from the initial bolus dose of ve-curonium has begun, muscle relaxation can be maintained with an infusion of vecuronium at a mean steady- state rate of 1.2 $\mu g/kg/min^{-1}$. When this infusion rate is stopped, mean recovery time to 25% of initial twitch height is 12.7 minutes (Ali et al., 1988).

Vecuronium is normally highly dependent on hepatic function for excretion (Bencini, Houwertjes, & Agoston, 1985). When high-dose vecuronium (0.2 mg/kg) is administered to patients with cirrhosis of the liver, decreased plasma clearance and increased elimination half-time are seen (Lebrault et al., 1985). When similar doses of vecuronium are administered to patients with cholestasis who are undergoing biliary surgery, an increased duration of action is noted (Lebrault, Duvaldestin, Henzel, Chauvin, & Guesnon, 1986). When lower doses of vecuronium (0.1 mg/kg) are given to patients with cirrhosis of the liver, the elimination half-time is the same as that of normal patients (Bell, Hunter, Jones, & Utting, 1985). These lower doses of vecuronium given to patients with cirrhosis are most likely cleared by compensatory renal excretion. Under normal conditions, about 30% of an administered dose of vecuronium is excreted in the urine as unchanged drug or drug metabolites in the first 24 hours (Bencini et al., 1986). In patients with end-stage renal disease, compensatory hepatic excretion of vecuronium occurs and no significant increase in duration of action is noted, and vecuronium can be used safely in patients with renal failure (Bencini et al., 1986).

The cumulative effects of vecuronium are clinically insignificant. Incremental doses given at consistent points of twitch recovery produce the same duration and intensity of neuromuscular blockade each time they are given (Fahey et al.,1981). The differences in potentiation by halogenated agents and effects of concentration changes are less pronounced in vecuronium than in the parent compound pancuronium. Potentiation of vecuronium muscle relaxation under steady-state isoflurane and enflurane is potentiated to a degree only 20% to 30% greater than that noted with halothane (Rupp, Miller, & Gencarelli, 1984).

CARDIOVASCULAR EFFECTS. Vecuronium has not been associated with any significant hemodynamic changes, histamine release, or autonomic ganglia–blocking properties. Doses 20 times greater than those required for neuromuscular blocking produced no cardiovascular changes in dogs or cats (Marshall, McGrath, Miller, Docherty, & Lamar, 1980). In humans anesthetized with halothane in doses of 0.28 mg/kg (12 × ED_{90}), no changes in heart rate or arterial blood pressure were noted (Morris et al., 1983). As has been noted with pipecuronium and doxacurium, the bradycardic effects of narcotic agents are more intense when used with vecuronium.

USE IN PREGNANCY. Vecuronium has been used safely in patients undergoing cesarean section without harmful effects to the fetus. If succinylcholine is contraindicated for reasons other than pseudocholinesterase abnormalities, mivacurium may be a more reasonable choice than vecuronium or atracurium.

Rocuronium

CHEMICAL PROPERTIES. Rocuronium is a competitive nondepolarizing muscle relaxant with a steroidal structure and is a desacetoxy derivative of vecuronium (Fig. 21–9). It has a rapid to intermediate dose-dependent rate of onset and an intermediate duration of action. The molecular weight of rocuronium is similar to that of vecuronium; however, estimates of rocuronium's potency indicate it is seven to eight times less potent than vecuronium. When equipotent doses of rocuronium and vecuronium are administered, rocuronium presents a greater mass of drug molecules to bind competitively to ACh receptors at the neuromuscular junction. The principle of drug mass and pharmacokinetics of receptor binding largely explains the more rapid onset of rocuronium than vecuronium. In addition, the high unbound fraction of rocuronium in the plasma results in more free drug (Wierda & Proost, 1995). The lower potency of rocuronium most likely results in lower affinity drug receptor interaction, allowing for easier removal of drug from the receptor site. Thus the greater drug mass of rocuronium results in a faster onset than vecuronium. However, lower potency or affinity of binding is partially responsible for the similar duration of action that is noted with equipotent doses of rocuronium and vecuronium.

PHARMACOKINETICS AND DOSAGE. The estimated ED_{95} for rocuronium is 0.3 mg/kg (Hofmockel & Benad, 1995; Prien, Zahn, Menges, & Brussel, 1995). Recommended intubation doses are from a low of 0.45 mg/kg up to 1.2 mg/kg. Rocuronium at a dose of 0.6 mg/kg produces satisfactory intubating conditions within 40 ± 10 seconds. However, time to 90% twitch recovery for rocuronium at this dose is an average of 2 to 3 times the 11 minutes to 90% twitch recovery noted with succinylcholine (Hofmockel & Benad, 1995). Using a priming dose of 0.06 mg/kg followed by an intubating dose of 0.24 mg/kg can produce good to excellent intubating conditions within 51 ± 11 seconds and time to 90% twitch recovery of 15 ± 3 minutes (Hofmockel & Benad, 1995). Initial maintenance infusion rates of 0.01 to 0.15 $\mu g/kg/min$ are common. The primary benefit of rocuronium over vecuronium probably is its more rapid rate of onset. Rocuronium's rapid rate of onset partially fulfills the search for a nondepolarizing muscle relaxant to replace succinylcholine in rapid-sequence inductions. At the time of this writing, the product manufacturer does not recommend rocuronium as a replacement for succinylcholine in cesarean section patients requiring rapid sequence intubation. When using succinylcholine, the inability to intubate successfully is associated with the capability to spontaneously ventilate the patient for a short time with cricoid pressure, to allow rapid return of spontaneous ventilation, and to wake the patient up and intubate with some form of awake intubation. When using nondepolarizing muscle relaxants, including rocuronium, this luxury does not exist.

CARDIOVASCULAR EFFECTS. As noted with vecuronium, rocuronium is not associated with any significant cardiovascular effects or histamine release (Naguib, Samarkandi, Bakhamees, Magboul, & el-Bakry, 1995).

Atracurium Besylate

HISTORY. Atracurium besylate (hereafter referred to as atracurium) (Fig. 21-9) was first synthesized by Stenlake, Waigh, Urwin, Dewar, and Coker (1983), who concentrated on producing a muscle relaxant that would be able to use the Hofmann elimination pathway for spontaneous breakdown of quaternary ammonium compounds at physiologic temperature and pH. This was not an easy process because chemical breakdown of quaternary ammonium compounds usually occurs at the boiling point of water in strong alkaline solutions. Initial pharmacologic studies were conducted by Hughes and Chapple (1981), and atracurium was first used clinically in 1979 (Hunt, Hughes, & Payne, 1980).

CHEMICAL PROPERTIES. Atracurium is a *bis*-quaternary ester competitive nondepolarizing neuromuscular blocking agent. A unique feature of atracurium is that under normal physiologic conditions renal or hepatic function is not required for its metabolism. The normal elimination half-time of atracurium is unchanged by renal (deBros et al., 1986) or hepatic failure (Bell et al., 1985). Chemical breakdown and elimination of atracurium take place by the Hofmann elimination process, which is the removal of a beta hydrogen and the disruption of an alpha C-N bond, and by ester hydrolysis in plasma by nonspecific esterases and not pseudocholinesterase (Fig. 21-9). To minimize the Hofmann elimination process under storage, atracurium is buffered to a pH of 3.25 to 3.65 and maintained under refrigeration at 5°C. When refrigerated, atracurium has a loss of potency of only approximately 6%/year; if atracurium is not refrigerated, the loss is approximately 5%/month.

Hofmann elimination breakdown of atracurium yields a monoacrylate and laudanosine, which is a tertiary amine that can enter the brain. Ester hydrolysis of atracurium yields a quaternary acid and a quaternary alcohol, both of which can be further metabolized by the Hofmann elimination process to yield laudanosine. Studies have indicated that laudanosine can cause seizures in dogs (Chapple, Miller, Ward, & Wheatley, 1987), and evidence of arousal on EEG has been noted after atracurium 1 to 2.5 mg/kg was given to dogs (Lanier, Milde, & Michenfelder, 1985). Transient reductions in blood pressure of 14% were noted after 1-mg/kg doses of laudanosine were given to dogs under halothane anesthesia (Hennis, Fahey, Canfell, Shi, & Miller, 1986). However, the atracurium or laudanosine doses given to laboratory animals in the previously mentioned studies are far greater than could ever be administered clinically. Similar neurologic side effects or cardiovascular findings have not been noted in acute care patients receiving atracurium infusions for 38 to 219 hours, which is longer than even the longest operations (Yate et al., 1987).

PHARMACOKINETICS AND PHARMACODYNAMICS. The average ED_{95} dose of atracurium is 0.20 mg/kg and produces its maximal effect in approximately 4 minutes with spontaneous recovery of 95% of twitch height in 44 minutes (Basta et al., 1982). In equipotent $1 \times ED_{95}$ bolus doses, both vecuronium and atracurium can generally be reversed within 20 minutes. Doses of 0.5 mg/kg produce a more rapid onset to maximal block in 2.5 minutes and a recovery to 10% of T_1 height within 40 minutes (Caldwell, Heier, et al., 1989), a point that allows for easy reversal of atracurium with neostigmine or edrophonium. The time to spontaneous 90% recovery of twitch height was 66 minutes (Caldwell, Heier, et al., 1989). Attempts to speed onset time and use atracurium rather than succinylcholine for intubation have relied on the priming principle and a bolus dose of $2.5 \times ED_{95}$ (0.5 mg/kg), the maximal dose not associated with significant histamine release. One priming technique involves a 0.06- to 0.08-mg/kg priming dose, and after 3 minutes the remaining 0.5-mg/kg dose is given (Haguib, Abdulatif, Gyasi, Khawaji, & Absood, 1987).

After signs of recovery from initial bolus of atracurium are evident (10% recovery of T_1 height), adequate muscle relaxation can be maintained with a mean steady-state atracurium infusion of 7.9 μg/kg/min^{-1} (Ali et al., 1988). With this infusion rate, 25% T_1 recovery can be expected within 12.5 minutes after the atracurium infusion is discontinued (Ali et al., 1988).

Both atracurium and vecuronium have been associated with slight evidence of cumulative effect (Fahey et al., 1981) with the effect of atracurium being even less noticeable than that of vecuronium; neither one of these has been associated with significant clinical cumulative effects. If succinylcholine is used for intubation, it may be desirable to reduce the initial atracurium dose to

0.3 mg/kg. Incremental doses of atracurium to maintain satisfactory muscle relaxation range from 0.05 to 0.1 mg/kg every 15 to 30 minutes.

Halogenated agent potentiation of the intermediate-acting muscle relaxants is not as agent or dose sensitive as are the long-acting muscle relaxants. With steady-state concentrations of isoflurane and enflurane, approximately 30% potentiation of atracurium is noted, and 20% potentiation is noted with halothane.

CARDIOVASCULAR EFFECTS. The potential for cardiovascular changes with atracurium is less than with D-tubocurarine or metocurine. When cardiovascular effects are noted, they are transient and associated with histamine release. Atracurium given in rapid bolus doses up to $2 \times ED_{95}$ (0.4 mg/kg) are not associated with changes in heart rate or blood pressure (Basta et al., 1982). When atracurium was given at doses of $3 \times ED_{95}$, the heart rate increased by 8.3% and the MAP decreased by 21.5%; these changes were evident in 60 to 90 seconds and disappeared within 5 minutes (Basta et al., 1982). Cardiovascular changes and histamine release with atracurium are related to the total dose and rate of administration. A dose of 0.8 mg/kg given over 5 seconds produced a 25% reduction in blood pressure, and slower injection of the same dose over 75 seconds or antihistamine pretreatment results in significant reduction of blood pressure and histamine changes (Scott et al., 1986).

USE IN PREGNANCY. Atracurium has been used safely in obstetric anesthesia. The fetal umbilical venous blood levels of atracurium were found to be below the sensitivity of the assay (Frank, Flynn, & Hughes, 1983).

cis-Atracurium Besylate

CHEMICAL PROPERTIES. *Cis*-atracurium besylate (hereafter referred to as *cis*-atracurium) is one of the stereoisomers of atracurium (Fig. 21–9). The *cis-cis* isomer, *cis*-atracurium is more potent than atracurium and has an ED_{95} of 0.05 mg/kg (Belmont, Beemer, Bownes, Wastila, & Savarese, 1993; Lien et al., 1995). *Cis*-atracurium is a nondepolarizing muscle relaxant with intermediate duration of action and noncumulative effects. The primary benefit of *cis*-atracurium over atracurium is that it is not associated with histamine release or significant cardiovascular effects. In doses equal to 8 to 40 times ED_{95}, no release of histamine or significant cardiovascular effects were demonstrated in clinical patients or rhesus monkeys (Belmont et al., 1993; Lien et al., 1995; Wastila, Maehr, Turner, Hill, & Savarese, 1996). *cis*-Atracurium is associated with less potential for the production of the metabolite laudanosine, a minor problem in long-term use of atracurium.

Because *cis*-atracurium is more potent than atracurium, less drug substrate is present to be metabolized to final metabolites such as laudanosine (Boyd, Eastwood, Parker, Hunter, 1996).

PHARMACOKINETICS AND PHARMACODYNAMICS. With an ED_{95} of 0.05 mg/kg, *cis*-atracurium is 2.5 times more potent than atracurium (Boyd et al., 1996). The recommended intubation dose of *cis*-atracurium is 0.15 to 20 mg/kg (Belmont et al., 1995, 1996). Intubation doses of 0.1 mg/kg produce maximum block which is noted in 5.2 minutes. By increasing the intubation dose of *cis*-atracurium to 0.4 mg/kg, onset of maximum block is noted in 1.9 minutes (Belmont et al., 1995). Infusion doses of *cis*-atracurium generally range from 1 to 3.0 µg/kg/min (Boyd et al., 1996; Brandon et al., 1989; Prielipp et al., 1995). After a mean population infusion rate of 3 µg/kg/min for an average period of 37 hours, the time to reach a TOF ratio of 0.7 was 60 minutes (Boyd et al., 1996). Current prescribing information recommends limiting the dose given to children older than the age of 2 years to 0.1 mg/kg. At equipotent doses, the pharmacokinetics of onset of neuromuscular block and rate of elimination of *cis*-atracurium are similar to those of atracurium. The mechanism of elimination of *cis*-atracurium is the same as for atracurium and follows the Hofmann elimination process, which does not depend on plasma pseudocholinesterase levels or hepatic or renal function. Clinically, *cis*-atracurium is a muscle relaxant that has less potential for clinical complications than does the parent compound.

Short-Acting Nondepolarizing Muscle Relaxants

Mivacurium Chloride

CHEMICAL PROPERTIES. Mivacurium chloride (hereafter referred to as mivacurium) is a synthetic *bis*-benzylisoquinolinium diester that is structurally related to atracurium (Fig. 21–9). It is a competitive nondepolarizing neuromuscular blocking agent that is hydrolyzed by plasma cholinesterase, but not true cholinesterase. Mivacurium is not subject to spontaneous hydrolysis in the absence of pseudocholinesterase.

PHARMACOKINETICS AND PHARMACODYNAMICS. Estimates of ED_{95} doses of mivacurium are variable between investigators who were all using nitrous oxide–narcotic anesthesia. The range is from a low of 0.058 mg/kg (Brandon et al., 1989), to 0.067 mg/kg (Caldwell, Kitts, et al., 1989), 0.075 mg/kg (Basta et al., 1982), and the highest estimate was 0.08 mg/kg (Savarese et al., 1989). The most commonly accepted mean ED_{95} would be 0.075 mg/kg in nitrous oxide–narcotic anesthesia. Both potency and duration of mivacurium are increased by halogenated anesthetics, and under stable enflurane anesthesia the ED_{95} was reduced to 0.052 mg/kg (Caldwell, Kitts, et al., 1989). During nitrous–oxide narcotic anesthesia the mean time to complete block was not dose dependent at doses of 0.15 mg/kg, 0.20 mg/kg, or 0.25 mg/kg; the mean time to achieve complete block was 2.5, 2.4, and 2.7 minutes, respectively. The mean time to 10% recovery of twitch height is dose dependent at 15.6, 18.0, and 20.6 minutes, respectively, from the lowest dose to the highest dose (Basta et al., 1982). When a patient has demonstrated 10% recovery of twitch height, mivacurium is reversed easily. Even if reversal is not attempted, mean time to 95% recovery of twitch height occurs in 26.9 minutes (Ali et al., 1988).

In a study by Ali et al. (1988), patients were intubated with approximately 1.5 to 3 × ED_{95} doses of mivacurium; patients were maintained under enflurane anesthesia and were allowed to recover to a twitch height of 18.2%. A mivacurium infusion was started at a rate of 8.4 μg/kg/min^{-1} for the first 15 minutes and then reduced to a rate of 6.6 μg/kg/min^{-1} to maintain 90% to 99% twitch suppression. At the end of infusions of up to 2 hours, no cumulative effects were noted and the mean time for recovery of T_4-to-T_1 ratio greater than 70% was 17 minutes without reversal. When edrophonium or neostigmine was given at the time the infusion was terminated, the T_4-to-T_1 ratio became greater than 70% within 8.2 minutes of edrophonium 0.75 mg/kg administration and 11.2 minutes with neostigmine 0.04 mg/kg. Essentially, rates of recovery from comparable levels of twitch suppression with either single bolus or steady-state infusion are similar. When infusions of mivacurium are used in nitrous oxide–narcotic anesthesia, the mean rate of infusion necessary to maintain a 95% suppression of twitch height is 8.3 μg/kg/min^{-1} (Ali et al., 1988), which is greater than the 6.6-μg/kg/min^{-1} rate during enflurane anesthesia (Goldhill et al., 1991). The equipotent doses of mivacurium have approximately half the duration of vecuronium or atracurium.

In vitro studies have shown that mivacurium is metabolized in a first-order process by pseudocholinesterase and not true cholinesterase, with a $t_{1/2}$ for elimination of 5.3 minutes compared to the $t_{1/2}$ for elimination of succinylcholine by pseudocholinesterase being 2.3 minutes. The rate of hydrolysis of mivacurium by pseudocholinesterase is 70% as fast as for succinylcholine (Cook et al., 1989). Chemical inhibition and qualitative or quantitative abnormalities of pseudocholinesterase prolong the action of mivacurium.

Attempts to speed the onset of paralysis using 4 × ED_{95} (0.30 mg/kg) along with a priming technique produce excellent intubation conditions within 60 seconds (Savarese, Ali, Basta, Embree, & Risner, 1982). Rapid injection of large doses of mivacurium has been associated with transient histamine release and hypotension.

CARDIOVASCULAR EFFECTS. Mivacurium in doses of 0.10 mg/kg or less given IV in 10 to 15 seconds are not associated with facial flushing, significant hemodynamic changes, or histamine release. At doses of 0.25 mg/kg, there is a high incidence of facial flushing associated with increases in plasma histamine and a transient mean reduction in arterial pressure from baseline of 13%. The incidence of facial flushing, hemodynamic changes, and histamine levels associated with mivacurium doses of 0.10 mg/kg given over 10 to 15 seconds could be equivalent to a dose of 0.25 mg/kg if it was given over a 60-second period (Savarese et al., 1989).

Mivacurium is a nondepolarizing agent that is not associated with many of the potential complications of succinylcholine. Its relatively rapid rate of onset and short duration of action should allow for its use in many situations where succinylcholine would have been the drug of choice in the past.

Drug Interactions With Nondepolarizing Muscle Relaxants

Potent Inhalation Anesthetics. The most common drug interaction with nondepolarizing muscle relaxants is the well-documented capability of potent inhalation anesthetics to potentiate all nondepolarizing muscle relaxants to varying degrees. In current clinical practice isoflurane is slightly more potent than enflurane, and both agents are more potent than halothane (Ali & Savarese, 1976). The mechanism of potentiation is probably due to a combination of CNS effects and effects in the postsynaptic surface or in the muscle. Discussion of inhalation agent effects on specific nondepolarizing agents has been included in the presentation of each agent.

Antibiotics. The aminoglycoside antibiotics have both pre- and postjunctional effects that potentiate nondepolarizing muscle relaxants. Aminoglycosides are thought to have an effect similar to that of magnesium, which decreases calcium availability and ACh release (Sokoll & Gergis, 1981). Calcium's ability to only partially reverse the effects of the aminoglycosides demonstrates the existence of both the pre- and postjunctional effects of these agents. Polypeptide antibiotics (polymyxin) have potent neuromuscular blocking properties of their own that are thought to be related to a local anesthetic-like action.

Local Anesthetics. The fast sodium channel–blocking capability of local anesthetics can depress all electrically excitable tissues in a dose-dependent fashion. This action results in decreased transmission of action potentials, the release of neurotransmitter, stabilizing effects on postjunctional membranes, and excitability of muscle cells. Nondepolarizing neuromuscular blockade can be potentiated by all local anesthetics (Matsuo, Rao, Chaudry, & Foldes, 1978).

Anticonvulsants. Phenytoin therapy has been reported to increase the dose of pancuronium, vecuronium, and metocurine necessary to produce satisfactory muscle relaxation (Plotkin & Ornstein, 1986). Carbamazepine has also been reported to produce increased dose requirements for pancuronium (Roth & Ebrahim, 1987).

Diuretics. Furosemide in low doses (<10 µg/kg) potentiates nondepolarizing agents, whereas in high doses (1–4 mg/kg) it antagonizes nondepolarizing agents (Azar, Cottrell, Gupta & Turndorf, 1980; Scappatici, Ham, Sohn, Miller & Dretchen, 1982). It is thought that low-dose furosemide inhibits a protein kinase that decreases cAMP and transmitter release, whereas high doses inhibit phosphodiesterase, which increases cAMP and transmitter release. The mechanism of action for potentiation of muscle relaxants by high-dose furosemide is similar to that reported for aminophylline. Mannitol, a substance that is filtered by the glomerulus and not reabsorbed by the renal tubule, has no direct effect on nondepolarizing relaxants because it does not affect glomerular filtration rates and muscle relaxant excretion (Matteo, Nishitateno, Pua, & Spector, 1980). Although the biphasic effects of furosemide on muscle relaxants have been reported, measurable effects in routine clinical practice may be difficult to observe.

Ionic Effects. Acute changes in potassium concentration alter the transmembrane potential, whereas chronic changes in potassium concentration allow for equilibration of intracellular and extracellular concentrations of potassium and cause no net change in transmembrane potential. Acute hypokalemia produces increased transmembrane potential, and it is more difficult to depolarize a neuron, thereby reducing transmitter release and potentiation of nondepolarizing muscle relaxants. Acute increases in extracellular potassium decrease transmembrane potential, making it easier to depolarize a neuron and increasing transmitter release and reduction in effectiveness of nondepolarizing muscle relaxants.

Increased serum concentrations of magnesium reduce neurotransmitter release presynaptically and reduce the sensitivity of the postjunctional membrane to the neurotransmitter. Magnesium has been shown to potentiate the effects of nondepolarizing muscle relaxants (Ghoneim & Long, 1970).

The effects of lithium are controversial. In a single case report, lithium was found to potentiate muscle relaxation from pancuronium administration (Borden, Clarke, & Katz, 1974). Other evidence indicates that lithium has a negligible effect on the degree of muscle relaxation produced with pancuronium or D-tubocurarine (Waud, Ferrell, & Waud, 1982).

Age and Nondepolarizing Muscle Relaxants

Geriatric Patients. Prolonged duration of action with long-acting nondepolarizing muscle relaxants in elderly patients usually is related to decreased renal or hepatic clearance. Decreased elimination and prolonged duration of action have been demonstrated for the long-acting nondepolarizing muscle relaxants (Matteo et al., 1985). The dose–response curves for elderly and young patients receiving long-acting nondepolarizing muscle relaxants are similar (Matteo et al., 1985). These findings suggest that elderly and young patients require comparable doses of long-acting nondepolarizing muscle relaxants to achieve a given degree of paralysis and that effective paralysis lasts longer in elderly than in young patients. Newer intermediate- or short-acting nondepolarizing muscle relaxants such as atracurium or mivacurium may provide the advantage of more predictable duration of action in elderly patients.

Pediatric Patients. Remarkable differences in the pharmacokinetic data for D-tubocurarine exist between neonates vs adults: The volume of distribution is 0.74 and 0.31 L/kg, the elimination half-time is 174 and 89 minutes, and the ED_{50} plasma concentration is 0.18 and 0.53 $\mu g/mL^{-1}$, respectively. The rate of clearance is similar for neonates and adults 3.7 and 3 $mL/kg/min^{-1}$, respectively (Fisher et al., 1982). It is clear that neonates and infants are more sensitive to the effects of D-tubocurarine. However, the larger volume of distribution in neonates and children than in adults may offset the increased sensitivity to D-tubocurarine and result in similar doses being necessary to produce a given degree of neuromuscular blockade in both neonates and adults (Fisher et al., 1982). Because of the potential for greater variability in response in children, long-acting nondepolarizing agents often are given in increments of one half the adult ED_{95}, and blockade monitoring is used to titrate the dose to the desired effect.

Reversal of Nondepolarizing Muscle Relaxants

Pharmacologic Principles and Practical Considerations. The primary goal of pharmacologic reversal of muscle relaxants is to increase the concentration of ACh present at the myoneural junction. Increasing the concentration of ACh molecules relative to residual nondepolarizing muscle relaxant molecules can prevent binding of the muscle relaxant molecules with ACh receptors by simple mass action competition and allow reversal of residual paralysis. Anticholinesterase drugs are used to inhibit AChE; the resulting inhibition of ACh hydrolysis allows the buildup of ACh necessary to overcome the action of residual muscle relaxant molecules at the myoneural junction. Timely muscle relaxant administration is required to allow the residual concentration of muscle relaxant present at the synapse to be low enough to allow anticholinesterase-induced ACh buildup to compete effectively for available ACh receptor–binding sites. Measurement of peripheral nerve stimulation should show some evidence of spontaneous recovery from nondepolarizing muscle relaxant paralysis before reversal is attempted, and mechanical ventilation should be continued until some evidence of spontaneous recovery is present. None of the recommended doses of anticholinesterase agents are intended to reverse a 100% block successfully. Current anticholinesterase compounds in clinical use are not selective and inhibit both pseudocholinesterase and true cholinesterase. Nonselective inhibition of true cholinesterase allows the accumulation of ACh at all cholinergic synaptic regions both nicotinic and muscarinic. Although the accumulation of ACh at nicotinic cholinergic receptors of the myoneural junction is desirable in this process, the buildup of ACh at nicotinic cholinergic receptors of autonomic ganglia and muscarinic receptors in the autonomic nervous system is accepted as a necessary side effect of the reversal process. To prevent symptoms of a cholinergic crisis that would be similar to those seen with exposure to military nerve agents or organophosphate insecticides (ie, bradycardia, bronchoconstriction, salivation, urination, lacrimation, and defecation), an antimuscarinic agent such as atropine or glycopyrrolate is administered prior to or with the anticholinesterase compound. Antimuscarinic agents are effective in blocking the effects of ACh at muscarinic receptors at the effector origins of the parasympathetic nervous system, but they have not been effective at blocking the effects of ACh at nicotinic cholinergic receptors in the autonomic ganglia.

Available Anticholinesterase Compounds.
Drugs that inhibit AChE are chemically related to the naturally occurring compound eserine or physostigmine, an alkaloid derived from the calibar bean that was used historically by African tribes in witchcraft trials. To someone with a thorough understanding of the autonomic nervous system, the mental image of an individual forced to consume extracts of the calibar bean would be quite repulsive and was probably a significant emotional event for members of the tribes who witnessed this type of ordeal. Physostigmine (Fig. 21-10) is a tertiary amine and, as such, crosses the blood–brain barrier to produce predictable CNS effects. For this reason it is not used to reverse the residual effects of muscle relaxants, but it has

been used in anesthesia as an analeptic to reverse the effects of central anticholinergic syndrome. The synthetic anticholinesterase agents neostigmine, pyridostigmine, and edrophonium (Fig. 21-10) are quaternary ammonium compounds that cross the blood–brain barrier poorly. They are associated with minimal CNS effects and useful agents for reversal of residual muscle relaxant effects.

The organophosphate cholinesterase inhibitor echothiophate (Fig. 21-10) is used in medicine, and other organophosphate inhibitors of AChE are used either in military nerve agents (Taubun®, Saran®, Soman®, VX®) or in insecticides (Malithion®, Parathion®). Useful anticholinesterase compounds in anesthesia produce reversible inhibition of AChE. Organophosphate inhibitors of AChE result in covalent binding of organic phosphate to the esteratic site of the enzyme (Fig. 21-11), which requires hours to regenerate active enzyme or inhibition and may require days or weeks to be overcome by synthesis of new AChE enzyme. Untreated high-dose exposure to potent organophosphate toxins is potentially lethal since physiologically the living organism is not able to survive the toxic effects long enough to regenerate or synthesize active AChE enzyme.

Anticholinesterase Mechanism of Action.
The AChE enzyme can exist in five different states: (1) normally active without substrate present; (2) acetylated; (3) sterically inhibited; (4) carbamylated; and (5) phosphorylated. The enzyme acetylcholinesterase has two active sites, an anionic (negative) site and the esteratic site, which contain the amino acids serine and histidine that can interact to donate a pair of electrons to break ester bonds. Under normal conditions the cationic (positive) quaternary ammonium portion of ACh is attracted to the anionic region of AChE, whereas the esteratic site interacts with the ester bond between choline and acetate. The electrons transferred from the serine residue allow choline to split off, leaving acetylated AChE enzyme that cannot be enzymatically active until reactivated. Within microseconds hydrolysis splits off acetate from the acetylated enzyme, leaving regenerated or active AChE enzyme and free acetate (Fig. 21-12).

Edrophonium lacks a carbamate group and inhibits AChE by electrostatic interaction with the anionic site and hydrogen bonding at the esteratic site of AChE. The competitive reversible steric obstruction of AChE that edrophonium produces prevents interaction between AChE and substrate ACh. This action results in the accumulation of ACh as long as effective concentrations of edrophonium are present at the synapse (Fig. 21-13).

The anticholinesterase agents neostigmine, pyridostigmine, and prostigmine are carbamate-containing compounds. These carbamate ester cholinesterase inhibitors are competitive substrates for the AChE, and the

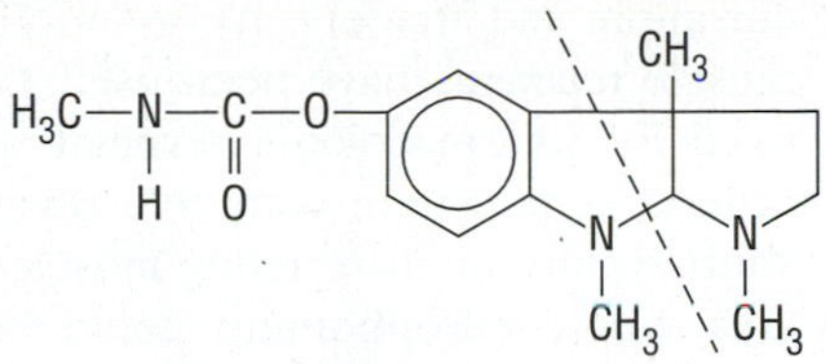

Figure 21–10. The chemical structure of some reversible and irreversible acetylcholinesterase inhibitors. The tertiary structure of physostigmine results in significant inhibition of acetylcholinesterase in the CNS. Physostigmine, neostigmine, and pyridostigmine produce reversible carbamylation of the esteratic site of acetylcholinesterase. Edrophonium, a hydroxy analog of neostigmine, lacks a carbamate group and is unable to carbamylate acetylcholinesterase enzyme. The interaction of the quaternary amine group of edrophonium with the anionic site of acetylcholinesterase inhibits the capability of acetylcholinesterase to hydrolize acetylcholine. Echothiopate is an organophosphate, irreversible inhibitor of acetylcholinesterase, and is commonly used as a topical miotic drug to treat glaucoma.

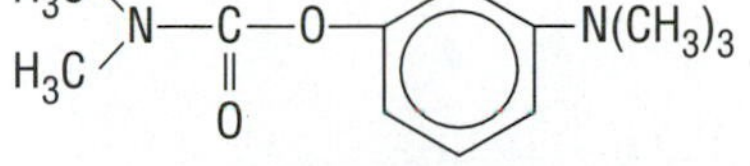

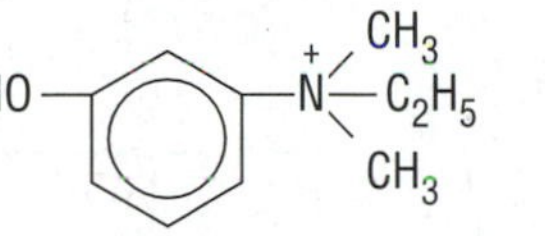

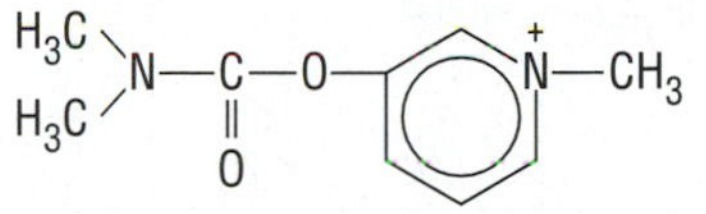

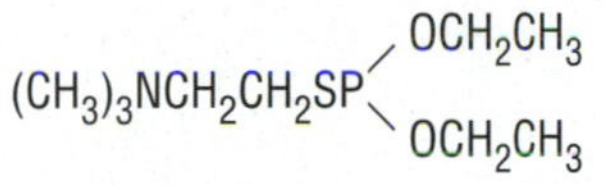

drug that binds to the AChE is metabolized by the esteratic site. Neostigmine and pyridostigmine interact with the anionic and esteratic site of AChE in the same manner as does ACh. When the esteratic site breaks the ester bond of carbamate-containing anticholinesterase agents, the carbamate portion of the molecule covalently binds to the esteratic site, resulting in a carbamylated AChE that is unable to breakdown ACh until the carbamate group is removed from the enzyme (Fig. 21–14). Unlike acetylated AChE, carbamylated enzyme is much more resistant to regeneration by hydrolysis and has a half-time for regeneration that is measured in minutes rather than microseconds for acetylated enzyme regeneration. Competitive inhibition of AChE with anticholinesterase agents is what many practitioners commonly think of when considering muscle relaxant reversal. The action of cholinesterase-inhibiting agents is more complex than simple AChE inhibition. Anticholinesterase drugs can generate antidromic action potentials and repetitive firing of motor nerve endings (Donati, Ferguson, & Bevan, 1983). Anticholinesterase agents are also capable of directly depolarizing motor nerve terminals and choliner-

gic receptors on the postsynaptic surface. These actions increase mobilization and release of ACh to the synapse at the myoneural junction and aid in competing for available binding sites on the alpha-subunits of the receptor to prevent binding of the depolarizing muscle relaxant. Anticholinesterase reversal of muscle relaxants is a combination of AChE inhibiton as well as direct pre- and postsynaptic effects of these agents.

The elimination of anticholinesterase agents depends on renal and hepatic function for elimination. Nondepolarizing muscle relaxants other than atracurium and mivacurium are also dependent on renal function for elimination. If anticholinesterase agents are used to reverse nondepolarizing muscle relaxants in patients with decreased renal function, the anticholinesterase drug should be eliminated as fast or faster than the muscle relaxant (Cronnelly, Stanski, & Miller, 1979; Cronnelly, Stanski, Miller, & Sheiner, 1980). This should make the occurrence of recurarization unlikely, leaving the remaining concern of a long-acting antimuscarinic agent to prevent the reappearance of muscarinic side effects. The entire question of recurarization in patients with renal disease

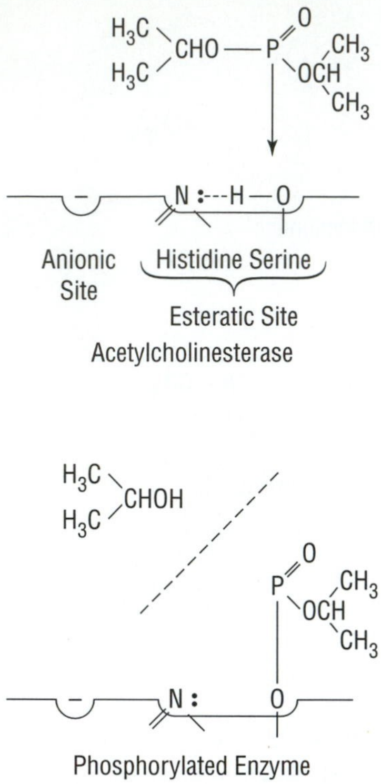

Figure 21–11. Organophosphate acetylcholinesterase drugs produce irreversible inhibition by forming a covalent bond at the esteratic site of the enzyme. The phosphorylated enzyme bond becomes more resistant to regeneration by hydrolysis due to "ageing," which involves the loss of alkyl side chains from the organophosphate molecule.

could be eliminated by choosing a muscle relaxant that does not depend on renal function for elimination.

Clinical Use of Specific Anticholinesterase Agents

EDROPHONIUM. In doses of 0.5 mg/kg edrophonium produces antagonism of residual nondepolarizing muscle relaxant paralysis that is equivalent in magnitude and duration to that seen with 0.043 mg/kg neostigmine (Cronnelly, Morris, & Miller, 1982). Because of edrophonium's rapid onset and lower potential for muscarinic side effects, atropine in doses of 7 µg/kg has been recommended to be given with edrophonium 0.5 mg/kg (Cronnelly, Morris, & Miller, 1982). If reversal with edrophonium is inadequate after the initial 0.5-mg/kg dose, an additional 0.25 mg/kg with atropine can be repeated. In cases where twitch height has returned to only 10% of control, 1 mg/kg edrophonium may be required to produce a rate of reversal that is equal to that for neostigmine (Rupp, McChristian, Miller, Taboada, & Cronnelly, 1986). Edrophonium is probably best suited for cases where TOF monitoring demonstrates the presence of 2 to 3 twitches with fade or where intermediate-acting (ve-

curonium and atracurium) or short-acting (mivacurium) muscle relaxants have been used. Controversy over the need for pharmacologic reversal when all monitoring criteria demonstrate complete reversal after the use of short- or intermediate-acting muscle relaxants may be an area where edrophonium could be helpful. Edropho-

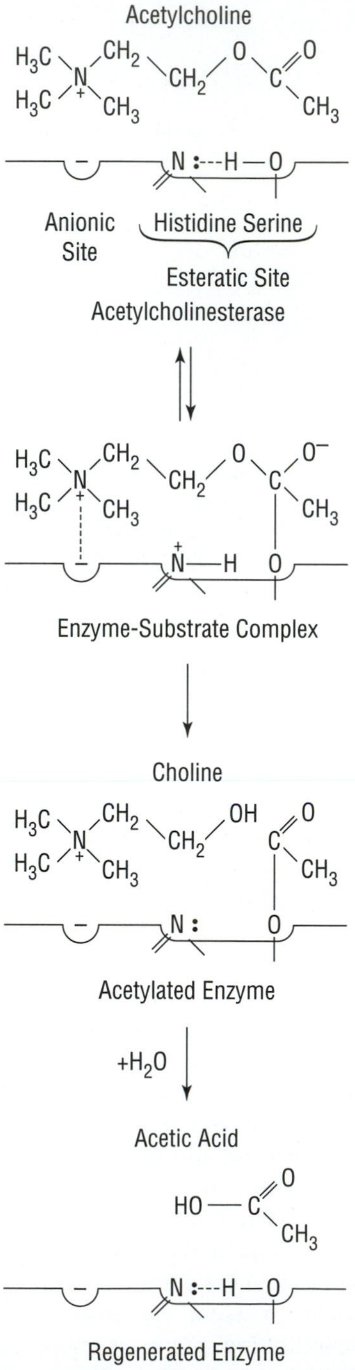

Figure 21–12. Hydrolysis of acetylcholine by acetylcholinesterase and the interaction of acetylcholine with the anionic and esteratic sites of the acetylcholinesterase enzyme. The third panel shows acetylated enzyme regenerated by hydrolysis in the fourth panel, resulting in free acetate and regenerated acetylcholinesterase.

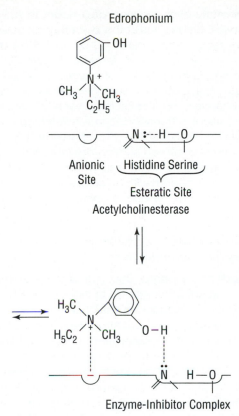

Figure 21–13. Interaction of edrophonium with the acetylcholinesterase enzyme.

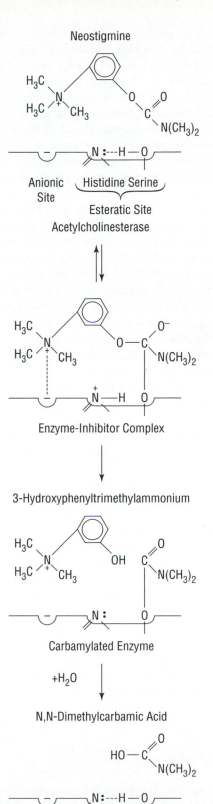

Figure 21–14. Interaction between neostigmine and the acetylcholinesterase enzyme. The breakdown of neostigmine by acetylcholinesterase results in carbamylated enzyme seen in panel three. Regeneration of active acetylcholinesterase enzyme by hydrolysis in panel four proceeds at a slower pace than does the regeneration of acetylated enzyme that was seen in Figure 21–12.

nium has the capability to reverse the subclinical effects of muscle relaxants, increase the margin of saftey for neuromuscular transmission, and reduce the potential for recurarization to the lowest point possible with minimal muscarinic side effects. Clinicians who, if only for litiginous reasons, believe that pharmacologic reversal of subclinical effects of nondepolarizing muscle relaxants is necessary may find edrophonium to be a reasonable choice. Onset of peak neuromuscular blocking antagonism is less than 5 minutes with edrophonium, whereas peak effects of neostigmine require 7 to 10 minutes (Cronnelly et al., 1982). It is difficult for this author to envision an efficient surgical team precise enough to justify the use of edrophonium based on a 2- to 5-minute shorter time to maximal reversal producing a significant difference in the patient's overall anesthetic time. Edrophonium has not been recommended for reversal with the new long-acting muscle relaxants pipecuronium or doxacurium due to either inadequate reversal or decreased safety margin of reversal and potential for recurarization.

NEOSTIGMINE. Neostigmine is an anticholinesterase drug that is suitable for reversal of all nondepolarizing muscle relaxants at any depth of residual paralysis as long as some evidence of spontaneous reversal is demonstrated by blockade monitoring. The usual dose of neostigmine is 35 to 40 µg/kg given with either 15 µg/kg atropine or 7.5 µg/kg glycopyrrolate. This dose may be repeated one time if satisfactory reversal is not evident after the initial dose. Maximal inhibition of AChE is achieved with neostigmine doses of 70 to 80 µg/kg; should this dose produce incomplete reversal, positive pressure ventilation to support respiration should be continued until neuromuscular blockade dissipates with time.

Glycopyrrolate's onset and duration of antimuscarinic action are better matched to the onset and duration of the anticholinesterase action of neostigmine or pyridostigmine. Simultaneous administration of glycopyrrolate with neostigmine or pyridostigmine produces reversal of residual paralysis with minimal change in heart rate (Salem, Richardson, Meadows, Lamplugh, & Lai, 1985). Glycopyrrolate is a tertiary amine and does not cross the blood–brain barrier to the degree atropine does to produce CNS depression. Patients who receive glycopyrrolate with neostigmine for reversal show more rapid arousal than patients who receive atropine neostigmine reversal (Sheref, 1985).

PYRIDOSTIGMINE. When compared with neostigmine and edrophonium, pyridostigmine is the anticholinesterase agent with the slowest onset time to maximum reversal (12–15 minutes) and the longest duration of action (Cronnelly et al., 1982). The average dose is 150 to 200 µg/kg and is given with either atropine 15 µg/kg or glycopyrrolate 7.5 µg/kg. As with neostigmine, this dose may be repeated one time if the first dose does not produce adequate reversal. If the second dose fails to produce complete reversal of residual paralysis, positive pressure ventilation should be used to support ventilation until time dissipates the effects of the muscle relaxant. During this time patient comfort must be ensured by providing analgesia and sedation if needed. When compared to neostigmine, pyridostigmine has been associated with a lower incidence of arrhythmias in the elderly.

▶ Case Study

A 28-year-old, 80-kg gravida 2 para 1, ASA 2E, white female presents to the labor unit for induction of labor with a diagnosis of postdates gestation at 41 weeks. The patient has a negative medical history with no preexisting medical or surgical conditions and no prior anesthetic administration. Admission laboratory findings show a hemoglobin of 11 g, hematocrit of 33%, and platelet count of 186 000 mm³. Induction of labor with pitocin infusion pro-

ceeds normally over a period of 5 hours to a point of 4 cm cervical dilation. It is at this point that an episode of persistent fetal bradycardia of 80 beats per minute develops. No improvement in fetal bradycardia is noted with maternal administration of oxygen at 10 L/min by face mask, termination of pitocin infusion, or maternal position change to right or left lateral or knee–chest position. The patient is transported immediately to the labor and delivery operative suite and prepared and draped for an emergency cesarean section delivery. During preparation for surgery the anesthesia history is obtained. The patient is premedicated with 30 cc of sodium bicitrate PO and lidocaine 75 mg IV prior to induction of general endotracheal anesthesia.

1. What general anesthetic, drug doses, and management are indicated?

Sodium thiopental 350 mg and succinylcholine 80 mg are administered to induce anesthesia using a rapid-sequence induction technique following preoxygenation. After verification of endotracheal tube placement, cricoid pressure is released and the surgical procedure commences. Anesthesia is maintained with nitrous oxide–oxygen in a 50%–50% mixture with 0.5% isoflurane until delivery of the infant. Three minutes after induction of anesthesia the infant is delivered with 1- and 5-minute Apgar scores of 5 and 9, respectively. For the remaining 15 minutes of operative time, anesthesia is maintained with nitrous oxide–oxygen mixture of 65%–35% with 0.5% isoflurane. Fentanyl 0.25 µg and 20 mg of a 0.2% succinylcholine infusion to facilitate closure are administered. On return of spontaneous ventilation with 100% O_2 and verification of antagonism of neuromuscular blockade with the peripheral nerve stimulator and sustained head lift for 5 seconds, the patient is extubated and transferred to the recovery room in stable condition. She is awake and oriented.

Thirty minutes after arrival in the recovery room, the patient's heart rate gradually increases from 100 to 149 beats per minute and her blood pressure decreases from 120/80 to 80/30 mmHg. Only 10 mL of urine output has been measured since the end of the operative procedure. Fundal massage only mildly improves poor uterine tone. However, fundal massage is accompanied by a large amount of bright bloody vaginal discharge. Continued pitocin infusion and 0.2 mg methergine IM fails to decrease vaginal bleeding. The hematocrit drops to 21%. The estimated blood loss from the cesarean section was 800 mL with intraoperative replacement of 1400 mL of Ringer's lactate solution. An additional 14-gauge peripheral IV infusion is started, and two 500-mL boluses of Ringer's lactate solution, two units of packed red blood cells, and 600 mL of 0.9% isotonic saline are administered. This produces a decrease in heart rate to 130 and the systolic blood pressure remains in the low 90 mmHg range with no improvement in urine output. Continued fundal massage produces large amounts of vaginal bloody discharge. In addition, blood was noted to be draining from the cesarean section incision. It is decided to take the patient to the surgical suite for an abdominal exploration.

2. Describe the anesthetic technique and muscle relaxant that might be selected for the second surgery.

   Anesthesia is induced with 50 mg of ketamine because of the patient's hemodynamic instability and 80 mg succinylcholine for rapid-sequence intubation with cricoid pressure. Anesthesia is maintained with 100% oxygen, 0.5% isoflurane, and intravenous fentanyl boluses as indicated by vital signs. Two milligrams of midazolam are administered IV for amnesia. Surgical exploration reveals a suprafascial hematoma of approximately 200 mL with no obvious site of bleeding and a large "boggy" uterus that is unresponsive to IM methergine or intrauterine hemabate. At this point, the surgical team decides to proceed with an emergency hysterectomy.

3. What change, if any, should be made in the selection of anesthetics and muscle relaxants?

   Because a longer surgical time than that needed for the cesarean section is anticipated, an intermediate-acting nondepolarizing agent is appropriate. When the peripheral nerve stimulator shows return of neuromuscular function to baseline TOF and tetanic stimulation without fade, neuromuscular blockade is induced with 0.05 mg/kg of vecuronium and maintained with a vecuronium bolus as needed according to the patient's response as measured by the peripheral nerve stimulator. Additional laboratory studies measured during the 2-hour surgical procedure reveal a PTT of 54 seconds with a control of 20 seconds, platelet count of 50 000 mm^3, fibrinogen of 100 mg/dL, and hematocrit of 25%. Estimated blood loss with the second procedure is 3000 mL, for which the patient receives an additional four units of packed red blood cells, 3 L of Ringer's lactate solution, 1.5 L of 0.9% isotonic saline, one unit of platelet concentrate, and one unit of fresh-frozen plasma.

4. Should neuromuscular blockade be antagonized at the end of the hysterectomy procedure, and, if so, what drug therapy should be considered?

At the completion of the surgical procedure, there is no indication to keep the patient on controlled ventilation postoperatively, so residual neuromuscular blockade is antagonized with a neostigmine–glycopyrrolate mixture based on the patient's ideal body weight. After full return of neuromuscular function following antagonism of the muscle relaxant, the patient is extubated and transported to the surgical intensive care unit. The patient is awake and oriented with a stable heart rate and blood pressure, but persistent oliguria of 15 to 30 mL/hr continues into the early postoperative phase. After a complicated intensive care admission that requires reintubation and positive pressure ventilation at the end of the first postoperative day and an exploratory laparotomy on the second postoperative cesarean section–hysterectomy day, the patient ultimately is discharged from the hospital without further complication.

Although this case could be used to make many excellent teaching points, it is presented in this chapter to emphasize the fact that succinylcholine continues to have a place in rapid-sequence induction, especially for the obstetric patient who presents for cesarean section or other operative procedures. It also illustrates the successful use of a nondepolarizing muscle relaxant for a subsequent procedure in the same patient.

▶ SUMMARY

Successful use of muscle relaxants requires adherence to three principles: acquisition of knowledge, vigilant monitoring, and titration of dose to desired effect. Comprehensive knowledge of the pharmacology of all muscle relaxants allows the practitioner both to choose the muscle relaxant best suited to the surgical procedure the patient will have and to assess the general medical condition of the patient. Frequent assessment of neuromuscular junction status with peripheral nerve stimulation monitoring allows rational decisions about the extent and nature of paralysis present and the necessity of additional muscle relaxant doses. Based on the results of vigilant monitoring, the size and timing of additional muscle relaxant doses can be titrated to produce adequate paralysis during the procedure and allow for some degree of spontaneous recovery prior to the time for reversal at the end of the anesthetic. With adherence to these principles, rapid reversal of residual paralysis is possible, a high margin of safety for neuromuscular conduction after reversal is present, and low or no incidence of recurarization is noted.

▶ KEY CONCEPTS

- In patients receiving neuromuscular blocking agents, loss of muscle strength is not noted until 75% of the available receptors are occupied by the muscle relaxant, and normal function returns when 25% of available receptors are available to interact with ACh.
- Clinical evaluation of adequate reversal of neuromuscular blockade includes the ability to sustain head lift, adequate vital capacity, negative inspiratory force, hand grasp, or the capability to keep the arms in an extended position.
- Train of four (TOF) monitoring is the most sensitive measure of neuromuscular function as measured by a peripheral nerve stimulator. The ratio between the amplitude of the fourth twitch (T_4) to the amplitude of the first twitch (T_1) often is used to determine the degree of nondepolarizing neuromuscular blockade. A ratio of T_4 to T_1 amplitude of 0.5 to 0.7 generally indicates satisfactory return of muscle function following administration of nondepolarizing muscle relaxants.
- Nondepolarizing blockade and competitive blockade are reversible processes that result from the drug binding competitively to the two alpha subunits of the ACh receptor, blocking the effects of ACh and preventing depolarization and neuromuscular transmission. Drugs in this class can be considered by duration of action: short-acting, intermediate-acting, and long-acting.
- Depolarizing neuromuscular blockade results when drugs with agonistic properties similar to those of succinylcholine depolarize the motor end-plate and generate an end-plate potential (EPP). The most commonly used drug in this classification is succinylcholine.
- Phase II block has occurred following succinylcholine administration, in which the normal depolarizing phase I block is converted to a nondepolarizing-type phase II block after excessive single doses or continuous infusions of succinylcholine for a long time. Although this type of block may be antagonized by anticholinesterase drugs, conservative clinicians may choose to support ventilation and let time reverse a phase II block.
- Succinylcholine is metabolized by pseudocholinesterase. Problems related to reductions in quality or quantity of pseudocholinesterase present to metabolize succinylcholine result in an unexpected prolongation of neuromuscular blockade after apparently normal doses of the drug.
- Liver dysfunction, pregnancy, and starvation or some eating disorders have been shown to reduce the amount of pseudocholinesterase produced. In addition, atypical enzymes have been reported in some individuals.
- Because succinylcholine produces muscle fasciculations with a release of potassium often increasing serum potassium levels about 0.5 to 1 mEq/L, use of this drug is generally contraindicated in patients who may have an elevated serum potassium level, such as burn patients or massive trauma patients.
- The popularity of nondepolarizing muscle relaxants for most procedures including induction of anesthesia has increased because of the ability of this class of drugs to be antagonized by anticholinesterase agents that allow ACh to accumulate at the synapse, promoting the return of normal neuromuscular function.

▶ STUDY QUESTIONS

1. What are the clinical variables to observe and measure when monitoring neuromuscular function? Compare the variables during induction, maintenance, and emergence from anesthesia.

2. What are the different characteristics of a nondepolarizing block, a depolarizing block, and a Phase II block? What is the physiologic significance of fade following train-of-four and tetanic stimulation and post-tetanic facilitation?

3. Why would a patient response to succinylcholine be prolonged? Describe two clinical situations.

4. Why is cisatracurium an appropriate drug for muscular relaxation in the patient with cardiac disease?

5. What is the pharmacologic mechanism of action of the anticholinesterase, edrophonium? What is the role of anticholinergic drugs during antagonism of neuromuscular blockade?

6. Why does the time of onset of neuromuscular blockade decrease with increasing doses of rocuronium?

KEY REFERENCES

Ali, H. H. & Savarese, J. J. (1976). Monitoring of neuromuscular function. *Anesthesiology, 45,* 216–249.

Ali, H. H., Savarese, J. J., Embree, P. B., Basta, S. J., Stout, R. G., Bottros, L. H., & Weakly, J. N. (1988). Clinical pharmacology of mivacurium chloride (BW B1090U) infusion: Comparison with vecuronium and atracurium. *British Journal of Anaesthesia, 61,* 541–546.

Ali, H. H., Savarese, J. J., Lebowitz, P. W., & Ramsey, F. M. (1981). Twitch, tetanus, and train-of-four as indices of recovery from nondepolarizing neuromuscular blockade. *Anesthesiology, 54,* 294–297.

Basta, S. J., Ali, H. H., Savarese, J. J., Sunder, N., Gionfriddo, M., Cloutier, G., Lineberry C., & Cato, A. E. (1982). Clinical pharmacology of atracurium besylate (BW33A): A new nondepolarizing muscle relaxant. *Anesthesia & Analgesia, 61,* 723–729.

Basta, S. J., Savarese, J. J., & Ali, H. H. (1988). Clinical pharmacology of doxacurium chloride: A new long-acting nondepolarizing muscle relaxant. *Anesthesiology, 69,* 478–486.

Boros, M., Szenohradszky, J., Marosi, G. Y., & Toth, I. (1980). Comparative clinical study of pipecuronium bromide and pancuronium bromide. *Arzneimittel-Forschung Drug Research, 30,* 389–393.

Bowman, W. C. (1980). Prejunctional and postjunctional cholinoceptors at the neuromuscular junction. *Anesthesia & Analgesia, 59,* 935–943.

Boyd, A. H., Eastwood, N. B., Parker, C. J., & Hunter, J. M. (1996). Comparison of the pharmacodynamics and pharmacokinetics of an infusion of cis-atracurium (51W89) or atracurium in critically ill patients undergoing mechanical ventilation in an intensive care unit. *British Journal of Anaesthesia, 76,* 382–388.

Brandom, B. W., Woelfel, S. K., Cook, D. R., Weber, S., Powers, D. M., & Weakly, J. N. (1989). Comparison of mivacurium and suxamethonium administered by bolus and infusion. *British Journal of Anaesthesia, 62,* 488–493.

Caldwell, J. E., Castagnoli, K. P., Canfell, P. C., Fahey, M. R., Lynam, D. P., Fisher, D. M., & Miller, R. D. (1988). Pipecuronium and pancuronium: Comparison of pharmacokinetics and duration of action. *British Journal of Anaesthesia, 61,* 693–697.

Caldwell, J. E., Heier, T., Kitts, J. B., Lynam, D. P., Fahey, M. R., & Miller, R. D. (1989). Comparison of the neuromuscular block induced by mivacurium, suxamethonium or atracurium during nitrous oxide–fentanyl anaesthesia. *British Journal of Anaesthesia, 63,* 393–399.

Cook, D. R., Stiller, R. L., Weakly, J. N., Chakravorti, S., Brandom, B. W., & Welch, R. M. (1989). In vitro metabolism of mivacurium chloride (BW B1090U) and succinylcholine. *Anesthesia & Analgesia, 68,* 452–456.

Donati, F., & Bevan, D. R. (1985). Antagonism of phase II succinylcholine block by neostigmine. *Anesthesia & Analgesia, 64,* 773–776.

Donati, F., Ferguson, A., & Bevan, D. R. (1983). Twitch depression and train-of-four ratio after antagonism of pancuronium with edrophonium, neostigmine, or pyridostigmine. *Anesthesia & Analgesia, 62,* 314–316.

Fahey, M. R., Morris, R. B., Miller, R. D., Sohn, Y. J., Cronnelly, R., & Gencarelli, P. (1981). Clinical pharmacology of ORG NC45 (Norcuron™): A new nondepolarizing muscle relaxant. *Anesthesiology, 55,* 6–11.

Foldes, F. F., McNall, P. G., & Borrengo-Hinojosa, J. M. (1952). Succinylcholine: A new approach to muscular relaxation in anesthesiology. *New England Journal of Medicine, 247,* 596–600.

Gissen, A. J. & Katz, R. L. (1969). Twitch, tetanus, and post-tetanic potentiation as indices of nerve–muscle block in man. *Anesthesiology, 30,* 491–497.

Griffith, H. R. & Johnson, G. E. (1942). The use of curare in general anesthesia. *Anesthesiology, 3,* 418–420.

Hughes, R. & Chapple, D. J. (1981). The pharmacology of atracurium: A new competitive neuromuscular blocking agent. *British Journal of Anaesthesia, 53,* 31–44.

Hughes, R., Ingram, G., & Payne, J. P. (1976). Studies on dimethyltubocurarine in anaesthetized man. *British Journal of Anaesthesia, 48,* 969–974.

Jones, R. J. (1980, April). Use of the peripheral nerve stimulator. *American Academy of Nurse Anesthetists Journal, 48,* 152–154.

Ka'rpa'ti, E., & Bir'o, K. (1980). Pharmacological study of a new competitive neuromuscular blocking steroid, pipecuronium bromide. *Arzneimittel-Forschung Drug Research, 30,* 346–354.

Katz, R. L. (Ed.). (1975). *Muscle relaxants.* Amsterdam: Excerpta Medica.

Larijani, G. E., Bartkowski, R. R., Azad, S. S., Seltzer, J. L., Weinberger, M. J., Beach, C. A., & Goldberg, M. E. (1989). Clinical pharmacology of pipecuronium bromide. *Anesthesia & Analgesia, 68,* 734–739.

Lebowitz, P. W., Ramsey, R. M., & Savarese, J. J. (1981). Combination of pancuronium and metocurine: Neuromuscular and hemodynamic advantages over pancuronium alone. *Anesthesia & Analgesia, 60,* 12–16.

Leighton, B. L., Cheek, T. G., Gross, J. B., Apfelbaum, J. L., Shantz, B. B., Gutsche, B. B., & Rosenberg, H. (1986). Succinylcholine pharmacodynamics in peripartum patients. *Anesthesiology, 64,* 202–205.

Naguib, M., Abdulatif, M., Gyasi, H. K., Khawaji, Y., & Absood, G. H. (1987). The pattern of train-of-four fade after atracurium: Influence of different priming doses. *Anesthesia & Analgesia, 66,* 427–430.

Rupp, S. M., McChristian, J. W., Miller, R. D., Taboada, J. A., & Cronnelly, R. (1986). Neostigmine and edrophonium antagonism of varying intensity of neuromuscular blockade induced by atracurium, pancuronium, or vecuronium. *Anesthesiology, 64,* 711–714.

Scott, R. P. F. & Savarese, J. J. (1985). The cardiovascular and autonomic effects of neuromuscular blocking agents. *Seminars in Anesthesiology, 3,* 319–334.

Taylor, P. (1985). Are neuromuscular blocking agents more efficacious in pairs? *Anesthesiology, 63,* 1–3.

Waud, B. E. & Waud, D. R. (1971). The relation between tetanic fade and receptor occlusion in the presence of competitive neuromuscular block. *Anesthesiology, 35,* 456–464.

Waud, B. E. & Waud, D. R. (1972). The relation between the response to "train-of-four" stimulation and receptor occlusion during competitive neuromuscular blockade. *Anesthesiology, 37,* 413–416.

REFERENCES

Agoston, S., Vermeer, G. A., Kersten, U. W., & Scaf, A. H. (1978). A preliminary investigation of the renal and hepatic excretion of gallamine triethoiodide in man. *British Journal of Anaesthesia, 50,* 345–351.

Ali, H. H. & Savarese, J. J. (1976). Monitoring of neuromuscular function. *Anesthesiology, 45,* 216–249.

Ali, H. H. & Savarese, J. J. (1980). Stimulus frequency and the dose response to D-tubocurarine in man. *Anesthesiology, 52,* 35–39.

Ali, H. H., Savarese, J. J., Embree, P. B., Basta, S. J., Stout, R. G., Bottros, L. H., & Weakly, J. N. (1988). Clinical pharmacology of mivacurium chloride (BW B1090U) infusion: Comparison with vecuronium and atracurium. *British Journal of Anaesthesia, 61,* 541–546.

Ali, H. H., Savarese, J. J., Lebowitz, P. W., & Ramsey, F. M. (1981). Twitch, tetanus, and train-of-four as indices of recovery from nondepolarizing neuromuscular blockade. *Anesthesiology, 54,* 294–297.

Azar, I., Cottrell, J., Gupta, B., & Turndorf, H. (1980). Furosemide facilitates recovery of evoked twitch response after pancuronium. *Anesthesia & Analgesia, 59,* 55–57.

Basta, S. J., Ali, H. H., Savarese, J. J., Sunder, N., Gionfriddo, M., Cloutier, G., Lineberry C., & Cato, A. E. (1982). Clinical pharmacology of atracurium besylate (BW33A): A new nondepolarizing muscle relaxant. *Anesthesia & Analgesia, 61,* 723–729.

Basta, S. J., Savarese, J. J., & Ali, H. H. (1988). Clinical pharmacology of doxacurium chloride: A new long-acting nondepolarizing muscle relaxant. *Anesthesiology, 69,* 478–486.

Beecher, H. K., & Todd, D. P. (1940). A study of deaths with anesthesia and surgery. *Annals of Surgery, 140,* 2–34.

Bell, C. F., Hunter, J. M., Jones, R. S., & Utting, J. E. (1985). Use of atracurium and vecuronium in patients with esophageal varices. *British Journal of Anaesthesia, 57,* 160–168.

Belmont, M., Beemer, G., Bownes, P., Wastila, W., & Savarese, J. J. (1993). Comparative pharmacology of atracurium and one of its isomers, 51W89, in rhesus monkeys. *Anesthesiology, 79,* A947.

Belmont, M. R., Lien, C. A., Quessy, S., Abou-Donia, M. M., Abalos, A., Eppich, L., & Savarese, J. J. (1995). The clinical neuromuscular pharmacology of 51W89 in patients receiving nitrous oxide/opioid/barbiturate anesthesia. *Anesthesiology, 82,* 1139–1145.

Bencini, A. F., Houwertjes, M. C., & Agoston, S. (1985). Effects of hepatic uptake of vecuronium bromide and its putative metabolites on their neuromuscular blocking actions in the cat. *British Journal of Anaesthesia, 57,* 789–795.

Bencini, A. F., Scaf, A. H., Sohn, Y. J., Meistelman, C., Lienhart, A., Kersten, U. W., Schwarz, S., & Agoston, S. (1986). Disposition and urinary excretion of vecuronium bromide in anesthetized patients with normal renal function or renal failure. *Anesthesia & Analgesia, 65,* 245–251.

Bennett, A. E. (1940). Preventing traumatic complications in convulsive shock therapy by curare. *Journal of the American Medical Association, 114,* 322–324.

Borden, H., Clarke, M. T., & Katz, H. (1974). The use of pancuronium in patients receiving lithium carbonate. *Canadian Anaesthesia Society Journal, 21,* 79–82.

Boros, M., Szenohradszky, J., Marosi, G. Y., & Toth, I. (1980). Comparative clinical study of pipecuronium bromide and pancuronium bromide. *Arzneimittel-Forschung Drug Research, 30,* 389–393.

Bowman, W. C. (1980). Prejunctional and postjunctional cholinoceptors at the neuromuscular junction. *Anesthesia & Analgesia, 59,* 935–943.

Bowman, W. C., Marshall, I. G., & Gibb, A. J. (1984). Is there feedback control of transmitter release at the neuromuscular junction? *Seminars in Anesthesiology, 3,* 275–283.

Boyd, A. H., Eastwood, N. B., Parker, C. J., & Hunter, J. M. (1996). Comparison of the pharmacodynamics and pharmacokinetics of an infusion of *cis*-atracurium (51W89) or atracurium in critically ill patients undergoing mechanical ventilation in an intensive care unit. *British Journal of Anaesthesia, 76,* 382–388.

Brandom, B. W., Woelfel, S. K., Cook, D. R., Weber, S., Powers, D. M., & Weakly, J. N. (1989). Comparison of mivacurium and suxamethonium administered by bolus and infusion. *British Journal of Anaesthesia, 62,* 488–493.

Brotherton, W. P., & Matteo, R. S. (1981). Pharmacokinetics and pharmacodynamics of metocurine in humans with and without renal failure. *Anesthesiology, 55,* 272–276.

Brown, B. R., & Crout, J. R. (1970). The sympathomimetic effect of gallamine on the heart. *Journal of Pharmacology and Experimental Therapeutics, 172,* 266–273.

Caldwell, J. E., Canfell, P. C., Catagnoli, K. P., Lynam, D. P., Fahey, M. R., Fisher, D. M., & Miller, R. D. (1989). The influence of renal failure on the pharmacokinetics and the duration of action of pipecuronium bromide in patients anesthetized with halothane and nitrous oxide. *Anesthesiology, 70,* 7–12.

Caldwell, J. E., Castagnoli, K. P., Canfell, P. C., Fahey, M. R., Lynam, D. P., Fisher, D. M., & Miller, R. D. (1988). Pipecuronium and pancuronium: Comparison of pharmacokinetics and duration of action. *British Journal of Anaesthesia, 61,* 693–697.

Caldwell, J. E., Heier, T., Kitts, J. B., Lynam, D. P., Fahey, M. R., & Miller, R. D. (1989). Comparison of the neuromuscular block induced by mivacurium, suxamethonium or atracurium during nitrous oxide-fentanyl anaesthesia. *British Journal of Anaesthesia, 63,* 393–399.

Caldwell, J .E., Kitts, J. B., Heier, T., Fahey, M. R., Lynam, D. P., & Miller, R. D. (1989). The dose–response relationship of mivacurium chloride in humans during nitrous oxide–fentanyl or nitrous oxide–enflurane anesthesia. *Anesthesiology, 70,* 31–35.

Carter, J. G., & Sokoll, M. D. (1981). Effect of spinal cord transection on neuromuscular function in the rat. *Anesthesiology, 55,* 542–546.

Chapple, D. J., Miller, A. A., Ward, J. B., & Wheatley, P. L. (1987). Cardiovascular and neurologic loss effects of laudanosine. *British Journal of Anaesthesia, 59,* 218–225.

Chatterji, S., Thind, S. S., & Daga, S. R. (1983). Lignocaine pretreatment for suxamethonium. A clinicobiochemical study. *Anaesthesia, 38,* 867–870.

Cohen, E. N., Corbascio, A., & Fleischli, G. (1965). The distribution and fate of D-tubocurarine. *Journal of Pharmacology and Experimental Therapeutics, 147,* 120–129.

Cook, D. R., Stiller, R. L., Weakly, J. N., Chakravorti, S., Brandom, B. W., & Welch, R. M. (1989). In vitro metabolism of mivacurium chloride (BW B1090U) and succinylcholine. *Anesthesia & Analgesia, 68,* 452–456.

Cook, J. H. (1981). The effect of suxamethonium on intraocular pressure. *Anaesthesia, 36,* 359–365.

Cronnelly, R., Morris, R. B., & Miller, R. D. (1982). Edrophonium: Duration of action and atropine requirement in humans during halothane anesthesia. *Anesthesiology, 57,* 261–266.

Cronnelly, R., Stanski, D. R., & Miller, R. D. (1979). Renal function and the pharmacokinetics of neostigmine in anesthetized man. *Anesthesiology, 51,* 222–226.

Cronnelly, R., Stanski, D. R., Miller, R. D., & Sheiner, L. B. (1980). Pyridostigmine kinetics with and without renal function. *Clinical Pharmacology and Therapeutics, 28,* 78–81.

Davies, A. O. (1983). Oral diazepam premedication reduces the incidence of post-succinylcholine muscle pains. *Canadian Anaesthesia Society Journal, 30,* 603–606.

deBros, F. M., Lai, A., Scott, R., deBros, J., Batson, A. G., Goudsouzian, N., Ali, H. H., Cosini, A. B., & Savarese, J. J. (1986). Pharmacokinetics and pharmacodynamics of atracurium during isoflurane anesthesia in normal and anephric patients. *Anesthesia & Analgesia, 65,* 743–746.

Del Castillo, J., & Katz, B. (1954). Quantal components of the end-plate potential. *Journal of Physiology, 124,* 560–573.

Denborough, M. A., Forster, J. F. A., Lovell, R. R. H., Maplestone, P. A., & Villiers, J. D. (1962). Anaesthetic deaths in a family. *British Journal of Anaesthesia, 34,* 395–396.

Donati, F., & Bevan, D. R. (1985). Antagonism of phase II succinylcholine block by neostigmine. *Anesthesia & Analgesia, 64,* 773–776.

Donati, F., Ferguson, A., & Bevan, D. R. (1983). Twitch depression and train-of-four ratio after antagonism of pancuronium with edrophonium, neostigmine, or pyridostigmine. *Anesthesia & Analgesia, 62,* 314–316.

Dorkins, H. R. (1982). Saxamethonium—The development of a modern drug from 1906 to the present day. *Medical History, 26,* 145–168.

Drachman, D. A. (1978). Myasthenia gravis. *New England Journal of Medicine, 298,* 136–142.

Edwards, R. P., Miller, R. D., & Roizen, M. F. (1979). Cardiac responses to imipramine and pancuronium during anesthesia with halothane and enflurane. *Anesthesiology, 50,* 421–425.

Elmqvist, D., & Quastel, D. M. J. (1965). Presynaptic action of hemicholinium at the neuromuscular junction. *Journal of Physiology, 177,* 463–482.

Emmott, R. S., Bracey, B. J., Goldhill, D. R., Yate, P. M., & Flynn, P. J. (1990). Cardiovascular effects of doxacurium, pancuronium and vecuronium in anaesthetized patients presenting for coronary artery bypass surgery. *British Journal of Anaesthesia, 65,* 480–486.

Everett, A. J., Lowe, L. A., & Wilkinson, S. (1970). Revision of the structures of (+)-tubocurarine chloride and (+)-chondrocurine. *Journal of the Chemical Society, D: Chemical Communications 16,* 1020–1021.

Fahey, M. R., Morris, R. B., Miller, R. D., Sohn, Y. J., Cronnelly, R., & Gencarelli, P. (1981). Clinical pharmacology of ORG

NC45 (Norcuron™): A new nondepolarizing muscle relaxant. *Anesthesiology, 55,* 6–11.

Fisher, D. M., O'Keefe, C., Stanski, D. R., Cronnelly, R., Miller, R. D., & Gregory, G. A. (1982). Pharmacokinetics and pharmacodynamics of D-tubocurarine in infants, children, and adults. *Anesthesiology, 57,* 203–208.

Foldes, F. F., McNall, P. G., & Borrengo-Hinojosa, J. M. (1952). Succinylcholine: A new approach to muscular relaxation in anesthesiology. *New England Journal of Medicine, 247,* 596–600.

Foldes, F. F., Nagashima, H., Nguyen, H. D., Duncalf, D., & Goldiner, P. L. (1990). Neuromuscular and cardiovascular effects of pipecuronium. *Canadian Journal of Anaesthesia, 37,* 549–555.

Foldes, F. F., Rendell-Baker, L., & Birch, J. H. (1956). Causes and prevention of prolonged apnea with succinylcholine. *Anesthesia & Analgesia, 35,* 609–613.

Frank, M., Flynn, P. J., & Hughes, R. (1983). Atracurium in obstetric anaesthesia. *British Journal of Anaesthesia, 55,* 113S–114S.

Futter, M. E. (1983). Prolonged suxamethonium infusion during nitrous oxide anesthesia supplemented by halothane or fentanyl. *British Journal of Anaesthesia, 55,* 947–953.

Gardier, R. W., Tsevdos, E. J., Jackson, D. B., & Delaunois, A. L. (1978). Distinct muscarinic mediation of suspected dopaminergic activity in sympathetic ganglia. *Federation Proceedings, 37,* 2422–2428.

Ghoneim, M. M., & Long, J. P. (1970). The interaction between magnesium and other neuromuscular blocking agents. *Anesthesiology, 32,* 23–27.

Gissen, A. J., & Katz, R. L. (1969). Twitch, tetanus, and post-tetanic potentiation as indices of nerve-muscle block in man. *Anesthesiology, 30,* 491–497.

Goldhill, D. R., Whitehead, J. P., Emmott, R. S., Griffith, A. P., Bracey, B. J., & Flynn, P. J. (1991). Neuromuscular and clinical effects of mivacurium chloride in healthy adult patients during nitrous oxide–enflurane anaesthesia. *British Journal of Anaesthesia, 67,* 289–295.

Greengard, P., & Kebabian, J. W. (1974). Role of cyclic AMP in synaptic transmission in the mammalian peripheral nervous system. *Federation Proceedings, 33,* 1059–1067.

Griffith, H. R., & Johnson, G. E. (1942). The use of curare in general anesthesia. *Anesthesiology, 3,* 418–420.

Gronert, G. A. (1980). Malignant hyperthermia. *Anesthesiology, 53,* 395–425.

Guy, H. R. (1984). A structural model of the acetylcholine receptor channel based on partition energy and helix packing calculations. *Biophysical Journal, 45,* 249–262.

Guyton, A. C. (1996). *Textbook of medical physiology* (9th ed.). Philadelphia: Saunders.

Harrington, J. R., Ford, D. J., & Striker, T. W. (1983). Myoglobinemia and myoglobinuria after succinylcholine in children. *Anesthesiology, 59,* A439.

Hennis, P. J., Fahey, M. R., Canfell, P. C., Shi, W. Z., & Miller, R. D. (1986). Pharmacology of laudanosine in dogs. *Anesthesiology, 65,* 56–60.

Hofmockel, R., & Benad, G. (1995). Time-course of action and intubating conditions with rocuronium bromide under propofol-alfentanil anesthesia. *European Journal of Anesthesia* (Suppl.11), September, 69–72.

Hubbard, J. I., & Wilson, D. F. (1973). Neuromuscular transmission in a mammalian preparation in the absence of blocking drugs and the effect of D-tubocurarine. *Journal of Physiology, 228,* 307–325.

Hubbard, J. I., Jones, S. F., & Landau, E. M. (1968). On the mechanism by which calcium and magnesium affect the release of transmitter by nerve impulses. *Journal of Physiology, 196,* 75–86.

Hughes, R., & Chapple, D. J. (1976). Cardiovascular and neuromuscular effects of dimethyltubocurarine in anaesthetized cats and rhesus monkeys. *British Journal of Anaesthesia, 48,* 847–852.

Hughes, R., & Chapple, D. J. (1981). The pharmacology of atracurium: A new competitive neuromuscularblocking agent. *British Journal of Anaesthesia, 53,*31–44.

Hughes, R., Ingram, G., & Payne, J. P. (1976). Studies on dimethyltubocurarine in anaesthetized man. *British Journal of Anaesthesia, 48,* 969–974.

Hunt, R., & de Taveau, M. R. (1906). On the physiologic action of certain cholin derivatives and new methods for detecting cholin. *British Medical Journal, 2,* 1178–1791.

Hunt, T. M., Hughes, R., & Payne, J. P. (1980). Preliminary studies with atracurium in anaesthetized man. *British Journal of Anaesthesia, 52,* 238P–239P.

Ivankovich, A. D., Miletich, D. J., Albrecht, R. F., & Zahed, B. (1975). The effect of pancuronium on myocardial contraction and catecholamine metabolism. *Journal of Pharmacy and Pharmacology, 27,* 837–841.

Jones, R. J. (1980, April). Use of the peripheral nerve stimulator. *American Academy of Nurse Anesthetists Journal, 48,* 152–154.

Jones, R. M., Pearce, A. C., & Williams, J. P. (1984). Recovery characteristics following antagonism of atracurium with neostigmine or edrophonium. *British Journal of Anaesthesia, 56,* 453–457.

Kalow, W. & Genest, K. (1957). A method for the detection of atypical forms of human serum cholinesterase. Determination of dibucaine numbers. *Canadian Journal of Biochemistry, 35,* 339–353.

Ka'rpa'ti, E., & Bir'o, K. (1980). Pharmacological study of a new competitive neuromuscular blocking steroid, pipecuronium bromide. *Arzneimittel-Forschung Drug Research, 30,* 346–354.

Katz, B. (1966). *Nerve, muscle and synapse.* New York: McGraw-Hill.

Katz, R. L., & Eakins, K. E. (1968). Mode of action of succinylcholine on intraocular pressure. *Journal of Pharmacology and Experimental Therapeutics, 162,* 1–9.

Katz, B., & Miledi, R. (1977). Transmitter leakage from motor nerve endings. *Proceedings of the Royal Society of London, 196,* 59–72.

Kopman, A. F., & Lawson, D. (1984). Milliamperage requirements for supramaximal stimulation of the ulnar nerve with surface electrodes. *Anesthesiology, 61,* 83–85.

Kreig, N., Crul, J. F., & Booij, L. H. D. J. (1980). Relative potency of ORG NC45, pancuronium, alcuronium, and tubocurarine in man. *British Journal of Anaesthesia, 52,* 783-787.

Lanier, W. L., Milde, J. H., & Michenfelder, J. D. (1985). The cerebral effects of pancuronium and atracurium in halothane-anesthetized dogs. *Anesthesiology, 63,* 589–597.

Larijani, G. E., Bartkowski, R. R., Azad, S. S., Seltzer, J. L., Weinberger, M. J., Beach, C. A., & Goldberg, M. E. (1989). Clinical pharmacology of pipecuronium bromide. *Anesthesia & Analgesia, 68,* 734–739.

Lebowitz, P. W., Ramsey, R. M., & Savarese, J. J. (1981). Combination of pancuronium and metocurine: Neuromuscular and hemodynamic advantages over pancuronium alone. *Anesthesia & Analgesia, 60,* 12–16.

Lebowitz, P. W., Ramsey, R. M., Savarese, J. J., & Ali, H. H. (1980). Potentiation of neuromuscular block in man produced by combination of pancuronium and metocurine or pancuronium and D-tubocurarine. *Anesthesia & Analgesia, 59,* 604–609.

Lebrault, C., Berger, J. L., D'Hollander, A. A., Gomeni, R., Henzel, D., & Duvaldest, P. (1985). Pharmacokinetics and pharmacodynamics of vecuronium (ORG NC45) in patients with cirrhosis. *Anesthesiology, 62,* 601–605.

Lebrault, C., Duvaldestin, P., Henzel, D., Chauvin, M., & Guesnon, P. (1986). Pharmacokinetics and pharmacodynamics of vecuronium in patients with cholestasis. *British Journal of Anaesthesia, 58,* 983–987.

Leighton, B. L., Cheek, T. G., Gross, J. B., Apfelbaum, J. L., Shantz, B. B., Gutsche, B. B., & Rosenberg, H. (1986). Succinylcholine pharmacodynamics in peripartum patients. *Anesthesiology, 64,* 202–205.

Lennon, R. L., Olson, R. A., & Gronert, G. A. (1986). Atracurium or vecuronium for rapid sequence endotracheal intubation. *Anesthesiology, 64,* 510–513.

LePage, J. Y., Malinovsky, J. M., Malinge, M., Cozian, A., & Pinaud, M. (1993). 51W89: Dose-response, neuromuscular blocking profile, and cardiovascular effects. *Anesthesiology, 79,* A945.

Lien, C. A., Belmont, M. R., Abalos, A., Eppich, L., Quessy, S., Abou-Donia, M. M., & Savarese, J. J. (1995). The cardiovascular effects and histamine-releasing properties of 51W89 in patients receiving nitrous oxide/opiate/barbiturate anesthesia. *Anesthesiology, 82,* 1131–1138.

Lindgren, L. & Saarnivaara, L. (1983). Effects of competitive myoneural blockade and fentanyl on muscle fasciculations caused by suxamethonium in children. *British Journal of Anaesthesia, 55,* 747–750.

Loffelholz, K. & Muscholl, E. (1970). Inhibition of parasympathetic nerve stimulation of the release of adrenergic transmitter. *Naunyn-Schmiedebergs Archives of Pharmacology, 267,* 181.

Longnecker, D. E., Stoelting, R. K., & Morrow, A. G. (1973). Cardiac and peripheral vascular effects of gallamine in man. *Anesthesia & Analgesia, 52,* 931–935.

Lowenstein, E. (1966). Succinylcholine administration in the burned patient. *Anesthesiology, 27,* 494–496.

Manchikanti, L., Grow, J. B., Colliver, J. A., Canella, M. G., & Hadley, C. H. (1985). Atracurium pretreatment for succinylcholine-induced fasciculations and postoperative myalgia. *Anesthesia & Analgesia, 64,* 1010–1014.

Marchand, P. (1957). A study of the forces productive of gastroesophageal regurgitation and herniation through the diaphragmatic hiatus. *Thorax, 12,* 189–202.

Marshall, R. J., McGrath, J. C., Miller, R. D., Docherty, J. R., & Lamar, J. C. (1980). Comparison of the cardiovascular actions of ORG NC45 with those produced by other non-depolarizing neuromuscular blocking agents in experimental animals. *British Journal of Anaesthesia, 52* (Suppl.), 21S–32S.

Mathias, J. A., Evans-Prosser, C. D. G., & Churchill-Davidson, H. C. (1970). The role of nondepolarizing drugs in the prevention of suxamethonium bradycardia. *British Journal of Anaesthesia, 42,* 609–613.

Matsuo, S., Rao, D. B., Chaudry, I., & Foldes, F. F. (1978). Interaction of muscle relaxants and local anesthetics at the neuromuscular junction. *Anesthesia & Analgesia, 57,* 580–587.

Matteo, R. S., Backus, W. W., McDaniel, D. D., Brotherton, W. P., Abraham, R., & Diaz, J. (1985). Pharmacokinetics and pharmacodynamics of D-tubocurarine and metocurarine in the elderly. *Anesthesia & Analgesia, 64,* 23–29.

Matteo, R. S., Nishitateno, K., Pua, K., & Spector, S. (1980). Pharmacokinetics of D-tubocurarine in man: Effect of an osmotic diuretic on urinary excretion. *Anesthesiology, 52,* 335–338.

Matteo, R. S., Pua, E. K., Khambatta, H. J., & Spector, S. (1977). Cerebrospinal fluid levels of D-tubocurarine in man. *Anesthesiology, 46,* 396–399.

Mazze, R. I, Escue, H. M., & Houston, J. B. (1969). Hyperkalemia and cardiovascular collapse following administration of succinylcholine to the traumatized patient. *Anesthesiology, 31,* 540–547.

McLeod, K., Watson, M. J., & Rawlins, M. D. (1976). Pharmacokinetics of pancuronium in patients with normal and impaired renal function. *British Journal of Anaesthesia, 48,* 341–345.

Merton, P. A. (1954). Voluntary strength and fatigue. *Journal of Physiology, 123,* 553–564.

Miller, R. D., & Way, W. L. (1971). Inhibition of succinylcholine-induced increased intragastric pressure by non-depolarizing muscle relaxant and lidocaine. *Anesthesiology, 34,* 185–188.

Minton, M. D., Grosslight, K., Stirt, J. A., & Bedford, R. F. (1986). Increases in intracranial pressure from succinylcholine: Prevention by prior nondepolarizing blockade. *Anesthesiology, 65,* 165–169.

Moore, G. & Williams, J. R. (1984, April). Monitoring of neuromuscular function of the facial nerve: A noninvasive technique. *AANA Journal, 52,* 171–172.

Morris, R. B., Cahalan, M. K., Miller, R. D., Wilkinson, P. L., Quasha, A. L., & Robinson, S. L. (1983). The cardiovascular effects of vecuronium (ORG NC45) and pancuronium in patients undergoing coronary artery bypass grafting. *Anesthesiology, 58,* 438–440.

Moss, J., Rosow, C. E., Savarese, J. J., Philbin, D. M., & Kniffen, K. J. (1981). Role of histamine in the hypotensive action of D-tubocurarine in humans. *Anesthesiology, 55,* 19–25.

Munger, W. L., Miller, R. D., & Stevens, W. C. (1974). The dependence of D-tubocurarine–induced hypotension on alveolar concentration of halothane, dose of D-tubocurarine, and nitrous oxide. *Anesthesiology, 40,* 442–448.

Naguib, M., Abdulatif, M., Gyasi, H. K., Khawaji, Y., & Absood, G. H. (1987). The pattern of train-of-four fade after atracurium: Influence of different priming doses. *Anesthesia & Analgesia, 66,* 427–430.

Naguib, M., Samarkandi, A. H., Bakhamees, H. S., Magboul, M. A., & el-Bakry, A. K. (1995). Histamine-release haemodynamic changes produced by rocuronium, vecuronium, atracurium, and tubocurarine. *British Journal of Anaesthesia, 5,* 588–592.

Pandey, K., Badola, R. P., & Kumar, S. (1972). Time course of intraocular hypertension produced by suxamethonium. *British Journal of Anaesthesia, 44,* 191–196.

Paton, W. D. M., & Zaimis, E. J. (1954) The methonium compounds. *Pharmacology Review, 4,* 219–253.

Perez, H. R. (1970). Cardiac arrhythmias after succinylcholine. *Anesthesia & Analgesia, 49,* 33–38.

Plotkin, C. N. & Ornstein, E. (1986). Resistance to pancuronium: Adult respiratory distress syndrome or phenytoin. *Anesthesia & Analgesia, 65,* 820–821.

Plotter, L. T.(1970). Synthesis and release of ^{14}C acetylcholine in isolated rat diaphram muscle. *Journal of Physiology, 177,* 463–482.

Prielipp, R. C., Coursin, D. B., Scuderi, P. E., Bowton, D. L., Ford, S. R., Cardenas, V. J., Jr., Vender, J., Howard, D., Casale, E. J., & Murray, M. J. (1995). Comparison of infusion requirements and recovery profiles of vecuronium and cis-atracurium 51W89 in intensive care unit patients. *Anesthesia & Analgesia, 81,* 3–12.

Prien, T., Zahn, P., Menges, M., & Brussel, T. (1995). $1 \times ED_{90}$ dose of rocuronium bromide: Tracheal intubation conditions and time–course of action. *European Journal of Anesthesia* (Suppl. 11), September, 85–90.

Riker, W. F. (1975). Prejunctional effects of neuromuscular and facilitory drugs. In R. L. Katz (Ed.), *Muscle relaxants* (pp. 59–102). Amsterdam: Excerpta Medica.

Roth, S. & Ebrahim, Z. Y. (1987). Resistance to pancuronium in patients receiving carbamazepine. *Anesthesiology, 66,* 691–693.

Rupp, S. M., McChristian, J. W., Miller, R. D., Taboada, J. A., & Cronnelly, R. (1986). Neostigmine and edrophonium antagonism of varying intensity of neuromuscular blockade induced by atracurium, pancuronium, or vecuronium. *Anesthesiology, 64,* 711–714.

Rupp, S. M., Miller, R. D., & Gencarelli, P. J. (1984). Vecuronium-induced neuromuscular blockade during enflurane, halothane, and isoflurane in humans. *Anesthesiology, 60,* 102–105.

Ryan, J. F., Kagen, L. J., & Hyman, A. L. (1971). Myoglobinemia after a single dose of succinylcholine. *New England Journal of Medicine, 285,* 824–825.

Salem, M. G., Richardson, J. C., Meadows, G. A., Lamplugh, G., & Lai, K. M. (1985). Comparison between glycopyrrolate and atropine in a mixture with neostigmine for reversal of neuromuscular blockade. *British Journal of Anaesthesia, 57,* 184–187.

Salem, M. R., Wong, A. Y., & Lin, Y. H. (1972). The effect of suxamethonium on the intragastric pressure in infants and children. *British Journal of Anaesthesia, 44,* 166–170.

Salt, P. J., Barnes, P. K., & Conway, C. M. (1980). Inhibition of neuronal uptake of noradrenaline in the isolated perfused rat heart by pancuronium and its homologues ORG 6368, ORG 7268, and ORG NC45. *British Journal of Anaesthesia, 52,* 313–317.

Savarese, J. J., Ali, H. H., & Antonio, R. P. (1977). The clinical pharmacology of metocurine: Dimethyltubocurine revisited. *Anesthesiology, 47,* 277–284.

Savarese, J. J., Ali, H. H., Basta, S. J., Embree, P. B., & Risner, M. E. (1987). Sixty-second tracheal intubation with BW B1090U after fentanyl–thiopental induction. *Anesthesiology, 67,* A351.

Savarese, J. J., Ali, H. H., Basta, S. J., Scott, R. P., Embree, P. B., Wastila, W. B., Abou-Donia, M. M., & Gelb, C. (1989). The cardiovascular effects of mivacurium chloride (BW1090U) in patients receiving nitrous oxide–opiate–barbiturate anesthesia. *Anesthesiology, 70,* 386–394.

Scappaticci, K. A., Ham, J. A., Sohn, Y. J., Miller, R. D., & Dretchen, K. L. (1982). Effects of furosemide on the neuromuscular junction. *Anesthesiology, 57,* 381–388.

Scott, R. P. F. & Norman, J. (1989). Doxacurium chloride: A preliminary clinical trial. *British Journal of Anaesthesia, 62,* 373–377.

Scott, R. P. F., Savarese, J. J., Basta, S. J., Embree, P., Ali, H. H., & Sunder, N. (1986). Clinical pharmacology of atracurium given in high dose. *British Journal of Anaesthesia, 58,* 834–838.

Scott, R. P. F. & Savarese, J. J. (1985). The cardiovascular and autonomic effects of neuromuscular blocking agents. *Seminars in Anesthesiology, 3,* 319–334.

Sheref, S. E. (1985). Pattern of CNS recovery following reversal of neuromuscular blockade: Comparison of atropine and glycopyrrolate. *British Journal of Anaesthesia, 57,* 188–191.

Shrivastava, O. P., Chatterji, S., Kachhawa, S., & Daga, S. R. (1983). Calcium gluconate pretreatment for prevention of succinylcholine-induced myalgia. *Anesthesia & Analgesia, 62,* 59–62.

Smith, G., Dalling, R., & Williams, T. I. R. (1978). Gastroesophageal pressure gradient changes produced by suxamethonium. *British Journal of Anaesthesia, 50,* 1137–1143.

Sokoll, M. D., & Gergis, S. D. (1981). Antibiotics and neuromuscular function. *Anesthesiology, 55,* 148–155.

Standaert, F. G., & Dretchen, K. L. (1981). Cyclic neucleotides in neuromuscular transmission. *Anesthesia & Analgesia, 60,* 91–99.

Stenlake, J. B., Waigh, R. D., Urwin, J., Dewar, G. H., & Coker, G. G. (1983). Atracurium: Conception and inception. *British Journal of Anaesthesia, 55* (Suppl.), 3S–10S.

Stirt, J. A., Grosslight, K., & Bedford, R. F. (1987). "Defasciculation" with metocurine prevents succinylcholine-induced increases in intracranial pressure. *Anesthesiology, 67,* 50–53.

Stoelting, R. K. (1972). The hemodynamic effects of pancuronium and D-tubocurarine in anesthetized patients. *Anesthesiology, 36,* 612–615.

Stoelting, R. K. (1973). Hemodynamic effects of gallamine during halothane–nitrous oxide anesthesia. *Anesthesiology, 39,* 645–647.

Stoelting, R. K. (1977). Comparison of gallamine and atropine as pretreatment before anesthesia induction and succinylcholine administration. *Anesthesia & Analgesia, 56,* 493–495.

Stoelting, R. K. & Peterson, C. (1975). Adverse effects of increased succinylcholine dose following D-tubocurarine pretreatment. *Anesthesia & Analgesia, 54,* 282–288.

Stoelting, R. K., McCammon, R. L., & Hilgenberg, J. C. (1980). Changes in blood pressure with varying rates of administration of D-tubocurarine. *Anesthesia & Analgesia, 59,* 697–699.

Sugimori, T. (1986). Shortened action of succinylcholine in individuals with cholinesterase C5 isoenzyme. *Canadian Anaesthesia Society Journal, 33,* 321–327.

Taboada, J. A., Rupp, S. M., & Miller, R. D. (1986). Refining the priming principle for vecuronium during rapid-sequence induction of anesthesia. *Anesthesiology, 64,* 242–247.

Tassonyi, E., Neidhart, P., Pittet, J. F., Morel, D. R., & Gemperle, M. (1988). Cardiovascular effects of pipecuronium and pancuronium in patients undergoing coronary artery bypass grafting. *Anesthesiology, 69,* 793–796.

Taylor, P. (1985). Are neuromuscular blocking agents more efficacious in pairs? *Anesthesiology, 63,* 1–3.

Taylor, P., Brown, R. D., & Johnson, D. A. (1983). The linkage between ligand occupation and response of the nicotinic acetylcholine receptor. In A. Kleinzeller & B. D. Martin (Eds.), *Current topics in membranes and transport* (Vol. 18, pp. 407–444). New York: Academic Press.

Thesleff, S., & Molg'o, J. (1983). A new type of transmitter release at the neuromuscular junction. *Neuroscience, 9,* 1–8.

Thompson, I. R., & Putnins, C. L. (1985). Adverse effects of pancuronium during high-dose fentanyl anesthesia for coronary artery bypass grafting. *Anesthesiology, 62,* 708–713.

Vercruysse, P., Bossuyt, P., Hanegreefs, G., Verbeuren, T. J., & Vanhoutte, P. M. (1979). Gallamine and pancuronium inhibit prejunctional and post-junctional muscarinic receptors in canine saphenous veins. *Journal of Pharmacology and Experimental Therapeutics, 209,* 225–230.

Viby-Mogensen, J. (1980). Correlation of succinylcholine duration of action with plasma cholinesterase activity in subjects with genotypically normal enzyme. *Anesthesiology, 53,* 517–520.

Wastila, W. B., Maehr, R. B., Turner, G. L., Hill, D. A., & Savarese, J. J. (1996). Comparative pharmacology of *cis*-atracurium (51W89), atracurium, and five isomers in cats. *Anesthesiology, 85,* 169–177.

Waud, B. E., Farrell, L., & Waud, D. R. (1982). Lithium and neuromuscular transmission. *Anesthesia & Analgesia, 61,* 399–402.

Waud, B. E., & Waud, D. R. (1971). The relation between tetanic fade and receptor occlusion in the presence of competitive neuromuscular block. *Anesthesiology, 35,* 456–464.

Waud, B. E., & Waud, D. R. (1972). The relation between the response to "train-of-four" stimulation and receptor occlusion during competitive neuromuscular blockade. *Anesthesiology, 37,* 413–416.

West, R. (1932). Curare in man. *Proceedings of the Royal Society of Medicine, 25,* 1107–1116.

Wierda, J. M., & Proost, J. H. (1995). Structure–pharmacodynamic–pharmacokinetic relationships of steroidal neuromuscular blocking agents. *European Journal of Anesthesia* (Suppl. 11), September, 79–80.

Wierda, J. M., Karliczek, G. F., Vandenbrom, R. H., Pinto, I., Kersten-Kleef, U. W., Meijer, D. K., & Agoston, S. (1990). Pharmacokinetics and cardiovascular dynamics of pipecuronium bromide during coronary artery surgery. *Canadian Journal of Anaesthesia, 37,* 183–191.

Wierda, J. M., Richardson, F. J., & Agoston, S. (1989). Dose–response relation and time course of action of pipecuronium bromide in humans anesthetized with nitrous oxide and isoflurane, halothane, or droperidol and fentanyl. *Anesthesia & Analgesia, 68,* 208–213.

Yate, P. M., Flynn, P. J., Arnold, R. W., Weatherly, B. C., Simmonds, R. J., & Dopson, T. (1987). Clinical experience and plasma laudanosine concentrations during infusion of atracurium in the intensive therapy unit. *British Journal of Anaesthesia, 59,* 211–217.

Pharmacology of Cardiovascular Drugs

Cathy Mastropietro

▶ PHARMACOLOGY OF CARDIOVASCULAR DRUGS

The wide variety of available cardioactive pharmacologic agents has increased the sophistication with which anesthesia practitioners can induce or manage hemodynamic alterations during surgery. These drugs are used in two different clinical modalities. They may be administered chronically prior to surgery or given acutely by intravenous route during the preoperative, perioperative, or postoperative periods. Selecting and administering the appropriate drug and its proper concentration to maximize the desired effect, but minimize side effects, create an interesting challenge to the anesthesia provider. The use of cardiovascular agents requires a strong understanding of the pharmacologic and physiologic responses of these drugs. Of particular concern and challenge is the readiness with which therapeutic effects change with dosage.

This chapter addresses the common agents used during perioperative management and their clinical applications. For the purposes of this review, the drugs are broken down into several categories: (1) sympathetic agonists, which include inotropes and vasopressors; (2) sympathetic antagonists, which include alpha- and beta-blockers, direct-acting vasodilators, antihypertensives, and calcium channel blockers; and (3) antiarrhythmics.

▶ INFLUENCE OF CARDIOACTIVE DRUGS

The majority of agents employed for hemodynamic control during anesthesia operate by modulating the effects of the autonomic nervous system. This mechanism of action allows for the ability to augment or reduce autonomic tone by use of selective agonists or antagonists. The effects of cardiovascular drugs on the autonomic nervous system are anatomically influenced. The sympathetic and parasympathetic efferents use acetylcholine (ACh) as the neurotransmitter at the ganglionic level, but they use different neurotransmitters at the neuroeffector junction. At the level of the spinal cord, the sympathetic fibers use norepinephrine (NE) at the effector site, whereas the parasympathetic fibers use ACh at both ganglionic and effector sites. With nerve stimulation, vesicles containing NE are mobilized to the cell membrane where NE is released into the synaptic cleft. At this level, presynaptic or postsynaptic receptors are stimulated, or the neurotransmitter is degraded by enzyme systems, or undergo uptake by local tissues. In addition to NE and ACh, adenosine triphosphate (ATP, recently found in neurotransmitter vesicles) may modulate the effects of sympathetic and parasympathetic nerve stimulation (Lincoln & Burnstock, 1990).

Adrenergic Receptor Pharmacology

Cardiovascular drugs produce their effects by interacting with specific receptors. Most available drugs used to control the cardiovascular system rapidly do so by means of direct and indirect receptors. Direct effects change heart rate (sinoatrial automaticity), myocardial contractility, conduction, and systemic vascular resistance. Indirect effects change cardiac output, stroke volume, and blood pressure (Reid, 1986). Although they are not the only receptors of importance in the cardiovascular system, they do produce critical responses in acute mediation of vasoconstriction and myocardial contractility. Agonists induce a response at the receptor site, whereas antagonists interact with and occupy the receptor site, thereby reducing or inhibiting the effects of the agonists. Several receptor subtypes responsible for the mediation of drug activity are classified according to location and effect. Although the classification of agonists serves as a useful means of explaining the clinical effects of cardiovascular drugs, the clinician should bear in mind that most drugs are not subtype specific and that effects are greatly influenced by dosage (Hoffman & Lefkowitz, 1996; Schwinn, 1994).

Alterations in Drug Disposition

Drugs produce effects according to their influence on drug plasma concentration. Pharmacokinetics and pharmacodynamics of drugs play critical roles in the clinical responses they produce, and various disease processes such as renal, hepatic, or cardiac contribute to individual variation in drug response. For the cardiac patient undergoing noncardiac surgery, these chronic conditions may significantly affect drug disposition; for the cardiac patient the critical influence on drug distribution is cardiopulmonary bypass (Schwinn, 1994; Wood, 1993).

Congestive Heart Failure

The patient with congestive heart failure (CHF) raises several challenging clinical concerns. Initially arterial blood pressure is maintained via reflex sympathetic stimulation accompanied by increases in plasma norepinephrine levels. This increase in sympathetic tone is thought to be responsible for the cardiac arrhythmias commonly found in CHF. As the disease progresses, myocardial failure decreases cardiac output, which ultimately reduces tissue organ perfusion. This alteration, especially in renal and hepatic tissue, affects the absorption, uptake, distribution, and metabolism of drugs. The volume of distribution is reduced because of alterations in blood flow, tissue perfusion, and clearance, resulting in increased plasma concentrations (Armstrong & Moe, 1994). It should be noted that in advanced stages of CHF hepatic clearance and plasma extraction of certain antiarrhythmics and local anesthetics are altered (Armstrong & Moe, 1994; Holley, Ponganis, & Stanski,

1984). Consequently, individual response variation is considerable and extreme caution must be exercised with drugs that have narrow therapeutic margins.

Cardiac Surgery: Cardiopulmonary Bypass

Changes in drug distribution produced by CPB are the result of changes in blood flow, protein binding, and hemodilution. Drug serum concentrations are decreased significantly at the onset of CPB because of these changes and then gradually increase because of decreased elimination. The reduction in elimination is due to impairment of renal and hepatic clearance from reduction in blood flow and hypothermia. Postoperatively, plasma protein binding is mildly affected; however, the concentration of a specific plasma protein, AG, rises significantly in the postoperative period following major cardiac surgery and directly affects the binding of some antiarrhythmics, local anesthetics, and beta-blockers (Wood, 1993).

► CARDIOACTIVE DRUGS

Sympathetic Agonists

Sympathetic agonists operate through two mechanisms, following the routes of sympathetic innervation and control. The intrinsic route operates from sympathetic fibers, which terminate in the systemic and pulmonary vasculature and in the heart at several sites, including the sinoatrial (SA) node, the atrioventricular (AV) node, and the Purkinje fibers responsible for transmission of the impulses to the ventricles (Merin, 1990). The primary neurotransmitter for the intrinsic route is norepinephrine, released at the site of the myoneural junction (Barques & Schwinn, 1991). In contrast, the hormonal or humoral route operates by releasing catecholamines from the adrenal medulla and has actions similar to those of the intrinsic route (Guyton, 1996). The primary neurotransmitter for the humoral route is epinephrine (Guyton, 1996; Merin, 1990) carried through the vascular tree after release from the adrenal medulla in response to stress.

Both sympathetic routes operate by enhancing the inotropic state of the ventricles, enhancing the rate of intrinsic depolarization in pacemaker cells and the development of arrhythmias. The effects on the peripheral vasculature increase dose dependently. Stimulation of the humoral route, which releases low concentrations of epinephrine, produces beta-mediated peripheral dilation, whereas releasing norepinephrine or higher concentrations of epinephrine results in an overriding alpha-mediated peripheral vasoconstriction. Development of an overriding alpha tone does not, however, eliminate beta-induced increases in inotropy, rate, and arrhythmogenicity.

The pharmacologic effects of sympathetic agonists occur via several mechanisms. Direct stimulation of sympathetic terminals may produce the corresponding beta or alpha effects, as is the case with direct-acting catecholamines. Alternately, indirect pathways may enhance the release of the sympathetic neurotransmitter or delay neurotransmitter breakdown and reuptake (Hoffman & Lefkowitz, 1996; Schwinn, 1994). Sympathetic agonists can be divided into three major groups: (1) catecholamines, which directly produce the classic graduated effects with increasing dosage; (2) inodilators, which indirectly produce increases in inotropy without increases in systemic vascular resistance at higher doses; and (3) vasoconstrictors, which directly mimic the vascular effects of norepinephrine or high-dose epinephrine. Although there is overlap between these groups, general patterns can be defined that direct their clinical application. Commonly employed agents, along with their doses and prominent clinical effects, are listed in Table 22–1.

Catecholamines

The catecholamines include four direct-acting agents: epinephrine, norepinephrine, dopamine, and isoproterenol. Except when used as emergency drugs, these agents are all generally employed as titratable continuous infusions. The first three are native sympathetic neurotransmitters; isoproterenol is a synthetic molecule. These agents all produce increases in inotropic state, in the rate of spontaneous depolarization in pacemaker cells, and in arrhythmogenicity. Their effects on systemic vasculature vary according to the specific drug.

Among these agents, epinephrine and dopamine demonstrate classic graduated response to increasing doses. Isoproterenol produces beta agonism, which increases inotropic state and heart rate without producing alpha-agonist systemic vasoconstriction. Norepinephrine produces primarily alpha-agonist increases in systemic vasomotor tone, with less effect on inotropic state and heart rate. An additional agent, ephedrine, produces its effects through an increase in the release of native catecholamine and operates as a weak neurotransmitter itself. It is generally used for bolus administration rather than as a continuous infusion.

Epinephrine

Epinephrine is predominantly an alpha-agonist in low dose. In therapeutic ranges beta effects predominate (Lawson, 1992). Clinical effects are rapid, usually occurring within 2 minutes and lasting 5 to 15 minutes after administration depending on the dose employed. In low doses (below 0.04 mg/kg/min) epinephrine produces increased inotropy, rate of spontaneous depolarization in the pacemaker cells, and arrhythmogenicity. As the dose is increased to the midrange (0.04 to 0.15 mg/kg/min), a gradual increase in systemic vascular resistance is noted with increased blood pressure. At high doses (over

0.15 mg/kg/min), alpha effects of increased vasomotor tone predominate, whereas beta-induced increases in inotropy eventually plateau (Larach & Solina, 1995). The arrhythmogenic effects of epinephrine increase with increasing dosage, as does the rate of spontaneous depolarization of the pacemaker cells. Hence, with increasing dosages, tachycardia and tachyarrhythmias become a prominent feature (Larach & Solina, 1995; Schwinn, 1994).

Norepinephrine

Norepinephrine (Levophed) also has potent direct alpha$_1$, alpha$_2$, and beta$_1$ actions, but no beta$_2$ properties. It has (Weiner, 1990b) similar onset and duration and operates through the intrinsic pathway similar to epinephrine in low doses, producing an increase in inotropic state and arrhythmogenicity (Chernow, Rainey, & Lake, 1984; Schwinn, 1994). In contrast to epinephrine, the hormonal effect of norepinephrine produces a direct increase in peripheral vasomotor tone, which is a prominent effect at all rates of administration. It generally is used in a titratable form with doses up to 0.1 mg/kg/min. In response to increased systemic pressure, slowing of the heart rate may occur as a reflex rather than a direct effect. Because the peripheral constrictor effects outweigh inotropic benefit, norepinephrine is seldom used in the clinical setting as an inotrope. Its use is generally restricted to that of a vasoconstrictor in patients demonstrating high cardiac output with unsatisfactory systemic pressures, and doses should be limited to the minimal effective dose.

Dopamine

Dopamine is itself a native sympathetic neurotransmitter and a precursor of both norepinephrine and epinephrine (Guyton, 1996; Raner et al., 1995). Dopamine is probably the most commonly employed catecholamine and maintains a physiologic profile slightly different from those of the other agents. It has a slightly slower onset than epinephrine, at 2 to 5 minutes for clinical effect, and a duration up to 10 minutes on termination of infusion. Dopamine is itself a native sympathetic neurotransmitter and a precursor in the formation of both norepinephrine and epinephrine (Guyton, 1996). Dopamine is a weaker inotropic agent than epinephrine and requires several times the dosage to produce similar effects. Part of the effects demonstrated by dopamine are indirect and are mediated by higher release of norepinephrine at the intrinsic terminals (Lawson, 1992). Hence, it demonstrates its greatest effect in the intact heart and has less potency in the denervated organ. Furthermore, long-term usage may result in decreased benefit, as native neurotransmitter stores are depleted and replaced by dopamine. At low doses (<5 mg/kg/min), it produces an increase in inotropy and in the rate of spontaneous depolarization of pacemaker cells, with only minimal increases in arrhythmogenicity. With progressive increases

TABLE 22–1. Commonly Used Sympathetic Agonists

Drug	Dosage (μg/kg/min)	Effect	Indications/Benefits[a]	Disadvantage
Epinephrine				
	0.0–0.4	Beta	Low CO, CHF, failure to wean from bypass, bradycardia	Atrial tachycardia
	0.04–0.1	Mixed beta/alpha	Low CO with low SVR	Arrhythmias (PACs, PVCs)
			Low arterial pressure with low SVR	As above
	>0.1	Alpha effects predominate	Profound hypotension low SVR, anaphylaxis	Induction of arrhythmias, vasoconstriction: reduced peripheral perfusion and metabolic acidosis
Isuprel				
	(All doses) 0–0.2	Beta-agonist	Bradycardia, CHF, low CO, pulmonary HTN, failure to wean from bypass	Profound peripheral dilation and systemic hypotension
Norepinephrine				
	(All doses) 0–0.2	Alpha-agonist	Profound hypotension from low SVR, failure to wean from bypass	Induction of arrhythmias, vasoconstriction: reduced peripheral perfusion and metabolic acidosis
Dopamine				
	0–3	Dopaminergic	Renal dilation, oliguria (renal)	
	0–5	Beta	Low CO, CHF, failure to wean from bypass	Atrial tachycardias, mild increase in PA pressure
	5–15	Mixed beta/alpha	Low CO with low SVR, low arterial pressure with low SVR	As above
	>15	Alpha effects predominate	Profound hypotension, low SVR, failure to wean from bypass	Peripheral vasoconstriction: reduced peripheral perfusion and metabolic acidosis, tachycardia
Dobutamine				
	0–15	Beta	Reduces PA pressure: failure to wean from bypass, CHF, low CO	Systemic hypotension in higher doses
	>15	Alpha effects demonstrated		
Amrinone				
	(All doses) 0–40	Beta	Reduces PA pressure: failure to wean from bypass, CHF, low CO	Systemic hypotension in higher doses

[a] CO, cardiac output; CHF, congestive heart failure; SVR, systemic vascular resistance; PACs, premature atrial contractions; PVCs, premature ventricular contractions; HTN, hypertension; PA, pulmonary artery.

in dosage to the midrange (5 to 15 mg/kg/min), it produces a gradual increase in systemic vascular resistance. At high doses (>15 to 20 mg/kg/min), alpha-induced peripheral vasoconstriction predominates.

In addition to its inotropic effects, dopamine demonstrates intrinsic renal and mesenteric vasodilator effects at low doses, mediated through specific dopaminergic receptors in the renal and mesenteric vasculature (Muhlbauer, 1996; Olsen et al., 1993). This may produce increases in renal blood flow and augment urinary output when the drug is used at low to intermediate doses. At high doses, the renal dilatory effect is overridden by the alpha-induced peripheral vasoconstriction (Muhlbauer, 1996; Olsen et al., 1993).

Isoproterenol

Isoproterenol was the first synthetic purely beta sympathetic agonist developed for clinical use in a continuous infusion. It has a rapid onset within 2 minutes and a slightly shorter duration of action than epinephrine, which may be related to the dose employed. It is generally titrated according to clinical response at rates up to 0.2 mg/kg/min. At all clinical doses, isoproterenol produces a pure beta-mediated increase in inotropic state (Lawson, 1992) that is otherwise similar to that of other catecholamines. Drawbacks include enhancement of arrhythmias and frequent tachycardias (Lawson, 1992). In addition, isoproterenol does not demonstrate any alpha effect on the peripheral and pulmonary vasculature

(Lawson, 1992). Hence, the effects on systemic pressure are unpredictable. When beta-induced inotropic benefits outweigh the reduction in systemic vascular resistance, blood pressure may be increased. When the beta-induced reduction in systemic vascular resistance predominates, systemic pressures may decline with its use. For these reasons, isoproterenol has found progressively less application in the management of the adult patient. It is a potent dysarrhythmogenic and is commonly used for maintaining heart rate in patients with SA node dysfunction (sick sinus syndrome, refractory bradycardia with secondary hypotension), in patients with cardiac transplant, or in managing pediatric patients in whom the systemic pressure is not maintained in the adult range (Waller, 1983).

Ephedrine

Ephedrine produces both direct and indirect effects. Its action is predominantly indirect by release of NE. Tachyphylaxis is common following repeated doses because of depleted stores of NE (Lawson, 1992). Ephedrine usually demonstrates an initial clinical effect within 2 to 5 minutes and lasts up to 15 minutes after a bolus administration. It also is taken up in the sympathetic nerve terminal, where it functions as a weak neurotransmitter in its own right (Lawson, 1992). It generally is used only in bolus doses of 2.5 mg to 10 mg for short-term hemodynamic support in the treatment of bradycardia and hypotension that follows mild myocardial depression in response to anesthetic agents.

Inodilators

Three drugs are included in the class of agents termed inodilators: dobutamine, amrinone, and milrinone. They combine positive inotrophy and vasodilation to produce their effects. These agents exert only mild beta-agonism directly; their mechanism of action depends on indirect effects as well and includes inhibition of the phosphodiesterase (PDE) enzyme system, specifically (PDE-III), that is responsible for the breakdown of endogenous catecholamine (George, Lehot, & Estanove, 1992; Rutman, LeJemtel, & Sonneblick, 1987). Thus, they produce increases in the inotropic state without increase in systemic vasomotor tone that accompanies administration of native catecholamine. These agents reportedly produce less frequent and less severe tachycardia, and are less arrhythmogenic than native catecholamine. In addition, they reduce pulmonary vascular resistance and may prove beneficial in the management of patients with pulmonary hypertension. Finally, inhibition of PDE-III provides a mechanism of action independent of direct beta-agonism, making these agents useful when managing patients with ventricular dysfunction who have been treated with beta-blocking agents.

Dobutamine

Dobutamine provides direct mild beta-agonism and possesses an indirect mechanism of action that may represent either norepinephrine accumulation or PDE-III inhibition (Olsen et al., 1993). It produces an increase in inotropic state with generally only mild increases in heart rate. Dobutamine is slower in onset than native catecholamine and requires 5 to 7 minutes to demonstrate clinical effects. Its duration of action is similarly extended to 10 to 12 minutes. Although there was initially less frequent tachycardia and less arrhythmogenicity reported with the use of dobutamine than with native catecholamine, mild increases in heart rate may be noted (Leirer & Unverferth, 1983; Olsen et al., 1993). Dobutamine is a relatively mild inotrope that requires a much higher dosage of epinephrine to produce similar increases in inotropic state. Reductions in systemic vasomotor tone and ventricular afterload augment the effects of increased inotropic state in the failing ventricle. The reduction in pulmonary vascular resistance may be proportionately greater than the increase in cardiac output, which results in a decrease in pulmonary artery pressure (Furman et al., 1982; Pank & Tinker, 1983). Dobutamine has none of the renal effects seen with dopamine. When high doses (over 15 to 20 mg/kg/min) are employed, a mild increase in systemic vascular resistance may be demonstrated, although profound systemic vasoconstriction is not noted with its use (Lawson, 1992; Leier, & Unverperth, 1983).

Amrinone

Amrinone is a mild direct beta-agonist, the physiologic effects of which have yet to be fully elucidated. Its effects are felt to be mediated primarily through inhibition of PDE-III (Rutman et al., 1987). Amrinone has an onset and duration of action similar to those of dobutamine. It produces increases in inotropic state with minimal increases in heart rate and no increase or a reduction in systemic vascular resistance. As amrinone acts primarily through enzyme inhibition, it is a comparatively weak inotrope and requires relatively high doses (up to 40 mg/kg/min) to produce inotropic increases similar to those obtained with epinephrine. Amrinone is an effective pulmonary vasodilator that decreases pulmonary vascular resistance as cardiac output increases. As amrinone is available in oral form, it is frequently used for prolonged management of the patient with congestive heart failure, for patients in coronary care units, and for patients prior to cardiac transplantation.

Milrinone

Milrinone is a newer PDE-III inhibitor that is 30 times more potent than amrinone. Its onset of action is faster than that of dobutamine or amrinone, and a greater decrease in peripheral vascular resistance is noted. It is used primarily to reverse low cardiac output syndrome in cardiac surgery patients, as it does not change heart rate or mean arterial pressure. Loading doses given during CPB are 37.5 to 50 μg/kg/min over 10 minutes (George, Lehot, & Estanove, 1992). Maintenance dose is 0.375 to 0.75 μg/kg/min.

Vasoconstrictors

The vasoconstrictors used in current clinical practice directly stimulate alpha receptors to produce an increase in systemic and pulmonary vasomotor tone. The result is increased systemic vascular resistance and an increase in corresponding arterial pressure when cardiac output is held constant. As a result of the increase in systemic arterial pressure, slowing of the heart rate may occur with their use through a reflex rather than a direct effect. Only two agents are commonly used in infusion form: norepinephrine and phenylephrine. A third agent, methoxamine, is generally used in bolus form rather than as a continuous infusion.

Norepinephrine

Norepinephrine has been discussed as a sympathetic agonist. It possesses direct sympathetic activity and is the primary neurotransmitter in the intrinsic sympathetic terminals in the myocardium. In infusion form at all doses up to 0.1 mg/kg/min, this effect is overshadowed by its role in the humoral route in which norepinephrine produces alpha-mediated increases in vasomotor tone. The overriding systemic alpha-agonism makes it more suitable as a vasoconstrictor than an inotrope. Hence, it is most commonly used for maintenance of systemic vascular resistance in the management of patients with high cardiac output and low systemic blood pressure.

Phenylephrine

Phenylephrine is a less potent vasoconstrictor that produces effects similar to those of norepinephrine when used at an approximately tenfold dosage. It has a rapid onset within 1 to 2 minutes and a duration of action of 5 to 10 minutes after termination of the infusion (Lawson, 1992). Phenylephrine is considered to be a pure alpha drug devoid of beta effects except at high doses producing alpha-mediated systemic vasoconstriction that increases with doses up to 1 mg/kg/min (Lawson, 1992). As with norepinephrine, its primary application is to manage patients with high cardiac output and low systemic arterial pressure. Phenylephrine provides effective, titratable increases in vasomotor tone and permits maintenance of normal systemic vascular resistance in most patients with pharmacologically induced reduction in sympathetic vasomotor tone.

Methoxamine

Methoxamine is a direct-acting predominantly alpha stimulant (Garcia-Sainz et al., 1985; Lawson, 1992) that produces little vasoconstriction. Primary effects are increased arterial resistance, increased afterload, and decreased flow. It is usually used in a single bolus dose of 5 mg and demonstrates an increase in systemic pressure within 2 minutes of administration (Lawson & Wallfisch, 1986). Methoxamine appears to be totally devoid of any beta effects (Lawson, 1992) and does not stimulate tachycardias or arrhythmias. Reflex bradycardia may follow its administration as a result of the increase in systemic arterial pressure. Because of its extended duration of action, methoxamine is not used as a continuous infusion.

Clinical Applications of Sympathetic Agonists

When employed in a physiologically sound fashion, inotropes and vasoconstrictors allow the practitioner to maintain both cardiac output and systemic blood pressure within a desired range. When the required preload is maintained, inotropic agents may be used to support the contractile state, the second determinant of stroke volume, and, therefore, cardiac output. When cardiac output is maintained, the use of vasoconstrictors permits adjustment of the systemic vascular resistance, which is the second determinant of systemic blood pressure. Appreciation of basic physiologic principles and pharmacologic actions of each of the agents will identify their individual applications.

The use of a catecholamine generally produces an increase in the inotropic state, along with mild to moderate increases in heart rate and progressive increases in vasomotor tone. These effects in combination permit the maintenance of both cardiac output and systemic arterial pressure. Ephedrine is frequently used to elicit both alpha and beta effects in the treatment of relatively mild myocardial depression. It provides effective short-term cardiovascular support when prolonged myocardial depression is not expected. In addition, its enhancement of sympathetic tone also may make ephedrine useful in accelerating SA node automaticity in the patient with SA node depression and secondary AV nodal electrical mechanism. This may prove beneficial in the management of patients with myocardial revascularization who fail to reestablish normal sinus rhythm on rewarming from the cold ischemia of cardioplegia.

Among the catecholamines used in continuous infusion, only isoproterenol is a pure beta-agonist, permitting the practitioner to increase heart rate and provide inotropic support without increasing systemic vascular resistance. It is primarily used to manage patients with profound hemodynamically significant bradycardia or patients who require inotropic support without increases in systemic vascular resistance. Isoproterenol may in fact produce profound beta-induced reductions in systemic vascular resistance at higher doses, and its lack of alpha activity makes it unsuitable as a sole agent for patients who require both inotropic support and maintenance of systemic vascular resistance. When isoproterenol is used to maintain heart rate in patients with reduced systemic vascular resistance, it may be necessary to use a second agent as a direct vasoconstrictor to maintain systemic vasomotor tone. Combined therapy with isoproterenol and phenylephrine or norepinephrine may permit maintenance of heart rate and inotropic state, while permitting the practitioner directly to augment systemic vascular resistance and therefore systemic pressures.

Although combined therapy with pure alpha- and beta-agonists is possible, it is more common practice to employ those catecholamines that produce the classic graduated response. Epinephrine and dopamine are frequently used to manage patients with poor cardiac output based on myocardial depression alone. In those patients, epinephrine is used for its direct action and by its role as the natural sympathetic neurotransmitter in the humoral sympathetic route. In contrast, dopamine is an effective sympathetic agonist with the additional benefit of renal vasodilation and improved renal blood flow. It is popular for both its direct cardiac effects and its systemic noncardiac action. However, because dopamine is a relatively less potent inotropic agent and part of its effect is indirect, it is less effective in maintaining the necessary alpha-mediated increase in systemic vascular resistance in patients with profound cardiovascular depression. Therefore, dopamine is used frequently in patients with comparatively mild myocardial depression and is useful in weaning patients from cardiopulmonary bypass or in treating the comparatively mild myocardial depression that may occur in the patient with compromised ventricular function when anesthetic agents that possess myocardial depressant effects are used. Epinephrine is used more frequently in patients with severe myocardial depression refractory to therapy with less potent agents such as dopamine and in patients who need both inotropic support and maintenance of systemic vascular resistance.

The role of the noncatecholamine sympathetic agonists is rapidly developing. Dobutamine, amrinone, and milrinone are all indirect-acting agents that depend on PDE-III inhibition for their effects and produce only weak direct sympathetic stimulation. These agents offer several advantages over the direct-acting sympathetic agonists. Each inodilator is an effective pulmonary vascular dilator that produces reductions in pulmonary vascular resistance that match or exceed increase in cardiac output. These agents may reduce pulmonary artery pressure and prove to be valuable in managing patients with acute increases in pulmonary pressure, unloading the right ventricle and maintaining cardiac output without increased risk of right ventricular failure. In addition, these agents provide inotropic support to the failing left ventricle without increasing systemic vascular resistance, which may prove undesirable in the patient with left ventricular failure. They are popular in the management of patients with chronic failure and high systemic vascular resistance whose cardiac function would be expected to deteriorate with further increases in afterload. In addition, the inodilators operate through an indirect action that bypasses direct stimulation of the sympathetic axis and are effective in treating ventricular failure in patients who are receiving beta antagonists chronically. They find application in acute management of the depressed ventricle as a primary inotropic agent or as a supplemental agent for patients who have demonstrated an inadequate response to a direct-acting catecholamine. In this fashion, dobutamine, amrinone, and milrinone frequently are employed in weaning patients from cardiopulmonary bypass who could not be weaned with only the use of direct-acting catecholamines. They also are useful in managing patients with ventricular failure after cross-clamping of the aorta and who need inotropic support without concomitant increase in systemic vascular resistance.

Vasoconstrictors provide a means of supporting systemic arterial pressure in those patients who maintain adequate cardiac output but demonstrate systemic hypotension secondary to reductions in systemic vascular resistance. They also are used in the management of patients who require higher-than-normal systemic vascular resistance to maintain coronary perfusion (eg, patients with left ventricular outflow obstruction from critical aortic stenosis). They are of little use in the patient with ventricular failure, because the increase in systemic resistance produces an increase in left ventricular afterload. Finally, vasoconstrictors may be used to autotransfuse effectively the patient with reduced vascular volume by augmenting vasomotor tone in venous capacitance vessels. This allows the practitioner to maintain preload, cardiac output, and systemic perfusion pressures while gradually increasing vascular volume. Vasoconstrictors may be useful in the volume-depleted patient on chronic diuretic therapy or in the patient with acute hemorrhage requiring emergency intervention. Because massive vasoconstriction reduces total systemic perfusion, these agents may cause hypoperfusion of selected organs with high doses and produce metabolic acidosis. Therefore they are not recommended for chronic therapy, except for those patients who demonstrate low systemic vascular resistance, such as the septic patient. Attention should be given to indices of systemic organ perfusion when they are used.

Sympathetic Antagonists

Sympathetic antagonists directly antagonize the systemic and cardiac effects of agonist agents. They operate through the sympathetic route to reduce inotropic state, slow heart rate, and reduce arrhythmogenicity by antagonizing beta-mediated effects, or they produce systemic dilation by antagonizing alpha-mediated vasomotor tone. In contrast to the agonist agents, most antagonists have very specific alpha- or beta-antagonist effects. Labetalol is the only agent that combines both alpha and beta antagonism. The majority of sympathetic antagonists have a far longer duration of action than their corresponding agonist agents and are not available for use as a continuous infusion. At present only one beta antagonist, esmolol, has a sufficiently short duration of action to be considered practical for use in continuous infusion.

Beta Antagonists

Two-beta antagonists are currently available that readily lend themselves to use in anesthetic practice: propranolol and esmolol. Both of these agents are effective in antagonizing the beta-mediated sympathetic effects. Therefore, they provide safe and effective means of slowing the heart, reducing arrhythmogenicity, and depressing the hyperdynamic ventricle. They are used most commonly to treat acute intraoperative hypertension and tachycardia, and they can be used to achieve similar goals. Esmolol has a very quick onset and is an extremely short-acting agent. This makes esmolol titratable and of use in acute management; it has too short a duration of action to provide long-term suppression of sympathetic stimulation. Propranolol, in contrast, has a slower onset combined with a prolonged duration of action. This makes it nontitratable for short-term management and, therefore, more suitable for long-term suppression. This combination of agents permits the practitioner to achieve short-term acute control of sympathetic overdrive, with the option of converting to long-acting activity when indicated.

Propranolol. Propranolol is a pure beta antagonist with a comparatively longer duration than esmolol. It finds clinical application primarily in three roles: reduction of heart rate in the tachycardic patient, treatment of hypertension, and as an adjunct in the treatment of malignant ventricular dysrhythmias refractory to standard therapy. Blood pressure reduction is the result of decreased cardiac output and renin release. The purpose for which propranolol is used generally determines the dose employed. To treat acute tachycardia, propranolol may be given in intravenous doses beginning at 0.1 to 0.25 mg and titrated to effect. Control of acute-onset tachycardia is generally achieved with a total dose of 1 to

2 mg, although a total dose of up to 5 mg may be employed in younger patients. In the management of sinus or atrial tachycardias, it generally depresses heart rate within 5 to 15 minutes. It has an extended duration of action, lasting 8 to 12 hours after administration (Hoffman & Lefkowitz, 1996). As a myocardial depressant, it finds application in the management of hypertension, but larger doses are required, usually in incremental doses of 0.25 to 0.5 mg. In patients who are on chronic betablocker therapy, larger initial doses may be employed. Control of ventricular hypertension generally is achieved with a total dose of 2 to 5 mg. When used for control of hypertension, propranolol generally demonstrates its clinical effect within 15 to 30 minutes, and its duration of action remains 8 to 12 hours. Because of its extended duration of action, however, it is not readily titratable, which makes it undesirable for short-term use. Initially CPB decreases propanolol levels by approximately 50% and then returns them to normal during bypass; however, they are elevated several hours postbypass so clinical effects must be closely assessed.

Esmolol. Esmolol is a rapid-acting, pure beta-antagonist with a rapid onset (approximately 2 minutes) and short duration of action (approximately 10 to 20 minutes), which makes it titratable (deBruihn et al., 1987; Gorczynski, 1985). This is particularly beneficial in the short-term management of sinus or atrial tachycardias or for use as an adjunct to standard antiarrhythmic therapy for patients with refractory ventricular dysrhythmias. It may prove beneficial in short-term management of the hyperdynamic ventricle, and its short duration of action permits rapid recovery from overdosage or quick return to baseline when used to treat overdose of sympathetic agonists. When used for treatment of tachycardia, graduated boluses of 10 mg permit the practitioner to titrate the effect of esmolol without producing severe reductions in heart rate or resultant bradycardia. Esmolol can be used in a continuous infusion. When so employed, it is recommended that a loading dose up to 500 mg/kg be used, then titrated to effect starting at a rate of 50 to 300 mg/kg/min (Lawson, 1992). At rates of up to 200 mg/kg/min, esmolol proves effective in controlling tachycardias; doses over 200 mg/kg/min have not been shown to offer any additional benefit. In infusion form, its rapid onset and rapid recovery can help adjust effect without prolonged cardiac depression after the infusion is over.

Alpha Antagonists

At present, only two agents are available for direct antagonism of alpha-mediated sympathetic effects: phentolamine and phenoxybenzamine. Both of these agents produce rapid reductions in alpha-mediated vasomotor tone and are effective in reducing systemic blood pressure; however, neither has an ultrashort duration of action, which makes them less popular to control systemic vascular resistance than the direct-acting vasodilators. For that reason, they find less application in broad practice. Both agents directly antagonize alpha-mediated systemic vasoconstriction.

Phentolamine. Phentolamine is a rapid-acting competitive antagonist of alpha$_1$- and alpha$_2$-receptors with an onset of 1 to 2 minutes when used in doses of 2 to 5 mg intravenously (Lawson, 1992). Its half-life is about 19 minutes (Armstrong & Moe, 1994). Tachyarrhythmias and hypotension are common side effects. Because it is less titratable than direct-acting vasodilators and has a longer duration of action, phentolamine finds little application in general practice, although, it still may be useful to manage acute hypertensive crisis in patients with autonomic hyperreflexia following spinal cord injury or paroxysmal hypertension in patients with pheochromocytoma (Lawson, 1992; Weiner, 1990a).

Phenoxybenzamine. Phenoxybenzamine is another direct alpha antagonist available only in oral form. As such, it has a slower onset of action than phentolamine and a half-life of 24 hours. It has little clinical application during anesthesia, but may be found as a preoperative treatment for patients with pheochromocytoma (Lawson, 1992).

Combined Antagonists

Labetalol. The combined alpha- and beta-antagonist effects of labetalol depend on the method of administration. It provides effective, readily titratable control of sympathetic tone with an approximate 1 to 7 ratio of alpha-to-beta blockade when used intravenously (Gold, Chang, & Cohen, 1982; Lawson, 1992). Labetalol proves effective to manage patients with transient hypertension and tachycardia, particularly during emergence from anesthesia (deBruihn et al., 1987). Labetalol has a rapid onset of action and usually reduces blood pressure within 5 minutes of intravenous administration. It generally is administered in doses beginning at 0.25 mg/kg and titrated in doubled doses at intervals of 5 to 10 minutes up to 300 mg to achieve the desired end point (Lawson, 1992). When used during the course of anesthesia, it is recommended that the drug dose be halved, which corresponds to an initial dose of 10 mg in the standard (70-kg) adult. It has a clinical duration of action of 16 to 18 hours. Labetalol may be administered in a continuous infusion, starting at a recommended dose of 2 mg/min (Lawson, 1992); however, because of its prolonged duration of action, it cannot be as tightly controlled as the direct-acting vasodilators and the rapidly metabolized beta-blocker esmolol.

Clinical Applications of Sympathetic Antagonists

The use of sympathetic antagonists during anesthesia is directed primarily to managing the hyperdynamic heart. Both beta antagonists are valuable in managing tachyarrhythmias and may be useful in acute-onset ventricular dysrhythmias that are unresponsive to or poorly controlled by standard antiarrhythmic therapy. Propranolol is frequently used in the management of patients with primary hypertension, both intraoperatively and as a chronic medication. The availability of the rapidly metabolized, short-acting beta-blocker esmolol has extended the usefulness of these agents for short-term management of hemodynamically significant tachycardias. When it proves necessary to convert to long-term suppression, it is possible to titrate esmolol dosage down while administering a longer-acting beta-antagonist such as propranolol. This allows the practitioner to achieve both immediate suppression without delay and long-term suppression without interruption. This method may be particularly useful in reducing arterial shear forces that may be increased during induced hypotension with direct-acting vasodilators such as nitroprusside. Thus, the combination of direct-acting vasodilators with short-acting beta-blockers may prove useful for aortic aneurysms suspected of dissection. Furthermore, the rapid titratability of esmolol makes it useful to treat catecholamine overdosage.

Because their beta-antagonistic effects may precipitate exacerbation of the underlying pulmonary dysfunction, it is recommended that beta-blockers be used with caution in patients with bronchospastic disease (Tattersfield & Harrison, 1983). It has been demonstrated that propranolol exacerbates pulmonary disease; esmolol appears to have less exacerbating effects (McDevitt, 1983). Similarly, beta-antagonists are not recommended for patients with primary ventricular failure, as they may exacerbate underlying ventricular dysfunction. In addition, they may markedly reduce blood sugar in the diabetic patient. Blood glucose should be carefully monitored when required (Hansten, 1980; Rizza, Cryer, & Hammond, 1980). Because of their synergistic effects, beta-antagonists should be used cautiously in patients receiving calcium channel blockers or digoxin (Lewis, 1983). Profound bradycardia can ensue when beta-antagonists in standard doses are given to patients receiving these agents.

Alpha-antagonists find comparatively less application in anesthetic practice. They may be used to manage patients with acute hypertension resulting from autonomic hyperreflexia following spinal cord injury or patients with uncontrolled pheochromocytoma. In the latter, it is recommended that alpha blockade be achieved before beta blockade, to prevent the development of heart failure when a depressed ventricle operates against excessive afterload. The availability of a variety of shorter-duration, rapidly titratable, direct-acting vasodilators such as nitroprusside has generally made control of systemic hypertension easier to achieve and maintain than the use of alpha-antagonists permits. Their application in anesthetic practice has therefore declined.

The combined alpha- and beta-antagonist labetalol provides rapid and effective control of hypertension and tachycardia, which is particularly effective in managing postoperative hypertension. This is particularly valuable in patients undergoing systemic vascular procedures such as carotid endarterectomy, in whom wide swings in pressure might otherwise be expected and in whom severe hypertension is to be avoided. Labetalol also may prove very effective as an adjunct in long-term control of postoperative hypertension in the general surgical population for up to 16 hours postoperatively (Malsch, Katonah, Gratz, & Scott, 1991).

Direct-Acting Vasodilators

At present, only three direct-acting vasodilators have broad clinical applications in the practice of anesthesia: nitroprusside, trimethaphan, and nitroglycerin. Both nitroprusside and nitroglycerin produce direct relaxation of the smooth muscle in vessels, although nitroprusside is more effective in low doses on the arterial tree and nitroglycerin is more effective in low doses on venous capacitance vessels. Trimethaphan has the additional effect of ganglionic blockade, which prevents increases in heart rate. The vasodilators are used primarily to control preload and afterload in anesthetic management, although nitroglycerin also is used to manage cardiac ischemia.

Nitroprusside

Nitroprusside is an extremely rapid-acting, short-lasting direct vasodilator. It has an onset of 1 to 2 minutes when administered in continuous infusion, and clinical effects last less than 5 minutes. It directly relaxes the smooth muscle in the vessel wall, causing both arterial and venous dilation that ultimately decreases systemic vascular resistance (Harrison & Bates, 1993; Stoelting, 1987a; Tinker & Michenfelder, 1980). It operates primarily on medium and small arteries and arterioles in low doses (<1.5 mg/kg/min), and it demonstrates progressively greater arterial dilation and dilation of venous capacitance vessels in higher doses up to 5 mg/kg/min (Lawson, 1992). It is not recommended that nitroprusside be used as a sole agent at doses in excess of 5 to 10 mg/kg/min or for prolonged maintenance because of the risk of cyanide toxicity (Lawson 1992; Lawson & Wallfisch, 1986; Tinker & Michenfelder, 1980).

Trimethaphan

Trimethaphan provides both direct-acting vasodilation and an accompanying autonomic ganglionic blockade (Lawson, 1992; Merin, 1990; Harioka, Hatano, Mori, & Toda, 1984; Knight, Lane, Hensinger, Bolles, & Bjoraker, 1983). It does cause histamine release, although this does not appear to have a significant impact on the production of hypotension (Fahmy & Sater, 1985; Merin, 1990). It generally is delivered as a continuous infusion with a starting dose of 1 to 2 mg/min, and it is titrated to control blood pressure in the desired range. It has a somewhat slower onset than nitroprusside, reaching clinical effect usually within 5 to 7 minutes, and the effects of ganglionic blockade are extended. However, systemic arterial pressure generally returns to the low normal range within about 10 minutes of discontinuation of the infusion because of metabolism by plasma pseudocholinesterases (Gerber & Nies, 1990).

Nitroglycerin

Nitroglycerin is a rapid-acting, short-lasting direct venodilator that affects primarily venous capacitance vessels in low doses (Lawson, 1992; Murad, 1990). It has a slightly slower onset than does nitroprusside (2 to 3 minutes) and a longer duration of action (5 to 10 minutes). At low doses (<1.5 mg/kg/min) it is an effective venodilator, reducing preload and pulmonary artery pressures. In higher doses (up to 5 mg/kg/min), it produces a progressive decrease in systemic resistance as well. In the recommended range, nitroglycerin has not been shown to have any toxicity (Murad, 1990). Nitroglycerin also has been shown to dilate the medium-sized coronary arteries, making it a mainstay in the treatment of myocardial ischemia.

Clinical Applications of Direct-Acting Vasodilators

All the direct-acting dilators are useful in managing patients with systemic hypertension or induction of deliberate hypotension, although nitroprusside is sometimes preferred for its more specific arterial action. Nitroglycerin may be used effectively in high doses for control of mild to moderate hypertension and is effective in managing mild to moderate degrees of pulmonary hypertension as well. Trimethaphan is useful in the management of hypertension and is sometimes preferred because its ganglionic blockade prevents the development of tachycardia that frequently accompanies rapid reductions in systemic arterial pressure (MacRae & Wildsmith, 1992; Simpson et al., 1996). In the management of hypertension nitroprusside is usually initiated at doses of 0.5 to 2 mg/kg/min and titrated to effect. Control of hypertension secondary to increased systemic vascular resistance usually is possible with doses less than 5 mg/kg/min. When doses greater than 5 to 10 mg/kg/min are required to manage primary hypertension in the patient who is not undergoing aortic cross-clamping, there is a risk of cyanide toxicity. To control hypertension in patients undergoing surgical cross-clamping of the aorta, doses in excess of 10 mg/kg/min may be required briefly during the interval of cross-clamping. In the clinical setting, higher doses have not resulted in any serious risk of toxicity. Nitroglycerin generally is used as a primary venodilator or to control pulmonary hypertension. In that capacity, it is useful in managing excessive preload in patients with congestive heart failure or in treating patients with volume overload in conjunction with diuresis. Nitroglycerin also may be used singly or in combination with nitroprusside in patients undergoing aortic cross-clamping. With infrarenal cross-clamping, nitroglycerin alone may prove effective in controlling hypertension. For patients undergoing procedures involving cross-clamping of the thoracic aorta, nitroglycerin does not prove as effective as nitroprusside in controlling hypertension during cross-clamping. It may, however, be used as an adjunct vasodilator to reduce preload and to unload the ventricle faced with excessive afterload.

Although trimethaphan has proven to be an effective arterial dilator, its ganglionic blockade lasts longer than the peripheral dilatory effect; this extended recovery time limits its use in patients susceptible to the hypotensive effects of ganglionic blockade. Because of the ganglionic blockade, it is effective in the management of hypertension and in reducing shear forces in patients with aortic dissection (Simpson et al., 1996), and it may be employed in that setting as an alternative to combined therapy with vasodilators and beta blockade. As it produces histamine release, trimethaphan may exacerbate symptoms in patients with bronchospastic disease, and it should be used with caution in that population.

Antihypertensive Agents

The antihypertensive agents are a mixed group with variable sites of action that are generally administered in bolus form to maintain blood pressure exclusively. In contrast to beta-antagonists, the actions of antihypertensive agents may center on centrally mediated control of hypertension, on peripheral vasomotor tone, or both. In contrast to the direct-acting vasodilators used in continuous infusion form, these agents have an extended duration of action and last several hours after a single bolus administration. A comprehensive listing of a variety of agents is provided in Table 22–2. Three drugs in this class find application during anesthetic management: hydralazine, methyldopa, and diazoxide.

Hydralazine

Hydralazine appears to produce an antihypertensive effect by direct peripheral vasodilation, possibly through release of endothelial factors (Lawson, 1992) that reduce systemic vascular resistance without producing myocardial depression (Lawson, 1992; Oates, 1996). In the patient with ventricular dysfunction, this may augment stroke volume and cardiac output. Hydralazine generally is administered in divided doses of 10 to 20 mg up to a total dose of 0.5 mg/kg (Lawson, 1992). The reduction in blood pressure is generally noted within 10 minutes, although peak reductions may not be noted for as long as 1 hour after administration. Tachycardia frequently accompanies the reduction in blood pressure after administration of hydralazine and may represent baroreceptor reflex or release of endogenous catecholamine (Azuma et al., 1987; Oates, 1996). Hydralazine appears to have a clinical half-life of 3 to 7 hours, though it may last up to 12 hours.

Methyldopa

Methyldopa appears to operate on the central axis by competing for metabolism with a natural transmitter to yield α-methylnorepinephrine or α-methylepinephrine, which operates as a weak false neurotransmitter producing central inhibitory alpha tone. Methyldopa also may produce a reduction in plasma renin activity. Because of its central action, onset is slow and may require up to 6 to 8 hours (Wright, Orozco-Gonzalez, Polak, & Dollery, 1982). It has a clinical duration of action of 10 to 16 hours after a single administration. The usual dose of methyldopa is 250 to 500 mg administered slowly. Because it has a slow onset, it usually is used only as maintenance in those patients receiving chronic therapy.

Diazoxide

Diazoxide operates directly on smooth muscle in the systemic arterial tree, promptly reducing systemic vascular resistance and arterial blood pressure (Lawson, 1992; Standen et al., 1989). The reduction in resistance may result in an increase in cardiac output, particularly in the patient with underlying left ventricular failure. Diazoxide is tightly protein bound, which makes it necessary to administer the drug intravenously as a rapid bolus to prevent complete binding of the administered dose (Lawson, 1992). Because of its protein binding, it is useful only for short-term control of hypertension. Diazoxide may be administered as a single rapid bolus of 150 to 300 mg or as a series of smaller divided boluses of 1 to 3 mg/kg at intervals greater than 5 minutes (Oates, 1996; Lawson, 1992). It has a rapid clinical effect, producing reductions in blood pressure within 5 to 10 minutes and peak effects within less than 30 minutes. The clinical duration of action is generally less than 12 hours (Lawson, 1992).

Clinical Applications of Antihypertensive Agents

The antihypertensive agents are generally used to manage patients who are on chronic antihypertensive ther-

TABLE 22–2. Antihypertensive Agents Employed during Anesthesia

Drug	Dose[a]	Latency	Duration	Side Effects
Diuretics				
Furosemide	20–40 mg IV	5–10 min	4 h	Hypokalemia, hypovolemia
Sympatholytics				
Alpha-methyldopa	250–500 mg SIV	20 min	24 h	Sedation, hepatitis, hemolytic anemia
Clonidine	0.2 mg in 10, mL NS per rectum	20 min	12–24 h	Sedation, dry mouth, withdrawal syndrome
Vasodilators				
Hydralazine	5–10 mg IV	15–20 min	4–6 h	Lupuslike syndrome, drug fever, rash
	10–40 mg IM	20–40 min		
Nifedipine	10 mg SIV	5–10 min	7 h	Headache, fluid retention
Verapamil	5 mg IV	2–5 min	4–6 h	Heart block, myocardial failure
Diazoxide	300 mg SIV	3–5 min	5–12 h	Decreased cerebral blood flow, hyperuricemia
Sodium nitroprusside	0.25–0.5 μg/kg/min	1–2 min	2–5 min	Cyanide toxicity, increased cerebral blood flow
Nitroglycerin		2–5 min	3–5 min	Headache, fluid retention

[a] Doses shown are for a 70-kg adult. IV, intravenous push; SIV, slow intravenous infusion; IM, intramuscular; SL, sublingual; NS, normal saline.
Source: Barash, P. G., Cullen, B. F., & Stoelting, R. K., (Eds.). (1989). Clinical anesthesia. *Philadelphia: Lippincott. Reprinted, with permission.*

apy or to control comparatively mild degrees of hypertension. Their relatively slow onset compared with direct-acting continuous-infusion vasodilators makes them less titratable, and their extended duration of action makes them less controllable. Hydralazine is useful for patients with acute hypertension not related to light anesthesia. It is an effective vasodilator for the patient expected to require treatment for hypertension for the first several hours following anesthesia when preoperative medications cannot be reinitiated. Likewise, it effectively reduces blood pressure in patients who require sustained control of systemic arterial pressure. It is synergistic when administered with titratable continuous-infusion agents. The rate of administration of infusion agents should be reduced to half the baseline when hydralazine is added to prevent severe hypotension from summated effects. Because the development of clinically significant tachycardias may accompany hydralazine-induced reductions in blood pressure, it is frequent practice to administer beta-blockers concomitantly to reduce myocardial oxygen demand. This may prove critical in the patient with symptomatic myocardial ischemia.

Diazoxide has a pattern of use similar to that of hydralazine. It finds application only for short-term maintenance during the perioperative period, and its use is not recommended for more than 10 days. It is generally employed only for the acute perioperative period. Patients receiving diazoxide may demonstrate increases in blood glucose levels, and diabetic patients should be monitored closely.

In contrast to other antihypertensive agents, methyldopa has a comparatively long onset and finds little application in short-term management of intraoperative hypertension. Its primary use in anesthesia is as a maintenance drug for those patients receiving methyl-

dopa as a chronic medication in the treatment of hypertension. Methyldopa may produce a positive Coombs test in patients (Gerber & Nies, 1990), leading to difficulty in establishing an accurate cross-match for compatible homologous blood. In general, when only the direct Coombs test is positive, a cross-match can be completed. When both direct and indirect Coombs tests are positive, cross-matching for compatible blood may be complex.

The advent of the rapid-onset continuous-infusion agents has reduced the use of antihypertensive agents for anesthesia because of the greater controllability of the former agents. Classic antihypertensive agents, however, should not be ignored. They may be used to establish and maintain prolonged reductions in blood pressure when desired. These agents are effective in producing a mild sustained reduction in systemic vascular resistance that can then be augmented by the use of reduced doses of the titratable agents when brief periods of profound hypotension are required or in reducing the requirement for direct-acting titratable vasodilators when sustained reductions in systemic vascular resistance and systemic pressure are required in the perioperative period.

Calcium Channel Blockers

Only two calcium channel blockers are currently in common anesthetic use: verapamil and nifedipine. These represent two different actions and applications. Calcium channel blockers have been grouped into two forms based on their blocking of the slow or fast calcium channels (Gagnon et al., 1982; Stoelting, 1987a); however, it is likely that both forms block the slow calcium channel. Calcium channel blockers may be used to control tachycardias, as in the treatment of supraventricular tachycardias, or vasomotor tone, as in the control of pulmonary artery hypertension or coronary spasm (Reves, 1984).

Verapamil

Verapamil is a calcium-entry blocker that provides effective treatment of supraventricular tachycardia (Haft & Habab, 1986; Lawson, 1992). It effectively blocks reuptake of calcium and prolongs the rate of spontaneous depolarization in pacemaker cells. It also appears to possess some alpha-blocking activity that reduces peripheral vasomotor tone, operating at the level of the resistance vessels (Tosone et al., 1983). Verapamil demonstrates only mild myocardial depressant effect in the normal heart; however, in the patient with ventricular dysfunction, the depressant effect may become clinically significant (Lawson, 1992). In doses of 2.5 to 5 mg intravenously it generally provides control of tachycardias, which is hemodynamically significant within 3 to 5 minutes (Lawson, 1992). Total doses of up to 10 mg may be required in young patients; elderly patients usually respond satisfactorily to a total dose of 5 mg. Verapamil has an initial redistribution half-life of about 4 hours and an elimination half-life of 2 to 5 hours, which may be extended in patients receiving chronic therapy (Murad, 1990; Raemsch & Sommer, 1983).

Nifedipine

Nifedipine is a calcium channel blocker that demonstrates little effect on the rate of recovery of slow calcium channels. It is of little benefit in controlling tachycardias. Nifedipine produces effective systemic and pulmonary artery dilation when administered in sublingual form. It also produces effective coronary artery dilation in the patient suffering from coronary artery spasm or Prinzmetals variant angina (Reves et al., 1982; Reves, 1984), and it is the treatment of choice for that condition. In addition, nifedipine appears to be effective in dilating internal mammary artery grafts that develop vasospasm, and it may be used for this purpose during myocardial revascularization. The usual dose of nifedipine is 0.1 to 0.25 mg/kg, which may be given sublingually, corresponding to 10 to 20 mg in the typical (70-kg) adult (Stoelting, 1987a). It has an onset of less than 5 minutes and a half-life of 1 to 2 hours (Lawson, 1992). At present, nifedipine is available only in the sublingual or oral form; however, current work is under way to prepare an intravenous form that will facilitate its use in clinical anesthesia.

Clinical Applications of Calcium Channel Blockers

Verapamil may be used during the course of anesthesia as an adjunct in the management of paroxysmal tachycardias. It is effective as a sole agent to control tachycardias;

however, with rapid administration marked decreases in systemic blood pressure may be seen because of its alpha-blocking effects and myocardial depression in response to calcium channel blockade. When declines in blood pressure are precipitous, as in the patient with impaired ventricular function, administration of calcium chloride titrated in increments of 100 to 250 mg may block myocardial depression and peripheral dilation without antagonizing the antiarrhythmic effects of the drug. Verapamil demonstrates no significant effect on coronary vasospasm, but it is not shown to be effective in controlling primary coronary spasm. It should be used with caution in conjunction with either beta-blocking agents or digoxin as the effects of these agents may be additive or synergistic and severe bradycardias may occur. However, it also has been used effectively to treat digoxin-induced ventricular arrhythmias (Rosen & Danil, 1980).

Nifedipine may be used preoperatively to manage coronary vasospasm. It is also useful in the patient with coronary artery spasm during surgery or to treat spasm of the internal mammary artery used as a coronary graft. As with verapamil, it should be used with caution in patients with primary ventricular dysfunction as it may demonstrate myocardial depressant effects that can be antagonized with calcium in incremental boluses. It also should be used with caution in patients receiving beta-blockers as it may be additive or synergistic. Because of its more potent pulmonary dilation, nifedipine may be effective in the management of patients with acute pulmonary hypertension in response to stress, such as aortic cross-clamping or acute left ventricular dysfunction.

Antiarrhythmic Agents

The antiarrhythmic agents represent a broad class of drugs with a variety of actions. Their primary use is to control ventricular or supraventricular arrhythmias during anesthesia. There is considerable overlap among antiarrhythmic agents, and a number of previously discussed agents are employed as antiarrhythmics. Sympathetic antagonists, particularly the beta-blockers, are used to control supraventricular tachycardias and may find application in the control of ventricular dysrhythmias that fail to respond to the usual antiarrhythmic therapy, as previously outlined. Calcium channel blockers, particularly verapamil, may be used to treat supraventricular tachycardias, as previously discussed. A comprehensive listing of antiarrhythmics is provided in Table 22-3. Six agents are typically used in anesthesia: the local anesthetics lidocaine and procainamide and bretylium, phenytoin, quinidine, and digoxin.

Local Anesthetics

Local anesthetics are used primarily to treat or control ventricular dysrhythmias. Two agents are typically used

TABLE 22–3. Pharmacology of Antiarrhythmic Agents

Class	Drug	Commonly Used Dosage	Elimination Half-Life	Therapeutic Plasma Level (μg mL^{-1})	Side Effects
IA	Quinidine	Oral: 200–600 mg q 6–8 h IV: 6–10 mg/kg over 30 min followed by 2–3 mg/min	6 h	2–6	Quinidine syncope, conduction disturbances, nausea, vomiting, diarrhea, thrombocytopenia, hypotension
	Procainamide	Oral: 250–1000 mg q 4 h (q 6 for sustained-release form) IV: 10–20 mg/kg over 20–40 min followed by 2–6 mg/min	2–4 h	4–12 (8–15, N-acetyl procainamide)	Conduction disturbances, nausea, diarrhea, fever, lupus syndrome, hypotension
	Disopyramide	Oral: 150–300 mg q 6–8 h IV: 2 mg/kg over 3–5 min	6–8 h	5–7	Cardiac depression, conduction disturbances, anticholingeric symptoms
IB	Lidocaine	IV: 1–2 mg/kg bolus followed by 20–40 μg/kg/min	1–2 h	2–5	Drowsiness, hallucination, seizures, paranoid ideation
	Tocainide	Oral: 400–600 mg q 8 h	13–15 h	4–10	Tremor, dizziness, ataxia, paresthesia, rash, hepatitis, nausea, vomiting
	Mexiletine	Oral: 150–300 mg q 6–8 h	10–20 h	0.75–2.0	Tremor, convulsion, dizziness, photosensitivity, dermatitis, hypotension, nausea, vomiting
	Phenytoin	Oral: 200–400 mg once daily IV: 50–100 mg every 5 min to maximum 1 g	24 h	10–18	Hypotension, vertigo, lethargy, dysarthria, gingivitis, macrocytic anemia, lupus, pulmonary infiltrates
	Moricizine (ethmozine)	Oral: 75–200 mg q 8 h	4–10 h		Dizziness, headache, pruritus
IC	Encainide	Oral: 25–75 mg q 6–8 h IV: 0.5–1 mg/kg over 15 min	3–4 h	0.01–0.02	Conduction disturbances, blurred vision, nystagmus, dizziness, ataxia, vertigo, paresthesia, nausea, proarrhythmic
	Flecainide	Oral: 100–200 mg q 12 h IV: 2 mg/kg over 10 min	18–20 h	0.2–1.0	Blurred vision, headache, lightheadedness, ataxia, proarrhythmic
	Lorcainide	Oral: 100–200 mg q 12 h IV: 1–2 mg/kg over 30 min	7–13 h (norlorcainide, 24 h)	0.05–0.3 0.08–0.3	Sleep disturbances, nightmares, tremor, hyponatremia, nausea, diarrhea
Unclassified					
	Propafenone	Oral: 100–300 mg q 8 h IV: 2 mg/kg over 15 min	4–8 h	0.5–2.0	Dizziness, metallic taste, conduction disturbances, nausea
II	Propranolol (β_1/β_2)[a]	Oral: 20–80 mg q 6 h IV: 0.5–1 mg q 2 min to maximum 6–10 mg	3–6 h	0.05–0.1	Depression, fatigue, atrioventricular block, bradycardia, myocardial depression
	Acebutolol (β_1/β_2)	Oral: 600–1200 mg once daily	24 h		As above
	Atenolol (β_1)	Oral: 50–200 mg once daily	24 h		As above
	Nadolol (β_1/β_2)	Oral: 40–240 mg	24 h		As above
	Timolol (β_1/β_2)	Oral: 20–60 mg	15 h		As above

continued

TABLE 22–3. Pharmacology of Antiarrhythmic Agents *(Continued)*

Class	Drug	Commonly Used Dosage	Elimination Half-Life	Therapeutic Plasma Level (μg mL^{-1})	Side Effects
III	Amiodarone	Oral: 800–1600 mg/d for 2 wk, then 200–600 mg/d maintenance IV: 5–10 mg/kg bolus over 5–15 min, then 800–1600 mg/d as a continuous infusion or in divided doses	13–60 d		Corneal deposit, gastrointestinal disturbances, altered thyroid function, interstitial pulmonary disease, peripheral neuropathy, bradycardia, conduction block, hepatic dysfunction
Unclassified					
	Bretylium	IV: 5–10 mg/kg bolus over 10–30 min, then 1–4 mg min^{-1}	6–8 h	0.8–2.0	Transient hypertension, sinus tachycardia, postural hypotension, proarrhythmic
IV	Verapamil	Oral: 80–160 mg q 6–8 h IV: 5–10 mg bolus, repeated after 10 min to a maximum of 20 mg Continuous infusion: 1–5 μg/kg/min	4–8 h	0.1	Cardiac depression, hypotension, atrioventricular block, asystole, edema, headache, constipation
	Diltiazem	Oral: 60–90 mg q 6 h	3–5 h		Edema, postural hypotension
Other agents					
	Digoxin	Oral: 1–1.5 mg in divided doses over 24 h for digitalization, 0.125–0.25 mg once daily for maintenance IV: 0.75–1 mg in divided doses over 24 h for digitalization	1.5 d	1–2	Anorexia, nausea, vomiting, diarrhea, malaise, fatigue, confusion, headache, colored vision, arrhythmias, aggravation of heart failure

[a] β_1/β_2, noncardioselective beta-blockers; β_1, cardioselective beta-blockers.
Source: Barash, P. G., Cullen, B. F., & Stoelting, R. K. (Eds.) (1989). Clinical anesthesia. Philadelphia: Lippincott. 1989; Platia, E. V. Management of cardiac arrhythmias. Philadelphia: Lippincott.

during anesthetic management: lidocaine and procainamide. Both appear to operate at the site of the Na–K channel to slow the rate of spontaneous depolarization and extend the refractory period in the conductive tissue. Hence, their action as antiarrhythmic agents parallels their action as anesthetic agents.

Lidocaine. Lidocaine appears to extend specifically the phase 4 period of depolarization in myocardial conductive tissue, thereby decreasing the rate of automaticity without producing significant changes in membrane function when used in the recommended therapeutic range (Bigger & Hoffman, 1990; Roden, 1996). When administered in the usual dose of 1 to 1.5 mg/kg, it generally produces a quelling of ventricular excitability within 1 to 2 minutes (Holley, Ponganis, & Stanski, 1984). Lidocaine has a short clinical duration, with a bolus dose lasting for no more than 10 to 15 minutes. Therefore, it is

generally continued as a prolonged infusion at a rate of 1 to 4 mg/min for long-term control of ventricular dysrhythmias. The appearance of continued ventricular ectopy may be treated with smaller boluses of 0.5 mg/kg and an increase in the rate of administration of the continuous infusion. Central nervous system (CNS) disturbances, such as drowsiness, hearing problems, disorientation, twitching, and convulsions, may occur.

Procainamide. Procainamide has a mechanism of action similar to that of lidocaine, but it also appears to produce electrophysiologic changes in the atria and AV node (Bigger & Hoffman, 1990; Roden, 1996). It appears to be a more potent suppressant of ventricular ectopy, but it is also a more potent myocardial depressant and produces peripheral vasodilation through ganglionic blockade (Bigger & Hoffman, 1990). For these reasons, procainamide seldom is used unless therapy with lidocaine alone has proven insufficient. Procainamide generally produces a clinical effect within 2 minutes and lasts 10 to 15 minutes after a single bolus. When administered as a bolus, it should be given slowly because of its myocardial depressant effect. It is recommended that no more than 50 to 100 mg be given in any bolus; a total of no more than 500 mg is recommended in divided boluses to control ventricular ectopy, although persistent ectopy may require a total loading dose of up to 1 gm (Roden, 1996). When administered as a continuous infusion, procainamide should be maintained at the rate of 2 to 6 mg/min (Zaidan & Barash, 1998).

Other Antiarrhythmics

Bretylium. Bretylium appears to accumulate in the sympathetic intrinsic nerve terminal blocking release of norepinephrine. This results in a predominance of alpha-adrenergic blocking effects (Bigger & Hoffman, 1990). Thus bretylium does not alter the depolarization of normal conductive tissue, but it does appear to restore the normal depolarization pattern in cells injured by ischemia or other events. It also may increase the duration of the action potential in conductive tissue. The administration of bretylium is associated with an early phase of increased catecholamine release that briefly aggravates ectopy, increases inotropy, and increases systemic vascular resistance (Bigger & Hoffman, 1990; Roden, 1996). This is followed by a second phase of suppression of sympathetic activity that produces the antiarrhythmic effects (Bigger & Hoffman, 1990; Roden, 1996). Therefore, bretylium generally is used only as an antiarrhythmic when other therapies such as the local anesthetics have failed to control adequately ventricular ectopy. The standard dose of bretylium is a 5- to 10-mg/kg bolus administered over several minutes up to 30 mg/kg. When ventricular ectopy persists, an additional bolus may be required for a total of 10 mg/kg (Bigger & Hoffman, 1990). Clinical effects are slow to appear, and peak effects in suppression of ventricular ectopy are not noted for up to 6 hours after administration, so that bretylium may be administered as intermittent slow boluses or may be maintained as a continuous infusion of 1 to 2 mg/min.

Quinidine. Quinidine generally is administered orally to treat arrhythmias resulting from states of enhanced atrial or ventricular automaticity, while enhancing the rate of transmission of impulses across the AV node (Bigger & Hoffman, 1990). It appears to reduce atrial and ventricular automaticity by extending phase 4 of depolarization and the duration of the refractory period by slowing the rate of depolarization and repolarization and reducing the amplitude of the action potential generated (Hoffman, 1990; Pritchett, 1992). The action on the AV node appears to be mediated by a direct anticholinergic effect that blocks vagal tone, which may also account for its mild myocardial depressant effect. Because it is usually administered orally, quinidine finds little direct application in anesthesia and is most frequently used in chronic maintenance therapy.

Phenytoin. Phenytoin is used most commonly as an anticonvulsant. Its ability to promote the efflux of sodium from the cell, resulting in a stabilization of the membrane potential, (Arky, 1997), also makes it useful in the management of atrial dysrhythmias. Because it continues to depress ventricular automaticity, it may not be recommended in patients with second- or third-degree heart block (Bigger & Hoffman, 1990). The standard dose of phenytoin is a 50- to 100-mg bolus administered every 5 minutes until desired effects are reached up to a total dose of 1 g (Bigger & Hoffman, 1990). A fast-flowing intravenous line should be used, as it will precipitate if not given proximally. It has a clinical effect within 5 minutes, and the duration of action appears to be up to 12 hours. Phenytoin may increase conduction across the AV node, enhancing the transmission of rapid atrial rates transiently (Bigger & Hoffman, 1990).

Digoxin. Digoxin is the only cardiac glycoside currently used in intravenous form to control atrial dysrhythmias. Digoxin produces alterations in both sympathetic outflow and vagal tone (Gillis & Onset, 1979; Vasalle, 1986). The latter produces a slowing of SA automaticity and conduction of impulses at the AV node, and it is the basis for the use of digoxin in controlling the ventricular response rate in patients with atrial fibrillation. Digoxin also may be used as an inotropic agent in the patient with congestive failure, in whom it increases the sympathetic tone and reduces systemic vascular resistance (Ferguson et al., 1989). The effects of digoxin administration on ventricular response rate may be seen within 5 to 30 minutes of administration of a 0.25-mg bolus intravenously. Repeated doses may be necessary to establish a therapeutic response in the patient who has not been previously digitalized. Peak effects may not be seen for up to 4 to 6 hours (Bigger & Hoffman, 1992). In the patient receiving digoxin preoperatively, supplemental doses of 0.125 to 0.25 mg may be sufficient. It has a clinical half-life of up to 2 days, which is variable depending on the patient's condition (Bigger & Hoffman, 1992). Because of the sympathetic axis stimulation, digoxin also may predispose the patient to ventricular ectopy.

Clinical Applications of Antiarrhythmic Agents

The use of antiarrhythmic agents is determined by the appearance of atrial or ventricular ectopy. The management of ventricular ectopy or fibrillation generally is predicated on the use of local anesthetics. Of those, lidocaine generally is preferred because it appears to produce less myocardial depression than procainamide and has fewer drug reactions. Management of refractory ventricular ectopy or fibrillation may incorporate the use of beta-antagonists, such as propranolol, to suppress sympathetic tone and augment the effects of the local anesthetics.

Alternately, the use of bretylium permits the practitioner to quell ventricular ectopy without suppressing the normal mechanism for depolarization in myocardial conductive tissue. Bretylium, however, does have an associated interval of sympathetic discharge, during which the patient may demonstrate hyperdynamism and increased irritability. It is not generally used unless previous efforts at therapy have failed and ventricular fibrillation persists despite the use of local anesthetics and countershock.

The use of quinidine allows control of atrial and ventricular dysrhythmias effectively, although its myocardial depressant effects may reduce ventricular function in the impaired ventricle. It should be used with caution in patients with atrial flutter as it does enhance transmission across the AV node and may predispose to rapid ventricular response rates in that situation. It also should be used cautiously in the presence of incomplete AV block. Administration of quinidine has been shown to increase the serum digoxin level in patients receiving both agents, and it should be used with caution in that patient population.

Phenytoin allows the practitioner to control atrial arrhythmias, although the use of calcium channel blockers and beta-antagonists has made this application less common. To manage atrial tachycardias, verapamil and beta-antagonists offer a more rapid control of rate and are preferred. Phenytoin does block the effects of digoxin at the level of the AV node, making it an effective treatment for digoxin-induced bradycardia or dysrhythmias. Phenytoin does cause an increase in blood glucose levels; therefore, diabetic patients should be monitored closely when it is employed.

The use of digoxin both to treat congestive heart failure and to control ventricular response rates in the patient with atrial fibrillation or flutter is well established. In the patient with new-onset atrial fibrillation, digoxin may quell atrial irritability and reestablish a sinus mechanism. For this reason, some practitioners use digoxin prophylactically in patients undergoing pneumonectomy, a population in which there is a high incidence of new-onset atrial fibrillation in response to the increased pulmonary artery pressures. In the patient with long-standing atrial fibrillation, digoxin reduces AV node transmission of the electrical impulse that parallels plasma level, permitting the practitioner to control the ventricular response rate effectively. Caution should be

used in the treatment of atrial flutter with digoxin as there is a narrow threshold at which the corresponding AV block must be maintained. Conversion of a 3:1 or 4:1 block allows the maintenance of a ventricular rate of 100 to 75 beats per minute, whereas increases in the dose of digoxin may easily convert the 4:1 to a greater ratio resulting in significant bradycardia. For that reason, the availability of continuous monitoring is paramount, and treatment of bradycardia with either pacing or phenytoin may be indicated. Digoxin may predispose to ventricular dysrhythmias, particularly in the presence of associated electrolyte disturbances. As these ventricular dysrhythmias generally are difficult to convert, it is important to follow the electrolyte profile in patients receiving digoxin, paying particular attention to the serum potassium level.

▶ CASE STUDY

A 66-year-old male is rushed to the operating room for emergency abdominal aortic aneurysm repair for impending rupture. Preoperative evaluation reveals that the patient underwent coronary artery bypass grafting 12 years before. A right carotid endarterectomy also was performed 3 months ago, and the left carotid artery remains 60% occluded. Chronic medications include digitalis, nitroglycerin patch, and aspirin. Upon admission to the operating room blood pressure is 90/60, heart rate 120, and respirations 32 per minute. The patient complains of severe back pain and is perspiring profusely.

1. What are the anesthetic implications for this case?

   This patient has systemic atherosclerosis with probable multiple organ involvement. Patency of coronary artery grafts should be questioned. In addition, a retroperitoneal tamponade from abdominal aortic aneurysm leak is probable. The goal of induction is a smooth course that avoids hypotension or hypertension. The goal of maintenance also is to control systemic blood pressure, prevent myocardial ischemia, and maintain adequate urinary output and thermal regulation.

2. What anesthetic protocol is best suited for this patient?

   Anesthetic management varies with the provider preference, emergent nature of the procedure, and risk factors. Initiate rapid-sequence induction with inhalation, narcotic, or combined anesthesia technique. In addition to routine monitoring, invasive monitoring that includes arterial and pulmonary artery pressures and central venous pressure should be instituted to guide fluid management. Large-bore intravenous catheters are warranted for judicious fluid and colloid administration. Precordial leads on the ECG are necessary for detecting myocardial ischemia. Fluid warmers should be part of the anesthetic care.

3. What pharmacologic agents would you use to support hemodynamics during episodes of hypotension or hypertension and aortic cross clamping? Provide rationale for each agent selected.

Because the goal of anesthesia is to maintain intravascular volume and protect the myocardium and kidneys, specific cardioactive drugs or combinations of these drugs are important components of the anesthetic regime. Therapy is initiated and titrated to effect according to the following parameters: heart rate, blood pressure, cardiac output pulmonary capillary wedge pressure, central venous pressure, ECG and urinary output. Prepare infusions of:

Nitroprusside: causes arterial and venous dilation decreasing systemic vascular resistance.
Nitroglycerine: low doses produce venodilator effects, reducing preload and pulmonary artery pressures; higher doses decrease systemic vascular resistance and dilate coronary arteries.
Dopamine: low dose produces positive inotropic and renal vasodilator effects.
Dobutamine: reduces vasomotor tone, and ventricular afterload. Reduces pulmonary vascular resistance; use is indicated in sudden increases in pulmonary pressure, unloading the right ventricle, and maintaining cardiac output

without increasing systemic vascular resistance.

4. Discuss bolus and/or drip doses of the cardioactive drugs identified in question 3.

Nitroprusside: 50 mg/250 mL (200 μg/mL); 0.1–8.0 μg/kg/min
Nitroglycerine: 50- to 100-μg bolus; 50–100 mg/250 mL (200–400 μg/mL); 0.1–7 μg/kg/min
Dopamine: 200 mg/250 mL (800 μg/mL); 2–10 μg/kg/min
Dobutamine: 250 mg/250 mL (1000 μg/mL); 2.5–5 μg/kg/min

▶ SUMMARY

Increases in the availability of intravenous agents have improved the sophistication and precision with which anesthesia providers can manage the hemodynamic profile of their patients. The effective use of these agents requires an appreciation of their basic pharmacologic and physiologic effects. Critical to this knowledge base is cognizance of the wide interpatient variation in drug response. Effective management of the unpredictable alteration in clinical response requires knowledge of dose effect of specific drugs and the ability to rapidly change that dosage. By applying principles of cardiovascular physiology and integrating the pharmacologic effects of the variety of agents available, complex cases can be more effectively and safely managed than previously possible.

▶ KEY CONCEPTS

- The majority of agents employed for hemodynamic control during anesthesia operate by modulating the effects of the autonomic nervous system. This mechanism of action allows for the ability to augment or reduce autonomic tone by use of selective agonists or antagonists.
- Cardiovascular drugs produce their effect by interacting with specific receptors. Direct effects change heart rate (sinoatrial automaticity), myocardial contractility, conduction, and systemic vascular resistance. Indirect effects change cardiac output, stroke volume, and blood pressure.
- Agonists induce a response at the receptor site, and antagonists interact with and occupy the receptor site, thereby reducing or inhibiting the effects of the agonists.
- Sympathetic agonists operate through two mechanisms: the intrinsic route from sympathetic fibers that terminate in the systemic and

pulmonary vasculature and in the heart at several sites including the sinoatrial (SA) node, the atrioventricular (AV) node, and the Purkinje fibers responsible for transmission of the impulses to the ventricles. The primary neurotransmitter for the intrinsic route is norepinephrine. The hormonal or humoral route operates by releasing catecholamines from the adrenal medulla. The primary neurotransmitter for the humoral route is epinephrine.
- The pharmacologic effect of sympathomimetics varies with dosage because of changes in type of receptor interaction with increasing concentrations.
- Sympathetic antagonists directly antagonize the systemic and cardiac effects of agonist agents. They operate through the sympathetic route to reduce the inotropic state, slow heart rate, and reduce arrhythmogenicity through antagonism of beta-mediated effects, or produce systemic dilation through antagonism of alpha-mediated vasomotor tone.

- Vasodilators are primarily used to control preload and afterload by directly relaxing smooth muscle in blood vessels.
- The action of antihypertensives is through central mediation of control of blood pressure, on peripheral muscle tone, or both.
- Calcium channel blockers are classified as slow or fast channel blockers and are used to control supraventricular tachyarrhythmias, vasomotor tone, pulmonary artery hypertension, or coronary spasm.
- Pulmonary artery catheter measurement of atrial filling pressures, cardiac output, and systemic and pulmonary vascular resistance is recommended to determine the benefit-risk ratios of drug therapy, particularly when sympathomimetics are used.

▶ STUDY QUESTIONS

1. What are the direct and indirect effects of drug receptors?

2. Distinguish between the receptor subtypes responsible for mediation of drug activity.

3. What are the mechanisms of action of sympathetic agonists?

4. What is the primary clinical application of direct-acting vasodilators in anesthetic protocols?

5. How do calcium channel blockers exert their pharmacologic effects?

KEY REFERENCES

Hoffman, B. B., & Lefkowitz, R. J. (1996). Catecholamines, sympathomimetic drugs, and adrenergic receptor antagonists. In J. G. Hardman, L. E. Limbird, P. B. Molinoff, R. W. Ruddon, & A. G. Gilman (Eds.), *Goodman & Gilman's The pharmacologic basis of therapeutics* (9th ed., pp. 199–248). New York: McGraw-Hill.

Larach, D. R., & Solina, A. R. (1995). Cardiovascular drugs. In F. A. Hensley & D. E. Martin (Eds.), *A practical approach to cardiac anesthesia* (2nd ed., pp. 32–95). Boston: Little, Brown.

Schwinn, D. (1994). Cardiac pharmacology. In F. G. Estafanous, P. G. Barash, & J. G. Reves (Eds.), *Cardiac anesthesia: Principles and clinical practice* (p. 21–65). Philadelphia: Lippincott.

Weiner, N. (1990a). Drugs that inhibit adrenergic nerves and block adrenergic receptors. In A. G. Gilman, T. W. Rall, A. S. Nies, & P. Taylor (Eds.), *Goodman and Gilman's The pharmacologic basis of therapeutics* (8th ed.). New York: Pergamon Press.

Weiner, N. (1990b). Norepinephrine, epinephrine, and the sympathomimetic amines. In A. G. Gilman, T. W. Rall, A. S. Nies, & P. Taylor (Eds.), *Goodman and Gilman's The pharmacologic basis of therapeutics* (8th ed., p. 145). New York: Pergamon Press.

REFERENCES

Arky, R. (1997). *Physicians desk reference* (51st ed., pp. 1967–1970). Oradell, NJ: Medical Economics Co.

Armstrong, P. W., & Moe, G. W. (1994). Medical advances in the treatment of congestive heart failure. *Circulation, 88,* 2941–2952.

Azuma, J., Sawamura, A., Harada, H., Awata, N., Kishimoto, S., & Sperelakis, N. (1987). Mechanism of direct cardiostimulating actions of hydralazine. *European Journal of Pharmacology, 135,* 137–144.

Barques, D. E., & Schwinn, D. A. (1991). New advances in receptor pharmacology. *Current Opinions in Anaesthesia, 486.*

Bigger, J. T., & Hoffman, B. F. (1990). Antiarrhythmic drugs. In A. G. Gilman, T. W. Rall, A. S. Nies, & P. Taylor (Eds.), *Goodman and Gilman's The pharmacologic basis of therapeutics* (8th ed.). New York: Pergamon Press.

Chernow, B., Rainey, T. G., & Lake, C. R. (1984). Catecholamines in critical care medicine. In M. G. Ziegler & C. R. Lake (Eds.), *Frontiers of clinical neuroscience. 2: Norepinephrine.* Baltimore: Williams & Wilkins.

deBruihn, N. P., Reves, J. G., Croughwell, N., Clements, F., & Drissel, D. A. (1987). Pharmacokinetics of esmolol in anesthetized patients receiving chronic beta blockade therapy. *Anesthesiology, 66,* 323–326.

Fahmy, N. R., & Sater, N. A. (1985). Effects of trimethaphan on arterial blood histamine and systemic hemodynamics in humans. *Anesthesiology, 62,* 562–566.

Ferguson, D. W., Berg , W. J., Sanders, J. S., Roach, P. J., Kempf, J. S., & Kienzle, M. G. (1989). Sympathoinhibitory responses to digitalis glycosides in heart failure patients. Direct evidence from sympathetic neural recordings. *Circulation, 80,* 65–77.

Furman, W. R., Summer, W. R., & Kennedy, T. P., & Sylvester, J. T. (1982). Comparison of the effects of dobutamine, dopamine and isoproterenol on hypoxic pulmonary vasoconstriction in the pig. *Critical Care Medicine, 10,* 371–374.

Gagnon, R. M., Morissette, M., Priesant, S., Savard, D., & Lemire, J. (1982). Hemodynamic and coronary effects of intravenous labetalol in coronary artery disease. *American Journal of Cardiology, 49,* 1267–1269.

Garcia-Sainz, J. A. G., Molina, R. V., Corvera, S., Bahena, J. H., Tsujimoto, G., & Hoffman, B. B. (1985). Differential effects of adrenergic agonists and phorbol esters on the alpha-adrenoreceptors of hepatocytes and aorta. *European Journal of Pharmacology, 112,* 393–397.

George, M., Lehot, J. J., & Estanove, S. (1992). Haemodynamic and biological effects of intravenous milrinone in patients with a low cardiac output syndrome following cardiac surgery: Multicenter study. *European Journal of Anaesthesiology, 5* (Suppl.), 31–34.

Gerber, J. G., & Nies, A. S. (1990). Antihypertensive agents and the drug therapy of hypertension. In A. G. Gilman, T. W. Rall, A. S. Nies, & P. Taylor (Eds.), *Goodman and Gilman's The pharmacologic basis of therapeutics* (8th ed.), New York: Pergamon Press.

Gillis, R. A., & Onset, J. A. (1979). The role of the nervous system in the cardiovascular effects of digitalis. *Pharmacology Review, 31,* 19–97.

Gold, E. H. , Chang, W., & Cohen, M. (1982). Synthesis and comparison of some cardiovascular properties of some stereoisomers of labetalol. *Journal of Medicinal Chemistry, 25,* 1363–1370.

Gorczynski, R. (1985). Basic pharmacology of esmolol. *American Journal of Cardiology, 56,* 3F.

Guyton, A. C. (1996). The autonomic nervous system: The adrenal medulla. In C. Guyton (Ed.), *Textbook of medical physiology.* Philadelphia: Saunders.

Haft, J. I., & Habbab, M. A. (1986). Treatment of atrial arrhythmias: Effectiveness of verapamil when preceded by calcium infusion. *Archive of Internal Medicine, 146,* 1085.

Hansten, P. D. (1980). Beta blocking agents and antidiabetic drugs. *Clinical Pharmacology, 14,* 46.

Harioka, T., Hatano, Y, Mori, K., & Toda, N. (1984). Trimethaphan is a direct arterial vasodilator and an alpha-adrenoreceptor antagonist. *Anesthesia & Analgesia, 63,* 290–296.

Hoffman, B., & Bigger, J. T. (1990). Digitalis and allied cardiac glycosides. In A. G. Gilman, T. W. , Rall, A. S. Nies, & P. Taylor (Eds.), *Goodman and Gilman's The pharmacologic basis of therapeutics* (8th ed.). New York: Pergamon Press.

Holley, F. O., Ponganis, K. V., & Stanski, D. R. (1984). Effects of cardiac surgery with cardiopulmonary bypass on lidocaine disposition. *Clinical Pharmacology Therapeutics, 35,* 617–626.

Knight, P. R., Lane, G. A., Hensinger, R. N., Bolles, R. S., & Bjoraker, D. J. (1983). Catecholamine and renin angiotensin response during hypotensive anesthesia induced by sodium nitroprusside or trimethaphan camsylate. *Anesthesiology. 59,* 248–253.

Larach, D. R., & Solina, A. R. (1995). Cardiovascular drugs. In F. A. Hensley & D. E. Martin (Eds.), *A practical approach to cardiac anesthesia* (2nd ed., pp. 32–95). Boston: Little, Brown.

Lawson, N. W. (1992). Autonomic nervous system physiology and pharmacology. In P. G. Barash, B. F. Cullen, & R. K. Stoelting (Eds.), *Clinical anesthesia* (pp. 319–384). Philadelphia: Lippincott.

Lawson, N. W., & Wallfisch, H. K. (1986). Cardiovascular pharmacology: A new look at the pressors. In R. K. Stoelting, P. G. Barash, & P. G. Gallagher (Eds.), *Advances in anesthesia.* Chicago: Year Book Publishers.

Leier, C. V., & Unverferth, D. V. (1983). Drugs five years later. Dobutamine. *Annals of Internal Medicine, 99,* 490–496.

Lewis, J. G. (1983). Adverse reactions to calcium antagonists. *Drugs, 25,* 196–222.

Lincoln, J., & Burnstock, G. (1990). Neuroendothelial interaction in control of local blood flow. In J. B. Warren (Ed.)., *The endothelium: An introduction to current research.* New York: Wiley-Liss.

MacRae, W. R., & Wildsmith, J. A. (1992). Mixtures of sodium nitroprusside and trimethaphan for induction of hypotension. *Anesthesia & Analgesia, 74,* 781–782.

Malsch, E., Katonah, J., Gratz, I., & Scott, A. (1991). The effectiveness of labetalol in treating postoperative hypertension. *Nurse Anesthesia, 2,* 65–71.

McDevitt, D. G. (1983). Beta-adrenoceptor blocking drugs and partial agonist activity. Is it clinically relevant? *Drugs, 25,* 331–338.

Merin, R. G. (1990). Autonomic nervous system pharmacology. In R. D. Miller (Ed.), *Anesthesia* (3rd ed.). New York: Churchill Livingstone.

Mulbauer, B. (1996). The therapeutic effects of dopamine in acute kidney failure. *Anaesthetist, 45,* 657–669.

Murad, F. (1990). Drugs used for the treatment of angina: Organic nitrates, calcium-channel blockers and beta-adrenergic antagonists. In A. G. Gilman, T. W. Rall, A. S. Nies, & P. Taylor (Eds.), *Goodman and Gilman's The pharmacologic basis of therapeutics* (8th ed.). New York: Pergamon Press.

Oates, J. A. (1996). Antihypertensive agents and the drug therapy of hypertension. In A. J. G. Hardman, L. E. Limbird, P. B. Molinoff, R.W. Ruddon, & A. G. Gilman (Eds.), *Goodman and Gilman's The pharmacologic basis of therapeutics* (9th ed., pp. 781–809). New York: McGraw-Hill.

Olsen, N. V., Jensen, P. F., Espersen, K., Kanstrup, I. L., Plum, I., & Leyssac, P. P. (1993). Dopamine, dobutamine, and dopexamine. A comparison of renal effects in unanesthetized human volunteers. *Anesthesiology, 79,* 685–694.

Pank, J. R., & Tinker, J. H. (1983). Cardioactive drugs and their monitorable effects. *Seminars in Anesthesia, 11,* 268.

Pritchett, L. C. (1992). Management of atrial fibrillation. *New England Journal of Medicine, 326,* 1264.

Raemsch, K. D., & Sommer, J. (1983). Pharmacokinetics and metabolism of nifedipine. *Hypertension, 5* (Suppl. II), 1118–1124.

Raner, C., Biber, B., Henriksson, B. A., Lundberg, J., Martner, J., & Winso, O. (1995). Are the cardiovascular effects of dopamine altered by isoflurane? *Acta Anesthesiology Scandinavca, 39,* 678–684.

Reid, J. L. (1986). Alpha-adrenergic receptors and blood pressure control. *American Journal of Cardiology, 57,* 6E–12E.

Reves, J. G. (1984). The relative hemodynamic effects of calcium entry blockers: Uses and implications for anesthesiologists. *Anesthesiology, 61,* 3–5.

Reves, J. G., Kissin, I., Lell, W. A., & Tosone, S.. (1982). Calcium entry blockers: Uses and implications for anesthesiologists. *Anesthesiology, 57,* 504–518.

Rizza, R. A., Cryer, P. E., & Hammond, M. W. (1980). Adrenergic mechanisms of catecholamine action on glucose homeostasis in man. *Metabolism, 29,* 1155.

Roden, D. M. (1996). Antiarrhythmic drugs. In J. G. Hardman, L. E. Limbird, P. B. Molinoff, R. W. Ruddon, & A. G. Gilman (Eds.), *Goodman and Gilman's The pharmacologic basis of therapeutics* (9th ed., pp. 839–875). New York: McGraw-Hill.

Rosen, M. R., & Danil, P., Jr. (1980). Effects of tetrodotoxin, lidocaine, verapamil, and AHR-2666 on ouabain-induced delay after depolarizations in canine Purkinje fibers. *Circulation and Respiration, 46,* 117–124.

Rosen, M. R., Danil, P., Jr., Alonso, M. B., & Pippenger, C. E. (1976). Effects of therapeutic concentrations of diphenylhydantoin on transmembrane potentials of normal and depressed Purkinje fibers. *Journal of Pharmacology and Experimental Therapy, 197,* 594–604.

Rutman, H. I., LeJemtel, T. H., & Sonnenblick, E. H. (1987). Newer cardiotonic agents: Implications for patients with heart failure and ischemic heart disease. *Journal of Cardiothoracic Anesthesia, 1,* 59.

Schwinn, D. (1994). Cardiac pharmacology. In F. G. Estafanous, P. G. Barash, & J. G. Reves (Eds.), *Cardiac anesthesia: Principles and clinical practice* (pp. 21–65). Philadelphia: Lippincott.

Simpson, J. I., Eide, T. R., Newman, S. B., Schiff, G. A., Levine, D., Bermudez, R., D'Ambra, T., & Lebowitz, P. (1996). Trimethaphan versus sodium nitroprusside for the control of proximal hypertension during thoracic aortic cross-clamping: The effects of spinal cord ischemia. *Anesthesia & Analgesia, 82,* 68–74.

Standen, N. B., Quayle, J. M., Davies, N. W., Brayden, J. E., Huang, Y., & Nelson, M. T. (1989). Hyperpolarizing vasodilators activate ATP-sensitive K^+ channels in arterial smooth muscle. *Science, 245,* 177–180.

Stoelting, R. K. (1987a). Calcium entry blockers. In R. K. Stoelting (Ed.), *Pharmacology and physiology in anesthetic practice* (2nd ed.). Philadelphia: Lippincott.

Stoelting, R. K. (1987b). Peripheral vasodilators. In R. K. Stoelting (Ed.), *Pharmacology and physiology in anesthetic practice* (2nd ed.). Philadelphia: Lippincott.

Tattersfield, A. E., & Harrison, R. N. (1983). Effect of beta blocker therapy on airway function. *Drugs, 5* (Suppl. 2), 227.

Tosone, S. R., Reves, J. G., Kissin, I., Smith, L. R., & Fournier, S. E. (1983). Hemodynamic responses to nifedipine in dogs anesthetized with halothane. *Anesthesia & Analgesia. 62,* 903.

Vasalle, M. (1986). Cardiac glycosides: Regulation of force and rhythm. In R. D. Nathan (Ed.), *Cardiac muscle: The regulation of excitation and contraction.* New York: Academic Press.

Waller, J. L. (1983). Inotropes and vasopressors. In J. A. Kaplan (Ed.), *Cardiac anesthesia, vol. 2: Cardiovascular pharmacology.* New York: Grune & Stratton.

Wood, M. (1993). Pharmacokinetics and principles of drug infusions in cardiac patients. In J. A. Kaplan (Ed.), *Cardiac anesthesia* (3rd ed., pp. 557–584). Philadelphia: Saunders.

Wright, J. M., Orozco-Gonzalez, M., Polak, G., & Dollery, C. T. (1982). Duration of effect of single daily dose methyldopa therapy. *British Journal of Pharmacology, 13,* 847–854.

Zaidan, J. R. & Barash, P. G. (1998). Electrocardiography. In P. B. Barash, B. F. Cullen, & R. K. Stoelting (Eds.), *Clinical anesthesia* (3rd ed., pp. 1411–1419). Philadelphia: Lippincott.

Perioperative Management, Techniques, and Applications

Perioperative Monitoring

Ceil E. Vercellino and Leo A. Le Bel

The prime function of certified registered nurse anesthetists (CRNAs) is to ensure the safety and optimum physiologic well-being of patients undergoing anesthesia and surgery. Achieving these goals requires the CRNA's ongoing attention to a myriad of details. Studies repeatedly show that inattention and distraction during patient monitoring are major factors contributing to anesthesia morbidity and mortality. The maxim often used to characterize the nature of anesthesia practice, "Hours of boredom, moments of panic," reflects the central problem CRNAs face: that the tedium of routine can quickly lead to life-threatening catastrophes. For this reason the CRNA must pay continuous, conscientious attention to the patient and to the electronic and other monitors used to assess the patient's status. Vigilance is the watchword of anesthesia practice.

▶ GOALS AND TYPES OF MONITORING

Monitoring can be defined as *collecting data for the purpose of either establishing trends in a patient's status or for detecting the occurrence of adverse events.* Data collection can be intermittent, repeated, or continuous; the last being more common now because of computerization.

Monitoring can be classed into three broad categories:

1. *Observational.* Performed directly by the anesthesia provider relying only on his or her senses, (eg, visual observation of a patient's movement or skin color).
2. *Invasive.* Performed with electromechanical de-

vices inserted into a patient's body (eg, intraarterial catheter used to monitor blood pressure). Invasive monitoring involves the risk of tissue damage and complications not seen with other monitoring approaches.
3. *Noninvasive.* Performed with electromechanical devices that do not enter the patient's body, but that measure one or more physiologic parameters indirectly (eg, noninvasive blood pressure machine). Noninvasive monitors often are preferred, but not always practical. Monitoring can further be described as being sensory (visual, tactile, auditory, olfactory, or gustatory), physiologic, mechanical, or electronic.

Early anesthesia practitioners could rely only on their observational skills. Today, multifunction, computerized, electromechanical devices provide overlapping and redundant measures of physiologic function. For example, heart rate can be obtained simultaneously from an electrocardiograph, pulse oximeter, and precordial or esophageal stethoscope. Today CRNAs rely heavily on cutting-edge, high-technology, multifunction monitors. However, new anesthetists sometimes place too much reliance on monitors to warn them of problems. Because of their complexity, monitors can be plagued by technical problems or fail altogether, so the anesthetist must still independently evaluate a patient's status. Therefore, there is some truth in the adage "When all else fails, look at the patient!" Many a student has thought a patient in cardiac arrest when a dislodged electrocardiogram lead led to a straight line tracing. Under such circumstances, it is very reassuring to note a patient's pink color and to feel manually his regular, bounding pulse.

Monitoring Standards

Monitoring guidelines have been promulgated by both the American Association of Nurse Anesthetists (AANA), and the American Society of Anesthesiologists (ASA; see Tables 23-1 and 23-2). Both organizations have incorporated their guidelines into their practice standards. In a few instances, anesthesia monitoring requirements are mandated by state law, and health facilities sometimes impose their own additional monitoring requirements. Therefore, every anesthetist must know and adhere to the requirements of his or her practice locale or facility.

In the last few decades, more attention has been paid to intraoperative patient safety, anesthesia technology, and the ergonomic aspects of anesthesia equipment and monitors. The Anesthesia Patient Safety Foundation and the Society for Technology in Anesthesia are two organizations spearheading improvements in these areas. Manufacturers of anesthesia equipment also continue to improve the "user-friendliness" of their products.

Legal and Other Implications of Inadequate Monitoring

Comprehensive monitoring helps the clinician recognize those events likely to harm the patient and to do so in time to intervene with corrective measures. Inadequate monitoring can result in a patient's injury or death and involve the anesthetist in a career-damaging lawsuit. The question of what constitutes adequate monitoring varies with each case, but certain clear principles have evolved over time and are now widely accepted.

Certain human, environmental, and anesthesia practice factors can combine to reduce the effectiveness of monitoring efforts by distracting the anesthetist. A quiet, dark operating room environment, coupled with repetitious and routine activities, can lull the anesthetist into a trance-like, daydreaming state of mind. Alternatively, loud noises or activities can distract the anesthetist's attention by drawing the anesthetist's focus away from the patient. For example, conversing with surgical team members, listening to music, watching laparoscopic surgery on a television monitor, reading a book or newspaper, or doing crossword puzzles can be so engaging as to divert the anesthetist's mind and thereby cause early clues to changes in a patient's condition to be missed. Neophyte anesthetists are particularly prone to such distractions, either because they have a tendency to focus too intently on one narrow aspect of the case or because they are unfamiliar with, or overwhelmed by, the clamor of the operating room. *It is imperative that the anesthetist avoid all distractions and concentrate on the tasks at hand.*

A way to do this is continually to redirect one's conscious attention in a systematic fashion, sequentially focusing on the patient, the surgical procedure, the intra-venous solutions and suction containers, the anesthesia machine flow meters, the ventilator settings, and last, each monitor being used. The cycle is then repeated over and over again. Eventually, this approach helps the anesthetist make the pattern a regular part of his or her practice, but it does require conscious effort, constant attention, repeated practice, and considerable experience to gain the needed expertise. Beginning students should note that experienced supervising anesthetists do this even while engaging the student in conversation. It also is best to avoid detrimental practices, such as turning one's back on the patient and surgical procedure for long periods while looking only at the array of monitors sitting atop the anesthesia machine.

Two other problems detract from an anesthetist's ability to concentrate on proper patient monitoring: stress and fatigue. Stress occurs in many ways. There can be the stress of dealing with unfamiliar anesthesia situations or that of working with patients who have complex, multisystem disease. Such stresses are a normal part of anesthesia practice, and one gradually adapts to them. However, these can be distinguished from the personal physical and mental stresses the anesthetist brings to the operating room. Mild illness or moderate pain may not keep an anesthetist from being clinically functional, but trying to endure severe pain such as that from injured back or flu-induced gastrointestinal spasms can so divert the anesthetist's attention as to create a dangerous situation for the patient. Under such circumstances, the anesthetist should ask to be relieved.

Equally dangerous are the mental distractions an anesthetist brings to the operating room. The psychological stress of family and financial problems or other fears, worries, or anger can quickly upset an anesthetist's ability to function effectively. Difficult as it may be, the anesthetist must learn to leave such concerns at the operating room door. All anesthesia professionals owe their allegiance—and 100% of their attention—to their patient for the entire perianesthetic period.

Another factor that causes an anesthetist's concentration to lapse is fatigue. The recurrent electronic "beeps" of heart monitors or the regular pulsations of heart sounds heard through a precordial or esophageal stethoscope can numb the mind and make it less attentive. In addition, physical exhaustion brought on by lack of sleep or a protracted "on-call" period can fatigue the anesthetist and reduce his or her mental agility or ability to react quickly to an emergency.

Last, beginning anesthetists must recognize those circumstances that lead to lapses in monitoring. A mid-surgery change of anesthesia provider (eg, for lunch relief or other "breaks") is a particularly critical event that can have both positive and negative consequences. The relieving anesthetist brings a fresh perspective that can detect a developing problem and allow early interven-

TABLE 23–1. American Association of Nurse Anesthetists Patient Monitoring Standards

Basic to safe anesthesia care is the application of qualitative and quantitative monitoring which enables the anesthetist to administer anesthesia and evaluate its effect in a manner that optimizes desired responses while minimizing the risks of anesthesia. Fundamental to this endeavor is the use of multiple monitoring modalities, which play vital roles in assisting anesthetists to provide conscientious care to patients receiving anesthesia.

These patient monitoring standards are intended to assist the CRNA practitioner in providing consistent, safe anesthesia care. These standards apply to patients undergoing general, regional, or monitored anesthesia care for diagnostic or therapeutic procedures in designated anesthetizing locations. In extenuating circumstances, the CRNA must use clinical judgment in prioritizing and implementing these standards. All of these standards do not normally apply to epidural analgesia for labor or pain management therapy. The standards may be exceeded in any or all respects at any time at the discretion of the anesthetist, as required by individual patient needs.

While the standards are intended to encourage high-quality patient care, they cannot ensure specific patient outcomes. It is recognized that appropriately used monitoring modalities may fail to detect untoward clinical developments. Further, it is recognized by the AANA that under some circumstances certain monitoring standards may not be applicable. While this is a fact of practice, the omission of one or more monitoring standards should be documented and the reason stated on the patient's anesthesia record. Interruptions in monitoring may be unavoidable. Occasionally, the anesthetist must work at some distance from the patient because of an environmental hazard such as, but not limited to, radiation. Under such circumstances, provisions for monitoring the patient must be made and documented on the patient's anesthesia record. Adequate facilities must exist to enable remote patient monitoring. The standards are subject to review and revision from time to time, as indicated by technology and practice.

Anesthesia Providers

Continuous clinical observation and anesthetist vigilance are the basis of safe anesthesia care. The anesthetist, or nurse anesthesia student, shall be in constant attendance of the patient until the responsibility for care has been accepted by another qualified health care provider.

Patient Monitors

Ventilation

Purpose. To assess adequate ventilation of the patient.

Standard. Intubation of the trachea shall be verified by auscultation, chest excursion and confirmation of carbon dioxide in the expired gas. Controlled or assisted ventilation during the anesthetic shall be monitored continuously with an end-tidal CO_2 monitor. Additionally, spirometry and ventilatory pressure monitors may also be used.

Breathing system disconnect monitor: When the patient is ventilated by an automatic mechanical ventilator, the integrity of the breathing system must be monitored by a device that is capable of detecting the disconnection of any component of the breathing system. Such a device shall be equipped with an audible alarm which is activated when its limits are exceeded.

Oxygenation

Purpose. To assess adequate oxygenation of the patient.

Standard. Adequacy of patient oxygenation shall be monitored continuously with pulse oximetry. In addition to pulse oximetry, oxygenation shall also be monitored by observations of skin color, the color of the blood in the surgical field, and arterial blood gas analysis when indicated.

During general anesthesia, the oxygen concentration delivered by the anesthesia machine shall be monitored continuously with an oxygen analyzer with a low-oxygen-concentration limit alarm. An oxygen supply failure alarm system shall be operational to warn of low oxygen pressure to the anesthesia machine.

Circulation

Purpose. To assess adequacy of the cardiovascular system.

Standard. Blood pressure and heart rate shall be determined and recorded at least every 5 minutes. The patient's electrocardiogram shall be monitored continuously during the course of the anesthetic.

Circulation also shall be assessed by at least one of the following measures: digital palpation of pulse, auscultation of heart sounds, continuous intraarterial pressure monitoring, electronic pulse monitoring, or pulse oximetry.

Body Temperature

Purpose. To assess changes in body temperature.

Standard. Body temperature shall be intermittently or continuously monitored and recorded on all patients receiving general anesthesia; the means to monitor temperature shall be immediately available for use on all patients receiving local or regional anesthesia and used when indicated.

Neuromuscular Function

Purpose. To assess neuromuscular function.

Standard. The means to evaluate the patient's neuromuscular function by the use of a nerve stimulator shall be available immediately when neuromuscular blocking agents have been used.

Anesthesia Equipment

A complete equipment safety check shall be performed daily and an abbreviated check of all equipment shall be performed before each anesthetic is administered. All anesthesia machines and monitoring equipment shall conform to the appropriate national and state standards. An ongoing preventive maintenance program shall be established and enforced.

From Foster, S. D., & Jordan, L. M. (Eds.). (1994). Professional aspects of nurse anesthesia (pp. 110–111). Philadelphia: F.A. Davis. Reprinted with permission.

TABLE 23–2. American Society of Anesthesiologists Standards for Basic Anesthetic Monitoring

These standards apply to all anesthesia care although, in emergency circumstances, appropriate life support measures take precedence. These standards may be exceeded at any time based on the judgment of the responsible anesthesiologist. They are intended to encourage quality patient care, but observing them cannot guarantee any specific patient outcome. They are subject to revision from time to time, as warranted by the evolution of technology and practice. They apply to all general anesthetics, regional anesthetics and monitored anesthesia care. This set of standards addresses only the issue of basic anesthetic monitoring, which is one component of anesthesia care. In certain rare or unusual circumstances, 1) some of these methods of monitoring may be clinically impractical, and 2) appropriate use of the described monitoring methods may fail to detect untoward clinical developments. Brief interruptions of continual[a] monitoring may be unavoidable. *Under extenuating circumstances, the responsible anesthesiologist may waive the requirements marked with an asterisk (*); it is recommended that when this is done, it should be so stated (including the reasons) in a note in the patient's medical record.* These standards are not intended for application to the care of the obstetrical patient in labor or in the conduct of pain management.

Standard I

Qualified anesthesia personnel shall be present in the room throughout the conduct of all general anesthetics, regional anesthetics and monitored anesthesia care.

Objective

Because of the rapid changes in patient status during anesthesia, qualified anesthesia personnel shall be continuously present to monitor the patient and provide anesthesia care. In the event there is a direct known hazard, e.g., radiation, to the anesthesia personnel which might require intermittent remote observation of the patient, some provision for monitoring the patient must be made. In the event that an emergency requires the temporary absence of the person primarily responsible for the anesthetic, the best judgment of the anesthesiologist will be exercised in comparing the emergency with the anesthetized patient's condition and in the selection of the person left responsible for the anesthetic during the temporary absence.

Standard II

During all anesthetics, the patient's oxygenation, ventilation, circulation and temperature shall be continually evaluated.

Oxygenation

Objective. To ensure adequate oxygen concentration in the inspired gas and the blood during all anesthetics.

Methods

1. Inspired gas: During every administration of general anesthesia using an anesthesia machine, the concentration of oxygen in the patient breathing system shall be measured by an oxygen analyzer with a low oxygen concentration limit alarm in use.*
2. Blood oxygenation: During all anesthetics, a quantitative method of assessing oxygenation such as pulse oximetry shall be employed.* Adequate illumination and exposure of the patient are necessary to assess color.*

Ventilation

Objective. To ensure adequate ventilation of the patient during all anesthetics.

Methods

1. Every patient receiving general anesthesia shall have the adequacy of ventilation continually evaluated. While qualitative clinical signs such as chest excursion, observation of the reservoir breathing bag and auscultation of breath sounds may be useful, quantitative monitoring of the carbon dioxide content and/or volume of expired gas is strongly encouraged.
2. When an endotracheal tube or laryngeal mask is inserted, its correct positioning must be verified by clinical assessment and by identification of carbon dioxide in the expired gas. Continual end-tidal carbon dioxide analysis, in use from the time of endotracheal tube/laryngeal mask placement, until extubation/removal or initiating transfer to a postoperative care location, shall be performed using a quantitative method such as capnography, capnometry or mass spectroscopy.*
3. When ventilation is controlled by a mechanical ventilator, there shall be in continuous use a device that is capable of detecting disconnection of components of the breathing system. The device must give an audible signal when its alarm threshold is exceeded.
4. During regional anesthesia and monitored anesthesia care, the adequacy of ventilation shall be evaluated, at least, by continual observation of qualitative clinical signs.

Circulation

Objective. To ensure the adequacy of the patient's circulatory function during all anesthetics.

Methods

1. Every patient receiving anesthesia shall have the electrocardiogram continuously displayed from the beginning of anesthesia until preparing to leave the anesthetizing location.*
2. Every patient receiving anesthesia shall have arterial blood pressure and heart rate determined and evaluated at least every five minutes.*
3. Every patient receiving general anesthesia shall have, in addition to the above, circulatory function continually evaluated by at least one of the following: palpation of a pulse, auscultation of heart sounds, monitoring of a tracing of intraarterial pressure, ultrasound peripheral pulse monitoring, or pulse plethysmography or oximetry.

Body Temperature

Objective. To aid in the maintenance of appropriate body temperature during all anesthetics.

Methods. There shall be readily available a means to continuously measure the patient's temperature. When changes in body temperature are intended, anticipated or suspected, the temperature shall be measured.

---

[a] Note that "continual" is defined as "repeated regularly and frequently in steady rapid succession" whereas "continuous" means "prolonged without any interruption at any time." *From American Society of Anesthesiologists (1997). 1997 directory of members (pp. 394–395). [Approved by House of Delegates on October 21, 1986, and last amended on October 23, 1996, became effective July 1, 1997.] Park Ridge, IL: Author. Reprinted with permission.*

tion, especially if the relieving anesthetist meticulously checks and independently evaluates the patient's status. Conversely, if the relieving anesthetist gets no report on the patient and fails to evaluate the patient independently, deleterious changes can be missed. Guidelines for performing an anesthesia provider exchange are as follows:

1. *Report.* The current anesthetist provides a summary report that includes:
   a. Patient status (pathophysiology and ASA category)
   b. Procedure and course of surgery
   c. Anesthesia plan, course, and problems (eg, hypotension, dysrhythmias, bronchospasm)
   d. Medications and time of last dose (eg, narcotics; sedatives, muscle relaxants, and antibiotics)
   e. Fluid, blood loss, and urine output status
   f. Airway and ventilatory status and problems (ie, ETT size and depth)
   g. Information on unusual or important aspects of the case
2. *Assess.* The relief provider independently assesses and verifies the patient's:
   a. Airway and ventilation status
   b. Circulatory status
   c. Fluid status
   d. Other pertinent data
3. *Monitor.* Both providers review each patient monitor.
4. *Document.* The exchange is documented on the anesthesia record.

You can recall these steps with the acronym RAM-D (Report, Assess, Monitor, Document).

Monitoring Practices

What constitutes adequate monitoring varies with each case, but certain widely accepted principles have evolved and are set out here. Beginning practitioners should familiarize themselves with these principles and incorporate them into their work routine.

All patients, whether undergoing monitored anesthesia care with sedation or a general or regional anesthetic should have their basic physiologic parameters monitored. At a minimum, every patient should be monitored for heart function (rate, rhythm, blood pressure, and electrocardiography); temperature (peripheral or core-depending on access); respiratory function (rate, depth, and pattern); fluid status (fluids administered, urine output, blood loss, etc.); oxygen saturation (by finger pulse oximetry and plethysmography); neuromuscular tone (tactilely or with a peripheral nerve stimulator); respiratory end-tidal carbon dioxide level (by capnography); and correct type and concentration of inhalation

and intravenous agents; and proper functioning of anesthesia equipment.

Ideally, monitor leads should be placed and baseline vital signs taken *before* a patient receives any medication or is otherwise subjected to changes apt to disturb his or her physiologic status (eg, surgical positioning). Only by taking baseline readings can one make sense of changes. A blood pressure of 80 systolic has more meaning compared to a beginning blood pressure of 120 than it has as an isolated reading. With no baseline reading as a reference, the anesthetist cannot correctly interpret the 80 systolic reading.

The type, extent, and placement of monitors will depend on the patient's physiologic status, the contemplated surgical procedure, and the needs of the surgeon. This means, for example, that even when desired, it may not be feasible to use a precordial electrocardiogram (ECG) lead or to place a lead across a point where the surgeon will make his incision. It also means that one may have to substitute rectal or bladder temperature monitoring for esophageal temperature monitoring, even though an esophageal probe would be a better measure of "core" temperature.

All monitoring devices reasonably anticipated to be used during surgery, including ancillary, alternative, or backup equipment, should be at hand and checked out before use. The anesthetist should check all needed monitoring equipment at the start of the day. This is usually done when checking out the anesthesia machine. After surgery starts is not the time to discover that equipment is malfunctioning; that a needed attachment is missing; that a large cuff rather than a medium one is needed; or that no working backup monitor is available. However, there are occasions when a need for an unanticipated monitor arises (eg, need for a glucometer to check a patient's blood sugar) or when an unexpected change in a patient's condition (or the requirements of anesthesia or surgery) creates a need for a monitor that the anesthetist could not have reasonably anticipated ahead of time. In such circumstances, one must adapt by having the circulating nurse or another individual procure the necessary equipment, although these individuals should not be routinely used for this purpose. It distracts them from their obligations and responsibilities. However, it is equally obvious that the anesthetist should not leave the patient unattended to procure the needed equipment.

Monitors are placed first and removed last. With the exceptions of administering oxygen and placing an intravenous catheter, this principle should be adhered to religiously if patient safety is to remain uncompromised. In the past several years, the reforms induced by managed health care have led to increasing pressure for time-efficient use of operating rooms and for rapid case turnovers. This in turn has led to two deleterious practices that compromise patient safety: *rushed inductions* (where monitors are placed at or after the time anesthesia is induced), and *premature removal of monitors* at the time of emergence and extubation. Neither practice can be logically rationalized to exculpate an anesthesia provider from liability for any mishap or injury arising from inadequate monitoring during these crucial periods. Practitioners, even if pressed to be more efficient, will still be held to a standard of care that requires full and accurate patient monitoring.

Any monitor suspected or known to be inaccurate or malfunctioning should be immediately removed from service; and no monitor should be adapted for a purpose it was not intended to perform. It should be patently obvious that making life-or-death clinical decisions based on equipment known to be unreliable is an irrational and indefensible thing to do. *Beginning practitioners should recognize that most anesthesia-related problems are mechanical in nature, not the result of physiologic changes.* That is, problems usually occur because of misapplied, kinked, twisted, disconnected, or incorrectly set equipment. Anesthetists frequently encounter situations where they identify and correct equipment-related problems. This requires identifying the likely cause of a problem. A wrong decision can lead either to: (1) a delay in correcting a real physiologic change, or (2) inappropriate treatment of a patient because of a wrong conclusion about an equipment malfunction.

For example, is a patient's sudden fall in blood pressure a real decrease or due to a loose, partially disconnected blood pressure cuff? A decision must be made about which situation exists. If the anesthetist correctly determines that the fall in blood pressure is real, administering a vasopressor might be appropriate. If the blood pressure decrease is real, but the anesthetist attributes it to an equipment malfunction, there will be a delay in treating the patient while an attempt is made to correct the nonexistent problem. This delay can have adverse consequences for the patient. Conversely, if the fall in blood pressure is not real, but is due to equipment malfunction, administering a vasopressor could lead to a dangerous rise in blood pressure, especially if the patient has a history of hypertension. Even where the anesthetist correctly concludes that the blood pressure drop is due to equipment malfunction, there can be consequences for the patient since the blood pressure monitor is now unreliable and the anesthetist must waste valuable time finding and correcting the cause of the malfunction. In sum, each decision by the anesthetist, whether right or wrong, has repercussions for the patient, so it becomes essential to reduce the likelihood of equipment failure or malfunction. Periodic maintenance by service representatives or hospital biomedical personnel is necessary to ensure that monitoring equipment functions properly when needed. Yet, despite such checks, equipment-related problems occur frequently.

All significant changes in monitor readings should be immediately verified. When a sudden change in the readings of any monitor occurs, it is wise immediately to recheck the reading to ascertain its accuracy. Occassionally, for a variety of reasons, single readings are erroneous. If subsequent readings continue the pattern that existed before the erroneous reading, the single erroneous reading should be disregarded. If subsequent readings confirm the change, it becomes increasingly likely that the change is real. In that case, there is a stronger rationale for instituting corrective measures when treatment is indicated. However, not all changes, even negative ones, necessarily require treatment. For instance, a downward trend in blood pressure is common once anesthesia has been induced. If the change is moderate and stabilizes, no treatment is indicated. Pharmacologic or other interventions are required only if the changes are significant, unanticipated, or otherwise indicative of a serious physiologic disruption.

The anesthetist must evaluate the data comprehensively from all monitors in use and document trends and significant changes on the anesthesia record. When indicated, the anesthetist must be willing and prepared to institute such additional monitoring as may be indicated by a patient's condition or required by the surgical circumstances. Inexplicable changes reflected by monitors can indicate serious, even life-threatening, changes in the patient's status that require the immediate attention of the anesthetist and, if necessary, the help of others. Whenever a concern cannot be immediately resolved, extra help or advice should be sought. No anesthetist should be too proud to ask for help.

▶ THE ANESTHETIST AS MONITOR

Using nothing more than the five senses, an anesthetist can monitor many basic physiologic parameters to enhance patient safety and help direct the course of the anesthetic. Visual and auditory senses provide the most information, but even taste, touch, and smell can make important contributions to patient monitoring. Visual senses help an anesthetist detect or determine a variety of indicators specific to the patient and the environment. These include patient color (eg, hyperemia, cyanosis); patient movement; rate, depth, and patterns of breathing; eye signs (eg, pupillary reflexes, ocular muscle movements); oral and nasal patency; color and condition of tissues (skin, mucous membranes, etc); dental status, jaw size and angles; signs of airway obstruction (eg, tracheal tug, suprasternal and intercostal retractions); limitations in patient movement; presence of some prosthetics; bleeding; rate of return of blood flow after blanching the skin or an appendage; some medical conditions (eg, torticollis, strabismus, hyper- or hypothyroidism, gigantism); diaphoresis or skin dryness that can establish a patient's state of hydration or hyper- or hypothermia, facial twitching or other indices of impending convulsions; color coding of syringe labels, inhalation agent flowmeters; functioning of ventilator bellows and electronic monitors; progress of surgery; retching and other signs of impending regurgitation; urine output, blood loss, and fluid administration; placement and displacement of intravenous catheters; invasive catheters and tubes; airway equipment, monitoring leads, and other device responses to monitors, such as peripheral nerve stimulators.

Hearing can help detect or determine airway obstruction, (eg, stridor, "crowing"); abnormal noises such as leaks from the anesthesia circuit or the whine of malfunctioning motors; course of surgery (by tracking the conversation of the surgical team); and warnings sounded by various monitor alarms. Use of a stethoscope or other device will advise of abnormal heart, lung, and abdominal sounds; the rate, depth, and pattern of a patient's breathing (and the presence of rales, rhonchi, rubs, etc.); and patient conditions such as a bronchitic cough or groaning from pain.

Touch (tactile sense) can be used to assess the rate, strength, and pattern of a patient's pulse (peripheral and precordial); asymmetric breathing patterns; the presence of abnormal masses; the presence of deep-tendon reflexes; a patient's passive range of motion; diaphoresis, dry skin, tremors, and increased or decreased body temperature; pressure felt by hand ventilation or on a needle or syringe plunger (such as when performing a subarachnoid [spinal] block or determining "loss of resistance" technique when performing an epidural block); determine the rate, volume, and force of a patient's exhalations; determine a patient's jaw angle to maintain a patent airway and the proper position of an endotracheal tube cuff; and bladder or stomach distention.

Smell can help detect patient body and breath odors caused by various conditions (eg, diabetic ketoacidosis, lung abscesses, alcohol intoxication); inhalation agents being administered from a vaporizer and anesthesia breathing circuit (or leaks from the circuit); the presence of patient infectious processes (eg, wound abscesses); the identity of aromatic compounds; and smoke or other signs of danger. Taste is useful to determine the identity of compounds (by their sweet, salty, or acid taste).

▶ UNDERSTANDING ELECTRONIC MONITORS

Basics

Electronic monitoring devices have become a mainstay of anesthesia practice. The array of screens, dials, knobs, and buttons confronting the anesthetist is confusing and intimidating, even for experienced clinicians. Understanding how a monitor works can be useful in diagnosing and troubleshooting problems; but learning the operational intricacies of a single monitor can be challenging, especially when multiple, cutting-edge technologies are involved. To appreciate how a given monitor functions, the anesthetist should first review its operating manual. If more information is needed, other anesthesia (and nonanesthesia) references should be consulted. It may be necessary to contact biomedical personnel or manufacturer representatives to find needed answers.

At a minimum, beginning practitioners should understand how the components common to most medical electronic monitors work. The components found in most monitors are similar. Moreover, the relationships between various electronic components tend to remain the same from monitor to monitor, regardless of the parameter being measured (ie, temperature, pulse rate, blood pressure).

Monitors typically include the following components or circuits:

- *Power supply.* Provides direct current (DC) electrical power to each circuit in the monitor, either directly from a battery or by converting alternating current (AC) electricity from a wall outlet.
- *Sensing device.* A probe inserted in, or attached to, a patient. It detects changes in the parameter being measured (eg, heat or pressure). The changes alter the electrical resistance in the measurement circuit. These fluctuations in resistance are then converted electronically to useful measurements.
- *Amplifier circuits.* Increase the intensity of a signal detected by sensing devices to levels that are more easily measured.
- *Suppression circuits.* Detect and diminish or eliminate unwanted stray electrical interference such as that from a cautery unit.
- *Measurement circuits.* Based on an electrical circuit known as a Wheatstone bridge. The bridges, which operate on the basis of Ohm's law, measure changes in electrical resistance detected by a sensing probe. To do this, the bridge uses three fixed resistances and one variable resistor. The value of the variable resistor changes with alterations in the measured parameter. The variable resistor changes are then converted to useful measurements.
- *Balancing circuits.* Used to set the scale of the measurement circuit. Sometimes called nulling or "zeroing" circuits, they are used to set the measurement scale to a starting point of zero.

- *Multiplier and divider circuits.* Take amplified signals and multiply or divide them by a factor of 10, thereby allowing the signal to be read on a scale of (for example) 0 to 3, 0 to 30, or 0 to 300.
- *Display circuits.* Show the calculated measurements on a meter, graph, digital display, or screen.

Macro- and Microshock Hazards

Today's surgical procedures require the use of multiple electrical devices. It is not uncommon to have a dozen or more in use concurrently on one surgical case. Some only generate low voltages, but others produce potentially lethal electrical charges. All operating room electrical equipment can be a source of injury to patients or staff. This includes lasers, x-ray equipment, electric operating room tables, microscopes, headlamps, fluid pumps, endoscopic equipment, monitors, and calculators. In particular, electrocautery units are a very likely source of injury because they generate high currents and require that a conductive pad attached to the patient be wired to an electrical ground. This provides any stray electricity the necessary pathway needed to complete a shock circuit (Le Bel, 1992).

Two types of electrical injuries are recognized. The first is *macroshock* injury, where a significant electrical charge, usually arising outside the body, is transmitted from its source, through the whole body, and discharged to some form of electrical ground. The second is *microshock* injury, where an electrical charge, either strong or weak, arises in conductors near the heart (eg, indwelling electrodes, pacemaker leads) and is transmitted across the heart. This disrupts the heart's normal electrical system and causes either dysrhythmias or cardiac arrest, or standstill (Le Bel, 1992).

How the body or body tissues react to electricity depends on four concepts: (1) that human tissue easily conducts electricity; (2) that tissues in contact with electrical circuits become part of the circuit; (3) that the type, amount, and path of electric current determine the extent of tissue injury; and (4) that all electricity seeks a nonresistive path to an electrical (earth) ground with zero potential (ie, no imbalance between positive and negative charges).

Under appropriate conditions, electric shocks can cause central nervous system disruption, cardiac dysrhythmias, asphyxiation, burns, and death. How much injury occurs depends on the magnitude of the electric charge and its current density (ie, the rate and direction it passes cross-sectionally through tissues). The highest current densities cause the most damage, and the electric charge is normally distributed and dissipated in cone fashion from the contact (entry) point through adjoining tissues.

Skin injuries are the most common form of injury because the skin is typically the entry and exit point for the charge. The skin also has some inherent resistance that varies with the amount of moisture present. Moisture alters skin conductivity as much as a hundredfold. With high tissue resistance, injuries are usually worse.

Body mass helps determine the total resistance a body exhibits as an electrical charge passes through it. The extent to which specific tissues conduct electricity varies, but the heart is the organ most susceptible to injury. In macroshock, the amount of current reaching the heart is attenuated because the charge passes through a wide area, so the likelihood of death is reduced somewhat. Still, some current reaches the heart and a current of 100 mA is enough to disrupt heart function. With microshock, the impulse source is usually at or near the heart. Current density is very high because the charge passes through a narrow path, even if the current flow is relatively small. Under these circumstances, ventricular fibrillation, cardiac arrest, and death can occur with as little as 20 μA of current flow.

Sources of Injury

Leakage current is a term referring to electricity that is unintentionally conducted through the body (or electrical equipment). Some leakage (typically below 1000 μA) is present in most electrical equipment. This is below the threshold level of perception and is not a major cause of concern.

Two major factors that do impact the extent of tissue injury are the type of current (either alternating current, AC, or direct current, DC), and its frequency. For example, AC of either high or low frequency produces heat and burns; but low-frequency AC is more likely to stimulate nerve and muscle tissue to paralyze chest muscles and lead to death by asphyxia. Unfortunately, low-frequency 60-cycle AC is not only the most common form of electricity in daily use, but also is ideally suited for causing such muscle paralysis. Direct current is less problematic but, again, under the right microshock conditions, it can cause death.

In general, a current of 1 mA causes skin tingling (perception threshold); of 16 mA causes individual to "let go" of the source;* and of 50 mA causes pain, loss of consciousness, and mechanical injury; and of 100 mA causes ventricular fibrillation. (All these currents can be generated from a typical wall outlet, 120-V, 60-cycle electrical source.) Two points of contact are needed for an electric shock to occur, a current source and a

---

* "Let go current" will cause the individual to drop the source of electricity, but it also causes flexor muscle paralysis, and if the individual has a good grasp of the source, the paralysis may make it impossible for the individual to release his grip. This is why one should shut off the source of electricity or remove the shock victim from the source with a nonconductive material (eg, wood plank), before attempting resuscitation (Lake, 1994).

ground point. Any electrical equipment found in an operating room can be a shock source, especially if it is malfunctioning. The presence of liquids adds to the hazard because substances like saline or blood facilitate electrical conduction. Once in contact with the source, one merely has to touch a conductor to ground to complete the circuit and receive a shock. Because the electrical appliances used in the operating room all have three-wire conductors in their plug-in cords, one of which is a ground, it is easy for a shock circuit to be completed. Actual contact may be unnecessary if the electrical field is highly charged. Simply drawing one's hand near can cause the electrical impulse to arc over and cause harm.

The situation is somewhat different where an operating room's electricity is provided through isolation transformers. These devices take electricity from its wire-conducted source and induce an electrical field that then transforms it to an "isolated" electrical circuit through a separate wiring system that delivers it to the operating room outlets. Now for a shock to occur, an individual must grasp three sources, both sides of the active electrical lines and ground before a shock circuit is complete. This reduces the likelihood of serious or fatal electrical injuries, but does not completely eliminate shock hazards. Isolation transformers were required when operating rooms used explosive anesthetic agents, but today, those agents have been abandoned. Few, if any, hospitals still use isolated systems. Most hospitals now have standard electrical systems that must still conform to local building and safety codes, including the national electrical code (NEC) and the National Fire Protection Association (NFPA) standards.

The differences in electrical charges that can arise between dissimilar items leads to the production of "static" charges. These, too, were once potential sources of ignition for explosive anesthetics, a danger that no longer exists. However, static charges still "zap" the unwary. For this reason, the anesthetist or a patient can occasionally get a "static shock." Though quite stimulating, such shocks are brief and do not cause serious injury. However, in the presence of volatile fumes, they could still be an ignition source. A few such cases still are occasionally reported.

Prevention

Many preventive measures can be taken to reduce electrical injuries. Foremost, all electrical equipment should be checked and evaluated by biomedical personnel before being used in the operating room. It also should undergo periodic reevaluation on a scheduled basis. Each device should be used according to manufacturer recommendations and standard operating room practices. Prior to every use, a visual inspection should be carried out to ensure that electrical cords are not frayed and that all plug-in items, such as grounding wires, are correctly secured. If at any time an alarm on the device indicates a malfunction, the equipment must be checked out. If the problem is not immediately correctable, the equipment should be removed from service until repaired and reevaluated. All repairs should be carried out by manufacturer representatives or certified hospital biomedical personnel, not by anesthesia personnel.

Electromechanical devices (eg, electrodes, probes, extensions, grounding pads also must be used properly. Electrocardiogram sensors, electrocautery grounding pads, and the like should not be placed over bony areas or scars. If required, appropriate jellies, conducting liquids, or lubricants should be applied carefully and not overused. Grounding pads, in particular, should be placed as far away from other electrical conductors as practical. All cords should be checked for intact insulation. Plugs should be placed securely into their correct receptacles. Cross-changing wiring between pieces of equipment should be avoided. No liquids should be placed on the top of equipment as a leak might quickly reach internal electrical circuits, causing them to short out. For this reason, all devices have fuses or circuit breakers that immediately shut down the device as soon as a short circuit occurs. Otherwise, a macroshock hazard could be created as live current flows through the unit (Le Bel, 1992).

Unapproved extension cords should not be used. Where a two-conductor extension cord is used with a device requiring a three-conductor cord, the path to ground is interrupted and poses a dangerous situation. Wires of various electrical equipment should not cross, especially those of cautery devices. If precautions are taken, serious electrical injuries can be avoided.

▶ MONITORING THE RESPIRATORY SYSTEM

Pulse Oximetry

With the possible exception of the electrocardiograph (ECG), no other single anesthesia monitor has had as profound an impact in clinical practice as the pulse oximeter. With the end-tidal capnograph, the two monitors have reduced anesthesia-related morbidity and mortality so significantly that professional liability (malpractice) insurance rates are lower for providers who routinely use both.

History and Operation

Pulse oximeters are not new. They were developed by Matthes, Squires, and others in the 1930s and introduced to clinical practice by Wood in the 1940s. The first anesthesia article on intraoperative use of the monitor appeared in 1951. However, these early devices were bulky, awkward to use, and subject to various interferences and calibration problems that made their use on patients impractical. In the 1970s, Takuo Aoyagi created the first dual wavelength oximeter. Further refinements (eg, microprocessors, solid-state components, light-emitting diodes, and advanced photodetection technologies) led to practical-size, high-reliability, cost-effective oximeters that by the mid-1980s, readily were accepted into clinical practice. Apart from intraoperative monitoring, pulse oximeters can be used to assess a patient's circulatory status; to monitor patients sedated for nonsurgical diagnostic and therapeutic procedures; to transport patients between locales; and to monitor routinely in presurgical holding areas and postanesthesia care units (PACU/Recovery Room; Kirby, & Gravenstein, 1994).

Pulse oximeters detect changes in arterial blood oxygen saturation (SpO_2). The changes in oxygen level are immediately detectable so the anesthetist can take corrective action to prevent hypoxemia by adjusting the patient's delivered oxygen concentration or other measures. Oximeters rely on sensing probes that emit red and infrared wavelength light across a point of pulsatile arterial blood flow. The sensor then measures the shifts that result from the absorption of those light waves by oxygenated and unoxygenated (reduced) hemoglobin in the blood. The measurements are founded on the Lambert–Beer law that describes how light transmitted through clear solutions varies with the amount (concentration) of solute present.

Oximeter sensor probes are made for use on the ear and nose, but the one most commonly employed is a clothespin like device that is simply clipped over a finger or toe digit at the nailbed. A self-adhering wrap-around sensor also is available. The artery's pulsatile flow causes minute changes in the transmission of light that can be detected, amplified, and converted (by electronic means) to provide an indirect measure of oxygen saturation level. Changes in light transmission caused by nonpulsatile tissues (eg, bone, skin) are ignored. A person's skin color does not generally interfere with readings, but the presence in the blood of abnormal hemoglobin may.

Currently used oximeters provide an oscilloscopic readout of the arterial pulse waveform and a reading of heart rate. These are useful for verifying the same measurements as those provided by other monitors (eg, arterial line, electrocardiograph). In some instances, the presence of a large dicrotic notch on the pulse oximeter waveform can result in two "beats" being registered for each arterial pulsation, leading to an erroneous reading that is double the actual heart rate.

There are two types of oximeters: transmission and reflectance. The first works by emitting and detecting changes in light at two different wavelengths: a red light of 660 nm that is absorbed by unoxygenated (reduced) hemoglobin, and a second at either 910 or 940 nm that is absorbed by oxyhemoglobin (oxygenated blood). The differences in light transmission are then converted to saturation readings. This is the type commonly used in anesthesia practice. In reflective oximetry, light reflected back from perfused tissues is used to determine the oxygen saturation level.

Variables in Using Pulse Oximetry

A number of problems are common with pulse oximeters. The most frequent is malposition of the sensor device. Twisting of the probe on the digit, disconnection, or accidental removal of the probe during the course of surgery all occur with some regularity. Whenever saturation readings are not as expected, the anesthetist should first check for correct probe placement. Limb movement can lead to erroneous readings, although much work has been done toward making probes less sensitive to the effects of motion. When the sensor is placed on a digit of the arm or leg on which a blood pressure cuff is used, readings will be undetectable whenever the cuff is inflated and limb circulation is obliterated. For this reason, most anesthetists place the sensor probe on a finger of the arm or hand in which the intravenous line has been placed and opposite that of arm where the blood pressure cuff is placed so that cuff compressions do not interfere with either pulse oximetry readings or the free flow of intravenous solution.

Another source of erroneous readings relates to a patient's use of nailpolish or synthetic nails. Dark colored nail polish can lower readings. Other colors, including opaque polishes, reduce light transmission and result in erratic readings. It is advisable to remove all nailpolish from the digit to be used for intraoperative monitoring. Patients with manicures may object to this. They should be advised of the safety aspects for removing the polish, or an alternative probe site should be selected. If only one nail is cleaned for oximeter probe placement, the anesthetist runs the risk that if a problem occurs intraoperatively there will not be a readily available back up site for the probe. Removing all nail polish is preferred. This makes every digit available for monitoring.

Patient temperature is another variable. In excessively warm patients, venous dilation in the area of the probe can interfere with readings. This is sometimes called the penumbra (shadow) effect. Moving the probe to a site with larger arterial pulsations resolves the problem. More problematic are patients who are hypothermic or in shock. These conditions shunt blood away from the body periphery to maintain adequate central circulation to vital organs such as the heart, liver, and spleen. The resulting intense vasoconstriction leads to severely inaccurate readings or loss of readings altogether. These problems are worse in severely obese individuals, those with cardiovascular disease, and persons suffering from acute accidental hypothermia. In some instances, readings can be maintained by topical administration of nitroglycerin paste or blocking the digit with local anesthetic. Both approaches help maintain digital blood flow.

Oximetry readings also can be influenced (high, low, or erratic readings) by ambient electromagnetic signal sources, such as magnetic resonance imaging (MRI), surgical electrocautery units, and even local light sources. The latter can be avoided by covering the probe with an opaque cover. Some oximeters provide a default reading (typically 85%) to indicate that the unit is being subjected to interference. Improvements in oximeters have greatly enhanced the stability and reliability of readings despite the proximity of interference sources.

Another problem area anesthetists must be familiar with is that of erroneous oximeter readings due to the presence of abnormal hemoglobin or the intravascular injection of dyes. Oximeter readings can be abnormal whenever a patient has abnormal hemoglobin or is administered indigo carmine, indocyanine green, methylene blue, or another drug that creates a temporary methemoglobinemia. Methylene blue is especially problematic because it both creates and treats methemoglobinemia and, concurrently, causes cardiac depression and a lowering of cardiac output. Heavy smokers or those with carbon monoxide poisoning tend to have falsely elevated readings because of the high carboxyhemoglobin content of their blood.

Transcutaneous Oxygen Analyzers

The goal of all anesthetics is to maintain optimum physiologic homeostasis. Therefore, it would be useful continuously to monitor a patient's intracellular environment, especially concentrations of oxygen and carbon dioxide. In the early 1970s, a monitor was introduced to clinical practice that made possible the noninvasive measurement of tissue oxygen levels by sensors attached to the skin. The transcutaneous oxygen analyzer was based on the principle of the Clark electrode used in blood gas analysis (Scurr, Feldman, & Soni, 1990).

Transcutaneous oxygen monitoring was briefly popular as a clinical modality in the 1970s, but problems later surfaced that limited its routine use. For example, proper functioning required heating of the probe device. This led to incidents of skin burns, particularly in infants and children, patients for whom this type of monitoring was particularly suited. Today, transcutaneous monitoring is reserved for situations with clear indications for its use. As technology evolves, it may become possible to track intracellular activity routinely. The information could then activate computer-driven anesthesia-delivery systems, such as intravenous drug pumps. Though it is unlikely that such systems will be developed soon, some

anesthesia practitioners think they might one day allow minute-to-minute control of anesthetic depth using an absolute minimum amount of agents.

End-Tidal Carbon Dioxide (CO_2) Monitoring (Capnography)

An important recent anesthesia monitor is the capnograph (from the Greek words for smoke, *kapnos,* and writing, *graphein*). It measures the level of carbon dioxide a patient exhales with each breath. Because the volume of air moved in a single breath is called the tidal volume, and because the capnograph measures the partial pressure of the carbon dioxide gas breathed out during exhalation, the measurement of end-tidal carbon dioxide is abbreviated as $PETCO_2$. Capnography is useful to detect respiratory arrest, mechanical disconnections of the anesthesia circuit, and changes in alveolar dead space and to assess the correct placement of endotracheal tubes. Along with other data, it can be used to determine changes in pulmonary blood flow, the likelihood of embolism, and mechanical problems with the anesthesia machine delivery circuit (Kirby & Gravenstein, 1994).

The gas can be sampled from the mainstream anesthesia gas flow or by a sidestream port, either of which must be located close to the patient's mouth, usually at the delivery circuit elbow or Y-piece. In mainstream sampling, gases pass through a detection device (cuvette) and sampling tends to be more accurate. Sidestream sampling collects the gas sample near the patient's mouth, but the sample has to be delivered to a measuring chamber in the capnograph monitor. This can cause a brief delay in obtaining a reading, which, itself, may then be slightly less accurate because of some gas mixing.

Capnograph Waveform

Exhaled carbon dioxide levels can be displayed on a monitor screen or chart recording. A normal recording (Fig. 23–1) typically has a near-rectangular appearance with a baseline, upslope, alveolar plateau, and a downslope (Kirby & Gravenstein, 1994). The first portion of the tracing is a flat baseline that occurs during inspiration. Next comes the ascending slope that represents the exhaled carbon dioxide. The slope then plateaus (usually evenly at its highest level) until the next breath causes the carbon dioxide level to fall. The waveform displays the concentration of CO_2 (height) for the time duration of exhalation (width of tracing). The terminal portion of the alveolar plateau generally reflects the highest reading, and the numerical readout of the CO_2 level (capnometer) usually is made at this point. Some units register high readings at other points during exhalation. Most capnograph monitors used today also register the (minimal) carbon dioxide level at the start of inspiration so that a correlation can be made between inspired and exhaled levels.

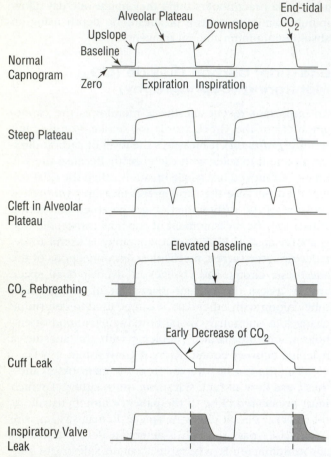

Figure 23–1. Normal and abnormal capnograph tracings. *(From Kirby, R. R., & Gravenstein, N. [Eds.]. [1994]. Clinical anesthesia practice [p. 351]. Philadelphia: Saunders.)*

Uses of Capnography

The two most important uses of the capnograph to the anesthetist are (1) to assess the adequacy of patient ventilation, especially the status of lung ventilation and perfusion; and (2) to determine the correct placement of endotracheal tubes. Whatever their cause, significantly elevated carbon dioxide levels indicate serious problems that, if uncorrected, can lead to a patient's death. Astute clinicians use the capnograph to detect problems before serious consequences occur. Elevations can be caused by lung dysfunction (eg, asthma, COPD); disease-induced elevations of carbon dioxide production (eg, malignant hyperthermia); depression of central respiratory centers by anesthetics or narcotics; neuromuscular blockade; neuromuscular diseases that affect respiration (eg, muscular dystrophy; Guillain–Barré syndrome); and airway or anesthesia circuit obstruction. Reduced levels are seen with embolism, hyperventilation, hypothermia, and situations that promote alkalotic states (Kirby & Gravenstein, 1994).

Two potentially fatal conditions that may first be indicated by capnographic changes are pulmonary em-

bolism (decreased $ETCO_2$) and malignant hyperthermia (significant CO_2 elevations). The monitor can also help discover previously undetected pathology, such as cardiac shunts; exhausted soda lime; adequacy of fresh gas flow in nonrebreathing systems; patient hyper- or hypoventilation; absorption of gases used to distend the abdominal cavity during laparoscopic procedures; and identification of anesthesia circuit problems, such as damaged unidirectional valves.

The capnograph's greatest impact has been in assessing the proper placement of endotracheal tubes. Transmitted breath sounds can fool an anesthetist auscultating a patient's chest after endotracheal intubation, the presence of an end-tidal carbon dioxide tracing virtually ensures that the tube is correctly placed and has not been inserted inadvertently into the esophagus. In this way, capnography has markedly decreased the incidence of unrecognized esophageal intubations and their associated brain injuries and deaths. However, one must get strong, repeated tracings to confirm that the tube is in the trachea. The presence of an initial slight carbon dioxide trace that then disappears is inadequate. Such a tracing can be due to an esophageal intubation and the presence of a small amount of carbon dioxide in the stomach from swallowed air. An anesthetist who erroneously relies on such a tracing as assurance of correct tube placement is headed for disaster. Strong end-tidal CO_2 tracings help confirm that the tube is in the trachea, but they neither warn nor protect against inadvertent endobronchial intubation.

Capnograph readings illustrating the least amount of mechanical interference are obtained in healthy, well-anesthetized, well-paralyzed, unobstructed patients who are mechanically ventilated. Experienced anesthetists can achieve a nearly identical waveform with manual (hand) ventilation. To achieve this level of proficiency, beginning anesthetists should use the capnograph to learn how properly to hand-ventilate a patient. Practicing manual compression of the rebreathing bag while watching the capnograph tracing helps educate the hand of the anesthetist. That is, one can get a sense of the volume, pressure, and rate of ventilation needed to achieve a near-normal tracing. Eventually, the proficient anesthetist can faithfully reproduce the waveform without looking at the capnograph. Additional verification of the adequacy of hand ventilation can be obtained by observing the measured tidal volume.

Capnograph waveforms vary with a patient's physiology, the rate and volume of respiration, ventilator settings, level of muscle paralysis, presence of respiratory disease, and other factors. Analyzing waveforms requires an understanding of how these factors interact, especially if the anesthetist needs to make corrective changes in the pattern of ventilation. Commonly seen variations of the normal capnograph pattern include elevated baselines (due to CO_2 rebreathing); dips in the alveolar plateau (sometimes called *curariform clefts*) that reflect inadequate muscle relaxation and movement of the diaphragm due to breathing efforts; and steep upslopes or downslopes that reflect lung disease, obstructions to breathing, or other such problems. Cardiac-induced variations in pulse waveforms also occur (cardiac oscillations).

How Capnographs and Other Anesthetic Gas Monitors Operate

End-tidal carbon dioxide levels can be measured by various means, including infrared light absorption; Raman and photoacoustic spectroscopy; and mass spectrometry. Most stand-alone monitors rely on infrared light absorption because carbon dioxide readily absorbs infrared light (frequency of 4.3 µm) and readings are made by comparing a sample of gas drawn from the breathing circuit to an internal, sealed gas sample of known concentration. The same technique can be used to measure concentrations of inhaled anesthetic gases; however, the operator must select on the monitor which agent is to be measured or readings will be inaccurate. A similar identification of anesthetic agents can be made with pairs of piezoelectric quartz crystals: One is coated with an oil that absorbs the agent, and the other serves as a reference electrode. Agents are identified from the difference in the measured frequency response of the two quartz crystals (Gal, 1994).

With Raman spectroscopy the gas sample is illuminated by a laser beam that re-emits the light at a different wavelength, the frequency of which is used to identify the agent. In mass spectroscopy, sampled gases are ionized within a vacuum chamber and the resulting particles are subjected to a magnetic field that separates them on the basis of their charges and masses, whose patterns identify specific agents.

Each of the aforementioned techniques vary in cost, ease of use, required frequency of calibration, advantages, and disadvantages. Two common problems can lead to erroneous readings. The first is the mixing of sample gases with other (diluent) gases, such as oxygen and nitrogen, especially ones that are nonpolar. The other problem is that of "contamination" of the sample by exhaled water vapor. Avoiding the latter problem usually means taking countermeasures, such as using in-line hydrophobic filters in the gas sample collecting tubing or, sometimes, coupling these with the use of Nafion tubing, a special tube made of a tetrafluoroethylene copolymer that adsorbs the water vapor (as well as any ethers, ketones, or alcohols that may be present) without affecting other gases. The exhaled water vapor passes through the tubing and is then evaporated.

Because Nafion tubes do not work well with water droplets, the tubing should be placed nearest the anesthesia circuit where the water remains in vapor form rather than near the gas analyzer where condensation and droplet formation occurs. Other techniques can help remove water vapor from the anesthesia circuit before the gas sample is withdrawn for analysis. These include heating exhaled gases to promote evaporation and using an "artificial nose" device in the anesthesia circuit that is designed to retain exhaled humidity. Drying exhaled water vapor before gas analysis can affect readings, especially where the reading is made against a standard reference gas sample on the basis of the gas's concentration (eg, 5% carbon dioxide sample) or its partial pressure (subject to changes in local atmospheric pressure). Depending on whether or not the readings compensate for the loss of water vapor, two different readings can be obtained. The readings can be erroneous if the correct factors (eg, atmospheric pressure) have not been taken into consideration. Other problems affecting gas sampling include sampling from line leaks that entrain other gases and sampling from partially dried gas samples. These sampling problems lead to artifactual changes in capnograph readings and to disparities in measured exhaled and arterial blood carbon dioxide levels.

Chemical Carbon Dioxide Detectors

Although they are not practical for routine intraoperative monitoring, chemical CO_2 detectors are useful for out-of-operating room verification of endotracheal tube placement. They function by inducing a pH-dependent color change in an indicator dye. The color change, visible through the detector's transparent plastic container, is triggered by the patient's exhaled carbon dioxide. Attaching the device to the endotracheal tube connector while manually or mechanically ventilating the patient is all that is required to make the device functional. Chemical detectors are used primarily as an adjunct to cardiopulmonary resuscitation efforts. They also are used to confirm capnography readings in the operating room, although their usefulness there is limited. The devices that add dead space to the circuit are of limited use (5–10 minutes) and cannot provide quantitative information about the levels of exhaled carbon dioxide. They sometimes are awkward to use and may not be readily at hand when needed. Despite their problems, chemical detectors provide useful visual confirmation to everyone present that a just-placed endotracheal tube is, indeed, in the trachea rather than in the esophagus.

Mass Spectrometry: General Principles

Currently, the mass spectrometer (MS) is the only commercially available device that analyzes respiratory gases, including carbon dioxide, oxygen, nitrogen, and the anesthetic gases halothane, enflurane, and isoflurane. The MS provides both numerical displays as percentages and millimeters of mercury and graphic displays of inspired and expired concentrations of these respiratory gases. Approximately 30% of the operating rooms in this country use a mass spectrometer.

Normally the mass spectrometer is used in several operating rooms simultaneously. These areas are usually within 150 ft of the central unit. Each area has a gas-sampling outlet and a computer terminal that receives information from the MS. The anesthetist installs an elbow connector at the Y-piece with an attached sampling tube that transports the gas to the central unit. Sampling of respiratory gas depends on a number of factors, such as distance from the MS, the number of rooms being sampled, and room priority. Because of the lag time between aspiration of the sample and display of the recorded value, breath-to-breath analysis of respiratory gases is not possible. Research is ongoing to produce an MS that displays breath-to-breath analysis of end-tidal CO_2 that continues in the event the central unit malfunctions. A centrally located printer provides a hardcopy record of the data for inclusion in the anesthesia record. Also available are single, self-contained, free-standing units that provide sampling of a range of physiologic and anesthetic gases for a single operating room.

The MS alerts the clinician to acute or potentially dangerous anesthetic conditions, such as equipment failure, initial stages of malignant hyperthermia, and ventilator disconnection. Equipment failures identifiable by MS include malfunctioning valves in circle absorber systems, exhausted soda lime, malfunctioning pop-off valves, and errors in polarographic oxygen sensors. The MS also can be used clinically to diagnose hyperventilation, hypoventilation, and residual muscle relaxation. The information supplied by the MS regarding the inspired and expired concentrations of volatile anesthetic helps the clinician assess uptake and distribution of these agents and promotes a more timely recovery from anesthesia. In addition, by measuring inspired concentration, the MS can reveal when a vaporizer is malfunctioning or when it does not contain the correct agent. Because presence of an end-tidal concentration of nitrogen is a sensitive indicator of the presence of air in the pulmonary or cardiovascular system, air embolus by this method is detected 30 to 90 seconds faster than by changes in precordial Doppler sounds (Matjasko, Gunselman, Delaney, & Mackenzie, 1986).

The greatest potential for the MS is to integrate all monitoring functions into a centralized alarm system that directs the anesthetist to the source of the problem. Cooper, Newbower, and Kitz (1984) found that equipment failures accounted for 5% of adverse anesthetic outcomes; approximately half of these incidents would have been detected by mass spectrometry. The functions of the individual monitoring devices discussed earlier can all be performed by the MS. It provides a reliable backup

system to the individual monitors employed; however, because of the reporting time lag in gas analysis, additional monitoring devices such as the oxygen analyzer, disconnect alarms, and low-flow alarms still are critical to detection problems early.

▶ MEASURING BODY TEMPERATURE (THERMOMETRY)

It is now standard anesthesia practice to measure every patient's body temperature in some fashion. The goals of thermometry are to detect significant or rapid deviations from normal body temperature and to guide attempts at controlling the patient's body temperature, either by warming or cooling. In the latter case, the anesthetist must actively manage both the patient's body temperature and the surrounding environment.

Heat Production and Elimination

Normal body temperature averages 98.6° (37°C) and is maintained within a narrow range of about 1 degree. To accomplish this, the body balances heat production and heat dissipation. Body heat is derived mainly through metabolic chemical reactions in skeletal muscle and the liver. Even at rest, heat production averages 75 kilocalories per hour, increasing to more than 600 kilocalories during periods of strenuous exercise (Kirby & Gravenstein, 1994).

Heat produced by body cells is carried away by blood to the central "core" portion of the body, where, to prevent the cellular damage that would occur with "overheating," the heat is dissipated by three mechanisms: conduction, convection, and radiation. With *conduction*, heat is transferred directly between tissues. *Convective heat losses* occur primarily in the lungs, where heat from the highly vascular lung tissues warms the air (or anesthetic gases) passing into and out of the tracheobronchial passages during respiration. Last, blood flowing to skin surfaces causes heat to be lost by *radiating* from body surfaces to the surrounding environment. This type of heat loss accounts for more than half of the body's heat losses and tends to be greatest at the scalp. For this reason, it has become a common anesthesia practice to wrap an anesthetized patient's head in plastic to reduce body heat loss during anesthesia. It is one method used to keep a patient normothermic.

One can gain a better appreciation for radiant heat loss by touching the forehead of a person who has a fever. Body heat can be dissipated more quickly by using measures that accelerate the removal of excess heat. Placing water-soaked sponges or towels on a patient's skin can, for example, cool a patient down more quickly because water has a high specific heat that enables it readily to absorb large amounts of heat. Cooling also can be accelerated by placing the patient on cooling blankets or in an air-conditioned environment. Both methods facilitate convective and conductive heat losses.

Central control of thermoregulation occurs in specialized centers of the anterior and posterior hypothalamus. There, alterations in perceived temperature occur either as a result of changes in the temperature of blood bathing the hypothalamic region or because of sensory nerve impulses arriving at the posterior hypothalamus from skin thermal receptors. These signals initiate changes in the anterior hypothalamus to control either heat production or loss. A temperature increase causes sweating and dilation of peripheral vessels to dissipate heat (to more than 650 kilocalories/h), whereas decreases in temperature promote shivering that increases heat production.

Other factors also play a role. Heat production can be affected by sympathetic nervous system stimulation and exercise. Heat loss is affected by the rate of sweat production, environmental humidity (see below), and surrounding air temperature and flow. Newborns and young infants have special temperature-regulating problems and needs. A discussion of these is beyond the scope of this chapter, but more information can be found in texts on anesthesia for pediatric surgery.

Affects of Hyper- and Hypothermia

Excesses of body temperature (either hyperthermia or hypothermia), have physiologic consequences. Temperature elevations facilitate metabolic and respiratory acidosis and cause a significantly higher need for oxygen. As a consequence, the cardiac and respiratory systems must work harder. This, too, causes more heat production and a further demand for oxygen. If severe enough, this vicious circle of events can cause a downward spiral in the patient's metabolic processes that ends in death.

Hypothermic conditions decrease oxygen consumption, but can lead to discomfort and shivering that reflexively causes oxygen demand to rise by more than 500%. Metabolic processes, including drug metabolism, are decreased. The heart's contractility is impaired and the drop in temperature, if great enough, leads to ventricular fibrillation. Other organs suffer decreased perfusion because of intense vasoconstriction. In the brain, both blood flow and oxygen consumption are reduced. For this reason, controlled hypothermia may benefit patients undergoing intracranial surgery. However, in uncontrolled circumstances, severe hypothermia can lead to central nervous system (CNS) depression, coma, and death. Other effects of hypothermia include thrombocytopenia; shifting of the oxyhemoglobin dissociation curve to the left; blood sugar elevation due to sympathetic nervous system stimulation; and delayed emergence from anesthesia. This last change is especially likely if the patient's hypothermia is inadvertent and unrecognized, a problem further compounded by the fact that hypothermia increases the solubility of inhaled anesthetic gases in blood. This phenomenon deepens the level of anesthesia even if the delivered anesthetic concentration remains the same. This occurs because of a principle from physics (Henry's law) that states that the solubility of a gas is inversely related to temperature.

The Concept of Core Temperature

Most medical personnel have taken a patient's temperature by using a mercury-filled glass thermometer placed under the tongue (first used in 1776 by Hunter). Until recently, this method was considered the best measure of a patient's central, or "core," temperature. With time, other methods for measuring temperature developed, including rectal, bladder, axillary, skin, esophageal, and tympanic approaches. As these were compared, it became evident that body heat (temperature) is not uniformly distributed throughout the body, which raised the question of which method best reflects body temperature.

As noted, the hypothalamus is responsible for thermoregulation. Therefore, it would seem reasonable to consider this area of the brain as best reflecting "core" temperature. The problem is that temperature in the hypothalamic region can be measured indirectly only with a probe placed in the ear canal and against the tympanic membrane (eardrum). This technique, while feasible, is not without problems. It does not reflect changes occurring at or near the central part of the body either, where the heart and lungs are located. Thus, although one sometimes hears the term *core temperature* used to refer to tympanic membrane temperature, this method does not provide a complete picture of the body's heat production.

The term *core temperature* also is used to refer to the temperature in the mediastinal area, where blood flow through the heart and lungs is highest. There are numerous advantages to using measurements in this region as being truly representative of core heat production. These include the fact that the heart and lungs generate heat themselves in doing their work; that blood flow in the area is very high; that temperature changes are quickly reflected to nearby tissues; and that accessing an esophageal probe close to the mediastinal area is relatively easy. Other methods are not as quickly reflective of changes or as good an index of the maximum amount of heat being produced. For example, rectal probe measurements may lag by several degrees and several minutes in the temperature of the mediastinal area. This difference can be critical when dealing with a situation of runaway heat production that can prove fatal, such as occurs with malignant hyperthermia. Additional factors affect the accuracy of readings, such as when a rectal probe becomes embedded in feces within the colon.

Therefore, it becomes clear that each monitoring method has some aspect that makes it a less than ideal indicator of the body's ability to generate heat or for accurately and quickly reflecting moment-to-moment changes in heat production. Despite this, most clinicians use the term *core temperature* to refer to the changes measured by an esophageal probe placed near the mediastinal region. This is the definition used in this chapter.

Temperature Monitors

The technology used in temperature monitors can be classed into the following groups: liquid crystal devices, infrared sensors, and those which use thermistors or thermocouples.

Liquid Crystal Devices

Liquid crystal devices are available in a number of forms. All rely on an adhesive-type backing to adhere the device to the skin, usually on the forehead, neck, or upper chest, where skin blood flow is high. Advantages include their cheap cost, ease of use, and suitability as backups to other types of temperature monitors. Disadvantages include their narrow range (typically 5–6°C), slow response times, adhesives that do not always stick, easy displacement by movement, and possibile patient sensitivity to the adhesive. In addition, they can be difficult to read if lighting is poor and are subject to erroneous readings if devices such as heating lamps are used to warm the patient. Measurements with liquid crystals do not always correlate well with readings by other methods. However, they are somewhat useful to detect blood flow changes to an extremity after regional sympathetic blockade with a local anesthetic (Lake, 1994).

Infrared Thermometry

All hot surfaces give off infrared radiation that can be detected by special sensors. In theory, one could use such a device to measure body temperature from skin emissions of heat. However, this would not adequately reflect core temperature. Nonetheless, infrared thermometers are used to measure ear canal tympanic membrane temperature, which is considered to be a reasonably accurate reflection of hypothalamic temperature. The device resembles an otoscope-like "gun" with an attached ear speculum over which a disposable paper cover is placed. The device is then carefully inserted into the patient's ear and aimed at the tympanic membrane. When the activating button is pushed, a temperature reading is available on the built-in digital readout display within 5 seconds. The measurement is made by registering the eardrum's emitted heat. The thermometer does not, however, come in contact with the eardrum, making this the only thermometric device that does not require direct contact with patient tissues.

Advantages of infrared thermometers are their (relatively) inexpensive costs, ease of use, and minimal likelihood of tissue injury if used properly. The major disadvantage is that only intermittent readings are possible. The device cannot be left in the ear to provide continuous readings. Erroneous (lower) readings may be obtained if the scope is misdirected at the walls of the ear canal rather than the tympanic membrane.

Mechanical temperature devices comprised of a central cotton-tipped sensor in the center of multiple plastic prongs (to keep the tip in place) have been used in the ear canal. These thermistor devices relied on direct contact with the tympanic membrane. They were abandoned in favor of easier-to-use infrared devices and also because of the high incidence of perforated eardrums and other complications.

Thermistors and Thermocouples

Thermistor is the name given to a resistorlike sensor that connects to a Wheatstone bridge–based monitor circuit. Readings are made in the manner described in the section on monitor electronic circuits. *Thermocouples* are devices made of bimetallic metals that expand or contract at different rates as temperature varies, causing alterations in each metal's ability to conduct electrical impulses, a difference that can be measured and converted to a temperature reading. Today, both types of devices are cheap, easy to use, and (usually) disposable.

In the past, probe devices for electronic thermometers incorporated needle or glass elements that caused injuries. Today, probes are usually made of flexible wires embedded in a nontoxic, flexible, waterproof material such as plastic. They are sometimes color-coded to indicate the intended monitoring modality (eg, esophageal or rectal).

Temperature-Monitoring Sites

Temperature-monitoring sites used clinically include the tympanic membrane, nasopharynx, oral cavity, esophagus, spinal cord, thoracic tissues, abdominal tissues, myocardium, pulmonary artery, bladder, rectum, and skin. Myocardial temperature measurements typically are made only during the course of open-heart surgery. Pulmonary artery temperature measurements generally are assessed in cardiothoracic surgery or when cardiac output is being measured. Spinal cord, thoracic, and intraabdominal temperature measurements have limited applicability for routine intraoperative monitoring and are not covered in this chapter.

Skin

Although skin blood flow is a major mechanism for heat dissipation, skin temperature monitoring has limited clinical usefulness. Skin temperatures lag behind core temperature and are subject to inaccuracies due to the skin's exposure to air; to covering of the skin by body oils, ointments, surgical prep solutions, and sweat; and to the lack of suitable probes. Adhesive-backed temperature monitors that use liquid crystal technology are used routinely as backups for other forms of intraoperative monitoring or for primary monitoring in awake patients undergoing minor surgery with monitored anesthesia care. They are placed on the patient's forehead, neck, or upper chest. Some monitors use a "banjo" probe taped to the skin as a sensing device. The probe is named for its banjolike appearance. Banjo probes, and some probes designed for esophageal or other monitoring modalities, sometimes can be used for skin temperature monitoring by placing them underneath the patient. The sensor must lie between the patient and the operating room table. If this is done, the anesthetist must make sure the probe does not harm the patient's skin. It also is important that the patient not be lying on either a wet operating room table sheet or on a warming blanket placed under the table cover. In either situation, readings will be grossly inaccurate. Skin temperature probes may be better placed in the axilla or groin areas, but care must be taken to avoid skin irritation.

Oral

As described in the section on core temperature, the oral cavity is the site first and most traditionally used for temperature monitoring. However, despite their ease of use and near-universal employment, mercury-filled glass thermometers were not without problems. They required "shaking down" the mercury to a baseline level and were influenced by other factors, including cold or hot fluid ingestion before a reading, mouth breathing, and crying. There also was the ever-present danger of breakage with consequent spillage of mercury into the mouth area where it could be swallowed or aspirated. These problems were particularly likely in children and uncooperative patients. Today mercury-based thermometers have no practical use in anesthesia settings. Intraoral measurements could be taken intraoperatively with a thermistor-type probe, but the more common and practical approach is to use esophageal temperature probes.

Nasopharynx

The advantages and disadvantages of intranasal temperature monitoring are largely the same as those for intraoral monitoring. If used, the probe should be inserted no further than the posterior pharynx. One advantage of a nasal probe is that, like a tympanic membrane sensor, it better reflects brain temperature because the probe tip lies near the internal carotid artery. This approach also is useful when continuous monitoring is desired, but esophageal or other routes are inaccessible. However, measurements can be affected by air movement through the nasal passages. The major drawback of nasopharyngeal probes is possible damage to tissues. Extreme care must be taken in inserting even a well-lubricated probe tip into the nose, especially if the patient has a bleeding disorder or is on anticoagulants. Epistaxis is common and can be difficult to manage. To keep the temperature probe from irritating nasal tissues, it is useful to tape the probe at the skin just below the nares. At no time should the probe be forced in.

Esophageal

Esophageal temperature probes generally combine an esophageal stethoscope device and thermistor probe into a single, catheter-type unit. The tip is lubricated and inserted into the mid- to lower third of the esophagus after oral intubation has been accomplished. If the esophageal probe rests high in the esophagus, readings may be erroneous because of air movement in the adjacent trachea. Readings in the lower esophagus more accurately reflect core temperature. Esophageal probes have a connector that attaches to the temperature-measuring box. The box typically is battery operated and has a digital readout that expresses the patient's temperature in either fahrenheit or centigrade degrees. For convenience, many such units simultaneously monitor temperature from two separate sources (eg, esophagus and bladder). The stethoscope portion of the catheter can be connected to the anesthetist's earpiece for continuous monitoring of heart and breath sounds.

Esophageal probes are extremely useful clinically. They best reflect central (mediastinal) core temperature, are easy to use, highly reliable, disposable, cheap, and minimally damaging to tissues if inserted with care. However, they can become kinked, or the internal wires connecting the distal probe and the temperature box can suffer damage. The plug that connects to the monitor box can become disconnected and readings can become inaccurate (eg, irrigation of the chest cavity with warm fluids or induced hypothermia).

Bladder

Some Foley catheters incorporate a temperature probe into their design in much the same fashion as do esophageal stethoscopes. This approach is useful when the patient will have an indwelling catheter in place for an extended period during and after surgery. Readings with a bladder thermometer are an acceptable reflection of core temperature and are less problematic than temperatures taken with a rectal probe. Bladder readings can be affected by warm or cold irrigations of the abdomen or bladder.

Rectal

Rectal temperature monitoring can be a useful backup to other approaches, but a number of problems plague this method for primary temperature monitoring intraoperatively. Probes are difficult to place and position because they can perforate or damage rectal mucosa. Probe tips can become embedded in feces, thereby making readings unreliable. As with bladder probes, rectal measurements are influenced by fluid irrigations of the lower abdomen. Last, probes can be easily contaminated, even if the probe tip is covered with a latex glove or other covering. Removing the probe makes it possible also to contaminate the surroundings with fecal material.

Adjuncts to Intraoperative Management of Patient Temperature

It is increasingly appreciated that effective temperature management plays a crucial role in preventing surgical complications, in reducing the incidence of nosocomial infections, and in saving the lives of trauma victims. A number of devices and techniques have been developed to manage a patient's temperature in the perioperative period. These are briefly noted here, but a full discussion of their merits can be found in applicable chapters of this text. Most of the measures are directed toward preventing inadvertent hypothermia, but some techniques also can be used to cool hyperthermic patients.

One easy approach to temperature management simply is to maintain room temperature at a higher-than-normal level. Studies that try to balance comfortable temperatures for operating room personnel with ambient temperatures that reduce the rate of cooling in anesthetized adult patients have shown mixed results. However, warming the operating room seems clearly more beneficial when dealing with pediatric patients because they are especially susceptible to intraoperative hypothermia. Two useful techniques for keeping these patients warm are to perform surgery on a neonatal warming unit and to use infrared heating lamps. Both provide radiant heat to keep the patient warm.

Useful for all age groups is the technique of warming intravenous fluids. A number of devices are available. Some function effectively, even when large volumes of fluids, including blood, are administered rapidly. Warming blankets also can be placed on the operating table, underneath a covering drape. These connect to a power unit that circulates water at a preset temperature through the blanket to warm the patient. Some also can cool hyperthermic patients by circulating an alcohol and water mixture through the blanket. One problem with blankets that circulate water is their susceptibility to damage and leakage. Thermal barriers can be placed over patients, including aluminum foil–type coverings and covers made of special heat-retaining materials. One easy technique is to cover the patient's head in a clear plastic drape once intubation has been accomplished as large amounts of body heat are dissipated from the scalp.

Clear plastic is used so that the anesthetist can continue to observe the patient.

Delivering anesthetic gases through an in-line humidifier that warms and moisturizes the inhaled anesthetic gases is another useful technique. Such units are highly effective in maintaining a patient's body temperature during surgery, but care must be taken to measure the temperature of the inspired gases if lung injuries due to overheated gases are to be avoided. A related approach is to use an "artificial nose" in the anesthesia delivery circuit near the point at which gases are delivered to the patient. Although not highly effective, they do help reduce evaporative losses from the patient's lungs during ventilation. Lavaging the abdominal and thoracic cavities with warm sterile saline can help restore core temperature quickly. This procedure must be carried out by the operating surgeon. In emergency situations where the patient's abdominal and thoracic cavities are not open, gastric lavage of warmed irrigating fluids delivered through a nasogastric tube can be effective.

Simply covering a patient with warmed sheets or towels is a good way to make a patient more comfortable and to reinforce the sensation of "feeling warm." However, this approach has limited usefulness for helping maintain a patient's core temperature. The device increasingly relied on to maintain a patient normothermic intraoperatively is the warm air convection blanket. These devices deliver warmed air to the patient through a paper blanket that has a large number of small holes on one side. The air temperature is preset. Blankets are made for upper torso, lower torso, or whole-body warming; some are made for use with a single limb. The blankets are configured to the patient's torso and held in place with an adhesive located along the blanket edges. These devices are highly effective for keeping a patient normothermic, especially when used with warmed intravenous fluids and other warming modalities. An advantage convection blankets have over water blankets is that tearing does not render them inoperable.

Environmental Temperature

Humidity and Barometric Pressure

When one talks of environmental temperature, one must also consider the issue of humidification; that is, the amount of water contained in the surrounding air. There are two types of humidity: absolute and relative. *Absolute humidity* is defined as the maximum amount of water (saturation) a given volume of air can hold, expressed in grams per liter. *Relative humidity* is defined as the actual degree of saturation a given volume of air contains. It is expressed as a percentage of absolute humidity. When a volume of moist air is cooled to a point where its water precipitates, we call that temperature the dew point (Le Bel, 1992).

Measuring humidity is called hygrometry. To measure the humidity level, one uses a dual thermometer device, one of which is connected to a wick immersed in water. In dry weather, the water rapidly evaporates to cause a decrease in temperature. This drop is read in comparison to the other thermometer. If the humidity is high, the temperature difference will be small, but if humidity is low, the differences in temperature will be wider. Moisturizing air actually makes it lighter as water molecules replace the heavier (diatomic) molecules of nitrogen and oxygen. This reduces the barometric pressure of the surrounding atmosphere. How much water saturation occurs in a given environment depends on the temperature, amount of water available, and barometric pressure. In proper amounts humidity makes the atmosphere seem more comfortable and cooler. It also reduces the likelihood of fires and static sparks that could serve as an ignition source for flammable materials. *Barometers* are devices that measure the pressure generated by the atmosphere. Also called *manometers,* they come in several varieties. Liquid manometers rely on a tube filled with mercury, the level of which rises or falls as barometric pressure changes. Water manometers exist, but are impractical. Water's lower density (compared to mercury) would make their size unmanageable. Aneroid barometers are dry. Changes in atmospheric pressure move a rubber diaphragm that, through gears and levers, cause a corresponding change in the pressure reading indicated by a needle and scale device. One aneroid manometer is a Bourdon gauge, which tells us the pressure within anesthesia gas cylinders.

Atmospheric pressure and humidity were once critical to operating room safety when explosive anesthetic agents such as ethers and cyclopropane were used. They have lost this significance, but they are still important factors in providing a comfortable work environment. Humidification of gases continues to be important for both anesthesia practice and respiratory therapy.

▶ MONITORING THE CARDIOVASCULAR SYSTEM

No other area of anesthesia practice has undergone such rapid development since the late 1970s as has cardiovascular monitoring. During that time, monitoring has progressed from blood pressure cuffs using a mercury manometer and palpation of a peripheral pulse to the availability of oximetry, multiple venous and arterial pressure monitors, and calculations of cardiac output. In terms of definition, all modalities of monitoring the cardiovascular system are used as indices of the adequacy of blood flow and oxygenation to critical organs. A variety of devices are employed for specific assessment of cardiac output, perfusion pressure, and other parameters of

organ perfusion and oxygenation. This section presents an overview of the variety of hemodynamic monitoring devices available and describes their use and how to interpret the data they offer (Foster & Reeves-Viets, 1992).

Hemodynamic monitoring usually assesses four critical parameters: (1) the electrical mechanism of myocardial contraction; (2) intravascular or intracavitary pressures; (3) net forward flow; and (4) adequacy of organ perfusion. For those purposes, the usual clinical monitors include continuous electrocardiogram (ECG); measurement of arterial, venous, or chamber pressures with invasive or noninvasive techniques; calculation of cardiac output with a thermodilution technique via pulmonary artery (Swan–Ganz) catheter; and assessment of perfusion with mixed venous and/or peripheral arterial pulse oximetry.

The ECG remains the most uniformly applied monitor in anesthesia. Continuous ECG monitoring permits the practitioner to assess the electrical mechanism and rate and demonstrates dysfunctional rhythms that would have a deleterious effect on cardiac output. The ECG monitors employed in anesthesia generally are either three- or five-lead systems. Both rely on measurement of electrical impulses using silver–silver chloride gel electrodes that may be placed either on the limbs or over the precordium to assess selected regions of the heart. Impulses are measured from a negative ground electrode to a second, distant positive reference electrode. The resulting electrical impulse is then transmitted to the monitor for display. The relationship between the electrical impulse generated and cardiac activity in the atria and ventricles is demonstrated in Figure 23–2.

The standard, color-coded electrode assignment is as follows: white to right upper limb, black to left upper limb, green to right lower limb, red to left lower limb, and brown to the precordial lead. In the three-lead system, only the right upper limb and left upper and lower limb electrodes are used to assess limb leads 1, 2, and 3 (Fig. 23–3). Summation of the limb leads as a ground with a unipolar limb electrode for reference permits the assessment of leads R, L, and F (Fig. 23–4). A precordial reference electrode allows electrical activity over selected regions of the ventricles and across the septum. These are the *V* leads 1 to 6.

The normal electrical mechanism of the heart begins at the level of the sinoatrial (SA) node, located at the juncture of the superior vena cava and the right atrium. Impulses are transmitted from the SA node through the atria by way of Bachmann's bundles and traverse the atria to the atrioventricular (AV) node located in the septum. Propagation of the impulse across the AV node permits depolarization of the ventricles through a single right and dual left anterior and posterior bundle branches and the Purkinje system.

The elements of the cardiac cycle may be demon-

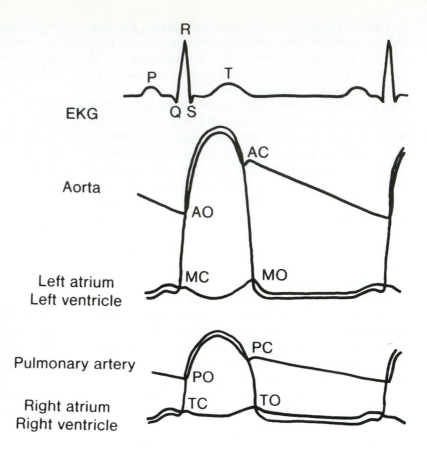

Figure 23–2. Correlation of the electrical and mechanical activities of the heart. AO, aortic opening; AC, aortic closure; MC, mitral closure; MO, mitral opening; PO, pulmonic opening; PC, pulmonic closure; TC, tricuspid closure; TO, tricuspid opening. A vertical line at any point gives the simultaneous events occurring at that time. *(From Burnside, J. W. [1981]. Physical diagnosis [16th ed., p. 154]. Baltimore: Williams & Wilkins. Reprinted with permission.)*

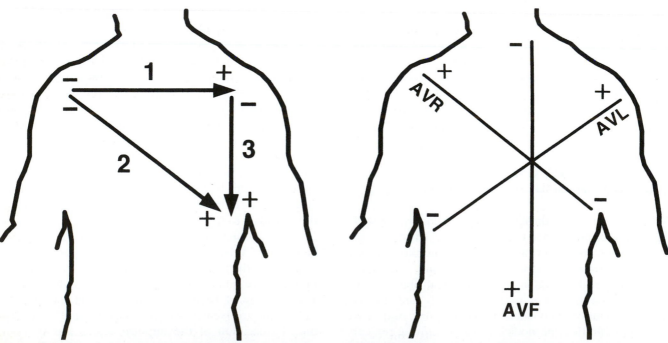

Figure 23–3. Electrode placement for ECG limbs leads 1,2, and 3. The − refers to negative electrode, the + to positive electrode. *(From Burnside, J. W. [1981]. Physical diagnosis [16th ed.]. Baltimore: Williams & Wilkins. Reprinted with permission.)*

Figure 23–4. Axes defined by ECG leads AVR, AVL, and AVF. The − is negative, the + positive. *(From Burnside, J. W. [1981]. Physical diagnosis [16th ed.]. Baltimore: Williams & Wilkins. Reprinted with permission.)*

strated with varying ease depending on the lead chosen. Limb lead 2 is most commonly used to identify the P-wave; the precordial leads may be used to assess ischemic changes. With a three-lead system, relocating limb electrodes allow an approximation of precordial leads. Placing the left upper limb electrode in the V-5 position and monitoring the AVL lead will approximate a V-5 precordial lead. The modified chest lead 1 (MCL-1) permits approximation of any of the selected precordial leads by placing the left upper limb electrode near the shoulder or under the clavicle and the left lower limb electrode in the selected precordial lead position and monitoring on lead 3. When choosing leads for continuous monitoring, it is useful to remember that leads 3 and AVF display greater variation in amplitude with the respiratory cycle than do other leads. Evaluating the information provided by ECG analysis provides a variety of parameters. Heart rate is directly measured. Disturbances in the electrical mechanism, including abnormal origin of rhythm, disturbances in synchronicity, appearance of ectopic beats, and evidence of myocardial ischemia or infarction may be demonstrable. Finally, ECG analysis may provide clues to electrolyte abnormalities or toxic responses to various anesthetic agents. Guidelines for rapid analysis of ECG activity are valuable to the practitioner. Although complete and detailed analysis is difficult in clinical practice, a simplified diagnostic scheme follows (Table 23-3).

The normal sinus mechanism produces synchronous depolarization of the atria, followed by the ventricles. Although the rhythm generally is regular, it is normal to note a pattern of variation in the beat-to-beat interval that corresponds with the respiratory cycle. That variation may be accentuated in the healthy young patient and should not be mistaken for the irregularly irregular rhythm of atrial fibrillation. The normal rate of depolarization in the SA node produces a resting heart rate of about 70 beats per minute in the typical adult that masks the intrinsic rates of 40 to 60 for the AV node or 30 to 40 for intrinsic ventricular depolarization.

Atrial dysrhythmias may present as prematurities, tachycardias, flutter, or fibrillation. Premature atrial contractions generally present with anomalous p-wave morphology and a shortened P-P interval and may have a shortened P-R interval. Atrial tachycardias present with a 1:1 ratio between the P-wave and QRS complex, although the P-wave may be superimposed on the T-wave when the heart rate is rapid, making identification difficult. The P-R interval may be decreased with rapid ventricular responses. Although the QRS complex generally is normal in appearance, aberrant ventricular conduction or the presence of a rate-dependent bundle branch block may mimic the appearance of ventricular tachycardia, unless P-waves are identified. Atrial flutter generally presents with a regular rhythm and conduction of only a

TABLE 23–3. Clinically Relevant Clues from Electrocardiographic Analysis

Possible Condition	Indication on ECG
Hyperkalemia	Appearance of tall "tented" T-wave
	Appearance of wide, bizarre QRS complex merging with T-wave
	Disappearance of p-wave
	Ventricular extrasystoles, fibrillation, or asystole
Hypokalemia	Flattening or inversion of T-wave
	Increase in P-R interval
	Depression of ST segment
	Appearance of U wave
	Apparent prolongation of Q-T interval (a normal Q-U interval)
	Atrial, ventricular extrasystoles, ventricular tachycardia
Hypercalcemia	Reduction in Q-T$_c$ interval[a]
	Blending of T with QRS
Hypocalcemia	Prolongation of Q-T$_c$ interval[a]
Hypomagnesemia	Prolongation of Q-T$_c$ interval[a]
Venous air embolism	Rightsided heart "strain" pattern
	Atrial and ventricular extrasystoles

[a]The Q-T interval varies with heart rate and, when corrected for a heart rate of 60 beats per minute, is signified "Q-T$_c$" (Q-T$_{corrected}$).
From Kessin, M., Schwartzchild, M., & Bakst, H. (1948). A nomogram for rate correction of the QT interval in the electrocardiogram. American Heart Journal 35, 990–992. Reprinted with permission from Gray, T. C., Nunn, J. F., & Utting, J. E. (Eds.). (1980). General anaesthesia (4th ed., vol. 1, 613; vol. 2, p. 1002). Boston: Butterworths.

fraction of the atrial rate of 300 beats per minute. The degree of block may vary according to the responsiveness of the AV node. With a 2:1 AV block, atrial flutter may mimic sinus tachycardia as the nonconducted P-wave is hidden in the preceding T-wave. Atrial fibrillation presents with the appearance of the classic jagged baseline representing "F-waves" that are irregular in both form and frequency. As conduction across the AV node is inconsistent, the rhythm is irregularly irregular.

Atrioventricular conduction abnormalities may appear either as dissociation or as junctional or nodal dysrhythmias. The latter may appear as premature complexes or as escape beats in the presence of severe sinus bradycardia. The P-wave may not be present or may follow the QRS complexes. Shortened P-R intervals that may appear with an aberrant atrial focus should not be confused with an actual nodal rhythm. The former represents an atrial focus near the AV node; the latter represents a failure to maintain normal sinus or atrial mechanisms entirely. Premature complexes usually occur at an accelerated rate with a shortened R-R interval. Junctional escape beats usually occur with sinus bradycardia when the sinus mechanism fails to maintain a resting rate above the normal AV nodal rate of 40 to 60 beats per minute. Several AV conduction abnormalities may be present. Each represents a block at one or another level in the conduction system. A first-degree block with an extended P-R interval represents a delay in conduction of the impulse generated in the SA node across the atria to the AV node and is generally not clinically significant in early stages. A second-degree block may present in two forms. Type I (Wenkebach) represents progressive failure of the AV node to transmit an impulse and shows a progressive lengthening of the P-R interval with eventual failure to conduct an atrial impulse. Rhythm is regularly irregular. Type II block generally occurs in the ventricular conductive pathway as spontaneous failure to propagate an impulse. Therefore, it occurs without a progressive lengthening of the P-R interval. When the conduction block occurs in the bundle branches, the QRS may be widened. A third-degree block presents a complete dissociation of the atrial and ventricular mechanisms, in which each chamber beats at its own intrinsic rhythm without any coordination. Often, QRS complexes and P-waves are normal, but unrelated. Ventricular response rates depend on the site or origin of the ventricular mechanism.

Ventricular dysrhythmias occur in four primary forms. Premature ventricular complexes (PVCs) are defined as ventricular contractions that appear prior to the next normally conducted beat. The QRS complex generally is broad and abnormal in conformation. It generally is reversed in polarity to the normal QRS complex. As it is associated with a refractory pause in the AV node, there is a compensatory pause following a PVC. Fixed, unifocal PVCs are more frequently benign. Multiform PVCs, multiple PVCs in sequence, and those occurring near the preceding T-wave predispose to ventricular tachycardia and are thus of greater concern. Ventricular tachycardia is defined as more than three ventricular prematurities in sequence with a rate greater than 100 beats per minute. Arterial pressure may or may not be transmitted, depending on the rate of ventricular filling. Morphology of the QRS complex is broad, generally inverted, and similar to that of PVCs. Ventricular fibrillation presents as a highly irregular rhythm with no discernible pattern. There is no effective forward arterial flow with ventricular fibrillation. Finally, bundle branch blocks may occur in conduction of the impulse to the ventricles. These represent failure to conduct the wave of depolarization in the normal antegrade fashion, with conduction in a retrograde manner from a point distal to the block. Hence, the QRS complex is broad and atypical. A single bundle branch block generally is benign, and the pattern may appear in patients with ventricular hypertrophy or discrete conduction abnormalities. Bundle branch blocks involving the right bundle and left anterior branch generally are benign, and only 10% progress to complete AV block. Right bundle branch block and left posterior hemiblock carry a 90% incidence of progression to complete AV block and are conse-

quently more grave. Analysis of the ECG complex provides evidence of a variety of pathologies. Ischemic changes present in the form of ST segment depression with depression greater than 2 mm considered critical. Myocardial injury may be demonstrated by the presence of ST segment elevation in the early phase or the presence of Q-waves associated with old infarction.

Pressure Monitoring

Monitoring pressure provides the most common mechanism for assessing volume status and circulatory adequacy. A variety of methods of measurement are employed and can be broken down into noninvasive and invasive systems. In general, the clinical practice is to employ noninvasive measurements of arterial pressure for intraoperative monitoring of healthy patients undergoing routine procedures and invasive techniques to measure arterial, venous, or chamber pressures in patients with selected disease states and for selected surgical procedures for which additional information is required for clinical management. For example, a patient with a history of coronary artery disease who is to undergo a carotid endarterectomy would require an arterial line and potentially a pulmonary artery catheter.

Noninvasive Monitoring

The accepted standard for monitoring arterial blood pressure during routine cases on healthy patients is the noninvasive technique. Two general methods may be employed: (1) manual techniques using either sphygmomanometer or mercury column with auscultation; (2) automated systems that operate on an oscillometric technique. Each of these has applications and selected drawbacks, and both are well described (Table 23–4).

TABLE 23–4. Factors Affecting the Accuracy of Indirect Blood Pressure Measurements

Factor	Consequence
Hearing ability	Variable sensitivity to Korotkoff sounds
Stethoscope	Design and positioning determines intensity of sounds
Touch	Variable sensitivity to pulse palpation
Cuff size	Falsely high BP—too small or loose-fitting cuff [a]
	Falsely low BP—too large a cuff
Aneroid manometer	Inaccurate BP with improper calibration
Deflation of sphygmomanometer	Falsely low BP—too rapid deflation
Oscillometry	Imprecise detection of first and last oscillations, indicating systolic and diastolic pressures, respectively

[a] BP, blood pressure.
From Hug, C. C., Jr. (1986). Monitoring. In R. D. Miller (Ed.), Anesthesia (2nd ed., vol. 1, pp. 411–463). New York: Churchill Livingstone. Reprinted with permission.

Auscultatory methods generally employ the upper extremities as the site for measurement, largely for sake of convenience. Lower-extremity cuffs also may be employed, although the inability to auscultate Korotkoff sounds readily limits their application. The auscultatory technique requires turbulent flow in the artery to produce the Korotkoff sounds that form the basis for determining systolic and diastolic pressures. The first sound heard represents the systolic pressure, and the point at which sounds are lost represents the diastolic pressure. In those instances where auscultatory sounds are continued to zero, the point at which a distinct diminution in auscultated sounds is noted is taken as the actual diastolic pressure.

Physiologic changes that alter the distensibility of the arterial wall may alter the readings obtained from auscultatory or oscillometric techniques. Thus, extremes of body temperature with consequent vasoconstriction or vasodilation may reduce the accuracy of measurement, as may the use of vasoconstrictors or vasodilators. This is particularly true with auscultatory methods, and less so with ultrasonic systems such as Dinamap- or Doppler-detected pulses. Likewise, stiffening of the arterial walls with progressive atherosclerosis may reduce the ability to auscultate pressure.

A final drawback of noninvasive techniques for measuring arterial pressure is their relatively cumbersome and time-inefficient operation. Noninvasive techniques provide only intermittent measurements of arterial pressure and require varying time intervals to obtain measurement. In comparison, invasive techniques provide immediate, beat-to-beat analysis. Hence, in complex cases or cases that include significant disturbances in normal pulsatile flow, noninvasive techniques are unsuitable.

Invasive Monitoring

Vascular cannulation provides the practitioner with the ability directly to measure pressures in the peripheral arterial or venous system, as well as chamber and central venous or pulmonary artery pressures. The availability of vascular and chamber pressure measures increases precision in assessment of hemodynamic and volume status. The techniques for transducing vascular pressures remain constant regardless of the vessel or chamber, although interpreting the information gained from cannulation depends on the particular monitoring modality selected for evaluation.

Mechanisms of Transducing. Mechanically, the system for transduction of pressures should be the same whether transducing high-pressure arterial or lower-pressure venous sites. The system should include a stiff, low-compliance pressure tubing connecting the vascular cannula to a pressure-sensing diaphragm. Transduction of the physical pressure wave to that diaphragm pro-

duces bending of the diaphragm, resulting in a small volume change in response to the applied change in pressure (Lee, 1981). The arterial compliance measurement should be 0.01 mm^3/100 mmHg pressure; that for venous compliance should be 0.1 mm^3/100 mmHg pressure. Three forms of transducers are generally employed in translating the pressure waveform into an electrical waveform: (1) electromagnetic; (2) capacitive; and strain (3) gauge transducers (Mishin & Jones, 1986).

In *electromagnetic transducers,* the diaphragm moves a soft iron core between the primary and secondary coils of a transformer. An alternative current passing through the primary coil sets up an alternative magnetic field, which in turn induces a current in the secondary coil that is modified in amplitude by the extent to which the iron core concentrates the magnetic field through the coils.

In *capacitative transducers,* the diaphragm forms one plate of a capacitor. As the capacitor is incapable of transmitting a unidirectional current, an alternative current is used to energize it. The impedance of the transducer changes with the displacement of the two plates of the capacitor, creating the changes in current that are later interpreted as the waveform in display.

In *strain gauge transducers,* the sensing elements are composed of electrically conductive elastic materials that respond reversibly to pressure deformation with a change in electrical resistance. That resistance is converted into a voltage signal by connecting the elements in the form of a Wheatstone bridge circuit. The elements are assembled in the transducer so that two elements are stretched and two compressed by the physical pressure applied to the diaphragm, with each pair being incorporated into the opposite sides of the bridge. A stable, unidirectional voltage is then applied across the bridge. The output voltage is proportional to the physical pressure applied and to the excitation voltage. Characteristically strain gauge transducers tend to drift electrically when first connected to a voltage supply because the current produces a heating effect on the strain gauge elements themselves. This drift usually settles within 15 minutes as temperature stabilizes in the elements of the strain gauge after which pressure measurements remain reliable.

Frequency responses in transducer systems should be at least 1.5 times the fastest component being measured. The frequency response of the arterial trace is normally 20 to 30 Hz, whereas that of the transducer is normally 150 to 1000 Hz (Hunter & Eastwood, 1986). Air in the tubing or stopcocks and longer tubing between the vessel and the transducer can lower the frequency response. These waveforms may approach the frequencies encountered in the vascular waveform and are particularly demonstrated in the systolic upstroke. The resulting distortion, commonly referred to as *ringing,* may produce an overshoot in measurement of systolic pressure.

An alternative was employed prior to the current, reliable, and easily managed monitoring systems that still provides an effective means of monitoring systemic pressure when the clinician is unable to readily access a monitoring screen, as during transport, or in selected sites external to the operating theater. By connecting the arterial line through an extension to a stopcock and a second extension to an aneroid manometer, one can identify the mean arterial pressure, which provides important clinical information about perfusion pressure. This system, however, does not provide immediate waveform analysis or information regarding the true systolic or diastolic pressures.

The Arterial Waveform. Physically, the conduction of an arterial waveform is not exclusively related to the flow of blood within the vessel (Brunner, 1978). The waveform demonstrated on the monitor represents a summation of the force of blood flow through the vessel and the propagation of the elastic forces in the wall of the vessels themselves. The left ventricular pulse wave travels at a speed of 10 m/s, in contrast to the aortic elastic recoil wave, which travels at 0.5 m/s (Remington, 1960).

Arterial pressure waveforms represent events of the left side of the heart that transfer to the systemic circulation. Arterial pressure has two phases, systole (ventricular events) and diastole (atrial events and ventricular filling). In the arterial pressure waveform, the systolic phase is demonstrated by the sharp upstroke, which represents the opening of the aortic valve and rapid ejection of blood into the aorta from the left ventricle. The decline in the waveform after peak pressure is achieved secondary to the runoff in the arterial tree. The subsequent fall in aortic pressure causes the closure of the aortic valve that results in the dicrotic notch. The diastolic phase ensues and is represented by the falling waveform after the notch (further runoff into the peripheral arterial tree).

In general, as the pressure wave is measured progressively farther from the heart in the normal vascular tree, there is a delay in the transmission of the waveform, a steeper inotropic upstroke, and loss of the dicrotic notch. This results in a steeper, more peaked systolic upstroke. This altered waveform results in part from the fact that peripheral arteries include proportionately less elastic fiber in the arterial wall, making them stiffer and less compliant. Furthermore, tapering of the vessel diameter as the artery proceeds peripherally serves to amplify the arterial waveform, in a fashion similar to the manner in which the ear trumpet amplifies sound waves (Bruner, Krenis, Kunsman, & Sherman, 1981; O'Rourke, & Taylor, 1966) (Fig. 23–5).

Physiologic abnormalities can be identified in the

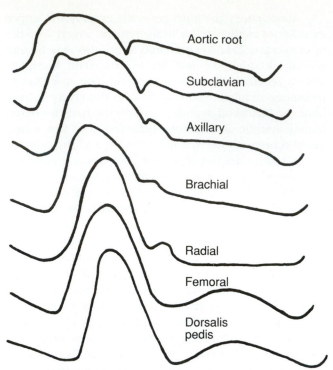

Figure 23–5. Arterial waveforms at different anatomic locations. *(From Blitt, C. D. [1985]. Monitoring in anesthesia and critical care medicine [p. 50]. New York: Churchill Livingstone. Reprinted with permission.)*

arterial pressure waveform. In the event of a premature ventricular contraction, lack of appropriate filling of the left ventricle will result in a depressed morphology and decreased amplitude of the waveform of the ventricular contraction. Hypertension is seen as exaggerated and increased amplitudes of the peak pressures of systole and diastole.

In the face of aortic insufficiency (regurgitation) the arterial waveform reveals a wide pulse pressure with an increased systolic and decreased diastolic pressure with an absent dicrotic notch. In contrast, the condition of aortic stenosis reveals a narrow pulse pressure secondary to an obstructed outflow tract (Fig. 23–6). The obstruction to flow causes a decrease in the rate of rise of the upstroke of systole and alters the dicrotic notch as there is ineffective aortic valve closure. This waveform also represents a decreased stroke volume. Similarly hypotension appears as a dampened waveform. The anesthetist is responsible for assessing these variables and correlating the data to make the appropriate diagnosis. It also is necessary to confirm this information with a second source of data, such as a manual or automatic blood pressure.

The arterial waveform reveals the effects of vasodilator therapy through an increased rate of rise of upstroke due to a decrease in impedance to flow, which

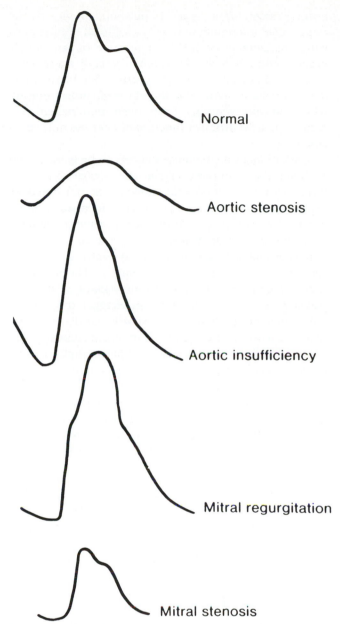

Normal

Aortic stenosis

Aortic insufficiency

Mitral regurgitation

Mitral stenosis

Figure 23–6. Arterial waveforms: normal and with valvular disease. *(From Burnside, J. W. [1981]. Physical diagnosis [16th ed., p. 149]. Baltimore: Williams & Wilkins. Reprinted with permission.)*

also contributes to a more pronounced runoff. The presence of atherosclerotic arterial occlusive disease may reduce all these components, resulting in a reduction in the measured pressure distal to the site of occlusion. The presence of aneurysmal dilation of the major vessels may blunt the systolic upstroke in the peripheral arteries, as well as form a "buffer zone" in the vascular tree that reduces the transmitted pressure in the peripheral artery.

Interpretation of Arterial Monitoring. In clinical practice, the usual information obtained from arterial monitoring is the systemic blood pressure, although

other information is applicable from arterial waveform monitoring. As indicated, if there is no damping or ringing that would alter the measured pressure, the pressures measured by arterial cannulation are presumed more reliable than those obtained from noninvasive means of monitoring. In nonphysiologic states, such as induced hypotension, extremes of temperature, or nonpulsatile flow such as seen in conjunction with cardiopulmonary bypass, measurement of intraarterial pressures may be the only reliable means of measuring systemic pressure.

Despite the fact that there is no absolute correlation between arterial pressure or waveform and cardiac output or other indices of perfusion, a variety of information can be gained by observing and analyzing the arterial waveform. Although these indirect indices are not absolute, they provide valuable clues in managing patients with arterial monitoring. When assuming that there is no mechanical cause for damping or ringing, the upstroke provides an index of the contractile mechanism, or inotropic state, of the left ventricle. Stroke volume also may be estimated by the area under the waveform, although not in a quantifiable fashion. Comparing the arterial waveform with the respiratory cycle may demonstrate fluctuations in arterial pressure in conjunction with respiration. Fluctuations in excess of 10 mmHg are considered abnormal and may represent vascular hypovolemia (Burnside, 1981). Furthermore, the dicrotic notch may be seen to fall with the development of hypovolemia. Caution should be employed in making absolute guides of changes in arterial waveforms, as the physiologic impact of anesthetic agents on hemodynamics includes the reduction of inotropic state, peripheral arterial dilation, and shunting of flow. Therefore, changes should be compared between two similar intervals. Waveforms observed prior to induction and volume shift should not be relied on solely as evidence of the development of hypovolemia following stabilization postinduction. It also should be noted that aortic valvular lesions may produce typical abnormalities in the confirmation of the arterial waveform, making interruption, without a baseline prior to induction of anesthesia or any physiologic change during the course of anesthesia, unreliable.

Cannulating the Artery. When cannulating vessels, it is important to consider the physical nature and structure of both the catheter and the monitoring system. In general, the smaller the catheter used in proportion to the lumen of the vessel, the lower the incidence of vascular thrombosis. The material composition of the catheter determines other physical characteristics. Being stiffer, polypropylene proves more resistant to kinking. In contrast, Teflon is less stiff and more prone to kinking, but is more widely used because it is least thrombogenic (Brown, Sweeney, & Lumley, 1969). It should be noted that as many as 20% of 20-gauge Teflon arterial catheters kink within 24 hours of placement (Bedford, 1977). Finally, the size of the catheter used determines the likelihood or degree of ringing that occurs. Smaller-gauge catheters demonstrate less ringing when transmitting the waveform.

The site, technique, and route employed for cannulation also determine the incidence of complications. Localized infection rates of 4% to 6.5% are reported. *Staphylococcus epidermidis* is the most common agent (Bedford, 1977; Pinilla, Ross, Martin, & Crump, 1983). In catheters inserted via cutdown, the rate increases to 30% to 39% for catheters in place for more than 4 days. Local antibiotic treatment is effective in reducing the infection rate. Catheters treated at the puncture site with iodophor demonstrated a 2.2% incidence of infection, compared with 3.6% for triple-antibiotic preparation and 6.5% for controls (Hayes, Morello, Rosenbaum, & Matsumoto, 1973). Some commercial systems purport to act as biologic filters and usually are impregnated with antibiotic material. They may be placed about the catheter or over the catheter for insertion under the skin surface. Data on whether these systems prevent sepsis have not yet been conclusive, particularly in short-term cannulations.

In sharp contrast to many other studies, one group demonstrated that the use of 18- to 20-gauge propylene catheters for periods not to exceed 48 hours in patients with no history of peripheral small-vessel disease such as Raynaud's had no associated, significant complications (Slogoff, Keats, & Arlund, 1983). Furthermore, there was no predictive value in the Allen test, based on a total of 16 patients with an abnormal Allen test on examination prior to cannulation. Nevertheless, it is generally recommended that an Allen test be performed prior to cannulating a radial artery and that an alternate site be chosen, if possible, when filling from the ulnar artery takes more than 5 seconds.

Interpretation of Central Venous Monitoring.

The interpretation of data from central venous monitoring depends on an appreciation of the physiologic basis for that particular monitor. In general, central venous pressure (CVP) is measured as an assessment of volume status. The purpose in monitoring volume status is to establish the patient's relative position on the typical volume/pressure curve or volume/cardiac output curve, which is the clinical correlate to the Frank–Starling curve. The normal patient demonstrates a roughly linear relationship between vascular volume and CVP within a limited physiologic range.

As CVP measurements in the normal population cover a broad range, absolute values are not reliable guides to volume status. Each patient operates within an individualized, normal range. Central venous pressure measurements outside that range may represent extremes of volume for the single patient, yet still be within

normal range for a larger population, or vice versa. Hence, CVP in conjunction with additional nonhemodynamic parameters such as maintenance of satisfactory urinary output help assess normovolemia. Measurements taken within that range may be presumed to be rough indices of volume status and, therefore, of cardiac output, when no interventions have been undertaken that would impair ventricular function or alter the normal relationship.

Additional valuable information can be gained from analyzing the venous waveform. The normal CVP waveform, with its component elements, is illustrated in Figure 23–7. The a-wave represents the wave of atrial contraction. In the normal patient, it remains a comparatively low-amplitude wave. In the case of ventricular nondistensibility, however, this atrial contraction occurs against an incompletely relaxed ventricle. The additional pressure generated by contraction against a stiff, unyielding ventricle presents as an exaggerated a-wave, which may be the first clue to ventricular diastolic dysfunction. This can be seen with tricuspid stenosis, right ventricular failure, pulmonary hypertension, or pulmonary stenosis. Furthermore, a-wave amplitude is exaggerated with the development of a nodal mechanism. The a-wave also is exaggerated with any dysrhythmia that results in a loss of synchronization between the atria and the ventricle (such as AVD). In the presence of atrial fibrillation, the a-wave is lost in the CVP waveform. Late

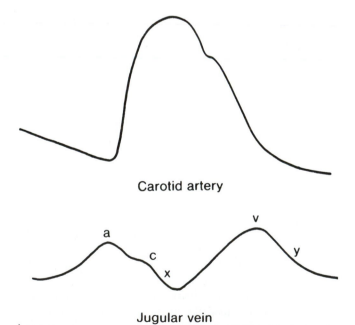

Figure 23–7. Typical central venous pressure waveform in the jugular vein. a, atrial contraction; c, tricuspid valve closure (may be seen only in right atrial pressure tracings); x, atrial relaxation and filling; v, ventricular contraction; y, tricuspid valve opening and ventricular filling. *(From Burnside, J. W. [1981]. Physical diagnosis [16th ed.]. Baltimore: Williams & Wilkins. Reprinted with permission.)*

in the cardiac cycle, the v-wave appears as a reflection of the force generated during ventricular contraction and the rapid filling of the atria. The amplitude of the v-wave may be grossly exaggerated in the presence of tricuspid regurgitation. Changes in the amplitude of the v-wave may serve as a rough index of the degree of regurgitation, and amplitude should return to normal when the cause for regurgitation is corrected.

Interpretation of Pulmonary Artery Monitoring.

The pulmonary artery is monitored with a Swan–Ganz catheter. This long, flexible, balloon-tipped catheter is designed to drift with blood flow from the point of insertion into the central circulation. It has a distal port at the tip of the catheter, which is protected when the balloon is inflated with the recommended 1.5 mL of air. A proximal port, located 30 cm from the tip of the catheter, provides a site for measuring central venous pressure when the catheter is inserted into a normal-size adult. A thermistor probe is located in the tip of the catheter to cannulate cardiac output by thermodilution. In more recent developments, continuous measurement of mixed venous oxygen saturation is available via this catheter. The final common pathway is through the right atrium and ventricle into the pulmonary artery, where pressure and other measurements are made.

A variety of information is available from a Swan–Ganz catheter. These measurements may be direct measurements, calculated parameters made using only the Swan–Ganz, or integrated parameters calculated from information derived from alternate invasive modalities. For this reason, sophistication in the management and interpretation of data derived from the Swan–Ganz catheter is critical to managing complex cases. A table of normal Swan–Ganz values can be found in Table 23–5.

Directly Measured Parameters.

Parameters directly measured with the Swan–Ganz catheter typically include CVP, pulmonary artery pressure, wedge pressure, and injectate and patient core temperatures. In sequence, these offer indices of right ventricular preload, integration of cardiac output and pulmonary vascular resistance, and index of left ventricular preload. Recent developments add the potential for measurement of mixed venous oxygen saturation. When interpreting data obtained from a Swan–Ganz catheter, the practitioner should consider the individual patient's hemodynamic and cardiac status. Other factors that alter interpretation of pressure data derived from the Swan–Ganz include valvular dysfunction, vascular and chamber compliance, ventricular function, and alterations in the normal electrical conduction pattern.

Clinical Interpretation of Data.

Valvular dysfunction may make pressure data derived from the Swan–

TABLE 23–5. Normal Resting Hemodynamic Values

	Systolic	Diastolic	Mean
Pressure (mmHg)			
Right atrium	—	—	−2 to +6
Right ventricle	15–30	0–8	5–15
Pulmonary artery			0–12
Left atrium			0–12
Left ventricle	100–140	60–90	70–105
Volume			
Left ventricle			
End-diastolic	70–95 mL m^{-2}		
End-systolic	24–36 mL m^{-2}		
Performance			
Cardiac index	2.5–4.2 L min^{-1} m^{-2}		
Stroke volume index	50–70 mL/m^{-2}		
Ejection fraction	0.67 ± 0.08 (SD)		
Resistance			
Pulmonary vascular	20–120 dyn · s cm^{-5}		
Systemic vascular	770–1500 dyn · s cm^{-5}		
Oxygen measurements			
Oxygen consumption	110–150 mL min^{-1} m^{-2}		
Arteriovenous oxygen difference	3–5 mL dL^{-1} blood		
Valve measurements			
Aortic valve area	2.6–3.5 cm^2		
Mitral valve area	4.0–6.0 cm^2		

From Nunn, J. F., Utting, J. E., & Brown, B. R. (1980). General anaesthesia (5th ed., p. 474). Boston: Butterworths. Reprinted, with permission.

Ganz catheter less reliable as a measure of ventricular preload. Regurgitant valvular lesions produce a retrograde v-wave that artificially elevates the upstream vascular pressure measurement (Fig. 23–8). Hence, actual ventricular preload may be substantially lower than the measured pressures indicate. Stenotic valvular lesions reduce the orifice across which blood flows during the diastolic filling interval, requiring higher atrial pressures to generate sufficient flow across the valve to maintain ventricular filling volume. As a result, increased CVP or wedge pressures may follow the degree of stenosis and may not reflect actual ventricular preload directly.

Vascular and chamber compliance also may affect the interpretation of pressure data derived from central venous and pulmonary artery monitoring. Vasodilators such as nitroglycerine may produce increases in venous or pulmonary artery compliance, resulting in lowered pressures, without reducing the actual vascular volume or flow. Conversely, vasoconstrictors and physiologic derangements such as hypoxemia and hypercarbia may

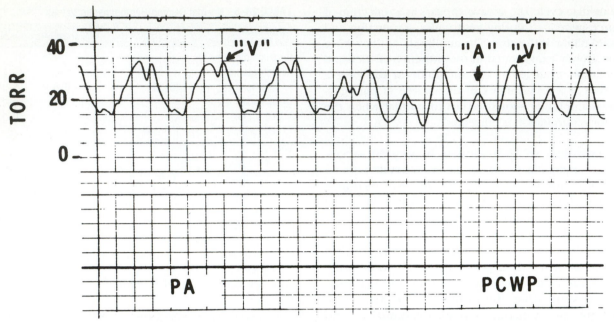

Figure 23–8. v-Wave morphology in pulmonary artery wedge tracing. PA, pulmonary artery; PCWP, pulmonary capillary wedge pressure; "V," v-wave; "A," a-wave. *(From Hug, C. C. [1986]. Monitoring. In R. D. Miller [Ed.],* Anesthesia *[2nd ed., p. 451]. NY: Churchill Livingstone. Reprinted with permission.)*

produce increases in measured pressures without actually altering the vascular volume or flow. Similarly, changes in chamber compliance may alter the normal volume–pressure relationship. Hypertrophy, ischemia, use of inotropic agents, and increases in afterload all may reduce ventricular compliance and make pressure data less reliable as guides to ventricular filling volume.

Although alterations in valvular and vascular status disrupt the typical pressure–volume relationship, each patient follows an individualized clinical Starling curve. Therefore, certain guidelines may be developed to support clinical decisions based on expected pressure alterations with selected lesions. Patients with long-standing systemic hypertension or outflow obstruction generally require higher filling pressures to maintain preload in a less compliant ventricle. Aortic insufficiency results in left-ventricle dilation and hypertrophy. Higher diastolic pressures reflect the degree of regurgitant flow, as insufficiency exposes the left ventricle to aortic root pressures. Hence, patients with long-standing hypertension or aortic valvular dysfunction may require a wedge pressure as great as 16 to 18 torr to maintain adequate left ventricular filling volume for a suitable cardiac output. Patients with mitral stenosis may require higher-than-normal atrial pressures to generate sufficient flow across a constricted valve area for adequate left ventricular filling. Thus, a wedge pressure of 18 to 22 torr may be required to maintain a suitable cardiac output. Patients with mitral insufficiency frequently demonstrate a regurgitant v-wave in the pulmonary artery tracing, making it impossible to obtain a wedge tracing. Estimating re-

ductions in the magnitude of the v-wave may provide a crude guide to improving forward low, provided that the cardiac output remains constant. Because the Swan–Ganz follows the venous circulation into the pulmonary circulation, its use is not generally recommended in patients with stenotic valvular lesions involving the right side of the heart. In patients with right-sided valvular insufficiency, it may prove difficult to pass the Swan–Ganz. Still, data derived from the wedge will be accurate, although data gathered on right-sided filling pressures will be subject to the same errors described for the left ventricular and pulmonary artery or wedge pressures.

As would be expected, patients with a history of ventricular dysfunction also frequently have a dilated and less compliant ventricle and require higher-than-normal filling pressures. As a result, it is typical to find that patients with chronic left ventricular dysfunction require a wedge pressure as great as 18 torr to maintain adequate filling pressures for a suitable cardiac output. Similarly, patients with chronic right ventricular dysfunction or pulmonary hypertension may require elevated filling pressures as evidenced by CVP measurements that may exceed 20 torr; however, those filling pressures may be limited to the right side, and left ventricular filling pressures may remain relatively normal. As the prognosis for patients with chronic pulmonary hypertension is ominous, it becomes critical to monitor right-sided filling pressures, and assessing right ventricular function may prove the most critical determinant of successful management.

Finally, conduction defects may alter the normal volume–pressure relationship. In general, it may be deduced that abnormalities in conduction, particularly those that disturb the normal pattern of atrioventricular synchronicity, result in the need for increased filling pressures. Patients with mitral stenosis frequently maintain a rhythm of atrial fibrillation, in which no atrial kick is present to augment left ventricular filling. Atrial "kick" also is lost in patients with a nodal rhythm or those with a paced ventricular mechanism. As a compensatory measure, elevated atrial pressures may be reflected as an increased CVP or wedge pressure, and patients may require higher venous or atrial pressures to maintain normal ventricular filling volumes. Patients with paced or nodal mechanisms generally maintain suitable cardiac output with a wedge pressure of about 16 torr, whereas patients with atrial fibrillation may require a wedge pressure of 18 to 22 torr. The amplitude of the normal a-wave of atrial contraction is higher in patients with nodal mechanisms, as the atria contract against a closed atrioventricular valve. Patients with acutely induced nondistensibility, as occurs in the presence of myocardial ischemia, also may demonstrate an exaggerated a-wave amplitude.

Oximetric Measurements.

The development of the oximetric Swan–Ganz has offered an additional benefit in invasive monitoring. The measurement of mixed venous oxygen saturation provides additional information on the global adequacy of circulatory function. The normal patient extracts approximately 25% of available oxygen in the awake, resting state. This corresponds to a mixed venous oxygen saturation of approximately 75% or a mixed venous Po_2 of about 40 torr. Reductions in mixed venous oxygen saturation provide a relatively sensitive index of global oxygen balance. Disturbances that decrease mixed venous oxygen saturation may result from decreased oxygen-carrying capacity through reductions in cardiac output with ventricular dysfunction, reductions in circulating hemoglobin levels as seen with acute bleeding, or increases in systemic oxygen utilization as seen in the toxic or septic patient.

Anesthesia accommodating the use of muscle relaxants produces a shunting of blood from the muscle bed and eliminates the work of breathing, which reduces oxygen utilization and increases the mixed venous oxygen saturation. A typical mixed venous oxygen saturation for the anesthetized, mechanically ventilated patient is 85% to 90%. Progressive decreases in body temperature, whether from deliberate induction of hypothermia or passive dissipation of heat into a cold operating room, account for progressive reductions in oxygen utilization and increases in mixed venous saturation, when cardiac output and hemoglobin concentrations remain constant. Thus, by incorporating factors of cardiac output, hemoglobin concentration, and oxygen-carrying capacity, the clinician can approximate the appropriate mixed venous oxygen saturation for the anesthetized patient.

Calculated Parameters.

In addition to those pressure parameters measured directly, the use of a Swan–Ganz permits the calculation of a variety of derived parameters. The most commonly employed calculation is the cardiac output. Cardiac output most often is calculated by a variety of available self-contained units, using an algorithm that employs the measured difference in temperature across time; hence the term *thermodilution cardiac output*. Alternative methods of measuring cardiac output, such as dye dilution, are relatively more cumbersome and less adaptable to the clinical setting. Calculations of cardiac output using the classic Fick method require assumptions about oxygen use that are not valid in the anesthetized, mechanically ventilated, and frequently hypothermic patient. For those reasons, current standards in clinical practice support the use of the thermodilution cardiac output technique derived from a Swan–Ganz catheter.

Measurement of cardiac output with a Swan–Ganz thermodilution catheter necessitates a variety of assumptions, and these incorporate potential measurement errors. These include the speed of the injection, error in volume of injectate, discrepancies in the temperature gradient between the patient and the injectate, and internal error of measure. Slow injection of excessive volumes may produce erroneously low output readings, as may reductions in the difference between the temperature of the patient and the injectate or the use of warmer injectate than incorporated in the coefficients dialed into the output computer. In contrast, too-rapid injection, lower-than-indicated volumes, extreme differences in temperature, and colder-than-indicated injectate tend to magnify cardiac output calculation. Finally, the error of measure makes absolute interpretation of cardiac output measurements unreliable. Within the normal range of cardiac output, the error of measure may be accepted as approximately 10%. As cardiac output deviates more than one standard deviation from the mean, the error in measure increases. At measurements greater than two standard deviations from the mean, the error of measure may approach 50%. In general, error of measure increases more rapidly in measurements below the mean, making low cardiac output measurements less reliable than correspondingly high measurements. For those reasons, most experienced clinicians rely heavily on trends in cardiac output rather than absolute calculations and use collateral data such as arterial blood gases, acid–base balance, and mixed venous oxygen saturation to judge the adequacy of systemic circulation and oxygenation.

Finally, it must be remembered that the thermodilution cardiac output technique actually measures right ventricular cardiac output. Thus, the clinician assumes that right and left ventricular outputs are consistently and directly related. In the normal state, that assumption remains accurate. In patients with ventricular failure, however, that rule is violated. Acute left ventricular failure does not result in an immediate decrease in right ventricular output, and other indices of left ventricular function, such as changes in wedge pressure or waveform analysis, may prove necessary to obtain a more complete analysis.

Integrated Calculations. A variety of integrated calculations can be made when the cardiac output is estimated with the thermodilution technique. Both systemic and pulmonary vascular resistances may be calculated using the formula in Table 23-6, which also lists normal values. These determinations may support the decision to employ vasodilators or vasoconstrictors. They also may indicate the requirement for therapy in the patient with left ventricular failure or direct the management of patients requiring higher-than-normal systemic vascular resistance to maintain coronary perfusion such as patients with ventricular hypertrophy. The development of a variety of drugs that are effective pulmonary dilators has made it possible to manage the patient with pulmonary hypertension with greater sophistication than previously possible by using integrated parameters.

In addition to vascular resistances, it is possible to gather an estimate of the ventricular stroke work from calculations provided by the Swan–Ganz catheter. The stroke work indices outlined in Table 23–6 allow the clinician to estimate the workload against which either ventricle is operating by incorporating indices of preload, afterload, and stroke index. For these calculations, it is necessary to convert absolute stroke volume to stroke index, by dividing the stroke volume by the patient's body surface area (BSA) in square meters. That area can be approximated from a variety of nomograms that use the patient's height and weight, as that shown in Figure 23-9. The use of BSA-adjusted figures permits adjustment for the individual patient's relative size, which is not other-

TABLE 23–6. Parameters Derived from Invasive Monitoring

Formula	Normal Value
$SV = \dfrac{CO}{HR} \times 1000$	$60\text{–}90 \text{ mL beat}^{-1}$
$SI = \dfrac{SV}{BSA}$	$40\text{–}60 \text{ mL beat}^{-1} \text{m}^{-2}$
$LVSWI = 1.36 \times \dfrac{(\overline{MAP} - \overline{PCWP}) \times SI}{100}$	$45\text{–}60 \text{ g} \cdot \text{m m}^{-2}\text{beat}^{-1}$
$RVSWI = 1.36 \times \dfrac{\left(\overline{PAP} - \dfrac{100}{CVP}\right) \times SI}{100}$	$5\text{–}10 \text{ g} \cdot \text{m m}^{-2}\text{beat}^{-1}$
$SVR = \dfrac{(\overline{MAP} - \overline{CVP}) \times 80}{CO}$	$900\text{–}1500 \text{ dyn} \cdot \text{cm}^{-5}$
$PVR = \dfrac{(\overline{PAP} - \overline{PCWP}) \times 80}{CO}$	$50\text{–}150 \text{ dyn} \cdot \text{s cm}^{-5}$

SV, stroke volume, CO, cardiac output; HR, heart rate; BSA, body surface area; LVSWI, left ventricular stroke work index; $\overline{MAP}$, mean arterial pressure; $\overline{PCWP}$, mean pulmonary capillary wedge pressure; RVSWI, right ventricular stroke work index; $\overline{PAP}$, mean pulmonary artery pressure; $\overline{CVP}$, mean central venous pressure; SVR, systemic vascular resistance; PVR, pulmonary vascular resistance; SI, stroke index. *Note:* All of these parameters are rapidly derived in both the operating room and intensive care unit using programmable portable calculators available at the present time.

From Hug, C. C. (1986). Monitoring. In R. D. Miller (Ed.), Anesthesia, (2nd ed., p. 453). New York: Churchill Livingstone. Reprinted with permission.

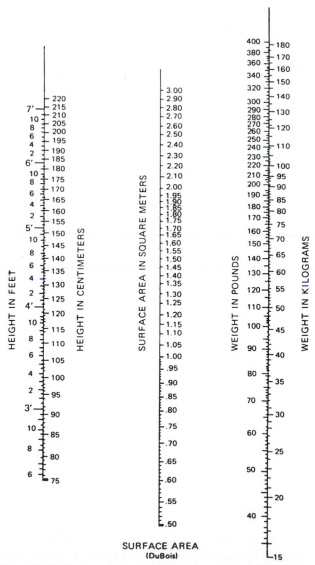

Figure 23–9. Body surface area nomogram. *Source: from DuBois, D., & Dubois, E. F. (1916). Clinical calorimetry. A formula to estimate the approximate surface area if height and weight are known. (From* Archives of Internal Medicine, 17, *863.)*

wise addressed in calculation. As it is inherently obvious that a 90-kg patient requires greater cardiac output and correspondingly higher indices than a 60-kg patient, or that a tall, muscular 70-kg patient requires a greater cardiac output than a short, obese 70-kg patient, the conversion of absolute calculations to indices provides a more precise and meaningful estimate of cardiovascular function.

The single drawback to these increasingly complex integrated calculations is the accumulation of error of measure with each successive calculation. It must be remembered that cardiac output itself is a calculated parameter subject to inherent assumptions. Violation of these assumptions makes the calculated result less reliable. In similar fashion, each of the successive derivations of additional integrated indices depend on assumptions for greater accuracy. With each additional calculation, these indices are rendered less reliable as absolute measurements. That progressive accumulation of error in measure may make values that are far outside the norm less reliable as absolute indicators; however, trends and the use of collateral supportive data and measurements supplement their use in clinical practice and form the basis for decisions in clinical management.

Echocardiography and Transesophageal Echocardiography

Echocardiography and transesophageal echocardiography (TEE) are based on the principles of ultrasound imaging. A generator produces an ultrasound pulse that then directs the beam through a medium (the heart), whereby the transducer analyzes the reflected echoes of the various objects along the path of the beam. Sound waves travel in a straight line as long as they are in a homogenous medium. When they reach the interface of two different media densities, the sound wave undergoes physical changes. Normally, the acoustic impedance is a product of velocity and medium density. The difference in the distortion of the sound waves depends on the differences in the acoustic impedances. The angle of incidence of the beam direction also is altered, and some of the sound wave is reflected and some of the wave is refracted. These differences are represented in pictoral fashion on a screen. The reflected echo waves of varying intensities return at different intervals. The time of reception of the electronic signals that the reflected echoes generate are analyzed to estimate depth of location provide information on tissue characteristics (ie, valve versus muscle) (Obeid, 1992).

Because the heart is located deep in the chest with multiple interface layers, usually there are significant impediments to external ultrasound imaging. Hence, the transesophageal echocardiogram was developed. A special monitor (an endoscope with an ultrasound trans-ducer replacing the light source) is placed into the esophagus at the level of the left atrium. Because the esophagus lies right behind the heart, in this position the skin, ribs, or chest wall do not interfere with the cardiac image. The ultrasound beam travels a shorter distance with a higher frequency, allowing better image resolution and imaging of the entire thoracic aorta, pulmonary veins, vena cava, and atrial appendages.

A TEE probe is placed after the patient is anesthetized under general anesthesia and intubated. It is useful in patients who are obese, or have a heavily muscled chest wall, or suffer from chronic obstructive pulmonary disease (the lung hyperexpansion interferes with regular echocardiography). It is a valuable monitor for evaluating cardiac and valvular function, especially during heart surgery. Perivalvular and valvular leaks were identified prior to coming off bypass (Jawad, 1996). Transesophageal echocardiography also can be used to evaluate congenital and wall motion abnormalities; monitor patients with significant heart disease undergoing noncardiac surgery (beat-to-beat evaluation of cardiac performance, preload, fluid balance, and wall motion parameters); identify the location and extent of diseases of the aorta, in particular, dissections, thrombus formation, and atherosclerotic plaques; help diagnose pericardial disease, effusions, or tamponade; detect ventricular abnormalities in relation to ischemic events and ventricular distensibility secondary to volume changes; detect intracardiac air in neurosurgery and emboli in orthopedic procedures; determine anesthetic drug effects on cardiac function (ie, shock, aortic cross-clamp, and surgeries with significant fluid shifts, such as liver transplantations or colon resection); and to detect prosthetic valve dysfunction. Transesophageal echocardiography is contraindicated in patients with esophageal disease and/or active stomach ulcers. However, it does not interfere with the surgical field.

Two Dimensional Echocardiography. Two-dimensional echocardiogaphy is based on the ability of a single ultrasound beam to move along the length of a large object, creating multiple images that are then superimposed to obtain a cross-sectional image. When multiple ultrasound beams are generated side by side, the whole length of the object can be imaged, giving a two-dimensional echo or cross-sectional echo. This mode of echocardiography also is employed to visualize cardiac function.

▶ MONITORING THE NERVOUS SYSTEM

The Electroencephalogram

Electroencephalogram (EEG) monitoring is the oldest form of clinical monitoring. It has been available since the 1930s (Gibbs, Gibbs, & Lennox, 1937). Both EEG and evoked potential (EP) monitoring provide information on the depth of anesthesia, integrity of neural pathways, presence of cerebral ischemia, and cerebral cortex function (Friedman, Theisen, & Grundy, 1989). Whereas EEG and EP monitoring were once considered laborious and complicated, significant efforts have been made to make this technology user-friendly, especially with the advent of bispectral index.

Electroencephalogram and Electrical Activity

The EEG is a strip-chart recording that measures the electrophysiology of brain cell activity. It is a continuous recording of the voltage and amplitude of the electrical signals obtained by scalp electrodes plotted on a graph of voltage versus time. The electrical activity of the brain is measured in microvolt differences in the electrical potentials (resting cell potential and action potential) produced by the granular layer of the cerebral cortex (versus the millivolt differences in the electrocardiogram). The granular layer is populated by pyramidal cells whose dendritic trees lie perpendicular to the cerebral cortex. The EEG is then generated by excitatory and inhibitory postsynaptic potentials that summate on these dendritic trees.

The EEG represents spontaneous intrinsically occurring brain activity, as compared to evoked potential (EP) monitoring, that requires the application of a specific stimulus, to which there is a certain elicited response. The EEG electrode can detect simultaneously the activity of many cells that usually lie somewhat far from the electrode, far from the site of origin. This is called a *field potential.* The *evoked potential* electrodes monitor specific locations along a nerve tract. The evoked potential is then described as either a *near-field* or *far-field* potential, depending on the relationship of the electrode to the monitoring site.

Physiology of Electroencephalographic Monitoring

The spontaneous electrical brain cell activity is created by the difference in the resting electrical potential of a neuron, which is a negative 50 to 100 mV, and the action potential, which is a positive 30 mV. Electroencephalographic activity is rhythmical (regular and sinusoidal), and based on the synchronized impulses from a central pacemaker formed by thalamic projection neurons and thalamic interneurons. These neurons either inhibit or excite other projection neurons at a rate of about 10 Hz. This rhythmical activity can be interrupted or facilitated by changes in the midbrain reticular activating system (MRAS). The MRAS receives input from all sensory systems and cortical areas and outputs to the cortex through direct connections and relays to the dien-

cephalon. Rhythmical activity can be facilitated by lower brainstem structures that inhibit the desynchronous effect of the ascending RAS. Rhythmical activity can be interrupted by MRAS overriding the input from the cortex and diencephalon.

Lead Systems.   Two lead systems are used to monitor EEG activity, bipolar and unipolar. *Bipolar* systems measure the difference in potential voltage between two scalp electrodes. The electrodes used are the standard silverplated contact electrodes applied with collodian gel. *Unipolar* systems measure the difference in potential voltage between one scalp electrode (active) and one electrode elsewhere on the body (reference). The frequency is measured in hertz. The distribution of the brain waves is classified under three terms: (1) widespread/diffuse/generalized: waves of activity that occur over the entire head; (2) lateralized: activity on one side of the head; and (3) focal: activity restricted to one or a few electrodes.

The scalp arrangement of electrodes follows the international 10-20 system. This is a system of lines that run across and along the head and intersect at intervals of 10% to 20% of their total length (Fig. 23–10). The letters indicate location, and the numbers indicated the distance from the midline. Increasing numbers represent increasing distances from the midline (except the temporal Fp leads, which increase in number from front to back). Numbers on the left are odd, and those on the right are even. Letters indicate location by anatomic reference: F, frontal; Fp, prefrontal; C, central; P, parietal; O,

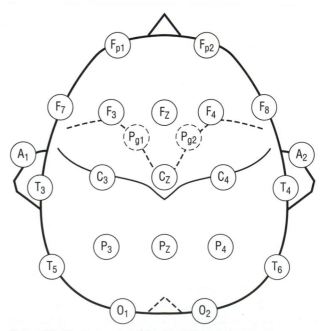

Figure 23–10. International 10–20 EEG lead placement.

occipital; A, auricular; Z, midline. There are three major reference points: (1) the nasion: bridge of the nose directly under the forehead; (2) the inion: the bony protuberance in the middle of the back of the head; and (3) the preauricular point: the depression of bone in front of the ear canal.

The most commonly used lead system in the operating room is a single channel that is either biparietal or frontotemporal. This system only displays global insults, however (Friedman, 1989). To simplify the waveform, the amplified subtraction method is employed. This method removes artifact and amplifies the signal. Another common method of recording is the power spectral array and compressed spectral array, which converts the recording of voltage versus time to a power versus frequency scale (Bickford et al., 1972) (Fig. 23–11).

Electroencephalographic Rhythms

There are four basic EEG rhythms (Fig. 23–12): delta, theta, alpha, and beta. They are described by amplitude, frequency, waveform, distribution, persistence, repetition, phase relation, reactivity, and timing. Delta rhythms are from 1 to 4 Hz and occur during deep sleep, deep anesthesia, or states of compromised or pathologic neurologic function. Theta waves occur at 4 to 8 Hz and are produced during drowsiness and general anesthesia. Alpha waves occur at 8 to 13 Hz and are the most dominant wave of the occipital region when the eyes are closed. Alpha waves are blocked when the eyes are open, with mental activity or by a startle response (Fig. 23–13). They often are seen over the entire cortex during moderate to deep anesthesia or coma. Finally beta waves occur at 13 to 40 Hz and are produced during the alert state with eyes open, during light anesthesia or mental activity (Friedman et al., 1989).

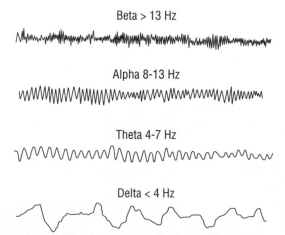

Figure 23–11. EEG waveforms. *(From Daube, J. R., Sandok, B. A., Reagan, T. J., et al. [1978]. Medical neurosciences [p. 50]. Boston: Little, Brown. Reprinted with permission.)*

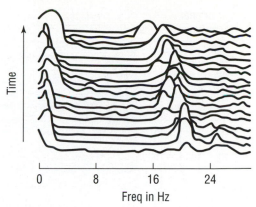

Figure 23–12. Compressed spectral array EEG: time versus frequency.

Physiologic Changes and Their Correlation to Electroencephalographic Rhythms

The EEG rhythms correlate well with cerebral blood flow even under general anesthesia (Friedman et al., 1989). If cerebral blood flow decreases with hypotension, the earliest EEG change is a decrease in the voltage of beta activity (Fig. 23–14). Delta rhythms appear as consciousness is lost. In patients who have impaired or reset autoregulatory mechanisms, the EEG changes will occur at higher pressures than what is normally considered hypotension. In the event of hypoxia, EEG activity in general slows and the amplitude decreases (Rossen, Simonson, & Baker,

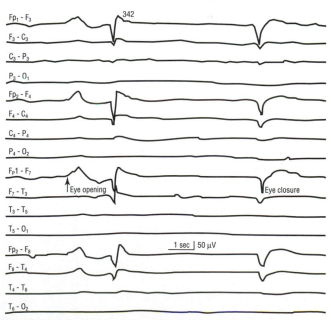

Figure 23–13. Alpha waves blocked with eyes open, eyes closed. *(From Dr. Eduardo Rubenstein, Professor, UCLA School of Medicine, Department of Anesthesiology, 1997. Reprinted with permission.)*

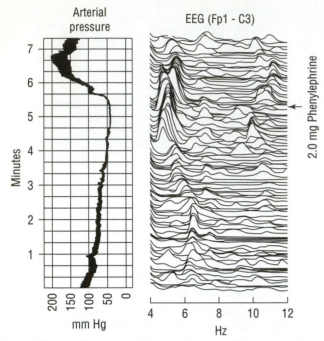

Figure 23–14. The effect of hypotension on EEG waves. Global ischemia, as observed during transient, severe hypotension is associated with a well-defined slow-wave, high-voltage pattern. *(From Dr. Eduardo Rubenstein, Professor, UCLA School of Medicine, Department of Anesthesiology, 1997. Reprinted with permission.)*

1961). The initial manifestation is frontal alpha activity and reflects changes in high-energy phosphate stores that are depleted during acute hypoxia. In procedures such as carotid endarterectomies, coronary artery bypass grafting, or deliberate hypotension, the EEG can be of valuable assistance in detecting cerebral ischemia.

In carotid endarterectomy procedures, there is ipsilateral slowing with loss of high-frequency activity. The

changes take approximately 1.5 to 2 minutes to develop, and if they last for less than 10 minutes, serious sequelae usually will resolve with reperfusion (Friedman et al., 1989). During CABG and neurosurgical procedures, EEG slowing can result from hypothermia, hypocapnia, electrolyte disturbances, or a need to raise perfusion pressure. During hypocarbia, EEG waves slow, but have increased amplitude and dominant frequencies are in the 4- to 6-Hz range. Changes in anesthetic depth are more apparent with hypocarbia. During episodes of hypercarbia, an arousal pattern is seen in the EEG. At carbon dioxide levels greater than 25%, there is a cessation of rapid activity (Wyke, 1957), and the brain becomes electrically silent at levels greater than 80% (Betz, 1974). If a condition of hypoglycemia is present, there is a loss of alpha activity. Continued hypoglycemia slows EEG waves to a delta rhythm. Hyperglycemia does not significantly alter the EEG (Friedman et al., 1989).

Anesthetic Effects on the Electroencephalogram

All anesthetics have some effect on the EEG waveforms (Fig. 23–15), and some drugs having more effects than others (Newfield & Cottrell, 1991; Table 23–7). For each particular surgery and anesthetic, the needs of the surgery and the effects of the anesthetic on the EEG must be correlated to optimize the analysis of the patient's condition. Knowledge of the anesthetic effects on the EEG is useful to correlate EEG waveforms and determine anesthetic depth. The EEG can be useful in assessing the status of brittle patients, demonstrating satisfactory amnesia and sufficient depth for unconsciousness. It can assist in deciphering hyperautonomic states versus light anesthesia and in planning emergence from long neurosurgical cases. Moreover, EEG monitoring evaluates the level of induced brain coma with high-dose barbiturates.

Figure 23–15. EEG patterns and the effect of anesthesia. The EEG clearly changes as a function of depth, and several levels have been defined as a function of waveform patterns. *(From Dr. Eduardo Rubenstein, Professor, UCLA School of Medicine, Department of Anesthesiology, 1997. Reprinted with permission.)*

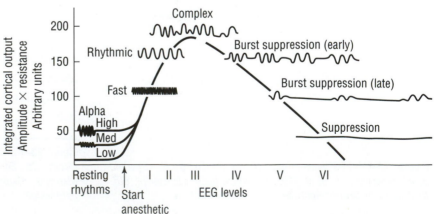

TABLE 23–7. Anesthetic Effects on the EEG

Premedications
   Benzodiazepines. Increase the 20- to 40-s activity in moderate to low
      doses; higher doses increase the proportion of slow-wave activity.
   Neuroleptics (phenothiazines, thioxanthines, butyrophenones). Increase
      the amount of alpha activity with a shift to the lower range; increase
      voltage of slow-wave activity; high doses result in slow, sharp waves.
General Anesthetics
   Thiopental. Increases beta activity but with increasing plasma
      concentrations produces high voltage slow waves; highest doses of
      barbiturates produce suppression of all EEG activity; can be titrated to
      dose-related responses of burst suppression cycles.
   Ketamine. Produces a complex pattern of enhanced beta activity, slow
      waves, and paroxysmal activity.
   Etomidate. Appears like barbiturate waveforms without the beta activity.
   Nitrous oxide. Rapidly desynchronizes the EEG; in a nitrous-narcotic
      technique produces well defined mid-voltage beta background waves
      alternating with low-voltage slow waves in proportion to narcotic dose.
   Narcotics. High doses produce high amplitude slow waves.
   Halogenated inhalation agents. Enhance beta rhythms: nitrous >
      isoflurane > enflurane > halothane; decrease voltage with increasing
      depth, finally producing slow waves with increasing voltage.

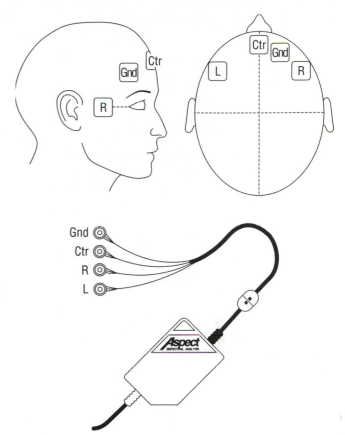

Figure 23–16. Bispectral analysis and two-channel recordings. Gnd, ground; Ctr, center; R, right; L, left. *(From Aspect Medical Corporation. Reprinted with permission.)*

Bispectral Analysis and Bispectral Index and Anesthetic Depth

The bispectral analysis is a signal processing technique from an EEG derivative recorded from a bispectral montage. Bispectral analysis is a four-lead, two-channel EEG rhythm analysis that compares and quantifies nonlinear functions between two EEG waveforms that occur simultaneously (Fig. 23–16). Bispectral analysis is able to quantify both frequency and power (linear components), as well as phase and harmonic (nonlinear components) segments of the EEG, thereby analyzing the interfrequency phase relationships (Sigl & Chamoun, 1994). By analyzing and comparing the relationship between phase and amplitude of the two waveforms and how frequently they occur, a correlation can be derived to determine the degree of hypnotic component of the anesthetic.

   Total anesthesia has several components. Those components are amnesia, hypnosis, muscle relaxation, analgesia, and areflexia. The depth and quality of the hypnotic component of anesthesia have been correlated to a scale, the bispectral index (BIS), via a complex mathematical formula (Fourier analysis) that converts the waveforms to a single-number digital reading. This number is able to quantify deviations from normal EEG rhythms (Fig. 23–17). The BIS allows a direct measurement of the brain's repsonse to stimulation and its level of hypnosis or state of unconsciousness (Fig. 23–18). The BIS is best able to track the patient's clinical responses of loss of consciousness. It has been shown to be a more accurate predictor of patient movement to skin incision than standard power-spectrum parameters or plasma propofol concentrations (Kearse, Manberg, & Chamoun, 1994). Ultimately, the BIS monitor allows for more accurate and safe titrations of anesthetics to produce reliable levels of unconsciousness.

   The BIS number increases as the anesthetic dose decreases (as the patient gets lighter or more awake/conscious, the number goes higher) or as the level of surgical stimulation increases. A lower BIS number means that the patient is more asleep (unaware), and the BIS number decreases as the anesthetic dose increases, or as surgical stimulation decreases. Because opioids do not influence state of consciousness at analgesic concentrations, they do not alter the BIS number (Kearse, Manberg, & Debros, 1994). Also, the BIS does not monitor muscle relaxation, so it does not indicate the level of paralysis, as would a peripheral nerve stimulator.

Evoked Potential Monitoring

An evoked potential (EP) is an EEG waveform that results from exogenous stimulation. Evoked potential monitoring is a test of neural function that involves the progressive activation of different levels of organization within the CNS in response to brief sensory stimuli first described by

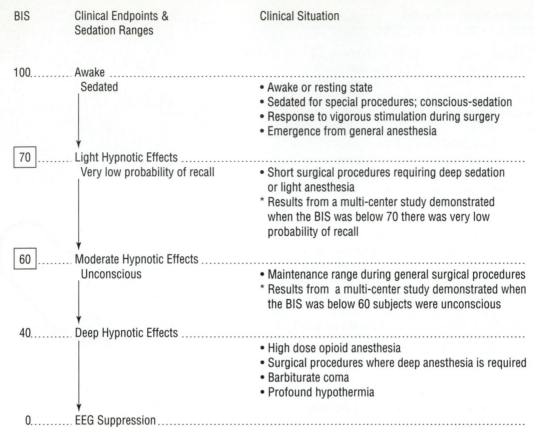

BIS | Clinical Endpoints & Sedation Ranges | Clinical Situation

100 .... Awake
          Sedated

- Awake or resting state
- Sedated for special procedures; conscious-sedation
- Response to vigorous stimulation during surgery
- Emergence from general anesthesia

70 .... Light Hypnotic Effects
          Very low probability of recall

- Short surgical procedures requiring deep sedation or light anesthesia
* Results from a multi-center study demonstrated when the BIS was below 70 there was very low probability of recall

60 .... Moderate Hypnotic Effects
          Unconscious

- Maintenance range during general surgical procedures
* Results from a multi-center study demonstrated when the BIS was below 60 subjects were unconscious

40 .... Deep Hypnotic Effects

- High dose opioid anesthesia
- Surgical procedures where deep anesthesia is required
- Barbiturate coma
- Profound hypothermia

0 .... EEG Suppression

Figure 23–17. BIS range guidelines and BIS scale. Ranges are based on results from a multicenter study of the BIS involving the administration of four commonly used anesthetics—propofol, midazolam, alfentanil and isoflurane. *Anesthesiology* 1995; 83(3A): A195, A374, A506. Note: Anesthesia is composed of many components. The BIS reflects the level of consciousness. To assess responsiveness, the degree of surgical stimulation and level of analgesia must be taken into consideration. BIS values and ranges assume that the EEG is free of artifacts that can affect its performance, i.e. ECG and EMG artifacts. *(From Aspect Medical Corporation. Reprinted with permission.)*

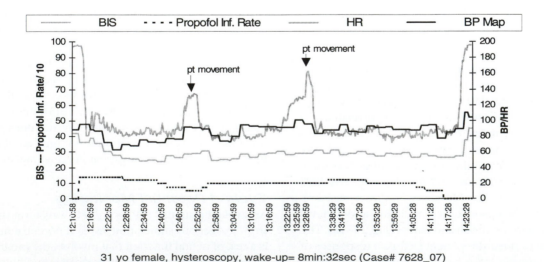

31 yo female, hysteroscopy, wake-up= 8min:32sec (Case# 7628_07)

Figure 23–18. BIS and patients' response to stimulation. *(From Aspect Medical Corporation. Reprinted with permission.)*

Caton in 1875. Evoked potentials are a common clinical diagnostic method for both peripheral and central neurological dysfunction. They are simpler to analyze and more easily automated than EEG recordings. They are used in the operating room to monitor the entire somatosensory pathways from the peripheral receptors to the cortex in orthopedic, vascular and neurosurgical procedures (Friedman et al., 1989). Examples include peripheral nerve trauma; aneurysms/arteriovenous malformations; cardotid endarterectomy; spinal surgery; aortic surgery; and posterior fossa surgery. Changes in amplitude and latency (the time required for a potential to reach a specific location) of the potentials evoked by nerve stimulation of the limbs alert the surgeon to possible nerve dysfunction, circulatory impairment, or excessive accidental retraction of structures within the nervous system. Changes related to anesthetic agents or hemodynamic function must be ruled out in correlation to EP changes.

There are two types of EP responses: near field and far field (Jacobson & Tew, 1987). *Near-field potentials* are recorded from sites generated relatively close to the recording electrode (active electrode). They have intermediate or long latency periods and greater amplitudes than far-field potentials. *Far-field potentials* are generated at a distance from the reference electrode. They have shorter latencies than near-field potentials.

There are generally three types of sensory stimulation used to elicit an EP: visual, brainstem auditory, or somatosensory. The signal is recorded from the skin surface over the area of interest. The EP is time locked to the stimulus to serve as the event marker for the waveform. The waveforms of EPs have both positive and negative peaks that appear at distinct latencies. The waveform potentials are divided into early- (<30 milliseconds), middle- (30–70 milliseconds), and long-latency (70–500 milliseconds components (Celesia, 1987). Somatosensory evoked potentials (SSEPs) reflect the transmission of sensory information from receptors through the peripheral nerves, plexus, spinal cord, brainstem, midbrain, pons, and thalamus to the sensory cortex (Grundy, 1995) (Fig. 23–19). Brief 0.1- to 0.5-millisecond stimulations are delivered at 5-second intervals over the median, peroneal, or tibial nerve and elicit potentials over the contralateral somatosensory cortex. Any interruption of the conduction pathway at any point from peripheral nerve to the cortex can abolish the cortical SSEP. The SSEPs are most frequently used for spinal cord surgery, study of peripheral nerve function, diagnoses of spinal cord, brainstem, and cortical lesions, scoliosis surgery, and intraoperative identification of the somatosensory cortex during posterior fossa surgery. They also can be used to diagnose multiple sclerosis (Jacobson & Tew, 1987).

Visual evoked potentials (VEPs) function with the same physical properties as SSEPs because visual stimulation affects the visual pathways. Visual EPs occur when light strikes the retina and gets changed into nerve impulses that get processed at successive synaptic levels

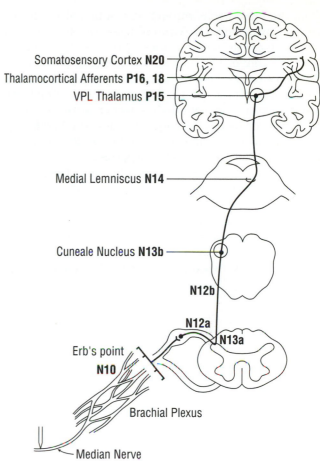

Figure 23–19. Somatosensory evoked potentials. *(From Friedman, W. A., Thiesen, G. J., & Grundy, B. L. [1989]. Electrophysiologic monitoring of the nervous system. In R. K. Stoelting, P. G. Barash, & T. J. Gallagher [Eds.],* Advances in anesthesia. *Chicago: Yearbook. Reprinted with permission.)*

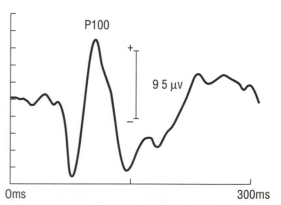

Figure 23–20. Visual evoked potentials. This visual evoked potential was generated by pattern shift stimuli with the typical positive response at 100 ms after stimulation. *(From Friedman, W. A., Thiesen, G. J., & Grundy, B. L. [1989]. Electrophysiologic monitoring of the nervous system. In R. K. Stoelting, P. G. Barash, & T. J. Gallagher [Eds.],* Advances in anesthesia. *Chicago: Yearbook. Reprinted with permission.)*

from the optic nerve, through the optic chiasm, to the lateral geniculate body (Grundy, 1995; Fig. 23–20). They can demonstrate abnormalities in the eye, optic nerve, optic chiasm, or the pathways continuing posterior to the visual cortex. Visual EPs are altered by multiple sclerosis, coma, hydrocephalus, and some forms of epilepsy. They are elicited by light flashes over closed eyelids from light-emitting diodes in opaque goggles. The EP/EEG signal is recorded from the occipital cortex against the vertex. Visual EPs have long latency periods.

Brainstem auditory evoked potentials (BAEPs) are produced when filtering clicks or tone bursts are delivered to the ear by acoustically shielded earphones or by ear insert transducers (Grundy, 1995). This produces short-latency subcortical potentials that are far-field responses recorded from electrodes on the vertex and earlobe. Mostly BAEPs are used to assess hearing in infants,

coma victims, and the elderly. They can detect abnormalities in nerve function resulting from multiple sclerosis, mass lesions such as acoustic neuromas, ischemic lesions like pontine infarction, and brainstem tumors (Friedman et al., 1989). The typical BAEP waveform has seven positive vertexes (Grundy, 1995). Each vertex represents a unique anatomic location: peak I, extracranial auditory nerve; peak II, intracranial auditory nerve and or cochlear nerve; peak III, superior olive; peak IV, lateral lemniscus; peak V, inferior colliculus; peak VI, thalamus; and peak VII, thalamocortical radiation (Fig. 23–21). Mid-latency potentials represent activity in the auditory projection area. Long latencies appear bilaterally and originate in the frontal association cortex. Changes in the latency and amplitude of early peaks may reflect effects on the cochlear nerve, changes in later peaks may reflect excessive retraction on the brainstem. Waves of BAEP

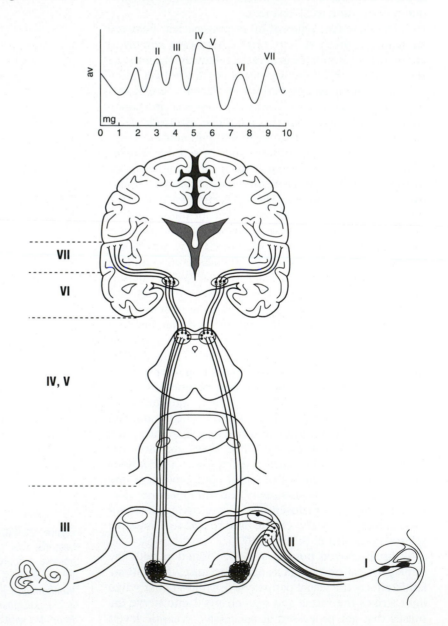

Figure 23–21. Brainstem auditory evoked potentials. *(From Friedman, W. A., Thiesen, G. J., & Grundy, B. L. [1989]. Electrophysiologic monitoring of the nervous system. In R. K. Stoelting, P. G. Barash, & T. J. Gallagher [Eds.],* Advances in anesthesia. *Chicago: Yearbook. Reprinted with permission.)*

also reflect auditory and brainstem function during posterior fossa surgery. Moreover, BAEPs show changes with eighth cranial nerve retraction (Friedman et al. 1989). Recent studies show that BAEPs, especially while monitoring the mid-latency auditory evoked potentials, are promising as indicators of the depth of anesthesia (de Beers et al., 1996; Davies, Mantzaridis, Kenny, & Fisher, 1996).

Evoked potentials are affected by temperature (increase in latency with no change in amplitudes), blood pressure (mild attenuation with hypotension), hypercapnia and hypocapnia, anesthetic agents (especially local anesthetics), and muscle relaxants. Hypothermia results in progressive latency increases for all EPs.

Anesthetic Effects on Evoked Potentials. In low doses barbiturates have no significant effects on early SSEP latencies or amplitudes. Moderate to high doses of barbiturates have measurable effects at the mid-latency period, and later peaks are much more sensitive, showing attenuation, delays, and alteration in waveform morphology (Grundy, 1990). Barbiturates can be used for short- or intermediate-acting latency recordings. Narcotics can be used for short- and intermediate-latency potentials. Nitrous oxide needs to be avoided in middle-ear surgeries, but it preserves spinal SSEPs (Friedman et al., 1989). In both the upper and lower extremities, EPs are attenuated by nitrous oxide. Halogenated inhalation agents decrease amplitudes and are to be avoided with intermediate latencies, although they do not affect short-latency potentials. Muscle relaxants have no direct effect on EPs. Last, diazepam will diminish long-latency potentials. In SSEPs modulated by midbrain reticular formation, longer-latency potential waveforms are diminished.

Surgeries Where Evoked Potential Monitoring Is Used. Evoked potential monitoring is commonly used during repair of peripheral nerve trauma for the differential diagnoses of neurapraxic, axonometric or neurometric lesions; for cerebral aneurysms and/or arteriovenous malformations to help determine vessel sacrifice; for brainstem strokes to detect basilar artery perfusion; in carotid endarterectomies to help decide whether or not to shunt; in spinal surgery and aortic surgery to determine spinal cord function and spinal cord tumor resection; and in posterior fossa surgery, acoustic neuroma resection, and microvascular decompression to prevent nerve trauma.

Electromyography

Electromyography (EMG) measures the electrical versus the mechanical response of skeletal muscles. It measures overall muscle activity by opening the electrical activity of the whole muscle rather than the contractile activity. Studies of nerve conduction are performed to evaluate suspected neuromuscular diseases and to objectify pathophysiologic changes of the nerves (Sethi & Thomson, 1989). They can document any peripheral nerve dysfunction, its location, and distribution. Surface electrodes are applied (active, reference, and ground) to the affected area. A stimulator generates an electrical pulse with a square wave that will depolarize the nerve in both directions from the point of stimulation, so that near-nerve recordings of nerve action potentials can be made. The different levels of nerve function can be differentiated, from sensory, to motor, mixed nerve conduction and sympathetic skin responses.

Neuromuscular Monitoring

A neuromuscular monitor, or peripheral nerve stimulator, evaluates the mechanical responses of neuromuscular function through an external electrical stimulus by a nerve stimulator over a peripheral nerve. Mechanical responses are less sensitive than electrical responses (Grundy, 1995), but far easier to perform in the operating room. Neuromuscular monitoring is discussed extensively in Chapter 21. The basic patterns of neuromuscular monitoring responses are single-twitch, train-of-four, tetanic, and post-tetanic stimulation. There is a single attachment of a pair of electrodes that produces a square-wave pattern in the previously described patterns. Each response represents a different level of neuromuscular function, and is especially helpful in determining the dose and effect of neuromuscular blocking and reversal agents. One distinct difference between the two types of muscle monitoring is that mechanical twitch response is capable of producing a post-tetanic potentiation twitch, whereas EMG monitoring is not.

Intracranial Pressure Monitoring

Normal intracranial pressure (ICP) is 5 to 14 mmHg. The ICP may increase as a result of cranial-cerebral trauma, tumor, subarachnoid hemorrhage, neurosurgery, or cerebrovascular occlusive disease. Monitoring ICP is a method to measure brain pressure directly. Intracranial pressure monitoring involves the surgical placement of (1) a subarachnoid bolt through a burr hole; (2) an intraventricular catheter through a burr hole into a lateral ventricle; (3) an epidural transducer where a transducer with a pressure sensitive membrane is placed onto the dura; or (4) measuring the topical pressure of the anterior fontanelle. All of the transducers are then connected to sterile pressure tubing filled with sterile saline and then to a digital monitor that provides a single digital readout.

The cerebrospinal fluid (CSF) wave is pulsatile and exhibits cycles with both respiratory and cardiac variation. An increase in ICP results is a decrease in cerebral perfusion (causing therefore cerebral hypoxia), to which the body's response is to increase the blood pressure to provide cerebral blood flow. This mechanism of action becomes a vicious cycle that results in cerebral edema and hypoxia. Therefore, all ICP measurements greater than 20 mmHg must be treated. The waveform is described in one of two ways: the first is the presence of a-waves that have a sharp rise, a plateau, and are then followed by a sharp fall (Warner & Sokoll, 1995). A-waves are associated with a negative prognosis and indicate a severe disease state. In contrast, b-waves have a lower amplitude, shorter duration, and are not associated with a negative prognosis. The first two previously mentioned devices allow CSF drainage to decrease ICP. Otherwise, other measures must be employed, such as mechanical hyperventilation, vasodilator therapy, or diuresis.

Transcranial Doppler

A transcranial Doppler is a probe that estimates the velocity of cerebral blood flow by utilizing the Doppler shift principle. Following ultrasonic penetration of the temporal bone (the middle cerebral, anterior, and posterior arteries), the orbit (ophthalmic artery), or the foramen magnum (intracranial vertebral and basilar arteries), the low-frequency waves reflect off erythrocytes in the basilar arteries. The Doppler signal is displayed on an oscilloscope as a wave pattern after it has undergone spectral analysis. This method helps assess intracranial arterial occlusions and ipsilateral carotid artery blood velocity. It is used to diagnose cerebral emboli and to evaluate the velocity of blood flow after recannulation. It can potentially help diagnose decreased cerebral perfusion early (Stiff & Caplan, 1995). It is not yet common in the operating room.

▶ CASE STUDY

A 62-year-old, 5′10″ tall, 230-lb (105-kg) African American male is to undergo open prostatectomy for carcinoma. He is ASA risk category IV for obesity. He has an ongoing 40-pack-year smoking history; hypertension treated with lisinopril; one episode of sickle cell crisis 10 years before admission; a poorly documented myocardial infarction (MI) 1 year ago; and nonspecific ST-T wave changes on ECG. Anesthesia is to be induced with propofol with vecuronium as the muscle relaxant. He is to be orally intubated and mechanically ventilated for the 2.5-hour surgery.

1. What monitoring parameters should be used?

   First, all basic monitoring must be utilized, including temperature, pulse oximetry, end-tidal carbon dioxide, electrocardiogram, blood pressure, foley catheter, and precordial stethoscope. Considering the patient's history of myocardial infarction, using at least a five-lead ECG with a V5 lead would be appropriate. Because of the history of hypertension, blood pressure monitoring would be most effective with an arterial line for accuracy and precise determination of arterial pressure. An arterial line also would allow frequent arterial blood gas sampling, which is necessary secondary to the patient's history of obesity, smoking, and sickle cell disease. After induction the precordial stethoscope can be replaced with an esophageal stethoscope with a temperature probe to optimize listening to heart and breath sounds and to providing core temperature monitoring.

   Second, given the nature of this surgery, which may lead to significant fluid shifting, potentially large blood loss, and given the patient's history of MI, a central venous monitoring line would be useful. The CVP line will assist in maintaining optimal fluid balance, cardiac filling pressure, and provide large vein access for blood/fluid or drug administration. This monitoring line also can be easily converted to a pulmonary artery catheter intraoperatively or postoperatively in case cardiac decompensation and the need to evaluate cardiac chamber pressures develop.

2. Should invasive monitors be placed prior to induction?

   It is not necessary to insert the central venous cathether for CVP monitoring prior to induction, but the arterial line should be inserted preoperatively to monitor blood pressure closely during induction.

3. What noninvasive monitors can be used?

   The pulse oximeter, end-tidal CO$_2$ monitor, automatic blood pressure device, ECG, and precordial stethoscope can all be used to monitor this patient.

4. What changes could be expected on the pulse oximeter and capnograph based on the patient's medical history and planned anesthetic?

   Smoking and obesity will produce hypoxemic and hypercarbic changes in baseline values. The pulse oximeter may have a dampened waveform because of the thickened skin of the fingers of the patient from chronic hypoxia. The capnograph will exhibit a decreased rate of rise and a slant in the upstroke of the first phase (exhalation). Because the surgical procedure is in the lower abdomen, there should be little effect on diaphragmatic movement. Mechanical ventilation may help compensate for some of the physiologic changes.

5. How should the patient's body temperature be measured through surgery, and what measures can be taken to keep the patient normothermic through surgery?

   The core temperature can be monitored most easily with an esophageal temperature probe. Hypothermia causes stress and can exacerbate the sickle cell condition. Effective warming measures include using a warm, moist humidifier in the breathing circuit, intravenous fluid warmer, and continuous forced-air heating blanket to the periphery and wrapping the head in a warmth-retaining material.

▶ SUMMARY

It is incumbent on all anesthetists to become quite familiar with the written standards of care expected of every provider. Should logistic barriers arise that do not allow using these standards (even if only on a temporary basis), notation should be made on the patient's record with a thorough, written justification. Under no circumstance should an elective case proceed without full monitoring equipment available, functional, and usable. Periodic checks and maintenance records of all equipment and the machine should also be documented in departmental files. Lack of appropriate monitoring or documentation or inability to interpret competently the data obtained may imply practitioner negligence. The technology of monitoring has increased substantially since the late 1980s as concerns for patient safety under anesthesia have justifiably increased. Still, vigilance remains the strongest defense in protecting patients from deleterious outcomes.

▶ KEY CONCEPTS

- Comprehensive monitoring helps the anesthetist recognize those events likely to harm the patient and to do so in time to intervene with corrective measures. It is imperative that the anesthetist avoid all distractions and concentrate on the tasks surrounding the anesthetic. Stress and fatigue detract from the ability to concentrate on proper patient monitoring.
- The anesthetist should continually redirect conscious attention in a systematic fashion; sequentially focusing on the patient, the surgical procedure, the intravenous solutions and suction containers, the anesthesia flow meters, the ventilator settings, and last, each monitor being used.
- Basic physiologic parameters that should be monitored for all cases include: heart function, body temperature, fluid status, oxygen saturation, respiratory end-tidal CO_2, correct type and concentration of inhalation agents, and proper functioning of anesthesia equipment. Monitors should be placed and vital signs recorded before the patient receives any medications. Monitors are placed first and removed last.
- Typical components of monitors used in anesthesia include a power supply, a sensing device, amplifier, suppression, measurement, balancing, multiplier and divider circuits. Electrical injuries resulting from monitoring equipment can be macroshock (significant electrical charge usually coming from outside the body) or microshock (strong or weak charge that arises in conductors near the heart and are transmitted across the heart).
- Core body temperature generally is measured by an esophageal probe near the heart region. Sites used clinically to monitor temperature in the perianesthetic period include the tympanic membrane, nasopharynx, oral cavity, esophagus, spinal cord, thoracic tissues, abdominal tissues, myocardium, pulmonary artery, bladder, rectum, and skin.
- Effective patient temperature management plays a crucial role in preventing surgical complications, reducing the incidence of nosocomial infections and saving the lives of trauma victims. Most measures are directed toward preventing inadvertent hypothermia, but some techniques also can be used to cool hyperthermic patients.
- The ECG is the most uniformly accepted monitor in anesthesia practice. Continuous ECG monitoring allows the anesthetists to assess the electrical mechanism and rate of the heart and illustrates dysfunctional rhythms that would have a deleterious effect on cardiac output. The ECG monitors employed in anesthesia practice are generally either three- or five-lead systems.
- Monitoring pressure is a mechanism for assessing volume status and circulatory adequacy. The methods used are noninvasive (manual or automatic) and invasive (vascular cannulation for either arterial, central venous, or pulmonary artery pressures).
- Echocardiography and transesophageal echocardiography (TEE) are based on the principles of ultrasound imaging. Transesophageal echocardiography is a valuable monitor for evaluating cardiac and valvular function, especially during heart surgery.
- Bispectral analysis is a signal-processing technique from an EEG derivative recorded from a bispectral montage. Bispectral analysis quantifies both frequency and power (linear), as well as phase and harmonic (nonlinear) segments of the EEG, thereby analyzing the interfrequency phase relationships. A correlation can then be derived to determine the degree of hypnotic component of the anesthetic.

▶ STUDY QUESTIONS

1. What problems detract from an anesthetist's ability to provide safe monitoring, and what are the legal consequences of inadequate monitoring?

2. What are the principles of safe anesthesia monitoring, and how does an anesthetist use the basic senses of hearing, sight, touch, smell, and taste to enhance monitoring?

3. What factors cause abnormal or loss of readings when using pulse oximetry, capnography, chemical carbon dioxide detectors, and thermometers?

4. What are the principal EEG waveforms and the effects each anesthetic has on the waveform during anesthesia?

5. How is evoked potential monitoring used in surgical and anesthesia practice, and what are the effects of each anesthetic on the waveform?

6. What pathophysiologic states can be identified with central venous and pulmonary artery pressure monitoring?

7. Why are there minimum requirements for monitoring perioperatively?

KEY REFERENCES

Blitt, C. D., & Hines, R. L. (Eds.). (1995). *Monitoring in anesthesia and critical care medicine* (3rd ed.) New York: Churchill Livingstone.

Eichhorn, J. H. (1998). Standards for patient monitoring. In D. E. Longnecker, J. H. Tinker, & G. E. Morgan, Jr. (Eds.), *Principles and practice of anesthesiology* (2nd ed., pp. 791–80). St. Louis: Mosby-Yearbook.

Goldman, J. M., & Strom, J. S. (1994). Respiratory monitoring. In R. R. Kirby & N. Gravenstein (Eds.), *Clinical anesthesia practice* (pp. 341–357). Philadelphia: Saunders.

Lake, C. L. (Ed.). (1994). *Monitoring for anesthesia and critical care* (2nd ed.) Philadelphia: Saunders.

Le Bel, L. A. (1992). Electronic and safety principles related to anesthesia. In W. R. Waugaman, S. D. Foster, & B. M. Rigor (Eds.), *Principles and practice of nurse anesthesia* (2nd ed., pp. 105–114). Norwalk, CT: Appleton & Lange.

Scurr, C., Feldman, S., & Soni, N. (1990). *Scientific foundations of anaesthesia: The basics of intensive care* (4th ed.) Chicago: Yearbook Medical Publishers.

Steifel, R. H. (1998). Electricity electrical safety, and instrumentation in the operating room. In D. E. Longnecker, J. H. Tinker, & G. E. Morgan, Jr. (Eds.), *Principles and practice of anesthesiology* (2nd ed., pp. 700–720). St. Louis: Mosby-Yearbook.

REFERENCES

Bedford, F. R. (1977). Radial arterial function following percutaneous cannulation with 18 and 20 gauge catheters. *Anesthesiology, 47,* 37.

Betz, E. (1974). The influence of changes of oxygen and carbon dioxide on the EEG, CBF and the energy rich substrates in brain tissue. In R. Cooper, (Ed.), *Influence on the EEG of certain physiological states and other parameters. Handbook of electroencephalography and neurophysiology* (p. 30). Amsterdam: Elsevier.

Bickford, R. G., Billinger, T. W., Fleming, N. I. (1972). The compressed spectral array: A pictoral EEG. *Proceedings of the San Diego Biomedical Symposium, 11,* 365.

Brown, A. E., Sweeney, D. B., & Lumley, J. (1969). Percutaneous radial artery cannulation. *Anesthesia, 24,* 532.

Bruner, J. M. R. (1978). *Handbook of blood pressure monitoring.* Littleton, MA: PSG.

Bruner, J. M., Krenis, L. J., Kunsman, J. M., & Sherman, A. P. (1981). Comparison of direct and indirect methods of measuring arterial blood pressure. Part 1. *Medical Instrumentation, 15,* 11–21.

Burnside, J. W. (1981). *Physical diagnosis* (16th ed., p. 49). Baltimore: Williams & Wilkins.

Caton, R. (1875). The electric currents of the brain. *British Medical Journal, 2,* 278.

Celesia, G. (1987). Clinical applications of evoked potentials. In E. Niedermeyer & F. Lopes da Silva (Eds.), *Electroenceophalography basic principles, clinical application and related fields* (2nd ed., pp. 665–684). Baltimore: Urban & Schwarzenberg.

Cooper, J. B., Newbower, R. S., & Kitz, R. J. (1984). An analysis of major errors and equipment failures in anesthesia management: Considerations for prevention and detection. *Anesthesiology, 60,* 34–42.

Davies, F. W., Mantzaridis, H., Kenny, G. N., & Fisher, A. C. (1996). Middle latency auditory evoked potentials during repeated transitions from consciousness to unconsciousness. *Anaesthesia, 51,* 107–113.

de Beers, N. A., Van Hooff, J. C., Brunia, C. H., Cluitmans, P. J., Korsten, H. H., & Beneken, J. E. (1996). Midlatency auditory evoked potentials as indicators of perceptual processing during general anesthesia. *British Journal of Anaesthesia, 77,* 617–624.

Foster, S. D., & Reeves-Viets, J. L. (1992). Perioperative monitoring. In W. R. Waugaman, S. D. Foster, & B. M. Rigor (Eds.), *Principles and practice of nurse anesthesia* (2nd ed., pp. 195–200). Norwalk, CT: Appleton & Lange.

Friedman, W. A., Theisen, G. J., & Grundy, B. L. (1989). Electrophysiologic monitoring of the nervous system. In R. K. Stoelting, P. G. Barash, & T. J. Gallagher (Eds.), *Advances in Anesthesia* (pp. 231–284). Chicago, IL: Yearbook Medical Publishing.

Gal, T. J. (1994). Monitoring the respiratory system. In C. L. Lake (Ed.), *Clinical monitoring for anesthesia and critical care* (2nd ed., pp. 223–225). Philadelphia: Saunders.

Gibbs, F. A., Gibbs, E. L., & Lennox, W. G. (1937). Effect on electroencephalogram of certain drugs which influence nervous activity. *Archives of Vort Medicine, 60.*

Grundy, B. L. (1990). Evoked potential monitoring. In C. D. Blitt (Ed.), *Monitoring in anesthesia and critical care medicine* (2nd ed., pp. 461–524). New York: Churchill Livingstone.

Grundy, B. L. (1995). The electroencephalogram and evoked potential monitoring. In C. D. Blitt & R. L. Hines (Eds.), *Monitoring in anesthesia and critical care medicine* (3rd ed., p. 428). New York: Churchill Livinstone.

Hayes, M. F., Jr., Morello, D. C., Rosenbaum, R. W., & Matsumoto, T. (1973). Radial artery catheterization by cutdown technique. *Critical Care Medicine, 1,* 151–152.

Hunter, F. P. & Eastwood, D. W. (1986). Manometry. In *Instrumentation and anesthesia* (p. 2964). Philadelphia: FA Davis.

Jacobson, G. P., & Tew, J. M. (1987). Intraoperative evoked potential monitoring. *Journal of Clinical Neurophysiology, 4*(2), 145–176.

Jawad, I. A. (1996). *A practical guide to echocardiography and cardiac doppler ultrasound* (2nd ed., pp. 70–85). Boston: Little, Brown.

Kearse, L. A., Manberg, P., & Chamoun, N. (1994). Bispectral analysis of the electroencephalogram correlates with patient movement to skin incision during propofol/nitrous oxide anesthesia. *Anesthesiology, 81,* 1365–1370.

Kearse, L. A., Manberg, P., & Debros, F. (1994). Bispectral analysis of the electroencephalogram during induction of anesthesia may predict hemodynamic responses to laryngoscopy and intubation. *Electroencephalography and Clinical Neurophysiology, 90,* 194–202.

Kirby, R. R., & Gravenstein, N. (1994). *Clinical anesthesia practice* (pp. 341–357). Philadelphia: Saunders.

Lake, C. L. (1994). Stethoscopy and thermometry. In G. L. Lake (Ed.), *Monitoring for anesthesia and critical care* (2nd ed., pp. 475–487). Philadelphia: Saunders.

Le Bel, L. A. (1992). Electronic and safety principles related to anesthesia. In W. R. Waugaman, S. D. Foster, & B. M. Rigor (Eds.), *Principles and practice of nurse anesthesia* (2nd ed., pp. 105–114). Norwalk, CT: Appleton & Lange.

Lee, A. P. (1981). Biotechnological principles of monitoring. *International Anesthesiology Clinics, 19,* 204.

Matjasko, J., Gunselman, J., Delaney, J., & Mackenzie, C. F. (1986). Sources of nitrogen in the anesthetic circuit. *Anesthesiology, 65,* 229.

Miller, R. D. (Ed.). (1986). *Anesthesia* (2nd ed., p. 467). New York: Churchill Livingstone.

Mishin, W. W., & Jones, P. L. (Eds.). (1986). *Physics for the anesthetist* (4th ed., pp. 489–499). Boston: Blackwell Scientific.

Newfield, P., & Cottrell, J. (1991). *Neuroanesthesia: Handbook of clinical and physiologic essentials* (2nd ed., pp 35–70). Boston: Little Brown.

Obeid, A. I. (1992). *Echocardiography in clinical practice* (pp. 310–324). Philadelphia: Lippincott.

O'Rourke, M. F., & Taylor, M. G. (1966). Vascular impedance of the femoral bed. *Circulation Research, 18,* 126.

Pinilla, J. C., Ross, D. F., Martin, T., & Crump, H. (1983). Study of the incidence of intravascular catheter infection and associated septicemia in critically ill patients. *Critical Care Medicine, 11,* 21–25.

Remington, J. W. (1960). Contour changes of the aortic pulse during propagation. *American Journal of Physiology, 199,* 331.

Rossen, R., Simonson, E., & Baker, J. (1961). Electroencephalograms during hypoxia in healthy men. *Archives of Neurology, 1*(5), 648.

Scurr, C., Feldman, S., & Soni, N. (1990). *Scientific foundations of anaesthesia: The basics of intensive care* (4th ed.). Chicago: Yearbook Medical Publishers.

Sethi, R. K., & Thompson, L. L. (1989). *The electromyographer's handbook* (2nd ed., pp. 26–42). Boston: Little, Brown.

Sigl, J. C., & Chamoun, N. G. (1994). An introduction to bispectral analysis for the electroencephalogram. *Journal of Clinical Monitoring, 10,* 392–404.

Slogoff, S., Keats, A. S., & Arlund, C. (1983). On the safety of radial artery cannulation. *Anesthesiology, 59,* 42.

Stiff, J. L., & Caplan, A. (1995). Monitoring modalities of the future. In C. D. Blitt & R. L. Hines (Eds.), *Monitoring in anesthesia and critical care medicine* (3rd ed.). New York: Churchill Livingstone.

Warner, D. S., & Sokoll, M. D. (1995). Monitoring intracranial pressure. In C. D. Blitt & R. L. Hines (Eds.), *Monitoring in anesthesia and critical care medicine* (3rd ed., pp. 529–541). New York: Churchill Livingstone.

Wyke, B. D. (1957). Electrographic monitoring of anaesthesia: Neuropharmacological aspects. *Anaesthesia, 12,* 157.

Positioning for Anesthesia and Surgery

Celeste G. Villanueva

Positioning the patient for a surgical procedure provides the surgeon with the maximum acceptable access to the operative field. Two equally important objectives of patient positioning are to allow access to the patient for the safe administration of anesthesia and to ensure the optimal physiologic function of all body systems. Proper positioning clearly contributes to the success of a surgical procedure and is an important factor in anesthesia-related morbidity and mortality.

Patient positioning is potentially an issue in two situations: when inadequate surgical posture compromises good exposure, thereby prolonging and possibly complicating surgery, or when the patient's position is so optimal in terms of exposure that the patient's physiologic limits are exceeded. The responsibility of adapting a position dictated by the operative procedure without compromising the patient falls primarily to the anesthetist.

A position-related anesthetic misadventure was documented as early as 1849 when an intraoperative death that was possibly attributable to a posture change. John Griffith, a 31-year-old U.S. seaman, received a chloroform anesthetic via an open mask technique in the sitting position. Soon after anesthetization, the patient was placed in the lateral position for a hemorrhoidectomy. The documented record of events indicates that directly after the posture change occurred, Mr. Griffith ceased to breathe and was pulseless. History also records that all efforts to restore the patient were ineffective (Little, 1960).

Alterations in the body's physiology caused by positioning patients for surgical procedures were the focus of study as early as 1933 (Dutton). The subsequent thirty years witnessed the publication of several landmark studies that correlated physiologic changes, particularly those involving the circulatory and respiratory systems, with varying surgical positions (Courington & Little, 1968; Henschel, Wyant, Dobkin, & Henschel, 1957; Slocum, Hoeflich, & Allen, 1947).

Since the 1960s Martin and his associates (Martin, 1997a, 1997b, 1997c; Martin & Warner, 1997) have contributed significantly to the body of knowledge pertaining to this basic, but often ignored, aspect of clinical practice. Their work has raised the level of understanding of positioning issues beyond anecdotal folklore to statistical assessments of huge patient databases. These types of studies are particularly timely in an era of patient risk management, performance improvement by care givers, and outcome analysis of anesthetic care.

Taking a different historical perspective of patient positioning, the continual evolution of new and innovative surgical techniques highly depends on the possibility of placing patients in extreme or nonanatomic positions that challenge the physiologic limits of the patient. Because of a greater understanding in the field of anesthesiology of the physiological consequences and management of patients in these "unusual" positions, patients can safely undergo newer procedures and surgical techniques can continue to evolve.

This chapter discusses the basic principles of safe positioning, conveys the importance of proper positioning from a medicolegal perspective, presents an overview of the alterations in body physiology caused by posture changes in general with emphasis on the circulatory, respiratory, and peripheral nervous systems, and presents common surgical positions along with the most important anesthetic implications entailed by each.

▶ PRINCIPLES OF SAFE POSITIONING

Basic Elements of Safe Positioning

The essential elements of safe patient positioning parallel what most practitioners consider basic components of the principles and practice of anesthesia: a strong theoretical knowledge base, forethought and organization, attention to detail, a collaborative effort, proper equipment, and vigilance.

An adequate fund of *knowledge* for proper positioning involves an understanding of the changes in body physiology, particularly in cardiopulmonary dynamics, that occur when a patient is placed in the various surgical postures. A solid grasp of the practical aspects of accomplishing certain positions also is necessary. Perhaps most critical is an awareness of the sometimes dire consequences of improperly positioning a patient. Last, an empathic awareness by the clinician of the discomfort associated with various surgical positions is extremely helpful. In many training programs, novice anesthetists are placed in each of the common postures to allow them to experience how difficult it can be to attain a comfortable and safe position without compromising operative exposure.

Forethought and *organization* refer to the careful planning of position changes by each member of the intraoperative team. This implies an adequate understanding of the logistics of the particular surgical procedure, the specific requirements of the operating surgeon, and the medical condition of the patient. Of critical importance, especially when attempting a complex position change, is the pharmacologic strategy developed by the anesthetist. A combination of agents, as well as the titration of their dosages and levels, is chosen based on the primary goal of circulatory and pulmonary stability. Proper planning also includes the development of a strategy for keeping intact the intravenous and monitoring lines, airway maintenance device, and all other devices attached to the patient during rotational position changes.

Safe positioning requires meticulous *attention to detail*. Moreover, attentiveness to detail is possible only when sufficient time is available and when involved personnel are focused on the procedure at hand. A common pitfall for many anesthesia students is to allow themselves to be rushed unprepared into a complex positioning sequence by an impatient surgical or anesthesia staff. It also is extremely important that all members of the positioning team be satisfied with every detail of the final posture of the patient prior to sterile preparation and draping of the surgical field. Any uneasiness that remains about aspects of the position or physiological status of the patient (as it relates to positioning) is greatly magnified after the surgical incision is made when access to the patient to correct a problem is difficult or impossible without a major disruption of the procedure (Colvin, 1987).

The importance of a *collaborative effort* by the positioning team—surgeons, anesthetists, nurses and technicians—cannot be overemphasized. Clear and continuous communication between members is the hallmark of a successful and efficient team. The question of who is ultimately responsible for properly positioning a patient for surgery can be hotly debated in legal circles, but the most correct and comprehensive answer is that all members of the team share this responsibility. Specific roles may vary between institutions and surgical practices. However, a reasonable generalization is that the anesthetist determines when the patient is physiologically prepared for a posture change and the actual pace and timing of the positioning maneuvers. The anesthetist takes direct physical responsibility for maintaining the stability of the head and neck and protecting the eyes and ears from trauma and the patency of the airway during all position changes.

The availability and functionality of the *proper equipment* necessary to achieve and maintain the proper position should be established prior to anesthetizing the patient and initiating a positioning process. In large, busy operating room suites this often represents the biggest challenge.

Vigilance is especially critical to avoid complications from positioning. Adequate anesthesia for surgical pain also implies that pain due to an uncomfortable position or a position that exceeds the patient's usual anatomic or physiologic limits is eliminated. In addition, the signs and symptoms of many position-related problems are not manifest on a monitor. Frequent visual inspection and palpation of the patient's body parts that are at risk are usually the best monitors for proper positioning.

Preanesthetic Evaluation

A preanesthetic positioning assessment focuses on the patient, the surgical procedure, and the positioning team. Identifying risk factors for positioning complications is the major objective of the preanesthetic assessment. An evaluation of the patient's cardiopulmonary reserve is critical, as the subsequent discussions of circulatory and respiratory alterations will make evident. Additional risk factors focus on the potential for position-related neuropathies. A study identified factors that were strongly predictive for the development of motor neuropathy in lower extremities (Warner, Warner, & Martin, 1994). These results can certainly be extrapolated to include risk for developing neuropathies in areas other than the lower extremities. The factors identified include a low body mass index (less than or equal to 20), increasing age, a history of smoking within 1 month of a surgical procedure, and preexisting diabetes or vascular disease.

Identifying and documenting preanesthetic musculoskeletal limitations and preexisting neurologic deficits or neuropathies are part of a thorough patient evaluation. The practice of incorporating a "dry run" of the specific surgical posture is a prudent undertaking, especially in situations where preoperative neuropathies exist. In this process, the awake patient places himself in the desired surgical position, communicating to the team the tolerable limits of his extremity and joint movements, and directing the placement of padding in potential problem areas.

Specific knowledge of the surgical procedure itself also is part of a preanesthetic evaluation. The best source of information in this matter is the primary surgeon involved in the case. Clarifying the exact purpose of the surgery (biopsy versus excision, partial versus total resection of an organ, diagnostic procedure prior to a therapeutic maneuver) is a perfectly reasonable request in an era when options concerning virtually every aspect of a procedure are numerous. Other useful bits of information are the likelihood of an intraoperative position change (or in some cases even a change in the operating table) and the anticipated duration of a case, as the duration of time spent in a particular extreme position has been found to correlate directly with the development of nerve damage (Warner, Warner, & Martin, 1994).

Assessing the preparedness of the intraoperative positioning team may seem too basic a concept to include in this discussion. However, a single experience with the anxiety produced when an inexperienced or inattentive team member fails to support the patient's limb or is unable to attach a critical stabilizing device is enough to convince most anesthetists that all team members should be ready prior to embarking on major position changes.

Postanesthetic Evaluation

The postanesthetic aspect of positioning principles is based on the importance of prompt recognition of complications to institute diagnostic procedures, consultations, and therapeutic measures. Major assessment points include hemodynamic stability, new-onset of sensory or motor neuropathies not explained by the anesthetic technique used, sustained or unexplained pain, and swelling, lacerations, or hematomas in a nonoperative site.

Evaluation of the Operating Table

There is a wide range of operating tables, ranging from basic, manually operated models to sophisticated, electronically controlled varieties. Specific tables are frequently used for certain surgical subspecialties and require a complete training session to be operated properly.

For the anesthetist in the early stages of training the best practice is to include a preoperative check of the surgical table as part of the daily setup routine. It is particularly important to determine the center of gravity of the table established for each procedure. Most operating rooms use tables whose tops move in relation to the stabilizing, fixed pedestal. Although this feature vastly improves access for radiologic equipment (fluoroscopes with C-shaped camera arms) underneath the table surface, an obese patient placed too far from the table's center of gravity may cause the entire unit to fall. In addition, a preoperative check of the table should include gaining familiarity with the specific workings of the table's control panel and ensuring the functionality of all of its moving parts. Realizing that a table is not functioning or that one is unable to manipulate the table because of lack of knowledge during the surgical procedure when the patient is already fully anesthetized predisposes to complications.

Armboards that are routinely attached to the surgical table and the padding used for various aspects of positioning often are viewed as mundane elements of positioning. However, their proper use is essential to avoid complications and provide quality care. The sections that discuss specific positions address proper placement of these items.

Another practice that will help ensure patient and provider safety is clearly to announce operating table position changes prior to instituting the change to allow all members of the surgical staff to protect the patient and themselves from the harmful consequences of moving table components.

▶ MEDICOLEGAL ASPECTS OF POSITIONING

A major source of professional liability in anesthetic practice continues to be patient injuries caused by related positioning-problems, most notably peripheral neuropathies. A retrospective study of a large closed claims database was undertaken to determine the frequency of nerve damage in the overall incidence of anesthesia-related injury (Kroll, Caplan, Posner, Ward, & Cheney, 1990). Fifteen percent of 1541 claims reviewed involved nerve injury directly related to anesthesia. Interestingly, the standard of care had been met in these nerve-related injury claims significantly more often than in claims not involving nerve injury, a finding that the authors of the study partly attribute to the unclear mechanism of the most common type of nerve injury (ie, ulnar neuropathy, which is discussed in a subsequent section of this chapter.)

In 1994 the major insurer of nurse anesthetists in the United States reported that nerve-related and arm- or shoulder-related events were the ninth and tenth, respectively, most common allegations made against CRNAs insured by their company during the 5 years prior to the report (St. Paul Medical Services, 1994). Although more recent data indicate that this statistic may not repeat itself in the subsequent 5 years (St. Paul Medical Services, 1997), it is clear that perioperative nerve-related injuries, correctly assumed to be most often related to positioning issues, should be of major concern to all anesthesia clinicians.

It has been clearly established (Stoelting, 1993) that anesthesia-related neuropathies can easily occur despite the use of "textbook" positioning. A clear message to the anesthetist in training certainly is to heed the basic principles and proper methods of positioning about to be discussed in the rest of the chapter and the lessons generated by innumerable malpractice cases involving positioning in anesthesia and surgery: Develop the habit of clearly and consistently documenting the measures taken to protect the patient adequately.

▶ THE PHYSIOLOGY OF POSTURE CHANGE

Prior to discussing the various surgical positions, it seems logical to examine the normal physiologic state of healthy, awake humans in the two positions in which we spend the majority of our lives, erect and supine. More specifically, what is relevant to the anesthetist is an understanding of the physiologic adaptations involved in changing from an erect to a supine position, as the majority of surgical procedures are done in some variation of the basic supine position. This discussion of physiologic adaptations focuses on the cardiovascular and pulmonary systems.

▶ CARDIOVASCULAR SYSTEM

The posture change from erect to supine in an awake, healthy individual is accompanied by a series of compensatory autonomic reflexes that provide circulatory homeostasis. The specific reflexes involved in maintaining a stable blood pressure and adequate tissue perfusion are the "low-pressure" reflexes, the arterial baroreceptor reflex, and the Bainbridge reflex.

The low-pressure receptors (also referred to as mechanoreceptors or cardiopulmonary receptors) are located in the great veins, the atria and the ventricles. They are components of a negative feedback system: an increase in intravascular volume stimulates the receptors to generate an increase in vagal activity via the medullary vasomotor center, resulting in a reflex inhibition of sympathetic outflow (O'Brien & Ebert, 1997). Conversely, a decrease in blood volume will cause sympathetic excitation. This physiologic response is distinct from, but works in concert with, the arterial baroreceptor reflex.

The arterial baroreceptor reflex originates in the pressure-sensitive receptors of the carotid sinus and aortic arch. These receptors send afferent impulses through the glossopharyngeal and vagus nerves to the medullary vasomotor center, which relays efferent sympathetic and parasympathetic outflow. Increased arterial blood pressure sensed by the baroreceptors ultimately results in increased vagal tone as well as diminished sympathetic activity, which leads to decreased heart rate and myocardial contractility.

The Bainbridge reflex involves an adjustment of heart rate in response to atrial volume; its baroreceptors are located in the right atrium and great veins. Changing from an erect to the supine position increases venous return because of gravitational changes. This increased atrial volume stimulates an increase in heart rate that serves to prevent blood from pooling in the veins, atria, and pulmonary system and to promote more effective left ventricular filling.

The cumulative effect of these aforementioned autonomic reflexes when activated by a postural change from upright to supine has been determined in two studies (Korner, 1971; Ward, Danzinger, & Bonica, 1966). There is a decrease in mean arterial pressure (systolic blood pressure is unchanged, diastolic pressure decreased), heart rate, and peripheral vascular resistance with a simultaneous increase in cardiac output and stroke volume (primarily due to the increased venous return).

The vigor of the protective cardiovascular reflexes just described is impaired by disease, injury, and anesthesia. Postural changes that normally cause little or no change in blood pressure and tissue perfusion will cause a significant fall in both blood pressure and perfusion in the anesthetized patient (Biddle & Caunady, 1990). This is especially true if the patient is repositioned in the immediate postinduction period. Clearly, an anesthetized individual with impaired cardiovascular reserve will be even less tolerant of the circulatory changes that accompany position changes.

The pharmacologic agents most commonly utilized in general anesthesia are volatile agents, barbiturates, benzodiazepines, which all depress the sympathetic response to position changes. The circulatory effect of this depressed response is a tendency for blood to pool in peripheral, dependent veins, decreasing venous return and cardiac output, with resultant hypotension. These sympatholytic effects of anesthetic drugs are dose related; the clinical corollary to this principle is to avoid dosages of drugs that will cause deep or even moderate levels of anesthesia prior to major position changes. Drugs with higher degrees of myocardial depression should, of course, be avoided until after the positioning process is complete.

Maintaining a minimal level of general anesthesia prior to a position change to prevent circulatory depression entails the risk of patient movement and therefore injury during positioning. If the anesthesia-induced depression of muscle tone is insufficient, muscle rigidity also can occur. The use of muscle relaxants prior to positioning is a common practice used to prevent either of the aforementioned events. However, this technique is not without its drawbacks. A relaxed and unprotected head and neck, joint, or limb is at higher risk for injury if it is inadequately controlled during positioning.

It also is not uncommon for a minimally anesthetized patient to become hypertensive during position maneuvering secondary to tracheal and joint stimulation. If an elevated blood pressure places the patient at increased cardiovascular risk, therapeutic measures should be anticipated and implemented prior to completing the posture change: increased doses of analgesics, titration of an antihypertensive agent that is appropriate for the patient, or judicious increases in the concentration of an inhalation agent.

Additional measures to prevent hypotension related to posture changes that should be instituted prior to positioning are (1) administration of a bolus of intravenous fluid to increase the intravascular volume; (2) application of compression (active or passive) devices to the lower extremities to minimize venous pooling; (3) institution of position changes gradually and carefully, allowing the depressed circulatory system slowly to adapt to postural changes. This is especially critical at the termination of surgery when intravascular volume shifts can adversely influence circulatory homeostasis.

Epidural and subarachnoid anesthetics result in a sympathetic blockade; hence, depending on the level of the blockade, avoiding hypotension with posture changes can be a challenge. The choice of local anesthetic (type, baricity, dose) as well as the timing and technique to achieve an anesthetic level (incremental dosing via a catheter versus a single dose) relative to the position change may be helpful to prevent a severe hypotensive episode. Judicious use of intravenous fluids and vasopressors, the mainstay of treatment for hypotension secondary to the sympatholysis of regional anesthetics, is particularly effective in these situations.

Respiratory System

A study has quantified the gravitational forces in the supine position on upper airway anatomy. In an awake individual the change from an erect to a supine position results in an increase in soft palate thickness and area, a decrease in the vertical length of the airway, and a 29% decrease in the oropharyngeal area (Pae, Lowe, & Sasaki, 1994). Clinically, this may have major implications for airway assessment and management. The following discussion on the effects of posture change on respiratory physiology is divided in terms of ventilation, perfusion, with some mention of specific lung volumes.

In normal respiration the lung expands in an inferior–superior direction as the diaphragm moves. Diaphragmatic movement in the supine position accounts for 66% of quiet ventilation; therefore, any limitation caused by a surgical position on the movement of this important respiratory muscle contributes heavily to any deleterious effect. In an awake, spontaneously breathing individual in the supine position, the abdominal contents limit excursion and force the diaphragm cephalad, reducing functional residual capacity (FRC) by approximately 800 mL (Lumb & Nunn, 1991). Total lung capacity (TLC) also is decreased. Froese and Bryan (1974) demonstrated that in a supine, anesthetized, spontaneously breathing state the diaphragm is placed further cephalad, and in an anesthetized, paralyzed state the diaphragm is pushed further still. Little (1960) noted that all of the common surgical positions do in fact restrict diaphragmatic movement.

In addition to diaphragmatic movement, thorax expansion plays a major role in normal ventilation. Mechanical interference with chest movement that limits lung expansion perhaps is the single most important effect of posture on respiration (Little, 1960). The following figures are extracted from Little's data. The percentages represent the degree to which the vital capacity (VC) decreased in healthy, awake subjects from a sitting position into the indicated common surgical positions. These percentages may be decreased further in the anesthetized individual:

Supine	9.5%
Reverse Trendelenburg	9%
Prone	10%
Lateral	10%
Jackknife	12.5%
Gallbladder	13.5%
Kidney	14.5%
Trendelenburg	14.5%
Lithotomy	18%

The concept of regional variations in ventilation (V) and perfusion (Q) should be familiar to a student of anesthesiology. The reader is encouraged to review these concepts in the classic textbooks and schematics of West (1995) when analyzing the effect of various position changes on respiration on an awake, spontaneously breathing individual. A simplistic view of regional perfusion is that blood flow essentially follows gravitational forces. The lower or dependent lung area will, generally speaking, be better perfused than the upper or nondependent lung areas. A similarly simplistic view of regional variations in ventilation is that ventilation decreases with distance up the lung. Stated differently, alveoli in lower, dependent lung areas have a smaller initial volume and a larger change in volume than those in the upper, nondependent lung areas. Hence, ventilation is greater in the dependent lung areas. Interestingly, radiologic evidence indicates that ventilation always is greater in the dependent portion of the lungs regardless of the surgical posture (Jenkins, 1968).

After summarily reviewing the changes in cardiorespiratory physiology involved in changing from the erect to the supine position in an awake individual and discussed how anesthesia disrupts the body's instinctual reflexes and mechanisms, the following statement should be noted. Changes related to positioning in cardiorespiratory dynamics in anesthetized patients are very difficult for the clinician to predict because an individual's response depends on a variety of factors, some of which are in a dynamic state themselves. These factors include the body habitus, the anesthetic drug levels at any given time, the patient's circulating volume, and whether ventilation is spontaneous or controlled.

Gastrointestinal System

In the supine position, esophageal sphincter tone increases (Babka, Hager, & Castell, 1973). This is a helpful natural counteraction to increased esophageal reflux tendencies in the supine state. The reflux is due to increased intragastric pressure. Not surprisingly, gastric emptying time also is significantly longer in the supine position (Hulme-Moir, Donnan, & McAlister, 1973). These physiologic findings provide strong rationales for rapid-sequence induction protocols.

Obesity constitutes one of the gravest hazards in anesthesia. Excess weight markedly restricts the diaphragm, with a reduction in the tidal volume (V_T) and functional residual capacity (FRC). Extreme obesity, therefore, exaggerates all of the deleterious effects of surgical posture and accelerates the clinical manifestations of respiratory insufficiency (Courington & Little, 1968). Further implications of obesity will be discussed in subsequent sections on the specific surgical postures.

Muscular System

A combination of general anesthesia and muscle relaxants produces complete muscle relaxation, as does sub-arachnoid anesthesia. This profound muscle relaxation causes the legs to lie flat on the operating table and unduly stretches ligaments and muscles of the lower spine. This stretch is responsible for most cases of backache in the postoperative period. Soft padding should be placed under the legs and back to prevent this discomfort.

The other important factor affecting the likelihood of backache is the duration of surgery. In cases lasting 1 to 60 minutes, 18% of the patients developed postoperative backache, whereas in those procedures lasting 181 to 240 minutes, 34% developed backache (Hicks & Koerbacher, 1992). The long-term effect of this finding is unclear.

▶ PERIPHERAL NERVE INJURIES ASSOCIATED WITH POSITIONING

Mechanisms of Injury

Peripheral neuropathies continue to persist as the most common, serious perioperative complications related to positioning. As such, a multitude of studies have been done, many of them attempting to elucidate the precise mechanism of a specific nerve group's injury. In truth, the etiologic factors in perioperative peripheral nerve lesions are complex and interrelated; they include preexisting medical conditions, the effects of anesthesia, in addition to intraoperative and postoperative positioning.

From a physiologic point of view, the most likely causes of nerve injury are section (intentional or inadvertent), compression, traction, and ischemia; the latter three are the ones most likely related to positioning. Compression injuries are the result of externally applied mechanical forces, a category that includes tourniquet compression, crush injuries, tumors, hematomas, edema, and increased intrafascicular pressure. Nerves that pass immediately adjacent to a hard structure (eg, the radial nerve as it courses around the humeral shaft) are particularly prone to this type of injury. Traction or stretching injuries can certainly be the result of positioning. Traction decreases the cross-sectional area of a nerve, raises the pressure in the nerve, and compresses the nerve's blood supply; this can lead to permanent damage and necrosis. Ischemic injuries occur when a peripheral nerve's blood supply is compressed or actually severed (as in femoral artery penetration or damage during cannulation).

A special mention should be made here concerning pneumatic arterial tourniquets in relation to peripheral nerve injuries as tourniquets are used extensively in the operating room; in some institutions, proper placement and monitoring of the tourniquet are considered the purview of the anesthesia team. The high pressure generated by tourniquets causes both compression and ischemic-type injuries to peripheral nerves. The degree of injury depends on both the quantity and duration of pressure; injury is related more to duration than to quantity (Nakata & Stoelting, 1997). It is customary to limit the tourniquet time to approximately 1 hour in the upper limb and 2 hours for the lower limb. If these time limitations are exceeded before the surgical procedure ends, temporary decompression of the tourniquet should be strongly considered to allow normal nerve conduction to be reestablished before reinflating the tourniquet.

The patient under general anesthesia is at higher risk of injury to peripheral nerves for two major reasons: (1) muscle tone is lost; and (2) the patient's perceptive sense of impending nerve damage (paresthesias, pain, or both) is absent.

The intent of this chapter is not to provide a detailed discussion of this important aspect of positioning, so the reader is referred to the works of Dylewsky and McAlpine (1997), Dawson and Krarup (1989), and Britt and Gordon (1964) for excellent reviews.

Brachial Plexus

The brachial plexus is by far the nerve group most vulnerable to damage from improper positioning. A 1988 study by Cooper, Jenkins, Bready, and Rockwood cited the overall incidence of this injury at 0.02%. Interestingly, this statistic was very similar to one generated by a similar study published 15 years earlier (Parks, 1973).

Stretching is the chief cause of damage to the brachial plexus. Many intraoperative maneuvers can produce stretching, but perhaps the most common are abduction and dorsal extension of the arm on an armboard at an angle of more than 60 degrees to the operating table. When the arm is extended to a maximum of 90 degrees and the hand is forcibly pronated, the brachial plexus is stretched across the humeral-clavicular joint, leading to injury (Figs. 24–1 and 24–2).

Suspension of the arm from the ether screen in any surgical position (most commonly occurs in the lateral decubitus) that produces an upper arm abduction greater than 90 degrees with the forearm pronated should be avoided (Fig. 24–3). The clinical picture in patients who have had a stretch injury to the brachial plexus usually is a relatively painless motor deficit commonly affecting the upper roots (C5-7). Surgical exploration is not indicated for this injury. The majority of patients recover within 3 months, although protracted and incomplete recoveries have been reported (Dawson & Krerup, 1989).

A brachial plexus injury distinctly related to the sternal retraction used in open-heart surgery has been studied by several investigators (Hanson et al., 1983; Lederman et al., 1982). According to the results of these studies, pain from the nerve lesion is a prominent feature, and recovery is long.

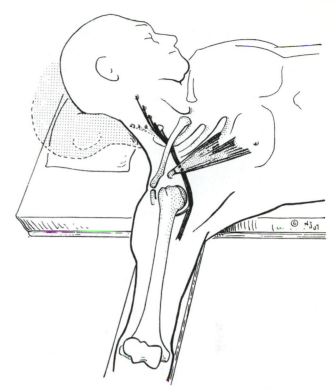

Figure 24–1. Nerve damage occurs when the brachial plexus is stretched when the arm is abducted, extended, and externally rotated and the head is deviated to the opposite side. *(Courtesy Department of Art as Applied to Medicine, Faculty of Medicine, University of Toronto.)*

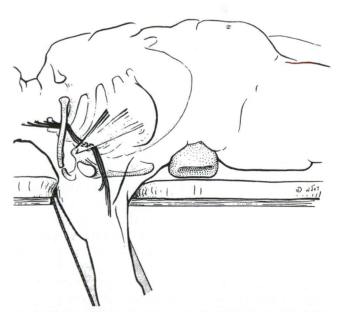

Figure 24–2. Damaging stretching of the brachial plexus around the tendon of pectoralis minor when the shoulder girdle falls back with the arm abducted, extended, and externally rated. *(Courtesy Department of Art as Applied to Medicine, Faculty of Medicine, University of Toronto.)*

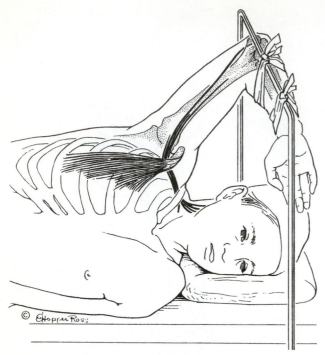

Figure 24–3. Stretching of the brachial plexus around the clavicle and tendon of pectoralis minor by fixation of the abducted arm to the frame of an ether screen is to be avoided. *(Courtesy Department of Art as Applied to Medicine, Faculty of Medicine, University of Toronto.)*

Ulnar Nerve

Perioperative lesions of the ulnar nerve are well recognized as a complication of surgery and anesthesia, and they often are the focus of litigation. The ulnar nerve is especially vulnerable to injury because it passes posteriorly under the medial epicondyle of the elbow. At the elbow, both the ulnar nerve and the ulnar collateral artery pass superficially through the cubital tunnel as they course from the arm to the forearm. Clinical manifestations of ulnar nerve damage include a "clawlike" hand, impaired adduction or abduction of the medial four digits, and a sensory deficit in the ulnar nerve distribution.

Wadsworth (1974) describes the cubital tunnel external compression syndrome, which is often cited as an explanation for the unexpected appearance of postoperative ulnar nerve palsy. Based on this perspective, ulnar nerve damage is a complication that can theoretically be prevented by proper arm positioning. If the arm is restricted to the patient's side, pronation (palms down) of the forearm prevents excess compression on the cubital tunnel. When the arm is abducted on a padded armboard, there is some disagreement regarding what constitutes proper position of the forearm, pronation or supination (palms up). Many practitioners believe that forearm pronation promotes cubital tunnel contact with

flat and/or hard surfaces (ie, the metal frame of the operating table), resulting in a more vulnerable ulnar nerve. However, forearm supination frees the cubital tunnel from compression, but may cause stretching of the brachial plexus and potential injury.

Compression of the ulnar nerve also may result when the elbow is allowed to sag slightly over the side of the side of the operating table or when the arms are folded across the abdomen or chest (Fig. 24–4).

With the forearm in either the pronated or supinated position, the cubital tunnel is best protected when sufficient padding is placed around the elbow and when the forearm is judiciously positioned. Some practitioners choose to alternate (when possible) the anesthetized patient's arm between the pronated and supinated position.

It is important for clinicians to recognize that the exact mechanism of ulnar nerve palsy has not been elucidated, that in fact multiple mechanisms can contribute to the problem. This situation prompts Stoelting (1993) to pose the question of whether ulnar nerve palsy is a preventable complication at all. Alvine and Schurrer (1987) propose that a preexisting subclinical ulnar neuropathy may be worsened by the effects of a surgical procedure. The large retrospective study of Warner, Warner, and Martin (1994) indicates that being male gr, extremes of body habitus, and prolonged hospitalization are risk factors strongly associated (despite proper positioning) with perioperative ulnar neuropathy. The clinical lessons implied by these studies is that a history of preanesthetic ulnar neuropathies should be elicited from the patient and documented, all positioning precautions should indeed be taken to prevent a perioperative ulnar neuropathy from developing. Preventive measures should be carefully documented.

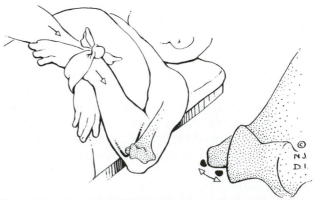

Figure 24–4. Ulnar nerve injury is caused by compression between the medial epicondyle of the humerus and the edge of the operating table. Inset: Anomalous position of ulnar nerve. *(Courtesy Department of Art as Applied to Medicine, Faculty of Medicine, University of Toronto.)*

Radial Nerve

When the arm is compressed between the body and the vertical bar of the ether screen or any other table attachment (eg, Bookwalter retractor) there is danger of damage to the radial nerve if the nerve is pinched between the screen and spiral groove of the humerus (Fig. 24-5). Clinically, radial nerve injury is manifested by wrist drop and the inability to extend the metacarpophalangeal joints due to paralysis of the extensor muscles in the forearm.

Peroneal and Saphenous Nerves

The most frequently damaged nerves of the lower extremities are the common peroneal and its distal branches and the saphenous (Warner, Martin, Schroeder, Offord, & Chute, 1994). The common peroneal nerve is injured in the lithotomy position when the legs are placed in stirrups. This posture causes the fibular neck to rest against the vertical bar of the lithotomy stirrup, thus compressing the nerve (Fig. 24-6).

Common peroneal neuropathies are manifested by foot drop, loss of dorsal extension of the toes, an inability to evert the foot, and sensory loss in the dorsal area of the foot. The major preventive measure is to place soft padding between the leg and the stirrup.

Saphenous nerve damage occurs in the lithotomy position when the legs are suspended lateral to the ver-

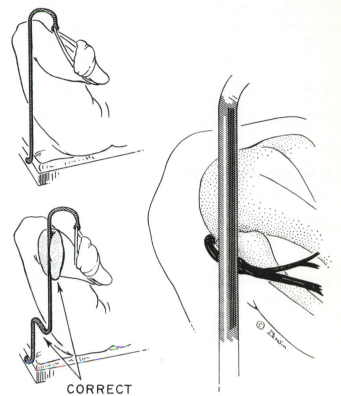

Figure 24–6. Common peroneal nerve compression between lithotomy stirrup and neck of fibula. This may be avoided by padding (see inset). *(Courtesy Department of Art as Applied to Medicine, Faculty of Medicine, University of Toronto.)*

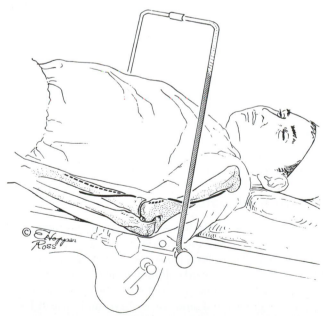

Figure 24–5. Damaging compression of the radial nerve between the humerus and an ether screen. *(Courtesy Department of Art as Applied to Medicine, Faculty of Medicine, University of Toronto.)*

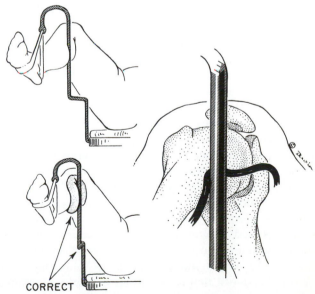

Figure 24–7. Saphenous nerve compressed between lithotomy stirrup and tibia. *(Courtesy Department of Art as Applied to Medicine, Faculty of Medicine, University of Toronto.)*

tical brace of the stirrup, potentially causing compression between the stirrup and the tibia (Fig. 24-7), or when excessive pressure on the medial aspect of the calf or tibial condyle is placed by the "knee crutch" stirrup.

Paresthesias along the medial and anteromedial aspects of the calf are the major symptoms of saphenous nerve lesions. Prevention also is accomplished by using soft padding between the legs and stirrup apparatus.

► BASIC POSITIONS USED IN ANESTHESIA AND SURGERY

Supine Position

In the traditional version of the supine position the patient is lying on her back with a small head support. The arms are either padded comfortably and placed alongside the patient's trunk or abducted on padded armboards. If the arms are positioned at the side, the palms should be turned down and the arms secured underneath a restraining sheet, usually the draw sheet beneath the patient. The cephalad border of the sheet should be placed above the elbows to the mid upper arms and tucked under the patient as opposed to under the mattress (Fig. 24-8).

If the arms are to be maintained abducted (which is often preferable to maintain access to intravenous lines and monitors), they should be placed on a padded armboard and positioned to protect the peripheral nerves of the upper extremity, as discussed.

The major weight-bearing areas in this supine position are the occiput, scapulae, spine, hips, and heels; these are all bony prominences whose overlying skin receives minimal subcutaneous protection and maximum pressure, ideal conditions for the development of ischemia. Padding these vulnerable areas helps disperse the pressure generated by the supporting surface against the body, allowing for more normal tissue perfusion. In the supine position it is especially easy to overlook the possibility of excessive or prolonged pressure against the occiput, which can cause alopecia. The anesthetist should pad the occiput sufficiently and reposition and/or massage the back of the head at regular intervals during lengthy procedures.

The "lawn chair" or "contoured" variation of the supine position is more physiologic than the traditional form discussed. It incorporates hip and knee flexion and slight head elevation (Fig. 24-9). This position not only redistributes weight, but also brings the knee joints and hips into a more neutral position, thereby decreasing pull or tension on muscles and nerves. The supine contoured position is advocated by Warner (1997) when the patient is required to lie awake and immobile for a long time.

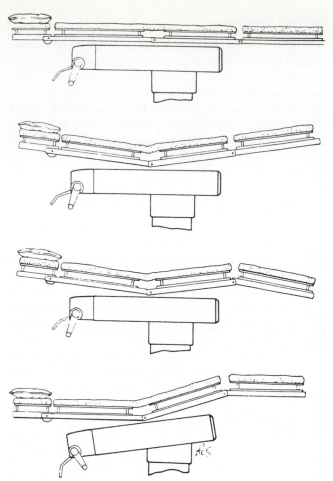

Figure 24–8. Supine position: head on small pillow, arm by side, well on mattress, with lift sheet extending above the elbow to provide support. *(Courtesy Department of Art as Applied to Medicine, Faculty of Medicine, University of Toronto.)*

During prolonged mask general anesthetic cases, in which incorrect hand position and pressure is applied, the optic nerve is at risk for damage because of direct, excessive pressure placed on the upper portion of the mask. If mask straps are improperly applied, the facial nerve, a portion of which passes around the mandibular rami, also is vulnerable to injury (Fig. 24-10).

Lithotomy Position

Since ancient times the lithotomy position has been used by both obstetrician and urologist. The designated term for this position comes from the fact that the ancient physicians who removed calculi (stones, *lithos*) from the urinary bladder did so in a patient whose position was upright, legs elevated, and knees bent and spread laterally. These physicians were called *lithotomists* and the procedural position *lithotomy* (Martin, 1997b, p. 47). Only in the nineteenth century has this posture been modified to a dorsal orientation and utilized by gynecol-

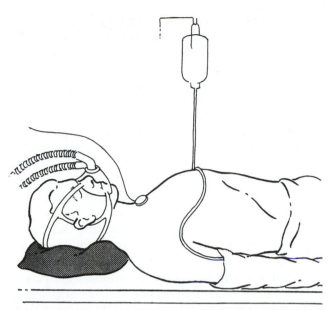

Figure 24–9. Supine position: Establishing the "lawn chair" position with hip and knee flexion and a pillow for the head. *(From Martin [1997]. Reprinted with permission.)*

ogists; it may have been the most convenient arrangement by which to visualize the reproductive tract of the female and conduct a bimanual examination.

The primary untoward effect of the lithotomy position on an anesthetized patient's circulatory system is manifested at the termination of the procedure as the pa-

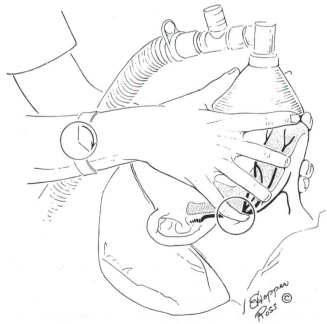

Figure 24–10. Motor root of facial nerve injured by traction on the angle of the mandible. *(Courtesy Department of Art as Applied to Medicine, Faculty of Medicine, University of Toronto.)*

tient is taken out of the lithotomy position. This maneuver may be accompanied by a dangerous lowering of the blood pressure, caused by too rapid a filling of the dilated peripheral vascular bed of the previously elevated extremities. The degree of hypotension is directly proportional to the amount of impairment of the vasoregulatory mechanisms of the upper and lower extremities, which in turn is predicated by the patient's cardiovascular reserve, the anesthetic level, duration of time spent in lithotomy, and the intravascular volume (Batillo & Hendler, 1993). Fortunately, the degree of hypotension also highly depends on the speed with which the lower extremity is lowered. The circulatory insult can be minimized or even eradicated by slowly, steadily lowering the legs and lightening the anesthetic level and restorating the intravascular volume beforehand.

A study by Little (1960) reveals that the vital capacity in the lithotomy position in awake, spontaneously breathing humans is reduced by 18%. However, Henschel et al., (1957) and Jones and Jacoby (1955) had established that tidal volume (VT) provides a better reflection of the respiratory condition of the anesthetized patient. Their data indicated that the lithotomy position caused a 3% decrease in VT, that an additional 10 degrees of head-down tilt caused a 14% decrease, and that a 20-degree head-down tilt caused a 15% decrease in VT. It also is well recognized that in lithotomy there is a correlation between the degree of thigh flexion on the abdomen and VT decreases (Walsh, 1994). A tenet of pulmonary function in patients under anesthesia is that ventilatory restrictions caused by the anesthetic state itself increase progressively during the course of the operation; if an already decreasing VT is further reduced by a certain posture (eg, lithotomy plus head-down tilt), the potential for general fatigue of the respiratory muscles becomes greater as time spent in the posture increases. From a clinical point of view, in the vast majority of patients major respiratory limitations produced by the lithotomy position can be corrected using an endotracheal tube and assisted or controlled ventilation.

Extremity-supporting devices attached to the frame of the operating table are needed to place the patient in the lithotomy position. The three most common configurations for these leg holders are the "candy cane pole" (Fig. 24–6), the "knee crutch," and the "knee crutch with an adjustable knee and foot support" (Fig. 24–11).

The candy cane pole should be used for relatively short procedures because the apparatus design (free swinging cloth slings for the feet) allows the lower extremities to move. The legs are thus easily displaced from their proper position either by operative team members who inadvertently push against the patient or the stirrups or by the patient (who may or may not be anesthetized). As described in the section relating to peripheral nerve injuries, the common peroneal and saphenous

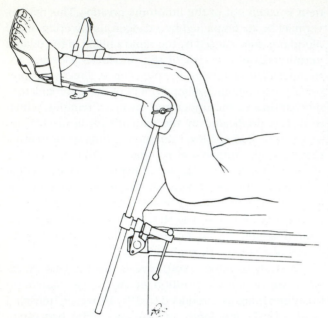

Figure 24–11. Lithotomy position: Note placement of legs into stirrups and buttocks on table. *(From Martin [1997]. Reprinted with permission.)*

nerves are at risk when the lithotomy position is established with the candy cane poles.

The advantage of the knee crutch with the leg and foot support is that it evenly distributes the weight of the lower extremity. Its proper use depends on team members who have the knowledge and take the time to adjust the hip, knee, and foot supports according to the patient's anatomy. The obturator, saphenous, and femoral nerves are all at risk when this particular leg holder is used because the weight of the legs within the support can cause compression of the aforementioned nerves. Compression syndromes have been well established as potential complications of several variations of the lithotomy position. Martin (1992), in an extensive review article, delineates some clear guidelines for anesthetists to employ to avoid this complication, including maintaining blood pressure at normal ranges for the patient as hypotension and loss of driving blood flow in elevated extremities facilitates the muscle compression and ischemic process.

There are several basic steps to place the patient in the lithotomy position. First, it is imperative that the equipment chosen be appropriate to the patient's length, body habitus, and range of both hip and knee joints. Second, if both extremities are to be placed in holders, both legs must be flexed and extended simultaneously to prevent a torsion injury to relaxed muscles and ligaments or joint and spinal injury, including hip disarticulation. Backache is not an uncommon postoperative complaint following lithotomy. Third, symmetrical

placement of both legs must be established in the holders, again to prevent rotational spine or joint injury. The anesthetist with a clear vantage point at the head of the surgical table often is consulted to determine whether the patient is symmetrically placed. Finally, the "takedown" maneuver of the lithotomy position entails a coordinated, smooth, slow lowering of the legs.

There are several options for proper arm placement in the lithotomy position: Both arms on padded boards; one arm on a board, the other placed across the chest; or both arms on the chest. The anesthetist must adhere to the precautions previously discussed when placing the arms on armboards. When positioning the arm or arms on the chest, care must be taken to ensure that the elbow does not rest on the metal edge of the operating table. Not only does this place pressure on the ulnar nerve, but also it inadvertently incorporates the patient into the electrocautery grounding site. The arm should not be acutely flexed across the chest. An angle of more than 100 degrees at the elbow can compromise the arterial supply to the lower arm and hand. Finally, placing the arm at the patient's side is discouraged. The fingers may potentially extend beyond the table break, become entrapped between the two table sections and, as the lower piece is raised when the surgical procedure is completed, result in damage to or even amputation of one or more fingers.

Head-Down Tilt

Interestingly in 1956 Inglis and Brooke stated "From the standpoint of the anesthesiologist, placing a patient in a head-down position has real problems and few assets." Yet in current anesthesia practice, despite the fact that most anesthesia providers continue to hold the same opinion as Inglis did in the late 1950s, the head-down tilt is used daily, frequently with the lithotomy position and a pneumoperitoneum, as required for laparoscopic surgery. The use of head-down tilt still presents real problems and a host of challenges to the anesthetist, primarily because of a variety of cardiovascular and respiratory insults.

The following represents a simplistic summary of the cardiovascular response of a healthy, normovolemic, anesthetized patient to minimal head-down tilt (MHDT), the term currently used to describe a tilt ranging from 10 to 20 degrees. The central blood volume is increased significantly (from 500 to 1000 mL). The rapid rise of hydrostatic pressure is sensed by the arterial baroreceptors, which stimulates the expected reflex vasodilatation and decreased stroke volume, resulting in decreased cardiac output and reduced perfusion of vital organs. The brain is especially vulnerable to decreased perfusion because a head-down tilt also increases cerebral venous pressure, compromising cerebral perfusion pressure.

Head-down tilt in patients with known or suspected intracranial pathology is absolutely contraindicated.

The vast majority of patients have an adequate cardiopulmonary reserve, and the physiologic challenge of the head-down tilt is met with normal compensatory responses. Assuming proper anesthetic management, patients tolerate the position well. In contrast, anesthetized patients with diminished cardiopulmonary reserve clearly do not tolerate a MHDT, as evidenced by right ventricular dilation, decreased right ventricular ejection fraction, and impaired oxygenation (Reich, Konstadt, Raissi, Hubbard, & Thys, 1989). Steep head-down tilt (SHDT), or approximately 30 to 45 degrees of tilt, has the potential to increase central blood volume and pulmonary blood flow enough to cause acute cardiac failure in normal individuals, hence the risk for failure in already compromised patients is quite significant. Furthermore, when returning to the horizontal position, the patient with decreased cardiovascular reserve will be very much at risk for a severe hypotensive episode. Limiting or eliminating SHDT in these patients is the best preventive measure for such untoward cardiac events. If one must be placed in MHDT, a slow, controlled shift of position, along with repetitive checks of the blood pressure facilitate the ability of compromised vasculature to adjust to a newly enlarged circulatory capacitance.

The potential for MHDT or SHDT to mask intraoperative blood loss has very important implications for the clinician. Unsuspected or underestimated hypovolemia will manifest as sudden hypotension when the patient is returned to the supine and horizontal position. Accurate fluid deficit calculation and appropriate and timely replacement are the key elements to avoiding this situation.

An allusion was made earlier to the frequent use of the head-down tilt during laparoscopic surgery. During recent years, advances in instrumentation and surgical technique have resulted in much more extensive, prolonged laparoscopic procedures, especially in the fields of gynecology and general surgery. These intraabdominal procedures require the establishment of a pneumoperitoneum. In addition, MHDT, SHDT, and various degrees of lithotomy are positions that the anesthetist commonly anticipates as part of the procedure. The cumulative effects of these factors on the patient's cardiopulmonary system represent the bulk of the anesthetic challenge. A 1989 study (Johannsen, Andersen, & Juhl) of healthy women undergoing elective diagnostic laparoscopies documents decreased stroke and cardiac indices (an average decrease of 42% for each index during periods of maximum hemodynamic stress) that were directly correlated to abdominal insufflation and head-down tilt. Despite these significant numerical changes, patients with healthy cardiac function tolerate such hemodynamic stresses, in part because anesthesia clinicians adhere to basic principles of safe positioning.

A recent study by Harris, Ballantyne, Luther, and Perrino (1996) of elderly patients with significant coexisting cardiopulmonary disease undergoing elective laparoscopic colectomies investigated cardiovascular performance with special emphasis on the response to SHDT. The magnitude of the adverse hemodynamic responses of these patients to the routine maneuvers of the procedure prompted the authors to recommend the use of pulmonary artery catheterization and/or transesophageal echocardiography in this setting. Most practitioners would agree that the prudent approach in this setting would be to establish clear benefits of proceeding with a laparoscopic approach (entailing obligatory placement in some degree of head-down tilt) over the risk of the procedure.

The respiratory effects of the head-down tilt are the result of the abdominal contents being pushed up against the diaphragm, the respiratory muscle that does most of the work of breathing under anesthesia. The workload of the diaphragm is greatly increased. In addition to lung ventilation it must lift the viscera, predisposing the patient to atelectasis. Pulmonary compliance, VT, and FRC also are diminished, resulting in increased work of breathing and varying degrees of ventilation–perfusion mismatch. Gravitational forces cause an increased pulmonary blood volume, contributing to the aforementioned decrease in pulmonary compliance.

The anticipated placement of an anesthetized patient in MHDT or SHDT obligates the anesthetist to insert an endotracheal tube and to use positive-pressure, controlled, mechanical ventilation. Judicious manipulation of ventilatory settings enables the delivery of adequate ventilation and oxygenation. The position of the endotracheal (ET) tube while the patient is in a head-down tilt must be monitored carefully. A tube previously well positioned in the trachea can enter the right mainstem bronchus after the patient is tilted head down as the abdominal and thoracic contents are pushed cephalad. The ET tube position should be checked after each positional modification, however minor, and periodically throughout the period in which the patient is in a head-down orientation.

Laparoscopic procedures require MHDT or SHDT and a pneumoperitoneum introduces an additional challenge to the anesthetist: an increased CO_2 load due to the continuous insufflation of gas must be excreted via ventilation to avoid hypercapnia and acidosis. According to Hirvonen, Nuutinen, and Kauko (1995), it seems more efficient to handle the increased ventilation requirement by increasing VT and keeping the respiratory frequency low.

The caveats discussed in the previous sections on preventing peripheral neuropathies secondary to positioning certainly apply to this position. An additional potential etiology of brachial plexus injury in the head-down tilt occurs when shoulder braces, attached to the surgical table, are used to prevent the patient from sliding in a cephalad direction. If shoulder braces are used, they should be placed laterally so that their pressure is on the area of the acromioclavicular articulation and not directly on either the clavicle or the root of the neck. A wide variety of options for securing the patient safely to the table in this position are explained comprehensively in Martin (1997a, pp. 95–124).

Lateral Decubitus Position

Lateral decubitus often is referred to as the standard thoracotomy position because it affords optimal exposure and access to thoracic structures. In addition to thoracic procedures, this position is utilized for cardiac, thoracovascular, and gastroesophageal surgeries. The flexed variation of the lateral decubitus is most commonly used in urologic procedures (nephrectomies); still other slight variations allow this position to be used in neurosurgical (craniotomies, laminectomies) and orthopedic (hip arthroplasties) procedures.

Utilizing the correct terminology when describing this position is helpful in protecting the patient and the care team from instituting a surgical intervention on the incorrect side of the patient. *Lateral, lateral decubitus,* and *lateral recumbent* are synonymous; the term generally used is *lateral decubitus. Right lateral decubitus* refers to a position in which the patient is lying on the right side and is appropriate for surgical procedures in which the left side is uppermost and vice versa.

An anesthetized patient in virtually all of the lateral positions exhibits a decrease in arterial pressure; the lowest pressures have been observed in the right lateral decubitus and the right lateral flexed decubitus variations. Cardiac output tends to remain stable in all of the lateral positions (Eggers, DeGroot, Tanner, & Leonard, 1963). The position-related blood pressure changes are attributable in most cases to a reduced systemic vascular resistance as opposed to decreased venous return. However, in the extreme flexed lateral position with the lower extremities markedly dependent, impaired venous return causes the decrease in arterial pressure.

Although most clinical studies have documented that cardiovascular compromise due to the lateral positions per se is uncommon, cardiovascular collapse during lateral positioning still is possible in the anesthetized patient. In addition, the lateral decubitus position causes a shift of the mediastinum toward the downside and rotates the heart on its axis, relative "anatomical" changes that can interfere with venous return and cardiac output.

The mechanical interference with thorax expansion caused by the lateral decubitus position in an anesthetized patient is manifested by a 10% to 14% decrease in tidal volume (Henschel et al., 1957), irrespective of a regional or general anesthetic. The effects of the lateral decubitus position on the respiratory system are traditionally discussed in terms of ventilation/perfusion (V/Q) ratios or mismatch. As a clinician, one is interested in V/Q ratios that are generated in the four scenarios listed in the next paragraph. To understand the changes in ventilation, remember that it is the mechanical efficiency of contraction of either the upper lung hemidiaphragm or the lower lung hemidiaphragm that confers preferential ventilation. In anesthetized states, the hemidiaphragm of the lower lung becomes mechanically less efficient and contracts less, and therefore ventilation is decreased.

- Scenario 1. In an awake, spontaneously breathing patient Q is greater in the lower lung because of gravitational flow while preferential V occurs in the lower lung, resulting in minimal V/Q mismatch.
- Scenario 2. In an anesthetized, spontaneously breathing patient with a closed chest Q is greater in the lower lung and V is greater in the upper lung, resulting in V/Q mismatch in both lungs.
- Scenario 3. In an anesthetized, paralyzed patient with a closed chest Q is greater in the lower lung, and, because paralysis and positive pressure ventilation further decrease the mechanical efficiency of the lower hemidiaphragm, V is even greater in the upper lung, resulting in increased V/Q mismatch.
- Scenario 4. In an anesthetized, paralyzed patient with an open chest Q is greater in the lower lung, and, because the upper lung is no longer restricted by the chest wall, it becomes even more compliant, greatly increasing ventilation, resulting in a further increase in V/Q mismatch.

From a practical point of view, any degree of V/Q mismatch predisposes the patient to hypoxia; understanding when and why a patient is at higher risk for this undesireable state provides the rationale by which the anesthetist will choose ventilatory parameters, whether or not paralysis is advantageous, as well as the percentage of oxygen to deliver. As it is not within the scope of this chapter, this discussion does not take into account the various techniques by which differential ventilation of either lung can be accomplished. The reader is referred to the works of Cohen (1995).

In the basic lateral decubitus position the patient is turned 90 degrees to the horizontal surface of the table and stabilized. Flexing the lower leg at the hip and knee while keeping the upper leg straight enhances stability; additional stabilizing devices include broad strips of non-elastic adhesive tape, velcro-type bands, or quick-release belts. All of these devices should be placed across the hips just below the iliac crest and across the shoulder and secured to the undersides of the operating table to ensure stability. Another alternative device to stabilize the patient is the bean bag (Vacu-Pac) that is shaped using a vacuum and placed beneath the patient as a molded support. Once the pelvics and thorax have been stabilized, the bony prominences of the lower extremities should be padded.

Proper placement of the arms in the basic position is important to adding stability, as well as protecting the upper extremity peripheral nerve groups. The downside arm usually is flexed and tucked under the pillow that supports the head. A small chest pad must be placed under the downside thorax just caudad to, but not in, the axilla; the purpose of this pad is to relieve pressure from the head of the downside humerus and to avoid compression of the brachial plexus. A covered, 1-L intravenous fluid bag frequently is used as a chest pad. This accessory is very commonly referred to as the axillary roll, a misnomer, that often is improperly positioned by uninformed individuals. During the final position check, the anesthetist must verify proper placement of the chest pad.

The upper arm usually is placed according to surgical needs. For nonthoracic procedures, there are several safe options: the arm can rest in an extended position on top of several pillows placed on an armboard positioned 90 degrees to the table, or the arm can be flexed at the elbow and extended to varying degrees and supported on a pillow that lies adjacent to the patient's face. Other options for upper-arm support in an elevated position are a double-deck ("airplane") armboard (Fig. 24-12), Mayo stand, or suspension from the ether screen. The use of the last three items often are discouraged because they greatly increase the susceptibility of upper-arm stretch or compression. With any of these options, body alignment must be maintained, brachial plexus stretch must be avoided, and adequate perfusion of both arms and hands must be ensured via pulse palpation, capillary refill check, or a pulse oximeter probe.

The flexed lateral decubitus (kidney) position is established by using the break between the upper and lower sections of the table. This break must be at the level of the iliac crest (Fig. 24-13). The "flex" in the table causes the lateral muscles to be stretched. The table can be placed in a head-up tilt, making the operative site parallel to the floor. The lower leg usually is slightly flexed, the upper leg remains extended, and a pillow or padding is placed between the two. Care must be taken not to allow the legs to overhang or touch the table's metal frame.

In any of the lateral decubitus positions, proper cervical spine alignment with head and neck support is crucial to prevent neck injury or brachial plexus injury via stretching of the upside neck (Fig. 24-14). The downside eye, ear, and facial nerve must be protected from excessive pressure or rough surfaces. Ocular damage to the downside eye is a particularly devastating complication considering it is highly preventable. Corneal abrasions are the result of careless eyelid protection, and retinal artery thrombosis (which can cause permanent blindness) is caused by excessive pressure on the downside eye.

Placement of a blood pressure–measuring device in the lateral decubitus position often is the focus of a preoperative planning session. If a noninvasive blood pressure (NIBP) cuff is to be used, the following principles should be recognized: (1) there is approximately a 32-mm Hg discrepancy in blood pressure between the two arms in the lateral position (the upper arm will indicate the lower of the two numbers); (2) the NIBP is more likely to be underestimated (relative to the true pressure of the heart or the brain) when the cuff is placed in the upper arm; some practitioners prefer this to minimize the risk of unrecognized hypotension, which may be more problematic than unrecognized hypertension; (3) placing the NIBP cuff on the downside arm may compress the axillary artery (Lawson & Meyer, 1997). Using an intraarterial catheter for direct measure-

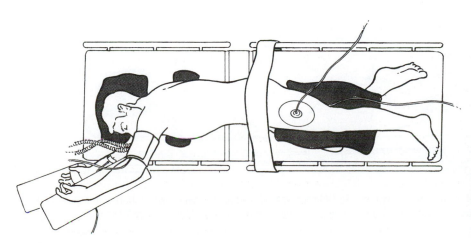

Figure 24-12. Lateral position. Note the placement of support, flexion of lower leg, extension of upper leg, separation by pillow, placement of IV catheter, grounding pad, blood pressure cuff, and strap across iliac crest. *(From Martin [1997]. Reprinted with permission.)*

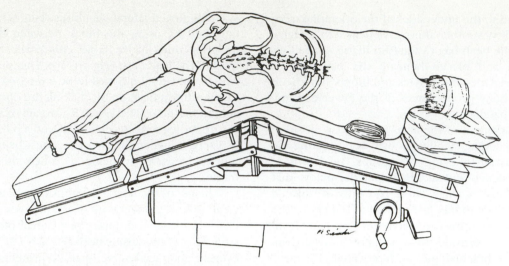

Figure 24–13. Kidney position. Note support of head, neck, and upper thorax, separation of legs by pillow and elevation of foot of upper leg, position of dependent flexed leg with foot on mattress, and position of nonelastic adhesive tape across iliac crest and under table to provide stable positioning. *(From Martin [1997]. Reprinted with permission.)*

ment of blood pressure is considered strongly when entry into the chest is anticipated. In most cases, either arm can be safely and effectively used, as placement of the calibrated transducer at the level of the heart is what determines the accuracy of the reading. The final decision usually depends on the practitioner's preference, as well as the caliber, condition, and accessibility of either of the radial arteries.

The basic features of the lateral turn sequence performed by a team are described, however; the reader

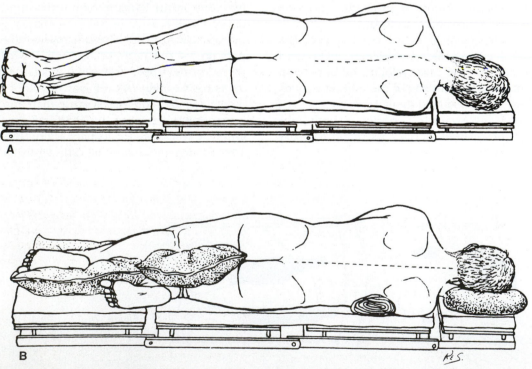

Figure 24–14. Spinal alignment in the lateral position. (**A**) Note the lack of support for head, upper thorax, and poor spinal alignment. (**B**) Proper support of head and upper thorax. *(From Martin [1997]. Reprinted with permission.)*

should note that the many fine details or variations of this sequence are best gained by demonstration and experience as well as studying a more in-depth reference text (Lawson & Meyer, 1997). The patient must be turned as a unit, and body alignment must be maintained at all times. A minimum of three people are required: a coordinator (the anesthetist) who supports and turns the head and neck and maintains the airway; one individual assigned to turn and support the shoulders and thorax; and one individual designated to turn and support the hips and legs. It is highly desirable to have a fourth team member to place the chest pad under the downside thorax, as the head, neck, shoulder, and thorax are slightly elevated and to place the appropriate padding while the patient is being secured to the table.

Prone Position

The prone position also is referred to as the *ventral decubitus,* or face-down, position. It is the most awkward for patients of all ages and sizes. There are numerous variations of this position: the Georgia, the Smith modification of the Georgia, the Overhold, and the Sellor-Brown, to name a few. In addition, several operating tables designed specifically for variations of the prone posture carry the designer's name.

In a healthy anesthetized individual, significant cardiovascular problems are unusual in the prone position, despite the usual depression of the normal compensatory autonomic reflexes. However, if the inferior vena cava (IVC) and the femoral veins are compressed, venous return can be severely compromised and cause a decrease in cardiac filling and hypotension. A compressed IVC forces venous return to occur through vessels that have lesser flow capabilities, often the venous plexus of the vertebral column (Walsh, 1994). Decreased stroke volume and cardiac index have been demonstrated in anesthetized prone patients (Backofen & Schauble, 1985). Generally speaking, if IVC and femoral vein compression are avoided, the untoward cardiovascular side effects of the prone position will be minimized.

If the patient's head is positioned below the level of the heart, venous pressure increases, causing increases in the carotid vasculature, increased intracranial pressure, venous congestion of the head and neck, and ocular edema. Improper positioning causes compression of the chest and abdomen and the work of breathing is greatly increased. Furthermore, mechanical ventilation may be associated with increased airway pressures and larger tidal volumes, potentiating the risk for pulmonary barotrauma (Martin, 1997c, pp. 155–196). The study by Pelosi et al. (1995) demonstrates that, if the position is accomplished properly, ensuring free abdominal and chest movement, lung and chest wall mechanics are not significantly altered, and lung volumes (VT and FRC) are

markedly improved, as is oxygenation. The same group of investigators (Pelosi et al., 1996) demonstrated a similar finding in obese (BMI greater than 30 kg/m^2) patients.

An essential feature of the classic, horizontal prone position is the ventral support device, either a chest roll or frame. The cephalad end of the support device should be placed just below the clavicles and should extend just to the iliac crest. Free excursion of the anterior thorax and the abdominal wall must be possible when the patient is pronated on the device. Placing the female breasts can be challenging, especially if they are large and pendulous. The question posed by the positioning team is whether to displace the breasts (relative to the ventral supportive device) medially or laterally. Although Martin (1997c, pp. 155–196) generally recommends a medial displacement, it is prudent to individualize this particular decision according to the patient's anatomy. The male genitalia should not be compressed or rotated.

The arms can be either extended above the head or placed alongside the torso. If the former option is chosen, the arms must be placed on well-padded armboards, which are positioned parallel to the table. The arms should be minimally abducted and the upper arm extended and the elbow flexed. The upper arm should be supported to the same elevation as the thorax to prevent pull and stretch on the brachial plexus. Padding should be placed so that there is no pressure on the axilla or the elbow. The presence of effective radial pulses should be palpated regularly. The option of placing the arms alongside the torso should be exercised in patients with known or suspected thoracic outlet syndrome (TOS), such as those with a history of inability to raise their hands above their head normally without experiencing numbness, tingling, or pain. Arms placed alongside the torso for any reason should have a restraining sheet that is snug enough to secure the arms, without compromising circulation. The usual vulnerable areas should be padded, and adequate radial pulses established.

Head and neck positioning must be approached with an extreme degree of care, followed by frequent checking for the development of untoward effects, especially in the downside eye, ear, facial structures, and nose. Injury to these structures can easily occur from protracted pressure from the weight of the head against the table surface. If there are no special headrests, the head should be supported and padded, turned slightly to one side, avoiding neck torsion. Extreme head or neck rotation may compress both the vertebral and carotid arteries and their branches. Managing a severely arthritic or unstable cervical spine represents a special challenge and should be extensively discussed with the entire positioning team prior to instituting a position change.

Padding should be placed under the iliac crests and knees, and the dorsum of the feet should be supported with several pillows. In kneeling variations of the prone position, the knees must be very well padded.

There are essentially two approaches to establishing the prone position: (1) pronating from the bed or cart to the operating table; or (2) pronating on the operating table. For the purposes of this discussion, a general endotracheal (ET) anesthetic will be assumed. The patient is anesthetized in the supine position. Postinduction, a type and level of anesthesia is established that maximally preserves autonomic reflexes, provides analgesia sufficient to withstand stimulation, and provides adequate muscle relaxation to allow for smooth movement of the patient. All monitoring leads and devices, intravascular lines, and urinary catheters should be secured and positioned to cause minimal entanglement. Careful attention must be paid to the manner in which the ET tube is secured to the patient.

Pronation of the patient from the cart to the table requires six individuals: the coordinator (anesthetist), two turners positioned at the free side of the cart, two receivers positioned at the free side of the surgical table, and one individual at the patient's foot. Prior to the actual positioning maneuvers, make sure that the table is completely set up with the selected supportive devices and positioning accessories and that all team members

are present and that their specific responsibilities have been assigned. The cart is moved parallel to and against the table, at equal height. The patient's arms are placed alongside the torso. Frequently, the patient is moved as a unit to the edge of the cart that approximates the table. The anesthetist, as the coordinator of the team, disconnects the ET tube from the anesthesia machine circuit and delivers the verbal signal to begin the position change. The receivers extend their arms in readiness for the patient as the turners rotate the patient sequentially from supine, to lateral, to prone. The goal is to move the patient on to the receivers' arms before it touches the table's surface. The anesthetist, stabilizing the patient's head and neck while ensuring the patency of the airway, keeps the head in the patient's sagittal plane. When the patient is lying in the receivers' arms, the head is gently turned in a preplanned position, and the circuit is reconnected to the ET tube. All monitoring and intravenous lines are checked for patency and function. The empty cart is then moved away from the operating table, where the entire team establishes the final position, as previously described.

The sequence of events for pronation of the patient on the operating table is illustrated in Fig. 24-15. The same preparatory steps described for moving from cart

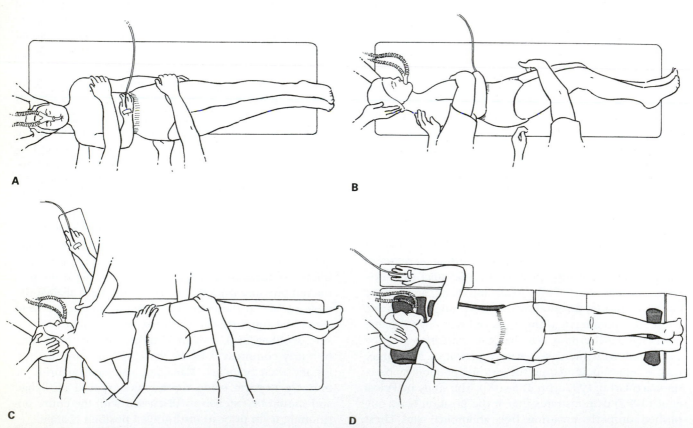

Figure 24-15. (A, B, C) Three people—one for head and coordinator, one for shoulder thorax, and one for hips and legs—turn patient as a unit. (D) Placement of supports. *(From Martin [1997]. Reprinted with permission.)*

to table are followed. The team, coordinated by the anesthetist, moves the patient in the supine position toward the turners' side of the table. Almost immediately, the patient is turned to the lateral position briefly, then pronated, after which the team members establish the final, proper posture.

Head-Elevated Position

The classic, high-sitting position is used in neurosurgery for occipital craniotomies and cervical laminectomies. The lower-sitting positions, more commonly called the "beach chair" or "barber chair" are used in head, neck, and shoulder surgeries.

The circulatory changes in the classic sitting position are due to the profound effect of gravity. Pooling of venous blood in the dependent periphery is increased by the vasodilatory and cardiac depressing effects of general anesthesia. The diminished venous return causes a 12% to 20% decrease in stroke volume and cardiac index, with a compensatory increase in both the pulmonary and systemic vasculature. Most notable is a 15% decrease in the cerebral perfusion pressure (Milde, 1997). This is problematic for patients with cerebrovascular disease, cervical spine changes, or longstanding hypertension.

Because of gravitational forces, respiratory mechanics and lung volumes are increased, as one would surmise. In fact, much less peak inspiratory pressure is required to expand the alveoli of an individual in the sitting position than in the supine position, favoring the development of hyperventilation and excessive hypocarbia. For neurosurgical patients or those with cerebrovascular disease, the resultant vasoconstrictive decrease in cerebral blood flow could be disastrous. In the sitting position, V/Q mismatch also can occur, as the upper-lung zones are far less perfused, yet more easily ventilated.

The risk of an air embolism in head-elevated positions is well established. When a surgical field is located higher than the level of the heart, a subatmospheric pressure differential is established, and air is more easily entrained into open venous channels, with subsequent entry into the central venous system. Current detection techniques are far more sensitive and can diagnose venous air embolism before catastrophic cardiopulmonary events transgress. For an in-depth discussion of venous air embolism, the reader is referred to Young (1994). Facial, tongue, and neck swelling can occur with the sitting position because of malposition of the endotracheal tube or oral airway, extreme neck flexion, or any condition that leads to decreased venous or lymphatic drainage.

The classic sitting position is shown in Fig. 24–16. A full description and explanation of this highly specialized position are beyond the scope of this chapter, and only the basic elements of the posture are outlined. The cervical, thoracic, and lumbar spine should be aligned.

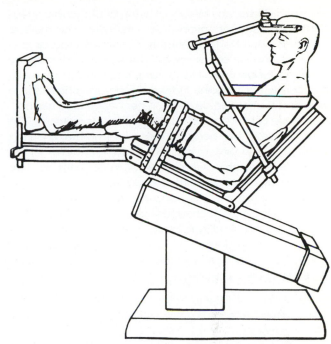

Figure 24–16. Park bench position. Head in skeletal holder, legs flexed and at heart level, with support hose to thigh level. Access to anterior thoracic wall. *(From Morgan, G. E., & Mikhail, M. S. [1996]. Clinical anesthesiology [2nd ed., p.455]. Stamford, CT: Appleton & Lange. Adapted with permission.)*

There are a wide variety of head-holding devices available; the frame is usually attached to the back section of the table so the head can be lowered rapidly, if required. The legs are positioned at the level of the heart and slightly flexed at the knees. The footboard should be padded and adjusted to prevent plantar flexion. Arms are crossed in the patient's lap with elbows flexed at 90 degrees or less to give the anesthetist access to intravascular lines and monitors. Access to the anterior thoracic wall also is maintained for monitoring and maneuvers related to a significant embolic event. Sufficient padding should be placed under the buttocks, knees, heels, and elbows.

▶ CASE STUDY

A 65-year-old female is scheduled for a left total hip arthroplasty. Her medical history is significant for hypertensive disease, well controlled with an ACE inhibitor. She denies any prior history of myocardial infarction, chest pain, or dyspnea on exertion; her exercise tolerance is difficult to ascertain because of the osteoarthritic pain she has been experiencing in her left hip. However, she used to tolerate moderate physical activity well. She has a remote smoking history (stopped smoking 20 years ago) and denies any history of asthma, bronchitis, pneumonia, or frequent urinary tract infections. Her medical history is negative for diabetes, peripheral vascular disease, or hepatic or neurologic disease. She denies any bleeding tendencies. Her osteoarthritis is symptomatic primarily in her hip joint. However, she does have some pain and decreased dexterity in her hands. She has normal range of motion and no pain in her cervical spine. On physical exam her heart sounds were normal and lung fields clear. Her airway was MP Class II, with normal TM distance. Laboratory values are within normal limits. Her chest x-ray revealed normal heart size and essentially clear lung fields. Her ECG showed normal sinus rhythm with nonspecific ST changes in the lateral leads. She weighs 65 kg, and her body mass index is 25. The patient will undergo a combination of epidural–general endotracheal anesthetic (ED–GETA) in the right lateral decubitus position.

1. Why is an ED–GETA technique appropriate (in the lateral decubitus position) for this procedure in this patient?

A regional anesthetic for total hip arthroplasties is preferred by both surgeons and anesthetists because of its clearly established benefits: decreased blood loss, decreased risk of thromboembolism, provision of postoperative analgesia, and avoidance of airway manipulation. However, placing the patient in the lateral decubitus position in an awake state often becomes very uncomfortable after 1 to 2 hours because of pressure on the patient's downside. Arthritic disease may increase the potential for discomfort. Furthermore, although an ED block at the level of the T10 dermatome is sufficient to relieve surgical pain, it is conceivable that a higher-level block may be attained in the patient; higher levels may compromise respiratory mechanics, especially in the lateral position. Therefore, the establishment of GETA at the onset (with the patient's airway accessible in the supine position) will obviate the need for airway manipulation in the lateral position and will prevent the patient from experiencing any degree of discomfort during the procedure. This particular patient appears to have a normal airway and a reasonable degree of cardiopulmonary reserve, making the benefits of GETA in this situation an acceptable risk. A caveat with the combined ED–GETA technique is that the potential for significant hypotension is increased; general anesthesia usually is kept at the minimal possible level.

2. What special respiratory function concerns does the lateral decubitus position entail?

The decrease in the patient's respiratory mechanics already has been mentioned. The use of positive pressure ventilation (PPV) certainly compensates for the decrease in the lung volumes. In addition, the anesthetized, paralyzed patient with a closed chest in the lateral position exhibits the potential for hypoxia due to V/Q mismatch. The lower (downside) lung is underventilated and relatively overperfused. Simultaneously, the upper lung is overventilated (increased compliance) and underperfused. Again, PPV delivered with an adequate inspired oxygen tension helps prevent a hypoxic state. After the patient is intubated, no muscle relaxants should be necessary from a surgical point of view as the epidural anesthetic provides a motor block. Keeping the diaphragm unparalyzed helps to decrease the V/Q mismatch of the lateral position.

Because this patient does not appear to have active pulmonary disease, one may hope that there will be no perioperative respiratory problems. However, total hip arthroplasties tend to promote large blood loss and overzealous fluid replacement could manifest as pulmonary congestion. Judicious management of fluids and ventilatory parameters will help prevent the occurrence of problems.

3. What risk factors does this patient exhibit for peripheral nerve injury? Which peripheral nerves are at risk for injury in the lateral decubitus position and why? What preventive measures must be taken for each nerve at risk?

With the exception of increasing age, this patient does not possess other risk factors identified for nerve injury. Her smoking history is noncontributory, and she does not have diabetes or peripheral vascular disease; her body mass index is well within normal range. In this case the position itself imposes the greatest risk for nerve damage.

In the lateral decubitus position the brachial plexus is at especially high risk for both compression and stretch injuries. Compression of the downside arm's brachial plexus occurs if the lower shoulder and arm are allowed to remain directly under the rib cage after assuming the lateral position. Proper placement of a chest pad (a device of sufficient bulk to support the chest wall, positioned just caudal to the axilla) is extremely helpful in preventing this complication. The upside arm's brachial plexus also is at risk for a stretch injury if upper-arm abduction is greater than 90 degrees or if cervical spine alignment is not properly attained. Excessive dorsal extension and lateral flexion of the neck cause the angle between the head and shoulder tip to widen, resulting in a stretched nerve bundle. Damage to the brachial plexus implies possible neurologic deficit to the nerves distal to the axilla. In addition, the ulnar and median nerves can be damaged by improper or careless management of the forearm of the downside arm.

In the lateral decubitus position the common

peroneal nerve in the lower extremity is at risk of injury because of inadequate padding between the lateral aspect of the downside leg and the operating table surface.

Excessive pressure can damage the facial nerve and its branches. Another devastating, but preventable, complication is retinal artery thrombosis. The proper choice and placement of the head support plus frequent monitoring of the downside eye is the best preventive measure for this complication.

4. Given the potential for hemodynamic instability (surgical blood loss in addition to position-related blood flow redistribution), where are blood pressure monitoring devices best placed?

The decision to use a direct blood pressure measurement via an intraarterial catheter (A-line) in addition to a noninvasive blood pressure device (NIBP) will depend on the customary practice of the institution and practitioner preference. This particular patient does not exhibit significant exercise-limiting cardiac or pulmonary disease, therefore the risk of an A-line placement might not balance the benefits (beat-to-beat measure of blood pressure, access for intraoperative lab draws) gained. However, the distinct possibilities for hypotensive events due to the anesthetic technique, the potential for blood loss, and the possible use of methylmethacrylate cement to place the prosthesis make a strong argument for placing an A-line.

Irrespective of the monitoring options chosen, the following principles are helpful in placing the monitor. Discrepancies (5–20 mmHg) between the readings of direct and indirect methods of blood pressure measurement are common; the direct A-line readings are invariably higher. Theoretically, the accuracy of the A-line readings should not be influenced by the choice of arm in which the line is placed. It is the placement of the calibrated transducer at the level of the heart that confers the veracity of the reading. Many practitioners prefer to use the radial artery of the downside arm for cannulation because its placement on an armboard allows the volar surface of the wrist to be exposed and the arm is placed on a stable, protected, and visible surface.

Many practitioners will place the NIBP cuff on the upside arm to eliminate any inaccuracy that a compressed axillary artery may transfer to a cuff reading. There often is a discrepancy between the NIBP readings in the upside versus the downside arm. Blood pressure measurements in the upside arm often are too low, which decreases the risk of unrecognized hypotension, making it another reason to place the cuff on the upside arm. From a practical point of view, the upper arm is the most accessible to monitor continually for proper cuff placement.

The clinical usefulness of a central venous line with monitoring (CVP line) in this situation also is debatable. The accuracy of a CVP reading in the lateral position is questionable because the usual external reference point for placement of the transducer is difficult to define and utilize consistently. The monitoring of CVP trends may be of benefit in this position.

▶ SUMMARY

All of the common surgical positions are potentially harmful because of both the cardiopulmonary challenges they present to an anesthetized patient and the peripheral nerve injuries they may cause. It is essential for the anesthetist to understand the physiologic basis of the hazards of positioning to protect the patient, while optimizing access to the operative site.

The ability to establish surgical positions in a safe and timely fashion entails both theoretical and practical knowledge regarding each position, planning and organizational skills, a consistent attention to detail, and the ability to coordinate the activities of the personnel involved in positioning the patient. Acceptable patient outcomes require continuous vigilance, with an eye for some of the positioning complications that tend to occur in long surgical procedure.

Positioning the patient in some of the routine surgical postures often becomes viewed as a mundane task, one in which a standard of care might easily be overlooked or omitted by any member of the positioning team. The anesthetist should assume the role of the enforcer of the standards of quality care.

▶ KEY CONCEPTS

• The most significant cardiovascular changes associated with positioning are related to the varying gravitational effects on the circulatory system. The normal autonomic reflexes that redistribute blood flow and provide circulatory homeostasis during posture changes are depressed under anesthesia, predisposing the patient to hypotension. Cardiovascular insults related to repositioning can be minimized or eliminated by implementing all position changes gradually and smoothly, with appropriate adjustments of anesthetic depth and intravascular volume prior to the change.

• The most significant pulmonary changes associated with positioning are related to the varying gravitational effects on respiratory mechanics and lung volumes. The most common surgical positions (supine and lithotomy) increase the work of breathing and decrease functional residual capacity and vital capacity in an awake state; anesthesia and muscle relaxation further diminish these lung volumes. Varying degrees of V/Q mismatch occur under anesthesia in most surgical positions. In most circumstances, positive pressure ventilation via an endotracheal tube adequately compensates for these alterations in respiratory function.

• A complete preanesthetic evaluation of positioning issues enables the anesthetist to incorporate into an anesthetic plan a pharmacologic strategy and logical sequence of events to establish the desired position. A thorough evaluation includes (1) the patient's habitus, cardiopulmonary reserve, and risk factors for peripheral neuropathies; (2) a precise understanding of the intent of the surgical procedure and how it relates to the position(s); and (3) the number of personnel available for assisting in positioning and the distinct roles assigned to each individual.

• Peripheral nerve injuries constitute the most common serious perioperative complication related to positioning. The relaxed state of muscles and ligaments under anesthesia, coupled with the unconscious patient's inability to perceive or communicate the feeling of discomfort caused by impending nerve damage, are the factors that place certain nerves at higher risk of injury. The nerves most vulnerable to injury are the brachial plexus, the ulnar and radial nerves, and the common peroneal nerve. Positioning and protecting the vulnerable nerve groups from traction, compression, or ischemia are the best ways to prevent neuropathies.

• Laparoscopy for intraabdominal procedures is used with increasing frequency. These procedures frequently require placing patients in lithotomy, often with the intermittent use of a steep head-down tilt. The presence of a pneumoperitoneum (abdominal insufflation of gas) potentiates the possibility of cardiovascular problems related to the lithotomy, head-down position. A patient's ability to tolerate this combination of physiologic challenges should be accurately assessed prior to instituting extreme degrees of any of these positions.

• Proper positioning of a patient entails a coordinated group effort. When establishing some of the more complex variations of the lateral, prone, or sitting positions, the anesthetist generally assumes the role of coordinator, taking responsibility for the timing, pace, and overall sequencing of the positioning maneuvers.

▶ STUDY QUESTIONS

1. What are the six tenets of proper positioning?

2. What factors can be identified during the preanesthetic evaluation that may place the patient at an increased risk for problems related to positioning?

3. What impact does posture have on the physiology of the cardiovascular, respiratory, gastrointestinal, and muscular systems?

4. What are the mechanisms of peripheral nerve injury associated with positioning, and which nerves are more commonly injured?

5. What are the concerns, advantages, and disadvantages of the commonly employed surgical positions, particularly in perianesthetic management?

KEY REFERENCES

Biddle, C., & Caunady, M. (1990). Surgical positions, their effect on cardiovascular, respiratory systems. *AORN Journal, 52*(2), 350–359.

Dornette, W. H. L. (1986). Compression neuropathies: medical aspects and legal implications. *International Anesthesiology Clinics, 24*(4), 201–220.

Martin, J. T., & Warner, M. A. (Eds.). (1997). *Positioning in anesthesia and surgery* (3rd ed.). Philadelphia: Saunders.

Walsh, J. (1994). AANA Journal Course: Update for nurse anesthetists—Patient positioning. *AANA Journal, 62*(3), 289–298.

REFERENCES

Alvine, F. G., & Schurrer, M. E. (1987). Postoperative Ulnar-Nerve Palsy. *Journal of Bone and Joint Surgery (Am), 69-A*(2), 255–259.

Babka, J. C., Hager, G. W., & Castell, D. O. (1973). Effect of body posture on lower esophageal sphincter pressure. *American Journal of Digestive Disease, 18*, 441–442.

Backofen, J. E., & Schauble, J. F. (1985). Hemodynamic changes with prone position during general anesthesia [abstract]. *Anesthesia & Analgesia, 64*, 194.

Battillo, J. A., & Hendler, M. A. (1993). Effects of patient positioning during anesthesia. *International Anesthesiology Clinics, 31*(1), 67–86.

Biddle, C., & Caunady, M. (1990). Surgical positions, their effect on cardiovascular, respiratory systems. *AORN Journal 52*(2), 350–359.

Britt, B. A., & Gordon, R. A. (1964). Peripheral nerve injuries associated with anesthesia. *Canadian Anaesthesia Society Journal, 11*, 514–536.

Cohen, E. (Ed.). (1995). *The practice of thoracic anesthesia.* Philadelphia: Lippincott.

Colvin, M. P. (1987). Patient position. In T. H. Taylor & E. Major (Eds.), *Hazards and complications of anesthesia* (pp. 379–391). New York: Churchill Livingstone.

Cooper, D. E., Jenkins, R. S., Bready, L., & Rockwood, C. A., Jr. (1988). The prevention of injuries of the brachial plexus secondary to malposition of the patient during surgery. *Clinical Orthopedics and Related Research, 228*, 33–41.

Courington, F. W., & Little, D. M., Jr. (1968). The role of posture in anesthesia. *Clinical Anesthesia, 3*, 24–54.

Dawson, D. M., & Krarup, C. (1989). Perioperative nerve lesions. *Neurological Review, 46*, 1355–1359.

Dutton, A. C. (1933). The effects of posture during anesthesia. *Anesthesia & Analgesia, 12*, 66–74.

Dylewsky, W., & McAlpine, F. S. (1997). Peripheral nervous system. In J. T. Martin & M. A. Warner (Eds.), *Positioning in anesthesia and surgery* (3rd ed., pp. 299–318). Philadelphia: Saunders.

Eggers, G. W. N., DeGroot, W. J., Tanner, C. R., & Leonard, J. J. (1963). Hemodynamic changes associated with various surgical positions. *Journal of the American Medical Association, 185*, 1–5.

Froese, A. B., & Bryan, A. C. (1974). Effects of anesthesia and paralysis on diaphragmatic mechanics in man. *Anesthesiology, 41*, 242–255.

Hanson, M. R., Breuer, A. C., Furlan, A. J., et al. (1983). Mechanism and frequency of brachial plexus injury in open-heart surgery: A prospective analysis. *Annals of Thoracic Surgery, 36*, 675–679.

Harris, S. N., Ballantyne, G. H., Luther, M. A., & Perrino, A. C. (1996). Alterations of cardiovascular performance during laparoscopic colectomy: A combined hemodynamic and echocardiographic analysis. *Anesthesia & Analgesia, 83*, 482–487.

Henschel, A. B., Wyant, G. M., Dobkin, A. B., & Henschel, E. O. (1957). Posture as it concerns the anesthesiologist: A preliminary study. *Anesthesia & Analgesia, 36*, 69–76.

Hicks, E. R., & Koerbacher, K. C. (1992). Positioning for anesthesia and surgery. In W. R. Waugaman, S. D. Foster, & B. M. Rigor (Eds.), *Principles and practice of nurse anesthesia* (2nd ed., pp. 221–232). Norwalk, CT: Appleton & Lange.

Hirvonen, E. A., Nuutinen, L. S., & Kauko, M. (1995). Ventilatory effects, blood gas changes, and oxygen consumption during laparoscopic hysterectomy. *Anesthesia & Analgesia, 80*, 961–966.

Hulme-Moir, I., Donnan, S. P., McAlister, J., & McColl, I. (1973). Effect of surgery and posture on the pattern and rate of gastric emptying. *Australian and New Zealand Journal of Surgery, 43*, 80–84.

Inglis, J. M., & Brooke, B. N. (1956). Trendelenburg tilt: An obsolete position. *British Medical Journal (London), II*, 343–344.

Jenkins, L. C. (1968). The interaction of drugs with particular reference for anesthetic practice. *Canadian Anaesthesia Society Journal, 15*, 111–117.

Johannsen, G., Andersen, M., & Juhl, B. (1989). The effect of general anesthesia on the haemodynamic events during laparoscopy with CO_2 insufflation. *Acta Anaesthesiology Scandinavica, 33*, 132–136.

Jones, J. R., & Jacoby, J. (1955). The effect of surgical positions on respiration. *Surgery Forum, 5*, 686–691.

Korner, P. I. (1971). Integrative neural cardiovascular control. *Physiology Review, 51*, 312–367.

Kroll, D. A., Caplan, R. A., Posner, K., Ward, R. J., & Cheney, F. W. (1990). Nerve injury associated with anesthesia. *Anesthesiology, 73*, 202–207.

Lawson, N. W., & Meyer, D. J. (1997). Lateral decubitus positions. In J. T. Martin & M. A. Warner (Eds.), *Positioning in anesthesia and surgery* (3rd ed., pp. 127–152). Philadelphia: Saunders.

Lederman, R. J., Breuer, A. C., Hanson, M. R., Furlan, A. J., Loop, F. D., Cosgrove, D. M., Estafanous, F. G., & Greenstreet, R. L. (1982). Peripheral nervous system complications of coronary artery bypass graft surgery. *Annals of Neurology, 12,* 297–301.

Little, D. M. (1960). Posture and anesthesia. *Canadian Anaesthesia Society Journal, 7,* 2–15.

Lumb, A. B., & Nunn, J. F. (1991). Respiratory function and rib cage contribution to ventilation in body positions commonly used during anesthesia. *Anesthesia & Analgesia, 73,* 422–426.

Martin, J. T. (1992). Compartment syndromes: Concepts and perspectives for the anesthesiologist. *Anesthesia & Analgesia, 75,* 275–283.

Martin, J. T. (1997a). Head-down tilt. In J. T. Martin & M. A. Warner (Eds.), *Positioning in anesthesia and surgery* (3rd ed., pp. 95–124). Philadelphia: Saunders.

Martin, J. T. (1997b). Lithotomy positions. In J. T. Martin & M. A. Warner (Eds.), *Positioning in anesthesia and surgery* (3rd ed., pp. 47–70). Philadelphia: Saunders.

Martin, J. T. (1997c). The ventral decubitus (prone) positions. In J. T. Martin & M. A. Warner (Eds.), *Positioning in anesthesia and surgery* (3rd ed., pp. 155–196). Philadelphia: Saunders.

Martin, J. T. & Warner, M. A. (Eds). (1997). *Positioning in anesthesia and surgery* (3rd ed.). Philadelphia: Saunders.

Milde, L. N. (1997). The head-elevated positions. In J. T. Warner & M. A. Warner (Eds.), *Positioning in surgery and anesthesia* (3rd ed., pp. 71–94). Philadelphia: Saunders.

Nakata, D. A., & Stoelting, R. K. (1997). Positioning the extremities. In J. T. Martin & M. A. Warner (Eds.), *Positioning in anesthesia and surgery* (3rd ed., pp. 199–222). Philadelphia: Saunders.

O'Brien, T. J., & Ebert, T. J. (1997). Physiologic changes associated with the supine position. In J. T. Martin & M. A. Warner (Eds.), *Positioning in anesthesia and surgery* (3rd ed., pp. 27–36). Philadelphia: Saunders.

Pae, E-K., Lowe, A. A., Sasaki, K., Price, C., Tsuchiya, M., & Fleetham, J. A. (1994). A cephalometric and electromyographic study of upper airway structures in the upright and supine positions. *American Journal of Orthodontics and Dentofacial Orthopedics, 106,* 52–59.

Parks, B. J. (1973). Postoperative peripheral neuropathies. *Surgery, 74,* 348–357.

Pelosi, P., Croci, M., Calapi, E., Mulazzi, D., Cerisara, M., Vercesi, P., Vicardi, P., & Gattinoni, L. (1995). The prone positioning during general anesthesia minimally affects respiratory mechanics while improving functional residual capacity and increasing oxygen tension. *Anesthesia & Analgesia, 80,* 955–960.

Pelosi, P., Croci, M., Calappi, E., Mulazzi, D., Cerisara, M., Vercesi, P., Vicardi, P., & Gattinoni, L. (1996). Prone positioning improves pulmonary function in obese patients during general anesthesia. *Anesthesia & Analgesia, 83,* 578–583.

Reich, D. L., Konstadt, S. N., Raissi, S., Hubbard, M., & Thys, D. M. (1989). Trendelenburg position and passive leg raising do not significantly improve cardiopulmonary performance in the anesthetized patient with coronary artery disease. *Critical Care Medicine, 17*(4), 313–317.

St. Paul Medical Services. (1994, July). *Nurse Anesthetist Update—A Special Report from The St. Paul.* St. Paul, MN: Author.

St. Paul Medical Services. (1997, July). *Nurse Anesthetist Update—A Special Report from The St. Paul.* St. Paul, MN: Author.

Slocum, H. C., Hoeflich, E. A., & Allen, C. R. (1947). Circulatory and respiratory distress from extreme positions on the operating table. *Surgery, Gynecology, and Obstetrics, 84,* 1051–1058.

Stoelting, R. K. (1993). Postoperative ulnar nerve palsy—Is it a preventable complication? [Editorial.] *Anesthesia & Analgesia, 76,* 7–9.

Wadsworth, T. G. (1974). The cubital tunnel and the external compression syndrome. *Anesthesia & Analgesia, 53,* 303–307.

Walsh, J. (1994). AANA Journal Course: Update for nurse anesthetists—Patient positioning. *AANA Journal, 62*(3), 289–298.

Ward, R. J., Danzinger, F., & Bonica, J. J. (1966). Cardiovascular effects of change of posture. *Aerospace Medicine, 37,* 257–259.

Warner, M. A. (1997). Supine Positions. In J. T. Martin & M. A. Warner (Eds.), *Positioning in anesthesia and surgery* (3rd ed., pp. 39–46). Philadelphia: Saunders.

Warner, M. A., Warner, M. E., & Martin, J. T. (1994). Ulnar neuropathy. *Anesthesiology, 81*(6), 1332–1340.

Warner, M. A., Martin, J. T., Schroeder, D. R., Offord, K. P., & Chute, C. G. (1994). Lower-extremity motor neuropathy associated with surgery performed on patients in a lithotomy position. *Anesthesiology, 81*(1), 6–12.

West, J. B. (1995). *Respiratory physiology—The essentials* (5th ed.). Baltimore: Williams & Wilkins.

Young, M. L. (1994). Posterior fossa: Anesthetic considerations. In J. E. Cottrell & D. S. Smith (Eds.), *Anesthesia and neurosurgery* (3rd ed., pp. 339–363). St. Louis, MO: Mosby.

Airway Management

W. Gray McCall

▶ AIRWAY MANAGEMENT

The airway is a major concern for the anesthesia provider. Regardless of whether the anesthetic is administered as monitored anesthesia care or as general or regional anesthesia, the provider bears full responsibility for maintaining the patient's airway. Airway management is not limited to the operating room suite and may include various areas outside the operating room, such as the emergency room, intensive care unit, or radiology department. The main goal of airway management is to recognize and promptly alleviate airway obstruction and to establish adequate alveolar ventilation.

Anatomy of the Upper Airway

To facilitate airway management and avoid potential obstacles, an understanding of the upper airway anatomy is essential. The upper airway consists of the nose, mouth, pharynx (nasopharynx, oropharynx, laryngopharynx), and larynx (Fig. 25–1). Both a nasal airway or a nasotracheal tube can be introduced into the nasal passageway to facilitate ventilation. The major nasal air passage lies beneath the inferior turbinate or conchae, which is covered with highly vascular mucous membrane. Before inserting a nasotracheal tube, a vasoconstrictor, such as cocaine or neosynephrine, should be administered to decrease the likelihood of epistaxis. Complications associated with use of the nasal passageway for airway management are:

1. Resistance to advancement due to
   a. Hypertrophied inferior turbinate
   b. Deviated nasal septum
2. Disruption of delicate nasal mucosa
3. Shearing of
   a. Adenoid tissue in children
   b. Tumor or polyps
4. Spread of infection to paranasal sinuses or lower respiratory tract
5. Puncture of soft palate
6. Puncture through mucosa of posterior nasopharyngeal wall

Once a nasal airway or nasotracheal tube passes through the posterior nare or choanae, the nasopharynx is entered. The nasopharynx communicates with the oropharynx. Located within the nasopharynx, in the path of a nasal airway or nasotracheal tube, lie the pharyngeal tonsils, more commonly referred to as the adenoids. More prominent in the pediatric patient, these tissues can hypertrophy to the point of interfering with air passage through the nasopharynx. This may predispose the patient to an obstructed airway once induction of anesthesia is initiated. When advancing the nasal airway or nasotracheal tube, avoid excessive forward pressure, which could potentially result in epistaxis and/or shearing of soft tissue.

The mouth is the other primary opening of the respiratory system. It is separated from the nasal cavity by the hard and soft palate. The combination of the soft and hard palate forms the floor of the nasal cavity and the roof of the oral cavity. When using the oral route for airway management, damage to the teeth, tongue, or lips can easily occur, primarily when pinching the tongue or lips between an oral airway and the teeth. During the preanesthetic evaluation, close attention should be paid to the teeth. If a loose tooth is present, inform the patient and, if the patient is a child, the parent and doc-

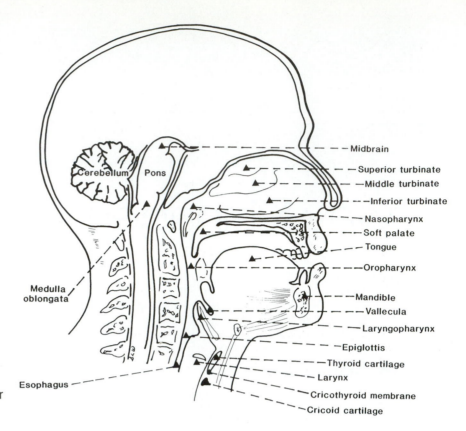

Figure 25–1. Sagittal section illustrating upper airway and superior portion of lower airway.

ument the abnormality in the medical record. At this time permission may be sought to pull the tooth or the child and parent should be advised of the possibility of accidental dislodgment. The presence of orthodontic appliances or dental prothesis must be established prior to induction. If a tooth or component of an orthodontic appliance or prothesis becomes dislodged during anesthesia, it must be recovered. If it cannot be located in the oral cavity, an x-ray must be taken to help establish the location of the tooth or appliance. If aspiration occurs, the tooth must be removed immediately, and bronchoscopy may be required to retrieve the foreign body in the airway.

The oropharynx extends from the soft palate to the base of the lingual surface of the epiglottis. Anatomical structures utilized as landmarks by the endoscopist include the soft palate, tongue, vallecula, and epiglottis. The palatine tonsils are located in the oropharynx and can increase in size, resulting in partial airway obstruction. The view of the endoscopist can be obscured by enlarged palatine tonsils. With severe enlargement of the palatine tonsils, the resultant partial airway obstruction can be confused with the signs and symptoms of epiglottitis. The second, third, and fourth cervical vertebrae are posterior to the oropharynx in adults. The laryngopharynx extends from the base of the tongue, at the level of the hyoid bone, to the opening of the esophagus, at the level of the cricoid cartilage. The fifth and sixth cervical

vertebrae are posterior to the laryngopharynx. The larynx is ventral to the laryngopharynx, which is continuous with the esophagus. The sensory innervation of the pharynx is through the glossopharyngeal nerve; motor innervation is through the vagus nerve.

The larynx is located in the anterior neck at the level of the third through the sixth cervical vertebrae. It extends from the laryngeal entrance to the lower border of the cricoid cartilage (located over the sixth cervical vertebra in adults). The larynx is composed of three unpaired cartilages and three paired cartilages (Fig. 25–2). The unpaired cartilages include the thyroid cartilage, the cricoid cartilage, and the epiglottis. The thyroid cartilage is the largest cartilage and is V-shaped. The anterior prominence of the thyroid is often called the Adam's apple. The thyroid cartilage is attached to the hyoid bone by the thyrohyoid membrane and to the cricoid cartilage by the cricothyroid membrane. The thyroid cartilage is the anterior attachment for the vocal cords. The cricoid cartilage consists of a ring that broadens into a platelike structure to form the lower and posterior border of the larynx. The cricoid cartilage is the only complete ring in the larynx and the narrowest portion of the upper airway in the pediatric patient. The epiglottis projects obliquely upward behind the tongue and in front of the entrance to the larynx. It covers the glottic opening to prevent entrance of solids and/or liquids into the airway during swallowing and respiration. The paired cartilages

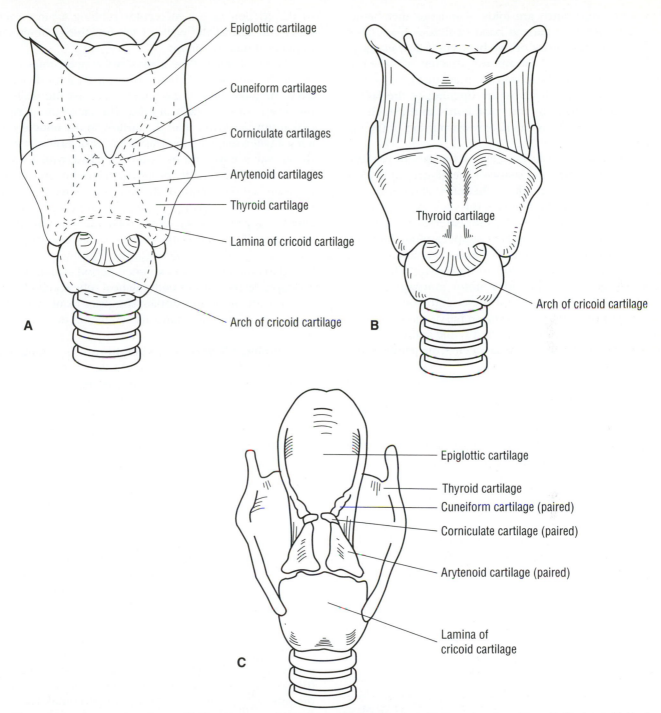

Figure 25–2. Laryngeal cartilages. (**A**) The nine laryngeal cartilages. (**B**) Anterior view. (**C**) Posterior view. *(From Hollinshead, W. H., & Rosse, C. [1985]. Textbook of Anatomy [4th ed., p. 51]. Philadelphia: Harper & Row.)*

are the arytenoid, corniculate, and cuneiform cartilages. The arytenoid cartilages are pyramidal in shape, sit on the cricoid cartilage, and each has a muscular process that is the insertion of the posterior and lateral cricoarytenoids. Each has a vocal process that is the posterior attachment of the vocal cords. The corniculate cartilages are cone-shaped structures situated in the posterior part of the aryepiglottic folds. Each is attached to the apex of an arytenoid cartilage. The cuneiform cartilages are elongated structures located slightly posterior to the corniculates at the base of the epiglottis.

Other structures located within the trachea include the aryepiglottic folds, which are folds of mucous membrane attaching the arytenoid cartilages to the epiglottis.

The false vocal cords are folds of mucous membrane, each attached to a narrow band of fibrous tissue. The true vocal cords consist of two bands of yellow elastic fibrous tissue. As noted, the anterior attachment is the thyroid cartilage and the posterior attachment is the arytenoids. The rima glottis is the opening of the larynx surrounded laterally by the vocal cords. In the adult airway, the rima glottis is the narrowest portion of the upper airway.

The nine intrinsic muscles of the larynx regulate and control the size and shape of the glottis. Table 25–1 lists their function and effect. The innervation of the larynx is composed of branches of the vagus nerve. The superior laryngeal nerve divides into external and internal branches. The external branch supplies motor innervation to the cricothyroid muscles, and the internal branch provides sensory innervation to the larynx. The recurrent laryngeal nerve provides motor innervation to all muscles of the larynx, except the cricothyroid muscles. Damage to the recurrent laryngeal nerve can occur during operative procedures on the thyroid and/or parathyroid glands. If unilateral damage occurs, the patient's presenting symptom will be hoarseness. If bilateral damage occurs, complete airway obstruction will occur and will require a tracheostomy or endotracheal intubation.

The trachea is a cartilaginous and membranous tube extending from the cords to the bifurcation at the carina to form the right and left mainstem bronchi. The trachea lies anterior to the esophagus, is protected anteriorly with cartilaginous rings, and its posterior wall is membranous. The average distance from the incisors to the vocal cords is 13 cm and the average distance from the vocal cords to the carina is 13 cm in the adult patient. The length of the upper airway has an impact on the distance the endotracheal tube can be advanced once the tip of the tube has passed between the vocal cords.

Physics of Airflow

The two main properties of gas flow within a tube are laminar flow and turbulent flow. Airway resistance is due to the friction of gas molecules rubbing against each other and against the walls of the breathing circuit, endotracheal tube, or airway.

During laminar flow, airway resistance comes from the molecules of gas rubbing or hitting each other and from the molecules of gas rubbing against the walls of the airway or endotracheal tube. Therefore, the peripheral airflow is slower than the airflow in the middle, creating a bullet-shaped flow. This behavior of airflow within the airway is governed by Poiseuille's Law, which states that resistance is directly proportional to the viscosity of the fluid and the length of the tube and is inversely proportional to the fourth power of the radius of the tube. During procedures such as microlaryngoscopy, utilizing an endotracheal tube with a small internal diameter, the increased resistance to flow can be a problem when allowed to continue for an extended period of time. When appropriate, the smaller endotracheal tube should be replaced with one of appropriate size prior to allowing the patient to attempt spontaneous ventilation during emergence.

Turbulent flow occurs when Reynold's number exceeds 2000. Reynold's number is a dimensionless number equal to the density of the fluid times the velocity of the fluid times the diameter of the tube divided by the viscosity of the fluid. Turbulent flow is a very chaotic and inefficient airflow pattern. In branching or irregular tubes or in very high flow in smooth tubes, the flow pattern results from laminar to turbulent flow. The critical flow rate is the point beyond which flow cannot be laminar because the frictional forces prevent the flow from being laminar. This concept is analogous to electrical resistance as described by Ohm's law. The flow of anesthetic gases in a 9-mm internal diameter endotracheal tube becomes turbulent when the flow exceeds approximately 9 L/min; the flow in a 15-mm-diameter trachea becomes turbulent at flows exceeding 15 L/min; and in the 22-mm internal diameter tubing of a breathing system, flow becomes turbulent when it exceeds 22 L/min. (Davis, Parbrook, & Kenny, 1995).

When a gas or a liquid flows within a tube, pressure is exerted against the side of the tube. As the speed of the flow increases, the pressure exerted on the walls of the tube will lessen. This is known as Bernoulli's law, and it applies to airway management when a venturi tube is utilized, as with atomizers and nebulizers when delivering drugs and aerosols or for humidifying anesthetic gases (Le Bel, 1992).

Airway Assessment

Routine evaluation of a patient's airway should include a review of the previous medical history and any airway difficulty encountered during previous general anesthesia. In assessing the airway of a patient, the patient should be viewed from the lateral and anterolateral posi-

TABLE 25–1. Muscles of the Larynx

Muscle	Function	Effect on Vocal Cords
Posterior cricoarytenoids (2)	Rotate arytenoids outward	Abduction
Lateral cricoarytenoids (2)	Rotate arytenoids inward	Adduction
Arytenoid (1)	Approximate arytenoids	Adduction
Thyroarytenoids (2)	Draw arytenoids forward	Relax and shorten
Cricothyroids (2)	Draw up arch of cricoid and tilt back its lamina	Tense and elongate

tions, and the neck should be palpated anteriorly and laterally. In addition, the patient should be instructed to extend his or her neck maximally. The mouth opening, teeth, and oral cavity also need to be inspected. Lateral neck x-rays or indirect laryngoscopy with a dental mirror may be useful diagnostic adjuncts.

Pharyngeal grading should be done with the patient seated opening his mouth as wide as possible and extending his tongue as far forward as possible while the observer looks at the patient at eye level and inspects the pharyngeal structures (Fig. 25–3). It is controversial whether or not the patient should phonate during the pharyngeal grading. In addition, if the patient arches the tongue, the view of the uvula will be obscured. The following lists the pharyngeal grading system proposed by Samsoon and Young (1987):

Grade I.   Soft palate, uvula, and pillars visible
Grade II.   Pillars obscured by base of tongue, but posterior pharyngeal wall visible below soft palate
Grade III. Soft palate only visible, posterior pharyngeal wall not seen
Grade IV.   Soft palate not visible

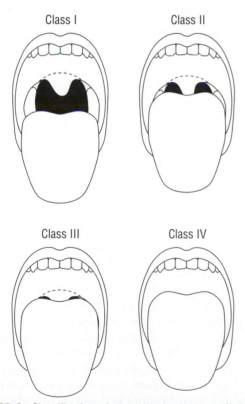

Figure 25–3. Classification of pharyngeal structures. Note that in Class III the soft palate is visible, but in Class IV it is not. *(From Samsoon, G. L. T. & Young, J. R. B. [1987]. "Difficult tracheal intubation: A retrospective study."* Anaesthesia, 42, *487. Copyright 1987 by Academic Press, London, and WB Saunders, London. Reprinted with permission.)*

One of the greatest criticisms of pharyngeal grading has been the problem of interobserver variation. In addition, pharyngeal grading has been shown in various studies to have a high false-positive rate that detracts from its usefulness. Frerk (1991) in his investigation of predicting difficult intubation, thought the combination of a second test in addition to pharyngeal grading was more successful in predicting difficult intubations. This second test consisted of measuring the thyromental distance with the head fully extended. The distance is measured between the prominence of the thyroid cartilage and the bony point of the chin. It is important when performing this test to ensure that the head is maximally extended to ensure reproducibility. The position also gives a measure of head extension that may be another important factor of importance in determining the ease or difficulty of intubation. The predictive value of pharyngeal grading alone resulted in a 43% false-positive rate ($n = 244$; Frerk, 1991). The predictive value of thyromental distance alone, taking a distance of 7 cm or less as a predictor of difficult intubation, resulted in a false-positive rate of 43%. When these two methods were combined, the false-positive rate was found to be 5% in the 244 patients participating in the study (Frerk, 1991). In patients who have both a pharyngeal grade of III or IV and a short thyromental distance (receding chin), intubation may prove to be difficult or not possible at all.

Benumof (1992) suggests three simple maneuvers to assess the airway: (1) the amount of space the tongue occupies in the pharynx; (2) the size of mandibular space (between the hyoid bone and the inner aspect of the mandible); and (3) the atlantooccipital extension. When the patient opens her mouth, does the tongue obscure the tip of the uvula and are the tonsillar pillars visible? If two fingers cannot fit between the hyoid bone and the inner aspect of the mandible, the probability that the larynx is anteriorly located is high. Being able to assume the sniffing position suggests that the oral, pharyngeal, and laryngeal axes can be aligned in a straight line. Table 25–2 lists factors characterizing the normal airway in adolescents and adults (Finucane & Santora, 1996).

If nasal intubation is planned, the nose should be examined. Potential anatomical abnormalities increasing the potential of complications and/or the level of difficulty of nasal endotracheal intubation include a deviated nasal septum or nasal polyps. To ascertain whether one nostril is more patent than the other, the patient should be instructed to blow forcefully through one nostril while the other is occluded. If appropriate, use the nostril with the least amount of obstruction first during the nasal endotracheal intubation.

Multiple anatomical factors contribute to the presence of a difficult airway. Table 25–3 lists the anatomic variations encountered in the operating room that can increase the difficulty in establishing an airway. When

TABLE 25–2. Factors Characterizing the Normal Airway in Adolescents and Adults

1. History of one or more easy intubations without sequelae
2. Normal-appearing face with "regular" features
3. Normal clear voice
4. Absence of scars, burns, swelling, infection, tumor, or hematoma; no history of radiation therapy to head or neck
5. Ability to lie supine asymptomatically; no history of snoring or sleep apnea
6. Patent nares
7. Ability to open mouth widely with temporomandibular joint rotation and subluxation (3 to 4 cm or two to three fingerbreadths)
8. Mallampati/Samsoon Class I
9. At least 6.5 cm (three fingerbreadths) from tip of mandible to thyroid notch with neck extended
10. At least 9 cm from symphysis of mandible to mandibular angle
11. Slender supple neck without masses; full range of neck motion
12. Larynx movable with swallowing and manually movable laterally
13. Slender to moderate body build
14. Ability to extend atlantooccipital joint (normal extension is 35°)

Source: Finucane, R. T., & Santora, A. H. (1996). Principles of airway management (p. 109). St. Louis, MO: Mosby. Copyright 1996 by Mosby. Reprinted with permission.

TABLE 25–3. Factors Associated with a Difficult Airway

1. Receding mandible (micrognathia)
   Distance between the lower border of the mandible and thyroid notch less than 6 cm
   Distance between prominence of thyroid cartilage and bony point of chin is less than 7 cm
2. Neck abnormalities
   Short, muscular neck
   Redundant soft tissue in upper airway causing obstruction
   Difficulty in mobilizing neck and tongue
   Rheumatoid arthritis with potential for subluxation
   Fractured, unstable cervical vertebrae
3. Morbid obesity, enlarged breasts, term or near-term pregnancy
4. Advanced rheumatoid arthritis with ankylosing spondylitis of C-spine
5. Protruding maxillary incisors and relative maxillary overgrowth
6. Poor mobility of mandible; mouth opens less than 40 mm or three fingerbreadths
7. Long arched palate associated with long, narrow mouth
8. Floppy epiglottis
9. Large distance from teeth to larynx
10. Short distance between the occiput and the spine of the atlas vertebrae
11. Trauma, deformity, burns, radiation therapy, infection, swelling; hematoma of the face, mouth, pharynx, larynx, and/or neck
12. Male gender
13. Age between 40 and 59 years of age
14. Thoracoabdominal abnormalities; kyphoscoliosis
15. Stridor, hoarseness
16. Inability to lie in supine position

Source: Miller, R. D. (Ed.), (1990), Anesthesia (3rd ed., p.1269). New York: Churchill Livingstone. Copyright 1990 by Churchill Livingstone. Liu, P. L. (Ed.) (1992). Basic principles of anesthesia care (p. 99). Philadelphia: Lippincott. Copyright 1992 by Lippincott. Finucane, B. T., & Santora, A. H. (1996). Principles of airway management (p. 110), St. Louis, MO: Mosby. Copyright 1996 by Mosby. Reprinted with permission.

confronted with a suspected difficult airway, the best option available is the topical anesthesia for the airways, mild sedation of the patient, followed by an awake intubation. If the practitioner is unable to visualize the anatomical structures necessary for direct placement of the endotracheal tube, alternative methods for establishing a secure airway are available. (Please refer to Management of the Difficult Airway.)

Pediatric Airway

Several anatomical features in the pediatric patient may have an impact on intubation. Endotracheal tube cuffs are not necessary in the pediatric patient because the cricoid ring, the narrowest orifice of the airway, provides an anatomical cuff. Upon placement of an uncuffed endotracheal tube, a leak should arise when 10 to 30 cm H_2O of inspiratory pressure is applied in a child 10 years old or less. If a leak occurs at less than 10 cm H_2O, the endotracheal tube needs to be replaced with a half-size larger tube. If a tight fit is present (no leak below 30 cm H_2O), the likelihood of submucosal edema or postintubation croup will be significantly increased. The too-large endotracheal tube should be replaced with one a half-size smaller. In the smaller pediatric airway, a small degree of edema can significantly increase the resistance to airflow. Other anatomical features that are specific to the pediatric patient include large head size relative to body size; a more horizontal, omega-shaped epiglottis; and right and left mainstem bronchi that bifurcate at the same angle. The distance from the lips to the carina in an

infant is approximately 13 cm, compared to 24 cm (female) and 28 cm (male) in the adult patient.

Preparation for Airway Management

When preparing a patient for general anesthesia, preoxygenation should be performed when possible. The theoretical objective of preoxygenation is to provide an oxygen-enriched environment within the functional residual capacity (FRC) of the patient. This can be accomplished by placing the mask over the patient's mouth and nose while monitors are being placed on the patient. Two key concepts of this technique must be kept in mind. First, oxygen must be turned on at the gas machine at a fresh gas flow rate greater than the minute volume of the patient. Second, an airtight seal must be established with the mask. If a leak occurs, entrainment of room air will diminish the efficacy of the maneuver. One reliable sign that preoxygenation is effective is when the reservoir bag moves synchronously with the patient's breathing. If preoxygenation is overlooked during the preparation of a patient prior to general anesthesia, four vital capacity breaths of 100% oxygenation immediately before induction will essentially provide the same reservoir of oxygen within the FRC.

Topicalization of the Upper Airway

Application of topical anesthesia to the upper airway is indicated when an awake intubation is planned or when the cardiovascular response to either laryngoscopy or surgical stimulation of the upper airway is undesirable. Many methods of applying topical anesthesia to the upper airway are available. A gargle of 4% topical lidocaine viscous is effective when only the oropharynx is to be anesthetized. A simple way to apply topical anesthesia to the upper airway is by using prepackaged aerosols. Another technique is to deliver the topical anesthetic via bulb nebulizer; the bulb of the nebulizer can be removed, and oxygen delivered from a flow meter can serve as the propellant (Fig. 25–4). Either 4% topical lidocaine or a combination of 4% topical lidocaine plus 0.5% tetracaine can be used with this type of nebulizer. If nasal intubation is planned, the addition of 1 : 200 000 epinephrine to the local anesthetic will help shrink nasal membranes. The topical anesthetic can be sprayed during slow advancement toward the vocal cords. Once topicalization is complete in the upper airway, the tip of the nebulizer can be curved and then directed toward the glottis. Then the patient should be instructed to take vi-

tal capacity breaths or to breathe in and out as fast as possible while the nebulizer is activated. The volume of either drug to be nebulized is 4 to 5 mL. A mixture of 2.5 mL each of tetracaine and 4% lidocaine or 4% intracardiac lidocaine provides intense surface anesthesia with a rapid onset.

Another simple method for providing surface anesthesia in the upper airway, including the epiglottis and trachea, consists of placing the topical anesthetic in a nebulizer ordinarily used to deliver bronchodilators. If an oral intubation is planned, use the mouthpiece that is provided with the nebulizer. Instruct the patient to take slow, deep breaths through the nebulizer and to exhale through the nose. When the maneuver is properly performed, the "fog" of the nebulized anesthetic can be visualized coming out of the nostrils during exhalation. As illustrated by the "fog" of the nebulized local anesthetic, not all of the local anesthetic is absorbed through the mucous membranes.

The use of 4% lidocaine ointment in the mouth provides good surface anesthesia. Apply a small amount of 4% lidocaine ointment (about the size of a robin's egg) onto the end of a tongue depressor and place it at the base of the patient's tongue. Instruct the patient to allow the ointment to melt into the back of his throat. After several minutes the patient may begin to cough. This is indicative that the patient is aspirating the ointment below the cords. This simple technique is very effective in providing topical anesthesia without using a specific

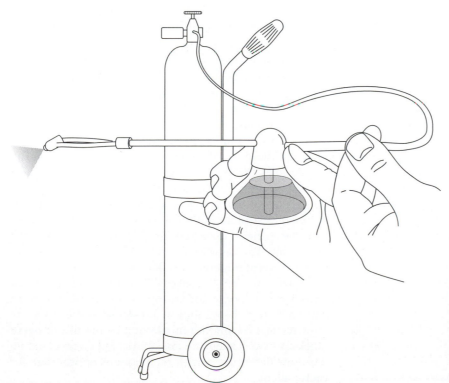

Figure 25–4. System for nebulizing local anesthetic prior to orotracheal or nasotracheal intubation. Digital occlusion of the hole in the oxygen tubing near the atomizer causes a fine mist of local anesthetic to be emitted from the atomizer when oxygen is flowing from the tank. *(From Barash, P. G., Cullen B F., & Stoelting, R. K. [1997]. Clinical anesthesia [3rd ed., p. 584]. Philadelphia: Lippincott-Raven. Copyright 1997 by Lippincott-Raven. Reprinted with permission.)*

piece of equipment, except a tongue depressor. A disadvantage of this technique is the increased amount of oropharyngeal secretions, which need to be suctioned. When performed properly, all of these topical anesthesia techniques can provide adequate anesthesia to the upper airway and can facilitate awake intubations with minimal discomfort to the patient.

The transtracheal block for awake intubations is another form of topical anesthesia. Lidocaine (4% topical) is the drug most frequently used; the total volume injected is 3 to 4 mL. The cricothyroid membrane is located and pierced with either a 23-gauge needle or a 22-gauge intravenous (IV) catheter (Fig. 25-5). During advancement of the needle through the cricothyroid membrane, aspiration of air confirms entrance into the trachea. If an IV catheter is used, advance the catheter to ensure that the catheter is completely within the trachea and then remove the needle and attach the syringe to the catheter. Instruct the patient to take a slow, deep breath, and before the end of inspiration inject the drug. The patient may cough at this point, which facilitates the spread of the local anesthetic upward, bathing the subglottic larynx and trachea. The amount of sedation plus the spread of the previous topical anesthesia will determine the strength of the cough. The transtracheal technique should never be used in the presence of disease or infection in the neck area or when an acute increase in intracranial pressure cannot be tolerated.

In summary, there are several guidelines concerning administration of topical anesthesia: (1) administer an adequate amount of local anesthetic; (2) do not allow secretions and/or blood to pool within the oropharynx; (3) allow time for the local anesthetic to work; and (4) complete the awake intubation, and/or retopicalize prior to the loss of anesthesia.

Nerve blocks

Transtracheal local anesthetic injection combined with glossopharyngeal nerve block and superior laryngeal nerve block can be used to provide intense anesthesia for procedures requiring instrumentation in the oropharynx. The following lists the areas anesthetized by the individual blocks:

> Glossopharyngeal nerve block
>> Posterior third of tongue
>> Uvula
>> Soft palate
>> Pharynx
> Superior laryngeal nerve
>> Laryngeal epiglottis
>> Vallecula
>> Vestibule
>> Aryepiglottic fold
>> Posterior rimaglottidis

The glossopharyngeal nerve block is performed bilaterally with the aid of a tongue depressor or laryngoscope blade depressing the tongue and thus stretching the tonsillar pillars. The laryngoscope blade will provide a source of light. The anatomic landmark is the palatopharyngeal fold (posterior tonsillar pillar). A 25-gauge, 3.5-inch spinal needle is used for this block, unless a glossopharyngeal nerve block needle is available. Direct the spinal needle behind the midpoint of the posterior tonsillar pillar, and aim it laterally and slightly anteriorly (Fig. 25-5). The needle is then inserted approximately 1 cm into the lateral pharyngeal wall and should lie very close to the glossopharyngeal plexus between the superior and middle pharyngeal constrictors. Each injection requires not more than 2 mL of local anesthetic solution. Lidocaine (1% to 2%) or mepivacaine (1% to 1.5%) provides excellent anesthesia for this block. Repeat the same procedure on the opposite side. If blood is aspirated, the block should be abandoned and the patient observed for hematoma formation. In addition to surface anesthesia, the glossopharyngeal nerve block inhibits the afferent limb of the gag reflex produced both by tactile and pressure sensation, but it preserves the patient's ability to swallow voluntarily.

As noted, the superior laryngeal nerve block provides anesthesia to the laryngeal surface of the epiglottis and the larynx down to the vocal cords. The superior laryngeal nerve is blocked as it divides into the smaller external branches and larger internal branch at the level of the superior cornu of the thyroid cartilage. A 23-gauge, 1-inch needle is used to perform this block. Begin by identifying the notch in the midline of the thyroid cartilage. Then move the index finger along the upper border of the thyroid cartilage over the thyrohyoid membrane, and move it laterally until the superior cornu of the thyroid cartilage is palpated. With the index finger tip resting on the superior cornu, the needle is directed immediately anterior to the finger and perpendicular to the skin in all planes (Fig. 25-6). The needle is advanced about 1 to 2 cm until the thyrohyoid membrane is pierced. There is a definite loss of resistance when the needle goes through the cartilage. Inject 2 mL of local anesthetic after careful aspiration. Like the glossopharyngeal nerve block, this block is performed bilaterally. If blood is aspirated, the block should be abandoned and the patient observed for the development of a hematoma. The disadvantages to these nerve blocks are (1) esophageal puncture; (2) damage to surrounding vascular structures; (3) hematoma formation; and (4) patient refusal. Nerve blocks and/or topical anesthesia can work extremely well. Using topical anesthesia (except for the transtracheal technique) in addition to the use of nerve blocks provides adequate anesthesia. Experience and indications determine which technique is appropriate for each patient.

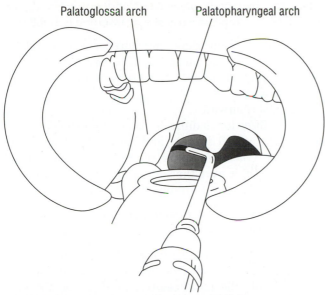

Figure 25–5. Anatomical landmarks for glossopharyngeal nerve block. *(From Barash, P. G., Cullen, B. F., & Stoelting, R. K. [1997]. Clinical anesthesia [3rd ed., p. 584]. Philadelphia: Lippincott-Raven. Copyright 1997 by Lippincott-Raven. Reprinted with permission.)*

Mask Ventilation

The most common problem encountered during mask ventilation is upper respiratory obstruction, usually due to soft-tissue collapse into the upper airway. During unconsciousness or light anesthesia, the base of the tongue relaxes against the posterior wall of the oropharynx, partially or completely blocking the patient's airway. A partial obstruction can be manifested by a snoring sound, very little movement of the reservoir bag, increased effort of respiratory muscles, and/or a rocking motion from the diaphragm expanding and chest retracting in an effort to ventilate. Additional methods quantifying ventilation are via end-tidal CO_2 measurement, pulse oximetry, and the respirometer.

A jaw lift, which will move the tongue away from the posterior pharyngeal wall, is the initial maneuver used to help correct the obstruction. Another alternative available is to position the fingers behind the temporomandibular joint and lift up (jaw thrust), resulting in a combination of chin lift–neck extension at the atlantooccipital joint. If the jaw thrust is unsuccessful, turning the head may ease the obstruction. When necessary, inserting an oral airway and/or nasal trumpet should relieve the obstruction (Fig. 25–7). One of the key points of mask ventilation is to avoid inspiratory pressures

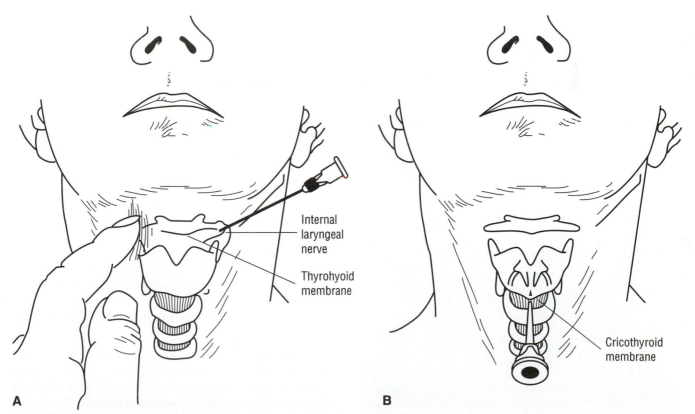

A

B

Figure 25–6. (**A**) Anatomical landmarks of superior laryngeal nerve block. (**B**) Anatomical landmarks of transtracheal instillation of local anesthetic. *(From Barash, P. G., Cullen, B. F., & Stoelting, R. K. [1997]. Anesthesia [3rd ed., p. 584]. Philadelphia: Lippincott-Raven. Copyright 1997 by Lippincott-Raven. Reprinted with permission.)*

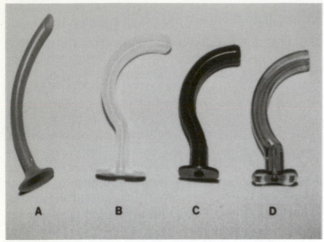

Figure 25–7. Pharyngeal airways. (**A**) Robertazzi nasopharyngeal airway. (**B**) Berman plastic oropharyngeal airway. (**C**) Guedel rubber oropharyngeal airway. (**D**) Guedel plastic oropharyngeal airway.

greater than 20 cm of H_2O. At higher inspiratory pressures, air can be forced into the esophagus and stomach. Figure 25-8 shows a proper mask fit. The purpose of the oropharyngeal and nasopharyngeal airway is to displace the tongue away, allowing the patient to breathe through (oral or nasal) or around the airway (oral). The oropharyngeal airway is efficient, but it is often difficult to insert

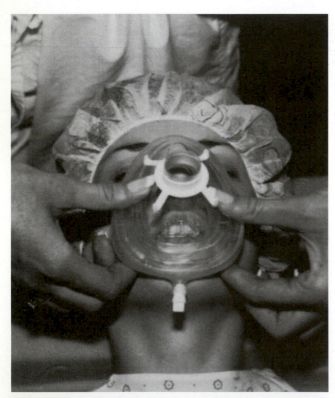

Figure 25–8. A good mask fit can be obtained by spreading the bottom of the mask and placing it on patient's chin before positioning the remainder of the mask.

when the patient is obstructed and not relaxed. The technique for oropharyngeal airway insertion is as follows:

1. Insert tongue depressor into oral cavity, and depress tongue anteriorly. The tip of the tongue depressor should extend beyond the base of the tongue.
2. Insert airway.
3. If insertion is difficult, rotate the oropharyngeal airway 180 degrees, and insert into the oral cavity. Once the distal tip of the oropharyngeal airway is over the soft palate, rotate the airway 180 degrees until the airway is inserted.

The technique for nasopharyngeal airway induction uses the following steps:

1. A soft lubricated airway should be used.
2. If time allows, the use of a vasoconstrictor within the nasal cavity may decrease the incidence or severity of nosebleed.
3. Carefully direct the nasopharyngeal airway between the floor of the nasal cavity and the inferior turbinate.
4. The sizes usually range between #28 French and #32 French.
5. Excessive force can result in a significant nosebleed that can aggravate airway obstruction.

During inhalation induction, the oropharyngeal or nasopharyngeal airway should be placed quickly to avoid a significant drop in the partial pressure of the anesthetic agent in the lungs. The following precautions should be observed during oropharyngeal airway insertion:

1. Check lips. Avoid pinching the lips between the teeth and the airway.
2. If the patient is edentulous or has full dentures, an oropharyngeal airway may not completely resolve the obstruction.
3. If the oropharyngeal airway is too short, the tongue may not be lifted away from the posterior pharynx.
4. Laryngospasm or gagging may occur if the oropharyngeal airway is too long.
5. Avoid using an oropharyngeal airway if a partial or permanent bridge or dental implants are present.
6. Avoid using a nasopharyngeal airway if coagulopathy is present.

Complications that can arise when using a face mask for prolonged ventilation include damage to the facial nerve from excessive pressure of the mask or pinching of ear lobes by tight head straps (Fig. 25–9). Eye care is extremely important when the mask is used during anesthesia. Options to protect the eyes include lubricating and taping them closed. In addition, eye patches pro-

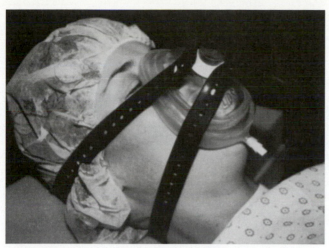

Figure 25–9. Proper mask fit with head strap attached.

vide another source of protection. If the eyes are left unattended or open during the anesthetic and a leak at the bridge of the nose develops, the potential for damage to the eyes increases.

In addition to an airway obstruction because of soft tissue collapse, coughing and laryngospasm can hinder adequate ventilation. Causes of cough and laryngospasm are (1) premature placement of an airway (oral or nasal); (2) sudden burst of a high concentration of pungent anesthetic agent; (3) secretions or blood on the vocal cords; (4) painful pharyngeal, laryngeal, or perioral stimulation (suction, airway, endoscopy, placement of endotracheal tube); and (5) inadequate anesthetic depth (stage II). Various maneuvers can be employed to prevent coughing and laryngospasm during the induction period. With the introduction of sevoflurane into clinical practice, an option is now available for a rapid inhalation anesthetic induction without significant coughing. Halothane can be used for inhalation induction, but, if the induction is rushed, patients tend to exhibit more breath holding, coughing, and laryngospasm. During inhalation induction, avoid forcing the endotracheal tube through the vocal cords to reduce the possibility of coughing and laryngospasm. Coughing and laryngospasm also can occur at the conclusion of the case or during extubation and emergence.

During emergence, the patient should be gently, but thoroughly, suctioned. Another useful maneuver to decrease the incidence of coughing and laryngospasm is to administer lidocaine 1 to 1.5 mg/kg intravenously. Manipulation of the airway should not occur until 3 full minutes after lidocaine has been administered to ensure the full benefit of this drug. A partial laryngospasm may present as a high-pitched crowing sound or absence of sound indicating complete glottic closure. Once laryngospasm occurs, multiple approaches can be taken to abort it:

1. Administer lidocaine 1 to 1.5 mg/IV or via ETT.
2. Inflate cuff of endotracheal tube with 4% topical lidocaine.
3. Partial laryngospasm.
   a. Slight positive pressure during inspiratory phase.
   b. Anterior mandibular displacement.
4. Complete laryngospasm, continuous positive airway pressure (CPAP) on the reservoir bag with 100% oxygen.
5. Succinylcholine 0.3 mg/kg; if succinylcholine has been used already, it may be necessary to give atropine first.

Laryngeal Mask Airway

The aim of the laryngeal mask airway (LMA) is to provide a relatively noninvasive method for airway management. The design was found to provide a clear airway if the following are true: (1) the LMA is correctly deflated to form a smooth flat wedge shape that would pass easily around the back of the tongue and behind the epiglottis; (2) protective reflexes are sufficiently depressed to permit smooth insertion; (3) the user has acquired the necessary skill.

Figure 25–10 describes the technique of LMA insertion. The fully inserted LMA lies with the mask tip resting against the upper esophageal sphincter, the sides facing the pyriform fossae, and the upper border under the base of the tongue. The epiglottis points up, above, or sometimes down and partially through the two aperture bars in the bowl of the mask. Inflating the cuff usually causes slight movement of the whole device upward as the expanding mask tip is partially squeezed out of the triangular-shaped base of the hypopharynx. The resulting position brings the glottic and LMA apertures in line with each other.

If the depth of anesthesia is not adequate during insertion, swallowing or laryngospasm may occur. The latter reflex explains why premature LMA insertion often is associated with complete inability to inflate the lungs until the laryngospasm is resolved. During emergence the laryngeal mask, if undisturbed, provokes very little stimulus and consequently can be left in place until protective reflexes have recovered to the point at which the patient can maintain the airway unassisted.

On the practical level, the most obvious advantage of the LMA is that it leaves both hands of the anesthetist free. Two clear dangers are due to the position of the laryngeal mask. First, because it does not penetrate sphincters, the LMA cannot prevent the effects of their inappropriate opening or closing. Hence the patient may still regurgitate and aspirate gastric contents because the LMA does not prevent passage of material into the larynx via the pyriform fossae. However, pharyngeal secre-

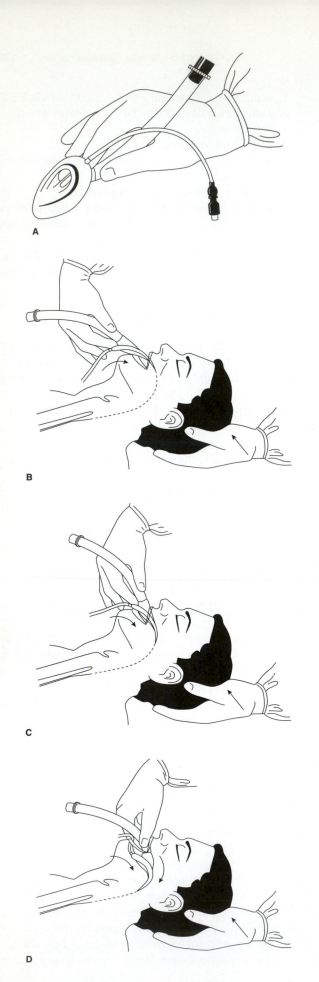

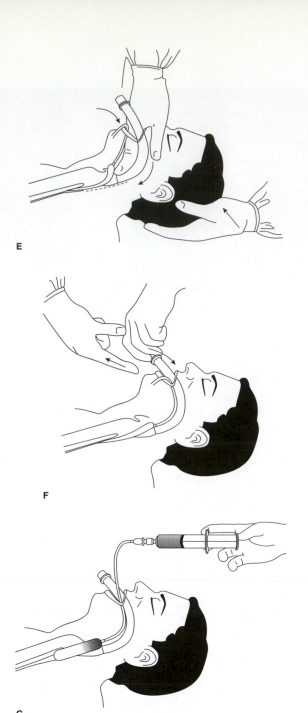

Figure 25–10. LMA insertion technique. (**A**) Recommended technique to hold the LMA like a pen, with the index finger placed at the junction of the cuff and the tube. (**B**) Under direct vision, press the tip of the cuff upward against the hard palate and flatten the cuff against it. (**C**) Use the middle finger to open the mouth by pushing the jaw downward. This will enable the index finger to enter further into the mouth during insertion. (**D**) Use the index finger to guide the LMA, and press backward toward the ears in one smooth movement. (**E**) Advance the LMA into the hypopharynx until a definite resistance is felt. (**F**) Before removing the finger, the nondominant hand is brought from behind the patient's head to press down on the LMA tube. (**G**) During cuff inflation, do not hold the tube as this may cause a postoperative sore throat. (*Reprinted with permission from Gensia, Inc.*)

tions or blood from the upper airway usually are effectively contained outside the mask. The glottic sphincter may close or laryngospasm may occur as a response to surgical stimulation at inadequate levels of anesthesia. The incidence of soreness of the pharynx postoperatively is not significantly different from that of using a face mask.

To complete the discussion of the laryngeal mask airway, contraindications and potential complications are presented. As noted, the LMA should not be routinely used in nonfasting patients unless their airway cannot be safely secured by other means. The LMA should not be used in the obese patient, in patients with hiatal hernia, or in those with a history of reflux or autonomic neuropathy, as well as pregnant patients over 14 weeks' gestation. The LMA is relatively contraindicated for patients with low pulmonary compliance, for example, pulmonary fibrosis or obesity or if inflation pressures greater than 20 cm H_2O are required. The inspiratory flow rate should be reduced to maximize gas entry. This instrument will not replace either the endotracheal tube or the face mask, but it certainly has earned its place as an alternative for airway management.

Ventilation via Endotracheal Tube

Preparation for endotracheal intubation requires a good knowledge of the anatomy of the upper airway, a moderate amount of technical skill, and the common sense to know when it is both appropriate and inappropriate to pursue intubation. Another important facet of successful intubation is to develop finesse in the technique. Intubation provides the following advantages: (1) reduces anatomic dead space by 50%; (2) provides patent upper airway; (3) helps prevent gastric aspiration; and (4) allows for positive-pressure ventilation of the lungs. Indications for tracheal intubation include anatomic features predisposing the patient to an inadequate mask fit and/or surgical requirements (ie, prone or lateral position). Other indications for tracheal intubation are preplanned postoperative ventilation, the potential for gastric aspiration, and the patient's general medical condition. The anesthetic requirements of an acutely ill patient can require the use of two hands by the anesthesia provider. Additional indications for tracheal intubation are:

Surgical procedures
  Neurosurgery
  Intraabdominal procedures
  Thoracotomy
  One-lung ventilation
  Prolonged need for postoperative ventilation (assisted or controlled ventilation, operative site in close proximity to or involving the head)
Position of anesthesia provider away from head of table

Prolonged duration of surgery (ie, neuromuscular blockade)
Adverse operative positions
  Trendelenburg position
  Extreme lithotomy position
  Lateral position, prone position, sitting position

During preparation for intubation, either orally or nasally, the required equipment must be available, clean, and in good working order. The equipment used during intubation consists of a laryngoscope and attachable blade, endotracheal tube, stylet, lubricant, and a syringe for the cuff. The straight (Miller) and curved (MacIntosh) are the two most commonly used laryngoscope blades (Fig. 25–11). These two laryngoscopes and other reusable laryngoscopes have a detachable blade, are easy to clean, have a bulb that can be placed distally to provide good lighting of the glottis, and are available in a variety of sizes. In addition, disposable laryngoscopes currently are available for one-time use.

The straight blade is designed to lift up the epiglottis to provide visualization of the vocal cords (Fig. 25-12). Because the laryngeal surface of the epiglottis is innervated by the vagal nerve (tenth cranial nerve), cardiac dysrhythmias may develop during endoscopy. The curved blade is designed to lift the epiglottis indirectly,

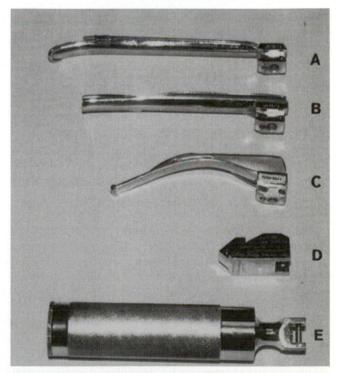

Figure 25–11. Laryngoscopes. **(A)** Miller blade (straight). **(B)** Wis–Foreggar blade (straight). **(C)** MacIntosh blade (curved). **(D)** Harlan lock. **(E)** Laryngoscopy handle with bar latch; batteries are inside cylinder, which is accessed by unscrewing the bottom of the handle.

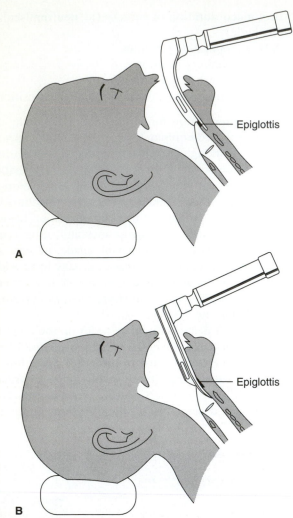

Figure 25–12. (**A**) When a curved laryngoscope blade is used, the tip of the blade is placed in the vallecula, the space between the base of the tongue and the pharyngeal surface of the epiglottis. (**B**) The tip of a straight blade is advanced beneath the epiglottis. *(From Barash, P. G., Cullen, B. F., & Stoelting, R. K. [1997]. Clinical anesthesia [3rd ed., p. 581]. Philadelphia: Lippincott-Raven. Copyright 1997 by Lippincott-Raven. Reprinted with permission.)*

as noted in Figure 25–12. During placement of the curved laryngoscope within the vallecula, stimulation of the glossopharyngeal nerve (ninth cranial nerve) has less potential to cause vagal-induced cardiovascular changes. An adequate depth of anesthesia will lessen the potential for any cardiovascular changes during laryngoscopy regardless of the type of laryngoscope being used. Laryngoscope handles operate on "AA," "C," and "D" battery sizes. A model also is available that uses only one "C" battery and has a shorter handle. This handle is designed to facilitate intubation for patients, such as extremely obese patients, whose anatomy restricts using a longer handle. Figure 25–13 illustrates the exposure of the vocal cords when using either a curved or straight laryngoscope

blade. Figures 25–14 and 25–15 illustrate the two most common head positions for intubation.

Endotracheal tubes are made of polyvinylchloride (PVC), a nontoxic, nonallergenic substance (Fig. 25–16). A manufacturer's "Z-79" label on an endotracheal tube indicates that the material has been implant-tested and found to be nontoxic to tissues. Standards for substance toxicity and tissue irritation are reviewed and revised by the American Society for Testing and Materials (ASTM) Committee F-29. A radiopaque strip facilitates verification of placement by x-ray. Two other common variations of endotracheal tubes include oral RAE and nasal RAE endotracheal tubes (Fig. 25–17). Another specialized endotracheal tube is the double-lumen tube that allows preferential ventilation of one lung during a thoracotomy. The internal diameter of the endotracheal tube sizes ranges from 2 to 10 mm in half-size increments. As the internal diameter of the endotracheal tube increases, resistance to airflow will decrease. This concept is important when the potential for postoperative ventilatory support exists. If the endotracheal tube chosen has too small an internal diameter for the size of the patient, the increased resistance may become acutely apparent during the weaning process. Placement of a size 7.5 endotracheal tube is appropriate for the majority of female patients, and an 8.5 is appropriate for the majority of male patients.

Historically, older, red-rubber endotracheal tubes were retrofitted with a cuff that had low volume and high pressure. Current cuffs on endotracheal tubes are high volume and low pressure to reduce the irritation and damage to the tracheal wall. Once the endotracheal tube has been correctly placed, an inspiratory pressure of 20 torr should be generated with the reservoir bag. At that point, the cuff should be inflated until no leak is heard. This technique may help avoid undue cuff pressure that can cause potential ischemia to the tracheal mucosa. If the cuff pressure is allowed to increase above mean capillary hydrostatic pressure (32 mmHg), mucosal ischemia can occur. One technique used to minimize the incidence of coughing during the immediate postoperative period is the use of 4% topical lidocaine to inflate the cuff instead of air. Over time, some of the lidocaine will leak out and anesthetize the tracheal mucosa that is in immediate contact with the cuff. This works especially well when intravenous lidocaine has been given to decrease the response to laryngoscopy.

Several methods are available to determine the length necessary to insert the endotracheal tube. With oral intubation, the endotracheal tube can be placed alongside the face and around to the cricoid cartilage. The distance from the teeth (gum line) to the midtrachea is between 18 and 22 cm. (If nasal intubation is planned, add 2 to 3 cm.) The average distance from the

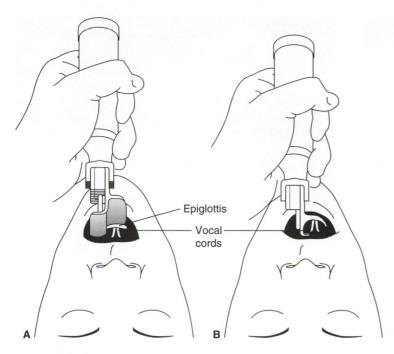

Epiglottis

Vocal
cords

A   B

Figure 25–13. **(A)** The curved laryngoscope blade is placed in the vallecula, and the vocal cords are exposed as the handle is lifted upward and forward. **(B)** A straight blade is advanced beneath the laryngeal surface of the epiglottis to expose the glottic opening. *(From Barash, P. G., Cullen, B. F., & Stoelting R. K. [1992]. Clinical anesthesia [2nd ed., p. 698]. Philadelphia: Lippincott-Raven. Copyright 1992 by Lippincott-Raven. Reprinted with permission.)*

teeth to the cords in an adult is 13 cm, and the average distance from the cords to the carina is 13 cm. The average distance from the lips to the carina is 24 cm. In the adult patient, once the cuff of the endotracheal tube has passed through the cords under direct visualization, the endotracheal tube should not be advanced anymore. When the practitioner is unable to visualize the cuff passing through the vocal cords, the advancement of the endotracheal tube should stop when the 20-cm mark is at the lips.

Other equipment that should be readily available includes a stylet of malleable firm metal to facilitate curvature of the endotracheal tube, water-soluble lubricant,

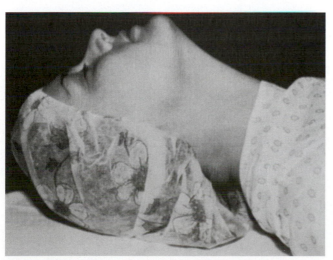

Figure 25–14. Classic Jacksonian position with gentle hyperextension.

suction apparatus, an oral airway to prevent the patient from biting the airway, adhesive tape to secure the endotracheal tube, and a stethoscope to auscultate the chest following intubation. If the stylet is used, avoid having the tip of the stylet at or beyond the Murphy's eye of the endotracheal tube. If the tip is allowed to enter the Murphy's eye or to extend beyond the orifice of the endotracheal tube, significant trauma could result when advancing the endotracheal tube. It is important to tape the endotracheal tube to the maxilla. If adhesive tape is inappropriate, either because of facial trauma, full mustache, or allergy to adhesive, gauze or umbilical tape can be used to secure the endotracheal tube. When placing the knot in the gauze or the tape, be careful not to incorporate the lips, as doing so will result in significant pain in the postoperative period. This method works especially well if the patient is expected to be in the prone position for a protracted period of time. Oral secretions can wet the tape or loosen the adhesive and contribute to an unexpected extubation!

If the endotracheal tube enters the esophagus on the initial attempt at intubation, the endoscopist can perform one of two maneuvers: either leave the initial endotracheal tube in place and attempt to intubate with another endotracheal tube or remove the endotracheal tube prior to the second attempt. If the patient needs to be ventilated prior to the second attempt, the endotracheal tube will have to be removed in order to obtain a proper mask fit, or a laryngeal mask airway may be inserted to provide oxygenation (Pace et al., 1994).

Endotracheal tubes generally maintain their curvature but can kink easily when warmed to body tempera-

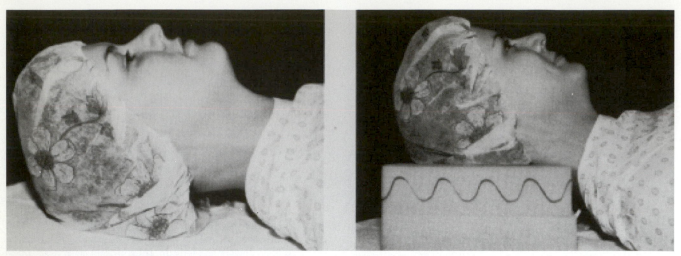

Figure 25–15. Positioning the head for endotracheal intubation. (Left) Sniffing or amended position. (Right) Classic, or Jacksonian, position.

ture. The weight of the breathing circuit or positioning over an oral retractor are common causes of kinking. Significant obstruction of the endotracheal tube due to kinking will be reflected as an elevated end-tidal CO_2, tachycardia, and decreased SpO_2 levels. Kinking can be prevented by using semirigid endotracheal tubes (armored or anode tubes) that have a coiled wire incorporated within the material of the tube. Another cause of either partial or complete obstruction is thick mucus secretions in the endotracheal tube. If complete obstruction occurs, the endotracheal tube should be replaced since suctioning the tube will only create a lumen the size of the suction catheter.

When the endotracheal tube is advanced too far distally in the adult patient, the tip will likely enter the right mainstem bronchus and a significant shunt will develop. If the endotracheal tube is not advanced far enough, the cuff may be located between the vocal cords when inflated. This will usually result in a leak at peak inspira-

tion, and, if more air is added to the cuff, the potential for vocal cord damage is apparent. Deflating the cuff and more distal advancement of the endotracheal tube will correct this problem. The steps for oral intubation follow:

1. Elevate operating table to appropriate position for the endoscopist. Position the head of the patient in the sniffing position. Adhere to Universal Precautions.
2. Open the mouth either by using the "scissor technique" or by hyperextension of the head.
3. Hold laryngoscope in left hand, introduce blade on the right side of mouth, and sweep the tongue left during advancement toward the midline.

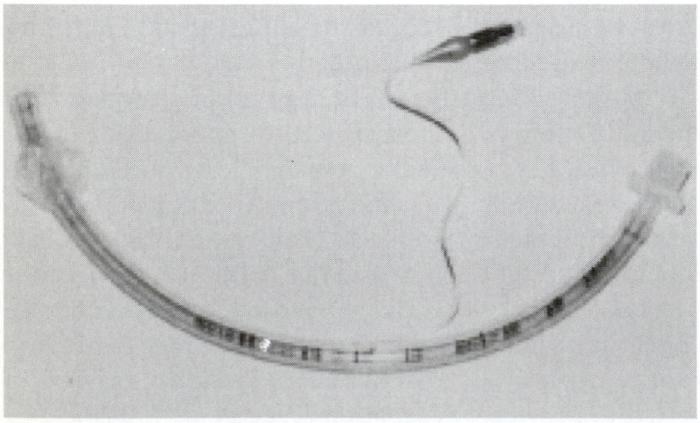

Figure 25–16. Disposable endotracheal tube with cuff and pilot balloon with valve.

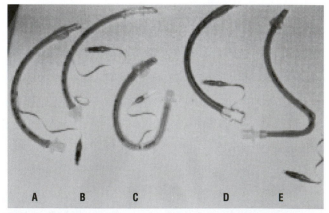

Figure 25–17. Variations of endotracheal tubes. Left to right: Traditional endotracheal tube. Endotrol by National Catheter, with plastic ring for deflecting the tip of the endotracheal tube. RAE tube for oral use. Disposable armored tube. RAE tube for nasal use.

4. If using a curved blade, direct the tip of the blade into the vallecula, and lift up and away (or forward). Hold the wrist rigid to avoid using the teeth as a fulcrum during the attempt at visualization. If the tip is inserted too deeply, the sphincter of the esophagus will be visualized. The blade can then be retracted and the triangular view of the vocal cords should appear. Visualization may be inadequate if a large, floppy epiglottis is present.

5. With a straight blade, direct the tip underneath the epiglottis, and lift upward and away. All other considerations as previously noted are identical.

6. Gently advance the tip of the endotracheal tube between the vocal cords. The appropriate depth to advance the endotracheal tube has been achieved once the cuff has passed the cords.

7. Inflate the cuff to occlusive pressure.

8. Begin ventilation, and verify correct placement by the continued presence of an $ETCO_2$ waveform and auscultation of the chest.

9. An oral airway may be inserted, followed by securing the endotracheal tube.

The multiple factors contributing to a failed intubation can be insufficient depth of general anesthesia; inadequate muscle relaxation; improper position of head; improper insertion of laryngoscope blade; unfamiliarity with anatomy, especially if distorted; and inexperience and lack of normal skill or dexterity. The most severe complication associated with failed intubation, either oral or nasal, is the development of hypoxia. Some clinicians lose their focus during the "failed intubation" scenario and forget to ventilate the patient with either a mask or laryngeal mask airway. The majority of hypoxic events can be avoided when the primary goal in airway management is to maintain ventilation, not intubation. The complications associated with endotracheal intubation are:

1. Aspiration
2. Laceration of the lips or gums
3. Dental damage
4. Laryngeal injury
5. Esophageal intubation
6. Inadvertent endobronchial intubation
7. Activation of sympathetic nervous system
8. Bronchospasm
9. Cardiac arrest
10. Death

The most reliable methods to confirm the correct placement of an endotracheal tube are observing the tip of the endotracheal tube pass through the vocal cords, a sus-tained $ETCO_2$ waveform, and confirmation by fiberoptic bronchoscopy.

Nasal Intubation

The primary indication for nasal intubation is when direct vision is not possible or when oral endotracheal intubation is potentially unsafe for the patient. Several indications for nasal intubation include ankylosis of the cervical spine or temporomandibular joint, fractured jaw, inability to flex or hyperextend the neck, and anatomical abnormalities such as a thick, muscular neck. Nasal intubations should be avoided if the patient has a nasal fracture, severe nasal obstruction, acute sinusitis, or a cerebrospinal leak due to head trauma.

Nasal intubations can be performed with the patient either awake or asleep. If an awake intubation is planned, topical anesthesia of the upper airway and sedation will provide minimal patient discomfort during the procedure. While sedating patients for an awake intubation, inhalation of 100% oxygen is preferred. A sedated, cooperative patient provides minimal stress for both the individual and the endoscopist. The most frequent complication associated with nasal intubation is epistaxis. The likelihood of this occurring can be lessened by the use of vasoconstrictors, such as cocaine, neosynephrine nose drops, or other over-the-counter nasal vasoconstrictors, lubricated nasal trumpets, warming of the nasotracheal tube, and the minimal use of force during the procedure. The procedure for nasal intubation is as follows:

1. Use topical anesthetic for the upper airway (awake technique). Use a vasoconstrictor to shrink nasal membranes.

2. Dilate nares with increasing sizes of nasal trumpets liberally lubricated (4% lidocaine ointment works well). Dilate with nasal trumpet one-half size larger than nasotracheal tube.

3. Gently insert the nasotracheal tube into the dilated naris. Follow the floor of the naris, being careful not to damage nasal turbinates. If resistance to forward movement is met, rotate the nasotracheal tube.

4. If the patient is spontaneously breathing, listen to breath sounds through the nasotracheal tube. (Consider placing an artificial nose on the proximal end of the endotracheal tube to avoid potential contamination from coughing.)

5. If breath sounds cease on forward movement of the endotracheal tube, retract till breath sounds are heard, and turn the patient's head opposite the nares being used to align the trachea with the nares. Another option is to retract the nasotracheal tube until breath sounds are again heard and inflate the cuff with 30 mL of air, lifting

the tip of the tube anteriorly. Advance the nasotracheal tube slowly and, when resistance is met, maintain slight forward pressure, deflate the cuff, and the endotracheal tube will enter the trachea. Magill forceps can be used if the above mentioned techniques fail under direct vision.

6. Instruct the patient to take a deep breath when attempting to advance the nasotracheal tube between the cords. During this time the vocal cords will be widely abducted. If a topical anesthetic was inadequate, placing the nasotracheal tube into the larynx will elicit a cough and rapid air movement. Prior to inducing the patient, inflate the cuff of the endotracheal tube, auscultate the chest for bilateral breath sounds, and monitor for continuous $ETCO_2$ measurement.

Measuring the length of a nasotracheal tube using external landmarks is illustrated in Figure 25–18. The occurrence of epistaxis will be greater if excessive force, rough insertion, lack of lubricant, or an excessively large nasotracheal tube are used. If the practitioner is unsuccessful in placing the nasotracheal tube and the patient requires ventilation, the practitioner should attach the breathing circuit to the nasotracheal tube, occlude the open naris, close the patient's mouth, and then ventilate. Another alternative is to remove the nasotracheal tube and ventilate with a mask. If nasotracheal intubation under direct visualization is planned while the patient is either awake or asleep and the tip of the nasotracheal tube cannot be directed between the vocal cords, the Magill forceps (Fig. 25–19) can facilitate the correct placement of the endotracheal tube. Avoid grasping the cuff or uvula when using the Magill forceps (Fig. 25–20). Once the tip of the tube is directed toward the glottis, an assistant is needed to advance the endotracheal tube, on

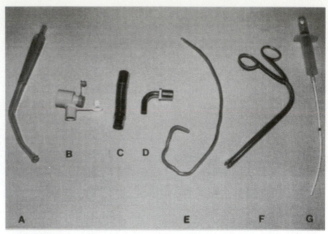

Figure 25–19. Additional airway equipment. (**A**) Tonsil suction. (**B**) Connector for use with fiberoptic bronchoscope. (**C**) Metal flex connector. (**D**) Metal curved connector. (**E**) Stylet. (**F**) Magill forceps. (**G**) Laryngeal-tracheal anesthesia kit.

command, into the trachea. The keys to successful nasal intubations are proper equipment, alignment of the nasotracheal axis to provide as nearly as possible a direct line from the posterior pharynx to the larynx, adequate sedation and topical anesthesia (if the patient is awake), and the finesse of the endoscopist.

Intubation During Emergent Conditions

The first priority during a rapid-sequence ("crash") induction (in addition to providing ventilation) is to protect the lungs from vomitus or regurgitation of gastrointestinal contents. The decision to perform a rapid-sequence induction should be balanced between the risk of losing control of the airway and the danger of

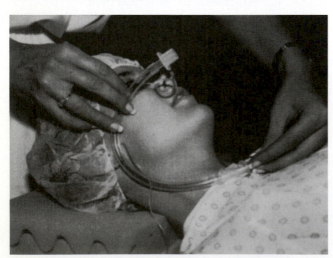

Figure 25–18. Measuring the length of a nasotracheal tube using external landmarks: suprasternal notch, earlobe, and naris.

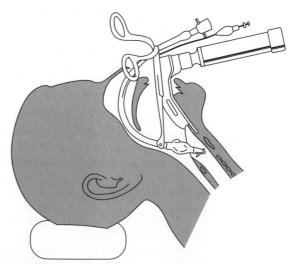

Figure 25–20. Magill forceps are used to grasp and direct the endotracheal tube during nasotracheal intubation. *(From Barash, P. G., Cullen, B. F., & Stoelting, R. K. [1997]. Clinical anesthesia [3rd ed., p. 585]. Philadelphia: Lippincott-Raven. Copyright 1997 by Lippincott-Raven. Reprinted with permission.)*

aspiration of gastric contents. Other anesthetic techniques, such as monitored anesthesia care or regional anesthesia, may be indicated if the patient is at high risk for aspiration. It is important to know that neither monitored anesthesia care nor a regional anesthesia technique guarantees the avoidance of aspiration. The following conditions increase the risk for gastric aspiration:

- Full meal within the last 8 hrs
- Active vomiting or nausea
- Surgically acute abdomen
- Pain from peripheral trauma
- Acute head injury
- Increased intraabdominal pressure (ie, pregnancy or obesity)
- Hiatal hernia with active reflux
- Esophageal obstruction
- Active pharyngeal bleeding (ie, epistaxis, post-tonsillectomy or hemorrhage)

One of the most important things when performing a rapid-sequence induction is to have all of the equipment readily available and in working order. The anesthesia machine must be checked, anesthetic drugs drawn up, suction at arms reach and properly working, and a dependable and functional intravenous line must be in place. The individual providing assistance should be positioned to the patient's right, facing the anesthesia provider. Prior to induction, preoxygenate the patient with 100% oxygen for at least 4 minutes. During this time the anesthesia provider should observe the reservoir bag of the gas machine collapsing and expanding with each breath of the patient. If there is no movement of the reservoir bag, a leak exists between the patient's face and the mask. Another preoxygenation technique is to have the patient take a minimum of four vital capacity breaths prior to induction. To increase the efficacy of this maneuver, a proper mask fit must be obtained. The patient can either be placed in reverse Trendelenburg, Trendelenburg, or neutral supine position prior to induction. The reverse Trendelenburg position uses gravity to decrease the incidence of passive regurgitation, and the Trendelenburg position allows regurgitated contents to pool in the pharynx and decreases the likelihood of their being aspirated into the trachea. The supine position facilitates the most rapid endotracheal tube insertion. The correct technique of cricoid pressure or Sellick's maneuver (Fig. 25–21) is to grasp the cricoid cartilage between the thumb and index finger and direct the cricoid cartilage posteriorly toward the vertebral body of C6, at a pressure of 44 newtons. An easier way to describe the amount of pressure to apply is that it would cause pain if it were applied to the bridge of the nose. Following a proper explanation to the patient of cricoid pressure, the assistant performs this maneuver, when requested, on the patient. Release of cricoid pres-

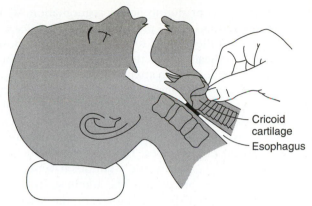

Figure 25–21. Cricoid pressure (Sellick's maneuver) is applied to occlude the esophagus and prevent aspiration of gastric contents. *(From Barash, P. G., Cullen, B. F., & Stoelting, R. K. [1997]. Clinical anesthesia [3rd ed., p. 585]. Philadelphia: Lippincott-Raven. Copyright 1997 by Lippincott-Raven. Reprinted with permission.)*

sure is done after verification of proper endotracheal tube placement or if ventilation by mask is not possible. If visualization of the glottis is difficult, consider applying external pressure on the thyroid cartilage while maintaining cricoid pressure.

When confronted with a patient at high risk for aspiration, the anesthesia provider can choose between either a rapid-sequence induction or a modified rapid-sequence induction. The difference between the two techniques is that with modified rapid sequence induction spontaneous mask ventilation is done before the initial attempt at intubation. During a rapid-sequence induction, after the patient has been preoxygenated, ventilation is not attempted until after proper endotracheal tube placement. If the attempt at intubation is unsuccessful and the patient's oxygen saturation begins to decrease, mask ventilation is indicated while the assistant maintains cricoid pressure. However, if a relatively long-acting nondepolarizing muscle relaxant is given to facilitate intubation followed by the ability to ventilate the patient, the potential for harm to the patient is present! This may be avoided by using a modified rapid-sequence induction.

A modified rapid-sequence induction differs from a rapid-sequence induction in that gentle mask ventilation is attempted following the loss of the lid reflex prior to the administration of a muscle relaxant. Inability to ventilate at this time is not due to the muscle relaxant. If the inability to ventilate is due solely to a rigid chest after an opioid has been administered, a muscle relaxant will alleviate this problem. The critical issue of a modified rapid-sequence induction is the obstruction created by cricoid pressure. Historically, the anesthesia provider has been comfortable with the fact that appropriate cricoid pressure will prevent gastric contents from entering the hypopharynx, except during active regurgitation. With active regurgitation, cricoid pressure should be released immediately and the patient turned to the lateral position with their head lower than their stomach. Conversely, it was felt that when attempting to ventilate prior to intubation air would immediately enter the stomach and the patient would vomit and aspirate. In fact, the obstruction created by properly applied cricoid pressure is a two-way valve that will remain competent to pressures greater than 20 cm of water. Thus, during a modified rapid-sequence induction, gentle attempts at ventilation following induction, but prior to the administration of a muscle relaxant, should have no impact on the risk of aspiration. The advantage of the modified rapid-sequence technique is the ability to ventilate the patient before administering a muscle relaxant. If the patient at risk for aspiration has significant redundant pharyngeal tissue, a muscle relaxant may actually worsen intubating conditions and an awake intubation may be the technique of choice other than a modified rapid-sequence induction.

A potential complication of cricoid pressure is esophageal rupture. If the patient begins to regurgitate actively, place the patient in a head-down position, turn the head to the side, and suction the oropharynx vigorously. As noted earlier, if active regurgitation is present, cricoid pressure should be released.

Extubation

Planning is as critical for extubation as it is for intubation. The anesthetic should be titrated to provide optimal conditions for extubation once the operative procedure is completed. Extubation should be done either while the patient is "deep" or "awake," never during stage II or the excitement stage of emergence. If the patient had a difficult airway or was induced with a "full stomach," their protective reflexes should be allowed to return completely prior to extubation. "Deep" extubation is indicated (1) for patients with reactive airway disease; (2) when "bucking" or straining on the endotracheal tube is undesirable (ie, hernia repair, craniotomy); and (3) to avoid the hypertensive and tachycardiac response associated with extubation. It must be noted that the risk of laryngospasm and aspiration is increased during a deep extubation if secretions are not properly suctioned prior to removal of the endotracheal tube. The following questions should be considered prior to deep extubation:

1. Did the patient require an awake intubation?
2. Did the patient require a (modified) rapid-sequence induction?
3. Is the bowel distended by blood or nitrous oxide?
4. Is a nasogastric tube in place?
5. Was placement difficult?
6. Does the patient have reactive airway disease?

Once the decision to extubate has been made, the following parameters must be considered to determine the appropriate timing of extubation:

1. Absence of uncoordinated movement (ie, rocking motion) between chest or abdomen during spontaneous ventilation
2. $SpO_2 > 90\%$ with an $FIO_2 > 40\%$
3. Respiratory rate > 8/min and < 30/min
4. Tidal volume > 5 mL/kg
5. Vital capacity breath > 10–15 mL/kg
6. Inspiratory force > −20 cm H_2O
7. TV/RR > 10
8. Fully reversed from muscle relaxant
   a. PNS, train-of-four with sustained tetanus
   b. Ability to lift head for 5 seconds
   c. Ability to raise arm and shoulder for 5 seconds
9. Level of consciousness stable or improving

If any doubts exist concerning the safety of the patient and immediate extubation, the patient should be taken to the Post Anesthesia Care Unit (PACU) and placed on a ventilator until conditions are suitable for extubation. The procedure for extubation is as follows:

1. Decrease opioids or gases gradually to maintain patient comfort.
2. At the appropriate time, stop the anesthetic and deliver 100% oxygen.
3. Suction the back of the oropharynx gently so as not to stimulate coughing, bucking, or spasm. Suction down the endotracheal tube only if indicated and with a new catheter. Suction for short periods, and use finger port off and on.
4. Tell patient to take a deep breath. If there are any doubts about reversal, ask patient to raise the head and hold it up for 5 seconds.
5. Have the patient take a deep breath or fill the lungs with oxygen from the reservoir bag. At the same time, deflate the cuff, close the pop-off valve, and extubate the patient.
6. Immediately following extubation, ensure that there is patent airway and no laryngospasm.

In addition to laryngospasm and aspiration other complications associated with extubation include transient vocal cord incompetence, glottic or subglottic edema, and pharyngitis or tracheitis. Laryngeal edema also can occur after extubation and can be treated with steroids (dexamethasone), racemic epinephrine, and ice packs placed over the patient's throat. During prolonged ventilatory support using an endotracheal tube, complications such as tracheal stenosis or tracheomalacia have been reported.

Difficult extubations can arise because of failure to deflate the cuff or oddities such as inadvertent suturing or wiring of the endotracheal tube. Another case scenario that occurs infrequently and that results in a difficult extubation is stapling of the distal tip of the endotracheal tube during pneumonectomy. If this occurs, the chest must be explored, the staples removed from the endotracheal tube, and the bronchus restapled. It is important to remember to pull the endotracheal tube back into the trachea prior to stapling of the bronchus in close proximity of the carina.

Management of the Difficult Airway

More than 85% of all respiratory-related closed malpractice claims involve a brain-damaged or brain-dead patient (Benumof, 1991). The inability to manage very difficult airways is responsible for 30% of deaths totally attributable to anesthesia. Worldwide up to 600 people are thought to die each year from intubation difficulties (Frerk, 1991). The cannot-ventilate-by-mask, cannot-intubate situation has been responsible for a previously irreducible 1% to 28% of all deaths associated with anesthesia (Benumof, 1990). The incidence of cannot-ventilate-by-mask/cannot-intubate is thought to range from 0.01 to 2 out of 10 000 anesthetics (Benumof, 1990). Figure 25–22 provides the frequencies of the best view obtainable with a laryngoscope.

Managing the difficult airway depends on recognizing a potential problem, the etiology of the problem, the patient's condition, the available equipment, familiarity of the operator with various techniques, and whether the difficulty was anticipated. Above all, ventilation and oxygenation must be maintained. As noted, patients do not die from failure to intubate but rather from failure to

oxygenate. The fundamental responsibility of the anesthesia provider is to provide adequate gas exchange.

An anticipated difficult airway is much easier to manage. The airway should be assessed before administering any anesthetic (general, regional, or monitored anesthesia care). The inability to intubate following a failed regional technique will only compound the problems faced by the anesthesia provider and can potentially result in a bad outcome for the patient. If significant maxillofacial trauma is apparent, the establishment of a surgical airway is indicated.

When confronted with a difficult airway, either anticipated or unanticipated, the main objective is to function in a calm and systematic manner. The American Society of Anesthesiologists' Difficult Airway Algorithm describes an organized approach to difficult airway management (Figure 25–23). This algorithm should be readily available on the anesthesia department's difficult airway cart. The following alternative methods of airway management can be used when confronted with a difficult airway:

> Noninvasive techniques
> > Laryngeal mask airway
> > Directional stylet
> > Light wand
> > Esophageal-tracheal combitube
> > Bullard laryngoscope
> > Fiberoptic intubation
> Invasive techniques
> > Needle cricothyrotomy with jet ventilation
> > Retrograde wire technique
> > Surgical airway

The inability to ventilate with a mask can be due to the lack of an oral or nasal airway, inadequate anesthesia, an opioid-induced rigid chest, improper positioning of the patient's head, and other factors. In most instances, intubation will not be difficult and will allow for ventilation. However, if the patient is already anesthetized and/or paralyzed and intubation is found to be difficult, avoid endless attempts at intubation. Change at least one component of your approach, as noted by the ASA Difficult Airway Algorithm. Alternative approaches to intubation include an attempt at nasal intubation, the laryngeal mask airway, a directional stylet, light wand, esophageal-tracheal combitube, a Bullard laryngoscope, and/or fiberoptic intubation. If the practitioner is unable to ventilate either by mask or laryngeal mask airway and attempts at intubation are unsuccessful, invasive techniques include needle cricothyrotomy with jet ventilation, retrograde wire technique, or a surgical airway. As attempts are made to establish the airway, the importance of anesthetic depth should not be forgotten. Avoid following the initial dose of succinyl-

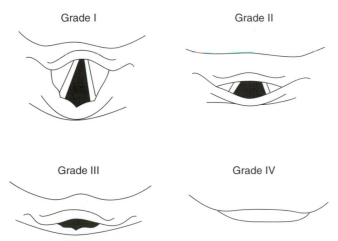

Figure 25–22. Best view obtainable at laryngoscopy, assuming correct technique. The frequencies apply to patients without neck pathology. Severe disease of the neck may produce a Grade IV view, but this rarely, if ever, occurs. The approximate frequencies are as follows: Grade I, 99%; Grade II, 1%; Grade III, 1/2000; Grade IV, less than 1/10^5. *(Courtesy of Circon Corporation.)*

1. Assess the likelihood and clinical impact of basic management problems:
   A. Difficult Intubation
   B. Difficult Ventilation
   C. Difficulty with Patient Cooperation or Consent

2. Consider the relative merits and feasibility of basic management choices:

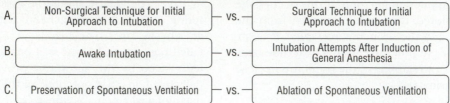

3. Develop primary and alternative strategies:

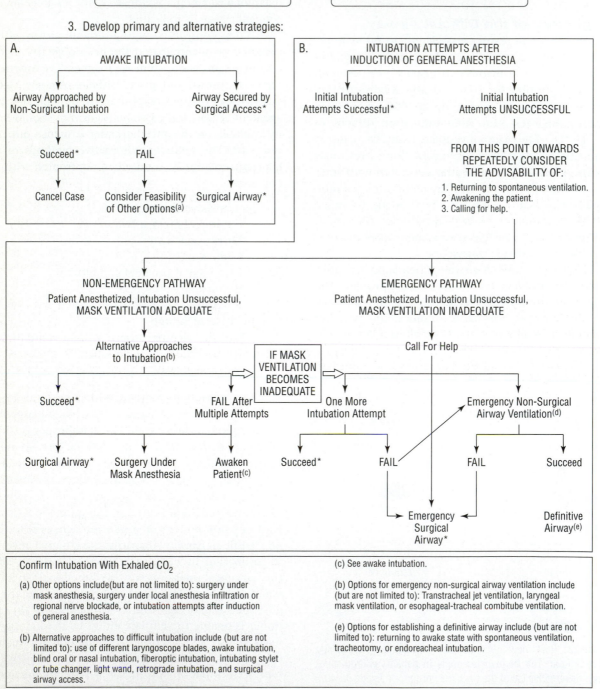

Figure 25–23. Difficult Airway Algorithm. *(From American Society of Anesthesiologists Task Force on Management of the Difficult Airway. [1993]. Practice guidelines for management of the difficult airway. Anesthesiology, 78, 597.)*

choline with a nondepolarizing muscle relaxant, especially if ventilation via mask or laryngeal mask airway is difficult. If able to ventilate but not to intubate, ask the question as to whether or not the case is amenable to ventilation by a mask or laryngeal mask airway. If not, the alternatives are to awaken the patient and proceed with an awake technique, cancel the case, or refer the individual to another institution. If risk of aspiration was an initial concern at the beginning of the case, maintain cricoid pressure until the patient is awake.

▶ CASE STUDY

In reviewing the anesthesia record from a previous surgery, the words "difficult airway" are found written in large red letters. The patient is scheduled for a total hip replacement because of degenerative osteoarthritis. She is not a candidate for a regional anesthetic because of her inability to be positioned comfortably for a long procedure from chronic pain associated with her arthritic condition.

1. How should the patient's airway be assessed?

   Ask the patient to open her mouth. Does the tongue obscure the tip of the uvula and are the tonsilar pillars visible? Can you place two fingers between the hyoid bone and the inner aspect of the mandible. If you cannot visualize these structures or have a two-fingerbreadth space, the probability of the larynx being located anteriorly is high. Evaluate the mobility of the patient's jaw and neck given the fact that she has degenerative arthritis.

2. What other measures might be used in evaluating this patient's airway?

   Obtain old medical records and ascertain how intubation was accomplished before. Learn from the experiences of others and avoid making mistakes by carefully assessing the patient and taking a good history as well as reviewing any old record describing previous attempts at intubation.

3. What equipment should the anesthetist have available?

   All standard airway equipment and working suction should be prepared and available. In addition, the difficult airway cart containing a variety of endo- and nasotracheal tubes, airways, laryngoscopes and blades, as well as local anesthetics, should be available. Review the difficult airway algorithm. Have a fiberoptic laryngoscope available. Discuss your plans with another anesthesia colleague or supervisor. It is prudent to have more than one anesthesia provider available whenever a difficult airway is suspected.

4. The patient has been evaluated and assigned a Mallampati Class III airway. Once all equipment is available in the operating room, how should the anesthetist proceed to establish the airway?

   Provide moderate sedation, use a topical anesthetic for the oropharynx, and attempt to visualize the cords. If unsuccessful, establish the airway prior to induction by using a different intubation technique, such as a fiberoptic technique. Avoid endless attempts at intubation. Change at least one component of the approach to intubation as noted in the difficult airway algorithm. Alternative aproaches to oral intubation would include nasal intubation, the laryngeal mask airway, a directional stylet, light wand, esophageal-tracheal combitube, a Bullard laryngoscope, and/or a fiberoptic approach, as previously mentioned.

5. The case has concluded and the patient is ventilating spontaneously but is not yet awake. Should this patient be extubated while deeply anesthetized? What other technique might be recommended?

   In patients whose airway has been assessed as difficult, it is optimal to have the patient fully awake with all reflexes intact prior to extubation. Because of the operative procedure performed (hip replacement), the anesthetist does not have to be concerned that the incision will be disrupted if the patient "bucks" or coughs upon awakening. In any case, the necessary equipment should be available in the event that reintubation becomes necessary.

▶ SUMMARY

Airway management is the primary function of the anesthesia provider and is not limited to the operating suite alone. The anesthetist may be called upon to manage the patient's airway in a variety of locations peripheral to the operating room, such as the emergency room, intensive care unit, or radiology department. The primary goal of airway management is to recognize and alleviate airway obstruction in order to provide adequate aveolar ventilation. Airway management requires knowledge and understanding of the anatomy of the upper airway in order to provide accurate airway assessment and subsequent appropriate airway management. The anesthesia provider must recognize anatomical differences between pediatric and adult patients in order to safely manage the airway. Knowledge of a variety of airway techniques is essential, including mask and intubation techniques and airway placement, as well as reducing the risk of aspiration. Successful management of the airway depends on recognizing potential problems and their etiology, assessing the patient's condition, having all appropriate equipment available and in working order, and on the anesthesia provider's adeptness and familiarity with various airway-management techniques. In all instances, the anesthesia provider must maintain adequate ventilation and oxygenation. Patients do not die from failure to intubate but rather from failure to oxygenate. The fundamental responsibility of the anesthesia provider is to provide adequate gas exchange.

▶ KEY CONCEPTS

- The main goal of airway management is to recognize and promptly alleviate airway obstruction and to establish adequate alveolar ventilation.
- If a tooth or component of an orthodontic appliance or prosthesis becomes dislodged during an anesthetic, it must be found.
- The cricoid cartilage is the only complete ring in the larynx and the narrowest portion of the upper airway in the pediatric patient.
- The nine intrinsic muscles of the larynx govern the size and shape of the glottis.
- If bilateral damage of the recurrent laryngeal nerve occurs, complete airway obstruction will occur and require tracheostomy or endotracheal intubation.
- The two main properties of gas flow within the airways are laminar flow and turbulent flow.
- Upon placement of an uncuffed endotracheal tube, a leak should arise when 10 to 30 cm H_2O of inspiratory pressure is applied in a child 10 years old or younger.
- The distance from the lips to the carina in an infant is approximately 13 cm, compared to 24 cm (female) and 28 cm (male) in the adult patient.
- One reliable sign that preoxygenation is actually occurring is the movement of the reservoir bag correlating with the patient's breathing.
- A topical anesthetic in the upper airway is indicated when an awake intubation is planned or when the cardiovascular response to either laryngoscopy or surgical stimulation of the upper airway is undesirable.
- The most common problem encountered during mask ventilation is upper respiratory obstruction, usually due to soft-tissue collapse within the upper airway.
- Avoid inspiratory pressures greater than 20 cm of H_2O during mask ventilation.
- The purpose of the oropharyngeal and nasopharyngeal airway is to displace the tongue anteriorly, allowing the patient to breathe through (oral or nasal) or around the airway (oral).
- Endotracheal intubation requires knowledge of the anatomy of the upper airway, a moderate amount of technical skill, and the common sense to know when it is both appropriate and inappropriate to pursue.

- Endotracheal tubes are made of polyvinylchloride (PVC), which is a nontoxic, nonallergenic substance.
- Obtaining adequate depth of anesthesia during laryngoscopy will lessen the potential for any cardiovascular changes during laryngoscopy irregardless of which laryngoscope is used.
- Nasal intubations should be avoided if the patient presents with a nasal fracture, severe nasal obstruction, acute sinusitis, or a cerebrospinal leak due to head trauma.
- When the endotracheal tube is advanced too distally in the adult patient, the tip will likely enter the right mainstem bronchus and a significant shunt will develop.
- The two most reliable methods confirming the correct placement of an endotracheal tube are to observe the tip of the endotracheal tube pass through the vocal cords and a sustained $ETCO_2$ waveform.
- The number-one priority during a rapid-sequence (crash) induction (in addition to providing ventilation) is to protect the lungs from vomitus or regurgitation of gastrointestinal contents.
- The correct technique of cricoid pressure is to grasp the cricoid cartilage between the thumb and index finger and direct the cricoid cartilage posterior toward the vertebral body of C6.
- Cricoid pressure should be released once proper endotracheal tube placement has been verified or if ventilation via mask is not possible.
- The advantage of the modified rapid-sequence technique is the ability to ventilate the patient prior to the administration of a muscle relaxant.
- Difficult extubations can arise because of failure to deflate the cuff or oddities such as inadvertent suturing or wiring of the endotracheal tube.
- Management of the difficult airway depends on recognizing a potential problem, the etiology of the problem, the patient's condition, the available equipment, familiarity of the operator with various techniques, and whether the difficulty was anticipated.
- The number-one priority of the anesthesia provider when confronted with a difficult airway is to provide ventilation for the patient, not intubation.

▶ STUDY QUESTIONS

1. What is the main goal of airway management?

2. What is the proper technique for preoxygenation prior to induction of anesthesia?

3. In what situations should nasal intubation be avoided?

4. What is the primary indication for a rapid-sequence induction?

5. Describe the two most reliable signs of correct placement of the endotracheal tube.

6. Discuss the proper techniques for endotracheal and nasotracheal intubation.

KEY REFERENCES

Benumof, J. L. (1990). Management of the difficult or impossible airway. *ASA refresher course lectures* (#163). Las Vegas: American Society of Anesthesiologists, Inc.

Benumof, J. L. (1991). Management of the difficult adult airway. *Anesthesiology, 75,* 1087–1110.

Benumof, J. L. (1992). Management of the difficult airway: The ASA algorithm. *ASA refresher course lectures* (#134, pp. 1–7). New Orleans: American Society of Anesthesiologists, Inc.

Finucane, B. T., & Santora, A. H. (1996). *Principles of airway management* (p. 109). St. Louis: Mosby.

Frerk, C. M. (1991). Predicting difficult intubation. *Anaesthesia, 46,* 1005–1008.

Pace, N. A., Gajraj, N. M., Pennant, J. H., Victory R. A., Johnson E. R., & White P. F. (1994). Use of laryngeal mask airway after oesophageal intubation. *British Journal of Anaesthesia, 73,* 688–689.

REFERENCES

Benumof, J. L. (1990). Management of the difficult or impossible airway. *ASA refresher course lectures* (#163). Las Vegas: American Society of Anesthesiologists, Inc.

Benumof, J. L. (1991). Management of the difficult adult airway. *Anesthesiology, 75,* 1087–1110.

Benumof, J. L. (1992). Management of the difficult airway: The ASA algorithm. *ASA refresher course lectures* (#134, pp. 1–7). New Orleans: American Society of Anesthesiologists, Inc.

Davis, P. D., Parbrook, D. G., & Kenny, G. N. C. (1995). *Basic physics and measurement in anaesthesia.* (4th ed., pp. 110–111). Oxford: Butterworth-Heinemann.

Finucane, B. T., & Santora, A. H. (1996). *Principles of airway management* (p. 109). St. Louis: Mosby.

Frerk, C. M. (1991). Predicting difficult intubation. *Anaesthesia, 46,* 1005–1008.

Le Bel, L. A. (1992). Principles of chemistry and physics in anesthesia. In W. R. Waugaman, S. D. Foster, & B. M. Rigor (Eds.), *Principles and practice of nurse anesthesia* (2nd ed., p. 79). Norwalk, CT: Appleton & Lange.

Pace, N. A., Gajraj, N. M., Pennant, J. H., Victory, R. A., Johnson E. R., & White, P. F. (1994). Use of laryngeal mask airway after oesophageal intubation. *British Journal of Anaesthesia, 73,* 688–689.

Samsoon, G. L. T., & Young, J. R. B. (1987). Difficult tracheal intubation: A retrospective study. *Anaesthesia, 42,* 487–490.

Fluid Therapy

Leon F. Deisering

Maintaining fluid balance is an integral part of the anesthetic management of the perioperative patient. Knowledge of body compartmental fluids, their changes, and the appropriate replacement therapy is essential. This chapter reviews all of the necessary components of fluid therapy.

► TOTAL BODY WATER

Water is the primary component of the human body. Total body water is approximately 42 L in an adult. The water content of the body varies with age, gender, and body habitus. In adult males 55% to 60% of the body weight is water, whereas in females water averages 45% to 50% of body weight (Stoelting & Miller, 1994).

Fat contains little water, and lean body mass has more body fluid. Obese persons have as much as 25% to 30% less total body water than do lean persons. Age also plays a significant factor in the amount of total body water a person has. As age increases, total body water decreases to a low of 52% for men and 47% for women. The opposite is true for infants. A full-term infant will have 70% to 80% total body water. This is illustrated in Table 26–1 (Jordan, 1992).

Total body water is divided into two major compartments: intracellular fluid (ICF) and extracellular fluid (ECF).

Intracellular Fluid

Intracellular fluid is the water contained within the different cells of the body. It makes up approximately 40% of body weight, or 28 L. The largest amount of ICF is located in the skeletal muscle mass. The ICF's principal cations are potassium and magnesium, and the principal anions are proteins and phosphates.

Extracellular Fluid

Extracellular fluid is the body water outside the cells. It constitutes 20% of body weight. Extracellular fluid helps maintain the internal environment of the body. It provides nutrients and removes wastes from the cells. It is further subdivided into two major types: the intravascular volume (plasma), which is about 5% of body weight, and the interstitial volume (fluid between the cells), which totals 15% of body weight (McCall, 1996).

Approximately 80% of the ECF is interstitial fluid. Intracellular fluid includes lymph, the extracellular portion of dense connective tissue, and the transcellular compartment. Transcellular water includes cerebrospinal, intraocular, synovial, peritoneal, and pericardial fluid.

The intravascular fluid or plasma portion of the ECF is the fluid portion of blood. Plasma interchanges with the interstitial fluid continuously, through pores, exchanging oxygen and other metabolic substances.

► REGULATION OF FLUIDS

The body attempts to maintain a homeostatic environment. The internal and external environments of the body fluids attempt to maintain stable conditions, in which the responses of compensatory mechanisms may be activated. The regulatory system assists in keeping the fluctuations of body fluids and electrolytes at a minimum. The internal environment is maintained by the kid-

TABLE 26–1. Approximate Values of Total Body Fluid as a Percentage of Body Weight in Relation to Age and Sex

| Age | Fluid (% body weight) | |
	Males	Females
Full-term newborn	70–80	70–80
1 year	64	64
Puberty to 39 years	60	52
40–60 years	55	47
>60 years	52	46

neys, lungs, brain, skin, and gastrointestinal tract. Situations such as surgical stress may alter the internal environment.

The body exchanges the fluid and electrolyte requirements on a daily basis. The average daily needs of a 60- to 80-kg adult male are outlined in Table 26–2. Daily water losses include 250 mL in the stool, 800 to 1500 mL as urine, and about 600 to 900 mL as insensible loss from the lungs and through the skin (Jordan, 1992).

Two variables help regulate body fluids. The sensation of thirst is the body's sensory drive for fluid replacement. The second variable associated with thirst is the secretion of antidiuretic hormone (ADH). A change in the tonicity of ECF inhibits the release of ADH, and water reabsorption by the renal tubules occurs. Many factors influence the thirst mechanism.

Water

Daily intake of water to the body is accomplished from two major sources: that ingested in the form of liquids or

TABLE 26–2. Water Exchange (60- to 80-kg man)

	Average Daily Volume (mL)	Minimal (mL)	Maximal (mL)
H₂O gain routes			
Sensible			
Oral fluids	800–1500	0	1500/h
Solid foods	500–700	0	1500
Insensible			
Water of oxidation	250	125	800
Water of solution	0	0	500
H₂O loss routes			
Sensible			
Urine	800–1500	300	1400/h
Intestinal	0–250	0	2500/h
Sweat	0	0	4000/h
Insensible			
Lungs and skin	600–900	600–900	1500

water in the food, which accounts for about 2100 mL a day of body fluids, and that synthesized in the body as a result of oxidation of carbohydrates, adding about 200 mL/day. This provides for a total of approximately 2300 mL/day of water intake. Fluid intake is highly variable and depends on individual variation, climate, habits, and level of physical activity.

Thirst, a conscious desire to drink water, is basically an emergency mechanism that points to a perceived water deficit. Intracellular dehydration will initiate this sensation by sending a signal to the thirst center, which is located in the hypothalamus. The mechanism is similar to that of the osmoreceptor cells triggering the secretion of ADH (Khraibi & Knox, 1995).

Hydrogen Bonding

One important property of water relates to its molecular structure and is termed hydrogen bonding. Water is composed of one oxygen and two hydrogen atoms. The configuration of a molecule of water is such that the two atoms of hydrogen are aligned to one side of the oxygen atom. This makes one side of the molecule relatively positive and the other relatively negative, giving the molecule a dipolar configuration. This configuration allows the hydrogen and oxygen to combine with the least expenditure of energy. It also facilitates the development of attractive forces between water molecules. The hydrogen atom of one water molecule becomes oriented toward the oxygen atom of another water molecule, forming a latticework arrangement. These weak hydrogen bonds account for the relative instability of complex proteins and help maintain amino acid peptide integrity for synthesis of new protein. Because water has polarity, it is an excellent solvent for other polar molecules, such as alcohols, but not for nonpolar substances, such as oils.

Hydrogen bonding helps account for many properties of water, such as a high boiling point and surface tension. Dissolving solutes in water will produce anions, cations, undissociated molecules or radicals, as well as changes in what are termed the *colligative properties* of water. Colligative changes are alterations in physical properties wrought by the disruption of water's normal structure. This disruption results in elevation of the boiling point, depression of the freezing point, lowering of the vapor pressure, and change in osmotic pressure (Fox & Whitesell, 1994).

Homeostasis

The body attempts to maintain a homeostatic environment. The internal and external environments of the body fluids attempt to maintain stable conditions, in which the responses of compensatory mechanisms may be activated. Surgical stress may alter the internal environment. The body exchanges fluid and electrolyte requirements on a daily basis. Insensible water losses occur from the lungs by the humidification of inspired air and through the skin by evaporation. Insensible loss can be greatly increased under hypermetabolic conditions, such as hyperventilation and fever. This loss through the breathing circuit during anesthesia is a major concern that must be considered, especially during long cases. The minimal amount of urinary output necessary to rid the body of the products of catabolism is 500 to 800 mL per day.

Osmosis

The most abundant substance to diffuse through the cell membrane is water. Normally, the amount that diffuses in the two directions across the cell membrane is precisely balanced, and little to no movement occurs. Consequently, the volume of the cell remains constant. Under certain conditions, a concentration difference of water can develop across the membrane. When this occurs, there is a net movement of water across the membrane, causing the cell to swell or shrink depending on the direction of movement. The process of net movement of water caused by a concentration difference of water is called *osmosis* (Guyton & Hall, 1996).

Osmolality

To measure the osmotic pressure of a solute, it is necessary to be able to determine the number of particles of the solute. The number of particles in a solute creates the osmotic pressure of a solution. The concentration or osmotic activity of a solute in terms of number of particles is expressed as osmoles. One osmole (osm) is 1 g molecular weight (GMW) of undissociated solute (Guyton & Hall, 1996). The particles of a solute may be a combination of several different kinds of nondiffusible ions and molecules in a given solution.

One GMW of a dissolved, nonionizing, nondiffusible solute equals 1 osm. One GMW of such a solute contains 6.02×10^{23} molecules (Avogadro's number). When there is a combination of several different kinds of solutes in a given solution, one GMW of each solute in the solution will be equal to the number of osmotically active particles. For example, sodium chloride will dissociate into two ions; 1 GMW of this solute will be equal to 2 osm because the number of osmotically active particles is twice as great (Waterhouse, 1992).

When a solution has 1 osm of solute dissolved in 1 kg of water, it is said to have an osmolality of 1 osmole per kilogram (1 osm/kg). A solution that has 1/1000 osm dissolved per kilogram has an osmolality of 1 milliosmole per kilogram (1 mOsm/kg). The normal osmolality of intracellular and extracellular fluids is about 300 mOsm/kg (Guyton & Hall, 1996).

Osmolarity

When measuring osmolality, it is necessary to measure solutions in terms of kilograms of water. In general, the osmole is too large a unit to express the osmotic activity of solutes in the body fluids. The solutions within the body are dilute solutions, making it more appropriate to express osmolar concentration in terms of osmoles per liter (osm/L) of solution. Therefore, osmolarity is the concentration of the particles of a solute in a solution and is generally expressed as osm/L of solution (Waterhouse, 1992).

Osmotic Pressure

Osmotic pressure is the precise amount of pressure required to prevent osmosis. It is equal to the amount of pressure that must be applied to prevent the net diffusion of water through a membrane and is expressed in millimeters of mercury (mmHg). Osmotic pressure is an indirect measurement of the water and solute concentrations of a solution. The higher the osmotic pressure of a solution, the lower the water concentration, and the higher the solute concentration of the solution (Guyton & Hall, 1996).

At normal body temperature, a concentration of 1 osm/L will cause an osmotic pressure of 19 300 mmHg in the solution. A concentration of 1 mOsm/L is therefore equivalent to an osmotic pressure of 19.3 mmHg. As stated, normal osmolality of the intracellular and extracellular fluids is about 300 mOsm/kg. Multiplying the osmotic pressure of 19.3 mmHg by 300 mOsm/kg will give a total calculated osmotic pressure for these fluids of 5790 mmHg, although the actual measurement is about 5500 mmHg. The difference is due to ions being attracted to one another and that are unable to create their full potential on osmotic pressure.

Oncotic Pressure

Oncotic pressure is the osmotic pressure due to the presence of colloids in a solution. In plasma, it is the force that tends to counterbalance the capillary blood pressure.

Milliequivalent Weights

A milliequivalent weight of an element is its weight in milligrams that is equivalent to or equal in combining weight to that of 1 mg of hydrogen:

$$1000 \text{ mg} = 1 \text{ g}$$
$$1 \text{ mg} = 0.001 \text{ g}$$
$$1000 \text{ milliequivalent weight (mEq)}$$
$$= 1 \text{ equivalent weight (GEW)}$$
$$1 \text{ mEq} = 0.001 \text{ GEW}$$

For NaCl:

> 1 GEW weighs 58 g
> 0.001 GEW weighs 0.058 g
> 1 mEq (weight) weighs 0.058 g
> 1 mEq weighs 58 mg

For H_2S:

> 1 GEW weighs 17 g
> 0.001 GEW weighs 0.017 g
> 1 mEq (weight) weighs 0.017 g
> 1 mEq weighs 17 mg

Milliequivalents are used to measure body concentrations of specific ions known as *electrolytes*. There is an optimum concentration of each electrolyte in each tissue or fluid compartment. Various laboratory tests of electrolytes are reported in milliequivalents because this is the only method by which specific laboratory results can be compared meaningfully with normal body electrolyte concentrations. In addition, electrolyte replacement therapy with drugs and intravenous fluids can be accurately determined by assessing the milliequivalent concentrations of various body fluids (Waterhouse, 1992).

Solutions

Solutions are intimate, homogeneous mixtures of two or more components. The components are made up of solutes and solvents. Solutions contain particles of about 0.05 to about 0.25 nanometer (nm) in diameter.

Solution Tonicity

Solution tonicity refers to the osmotic pressure of a solution relative to that of body fluids. The tonicity of solutions depends on the concentrations of impermeant solutes (Guyton & Hall, 1996). The terms *isotonic, hypotonic,* and *hypertonic* refer to whether the solutions will cause a change in cell volume.

Isotonic, Hypertonic, and Hypotonic Solutions

Isotonic or isosmotic solutions have an osmotic pressure similar to that of body fluids. Hypertonic or hyperosmotic solutions have an osmotic pressure that is greater than that of normal body fluids. Hypotonic or hypoosmotic solutions have an osmotic pressure that is lower than that of normal body fluids.

Some substances that are highly permeative can cause transient shifts in fluid volumes between the intracellular and extracellular compartments, but, over time, the concentration of these substances becomes equal between the two compartments and a steady state returns.

Normal Solutions

A 1 normal solution of any solute contains 1 GEW/L of solution; a 0.5 normal solution contains 0.5 GEW/L, or 0.5 mEq/mL of solution. One GEW of NaCl weighs 58 g; 58 g NaCl/L = 5.8% NaCl. A 1 molar solution of NaCl equals a 1 normal solution of NaCl (Waterhouse, 1992).

Molar Solutions

A 1 molar solution of any solute contains 1 GMW, or 1 mol/L of solution. The molar concentration of a solution is the number of moles or the fraction of 1 mol of solute present in 1 L of solution.

One GMW of dextrose ($C_6H_{12}O_6$) weighs 180 g: 180 g/L in an 18% solution. An 18% solution of dextrose in water ($D_{18}W$) is a 1 molar dextrose solution (Waterhouse, 1992).

Osmolarity of Solutions

To calculate the osmolarity of a solution, all the solute particles in a given volume of the solution must be counted.

Example 1. What is the osmolarity of 5.4% DW?

> 5.4% DW = 54 g of dextrose/L of solution
> 1 molar DW = 180 g/L

Therefore, the molarity of 5.4% DW is:

$$\frac{54 \text{ g}}{L} \div \frac{180 \text{ g}}{mol} = \frac{54 \text{ g}}{L} \times \frac{mol}{180} = \frac{0.3 \text{ mol}}{L}$$

As shown, 1 molar dextrose = 1 osmolar dextrose; 0.3 molar dextrose = 0.3 osmolar dextrose, or 300 mOsm/L, an isotonic solution (Waterhouse, 1992).

Example 2. What is the osmolarity of 5.4% dextrose in 0.87% sodium chloride? As shown in the previous example, the osmotic pressure of 5.4% DW is 300 mOsm/L.

> 0.87% NaCl = 8.7 g NaCl/L
> 1 molar NaCl = 58 g/L

The molarity of 0.87% NaCl is:

$$\frac{8.7 \text{ g}}{L} \div \frac{58 \text{ g}}{mol} = \frac{8.7 \text{ g}}{L} \times \frac{mol}{58 \text{ g}} = \frac{0.15 \text{ mol}}{L}$$

One molar NaCl equals 2 osmolar NaCl. Each molecule ionizes into two ions. Therefore, 0.15 molar NaCl = 0.3 osmolar NaCl, or 300 mOsm. The osmotic pressure of 5.4% dextrose in 0.87% NaCl is:

> 300 mOsm of dextrose/L
> + 300 mOsm of NaCl/L
> _____
> 600 mOsm/L, a hypertonic solution

Because the osmotic pressure of body fluids is about 0.3 osm/L, it is necessary to calculate the percentages of all injectable solutions to be sure that they are compatible with the body fluids.

Molar solutions are not necessarily the same as osmolar solutions: 1 GMW/L dextrose = 1 osmolar solution, but 1 GMW/L NaCl = 2 osmolar solution. Therefore, 0.3 molar (or 0.3 osmolar) dextrose solution = 0.3 (180 g)/L = 54 g/L = 5.4% DW, an isotonic solution, and 0.3 molar NaCl = 0.6 osmolar solution, which is hypertonic 0.15 molar (0.3 osmolar) NaCl = 0.15 (58 g/L) = 8.7 g/L = 0.87% NaCl, an isotonic solution (Waterhouse, 1992).

Saturated Solution

A solution that contains all the solute that it can at equilibrium is saturated. One that contains less than this amount would be an unsaturated solution.

Supersaturated Solution

A supersaturated solution contains solute in excess of what it would contain at equilibrium. These solutions are unstable because they are not in equilibrium. The excess solute may precipitate readily and quite rapidly when the supersaturated solution is agitated or any additional solute is added. Precipitation occurs until equilibrium is once again established in the solution.

Solvent

A solvent is a substance that dissolves the components of a solution. A solvent usually is present in a greater proportion than the solute in a solution.

Solute

A solute is a component of a solution and is the substance that is being dissolved by the solvent. A solute is usually present in a smaller proportion than the solvent in a solution.

Emulsions

Emulsions are colloidal dispersions that have charged particles. Ions are located on the surface of each particle, and all particles of a dispersion will bear like charges. Because like charges repel, particles in a colloidal dispersion tend to stay away from one another, preventing the formation of large particles that would settle out. Particle size in these dispersions range between 0.25 to 100 nm.

Suspensions

Suspensions are heterogeneous mixtures where components are not dissolved. Each component will separate from each other when left to settle. There is only a temporary dispersion of particles in the mixture. Particle size in suspensions are 100 nm or more (Masterson, Slowinski, & Stanitski, 1981).

► BODY FLUID CHANGES

Disorders of fluid balance can be categorized as disturbances of volume, concentration, and composition.

Volume Changes

Volume changes that occur within the body are either a volume deficit or a volume excess.

Volume Deficit

Extracellular fluid volume deficit frequently is referred to as fluid deficit, hypovolemia, or dehydration. An ECF volume deficit is due to a loss of water and electrolytes where there is a greater loss of fluid than there is intake of fluid. The hallmark of water deficit in the body is a plasma sodium concentration above 145 mEq/L (Stoelting & Dierdorf, 1993).

The body loses fluid via the kidneys, skin, lungs, and gastrointestinal tract. The skin loses water through perspiration, which varies widely with the temperature of the environment. Insensible loss of water through the skin occurs by evaporation. The loss of fluid from the lungs occurs at a rate of 300 to 400 mL every day. This loss can increase greatly with a higher respiratory rate and tidal volume. The body loses 100 to 200 mL of fluid daily through the gastrointestinal tract. Therefore, the average adult requires at least 2000 mL of water per day.

Extracellular fluid volume may be caused by vomiting, diarrhea, loss of nasogastric secretions, prolonged mechanical ventilation, and fistula drainage. During surgery, the patient loses a great deal of ECF by evaporation and blood and third-space losses as a result of surgical trauma. Other causes of ECF loss include burns, peritonitis, intestinal obstruction, and sequestration of fluid from soft-tissue injury.

Clinical manifestations of ECF volume deficit include dry mucous membranes and reduced skin turgor. When dehydration becomes more pronounced, a decrease in blood pressure, venous pressure, and urine output may be seen. Increased heart rate, weight loss, nausea and vomiting, weakness, and apathy also are signs of fluid deficit. Severe dehydration may lead to cardiovascular collapse, shock, inadequate perfusion of the kidneys, and severe kidney damage. The treatment for volume excess includes fluid administration, orally and/or parenterally (Jordan, 1992).

Volume Excess

Excess of ECF volume often is caused by fluid excess, which develops when fluid input exceeds output. The kidneys are unable to rid the body of excess water and electrolytes. Volume excess often develops when the body is overloaded by oral or parenteral administration of excessive quantities of fluid or as a result of renal failure. Excess ECF indicates an increase in both plasma and interstitial fluid volume.

The hallmark of water excess in the body is a plasma sodium concentration below 135 mEq/L (Stoelting & Dierdorf, 1993). Clinical manifestations of excess ECF include circulatory overload manifested by pulmonary hypertension, dyspnea, cyanosis, coughing, frothy sputum, elevated pulmonary artery pressures, ascites, peripheral edema, distended neck veins, moist rales, and increased central venous pressure and blood pressure.

The treatment for volume excess includes fluid restriction, administration of diuretics, restriction of sodium intake, administration of vasodilators, and positive-pressure ventilation (Jordan, 1992).

► ELECTROLYTES

Electrolytes are electrically charged particles within the body fluids. These charged particles are ions. The term *ion* describes chemical reactivity. Ions possess negative (anions) and positive (cations) charges. Intracellular fluid and ECF have different concentrations of ions.

Sodium

Sodium (Na) is the most abundant cation of the ECF and is the most important ion exerting osmotic pressure on the cellular membrane. Sodium is a primary determinant of ECF and water distribution. Sodium is regulated in part by the kidneys. It helps maintain the normal composition of ECF, as well as chemical–electrical equilibrium. Sodium also mediates action potentials within the nerves and muscles.

Sodium is regulated in the body by the secretion of antidiuretic hormone (ADH) and aldosterone. The secretion of ADH from the hypothalamic posterior pituitary causes an increase in water reabsorption by the kidneys that results in decreased urinary output and increased urinary concentration. The production and release of ADH are influenced by receptors in the anterior hypothalamus known as osmoreceptor cells. Osmoreceptors are sensitive to osmotic pressure of the plasma. An increase in ECF osmolarity (which also means an increase in plasma sodium concentration) causes these osmoreceptor cells to shrink. The shrinkage of these cells stimulates them to send nerve signals to the posterior pituitary gland, which stimulates the release of ADH (Guyton & Hall, 1996). The opposite sequence of events will occur when ECF becomes too dilute and osmolarity decreases.

Aldosterone is a mineralocorticoid secreted by the adrenal cortex. Its primary function is to promote transport of sodium and potassium through the renal tubular walls. Aldosterone will cause an increase in the absorption of sodium and the simultaneous excretion of potassium, primarily in the collecting tubule, thereby conserving sodium in the ECF.

Potassium

Most potassium within the body is found in the intracellular compartment, where it is the major cation. Its primary function is to transmit nerve impulses and to make muscles contract. Potassium moves freely between the intracellular and extracellular compartments. The sodium–potassium pump controls the movement of potassium between the cells and ECF. Two mechanisms that regulate potassium balance are (1) plasma potassium concentration and (2) aldosterone (Khraibi & Knox, 1995).

Plasma potassium concentration directly affects potassium excretion. Ninety percent of the filtered potassium is reabsorbed in the proximal convoluted tubule and loop of Henle of the kidney. The remaining 10% that reaches the distal convoluted tubule and the collecting ducts is regulated according to the level of potassium in the plasma. Elevated extracellular potassium concentration will cause the collecting duct cells to increase the uptake of potassium, and this leads to increased intracellular potassium. Increased intracellular potassium causes increased potassium secretion in the tubules and increased potassium excretion (Khraibi & Knox, 1995). This mechanism plays the dominant role in controlling potassium excretion.

Aldosterone also plays a major role in potassium balance. Aldosterone is the only factor that can maintain a simultaneous balance of potassium and sodium. Increased levels of potassium will cause aldosterone to be secreted. Aldosterone acts on the collecting ducts to increase potassium excretion.

Calcium

Calcium is the most abundant cation in the body. It is found in the protoplasm and is present in large proportions in bones and teeth. Calcium is involved with cellular permeability, neuromuscular activity, and normal blood-clotting mechanisms. Plasma calcium level is controlled through renal regulation.

Approximately 40% of plasma calcium is bound to plasma proteins. The remaining 60% consists of ionized calcium and is physiologically active. This ionized calcium is filtered at the glomerular capillaries. Of the 100% of the filtered calcium, only 0.5% to 2% actually remains in the urine and is excreted (Khraibi & Knox, 1995).

Parathyroid hormone also controls the level of ECF calcium. Any change in ECF calcium concentration will create a response from the parathyroid gland. A decrease in ionized calcium concentration of ECF increases the rate of secretion of parathyroid hormone. When the level of calcium ion concentration of the ECF increases, parathyroid hormone secretion is reduced. Parathyroid hormone stimulates calcium reabsorption in the kidney, decreasing urinary calcium excretion.

Calcitonin, a hormone produced by the thyroid gland, also affects plasma calcium concentration by reducing plasma calcium concentration. Calcitonin has only a weak effect on controlling calcium levels and is easily overpowered by the parathyroid hormone.

Magnesium

Magnesium serves as a catalyst for intracellular enzymatic actions. Magnesium is the second most abundant cation in the ICF compartment after potassium. Smaller amounts of magnesium are found in the ECF, where it is constantly filtered and regulated primarily by the kidneys. Increases in the extracellular concentration of magnesium depresses the nervous and skeletal muscular systems. The regulation and distribution of magnesium within the body parallel those of calcium (Khraibi & Knox, 1995).

Phosphate

Inorganic phosphate is the major intracellular anion and is involved in the conservation of the chemical energy used to drive chemical syntheses and muscle contractions and to maintain membrane potential. Organic phosphate occurs in many body constituents and is involved with intermediary metabolism. Phosphate excretion is regulated primarily in the proximal tubule. Parathyroid hormone will inhibit reabsorption and increase the excretion of phosphate (Khraibi & Knox, 1995).

► ALTERATIONS IN ELECTROLYTE CONCENTRATION

Sodium

Concentrations of sodium in the ECF normally range from 135 to 145 mEq/L. Levels above or below this range indicate an abnormality.

Hyponatremia

Hyponatremia is a low sodium concentration in the ECF, below 135 mEq/L. Hyponatremia may be caused by excessive loss of sodium from vomiting, diarrhea, diuretics, and through body cavities as seen in peritonitis, draining ascites, and burns. The most common cause of sodium deficit is excessive intake of water, which dilutes the serum sodium (Khraibi & Knox, 1995). The hyponatremic state lends itself to an osmotic shift out of the ECF compartment and into the ICF compartment. This shift causes fluid depletion in the ECF compartment and leads to hypovolemia. A severe shift of fluid causes cerebral edema, leading to the development of neurologic symptoms.

The clinical signs associated with hyponatremia resulting from sodium loss are weakness, confusion, nausea, vomiting, neurologic signs, postural hypotension, and lethargy. Some of the more serious neurologic symptoms that may develop are loss of reflexes, the Babinski sign, and seizures.

The treatment for sodium deficiency is aimed at restoring sodium in the ECF compartment. Oral sodium and/or intravenous fluid replacement of sodium with a hypertonic sodium chloride solution may be used to treat sodium deficiency (Jordan, 1992).

Hypernatremia

Hypernatremia exists when the plasma sodium concentration exceeds 145 mEq/L. The kidneys closely regulate total body sodium content, and excess accumulation of sodium occurs infrequently. Some conditions contribute to excess sodium in the body, such as decreased water intake, excessive loss of body fluids, increased aldosterone levels, excessive administration of sodium-containing fluids, and impaired renal function.

Signs of hypernatremia include furrowed tongue, restlessness, lethargy, increased deep-tendon reflexes, flushed skin, thirst, peripheral edema, ascites, and pleural edema. The treatment for excessive sodium consists of limiting sodium intake, facilitating excretion of sodium through diuretics and the administration of water (Jordan, 1992).

Potassium

The normal value for serum potassium is 3.5 to 5.5 mEq/L. The normal dietary intake of potassium is 50 to 100 mg daily; however, 80% of the potassium is excreted via the renal system, and the other 20% is lost through the bowel and sweat glands. The kidneys do not conserve potassium; therefore, a daily intake of potassium is vital for body function.

Hypokalemia

Hypokalemia can be defined as low serum levels of potassium of less than 3.5 mEq/L. Many of the causes of hypokalemia are iatrogenic. It is common in patients on diuretic therapy. Because hypertension is more frequent and often is treated with diuretics, the frequency of hypokalemia in surgical patients has increased. Other factors that contribute to hypokalemia are starvation; diarrhea; loss of body fluids, particularly gastric secretions; reduced renal absorption; and stressful situations such as fever, sweating, and thyroid storm. Prolonged administration of antibiotics also may lead to hypokalemia. Surgical patients tend to have increased potassium loss in the immediate postoperative period. Metabolic and respiratory alkalosis also increases the renal excretion of potassium. Hyperventilation of the lungs during anesthesia can produce acute hypokalemia due to changes in the distribution of potassium between the cells and extracellular fluid. The same mechanism will cause acute hypokalemia when a glucose-insulin infusion is given (Stoelting & Dierdorf, 1993).

The signs and symptoms of hypokalemia result from alteration of the body systems. The neuromuscular dysfunctions that are due to hypokalemia are anorexia, weakness, loss of muscle tone, and loss of muscle reflexes. The cardiovascular system displays signs such as a weak pulse, arrhythmias, decreased intensity of heart sounds, and decreased blood pressure. The electrocardiogram (ECG) shows a low, flattened T-wave, depressed S-T segment, and predominant U-wave (Fig. 26–1). Cardiac arrest may eventually follow. The gastrointestinal tract decreases peristaltic movement, and abdominal distention may result. A pseudodiabetic glycosuria may result because glucose cannot move across the cell membrane.

Treatment for hypokalemia includes potassium replacement and correcting the causes for the loss. Supplemental dietary potassium intake is useful if the hypokalemia is mild. In more severe situations, decreased potassium levels can be life-threatening and potassium may be given intravenously. Care is necessary in administering intravenous potassium. Too rapid an infusion of potassium is potentially dangerous. Patients should have ECG monitoring during potassium infusion and repeat plasma potassium measurements should be done every 12 to 24 hours. In cases of severe hypokalemia, replacement and restoration to normal serum levels may take days to weeks (Jordan, 1992).

Hyperkalemia

Hyperkalemia is an excess of plasma potassium above 5.5 mEq/L. A common cause of hyperkalemia is renal failure and the inability of the kidney to excrete potassium. Life-threatening situations such as crushing injuries, burns, and myocardial damage allow a sudden release of potassium into the ECF. This sudden release of potassium can lead to cardiac arrhythmia, a flaccid myocardium, and cardiac arrest. The administration of succinylcholine to patients with burns, spinal cord transection, or muscle trauma causes the release of intracellular potassium and a hyperkalemic state (Khraibi & Knox, 1995). Other factors associated with hyperkalemia include transfusion of old blood, adrenocortical insufficiency, and too rapid or excessive administration of potassium.

Signs and symptoms of hyperkalemia are associated with nerve and muscle function. The muscular systems demonstrate signs of weakness and flaccid paralysis. The myocardium becomes flaccid, and arrhythmias and cardiac arrest develop. The conduction system throughout the myocardium is affected, and the ECG demonstrates high, center T-waves. P-waves disappear, the QRS complex widens, and bradycardia develops (Fig. 26–2). Heart block may occur during a severe state of hyperkalemia. The gastrointestinal tract of a patient in a hyperkalemic state demonstrates signs of hyperactivity, such as nausea, vomiting, intestinal colic, and diarrhea.

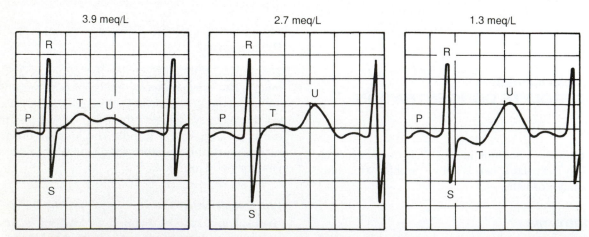

Figure 26–1. Electrocardiographic effects of hypokalemia. Note the progressive flattening of the T-wave, an increasingly prominent U-wave, increased amplitude of the P-wave, prolongation of the PR interval, and the ST segment depression. *(From Morgan, G. E., & Mikhail, M. S. [1996]. Clinical anesthesiology [2nd ed., p. 533], Stamford, CT: Appleton & Lange. Reprinted with permission.)*

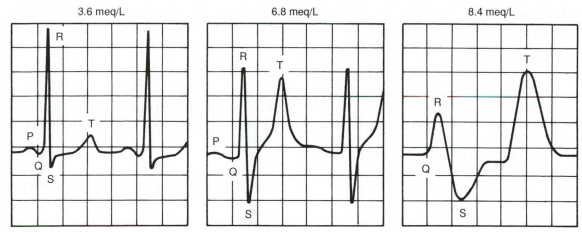

Figure 26–2. Electrocardiographic effect of hyperkalemia. Electrocardiographic changes characteristically progress from symmetrically peaked T-waves, often with a shortened QT interval, to widening of the QRS complex, prolongation of the PR interval, loss of the P-wave, loss of R-wave amplitude, and ST segment depression (occasionally elevation, to an ECG that resembles a sine wave, before final progression into ventricular fibrillation or asystole). *(From Morgan, G. E., & Mikhail, M. S. [1996].* Clinical anesthesiology *[2nd ed., p. 535]. Stamford, CT: Appleton & Lange. Reprinted with permission.)*

The treatment for hyperkalemia entails a reduction of serum potassium levels. Restriction of potassium administration and intake is one corrective measure. The use of cation-exchange resin will help facilitate the excretion of potassium. The treatment of severe hyperkalemia may include intravenous administration of calcium gluconate, sodium bicarbonate, and/or regular insulin. These forms of treatment facilitate the movement of potassium from the plasma into cells and serve as temporary control measures. Peritoneal dialysis and hemodialysis also can be used (Jordan, 1992).

Calcium

The normal daily intake of calcium is 1 to 3 g. The body cannot store calcium and daily consumption is necessary to sustain adequate levels in the body. The normal serum level of calcium is 8.6 to 10.5 mg/100 mL or 4.5 to 5.5 mEq/L. About 50% of serum calcium exists in the ionized form and is responsible for neuromuscular function.

Hypocalcemia

Hypocalcemia occurs when the plasma calcium concentration is below 8.6 mg/100 mL or 4.5 mEq/L. The more common causes of hypocalcemia are hypoparathyroidism, surgical removal of parathyroid glands, acute pancreatitis, vitamin D deficiency, renal failure, and decreased plasma albumin concentration (Stoelting & Dierdorf, 1993).

Signs and symptoms of hypocalcemia are shown by the central nervous system, heart, and neuromuscular function. The symptoms include tingling and numbness of the fingers, toes, and circumoral region; hyperactivity

of the deep-tendon reflexes; and mental confusion leading to convulsions. The ECG manifests a prolonged Q-T interval and S-T segment (Fig. 26–3). Many patients with hypocalcemia complain of skeletal muscle weakness, fatigue, and skeletal muscle spasms. Of concern to anesthetists is the possibility of laryngeal muscle spasm leading to airway obstruction, which can occur precipitously with the removal of the parathyroid glands.

Treatment is aimed at restoring calcium to normal levels. An intravenous infusion of calcium gluconate or calcium chloride should be considered when there are symptoms. In mild cases the calcium deficit can be treated with oral supplement and vitamin D (Jordan, 1992).

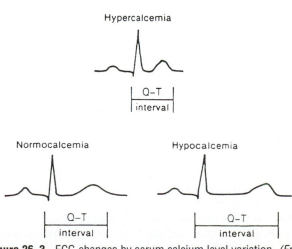

Figure 26–3. ECG changes by serum calcium level variation. *(From Wilson, R. F. [Ed.]. [1976].* Principles and techniques of critical care *[p. 26]. Philadelphia: Davis. Reprinted with permission.)*

Hypercalcemia

Hypercalcemia is present when the plasma calcium concentration is above 10.5 mg/100 mL or 5.5 mEq/L. Common causes of hypercalcemia are hyperparathyroidism, neoplastic disorders, overuse of calcium-containing antacids, vitamin D intoxication, and immobilization.

Signs and symptoms affect the central nervous system, gastrointestinal tract, kidneys, and heart. The symptoms most commonly seen are fatigue, anorexia, nausea, vomiting, urinary calcium stones, somnambulism, stupor, polydipsia, polyuria, and thirst. The ECG displays a shortened S-T segment and Q-T interval, prolonged P-R interval and a wide QRS complex (Fig. 26–3).

Treatment consists of hydration with saline, 0.45% or 0.9% solutions, to dilute the calcium concentration and to promote urinary excretion. Other treatment measures include the use of chelating agents, steroids, and hemodialysis (Jordan, 1992).

Magnesium

Normal extracellular levels of magnesium range from 1.5 to 2.5 mEq/L. A magnesium imbalance is not frequently seen. The normal dietary intake of magnesium is approximately 20 mEq daily.

Hypomagnesemia

Magnesium deficiency with a plasma concentration below 1.5 mEq/L is associated with chronic alcoholism, malabsorption syndromes, and vomiting and diarrhea.

The signs and symptoms of hypomagnesemia are characterized by neuromuscular and central nervous system hyperactivity. Coarse tremors, muscle cramps, hyperactive reflexes, tachycardia, paresthesias of the feet and legs, and arrhythmias are all clinical signs of magnesium deficiency. The ECG will demonstrate a prolonged P-R interval, wide QRS complex, S-T depression, and broadened and flattened T-waves.

The treatment focuses on restoring the magnesium levels. Oral administration of magnesium salts can be given for mild cases. Intravenous magnesium sulfate or magnesium chloride is necessary in more serious cases. Vital signs and patellar reflexes should be monitored during intravenous therapy (Jordan, 1992).

Hypermagnesemia

Hypermagnesemia occurs when the plasma concentration is above 2.5 mEq/L. Renal failure is one of the major causes of hypermagnesemia. Another common cause is iatrogenic, including the administration of magnesium sulfate to treat pregnancy-induced hypertension. Other contributing factors include Addison's disease, ketoacidosis, and hypothyroidism.

Clinical signs of hypermagnesemia include lethargy; loss of deep-tendon reflexes, which may progress to coma; flushing hypotension; depressed respirations; bradycardia; and ECG changes. The ECG displays an increased P-R interval, widened QRS complex, and a prolonged Q-T interval.

Treatment for severe hypermagnesemia is the administration of calcium gluconate or calcium carbonate to antagonize the action of magnesium. Diuresis also can be used to help lower the magnesium level (Jordan, 1992).

▶ FLUID AND ELECTROLYTE THERAPY

Parenteral Solution

The selection of parenteral solution should be based on the needs of the individual patient. The type and amount of parenteral solution should be carefully reviewed and estimated according to the physical status, weight, and cardiovascular status of the patient; daily maintenance requirements based on weight or body surface area; and the present fluid status of the patient prior to fluid therapy. Maintenance fluids provide replacement for normal fluid loss, such as loss via the lungs, urine, and skin. Maintenance fluids are isotonic. Replacement fluids are given to correct a loss of isotonic fluid from the body. The loss of isotonic fluid may include ascites and interstitial edema (Jordan, 1992). Table 26–3 can be used as a guide for the most appropriate fluid therapy for maintenance or replacement therapy.

Crystalloids are solutions that contain electrolytes dissolved in water or in dextrose and water. Commonly used crystalloid solutions are saline solutions and lactated Ringer's solutions. Crystalloid solutions determine the total osmotic pressure that balances water between the extracellular and the intracellular spaces (Litwack & Keithley, 1997).

Colloids are solutions that contain natural or synthetic molecules that are relatively impermeable to the vascular membrane. Colloids determine the colloid osmotic pressure that balances the distribution of water between the intravascular and the interstitial spaces (Litwack & Keithley, 1997). Albumin is an example of a natural colloid, and hetastarch and Dextran are synthetic colloids.

The decision to use a crystalloid or colloid solution during fluid therapy is based on the purpose of the therapy. Crystalloids commonly are used as maintenance fluids for normal losses or as replacement fluids to correct body fluid deficits. Colloids are used for fluid replacement and fluid resuscitation.

Perioperative Fluid Requirements

During the perioperative period, all surgical patients have the potential to develop fluid imbalance. The peri-

TABLE 26–3. Parenteral Fluids and Their Components

| Solution[a] | Type[b] | Components | | | | | |
		Na+	K+	Cl−	Ca++	Dextrose (g)	Lactate mOsm/kg
D₅W	M					5	252
D₅W 0.2% NaCl	R	34		34		5	321
D₅W 0.45% NaCl	M	77		77		5	406
D₅W 0.9% NaCl	R	154		154		5	506
D₅W/LR	R	130	4	109	3	5	525
LR	R	130	4	109	3		273
0.45% NS	M	77		77			154
0.9% NS	R	154		154			308

[a] D₅W, dextrose in water; D₅W 0.2% NaCl, 5% dextrose in one-quarter strength normal saline; D₅W 0.45% NaCl, 5% dextrose in one-half strength normal saline; D₅W 0.9% NaCl, 5% dextrose in normal saline; D₅W/LR, 5% dextrose in lactated Ringer's; LR, lactated Ringer's; 0.45% NS, one-half strength normal saline; 0.9% NS, normal saline. Na+, sodium; K+, potassium; Ca++, calcium.
[b] M, maintenance fluid; R, replacement fluid.

operative management of a surgical patient includes preoperative, intraoperative, and postoperative assessment and intervention (Achatz-Deresz, Cibula, & Emberson, 1992). The goal during this time frame is to maintain an optimal fluid balance and adequate tissue perfusion (McCall, 1996). All surgical patients have insensible fluid losses: evaporation from the respiratory tract, sweat, feces, and urinary excretion requiring fluid replacement. Certain conditions can increase these losses and requirements. A febrile patient, the size of the surgical incision, the type of surgical procedure, and the length of the surgery all influence insensible losses. The use of general anesthesia, the type of breathing circuits used, as well as the use of nonhumidified high gas flows will influence the amount of fluid loss during a surgical procedure. The anesthetist must consider all of these factors as well as the physical characteristics and medical condition of the patient when developing an anesthesia care plan (Jordan, 1992).

Preoperative Fluid Management

Fluid Deficit

Assessment of the preoperative fluid and electrolyte balance and subsequent management is necessary for successful surgical intervention. Observation and an accurate history of the patient's fluid intake are means of appraising a patient's fluid status. Areas of assessment should include the cardiovascular, respiratory, neurologic, integumentary, gastrointestinal, and genitourinary systems. Factors that will influence fluid imbalance include recent episodes of vomiting, increased nasogastric output, diarrhea, blood loss, decreased fluid intake, and extensive bowel preps. Recent weight loss, skin turgor, and the condition of the mucous membrane also may suggest the current fluid status of the patient (Jordan, 1992).

Estimating fluid deficit can be difficult and is best accomplished by evaluating clinical signs. A mild deficit represents approximately 4% of body weight, a moderate deficit 6% to 8%, and a severe loss 10%. Signs of ECF loss are manifested by tachycardia, dry mucous membranes, hypotension, furrowed tongue, apathy, oliguria, collapsed veins, poor skin turgor, cool and dry skin, and subnormal temperature (Jordan, 1992).

The majority of surgical patients have been fasting 6 to 8 hours prior to surgery. Therefore, patients coming to surgery are depleted of solutes and water as a result of normal body function. Generally, adult patients will have intravenous fluids started prior to induction of anesthesia to replace these losses and to provide access to the circulatory system (Jordan, 1992).

Maintenance Fluid Requirements

To determine perioperative fluid requirements, it is necessary to know the typical requirements for fluid maintenance. Table 26–4 lists the typical requirements in milliliters per kilogram per hour for the adult, child, infant, and neonate and helps determine both the maintenance fluid requirements for each hour the patient is in surgery and the amount of fluid deficit the patient is experiencing on arrival in the operating room suite. Another example for determining basic fluid maintenance requirements for a 24-hour period is outlined in Table 26–5.

TABLE 26–4. Typical Requirements for Maintenance Fluids

Age	Amount (mL/kg/h)
Neonate	3
Infant	4–6
Child	2–4
Adult	1.5–2

TABLE 26–5. Baseline 24-Hour Fluid Requirement

1–10 kg body weight	100 mL/kg
11–20 kg body weight	50 mL/kg
21 kg and above body weight	20 mL/kg

Example 1.

A 70-kg adult patient arrives in the OR suite after having been NPO for 8 hours. What is the patient's hourly maintenance fluid requirement?

Using Table 26–4	Using Table 26–5
1.5 mL/kg/h = 105 mL/h	10 kg × 100 mL = 1000 mL
	10 kg × 50 mL = 500 mL
	50 kg × 20 mL = 1000 mL
	24-h requirement = 2500 mL
	or 104 mL/h

The typical fluid maintenance requirements for this 70-kg adult would be 104 to 105 mL/h.

What would this patient's fluid deficit be after she has been NPO for 8 hours?

$$8 \text{ hours} \times 105 \text{ mL/h} = 840 \text{ mL}$$

The fluid deficit for this adult patient would be 840 mL upon arrival in the OR.

Replacing Fluid Deficit

After a patient arrives in the OR suite, an intravenous line is usually placed. Insensible loss and fluid deficit are replaced using the maintenance replacement guidelines mentioned previously. In most situations, lactated Ringer's solution or D_5W/LR are the solutions of choice. Replacement of the fluid deficit is usually accomplished in several hours. Table 26–6 offers guidelines that can be used for replacing the fluid deficit.

Example 2.

The 70-kg adult patient has a fluid deficit of 840 mL. Using Basic Formula #1, one obtains:

10 mL/kg × 70 kg = 700 mL	first hour
7 mL/kg × 70 kg = 490 mL	second hour
5 mL/kg × 70 kg = 350 mL	third hour
3 mL/kg × 70 kg = 210 mL	fourth hour
Total fluids = 1750 mL	

TABLE 26–6. Replacing Fluid Deficit[a]

Basic Formula #1	Basic Formula #2
10 mL/kg first h	1/2 total deficit first h
7 mL/kg second h	1/4 total deficit second h
5 mL/kg third h	1/4 total deficit third h
3 mL/kg fourth h	

[a] Hourly maintenance fluid requirements must be added to each hour of replacement time.

Using Basic Formula #2, one obtains:

1/2 total deficit	420 mL + 105 mL = 535 mL	first hour
1/4 total deficit	220 mL + 105 mL = 325 mL	second hour
1/4 total deficit	220 mL + 105 mL = 325 mL	third hour

The total fluid deficit is 1185 mL.

Intraoperative Fluid Management

Total fluid management of patients undergoing surgical procedures includes normal maintenance fluid, replacing fluid deficit, and intraoperative fluid management. The amount of fluid needed to maintain fluid balance in a patient receiving anesthesia and having a surgical procedure performed varies greatly. The amount of surgical stress and its influence on the fluid balance of the patient will vary dramatically not only between various surgical procedures but also during the same surgical procedure (Jordan, 1992).

A great deal of surgical stress is related to sequestration, or "third spacing." This can be defined as the body fluid volume that is neither ICF (first space) nor ECF (interstitial fluid + plasma volume, or second space), but rather is sequestered fluid that cannot interact with either the ICF or the ECF. Significant third-space loss can result from trauma, injury, ascites, burns, and other factors. It also can present in the peritoneum, bowel wall, and lumen of the gastrointestinal tract during abdominal surgery. The volume can be extremely variable and depends on the duration and the extent of the surgery or trauma. It makes fluid replacement management more difficult and must be taken into consideration while the surgery is ongoing. This fluid must be mobilized and must reenter the vascular space before excretion can take place; however, acutely it must be considered as fluid loss and replaced to maintain vascular volume (Stoelting & Miller, 1994).

Although surgical trauma losses are based on the various types of surgery, the same level of trauma does not occur during each hour of the surgical procedure. The first hour of a procedure may entail little trauma, whereas the second and third hours entail extreme trauma. Adjustments should be made based on the trauma level and the time involved, and the range of fluid replacement should match the surgical procedure. *Clinical judgment is very important.*

Calculating Third-Space Loss

Third space losses are based on the level of surgical trauma that occurs during surgery. Table 26–7 provides guidelines for determining the extent of surgical trauma.

Crystalloid Replacement

When crystalloid therapy is not adequate or loss of body fluids is such that replacing what has been lost is required, then colloid solutions are used. These consist of

TABLE 26–7. Third-Space Loss Calculation

1. Little or no surgical trauma means little or no third spacing. This type of surgery requires 0 to 1 mL/kg/h in addition to maintenance and deficit fluid volume requirements. Examples include microsurgery of the ear, ophthalmologic surgery, minor biopsies, minor extremity surgery, especially with the use of a tourniquet.

2. Minimal surgical trauma means minimal third spacing. This type of surgery usually requires 2 to 3 mL/kg/h in addition to maintenance and deficit fluid volume requirements. Examples of minimal trauma include some plastic surgery, tonsillectomy, laparoscopy.

3. Moderate surgical trauma means moderate third spacing. This type of surgery requires 4 to 6 mL/kg/h in addition to the maintenance and deficit fluid volume requirements. Examples of moderate trauma include, hernia repair, thoracotomy, and appendectomy.

4. Severe surgical trauma means severe third spacing. This type of surgery requires 7 to 10 mL/kg/h in addition to maintenance and deficit fluid volume requirements. Examples of severe trauma include bowel resection for obstruction, radical mastectomy, abdominal surgery.

TABLE 26–9. Implementation of Fluid Therapy Plan

1. Start an appropriate IV or IVs depending on the anticipated needs.
   18- to 20-gauge IV for average adult population
   14- to 16-gauge IV may be needed for more extensive cases
   Multiple lines may be necessary for transfusions, drips, etc.
2. Fluid volume preload the patient with a portion of the calculated NPO deficit with a maintenance type of solution.
3. Continue the maintenance solution to replace the NPO volume deficit.
   50% of the deficit should be replaced during the first hour of surgery.
   25% should be replaced during the second and third hour of surgery.
4. Administer the appropriate hourly volume of replacement type solutions in response to third-space losses appropriate for the surgical procedure.
5. Administer replacement type solutions (crystalloid) to replace the appropriate acceptable blood loss volumes (2 or 3 mL of blood lost).

blood and blood products. If blood loss is less than the amount calculated to require transfusion, such loss can be replaced by a crystalloid solution to maintain adequate fluid balance in the patient. The recommended guidelines for replacing fluid due to blood loss are (1) 2 mL of crystalloid solution for each 1 mL of blood loss without a Foley catheter; or (2) 3 mL of crystalloid solution for each 1 mL of blood loss with a Foley catheter in place. Blood and/or blood components are indicated when losses are greater than the calculated acceptable blood loss.

Table 26-8 provides a basic guideline for planning fluid management for individual patients during the perioperative period. Table 26-9 provides a basic step-by-step guide for implementing a plan of fluid management for individual patients.

Postoperative Fluid Management

In the Postanesthesia Care Unit (PACU) fluid evaluation should include the preoperative fluid status, the amount of fluid lost and given during surgery, and a clinical as-

TABLE 26–8. Fluid Therapy Plan

1. Evaluate the patient's physiologic status in terms of fluid needs.
2. Evaluate the surgical procedure in terms of anticipating third space sequestration.
3. Evaluate the anesthesia plan (techniques and agents to be used in terms of volume shifts and physiologic responses).
4. Calculate the daily fluid volume requirement based on the guidelines.
5. Calculate the hourly fluid volume requirement.
6. Calculate the NPO fluid volume deficit.
7. Calculate the acceptable blood loss limit.

sessment of vital signs and urinary output. Additional fluid loss in the PACU can result from bleeding at the surgical site, internal bleeding, evaporation, and loss through external draining devices. Signs of ECF deficit resulting from fluid loss are manifested primarily by circulatory instability. The replacement of fluids in the postoperative period often requires the use of hypotonic solutions and, as necessary, isotonic salt solutions combined with blood products to replace surgical losses.

Continuously monitoring the patient in the postoperative period includes assessing the blood pressure, heart rate, urinary output, level of consciousness, pupil size, airway patency, respiratory patterns, body temperature, and skin color.

► CASE STUDY

A 35-year-old, 5'4", 65-kg female, ASA 1, presented for hysterectomy. The patient was NPO since midnight, and the surgery began at 0800. The estimated blood loss (EBL) was calculated at 1500 mL. The surgery lasted 3 hours, and the blood loss was 200 mL in the first hour, 300 mL in the second hour, and 100 mL in the third hour. A Foley catheter was placed preoperatively and vital signs were stable throughout.

1. Calculate the daily fluid volume requirements for this case using the guidelines from the text.

   100 mL × 1st 10 kg = 1000 mL
   50 mL × 2nd 10 kg = 500 mL
   20 mL × 45 kg = 911 mL
   The daily volume requirements are 2400 mL/24 hours.

2. What would the hourly fluid requirements for this patient be?

2400 mL divided by 24 hours = 100 mL/h

3. Calculate the fluid deficit prior to the start of surgery.

NPO × 8 hours
100 mL/h × 8 hours = 800 mL of fluid deficit

4. Calculate third-spacing fluid requirements for moderate trauma in this patient.

Moderate trauma = moderate third spacing = 4 to 6 mL/kg/h replacement
4 to 6 mL/kg × 65 kg = 260 to 390 mL/h

5. What is the crystalloid replacement for a 200-mL blood loss during the first hour?

With a Foley catheter in place, 3 mL crystalloid for each millimeter of blood loss.
3 mL × 200 mL = 600 mL

6. What will be the total replacement volume of IV fluids needed for the first hour?

Hourly requirement = 100 mL
NPO replacement = 400 mL (1/2 calculated fluid deficit)
Third-space replacement = 325 mL
Crystalloid blood loss replacement = 600 mL
Total = 1425 mL first-hour fluid requirements

7. What will be the approximate total volume of IV replacement fluids for the second hour?

Hourly requirement = 100 mL
NPO replacement = 200 mL (1/4 calculated fluid deficit)
Third-space replacement = 325 mL
Crystalloid blood loss replacement (3 × 300 mL) = 900 mL
Total = 1525 mL 2nd-hour fluid requirements

8. What are the approximate third-hour replacement requirements for IV fluids?

Hourly replacement = 100 mL
NPO replacement = 200 mL (1/4 of calculated fluid deficit)
Third-space replacement = 325 mL
Crystalloid blood loss replacement (3 × 100 mL) = 300 mL
Total = 925 mL third-hour fluid requirements

9. What would the approximate total amount of IV fluid replacement be for this 3-hour procedure?

1425 mL (first hour)
1525 mL (second hour)
 925 mL (third hour)
3875 mL total fluid requirement for procedure

► SUMMARY

Accurate maintenance of fluid balance is a critical component of the anesthetic process. Knowledge of body compartmental fluids and of the importance of physical and chemical balance is essential to the perianesthetic planning process. Perianesthetic fluid management extends from the preoperative through the postoperative period and requires the anesthesia provider to consider fluid deficit and replacement preoperatively, fluid loss such as "third spacing" intraoperatively, and appropriate crystalloid replacement and fluid evaluation and replacement in the postoperative period. The fluid therapy plan remains a critical and essential component of the perianesthetic process and requires vigilance and continuous evaluation by the anesthesia provider.

► KEY CONCEPTS

- Maintaining fluid balance is an integral part of the anesthetic management of the perioperative patient.
- Water is the primary component of the human body.
- Total body water is divided into two major compartments: intracellular and extracellular fluid.
- The body attempts to maintain a homeostatic environment.
- Disorders of fluid balance can be categorized as disturbances of volume, concentration, and composition.
- Electrolytes are electrically charged particles within the body fluids.
- Alterations in electrolyte concentration can influence normal body functioning.

- The type and amount of parenteral solutions should be carefully evaluated.
- During the perioperative period, surgical patients have the potential to develop fluid and electrolyte imbalance.
- Determining perioperative fluid requirements is essential.
- Total fluid management for patients undergoing surgical procedures includes normal maintenance fluid, replacing fluid deficit, and intraoperative fluid management.
- Postanesthesia, fluid evaluation should include the preoperative status, fluid lost and given during surgery, clinical assessment of vital signs, and urinary output.

► STUDY QUESTIONS

1. How are fluid requirements calculated?

2. How is hourly fluid placement computed?

3. How is fluid deficit calculated prior to surgery?

4. Describe the process to calculate third-space fluid replacement for surgeries characterized as mild, moderate, and severe trauma.

5. What factors must be considered during the perianesthetic period to maintain electrolyte balance?

KEY REFERENCES

Achatz-Deresz, G., Cibula, K., & Emberson, H. (1992). Adult fluid replacement therapy. *Anesthesia Today, 4*(2), 14–17.

Khraibi, A. A., & Knox, F. G. (1995). Regulation of fluid and electrolyte balance. In R. A. Rhoades & G. A. Tanner (Eds.), *Medical physiology* (pp. 446–463). Boston: Little, Brown.

McCall, W. G. (1996). Physiological and practical considerations of fluid management. CRNA: *The Clinical Forum for Nurse Anesthetists, 7*(2), 62–70.

REFERENCES

Fox, M. A., & Whitesell, J. K. (1994). *Organic chemistry.* Sudbury, MA: Jones & Bartlett.

Guyton, A. C., & Hall, J. E. (1996). *Textbook of medical physiology* (9th ed., pp. 297–314). Philadelphia: Saunders.

Jordan, L. M. (1992). Fluid and electrolyte therapy. In W. R. Waugaman, S. D. Foster, & B. M. Rigor (Eds.), *Principles and practice of nurse anesthesia* (2nd ed., pp. 287–298). Norwalk, CT: Appleton & Lange.

Litwack, K., & Keithley, J. K. (1997). In J. J. Nagelhout & K. L. Zaglaniczny (Eds.), *Nurse anesthesia* (pp. 675–692). Philadelphia: Saunders.

Masterson, W. L., Slowinski, E. J., & Stanitski, C. L. (1981). *Chemical principles* (5th ed.). Philadelphia: Saunders.

Stoelting, R. K., & Dierdorf, S. F. (1993). *Anesthesia and coexisting disease* (3rd ed., p. 357). New York: Churchill Livingstone.

Stoelting, R. K., & Miller, R. D. (1994). *Basics of anesthesia* (3rd ed.). New York: Churchill Livingstone.

Waterhouse, M. (1992). Metric medical mathematics. In W. R. Waugaman, S. D. Foster, & B. M. Rigor (Eds.), *Principles and practice of nurse anesthesia* (2nd ed., pp. 39–56). Norwalk, CT: Appleton & Lange.

Blood and Blood Component Therapy

J. L. Reeves-Viets

The administration of blood components is a routine practice in contemporary medical care, and over 22 million components are expected to be administered annually (Wallace et al., 1993). The use of red blood cells and plasma components is common in many extensive operations, and in most institutions the majority of blood components are in fact administered in the perioperative period, usually by members of the anesthesia care team. The practice is in fact so common that it often masks the seriousness of the event. It should be remembered that transfusion of every individual homologous blood component still necessitates exposing the recipient to foreign proteins or cellular elements. Such exposures carry the risks of reaction, infection, and rejection. In that regard, transfusion of blood components is similar to organ transplantation in that the same risks are present, although at a lower incidence and lesser intensity.

This chapter introduces basic principles of blood and component therapy. Emphasis is on perioperative blood component therapy and on specific therapy for selected hematologic disorders. An overview of blood banking, including principles of blood typing, antibody screening, and cross-matching is presented, along with selected hemoglobinopathies and red cell dyscrasias. Essentials of hemostasis and coagulation are outlined, including the most commonly used laboratory and intraoperative tests for anticoagulation. Indications for the use of blood and component therapy and the management of transfusion therapy in the perioperative period are discussed. The risks of transfusion of blood components are reviewed, including transfusion reactions and

potential infectious hazards. Adjuncts to transfusion management are considered, including preoperative therapy to increase erythrogenesis and use of antifibrinolytics and platelet activators. Blood salvage and processing techniques and alternatives to transfusion also are considered.

▶ BLOOD TYPING, ANTIBODY SCREENING, CROSS-MATCHING

Blood volume in the normal adult is approximately 6% to 7% of the body mass in kilograms, or 60 to 70 mL/kg, based on age, sex, and body type. About 40% of blood volume is composed of formed elements, including red blood cells, white blood cells, and platelets suspended in the plasma fraction that includes serum proteins, which constitutes the other 60% of blood volume. Red blood cells (RBCs), being enucleate, are cellular elements incapable of further development. Their survival time after release into the circulation is approximately 120 days. Their principal function is to transport oxygen and to be a component of the buffer system and maintain acid–base balance. White blood cells (WBCs) are a heterogenous group that operate principally as defense mechanisms and produce inflammatory responses to antigenic stimuli, either phagocytizing foreign matter or producing antibodies in response to foreign antigens. Platelets represent small subcellular fragments that function in the initial stage of hemostasis. The average life span of platelets is generally 8 to 12 days (Spiess, 1990;

Williams, Beutler, Erslev & Lichtman, 1983). The principal plasma proteins of concern in blood component therapy include albumin and globulins and the procoagulant factors that facilitate the coagulation process. Indications exist to transfuse each of these elements individually, which accounts for the general practice of fractionating donated whole blood into components to promote more discrete therapy and to extend the availability of a scarce resource.

Because RBCs are enucleate and operate principally as a transport mechanism, they maintain viable function for an extended time when anticoagulated and stored in an appropriately cooled environment. Platelets and WBCs have a shorter survival time and are generally considered to be lysed or rendered ineffective within the first few days of storage, unless specially managed with continuous agitation for oxygenation and kept at higher room temperatures. Acellular plasma proteins are comparatively more stable, will tolerate prolonged storage, and may be frozen, which permits storage for extended periods. Fractionated products such as cryoprecipitate, Co-9, albumin, human globulins, antithrombin-III, and Factors 8 and 9 may be produced by recombinant technology or processed through fractionation and stored in frozen or anhydrous form for extended periods, depending on the nature of the element.

A wide variety of human blood types are determined by a series of genetically controlled moieties incorporated in or on the membrane of the red blood cell and other circulating formed elements, as demonstrated in Table 27–1. These may be identified by evaluating agglutination reactions between red cells of unknown type and selected antisera containing antibodies to known antigens. Exposure to incompatible antigenic moieties in administered components results in the development of antibodies in the recipient. These antibodies result in agglutination of the incompatible cellular elements and lysis with complement activation that follows. In more critical cases, lysis may be immediate and intravascular, representing a life-threatening event. In less critical cases, agglutinated red cells may be removed by the reticuloendothelial system, limiting their lysis in the systemic circulation. The presence of antibodies in donor plasma to selected antigens may be identified by evaluating agglutination reactions between unknown plasma and red cells known to contain selected antigens. In transfusion of blood components, it is important to identify those systems that are incompatible prior to administration and to recognize those interventions that may result in erroneous typing of either the patient or donor component to prevent administration of incompatible components.

Conceptually, three principal groups of blood types may be recognized. First, the ABO system is alloantigenic and demonstrates inherited isoagglutinins so that administration of incompatible components may result in immediate life-threatening reactions. Second, highly antigenic systems induce delayed antibodies on first administration with rapidly induced exaggerated responses on subsequent exposures. Last, low-antigenic systems result in delayed responses on first exposure and generally result in less exaggerated induced responses on subsequent exposures. Recent advances have increased the sophistication with which blood types can be identified, altering their nomenclature, and even permitting in some cases genetic analysis to determine the exact genetic site or sequences responsible for antigenicity.

ABO System

The ABO system is the most commonly recognized of human blood types and is the system generally responsible for the most serious threat when incompatible products are administered as alloantibodies are present for any ABO-incompatible cellular elements. Thus, the first exposure to incompatible ABO cellular elements results in an intravascular lytic response that may be life-threatening. Determination of ABO type is predicated on

TABLE 27–1. ISBT Blood Group Systems

System Name	System Symbol	ISBT Number
ABO	ABO	001
MNS	MNS	002
P	P1	003
Rh	RH	004
Lutheran	LU	005
Kell	KEL	006
Lewis	LE	007
Duffy	FY	008
Kidd	JK	009
Diego	DI	010
Yt	YT	011
Xg	XG	012
Scianna	SC	013
Dombrock	DO	014
Colton	CO	015
Landsteiner-Weiner	LW	016
Chido/Rodgers	CH/RG	017
Hh	H	018
Kx	XK	019
Gerbich	GE	020
Cromer	CROM	021
Knops	KN	022
Indian	IN	023

From Issitt, L. A. (1996). Blood group nomenclature. In Blood groups: Refresher and update *(p. 14). Bethesda, MD: American Association of Blood Banks. Reprinted with permission.*

the presence of a facilitating protein on the surface of the red cell membrane termed the H-receptor. This moiety facilitates the addition of an antigenic glycoprotein in which a difference of one sugar residue determines ABO type. The presence of N-acetylgalactosamine in the glycoprotein moiety directs type A red cells; the presence of galactose in the glycoprotein moiety directs type B red cells. Patients with neither moiety will not respond to corresponding antisera and will be typed as O; patients with both moieties will type as AB.

Type O red cells may generally be transfused into any ABO recipient as no antigenic site exists. Type A or B individuals will develop acute reactions to the corresponding incompatible cell types on administration, so that type A patients may receive only A or O red cells and type B patients may receive only B or O red cells. Type AB individuals may receive all red cell types in the ABO system. Type O patients can receive only type O red cells, as all others in the ABO system will be antigenically incompatible. Hence, type O red cells often are referred to as *universal donor cells* and are the red cells of choice for emergent administration when there is inadequate time for typing the patient's red cells prior to administration. Type AB patients are likewise often referred to as *universal recipients.*

In addition to the standard ABO system, there are subgroups that generally are not clinically significant. Type A red blood cells may be subcategorized into two component subtypes that are generally cross-compatible unless patients are subjected to repeated exposures. The complexity of these subgroups is beyond the scope of this review. Of particular concern is a small population of individuals who lack the enzymes catalyzing attachment of the antigenic moiety and the hydrogen-containing base to which those enzymes attach (Ganong, 1987). These patients, often termed Bombay-O, or null types, will appear on initial typing to be ABO type O. Because the H-substance is not present, these individuals are false type O and are actually antigenically outside the ABO system. True type O red cells will elicit an antibody response when administered to the Bombay-O individual. For these reasons, when clinical conditions permit, it is always appropriate to determine correct, complete blood type, and full cross matching even among patients who appear on initial typing and screening to be ABO compatible.

Highly Antigenic Systems

The Rh system agglutinogen-D, Kell, and Kidd Duffy systems are classic highly antigenic inducible antibody systems. In these systems presence of the antigen induces an antibody response from patients with the alternate or null type for that system. All groups have more than one genotype, and various combinations of genotypes are possible. Cross-reactivity between subtypes is variable and too complex for discussion in this chapter. In this overview, the most commonly known of the systems will be used. The Rh system actually is composed of several elements termed C/c, D, and E/e. As with other systems, the most antigenic of the sites is the D site, which occurs as a D^+ or D-null genotype. The presence of the D^+ antigen proves highly antigenic to individuals lacking the genetic locus for that protein (Colin et al., 1991). The presence of all these proteins on the surface of the red cell membrane results in the true Rh-positive red cell. Absence of all these elements represents the true Rh-negative state. Intermediate states, in which only part of the total Rh sequence is present, will produce intermediate types, as demonstrated in Table 27–2. These intermediate forms may type as Rh positive while eliciting little or no response from Rh-negative recipients, or type as Rh negative while still producing a response from true Rh-negative individuals. Therefore, it is the practice to identify Rh subtypes when completing a full blood type and cross-match. Rh-negative red cells may be used for transfusion to any patient as no antigenic factor exists, making Rh-negative cells the cells of choice for emergent administration when inadequate time for complete typing exists.

The development of antibodies in response to an initial exposure to highly antigenic red cell types generally takes 2 to 4 weeks. As a result, the agglutination and destruction of incompatible red cells usually are progressive and slow on the first exposure, and the process is not typically immediately life-threatening for the recipient. In the case of Rh incompatibility, the use of prepared hyperimmune anti-D antibodies such as Rho-Gam® can suppress the development of the recipient's antibody response and practically eliminate the antibody response if initiated immediately following exposure. A single 300 microgram dose of Rho-Gam® protects against

TABLE 27–2. Common Rh Haplotypes

Short Symbol (Gene)	CDE Term (Gene)	Short Symbol (Phenotype)	CDE Term (Phenotype)	Antigenic Specificities
R^1	CDe	R_1	CDe	C, D, e
r	cde	r	cde	c, e
R^2	cDE	R_2	cDE	c, D, E
R_o	cDe	R_o	cDe	c, D, e
r'	Cde	r'	Cde	C, e
r''	cdE	r''	cdE	c, E
R^z	CDE	R_z	CDE	C, D, E
r^y	CdE	r^y	CdE	C, E

From Issitt, L. A. (1996). Blood Groups Nomenclature. In Blood groups: Refresher and update (p. 15). Bethesda, MD: American Association of Blood Banks. Reprinted with permission.

the antigenic load of an estimated 15 mL of Rh-positive fetal blood (Hurd & Mioduvi, 1983). Thus, Rh-negative females are generally given suppression doses of Rho-Gam® following delivery of an Rh-positive fetus. Repeated exposure will result in a more rapidly developed antibody response and can result in an immediate intravascular lytic response that may be life-threatening. Because previous exposure may result in antibody production that remains rapidly inducible after plasma antibody levels decline, it is important to elicit or recognize potential exposures through transfusion, pregnancy, or other causes, specifically in known Rh-negative females.

Low-Antigenicity Systems

A host of lower-antigenicity systems produce delayed antibody responses, as with the highly antigenic systems. In contrast, however, the antibody response often is slower to develop and is seldom as exaggerated as in the highly antigenic groups. Because antibody production for the less antigenic systems is slower, agglutination usually is progressive and the incompatible red cells generally are cleared by the reticuloendothelial system. As a result, they commonly are less clinically significant in first exposures. The exception is the patient with multiple previous exposures, such as patients with blood dyscrasias or other malignancies who have required frequent transfusions, in whom antigen systems that would generally be considered clinically insignificant may acquire greater importance to prevent acute transfusion reactions.

Blood Typing, Screening, and Cross-Matching

Generally blood typing can be completed within minutes using the current technology and involves the evaluation of agglutination responses between unknown red cells and plasma with known antibodies, or unknown plasma and red cells with known antigens in a panel. The ABO and Rh type of an individual can be quickly determined, which eliminates the principal considerations in life-threatening transfusion reactions. Blood type may be misidentified when red cells are coated with foreign compounds that prevent the normal antigen–antibody binding process that produces agglutination. Use of synthetic colloid preparations, such as low-molecular-weight dextran, may render blood typing, screening, and cross-matching inaccurate.

Screening for other antigens or antibodies takes somewhat longer but can generally be completed within 30 to 45 minutes. Both patients and potential donor units may be screened for the presence of antibodies or antigens that would predict most incompatible transfusions. When screening for antibodies, plasma from the donor or patient may be matched against selected panels of prepared red cells with known antigenic moieties. By us-

ing a panel of red blood cells with known antigenic character, it is possible to determine whether antibodies exist in the plasma, and with subsequent testing, the nature of those antibodies may be elucidated. Red cells may be tested for antigenicity by using plasma with known antibodies that permits the identification of antigens on the red blood cell. However, it is important to remember that induced antibodies will decay over time if no subsequent exposures occur and that failure to demonstrate antibodies in a screening does not absolutely guarantee that transfusion reactions cannot occur when homologous red cells are administered. In addition, it is important to remember that typing is completed by using antigen–antibody reactions and subsequent agglutination to elucidate the patient's blood type. For that reason, low antibody levels in donor plasma may result in inadequate saturation of receptor sites on recipient cells to promote effective agglutination. In contrast, oversaturation of antigenic receptors in donor cells by high titers of antibodies in the recipient's plasma may prevent effective agglutination by overwhelming the receptor sites and effectively blocking red cell aggregation. A Coombs test involving the washing of cross-matched samples and saturation with antihuman antibody may uncover cross reactions that would be missed initially by simpler techniques. Finally, an additional group of agglutinins may produce agglutination of red cells at temperatures lower than 5°C. Known as cold agglutinins, they do not produce agglutination at normal temperatures and are thus of less importance, unless the surgical procedure involves the use of profound hypothermia (Mollison, 1987).

Cross-matching is a more complete process that includes mixing the recipient's plasma with donor red blood cells to identify the presence of antibodies in the recipient that would prove incompatible with donor red cells, as in a host-versus-graft response. In addition, it includes matching the recipient's red cells with donor plasma to identify the presence of unknown antibodies in the donor plasma to the recipient's red cells, as in a graft-versus-host response. These are completed both at room temperature and with warming to uncover any temperature-sensitive incompatibilities. Complete cross-matching is a more time-consuming process and requires approximately 1 hour to complete.

The relative efficacy of typing, screening, and cross-matching in identifying potential transfusion reactions is progressive. In previously unexposed individuals, typing alone will result in compatibility of 99.8%; addition of screening will increase compatibility to 99.94% of cases; addition of a complete cross-match will increase compatibility only to 99.95% (Walker, 1982). Because the majority of reactions are identifiable by typing and screening and further reductions in risk of transfusion by cross-matching are extremely limited, often only typing and screening are done when the likelihood of transfusion is remote (Boyd, Sheedy, & Henry, 1980; Mead, Anthony, & Sattler, 1980; Oberman, Barnes, & Friedman, 1978). A complete cross-match still is the standard of practice for patients who have clinically significant detectable antibodies, those in whom the likelihood of transfusion is probable, or for procedures in which blood loss might be predicted to be massive.

▶ HEMOGLOBINOPATHIES AND RED CELL DYSCRASIAS

In the normal adult, red cells represent an enucleate cellular end product of hematopoiesis in the erythrocytic line that occurs in the bone marrow. During the process of development and maturation, hemoglobin is formed and the nucleus decays, resulting in a cell incapable of further development or adaptation. Normal red cell survival time once released is about 120 days. In the fetus, red cells are produced principally in the liver and spleen, and the development of marrow as the principal source for hematogenesis begins after birth. Normal adult hemoglobin is composed of two alpha and two beta chains that form a complex incorporating iron as a means of binding oxygen for transport and delivery. Hemoglobin in the fetal red cell differs from adult hemoglobin in that the beta chain is largely replaced by a fetal gamma chain, which binds oxygen more tightly and favors transport and release of oxygen in the uterine environment. Fetal hemoglobin normally begins to be replaced before the end of gestation by beta chains. After birth, development of red cells becomes principally located in the marrow, and hemoglobin formation completes transformation to the normal adult hemoglobin structure incorporating alpha and beta chains as virtually the only hemoglobin chains in adult red cells. Red cells are released in response to erythrogenic stimuli to maintain adequate circulating red cell mass to meet the requirements for oxygen delivery. The amount of hemoglobin in the red cell may be affected by nutritional state, genetics, or environmental effects. Defects in the development of the red cells or in the formation of hemoglobin also may alter the viability of the red cell itself.

The formation of normal red cells requires erythropoietin stimulation to encourage the development of the erythrocytic precursors in the marrow. Failure to produce adequate erythropoietin in the kidney or a refractory state in the marrow will produce an inadequate hematogenic response and reduce the development and release of red cells. During the process of red cell development, vitamin B_{12}, folate, and iron all are required for the development of normal hemoglobin, and defects in transport or metabolism of these critical cofactors may result in abnormally low hemoglobin levels in the red

cells often seen as a macrocytic anemia. Hemoglobinopathies also may occur when genetic mutations alter the structure of the hemoglobin molecule, thereby reducing the efficacy with which hemoglobin binds and releases oxygen despite a normal red cell hemoglobin content. These also may alter the viability of the red cell as occurs with thalassemias or produce deformation in the structure of the red cell, as shown in patients with the sickle-cell trait. Deformation of the red cell limits the normal span of red cells and may actually produce microvascular obstruction and cellular ischemia when rigid red cells are unable to conform with the flow in the capillary bed. Morphologic red cell dyscrasias, in contrast, may not alter the efficacy with which oxygen is transported or released, but anomalous red cell formation reduces the uniformity of microvascular flow and may result in reduced red cell survival time.

Sickle cell factor develops when a genetic mutation alters the structure of the beta chain of the hemoglobin macromolecule by substitution of a single amino acid. Because it affects the beta chain, it does not affect the fetus, because fetal hemoglobin incorporates a gamma chain rather than a beta chain in the hemoglobin complex. This trait does not prevent the red cell from transporting or releasing oxygen until trigger factors create the development of polymeric hemoglobin complexes. Stresses or reductions in oxygen tension cause the hemoglobin to reconform, creating rigid macromolecular structures and deformation of the red cell. With repeated episodes, the red cell becomes permanently deformed, causing entrapment and breakdown of the affected red cell when the process is in the chronic, smoldering state. Accelerated breakdown reduces the red cell life span to approximately 5 to 20 days. In a crisis, a critical mass of red cells becomes affected and massive widespread deformation of red cells results in microvascular occlusion and tissue or organ ischemia. In exaggerated states, it may result in death unless early treatment is initiated.

An additional constellation of hemoglobinopathies are termed *thalassemias*. A diverse population of mutations exists, but they all share the common element of disparate underproduction of either the alpha or beta chains in the hemoglobin complex. In less severe cases of beta-chain thalassemias, substitution with a fetal gamma chain permits the generation of stable hemoglobin complexes, but excess alpha chains may precipitate in the red cell. Retention of the fetal form of hemoglobin may permit circulation of oxygen, although indices such as red cell volume are reduced and red cell survival time is lessened. In more severe forms of beta thalassemia and in alpha thalassemia, lack of appropriate hemoglobin chains can reduce the ability of the red cell to transport oxygen effectively, and the precipitation of unconjugated chains can result in destruction of the red cell even before it is released from the marrow. The most severe forms, particularly the alpha thalassemias, are incompatible with fetal or neonatal survival without immediate and continuous transfusion.

Anomalies in the structure of the red cell itself also can affect cell survival time. The abnormal protein structure of the red cell membrane can result in the development of a variety of morphologically abnormal red cells. Most common are spherocytic or elliptocytic red cells, although there are rarer pyropoikilocytic and stomatocystocitic forms. In all cases, the anomalous conformation results in red cells that lack the normal biconcave structure and that are more rigid and less able to adapt to the conformational changes that occur in the microcirculation in red cells of normal conformation. As a result, anomalously distorted red cells have reduced survival time and increased clearance by the reticuloendothelial system, which results in anemia in affected individuals. In mild cases, the increased clearance can be easily corrected and the hematologic profile can appear grossly normal. Crises may, however, occur, following even apparently mild-stress events in which increased clearance is not compensated and anemia ensues that may require transfusion. In more severe cases, chronic anemia can be profound and splenectomy may be required or periodic transfusion may be indicated.

► HEMOSTASIS AND COAGULATION

In the normal patient, a variety of mechanisms operate to maintain vascular stability and to repair any breach in the integrity of the vascular wall. Hemostatic defenses begin when physiologic mechanisms produce constriction and contraction of the vessel in response to injury, creating the first defense against excessive blood loss. In addition, coagulation occurs as platelet activation forms an occlusive plug in response to subendothelial factors and a fibrin network develops to stabilize the occlusive plug. Concomitant with activation of the coagulation process is activation of the fibrinolytic pathway, which controls the process, preventing widespread microvascular coagulation, and ultimately resolving the platelet and fibrin complex when vascular injury is repaired. In cases of extensive blood loss with depletion of the normal mechanisms or in cases with defective hemostatic mechanisms, it is important to understand the mechanism of hemostasis and to appreciate the supportive treatment necessary to reestablish hemostatic and coagulation competence.

Two pathways frequently are described for the coagulation process to occur. The intrinsic pathway is triggered by the contact activation system, which depends on Factor XII, whereas the extrinsic pathway is triggered by the tissue factor system, which depends on activated Factor VII. Although these pathways may be of value in the laboratory analysis of bleeding disorders, they have little actual clinical application because the intrinsic pathway is an in vitro mechanism and both pathways terminate by activating the coagulation cascade and forming organized thrombus. An understanding of the basic physiologic process of coagulation is necessary, and differentiation of causes of abnormalities in coagulation may generally be grouped into vascular defects, platelet defects, and plasma procoagulant deficiencies.

The initial vascular response to injury includes the release of thromboplastin and subendothelial activating factors, including endothelial stores of activated Factor VIII. Release of serotonin results in constriction of smooth muscle in the wall of the damaged vessel, which causes vascular constriction and contraction. Platelet activation is enhanced by the release of activated Factor VIII, permitting platelets to bind to subendothelial collagen at the site of injury. This forms the initial hemostatic plug as platelets undergo conformational change from the circulating spheroidal form to a spiculate form that offers sites for cross-bonding of the initial fibrin monomers. Subendothelial activating factors include thromboplastin, which initiates the conversion of prothrombin to thrombin and, in turn, facilitates the conversion of fibrinogen to fibrin monomers that bind at available sites on the platelet aggregate. In the final stage of clot formation, fibrin monomers are converted to polymers by cross-bonding that stabilizes and solidifies the fibrin plug. A complete list of coagulation factors and their characteristics is given in Table 27–3. It is important to remember that homologous blood components are anticoagulated by binding plasma calcium, an essential cofactor in the coagulation process at several points. Thus, supplementation of ionized calcium may prove necessary in cases of massive transfusion, generally with calcium chloride. Determining ionized calcium is recommended during rapid, massive transfusion to maintain normal coagulation activity, as well as to prevent the ventricular hypotonia or myocardial depression that may develop with acute hypocalcemia.

Serine proteases that catalyze the conversion of procoagulant proteins belong to a nonspecific family of proteases that also catalyze the lytic process of fibrin polymer breakdown. Antithrombin III operates as a modulator in the activity of proteases, specifically altering the activity of thrombin. In the initial phase of clot formation, platelet conformational changes create cusps in which proteases are released. The proteases released at the initial site of coagulum formation thus initiate the process of clot lysis. Lysis of organized clot may be identified by laboratory analysis of fibrin degradation products.

Reviewing several principal tests commonly used to assess coagulation parameters is valuable: bleeding time, prothrombin time (PT), partial thromboplastin time

TABLE 27–3. Hemostatic Factors

Factor	Name	Type	Site of Origin	Normal Level	Minimal Level (% NL)	Half-life (h)
Factor I	Fibrinogen	—	Liver	150–300 mg%	50–100	72–144
Factor II	Prothrombin	Protease	Liver	100 μg/mL	20–40	72–120
Factor III	Tissue factor	Cofactor	Vasculature	Unknown	Unknown	Unknown
Factor IV	Calcium ions					
Factor V	Labile factor	Cofactor	Liver	5–12 μg/mL	5–10	12–36
Factor VII[a]	Stable factor	Protease	Liver	0.5 μg/mL	30	4–6
Factor VIII c	AHF	Cofactor		0.2 μg/mL	30	10–18
Factor VIII vWF	von Willebrand	Adhesion	Endothelium Megakaryocytes Platelet α granule	10 μg/mL	30	10
Factor IX	Christmas	Protease	Liver	5 μg/mL	20–25	18–36
Factor X	Stuart–Prower	Protease	Liver	10 μg/mL	10–20	24–60
Factor XI	PTA	Protease	Liver	5 μg/mL	20–30	40–80
Factor XII	Hageman	Protease	Liver	30 μg/mL	0	60
Factor XIII	Fibrin stabilizing	Transamidase	Liver, platelets	15 μg/mL	1–3	150

[a] This is the only coagulation protein circulating in active form.

From Lake, C. L. (1995). Normal hemostasis. In C. L. Lake & R. A. Rogers (Eds.), Blood: Hemostasis, transfusion and alternatives in the perioperative period *(p. 4). NY: Raven Press. Reprinted with permission.*

(APTT), plasma fibrinogen level, platelet count, fibrin degradation products to include the D-dimer, and intraoperative measures of anticoagulation. An overview of a number of diagnostic laboratory tests is offered in Table 27–4. Each of these tests has different clinical applications in the determination to administer coagulation components, although little or no evidence has been demonstrated that the use of laboratory screening tests has any predictive or clinical value in patients who have no history of bleeding diathesis (Koutts, 1985; Ramsey, Arvan, Steward, & Blumberg, 1983; Rohrer, Michelotti, & Nahrwold, 1988). Thus, routine preoperative coagulation screens have little value in the normal and healthy population.

Bleeding time frequently is used to test the efficacy of the entire hemostatic cascade, beginning with the initial vascular response to injury. Normal values are usually 2 to 8 minutes, and extensions in bleeding time are noted in patients with abnormalities in the vascular component of hemostasis. Thus in patients with von Willebrand's disorder, increases in bleeding time may be noted. However, care must be taken in correctly performing the examination, and multiple factors may increase bleeding time. Because multiple factors are assessed and the test offers little specificity, it is seldom used as a clinical tool in detailed assessment of abnormalities in hemostasis. It may still be used in patients with known coagulation disorders to demonstrate a clinical index of the magnitude of the disorder, it has little demonstrated value as a preoperative indicator of the likelihood of bleeding problems (Burns, Billet, Frater, & Sisto, 1986).

Laboratory analyses of coagulation may prove useful in patients with no hepatic dysfunction. Plasma procoagulant factors II, V, VII, IX, X, XI, XII, and XIII and fibrinogen are produced in the liver. Likewise, the liver produces inhibitors to fibrinolysis, so that reductions in hepatic function may be revealed rapidly as coagulant factor supplies are reduced and inhibition of fibrinolysis is lost. In addition, the plasma half-life of procoagulants is short, from a few hours for Factor VII to a few days for fibrinogen, as shown in Table 27–3. Thus, hepatic dysfunction may result in severe coagulopathies for a host of reasons. In patients with evidence of hepatic dysfunction or known bleeding diathesis, laboratory analysis may be beneficial as an indicator of function.

Prothrombin time (PT) values are useful in assessing extrinsic pathway and depend on the activity of hepatic factors II, V, VIII, and X and fibrinogen, which depend on calcium for activation. The test frequently is used to determine the efficacy of anticoagulation in patients who receive long-term systemic anticoagulation with coumadin, which reduces the release of normal vitamin-K–dependent factors II, VII, IX, and X. Normal values must be adjusted to the individual laboratory but generally are 10 to 13 seconds. Extensions approximately 50% greater than the baseline generally are considered evidence of effective systemic anticoagulation without increased risk of spontaneous bleeding, whereas extensions above that level are associated with increased bleeding (Gazzard, Henderson, & Williams, 1975; Hull et al., 1982; Miller, Robbins, Tong, & Barton, 1971). When using PT values to direct acute reversal

TABLE 27–4. Profile of Hemostatic Screening Tests[a]

	Hemophilia A or B or Other Intrinsic System Deficiency or Inhibitor	von Willebrand Disease	Severe Acute Disseminated Intravascular Coagulation	Heparin	Warfarin	Final Common Pathway Deficiency or Inhibitor	Factor VII Deficiency or Inhibitor	Hypofibrino-genemia or Dysfibrino-genemia	Chronic Liver Disease
Platelet count	Normal	Normal	*Low*	Normal	Normal	Normal	Normal	Normal	Normal
Bleeding time	Normal	*Prolonged*	*Prolonged*	Normal	Normal	Normal	Normal	Normal	Normal
Fibrinogen (kinetic method)	Normal	Normal	*Low*	Normal	Normal	Normal	Normal	*Low* or normal	*Low* or normal
Thrombin time	Normal	Normal	*Prolonged*	*Prolonged*	Normal	Normal	Normal	*Prolonged*	Normal or pro-longed
Reptilase time	Normal	Normal	*Prolonged*	Normal	Normal	Normal	Normal	*Prolonged*	Normal or pro-longed
PT	Normal	Normal	*Prolonged*	Normal or prolonged	*Prolonged*	*Prolonged*	*Prolonged*	*Prolonged* or normal	*Prolonged*
PTT	*Prolonged*	*Prolonged*	*Prolonged* or normal	*Prolonged*	*Prolonged*	*Prolonged*	Normal	*Prolonged* or normal	*Prolonged* or normal

[a] The appropriate sequence of screening tests differs for critically ill patients with acquired bleeding defects and for patients who are seen for evaluation of possible mild congenital disorders. Late-stage defects with hypofibrinogenemia and delayed fibrin polymerization from degradation products are common in critically ill patients, whereas intrinsic system defects and platelet function abnormalities are common in congenital disorders. Patients with absence of α_2-plasmin inhibitor or factor XIII will have excess bleeding despite normal screening tests. Clot solubility in 5 M urea is abnormal in factor XIII deficiency, and patients with α_2-plasmin inhibitor deficiency will have a short clot lysis time.
From Smith, K. J. (1991). Coagulation mechanism. In E. C. Simon, T. L. Simon, & G. S. Moss (Eds.), Principles of transfusion medicine (p. 320). Baltimore: Williams & Wilkins. Reprinted with permission.

therapy in coumadin overdose or for urgent and emergent surgery, desired end points will be determined by the clinical situation. In patients receiving vitamin K or plasma to correct coumadin overdose without evidence of active bleeding, correction to the desired level of anticoagulation generally is the minimal goal. Correction of excessive anticoagulation with bleeding or prior to emergent surgery typically requires a value within no more than 3 to 4 seconds of normal baseline PT.

Partial thromboplastin time (APTT) values are useful in assessing the intrinsic pathway and depend on all factors except VII and XIII. Because the intrinsic pathway is assessed, APTT values may be used as an index of heparinization in patients undergoing long-term heparinization for several days. Like the PT, APTT values must be adjusted to the individual laboratory but generally are 28 to 38 seconds. In the clinical setting, APTT measurements may be used to determine the efficacy of anticoagulation in critical care settings. Because determining APTT is time-consuming and requires laboratory support, it is not an efficacious means of determining anticoagulation for operative purposes.

In general, abnormalities in the intrinsic pathway generally result in a normal PT and abnormal APTT. Factor VII deficiency may occur with the reverse pattern. Abnormalities in both PT and APTT may be indicative of other factor deficiency or the presence of inhibitors in the plasma. For that reason, additional testing may be done with the patient's sample mixed with normal plasma. When PT or APTT returns to normal, it is generally considered that a factor deficiency uncovered by that test has been normalized. Further discrete analysis may then expose the exact nature of the factor deficiency. However, clinical therapy may then be guided by the assumption of a factor deficiency, generally treatable with plasma products.

Plasma fibrinogen levels, platelet counts, and the presence of fibrin degradation products also may be obtained by laboratory analysis. Maintenance of adequate circulating platelet count and fibrinogen is discussed under the indications for transfusion of those products. Competition may occur in the presence of fibrin degradation products. Of the degradation products that may be isolated, the D-dimer is useful as an indicator of disseminated intravascular coagulation (DIC). Other fibrin degradation products may be present when fibrin monomers are cleaved, but the D-dimer only occurs when cross-bonding has occurred between fibrin monomers. Hence, the presence of D-dimers is indicative that effective clot formation has occurred and elevated levels indicate clot lysis or intravascular coagulopathy. When both PT and APTT values remain long in the mixed sample, it is generally an indicator of inhibitors such as fibrin degradation products following DIC.

Successful short-term heparinization during surgical procedures depends on the requirements of anticoagulation. For procedures involving cardiopulmonary bypass, measurements such as activated clotting time (ACT) may be used. Activated clotting time measurements assess the activity of the intrinsic system and depend on initiation of the clotting cascade by exogenous exposure to kaolin particles or diatomaceous material. Activation of the clotting cascade to produce an effective clot blocks rotation of a magnet in the test tube and activates the sensor. An extension of ACT from a normal of 150 seconds to values between 450 and 500 seconds generally is considered evidence of full systemic heparinization suitable for cardiopulmonary bypass, generally readily achieved by doses of 3 to 4 mg/kg or 300 to 400 units/kg of heparin. Caution should be used when interpreting ACT values during the use of aprotinin, as aprotonin is itself a serine protease inhibitor and may extend the ACT value slightly when using celite-activated tubes (deSmet et al., 1990; Harder, Eijsman, Roozendaal, van Oeveren, & Wildevuur, 1991) and proves synergistic in producing ACT extension in celite-activated tubes (deSmet, 1990; Dietrich, Conrad, Hebert, Levy, & Romero, 1990), but not with kaolin-activated tubes (Wang, Lin, Hung, & Karp, 1992; Wang, Lin, Hung, Thisted, & Karp, 1992). Thus many clinicians use kaolin-activated ACT measurements and extend the accepted value to 500 to 750 seconds.

An alternative is to use so-called heparin assay tests such as the Hep-Con. These systems employ algorithms based on age, sex, height, and weight to estimate the plasma volume. From that calculation, an estimated initial dose of heparin is recommended to establish an accepted plasma heparin level. Plasma levels of 2 to 4 units/mL heparin activity are generally considered to be suitable for cardiopulmonary bypass. Extension in coagulation times may be measured after administration of heparin to ensure adequate anticoagulation. In addition, the use of a gradated series of samples permits estimation of the plasma heparin concentration based on a heparin-protamine dose–response curve. Therefore, many of the same principles apply in the Hep-Con that apply in a regular ACT, as well as assumptions of the adequacy of procoagulant proteins, absence of antagonists other than heparin that compete in the coagulation process and ultimately the correct reversal ratio between

heparin and protamine. That ratio varies according to clinical or laboratory criteria across a range of approximately 0.9 to 1.3 mg protamine for every 1 mg or 100 units of heparin.

A variety of other laboratory examinations are available to establish the adequacy of the coagulation system, including thromboelastograph and sonoclot analysis. Both of these provide an estimate of coagulation activity based on clot development, strength, retraction, and, ultimately, breakdown. Neither of these tests is typically used in the operating room per se, and laboratory analysis is lengthy, which limits their application in the rapid decision making required in cardiovascular cases.

▶ INDICATIONS FOR TRANSFUSION AND MANAGEMENT IN THE PERIOPERATIVE PERIOD

A variety of blood components are presently available from donated whole blood, separated by fractionation at the time of collection or collected by apheresis techniques. An overview of the most commonly used blood components is listed in Table 27–5. These components have different general clinical indications and widely disparate storage times based on the character of the component and the available technology for storage. Differences in the character of stored whole blood and packed red cells are demonstrated in Table 27–6. These derive in part from the diluent effect of plasma on potassium released during storage, on the buffer effect induced by plasma, and on the presence of plasma glucose that provides substrate for reduced metabolic requirements in stored blood. Although these differences are generally not significant when administration of stored blood is slow, electrolyte abnormalities and less effective oxygen-carrying capacity are noted in patients who receive rapid

TABLE 27–5. Common Blood Components

Whole blood
Erythrocyte (RBC) preparations
Packed RBCs (plasma removed)
Leukocyte-poor RBCs (plasma and white cells removed)
Washed RBCs (plasma and other elements removed)
Deglycerolized RBCs
Frozen RBCs (plasma removed)
Plasma
Stored plasma
Fresh-frozen plasma
Platelets
Leukocyte concentration
Cryoprecipitate
Albumin
Factor concentrations

TABLE 27–6. Properties of Whole Blood and Packed Red Cell Concentrates Stored in Citrate Phosphate Dextrose Adenine-1 (CPDA-1)

Parameter	0	35 (Whole blood)	35 (Packed cells)
		Days of Storage	
pH	7.55	6.98	6.71
Plasma hemoglobin (mg/dL)	8.2	46.1	246.0
Plasma potassium (mEq/L)	4.2	27.3	76.0
Plasma sodium (mEq/L)	169	155	122
Blood dextrose (mg/dL)	440	229	84
2,3-Diphosphoglycerate (μM/mL)	13.2	<1	<1
Percent survival[a]	—	79	71

[a] Percent recovery of O_R-tagged red blood cells at 24 hours.
From Miller, D. (1990). Transfusion therapy. New York: Churchill Livingstone. Reprinted with permission.

administration of stored blood. An overview of the most commonly used plasma components is given in Table 27-7. The majority of factors used in the perioperative period include red cells either as packed red cells (PRCs) or whole blood (WB), fresh or frozen plasma (FFP), platelets, and cryoprecipitate.

Current technology permits the collection of whole blood and subsequent fractionation or of selected whole-blood components by apheresis, resulting in plasma or platelet collection equivalent to a number of individual fractionated whole-blood components. Availability of technology permitting fractionation and increased sophistication in blood component therapy encouraged the development of component-specific therapy for abnormalities, tailored to the individual patient's requirements. A variety of guidelines has been created for selected procedures or by organized groups for the administration and review of blood component utilization, creating a wealth of recommendations too complex for simple overview. This led to the formation of a consensus conference on blood component management, directed by the National Institutes of Health, to develop recommendations for blood component therapy (NIH, 1985, 1987, 1988). These guidelines were generally endorsed by the American Association of Blood Banks and have served as general guidelines since their inception. The consensus guidelines for managing blood component therapy are summarized in tabular form in each section on indications. Since their development in the 1980s, more generalized use of invasive monitoring and increased technology has provided even more sound physiologic indications to guide therapy.

Indications for Red Blood Cells

General historical recommendations for the transfusion of whole blood and packed red cells are demonstrated in Table 27-8. However, recent recommendations by an

TABLE 27–7. Platelet, Leukocyte, and Plasma Components

Blood Component	Clinical Indications	Approximate Composition		Shelf Life and Storage Temperature
		Plasma	**Platelets**	
Random donor platelet	Thrombocytopenia with hemorrhage, severe thrombocytopenia, functional platelet disorders with hemorrhage	30 mL (4°C) 50 mL (20–24°C)	$>5.5 \times 10^{10}$	48 h at 4°C 72 h at 20–24°C
Single-donor platelet concentrate by apheresis	Refractory to random-donor platelet concentrate, severe thrombocytopenia, hemorrhage with thrombocytopenia or functional disorder	300–500 mL	$3–8 \times 10^{11}$	24 h at 20–24°C
Leukocyte concentrate by apheresis	Severe neutropenia, fever, and infection unresponsive to antibiotics	300–700 mL	$3–8 \times 10^{11}$ (granulocytes $= 1 \times 10^{10}$)	24 h at 4°C or 20–24°C
Fresh-frozen plasma	Multiple coagulation deficiencies	200–275 mL	Nil	1 y at −18°C 24 h at 4°C
Single-donor plasma	Plasma expansion	200–275 mL	Nil	5 y at −18°C 24 h at 4°C
Cryoprecipitate	Factor VIII deficiency, factor XIII deficiency, von Willebrand's disease, hypofibrinogenemia	10–15 mL	Nil	1 y at −18°C 6 h at 20–24°C

From Kennedy, M. S. (1982). Essentials of immunohematology and blood therapy. In P. F. Zuspan & E. J. Quilligan (Eds.), A practical manual of obstetrical care. St. Louis, MO: Mosby. Reprinted with permission.

TABLE 27–8. Indications for Transfusion of Whole Blood, Packed Red Cells, and Washed Red Cells

Whole blood
    Acute massive blood loss in excess of 1500 mL or 25% of intravascular volume
    Hypovolemic shock
Packed red cells
    Normovolemic anemia
    Controlled major intraoperative blood loss
Washed red cells
    Neonatal or intrauterine transfusions
    Recurrent or severe allergic reactions to whole blood or packed red cell transfusion
    Selected immune suppressed patients

From Perez, W. E., & Viets, J. L. (1990). Transfusion and coagulation: An overview and recent advances in practice modalities. Part I: Blood banking and transfusion practices. Nurse Anesthesia, 1(3), 149–161. Reprinted with permission.

American Society of Anesthesiologists Task Force confirms that it is inappropriate to make assumptions on the indications for transfusion without interpreting the requirements with regard to the individual patient's condition (ASA Task Force, 1996).

As a general rule, it is reasonable to assume that for the otherwise normal patient, losses of 10% to 20% of the blood volume will be tolerated without critically compromising hemodynamic stability. Up to that loss, it is generally recommended that blood losses be replaced with crystalloid or colloid solution, as outlined in the chapter on fluid management. However, a more accurate and defensible approach considers the entire patient's condition and baseline hematocrit, then determines an acceptable blood loss to be tolerated. To do so, one can use a formula using estimated blood volume (EBV), baseline hemoglobin [Hgb(b)] and minimal tolerated hemoglobin [Hgb(m)]:

$$\text{Tolerated blood loss} = [\text{EBV}] \times \frac{[\text{Hgb(b)} - \text{Hgb(m)}]}{\text{Hgb(b)}}$$

Determining how low hemoglobin levels should be allowed to go depends on the patient's ability to maintain cardiac output and systemic arterial oxygen saturation. Cases involving patients who are Jehovah's Witnesses and who have refused all blood component therapy indicate that survival is possible with a circulating hemoglobin lower than 4 g/dL in otherwise healthy patients, although prolonged postoperative support is necessary and mortality is substantially increased. Coexisting medical conditions such as increased metabolic oxygen demand from hyperthermia or hypermetabolic states, systemic vascular occlusive disease, limited cardiac reserve, or pulmonary dysfunction can support the decision to transfuse to a circulating hemoglobin of up to 10 g/dL. Except in limited populations of patients with severe disease or profoundly limited cardiac or pulmonary reserves, there is little benefit with additional increases in hemoglobin over that limit.

The likelihood of continued blood loss beyond the tolerated minimal hemoglobin will determine which red cell–containing blood component is appropriate for use. If blood loss is expected to remain under 25% the estimated blood volume, or if the initial hemoglobin concentration is low, use of packed red cells may be indicated to treat isolated anemia without compromising hemostatic competence. With expected continued blood losses that exceed 25% of the patient's blood volume, whole blood may be recommended to help preserve the procoagulant mass. Blood losses that exceed the patient's blood volume will typically require the administration of whole blood and/or concomitant coagulation component therapy, as outlined in the sections on indications for plasma and platelets.

Historic practice has maintained that a minimum hemoglobin of 10 g/dL is required to optimize postoperative survival rates (Czer & Shoemaker, 1978). Based on oxygen-carrying capacity and rheology, which indicate that the most efficient laminar flows occur at this hemoglobin level, the practice has long been accepted as a standard. Current technology using pulmonary artery catheters to determine thermodilution cardiac output permits calculation of available oxygen-carrying capacity. Consideration of the patient's age, coexisting medical condition, physiologic reserve, and estimated metabolic oxygen demand permits estimation of the adequacy of oxygen delivery at a given hemoglobin level. In addition, the use of arterial blood gas monitoring and mixed venous oxygen saturation analysis through blood gas analysis or oximetry by pulmonary artery catheters permits assessment of oxygen-carrying capacity and metabolic utilization. These improvements in technology have been a principal reason for reducing the "trigger hemoglobin" at which transfusion is practiced even in critically ill patients (Dietrich, Conrad et al., 1990; Hebert et al., 1995; Kim, Brecher, Estes, & Morrey, 1993; Lorenta et al., 1993; Marik & Sibbald, 1993). Evidence suggests that even patients with limited cardiac reserve tolerate lower hemoglobin concentrations than historically recommended (Estafanous, 1986) and that reductions in hemoglobin to 7 to 8 g/dL generally are tolerated in healthy individuals in current practice. This is consistent with evidence that wound healing and recovery are achieved with oxygen extraction as low as 0.7 volumes per 100 mL, which permits dilution of hemoglobin to approximately one-third normal without reductions in wound healing (Hunt, 1988). Indications from clinical reports, usually involving patients who have refused blood transfusion, suggest that patients are capable of surviving even lower hemoglobin concentrations when metabolic oxygen demand is minimized. As a result, a variety of indices are now considered in making the determination to transfuse red cells or whole blood.

In general, whole blood is indicated only in patients suffering major blood loss. Because platelet counts and plasma fibrinogen levels remain within accepted limits until replacement of up to half the total blood volume in most patients, the population for which whole blood is indicated is limited. However, although current practice focuses on the use of fractionated therapy with packed red cells and plasma components, the use of whole blood in selected cases involving expected massive blood loss has been demonstrated to be associated with a marked reduction in total homologous blood component utilization while maintaining similar outcome profiles in hemoglobin and coagulation parameters (Reeves-Viets, Safi, et al., 1992; Reeves-Viets, Yawn, et al., 1992; Viets & Yawn, 1991). The scarcity of whole blood in current practice makes it effectively unavailable except by special request or when blood is collected from directed or autologous donation specifically for the individual patient. Packed red cell component therapy is, therefore, generally used when blood is required for patients in whom blood loss is gradual when the principal goal is to restore or manage circulating hemoglobin concentrations, and hemostasis remains mainly a matter of surgical technique or skill.

An additional means of determining the point at which transfusion is indicated is to calculate the oxygen-carrying capacity and estimate metabolic oxygen demand. Oxygen-carrying capacity is measured by using pulmonary artery catheters with thermodilution cardiac output (CO) capacity, analysis of circulating hemoglobin concentration and arterial oxygen saturation, according to the formula:

$$CcO_2 = [Hgb \times SpO_2 \times CO] + 0.003(PaO_2)$$

From a practical clinical standpoint, oxygen dissolved in the plasma fraction contributes too little to total oxygen-carrying capacity to be of value. Therefore, the principal determinants remain circulating hemoglobin concentration and the maintenance of arterial saturation and cardiac output. In calculating oxygen availability, it is necessary to remember that the last 25% of oxygen bound in the oxyhemoglobin complex remains effectively unavailable and that saturation below that level usually corresponds with tissue or cellular damage. Thus, the total available metabolic oxygen is less than the total calculated oxygen-carrying capacity using the formula provided. Estimates of metabolic demand require consideration of temperature, effects of anesthetic agents, and muscle relaxation.

As an alternative to repeated analysis and calculations based on assumptions of metabolic oxygen demand, the use of mixed venous oximetry with a pul-

monary artery catheter permits continuous analysis of the global oxygen supply–demand relationship. The benefit of continuous monitoring is balanced by the fact that a pulmonary arterial catheter is mandatory, as the only accurate global determinant of oxygen supply–demand is a true mixed venous arterial saturation taken from the pulmonary artery. Also, global monitors of oxygen supply–demand do not indicate specific end-organ oxygen balance. Thus selected high-extraction organs such as the heart and brain may develop signs of ischemia when selectively monitored, even though global indices appear normal or are not critically reduced. Not all patients are capable of maintaining increased cardiac output to meet metabolic oxygen demand in the awake state when anemic, which limits the effectiveness of mixed venous oximetry in the anesthetized patient as an indicator of global oxygen supply–demand in the awake, normothermic state. Nevertheless, by recalculating projected oxygen demand based on determinations of the effects of temperature and anesthetic agents, one can gain an estimate of the projected mixed venous oxygen saturation in the awake state. Evidence in patients undergoing cardiopulmonary bypass indicates that a mixed venous oxygen saturation of 50% is the cutoff at which discrete neurologic impairment begins to increase, and a similar increase in morbidity and mortality appears in patients in the critical care setting whose mixed venous oxygen saturation declines below 50%. The impact of short-term reductions below 50% and critical time period of mixed venous hypoxemia has not been determined. It is therefore reasonable to consider a mixed venous oxygen saturation of 50% to be the lowest preferred limit.

In selecting red cells for transfusion intraoperatively, the first choice remains red cells or whole blood determined to be compatible with a full typing and cross-match. When circumstances do not permit selection of fully compatible units, the use of packed red cells permits administration of units that could theoretically contain incompatible antibodies in the plasma. Most clinicians recommend the use of low-titer, Rh-negative, type-O packed red cells when transfusing in emergent situations that do not permit selection of fully compatible whole blood or red cells. Practically, the mass of antibody present in donor units would be insufficient to generate a clinically significant transfusion reaction if undetectable by current screening technology. For that reason, it is clinically practical to administer antigenically negative whole blood to patients positive for that blood type when cross-matched, fully compatible blood is not available.

Indications for Plasma

Plasma and plasma products seldom are indicated for a sole transfusion in the operating room, although historical consensus indications are provided as outlined in

Table 27–9. Use of whole blood when necessary for massive blood replacement provides sufficient plasma for normal coagulation as plasma procoagulant factors are relatively stable in stored blood. Factors V and VIII are unstable in stored blood and have shown substantial degeneration in plasma activity when blood is stored for more than 3 weeks (Miller, 1973), and although the importance is questioned, the levels do not decrease below the minimal plasma activity required to maintain effective coagulation. Use of packed red cells may necessitate plasma administration to maintain an adequate circulating mass of procoagulants in patients suffering massive blood loss and transfusion, as well as in selected factor deficiencies. Indications for emergent administration of plasma for replacement of factor deficiencies are given in Table 27–10.

The majority of coagulation factors need to be maintained at only about 30% of activity to maintain normal coagulation in the uncompromised patient, as shown in Table 27–3. Therefore, plasma is not required to maintain normal coagulation function in most cases. Maintaining a plasma fibrinogen level of 100 to 150 g percent generally is compatible with adequate coagulation and represents a reasonable target when analyzing the effectiveness of plasma replacement. In patients undergoing cardiopulmonary bypass and those with synthetic grafts of the aorta, plasma fibrinogen levels of 150 to 200 may be required. Those levels are generally readily maintained with the use of fresh-frozen plasma when operative blood losses begin to reach that of the patient's estimated blood volume. The ASA Task Force (1996) recommends that plasma be used only when blood losses exceed one blood volume and coagulation studies are not readily available, or for supplementation of coagulation factors to 30% of normal.

TABLE 27–9. Indications for Transfusion of Fresh-Frozen Plasma and Cryoprecipitate Concentrate

Fresh-frozen plasma
  Bleeding coagulopathy and factor deficiency due to
    Disseminated intravascular coagulation (DIC)
    Massive blood loss
    Severe hepatic dysfunction
  Congenital factor deficiencies of V or XI that have no currently available
    concentrates for treatment
  Treatment of mild congenital factor deficiencies such as Factor IX
  Antithrombin-III deficiency
  Reversal of coumadin/warfarin therapy
Cryoprecipitate concentrates
  Factor VIII deficiency
  DIC with hypofibrinogenemia
  Primary hypofibrinogenemia

From Perez, W. E., & Viets, J. L. (1990). Transfusion and coagulation: An overview and recent advances in practice modalities. Part I: Blood banking and transfusion practices. Nurse Anesthesia, 1(3), 149–161. Reprinted with permission.

TABLE 27–10. Emergency Replacement Therapy with Plasma for Miscellaneous Specific Coagulation Deficiencies

Disease	Loading Dose	Maintenance Dose
Hemophilia A[a] (factor VIII deficiency)	Not required	15 mL/kg every 8 h for 1–2 days and every 12 h thereafter
Hemophilia B[a] (factor IX deficiency)	60 mL/kg	7 mL/kg every 12 h
von Willebrand's disease[a]	Not required	10 mL/kg daily
Prothrombin deficiency	15 mL/kg	5–10 mL/kg daily
Factor V deficiency	20 mL/kg	10 mL/kg every 12 h
Factor VII deficiency	10 mL/kg	5 mL/kg every 6–24 h
Factor X deficiency	15 mL/kg	10 mL/kg daily
Factor XI deficiency	10 mL/kg	5 mL/kg daily
Factor XIII deficiency	5 mL/kg every 1 to 2 wk	Not required

[a] Specific factor concentrates are generally available and more effective and convenient than plasma in most situations. They may pose an increased risk for disease transmission.
From Wintrobe, M. M. (1979). Therapy of the hereditary coagulation disorders. In Clinical hematology (p. 1190). Philadelphia: Lea & Febiger. Reprinted with permission.

Selected cases support the use of plasma for chronic management, such as burn therapy or gastrointestinal losses of plasma protein in which massive volumes of plasma protein are lost. Because other forms of colloids are now available to maintain colloid osmotic pressure, the use of plasma as a volume expander is no longer considered an appropriate therapeutic alternative in most patients. However, synthetic volume expanders such as hetastarch are known to reduce platelet activity, particularly when used in large volumes. Thus the use of plasma may be indicated in patients expected to undergo massive blood losses or volume exchanges, as in cardiopulmonary bypass or thoracic aortic surgery, or those who have preexisting platelet dysfunction, such as patients with renal or hepatic dysfunction or failure. In those patients in whom platelet and plasma therapy is required, early use of plasma as opposed to synthetic volume expanders is favored by many clinicians.

Plasma therapy also may be initiated for emergent correction of coumadin overdose or to return coagulation studies to normal when inadequate time exists to reverse the effects with vitamin K prior to urgent or emergent surgery. In general, clinical practice indicates that the use of 10 to 15 mL/kg of fresh-frozen plasma is sufficient to reverse coumadinization and to produce a satisfactory coagulation profile. In addition, plasma may be used to correct deficiencies in antithrombin-III activity. Selected patients may demonstrate chronically low plasma AT-III activity, such as those receiving chronic heparin administration. Reductions in AT-III activity below

50% have been implicated in the failure to respond to the anticoagulant effects of heparin using laboratory tests as an indicator and also have been implicated in hypercoagulable states that may result in diffuse microvascular coagulopathies or early graft occlusion in patients undergoing vascular bypass procedures. With the use of prepared forms of purified AT-III now available, therapy for selected AT-III deficiency includes direct supplementation of the deficient factor rather than supplementation with plasma products. Finally, therapy with plasma is indicated in those patients in whom thrombolytic therapy has been initiated preoperatively. This scenario usually is limited to patients failing thrombolytic treatment for acute peripheral vascular occlusion and those failing thrombolytic therapy for myocardial ischemia who might require emergent peripheral vascular or coronary artery bypass. Because these patients are typically at greater risk to develop DIC, these components may be necessary to maintain hemostasis.

Because antibody levels decline in the serum unless there is repeated exposure after their initial formation and exposed individuals are discouraged from blood donation for 6 months to 1 year, antibody levels in donor plasma can generally be considered to be low. In clinical practice, the theoretic mass of antibody is so low in ABO-incompatible plasma that it represents no risk to the recipient, and plasma without detectable antibodies may be used regardless of the donor and recipient's blood types. As a result, transfusion of plasma with incompatible blood types generally is safe even within the ABO system. Still, whenever possible, only type-compatible plasma is administered to recipients as the administration of components to patients with incompatible blood types, particularly within the ABO system, that possess alloantibodies, is in theory susceptible to trigger a graft-versus-host immunologic response. Type AB, Rh-positive donors may be considered universal plasma donors since they possess no antibodies to type A, B, or Rh-positive red cells.

Indications for Platelets

Indications for the use of platelets are more complex and controversial than for red cells or plasma. Although historically accepted indications for platelet transfusion are shown in Table 27–11, the clinical setting also is a major determinant in the decision to transfuse platelets. Platelets may be indicated in patients whose circulating platelet counts are critically low and whose platelet function is impaired. Without intervention, patients with blood dyscrasias or hematopoietic dysfunction may readily tolerate platelet counts below 10 000/mm^3 without spontaneous bleeding but may require platelet support for surgical intervention only with platelet counts less than 10 000 to 50 000/mm^3 (Gaydos, Freireich, & Mantel,

TABLE 27–11.   Indications for Transfusion of Platelet Concentrates

Chronic thrombocytopenia with platelet count under 20 000
Thrombocytopenia with bleeding; platelet count under 50 000
Massive blood loss with platelet count between 75 000 and 100 000
Demonstrated thrombocytopathy
    Immature platelets
    Dysfunctional platelets
    Drug-induced platelet dysfunction
Disseminated intravascular coagulation

From Perez, W. E., & Viets, J. L. (1990). Transfusion and coagulation: An overview and recent advances in practice modalities. Part I: Blood banking and transfusion practices. Nurse Anesthesia, 1(3), 149–161.

1962). Because many patients with preexisting thrombocytopenia have received multiple platelet infusions previously, antiplatelet antibodies are present, and it is recommended that platelet administration be given preoperatively or even during the induction period. However, in normal surgical patients platelet counts below 50 000 to 75 000/mm^3 appear to be associated with a marked increase in the incidence of diffuse bleeding and coagulopathy (Miller, Robbins, Tong, & Barton, 1971). A platelet count under 50 000 is generally considered an accepted rationale for treating acutely induced thrombocytopenia with platelet infusion in keeping with the guidelines of the ASA Task Force (1996).

In contrast, platelet therapy is not indicated in patients with induced thrombocytopenia that may occur with heparin-induced antiplatelet antibodies because the administration of platelets in that circumstance may actually induce or worsen diffuse microvascular coagulation and occlusion. To manage patients with antiplatelet antibodies and to discern the nature and origin of those antibodies, obtaining a hematology consult is critical to determine platelet therapy. Administration of platelets in surgical procedures involving cardiopulmonary bypass was historically advocated by some clinicians. However, all controlled studies indicated that increased absolute platelet count before bypass did nothing to reduce component requirements after the bypass. For that reason, the use of platelets in patients undergoing procedures with cardiopulmonary bypass is no longer an accepted clinical practice. For patients undergoing procedures not involving cardiovascular bypass and who are on platelet inhibitor therapy, the decision to use platelets should be based on evidence of platelet function inhibition and clinical signs of diffuse surgical bleeding. Routine platelet administration is not considered to be indicated.

Recommendations of the ASA Task Force (1996) recognize that selected patients may demonstrate ineffective platelet activity despite apparently normal circulating platelet counts. Patients whose platelets are inactivated by metabolic disease, such as renal or hepatic dysfunction, those receiving antiplatelet therapy, such as aspirin to reduce the risk of coronary thrombosis, those receiving large volumes of synthetic colloids, and those undergoing cardiopulmonary bypass may demonstrate diffuse surgical bleeding with higher platelet counts. In those populations, platelet administration may be necessary to maintain adequate hemostatically effective platelets. Because platelet function tests are cumbersome and time-consuming, acute therapy in those patients may have to rely on clinical indices rather than laboratory analysis for ongoing operative management.

In determining the requirement for platelet therapy, general rules of thumb may be used to guide clinical decisions. In the normal patient, one individual platelet donor unit for every 7 to 10 kg body weight may be expected to increase the circulating platelet count by up to 10 000/mL. Repeated posttransfusion platelet counts are necessary to guide the efficacy of therapy, and the determination to continue platelet transfusion depends on clinical assessment as well as laboratory analysis. Because the majority of conditions that induce plasma loss also induce loss of platelets or their inactivation, there is little evidence to support the use of plasma without concomitant use of platelets as well.

The antigenic capacity of platelets is limited in normal operative administration, so that, for the majority of patients, antibody responses to platelet administration are not a critical consideration in their use. However, in patients with repeated exposures, specific antibodies to platelets may develop and require more exhaustive cross-matching to ensure that administered homologous platelets will not generate an immunologic response that would result in their immediate aggregation and inactivation. It is important to ascertain the nature of previous exposures in patients undergoing surgery where expected blood losses would necessitate coagulation factor replacement in order to identify those patients whose antibody status may complicate platelet administration.

Indications for Processed Plasma Preparations

A variety of processed plasma factors are available for discrete therapy in selected disease conditions. These are generally not employed as a first line of action in coagulation management, and their uses fall into three principal categories. In the first category are induced abnormalities in coagulation, including metabolic disorders that prevent the development or release of procoagulant factors and blood losses that require massive resuscitation, such as trauma, selected major vascular procedures, and intravascular coagulopathies. Patients with induced coagulation abnormalities generally are treated with plasma, because it contains the greater number of coagulant factors. In the second category are congenital ab-

normalities in coagulation resulting from the inability to produce or release procoagulant factors. These include congenital factor IX deficiency, absence or failure to utilize von Willebrand's factor or Factor VIII, and the hemophilias. A detailed discussion of these populations is beyond the scope of a basic chapter, but indications are listed in Table 27–12. The third group includes the use of albumin as a natural protein for use as a volume expander for patients who require chronic colloid therapy but for whom synthetic colloid expanders are not an appropriate clinical choice. When acute volume resuscitation with limited volumes of expanders is the clinical goal, many clinicians now elect to use synthetic colloid preparations that carry less risk of infection or immunologic response. The use of albumin in the perioperative period is decreasing because of the expense or cost.

The most commonly used plasma derivative in anesthetic practice is cryoprecipitate, which is obtained by cold-fractionated precipitation of plasma to remove those plasma proteins most critical in clot formation. Hence, cryoprecipitate is particularly high in fibrinogen and may be used when plasma therapy alone is insufficient to maintain satisfactory levels of fibrinogen. Because the majority of patients receiving adequate volume resuscitation with plasma will maintain satisfactory levels of fibrinogen as a result of plasma therapy alone, cryoprecipitate is generally indicated only for those patients with isolated hypofibrinogenemia, severe hepatic dysfunction with resultant failure to produce procoagulant proteins, and severe diffuse intravascular coagulopathies that may occur with dissection or rupture of aortic aneurysms, sepsis, massive transfusion, or the preoperative use of fibrinolytic therapy. In general, the cryoprecipitate requirements of patients with severe hypofibrinogenemia can be estimated by calculating plasma

TABLE 27–12. Blood Products for Treatment of Coagulation Factor Deficiencies

Fibrinogen deficiency	Cryoprecipitate Stored plasma
Factor V deficiency	Fresh-frozen plasma
Factor VII deficiency	Factor IX complex (II, VII, IX, X) Stored plasma
Factor VIII deficiency	Factor VIII concentrate (AHF) Cryoprecipitate Fresh-frozen plasma
Von Willebrand's disease	Cryoprecipitate Fresh-frozen plasma
Factor IX deficiency	Factor IX complex (II, VII, IX, X) Stored plasma
Factor XIII deficiency	Stored plasma

From Blajchman, M. A., Sheppard, F. A., & Perrault, R. A. (1979). Clinical use of blood, blood components and blood products. Canadian Medical Association Journal, 121, 33. Reprinted with permission.

volume and the total fibrinogen requirement in mg/dL, and assuming that each unit of cryoprecipitate will contain approximately 250 mg of fibrinogen. This usually corresponds to the infusion of one unit of cryoprecipitate for every 2 to 4 kg of body weight in patients demonstrating moderate to severe hypofibrinogenemia. Cryoprecipitate also may be used for acute supplementation of Factor VIII factors in patients with hemophilia A. The total dose of cryoprecipitate required may be calculated using the following equation:

$$\text{Factor VIII units infused} = \frac{(40 \text{ mL/kg plasma volume}) \times (\text{weight in kg}) \times (\% \text{ increase required})}{100}$$

when each unit of cryoprecipitate may be presumed to carry 80 to 120 units activity. However, because the majority of these processes are ongoing, it is critical to continue to monitor plasma fibrinogen levels after cryoprecipitate administration to ensure that adequate supplementation is achieved and the plasma levels of fibrinogen continue to be satisfactory.

Processed plasma derivatives carry no cellular elements and are generally derived from pooled serum from multiple donors (except cryoprecipitate). Any antibodies in the donor unit are removed during processing and may be given without considering donor–recipient incompatibility.

Risks of Transfusion Therapy

The risks of transfusion may be conceptually divided into two groups. The first group is immediate risk, which centers on the identification and treatment of hemolytic immunologic reactions to incompatible blood or nonhemolytic reactions that are usually due to preservative or foreign plasma antigens in the donor unit. The second group is delayed risk, which is principally focused on the infectious risks of transfusion based on the individual donor unit. The majority of infectious risks in the latter group are viral, including hepatitis, cytomegalovirus, and AIDS, although there is the potential for limited risk from blood contaminated with protozoal infections or bacterial contaminants in the collection process.

The relative risks of transfusion reaction to administration of incompatible components depend on the character of the incompatibility. A list of clinically significant antibodies and their associated transfusion-related reactions is offered in Table 27–13. The most critical reactions occur in the ABO system and in patients previously sensitized to highly antigenic blood types, such as Rh, who are transfused with incompatible red blood cells. These invoke an immediate, intravascular, lytic transfusion that may be life-threatening. Hemolytic transfusion reactions have been reported to occur in approximately 1 in 4000 to 1 in 6000 administrations (Pineda & Brzica, 1980), although the incidence of fatal hemolytic transfu-

sion reactions has been estimated at 1 in 500 000 to 1 in 800 000 (Linden & Kaplan, 1994). The risk of ABO-incompatibile hemolytic transfusion reactions is estimated to be approximately 1 in 33 000 units (Linden, Paul, & Dressler, 1992; Linden & Kaplan, 1994). The classic signs of hemolytic transfusion reaction of fever, chills, nausea, and headache may not be demonstrable under anesthesia, and the most common early signs under anesthesia include hemoglobinuria, hypotension, and the development of excessive bleeding or coagulopathies. Later signs may include renal dysfunction or failure and pulmonary complications, including respiratory distress syndrome. The release of red cell stroma in a hemolytic transfusion probably accounts for the development of renal dysfunction or failure after a hemolytic transfusion reaction, rather than free plasma hemoglobin. Haptoglobin is capable of binding up to 100 mg/dL of free hemoglobin, and the presence of free plasma hemoglobin alone does not appear to produce renal dysfunction.

The treatment of hemolytic transfusion reactions is supportive, as outlined in Table 27–14. Circulatory support may be necessary with inotropes and volume. Renal support with crystalloid administration and diuretics to maintain a urine output of 75 to 100 mL/h is recommended. Some clinicians advocate using sodium bicarbonate to alkalinize the urine and prevent the deposition of acid hematin in the distal renal tubules. Treatment of DIC that may accompany a hemolytic transfusion reaction is supportive, and coagulant factors can be administered as indicated by laboratory and clinical analysis.

Nonhemolytic transfusion reactions are generally due to foreign antigenic proteins or the preservative in stored homologous blood and occur in 1% to 5% of all transfusions (NIH, 1988). These generally are mild and result only in urticaria or rash, for which only symptomatic treatment is recommended with antipruritics such as diphenhydramine. More severe reactions may occur in patients who are IgA or IgE deficient and who develop antibodies in response to administration of homologous blood components containing normal IgA or IgE. These may result in classic anaphylactic reactions with hypotension, myocardial depression, and the development of laryngeal edema. Supportive therapy with epinephrine is recommended as with any anaphylactic reaction, and responses are generally seen with doses as low as 5 μg/kg (Stoelting, 1983). In these patients, transfusion with red cells known to be from IgA-free donors (Rustagi & Logue, 1990) or washed red cells from which all IgE is removed may be necessary (Giblett, 1980).

Other potential consequences of massive transfusion are citrate toxicity or electrolyte disturbances. The use of chelating agents for anticoagulation of stored donor blood and the characteristics of that stored blood indicate that hypocalcemia and hyperkalemia are potential events when transfusion of large volumes of red cells

TABLE 27–13. Selected Erythrocyte Antibodies: Clinical Implication and Probability of Finding a Compatible Donor

Antibody	Associated with[b] Hemolytic Disease of the Newborn	Hemolytic Transfusion Reaction	Probability of Finding Compatible Donor (%) White	African Americans[a]
Anti-A	Yes	Yes	56	69
Anti-B	Yes	Yes	85	76
Anti-A$_1$	?	Yes	53	52
Anti-A,B	Yes	Yes	45	49
Anti-D	Yes	Yes	15	8
Anti-C	Yes	Yes	30	68
Anti-C^w	Yes	Yes	99	100
Anti-E	Yes	Yes	70	98
Anti-c	Yes	Yes	20	1
Anti-e	Yes	Yes	2	2
Anti-M	Few	Few	22	30
Anti-N	Rare	?	28	26
Anti-S	Yes	Yes	45	69
Anti-s	Yes	Yes	11	3
Anti-U	Yes	Yes	0	<1
Anti-P^1	No	Rare	21	6
Anti-P	No	?	Extremely rare	
Anti-PP$_1$P^K	Rare	?	Extremely rare	
Anti-Lu^a	No	?	92	—
Anti-Lu^b	Mild	Yes	0.15	—
Anti-K	Yes	Yes	91	98
Anti-k	Yes	Yes	0.2	Rare
Anti-K$_p$^{a}	Yes	?	97.7	100
Anti-K$_p$^{b}	Yes	?	Rare	0
Anti-Js^a	Yes	?	100	80
Anti-Js^b	Yes	?	0	1
Anti-Le^a	No	Few	78	77
Anti-Le^b	No	?	28	45
Anti-Fy^a	Yes	Yes	34	22
Anti-Fy^b	Yes	Yes	17	77
Anti-Jk^a	Yes	Yes	23	9
Anti-Jk^b	Yes	Yes	28	57
Anti-Xg^a	No report		M, 34	—
			F, 11	—
Anti-Di^a	Yes	Yes	100	—
Anti-Di^b	Yes	Yes	0	—
Anti-Yt^a	No	Yes	0.2	—
Anti-Yt^b	No report		92	—
Anti-Do^a	?	Yes	33	—
Anti-Do^b	No report		17	—
Anti-Co^a	Yes	?	0.3	—
Anti-Co^b	No report		89	—
Anti-Sc1	No report		Very rare	—
Anti-Sc2	No report		99.7	—

[a] Blanks indicate insufficient data for reliable calculation of frequencies.

From the American Association of Blood Banking Technical Manual (1985); table from Bresher, M. E., & Taswell. H. F. (1991). Hemolytic transfusion reactions. In E. C. Rossi, T. L. Simon, & G. S. Moss (Eds.), Principles of transfusion medicine *(p. 626). Baltimore: Williams & Wilkins. Reprinted with permission.*

TABLE 27–14. Steps for the Treatment of Hemolytic Transfusion Reaction

1. *Stop the transfusion.*
2. Maintain the urine output at a minimum of 75 to 100 mL/h by the following methods:
   a. Generously administer fluids intravenously and possibly mannitol, 12.5 to 50 g, given over a 5- to 15-min period.
   b. If intravenously administered fluids and mannitol are ineffective, then administer furosemide, 20 to 40 mg, intravenously.
3. Alkalinize the urine; as bicarbonate is preferentially excreted in the urine, only 40 to 70 mEq/70 kg of sodium bicarbonate is usually required to raise the urine pH to 8, whereupon repeat urine pH determinations indicate the need for additional bicarbonate.
4. Assay urine and plasma hemoglobin concentrations.
5. Determine platelet count, partial thromboplastin time, and serum fibrinogen level.
6. Return unused blood to blood bank for recrossmatch.
7. Send patient blood sample to blood bank for antibody screen and direct antiglobulin test.
8. Prevent hypotension to ensure adequate renal blood flow.

are administered quickly. Plasma products carry the risk of hypocalcemia without the risks of hyperkalemia from red cell losses. Replacement of ionized calcium may be necessary, and measurements of potassium should be followed to identify hyperkalemia before it becomes clinically critical. In theory, a late-phase development of hypokalemia may ensue when citrate is metabolized to bicarbonate, creating alkalosis and secondary hypokalemia (Carmichael, Hosty, Kastl, & Beckman, 1984; Driscoll et al., 1987). However, this is not generally a clinical problem. Likewise, ammonia toxicity may occur, but this is an uncommon event, with the exception of patients who have severe hepatic dysfunction (Spear, Sass, & Cincotti, 1956).

Infectious risks of transfusion are generally not immediately immunologic and manifest with late development of viral, bacterial, or protozoal syndromes. Bacterial contamination is rare, and the development of sepsis from contaminated blood products in the United States is extremely rare due to testing and strict adherence to sterile technique during donation. Twenty-six deaths due to bacterial contamination were reported to the Food and Drug Administration between 1976 and 1985 (Sazama, 1985). Protozoal contamination in the United States is likewise extremely rare with an incidence estimated at 1 in one million (Dodd, 1992). Limitation of volunteer donors who have traveled outside the country to areas in which protozoal infection is endemic has virtually eliminated that hazard. As a result, the principal sources for infectious risk are now viral diseases. Three viral groups are principally involved: (1) cytomegalovirus (CMV); (2) the family of hepatitis viruses, including principally

hepatitis B and C; and (3) the retroviruses, including the human immunodeficiency virus (HIV) responsible for acquired immune deficiency syndrome (AIDS) and the human T-cell lymphotrophic virus (HTLV). The incidence of these viral transmissions initially proved difficult to estimate due to the low frequency and tremendous numbers of donors required to reach statistical significance. Thus the initial impetus to reduce the transmission of these viral diseases was directed to voluntary exclusion of blood donors, augmented later with increasingly sensitive and specific serologic testing. Recent meta-analysis by the Retrovirus Epidemiology Donor Study, or so-called REDS study (Schreiber, Busch, Kleinman, & Korelitz, 1996), has been able to provide more reliable estimates of the likelihood of transmission. The study suggests that recent additional testing is expected to reduce the likelihood of transmission by 27% to 72%.

The risk of CMV transmission is relatively less critical in the normal healthy patient. Estimates of CMV prevalence indicate that the majority of the adult population is antibody-positive to CMV. Patients undergoing solid-organ transplantation, those receiving obliterative therapy prior to bone marrow transplantation, and those who are CMV-negative and immunosuppressed may be at risk for developing CMV infection following transfusion. Therefore, it is recommended that these patients be transfused only with blood products that are tested as CMV-negative.

The risk of posttransfusion hepatitis has always remained the most common and clinically significant risk. The risks of developing icteric hepatitis were historically considered to be about 0.2% for each unit transfused, and the incidence of anicteric hepatitis was considered to be about five times higher (Miller & Brzica, 1986). The meta-analyses of the REDS study (Schreiber, Busch, Kleinman, & Korelitz, 1996) suggest that the likelihood of transmission of hepatitis B is roughly 1 in 63 000, whereas the likelihood of transmission of hepatitis C is roughly 1 in 103 000. The development of additional testing methods for both antigen and antibodies to hepatitis B and C is expected to reduce the likelihood of transmission even further. In identifying posttransfusion development of hepatitis, it is important to verify the character of the hepatitis incurred, as the incidence of non-A, non-B hepatitis in patients who were never transfused has been reported to be as high as 2.2% (Aach & Kuhn, 1980).

The risks of posttransfusion hepatitis are greater, but the public perception is that the greatest risk from blood transfusion remains the transmission of HIV and the development of AIDS. The identification of the AIDS syndrome in the early 1980s was followed shortly by an identification of the responsible virus. At that time, voluntary exclusion of high-risk donors led to an immediate reduction in the risk of transfusion-related transmission of HIV infection. The development and refinement of antibody testing, and more recently the development of antigenic testing for HIV have reduced the estimated risks of infection to roughly 1 in 500 000 (Lackritz et al., 1995; Schreiber et al., 1996). Nevertheless, HIV infection currently is believed to lead in virtually all cases to the eventual development of AIDS, which presently has a near-100% mortality despite supportive therapy and therapy to delay the onset of the syndrome. A similar retrovirus, human T-cell lymphotrophic virus (HTLV), shows a similar profile with estimated risks of transmission of 1 in 641 000 (Schreiber et al., 1996).

Public concerns about the safety of the homologous donor pool have led to an increased reliance on autologous or designated blood donation as an alternative to the general homologous pool. The use of autologous blood donation does decrease the risk of incompatibility and exogenous infections, but the same is not necessarily true for directed blood donors. Evidence gathered from analysis of designated donors has not consistently supported that perception, and the safety of designated donations has been challenged using markers for infectivity. The use of first-time donors as designated volunteer donors reveals a higher incidence of exclusion markers, including viral and biochemical exclusion markers in the units received (Kamel, Flynn, & Ballas, 1989; Kruskall, Popovsky, Pacini, Donovan, & Ransil, 1988; Owings, Kruskall, Thurer, & Donovan, 1989; Page, 1989). When previous volunteer donors alone are used for directed donation, the risk remains at the lowest limit. The use of designated donors for homologous blood products has not necessarily resulted in a truly safer homologous donor source. Finally, data supports the fact that the increased incidence of markers causes donor blood to be removed from the pool in first-time autologous donors and designated donors. This limits the value for their use in the cross-over pool if not used by the directed recipient (Cordell, Yalon, & Cigahn-Haskell, 1986; Grossman, Steward, & Grindon, 1988; Kamel, Flynn, & Ballas, 1989; Kruskall, Popovsky, Pacini, Donovan, & Ransil, 1988; Starkey et al., 1989).

Pharmacologic Adjuncts to Transfusion Therapy

Adjuncts are available to support patients who require transfusion of blood components. Preoperative measures include enhancement of hematogenesis through preoperative phlebotomy as an element of autologous predonation in conjunction with pharmacologic support with erythropoietin and essential cofactors required for the development of red cells. Intraoperative measures include pharmacologic support with antifibrinolytics and plasma or platelet activators.

Beneficial side effects to the practice of autologous predonation are the upregulation and increase in hematogenesis that result from acute blood losses incurred through phlebotomy. Evidence suggests that serial collec-

tion of donated whole blood caused a two- to three-fold increase in the rate of bone marrow activity during the first 2 weeks of donation (Hamstra & Block, 1969; Hillman & Henderson, 1969). In normal patients that increase in hematogenesis is sufficient to reduce the delay in red cell production and release in response to anemia following surgical blood losses. In patients with impaired nutritional status or hematogenesis, pharmacologic support for hematogenesis may prove useful. In patients with preexisting anemia, recombinant human erythropoietin may be administered along with supplemental vitamin B_{12}, thiamin, and iron. When used to induce increased hematogenesis, the recommended dose of recombinant erythropoietin is 200 to 300 units/kg of body weight (Goodnough, Verbrugge, Marcus, & Goldberg, 1994), far above the maintenance doses of 4 units/kg generally used to maintain erythrogenesis in patients with chronic mild to moderate anemia. Erythropoietin should be administered subcutaneously for more uniform plasma levels, and increases in erythrogenesis should be noted within approximately 1 week. Indices of increased erythrogenesis include higher hematocrit and reticulocyte counts. Reticulocytes, incompletely matured red cells with fragments of nuclear debris demonstrable under microscopy by differential staining, should represent less than 1% of the circulating red cell population in normal patients. With increased erythrogenesis, the reticulocyte count may reach 5%, which is indicative of a substantial increase in the rate of formation and release of red cells.

The advantage of treatment with erythropoietin is the increase in available red cell mass, but it requires preoperative coordination with multiple services, including the blood bank or donor center. It also involves potential delays that limit its application in patients undergoing urgent surgery and eliminate the preoperative value in emergent cases. Although they do not directly increase the availability of procoagulant proteins, increases in circulating red cell mass may permit the predonation of additional autologous whole blood or increased apheresis collection of plasma or platelets in the preoperative period. This therapy has been successfully in combination with intraoperative autologous sequestration in renal patients. It also has been useful in patients who are Jehovah's Witnesses and present with anemia and refuse blood component therapy or who are scheduled for elective thoracic aortic surgery or coronary artery bypass.

In addition to preoperative donation, pharmacologic support may reduce the inactivation of procoagulant factors in selected cases. A schematic representation of the effects of serine protease inhibitors is provided in Figure 27–1. Serine protease inhibitors may be indicated in patients with excessive bleeding during procedures on organs that increase fibrinolysis, such as surgical procedures on the brain and prostate. In addition, exposure

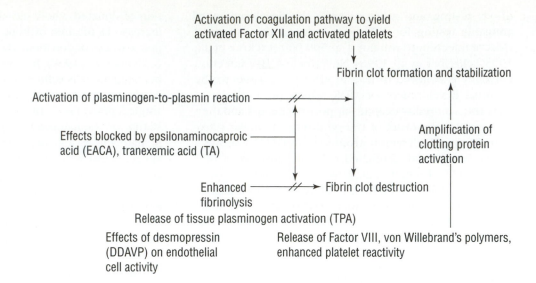

Figure 27–1.

to exogenous surfaces such as the cardiopulmonary bypass circuit is known to induce platelet and complement activation and to result in a degree of primary fibrinolysis. Although these are generally hemostatically insignificant, they may become a contributing factor to the development of coagulopathies in repeat operations or complex operations. For those patients, the use of antifibrinolytics may be recommended to reduce complement activation (Bennet, Yawn, & Migliore, 1987) and to bind active sites on the plasmin molecule and prevent its degradation of fibrin (Griffith & Ellamn, 1978).

Serine protease inhibitors may be used before, during, and after cardiopulmonary bypass to reduce primary fibrinolysis. Various protocols have been recommended, including use of epsilon-amino caproic acid (Amicar) in doses of 5 to 10 g or 75 to 150 mg/kg before bypass. This may be used in conjunction with infusions at 1 g/h or 15 mg/kg/h during bypass and up to 6 to 12 hours (Hardy & Desroches, 1992; Horrow, 1990; Verstraaete, 1985; Woodman & Harker, 1990) or supplemented with additional doses of 5 to 10 g administered with protamine. As an alternative, tranexamic acid may be used in a similar fashion. Because tranexamic acid is approximately five times as potent as Amicar, it is generally used in a loading dose of 10 to 15 mg/kg (usually 1 g) with infusion rates of 1 to 1.5 mg/kg/h (Czer et al., 1987; Horrow, 1990). Although there may be some use for antifibrinolytics in repeat operations, evidence of their effectiveness in other cases is inconclusive (Bick, 1985; Mammen, Koets, & Washington, 1984), and generally this practice has not been recommended. Indications for the use of serine protease inhibitors in treatment of DIC includes the risk of diffuse microvascular occlusion if fibrinolysis is halted when excessive coagulation activity is demonstrated. For that reason, the current therapeutic recommendation for treating DIC is

supportive therapy with coagulation components rather than serine protease inhibitors.

Another serine protease inhibitor is aprotonin (Trasylol), which was used initially in the treatment of patients with pancreatitis. Aprotonin is common in Europe where clinical reports indicate it reduces or eliminates activation of complement, reduces the degree of fibrinolysis by inhibiting plasmin and trypsin, and appears to inhibit both tissue and plasma kallikrein (Hardy & Desroches, 1992). In addition, it appears to preserve platelet function by preventing platelet activation during cardiopulmonary bypass. Preliminary reports concerning its use in the United States, however, included case reports of early graft occlusion in coronary artery bypass using the higher recommended dose of two million units as a loading dose, two million units in the cardiopulmonary bypass circuit and, one million units per hour during bypass, up to a total administered dose of six million units (Cosgrove et al., 1992). For that reason, many clinicians now favor a reduced dose half that of the original recommended dose. Indications for using aprotonin in cases not involving cardiopulmonary bypass have not been demonstrated, and aprotonin is currently used only for repeat operations involving cardiopulmonary bypass.

In addition to the serine protease inhibitors, drugs may be used that enhance the release of Factor VIII. This may potentially support or correct the lesion associated with von Willebrand's disorder, where the defect is inadequate subendothelial stores or ineffective release of Factor VIII in response to vascular injury. The drug 1-deamino-8-ᴅ-arginine vasopressin (DDAVP, or Desmopressin) promotes the release of the coagulant and high-molecular-weight portions of Factor VIII from endothelial stores, and it also may improve platelet function in patients with azotemia. DDAVP is recommended in a single dose of 0.3 µg/kg infused slowly, as it is a

TABLE 27–15. Effects of DDAVP in Treatment of Patients with von Willebrand's Disorder

Variant	Physiologic Defect	Effect of DDAVP
Type I	Low endothelial stores of Factor VIII complex	Little clinical effect
Type IIA	No endothelial stores of Factor VIII complex	No clinical effect
Type IIB	Endothelial stores of Factor VIII complex present	Massive release with potential for uncontrolled coagulation
Type III	Low endothelial stores of Factor VIII complex	Little clinical effect

From Viets, J. L., & Yawn, D. H. (1990). Transfusion and coagulation: An overview and recent advances in practice modalities. Part II: Pharmacologic adjuncts, cell salvage mechanisms, alternatives in blood donation. Nurse Anesthesia, 1(4), 206–220. Reprinted by permission of Appleton & Lange, Inc.

vasodilator (Johns, 1990), with a maximum dose of 0.6 μg/kg/day.

Patients with von Willebrand's disorder may belong to any of several groups that respond differently to the administration of DDAVP. It is therefore important to identify the nature of their defect prior to routine use of DDAVP, as outlined in Table 27–15. Patients who do not produce Factor VIII as Type IIA did not respond to DDAVP. Patients with reduced stores of Factor VIII as seen in von Willebrand's Type I and III may benefit from accelerated release. However, patients with normal endothelial stores of Factor VIII as seen in von Willebrand's Type IIB may respond to DDAVP with excessive release leading to uncontrolled coagulation and microvascular occlusion. For those reasons, the use of DDAVP generally is recommended only for patients with known platelet function abnormalities secondary to hepatic or renal disease (Agnelli, Berretine, deCunto, & Nenci, 1983; Watson & Keogh, 1983).

Blood Salvage

A variety of mechanisms may be used to reduce operative blood losses and the requirements for total homologous blood component administration. These have been undertaken for a variety of reasons, including patient anxieties about the safety of homologous donor blood, conservation of scarce blood component resources, and reduction in transfusion costs. Most of the initial work done with blood salvage systems was done in patients undergoing vascular and cardiac surgery, and these cases still account for as much as 90% of units of salvaged blood processed in some centers (Yawn, 1989). In general, there are two types of blood salvage systems. The first of these is a passive blood salvaging system that simply collects shed blood for direct retransfusion. The sec-

ond incorporates any of a variety of systems for processing scavenged blood that filter particulate debris, wash out any free hemoglobin and subcellular components, and resuspend the red cells in a balanced salt solution. Their differences are substantial and play a principal role in determining the appropriate form of blood salvage to be used for any procedure.

Passive blood salvage systems operate by interposing a collection cannister in suction lines from the surgical field intraoperatively or in suction tubes or drains in the postoperative period. Blood is collected under sterile conditions with concomitant administration of a heparinized saline solution to prevent clotting in the collection cannister. After collection is completed, the scavenged blood is simply readministered to the patient through a filter to remove particulate debris and platelet aggregates. The principal benefit in this system is its simplicity. Passive scavenging requires only that an appropriate scavenging system be interposed in the suction or drainage lines, and no special preparations are required prior to administration outside those used in normal transfusion recommendations. It is relatively simple and quick to utilize and can be employed by nursing personnel and members of the anesthesia care team without removing attention from other immediate tasks. Administration of protamine to reverse the effects of heparin used to anticoagulate scavenged blood is relatively low risk. For patients who might be at increased risk from protamine reaction, systems can utilize sodium citrate solutions rather than heparin. Citrate must be metabolized, but, in the volumes typically used in passive systems, the systemic effect of the volume of sodium citrate used is negligible and is treated with the administration of calcium chloride.

The character of the final product varies widely between passively scavenged blood and washed, processed red cells, resuspended in a normal saline solution, as demonstrated in Table 27–16. Collection of shed blood from drainage systems permits activation of the coagulation cascade prior to collection, while suctioning from the field generally removes shed blood before it has the opportunity to activate the coagulation cascade. The resultant collection is a heparinized collection of shed blood, which includes preservation of part of the procoagulant proteins in the plasma fraction. Fibrinogen levels around 90 g/dL, Factor VIII levels of 75% normal, and Factor V levels of 36% normal are reported, all of which are consistent with the requirements of normal hemostasis (Noon, 1978). Levels of AT-III and plasminogen, in contrast, are each reduced to about 45% normal and may represent a clinically significant reduction (Yawn, 1991). Platelet counts are reduced in passively collected blood to mean counts of 82 000 to 111 000 per μL, and, although they appear microscopically normal, they may be activated in the collection process and rendered ineffective hemostatically.

TABLE 27–16. Biochemical Characteristics of Salvaged Blood (Baylor Bowl)

Variable	Unprocessed		Processed	
	Mean ± SD	Range	Mean ± SD	Range
Na$^+$ (mEq/L)	137 ± 2.4	132–141	147 ± 2.4	143–150
K$^+$ (mEq/L)	4.4 ± 0.7	3.1–5.3	1.6 ± 1.5	0.8–2.3
Cl$^-$ (mEq/L)	111 ± 3.5	118–197	134 ± 3.3	127–139
CO$_2$ (mEq/L)	12 ± 2.6	7.0–16	5.4 ± 1.6	4.0–10.0
BUN (mg/dL)	11 ± 6.5	4.0–29	5.6 ± 3.2	2–14
Creatinine (mg/dL)	0.88 ± 0.32	0.4–1.5	0.44 ± 0.13	0.3–0.7
Glucose (mg/dL)	240 ± 118	71–457	127 ± 93	59–324
Cholesterol (mg/dL)	90 ± 36	3.5–142	29 ± 24	11–100
Triglycerides (mg/dL)	67 ± 54	11–198	19 ± 19	2–71
Ca^{++} (mg/dL)	5.7 ± 1.6	4.1–9.1	2.3 ± 0.5	1.2–3.1
Phosphorus (mg/dL)	1.94 ± 0.63	1.1–2.9	0.65 ± 0.22	0.3–0.9
Total protein (g/dL)	3.5 ± 0.53	2.3–4.4	0.91± 0.34	0.4–1.5
Albumin (g/dL)	1.94 ± 0.33	1.1–2.5	0.39 ± 0.11	0.2–0.6
Total bilirubin (mg/dL)	0.39 ± 0.11	0.3–0.6	0.11 ± 0.07	0.0–0.3
Alk. Pase (U/L)	55 ± 22	38–113	14 ± 4	7–21
GOT (U/L)	24 ± 22	9–93	9 ± 5	4–21
GPT (U/L)	48 ± 25	7–93	15± 9	1–30
LDH (U/L)	466 ± 160	139–690	214 ± 103	83–430
Uric acid (mg/dL)	3.8 ± 1.5	2.3–7.7	2.4 ± 2.2	0.6–6.9

Abbreviations: Alk. Pase, alkaline phosphatase; BUN, blood urea nitrogen; GOT, aspartate aminotransferase; GPT, alanine aminotransferase; LDH, lactate dehydrogenase.
From Yawn, D. H. (1991). Properties of salvaged blood. In H. F. Taswell & A. A. Pineda (Eds.), Autologous transfusion and hemotherapy (p. 200). Oxford: Blackwell Scientific. Reprinted with permission.

Suctioning from pools of blood produces less cellular damage and fragmentation than "skim suctioning" from surfaces on which blood slowly accumulates. Red cells undergo varying degrees of trauma depending on the suctioning process, but damaged or fractured red cells are a substantial part of the collected shed blood. Hemoglobin concentrations in passively collected blood range from 4.2% to 9.9%, whereas the hemoglobin of processed shed blood ranges between 14.1 g/dL and 17.19 g/dL (Yawn, 1991). Fractured red cells release red cell stroma and free hemoglobin into the plasma fraction, which carries the risk of renal or pulmonary injury with transfusion of massive volumes. Fracture of red cells also results in the release of intracellular electrolytes and hyperkalemia is a frequent development. For these reasons, the use of passively scavenged blood is generally not suitable for patients undergoing massive procedures in which substantial blood loss is to be expected. However, in procedures with limited blood loss, there is a role for the use of passively scavenged blood to reduce or eliminate the use of homologous component administration.

To correct some of the deficiencies encountered in passively scavenged blood, several systems are available for processing scavenged blood to remove debris and unwanted plasma components. Blood banks may be used when systems exist for distant processing of scavenged blood or portable systems may be used directly in the operating room for on-site processing. Operating rooms that routinely perform cases involving massive blood losses often maintain on-site portable systems for cell salvage and processing in the operating room that are operated by trained personnel dedicated to that role only. Since the risks of massive transfusion of unprocessed scavenged blood are numerous and severe, cell salvage and processing should be the responsibility of dedicated personnel rather than an added responsibility to other professionals on the nursing or anesthesia care team. Processing effectively removes any procoagulant proteins and platelets (Yawn, 1991), so that the system operates to reduce the total administration of homologous red cells only. The nature of washed and processed red cell suspensions also may vary according to the technique or equipment used, as demonstrated in Table 27–17.

Because cell damage and lysis are common in scavenged blood, the mass of salvaged processed red cells represents only a fragment of total surgical blood loss. In addition, resuspension in saline results in administration of a hypokalemic, hypocalcemic solution and may result in systemic hypokalemia or hypocalcemia when large

TABLE 27–17. Hematologic Characteristics of Blood Salvaged in Two Consecutive Series of Aneurysm Cases[a]

Variable	Before Processing		After Processing	
	Series 1	Series 2	Series 1	Series 2
Mean hemoglobin (g/dL)	6.0	7.6	14.1	17.9
Leukocytes (no./μL)	7600	6600	6600	11 000
Platelets (no./μL)	111 000	82 000	16 000	64 000
Mean corpuscular volume (μm³)	87	89	87	89
Free plasma hemoglobin (mg/dL)	2028	245	78	123

[a] Series 1, Latham bowl, $n = 20$; Series 2, Baylor bowl, $n = 11$.
From Yawn, D. H. (1991). Properties of salvaged blood. In H. F. Taswell & A. A. Pineda (Eds.), Autologous transfusion and hemotherapy (p. 195). Oxford: Blackwell Scientific. Reprinted with permission.

volumes of processed shed blood are used, requiring the selective treatment of electrolyte disorders or resuspension in a balanced salt solution. Although some clinicians are concerned with the possibility of reheparinization with processed shed blood, laboratory analysis has revealed no evidence of residual heparin in properly processed shed blood (Ulmas & O'Neill, 1981; Yawn, 1991). In addition, these systems also may use sodium citrate as an anticoagulant, which eliminates the problem of reheparinization.

Appropriate use of passive scavenging systems or processed shed blood for surgical procedures has resulted in a reduction in the total administration requirements for homologous blood products (Giordano et al., 1990, 1991; Hawlett, Popovsky, & Ilstrup, 1986). In cases involving slow, continuous loss of only minimal blood, the use of passive scavenging systems permits the return of scavenged red cells and a fraction of the coagulant factors without substantial risk from the stroma of fractured red cells. In cases with massive blood losses, the risks of end-organ damage to kidneys and lungs make the use of processing systems for shed blood the method of choice, although it returns only red cells and does mandate the use of procoagulant factors in those cases (Yawn, 1989).

Alternatives to Transfusion

Several techniques exist to reduce usage and exposure to homologous donor blood components. These include preoperative measures, such as predonation or limitation of the homologous donor pool by using directed donation and intraoperative measures such as controlled hypotension, hemodilution, and autologous intraoperative autologous donation or sequestration. The use of plasma-free hemoglobin and nonhemoglobin oxygen carriers

will be only briefly reviewed as these modalities are not currently approved for general practice. Jehovah's Witnesses, who may refuse all blood components categorically as a matter of religious principle, have served both as a stimulus to alternatives to transfusion and as a marker group that has demonstrated the physiologic limits to hemodilution and autotransfusion practices.

Since the late 1980s there has been an increasing interest in the practice of autologous or directed predonation of blood products prior to major surgery. Predonation of autologous blood offers several advantages to the patient that include elimination of the risks of immunologic transfusion reactions or exogenous viral infection from homologous blood products. When moderate blood losses are predictable and the incidence of transfusion warrants, predonation of autologous whole blood or packed red cells can reduce or eliminate the need for homologous blood components. With the development of apheresis techniques, it is now possible to separate plasma or platelet fractions in the late preoperative period for patients undergoing procedures in which the use of coagulant components is to be expected. These techniques have been used along with intraoperative autologous donation to reduce or eliminate the use of homologous blood components in complex aortic surgery. The increases in bone marrow activity already outlined may benefit patients, and the risk of autologous predonation is minimal. Even patients scheduled for cardiac surgery have undergone elective autologous predonation without evidence of increased risk for clinically significant cardiac events (Owings, Kruskall, Thurer, & Donovan, 1989).

Although it reduces the incidence of exogenous viral infections, autologous blood donation does not guarantee absolute safety. Microbial contamination may still occur, as with any donor blood, and transfusion reactions to anticoagulants or preservatives are still potential risks. However, because autologous predonated blood is seldom stored for long-term use and because collection and storage conditions must meet the same requirements as for homologous donor pool, inadvertent bacterial contamination is unlikely. Furthermore, because transfusion reactions to anticoagulants or preservatives are generally limited to urticaria and pruritis, they are not hemodynamically critical. Thus, the most likely risks of autologous blood transfusion reactions are minimal.

In addition to the potential increase in infectious markers invalidating units of designated or autologous blood, predonation of autologous blood also requires a reduplication of storage and isolation of the autologous blood components from the homologous donor pool to prevent misassignment of autologous units to other compatible patients. This creates additional expenses generated by sequestering autologous blood components for designated patients, and it requires increased available storage space. Even proponents of autologous predonation admit that increased demands and complexity make their collection and storage less practical unless strongly indicated (Goldfinger, 1989; Kruskall & Umlas, 1988). In addition, because potential autologous predonations generally are required to meet the same criteria for donation as the volunteer pool, blood bankers have expressed concerns about the liability of sequestering autologous blood components from the general pool, particularly if blood shortages become critical in emergent situations (Page, 1989). Using autologous predonated blood components also requires strict cooperation between the donor collection site and the operating team. Donor collections must be scheduled for specific component donation to prevent fractionation into packed red cells, which is the common practice. This fractionation may result in the loss of the plasma fraction, and differences in the character of donor packed red cells and whole blood are demonstrable over time, as described.

Autologous predonation may be used for patients whose blood losses are expected to be minimal to moderate; it may be combined with hematogenic therapy to support predonation in patients whose blood losses might be expected to be moderate to great; and it may be used in patients who require hematogenic therapy in order to support the physiologic demands of autologous predonation. The limiting factors in autologous predonation include the shelf life of the blood components and the tolerable limits of donation based on the patient's physical status. In healthy patients, the risks of autologous donation are few and are generally limited to mild orthostatic hypotension immediately after phlebotomy. Patients with coexisting disease, such as coronary artery disease, diabetes, or pulmonary disease may have a higher incidence of risk due to the limitations of their coexisting disease, but none of these represents a contraindication to autologous predonation in controlled circumstances.

Shelf life in stored blood components may limit the time during which autologous predonation may occur, although plasma can be frozen for an extended period and techniques do exist for freezing glycerolized red blood cells for extended storage. The use of frozen, glycerolized red cells requires additional coordination between the blood bank and the operating team because thawing and deglycerolizing red cells is a time-consuming process. Platelets cannot be frozen or stored for prolonged periods, but apheresis may permit collection of volumes of platelet-rich plasma up to 1 L shortly prior to surgery in many patients. Despite the complexities, the carefully calculated use of autologous predonation permits the collection of a moderate reserve of blood components in selected patients.

Another adjunct to autologous predonation is intraoperative autologous donation or sequestration. When autologous predonation is used in combination with intra-operative autologous donation, it may be possible to complete complex procedures without the requirement for homologous blood components, while maintaining similar outcomes. Intraoperative autologous blood donation is predicated on the fact that anesthesia and mechanical ventilation, in combination with the mild degrees of hypothermia generally noted under anesthesia, all reduce metabolic oxygen demand and permit tolerance of lower hemoglobin concentrations than are comfortably accepted by the awake, normothermic patient. This may permit phlebotomy of several units of fresh whole blood in the operating room, typically after induction of anesthesia with careful hemodynamic monitoring. These fresh autologous units may then be readministered as necessary in the course of the surgical procedure.

Two techniques may be used for intraoperative autologous donation. Normovolemic phlebotomy consists of the withdrawal of fresh whole blood while maintaining normal volume status with administration of crystalloid or colloids in the form of prepared plasma albumin or synthetic colloids. The use of synthetic plasma expanders may be discouraged because the synthetic starch colloids are known to reduce platelet effectiveness, which defeats the benefits of autologous donation of platelets. Multiple formulae have been used to determine the allowed blood volume that can be withdrawn. A simple formula is as follows:

$$\text{Volume available} = \frac{[\text{Hgb(initial)} - \text{Hgb(terminal)}]}{\text{Hgb(average)}}$$
$$\times [\text{Estimated blood volume}]$$

This technique provides a greater number of units with a progressively lower hematocrit and coagulation component as more units are drawn from progressively more hemodiluted patients.

Hypovolemic phlebotomy consists of withdrawal of a calculated permissible blood volume, while monitoring indices of hemodynamic stability and adequacy of systemic oxygen delivery. A simple formula for determining the allowed blood volume that can be withdrawn is as follows:

$$\text{Volume available} = \frac{[\text{Hgb(initial)} - \text{Hgb(terminal)}]}{\text{Hgb(initial)}}$$
$$\times [\text{Estimated blood volume}]$$

This technique provides fewer units of fresh whole blood, each unit having greater hematocrit and increased coagulation components. Because hypovolemic phlebotomy may be expected to result in significant hemodynamic changes, the practice frequently includes arterial cannulation for continuous blood pressure monitoring and use of oximetry with pulmonary artery catheters to assess mixed venous oxygen saturation. These monitoring modalities permit continuous assessment of the patient's condition and may determine the end point at which hypovolemic phlebotomy is terminated. The blood component requirements expected and the patient's individual hemodynamic status will determine which of these techniques is preferable.

Two different purposes may be met with these techniques. When blood loss is gradual and coagulation abnormalities are not expected or are induced intraoperatively, the principal uses of autologous donation are provision of red cells for adequate oxygen delivery and maintenance of an already normal coagulation cascade. Autologous predonation and intraoperative donation with normovolemic phlebotomy make available large volumes of stored and fresh whole blood that may equal or exceed the patient's initial blood volume. Blood may be retransfused as indices for transfusion are met intraoperatively, using blood gas analysis, mixed venous oxygen saturation monitoring, and serial hematocrit measurements. Determination of the sequence of readministration of predonated or intraoperatively donated units is of less consequence in that population.

In patients in whom coagulation abnormalities may be expected, autologous donation helps manage coagulation abnormalities as well as meet the requirements for circulating hemoglobin concentration and oxygen-carrying capacity. This proves useful in patients who will be anticoagulated intraoperatively. When used with autologous predonation, it is possible to use the oldest packed red cells or whole blood to meet transfusion needs for circulating hemoglobin during the early part of the procedure and to use fresh whole blood in the period when establishing hemostasis is imperative. When fresh whole blood is used, evidence suggests that fresh whole blood contains the hemostatic capacity of up to three to four individual plasma donor units and up to eight to ten individual platelet donor units (Lavee et al., 1989). Thus, peak hemostatic effect is achievable with heparin reversal.

Similar practices possibly may be beneficial in those who were on anticoagulant therapy preoperatively with coumadin. The practice of "leapfrogging" involves the administration of the oldest units to permit the phlebotomy of more units of fresh whole blood intraoperatively, which presumably would be hemostatically competent if laboratory analysis of anticoagulation indicates return to normal values. Thus, fresh whole blood donation is increased, and early transfusion may be achieved with older units that have diminished hemostatic benefit. Early administration of older units to a patient returned to hemostatic competence will not substantially reduce hemostatic capacity because coumadin is not a direct anticoagulant, as is heparin. Later administration of fresh whole blood collected after reversal of coumadin with vitamin K may permit maintenance of a more nearly normal coagulation profile. This, in combination with preoperative autologous platelet apheresis,

may in theory reduce the necessity of homologous component administration.

Work has been done to identify potential sources for oxygen-carrying capacity that would preclude the risks of red cell transfusion altogether. The use of red cells has been proven theoretically unnecessary for the transport of hemoglobin as technology has permitted effective separation of hemoglobin from cellular stroma. In some of the more successful work, stroma-free hemoglobin has been shown in experimental settings to provide adequate oxygen-carrying capacity to meet metabolic requirements in animal models (Moss, DeWoskin, Rosen, Levine, & Palani, 1976). Because limitations in total hemoglobin concentration were experienced based on increased colloid osmotic pressure, polymerization was used successfully to increase the total hemoglobin concentration without further increases in osmotic pressure (Sehgal, Gould, Rosen, Sehgal, & Moss, 1983). As a coincidental effect, polymerization also increased the plasma half-life from 6 hours to 46 hours (Sehgal, Rosen, Gould, Seghal, & Moss, 1983), which reduced the requirement for continuous infusion. Less success has been demonstrated when using perfluorochemicals, which have about 20 times the oxygen affinity of water. Initial work demonstrated the efficacy of perfluorochemicals in oxygen binding and transport, but limitations were noted in the ability to create a stable, soluble solution with a high enough percentage to meet the metabolic requirements for oxygen delivery without replacing the entire blood volume. Another drawback was the necessity to maintain continuous infusion until recovery of sufficient blood volume to maintain oxygen transport. Therefore, neither technique has proven effective in clinical settings to date.

▶ CASE STUDY

An otherwise healthy 46-year-old female presents for elective spinal fusion with rod instrumentation. The surgeon expects an operative time of at least 4 hours and typical blood losses are continuous throughout the procedure and usually reach 3 to 4 L. No history of bleeding abnormalities are demonstrated and laboratory analysis appears within normal limits, including a hemoglobin concentration of 11.7 g percent. The surgeon requests consultation to manage the patient, who has indicated that she will refuse surgery unless measures are taken to prevent the use of homologous bank blood.

1. What is the nature of the blood component therapy required?

   In this case, the blood loss requirements necessitate that circulating hemoglobin concentration and adequate circulating levels of procoagulants be maintained to permit normal hemostatic function. Because blood losses are gradual and continuous and no synthetic graft interface would be expected to increase procoagulant utilization, these requirements may be met with a combination of preoperative autologous blood donation and intraoperative phlebotomy for fresh whole blood in conjunction with mild hemodilution.

2. Which preoperative measures might optimize circulating blood volume and hemoglobin?

Preoperative treatment with erythrogenics would be indicated to increase the circulating red cell mass to facilitate the intraoperative phlebotomy of fresh autologous whole blood. In addition, withdrawal of autologous predonated whole blood will enhance the upregulation of the erythropoietic process and encourage new red cell formation.

3. What is the time interval required for preoperative optimization and preparation?

Treatment with erythrogenics and autologous whole-blood predonation can readily be accomplished within 2 weeks in the normal healthy patient.

4. Which tests will evaluate the efficacy of preoperative therapy?

Laboratory analysis should reveal an increased hemoglobin concentration and an increase in the circulating reticulocyte count as an index of increased erythrogenesis.

5. What perioperative measures are indicative to prevent homologous component administration and the tolerated intraoperative limits to trigger transfusion of autologous blood?

Perioperatively, the patient may undergo normovolemic phlebotomy to permit the acquisition of fresh whole blood for readministration during the procedure. Use of predonated autologous whole blood by "leapfrogging" will increase the yield of fresh autologous whole blood, and the total projected requirements could conceivably be met with accepted hemodilution and readministration of fresh autologous whole blood. A circulating hemoglobin of 7 to 8 g percent should be tolerated readily in the otherwise healthy individual and may be accepted as the transfusion trigger. Concentrations of 30% to 40% the normal circulating levels of procoagulants should permit a normal hemostatic mechanism. These can be accomplished by tolerating a lower circulating hemoglobin and assessing systemic oxygen delivery based on mixed venous oximetry and by laboratory analysis to determine circulating platelet counts and fibrinogen levels. By using intraoperative donated autologous whole blood in reverse

order, replacement with fresh whole blood will begin with units that have the least procoagulant levels and terminate in those with greatest hemostatic capacity at the end of the case when closure and final hemostasis are important. In addition, the use of intraoperative cell salvage and washing systems would reduce the total red cell losses and replacement requirements. Because blood losses are expected to be massive, passive scavenging would not be the preferred system. The recovery of procoagulants is poor and the readministration of subcellular fragments and red cell stroma poses potential systemic complications. Coordination of the planned erythrogenic support, predonation of autologous blood, intraoperative phlebotomy and hemodilution, planned systematic replacement of blood losses with autologous fresh blood, and intraoperative salvage and washing of shed blood should permit management of the expected blood losses without trespassing the limits of circulating hemoglobin and procoagulants required to meet systemic oxygen requirements and hemostatic competence in the otherwise normal patient.

▶ SUMMARY

The indications for using blood and component therapy are being reviewed because of multiple factors, including the public's perception of the risks of infection, more efficient utilization of a scarce natural resource, and the increased capacity of technology and medical support for alternatives to standard homologous donor component utilization. The decisions made on a daily basis to elect transfusion of blood components should be based on a firm understanding of the principles of balancing oxygen delivery and metabolic demand and the requirements for effective coagulation/hemostasis rather than a basic "cookbook" approach or application of strictly limited criteria. Guidelines on the use of blood components are useful only when employed with a basic understanding of the patient's underlying status or abnormalities induced, the character of the component required to correct any deficiency, and the most efficient means of meeting that requirement with the most efficacious use of limited resources. All judgments determining the use of blood components should incorporate the potential risks of transfusion and the demonstrable benefits to the patient for their justification. Application of the principles outlined in this chapter should permit the student to develop a justifiable and physiologically sound approach to management and decisions regarding transfusion of blood components that balances all these requirements in an individualized plan that best supports the needs of each unique patient.

► KEY CONCEPTS

- Essential concepts in blood component therapy include an appreciation of the immunologic and infectious risks of blood component therapy and an understanding of the physiologic determinants that justify using red blood cell versus whole-blood transfusion.
- The alternatives to standard homologous donor component administration include perioperative autologous donation/sequestration, proerythrogenic therapy in the preoperative period, hemodilution, the techniques of "leapfrogging," and coagulation management.
- The intraoperative autologous salvage of shed

blood, including passive collection systems and processing alternatives, must address the differences in character between shed blood, passively collected blood, and processed red cells and their respective risks and benefits versus those of directed donation.
- The indications for the use of plasma components include replacement of plasma colloid fractions, recognition of the plasma half-life and required activity of coagulation, factors for normal hemostasis, procoagulant components, including platelets and plasma, and specifically directed therapy for coagulation abnormalities, such as von Willebrand's disorder.

► STUDY QUESTIONS

1. What hemoglobin would you recommend as a "transfusion trigger," and what would be the factors determining your justification of that trigger?

2. What indices other than measurement of circulating hemoglobin might be used for a "transfusion trigger," and what are their justifications?

3. What practices can you recommend to the surgeon

and/or patient to reduce the risk of intraoperative blood component utilization?

4. What will be the determinants of the specific intraoperative blood/component management techniques you would recommend?

5. Would you recommend predonation with directed volunteer donor blood, and why or how would you justify your recommendations to the patient and surgeon?

KEY REFERENCES

Lake, C. L. & Moore, R. A. (Eds.). (1995). *Blood: Hemostasis, transfusion, and alternatives in the perioperative period.* New York: Raven Press.

Rossi, E. C., Simon, T. L., & Moss, G. S. (1991). *Principles of transfusion medicine.* Baltimore: Williams & Wilkins.

REFERENCES

Aach, R. D., & Kuhn R. A. (1980). Post-transfusion hepatitis: Current perspectives. *Annals of Internal Medicine, 92,* 539.

Agnelli,G., Berretine, M., DeCunto, M., & Nenci, G. G. (1983). Desmopressin induced improvement of abnormal coagulation in chronic liver disease. *Lancet, 1,* 645.

ASA Task Force. (1996). A report by the American Society of Anesthesiologists task force on blood component therapy. Practice guidelines for blood component therapy. *Anesthesiology, 84,* 732–747.

Bennet, R., Yawn, D. H., & Migliore, P. L. (1987). Activation of the complement system by recombinant tissue plasminogen activator. *Journal of American College of Cardiology, 10,* 627–632.

Bick, R. L. (1985). Hemostasis defects associated with cardiac surgery, prosthetic devices and other extracorporeal circuits. *Seminars in Thrombosis and Hemostasis, 11,* 249–279.

Boyd, P. R., Sheedy, K. C., & Henry, J. B. (1980). Type and screen: Use and effectiveness in elective surgery. *American Journal of Clinical Pathology, 74,* 694–699.

Burns, E. R., Billet, H. H., Frater, R. W. M., & Sisto, D. A. (1986). The preoperative bleeding time as a predictor of postoperative hemorrhage after cardiopulmonary bypass. *Journal of Thoracic & Cardiovascular Surgery, 92,* 310–312.

Carmichael, D., Hosty, K., Kastl, D., & Beckman, D. (1984). Hypokalemia and massive transfusion. *Southern Medical Journal, 77,* 315–317.

Colin, Y., Cherif-Zahar, B., Le Van, Kim C., Raynal, V., Van Huffel., V., & Carlton, J. P. (1991). Genetic basis of the RhD-positive and RhD-negative blood group polymorphism as determined by Southern analysis. *Blood, 78,* 2747–2752.

Cordell, R. R., Yalon, V. A., & Cigahn-Haskell, C. (1986). Experience with 11,916 designated donors. *Transfusion, 26,* 484–486.

Cosgrove, D. M., III, Heric, B., Lytle, B. W., Taylor, P. C., Novoa, R., Golding, L. A., Stewart, R. W., McCarthy, P. M., & Loop, F. D. (1992). Aprotinin therapy for reoperative myocardial revascularization: A placebo-controlled study. *Annals of Thoracic Surgery, 54,* 1031–1036.

Czer, L. S., & Shoemaker, W. C. (1978). Optimal hematocrit value in critically ill postoperative patients. *Surgery, Gynecology, and Obstetrics, 147,* 363.

Czer, L. S., Bateman, T. M., Gray, R. J., Raymond, M., Stewart, M. R., Lee, S. Goldfinger, D., Chaux, A., & Matloff, J. M. (1987). Treatment of severe platelet dysfunction and hemorrhage after cardiopulmonary bypass: Reduction in blood product usage with desmopressin. *Journal of American College of Cardiology, 9,* 1139–1147.

deSmet, A. A., Joen, M. C., van Oeveren, W., Roozendaal, K. J., Harder, M. P., Eijsman, L., & Wildevuur, C. R. (1990). Increased anticoagulation during cardiopulmonary bypass by aprotinin. *Journal of Thoracic & Cardiovascular Surgery, 100,* 520–527.

Dietrich, K. A., Conrad, S. A., Hebert, C. A., Levy, G. I., & Romero, M. D. (1990). Cardiovascular and metabolic response to red blood cell transfusion in critically ill volume-resuscitated nonsurgical patients. *Critical Care Medicine, 18,* 940–944.

Dietrich, W., Spannagl, M., Jochum, M., Wendt, P., Schramm, W., Barankay, A., Sebening, F., & Richter, J. A. (1990). Influence of high-dose aprotinin treatment on blood loss and coagulation patterns in patients undergoing myocardial revascularization. *Anesthesiology, 73,* 1119–1126.

Dodd, R. Y. (1992). The risk of transfusion-transmitted infection. *New England Journal of Medicine, 327,* 419–420.

Driscoll, D. F., Bistrian, B. R., Jenkins, R. L., Randall, S., Dzik, W. H., Gerson, B., & Blackburn, G. L. (1987). Development of metabolic alkalosis after massive transfusion during orthotopic liver transplantation. *Critical Care Medicine, 15,* 905–908.

Estafanous, F. G. (1986). Effects of different degrees of cardiac depression on hemodynamic responses to variable degrees of hemodilution. *Proceedings of the Cardiovascular Anesthesia Society Meeting.*

Ganong, W. F. (1987). *Review of medical physiology,* (pp. 442–443). Norwalk, CT: Appleton & Lange.

Gaydos, L. A., Freireich, E. J., & Mantel, N. (1962). The quantitative relation between platelet count and hemorrhage in patients with acute leukemia. *New England Journal of Medicine, 266,* 905–909.

Gazzard, B. G., Henderson, S. M., & Williams, R. (1975). The use of fresh frozen plasma or a concentrate of factor IX as a replacement therapy before liver biopsy. *Gut, 16,* 621–625.

Giblett, E. R. (1980). Blood groups and blood transfusion. In *Principles of internal medicine* (pp. 1573–1574). Boston: Little Brown.

Giordano, G. F., Dockery, J., Wallace, B. A., Donohoe, K. M., Rivers, S. L., Bass, L. J., Fretwell, R. L., Huestit, D. W., & Sandler, S. G. (1991). An autologous blood program coordinated by a regional blood center: A 5-year experience. Southern Arizona Regional Red Cross Blood Program, Tucson, Arizona. *Transfusion, 31,* 509–512.

Giordano, G. F., Wallace, B. A., AuBuchon, J. P., Stewart, D. K., Gonzales, A. A., & Pohlbeber, R. (1990). Intraoperative autotransfusion: A community program. *Hospital & Health Services Administration, 35*(1), 140–148.

Goldfinger, D. (1989). Controversies in transfusion medicine. Directed blood donations: pro. *Transfusion, 29,* 70–74.

Goodnough, L. T., Verbrugge, D., Marcus, R. E., & Goldberg, V. (1994). The effect of patient size and dose on recombinant human erythropoietin therapy on red blood cell volume expansion in autologous blood donors for elective orthopedic operation. *Journal of American College of Surgery, 179,* 171–176.

Griffith, J. D., & Ellamn, L. (1978). Epsilon amino caproic acid (EACA). *Seminars in Thrombosis and Hemostasis, 5,* 27–40.

Grossman, B. J., Steward, N. C., & Grindon, A. J. (1988). Increased risk of positive test for antibody to hepatitis B core antigen (anti-HBC) in autologous blood donors. *Transfusion, 28,* 283–285.

Hamstra, R. D., & Block, M. H. (1969). Erythropoiesis in response to blood loss in man *Journal of Applied Physiology, 27,* 503–507.

Harder, M. P., Eijsman, L., Roozendaal, K. J., van Oeveren, W., & Wildevuur, C. R. (1991). Aprotinin reduces intraoperative and postoperative blood loss in membrane oxygenator cardiopulmonary bypass. *Annals of Thoracic Surgery, 51,* 936–941.

Hardy, J. F., & Desroches, J. (1992). Natural and synthetic antifibrinolytics in cardiac surgery. *Canadian Journal of Anaesthesia, 39,* 353–365.

Hawlett, J. W., Popovsky, M., & Ilstrup, D. (1986, September). Minimizing blood transfusions during abdominal aortic surgery: Recent advances in rapid transfusion. *Tenth Annual Meeting of the Midwestern Vascular Surgical Society,* Indianapolis, Indiana.

Hebert, P. C., Wells, G., Marshall, J., Martin, C., Tweeddale, M., Pagliarello, G., & Blajchman, M. (1995). Transfusion requirements in critical care: A pilot study. *Journal of the American Medical Association, 273,* 1439–1444.

Hillman, R. S., & Henderson, P. A. (1969). Control of marrow production by the level of iron supply. *Journal of Clinical Investigation, 48,* 454–460.

Horrow, J. C. (1990). Desmopressin and antifibrinolytics. *International Anesthesiology Clinics, 28,* 230–236.

Horrow, J. C., Hlavacek, J., Strong, M. D., Collier, W., Brodsky, I., Goldman, S. M., & Goel, I. P. (1990). Prophylactic tranexamic acid decreases bleeding after cardiac operations. *Journal of Thoracic & Cardiovascular Surgery, 99,* 70–74.

Hull, R., Hirsh, J., Jay, R., Carter, C., England, C., Gent, M., Turpie, A. G., McLoughlin, D., Dodd, P., Thomas, M., Raskob, G., & Ockelford, P. (1982). Different intensities of oral anticoagulant therapy in the treatment of proximal vein thrombosis. *New England Journal of Medicine, 307,* 1676–1681.

Hunt, T. K. (1988). Perioperative anemia and wound healing. In *NIH Consensus Development Conference Proceedings,* (pp. 37–38). Washington, DC: U.S. Department of Health, Education, and Welfare.

Hurd, W. W., & Mioduvi, K. M. (1983). Selective management of abruptio placentae: A prospective study. *Obstetrics & Gynecology, 61,* 467.

Johns, R. A. (1990). Desmopressin is a potent vasorelaxant of aorta and pulmonary artery isolated from rabbit and rat. *Anesthesiology, 72,* 858–864.

Kamel, H. T., Flynn, J. C., & Ballas, S. K. (1989, November). Utilization of autologous and directed donations in a university hospital. *Laboratory Medicine,* 763–766.

Kim, D. M., Brecher, M. E., Estes, T. J., & Morrey, B. F. (1993). Relationship of hemoglobin level and duration of hospitalization after total hip arthroplasty: Implications for the transfusion target. *Mayo Clinic Proceedings, 68,* 37–41.

Koutts, J. (1985). Clinching the diagnosis: Assessment of hemostatic function. *Pathology, 17,* 643–647.

Kruskall, M. S., & Umlas, J. (1988). Acquired immunodeficiency syndrome and directed blood donations. A dilemma for American medicine. *Archives of Surgery, 123,* 23–25.

Kruskall, M. S., Popovsky, M. A., Pacini, D. G., Donovan, L. M., & Ransil, B. J. (1988). Autologous versus homologous donors: Evaluation of markers for infectious disease. *Transfusion, 28,* 286–288.

Lackritz, E. M., Satten, G. A., Aberle-Grasse, J., Dodd, R. Y., Raimondi, V. P., Janssen, R. S., Lewis, W. F., Notari, E. P., IV, & Petersen, L. R. (1995). Estimated risk of transmission of the human immunodeficiency virus by screened blood in the United States. *New England Journal of Medicine, 333,* 1721–1725.

Lavee, J., Martinowitz, U., Mohr, R., Goor, D. A., Golan, M., Langsam., J., Malik, Z., & Savion, N. (1989). The effect of transfusion of fresh whole blood versus platelet concentrates after cardiac operations. *Journal of Thoracic & Cardiovascular Surgery, 97,* 204.

Linden, J. V., & Kaplan, H.S. (1994). Transfusion errors: Causes and effects. *Transfusion Medical Review, 8,* 169–183.

Linden, J. V., Paul, B., & Dressler, K. P. (1992). A report of 104 transfusion errors in New York State. *Transfusion, 32,* 601–606.

Lorenta, J. A., Landin, L., DePablo, R., Renes, E., Rodriquez-Diaz, R., & Liste, D. (1993). Effects of blood transfusion on oxygen transport variables in severe sepsis. *Critical Care Medicine, 21,* 1312–1318.

Mammen, E. F., Koets, M. H., & Washington, B. C. (1984). Hemostasis changes during cardiopulmonary bypass surgery. *Seminars in Thrombosis and Hemostasis, 11,* 281–292.

Marik, P. E., & Sibbald, W. J. (1993). Effect of stored-blood transfusion on oxygen delivery in patients with sepsis. *Journal of the American Medical Association, 269,* 3024–3029.

Mead, J. H., Anthony, C. D., & Sattler, M. (1980). Hemotherapy in elective surgery. *American Journal of Clinical Pathology, 74,* 223–227.

Miller, R. D. (1973). Complications of massive blood transfusions. *Anesthesiology, 39,* 82.

Miller, R. D., & Brzica, S. M. (1986). Blood, blood components, colloids and autotransfusion. In R. D. Miller (Ed.), *Anesthesia* (2nd ed., pp. 1332–1353). New York: Churchill-Livingstone.

Miller, R. D., Robbins, T. O., Tong, M. J., & Barton, S. L. (1971). Coagulation defects associated with massive blood transfusions. *Annals of Surgery, 74,* 794–801.

Mollison, P. L. (1987). *Blood transfusion in clinical practice* (pp. 74–75, 330–350, 411–414, 454–513). Oxford: Blackwell Scientific.

Moss, G. S., DeWoskin, R., Rosen, A. L., Levine, H., & Palani, C. K. (1976). Transport of oxygen and carbon dioxide by hemoglobin-saline solution in the red cell-free primate. *Surgery, Gynecology, and Obstetrics, 142,* 357–362.

National Institutes of Health, Office of Medical Applications of Research. (1985). Fresh frozen plasma: Indications and risks. *Journal of the American Medical Association, 253,* 551–553.

National Institutes of Health, Office of Medical Applications of Research. (1987). Platelet transfusion therapy. *Journal of the American Medical Association, 257,* 1777–1780.

National Institutes of Health, Office of Medical Applications of Research. (1988). Perioperative red blood cell transfusion. *Journal of the American Medical Association, 260,* 2700–2703.

Noon, G. (1978). Intraoperative autotransfusion. *Surgery, 84,* 719–721.

Oberman, A. J., Barnes, B. A., & Friedman, B. A. (1978). The risk of abbreviating the major crossmatch in urgent or massive transfusion. *Transfusion, 18,* 137.

Owings, D. V., Kruskall, M. S., Thurer, R. L., & Donovan, L. M. (1989). Autologous blood donations prior to elective cardiac surgery. *Journal of the American Medical Association, 262,* 1963–1968.

Page, P. L. (1989). Controversies in transfusion medicine. Directed donations: Con. *Transfusion, 29,* 65–68.

Pineda, A. A., & Brzica, S. M. (1980). Hemolytic transfusion reaction. *American Journal of Clinical Pathology, 74,* 94.

Ramsey, G., Arvan, D. A., Steward, S., & Blumberg, N. (1983). Do preoperative laboratory tests predict blood transfusion needs in cardiac operations? *Journal of Thoracic & Cardiovascular Surgery, 85,* 564–569.

Reeves-Viets, J. L., Yawn, D. K., Safi, H. J., Childres, W. F., Kubicek, M. A., & Viets-Upchurch, J. M. (1992, November). Whole blood transfusion is associated with reduced component utilization during thoracic aortic surgery. [Abstract]. Annual Meeting of the American Association of Blood Banks. *Transfusion, 32*(suppl.), 28S.

Reeves-Viets, J. L., Safi, H. J., Childres, W. F., Viets-Upchurch, J. M., Kubicek, M. A., & Yawn, D. H. (1992, May). Whole blood revisited: Reduction in blood component usage during massive transfusion with whole blood usage. [Abstract]. Fourteenth Annual Meeting, Society of Cardiovascular Anesthesiologists, Boston, MA.

Rohrer, M. J., Michelotti, M. C., & Nahrwold, D. L. (1988). A prospective evaluation of the efficacy of preoperative coagulation testing. *Annals of Surgery, 208,* 554.

Rustagi, P. K., & Logue, G. L. (1990). Blood Transfusion. In J. Stein (Ed.), *Internal medicine* (pp. 999–1002). Boston: Little Brown.

Sazama, K. (1976). Reports of 355 transfusion associated deaths: 1976–1985. *Transfusion, 30,* 583–590.

Schreiber, G. B., Busch, M. P., Kleinman, S. H., & Korelitz, J. J.

(for the Retrovirus Epidemiology Donor Study). (1996). The risk of transfusion-transmitted viral infections. *New England Journal of Medicine, 334*(26), 1685–1690.

Sehgal, L. R., Gould, S. A., Rosen, A. L., Sehgal, H. L., & Moss, G. S. (1983). Polymerized pyridoxylated hemoglobin: A red cell substitute with normal O_2 capacity. *Surgery, 95,* 433–438.

Sehgal, L. R., Rosen, A. L., Gould, S. A., Sehgal, H. L., & Moss, G. S. (1983). Preparation and in vitro characteristics of polymerized pyridoxylated hemoglobin. *Transfusion, 23,* 148–152.

Spear, P. W., Sass, M., & Cincotti, J. J. (1956). Ammonia levels in transfused blood. J*ournal of Laboratory & Clinical Medicine, 418,* 702–707.

Spiess, B. D. (1990). Coagulation function in the operating room. *Anesthesiology Clinics of North America, 8,* 481–491.

Starkey, J. M., MacPherson, J. L., Bolgiano, D. C., Simon, E. R., Zuck, T. F., & Sayers, M. H. (1989). Markers for transfusion transmitted disease in different groups of blood donors. *Journal of the American Medical Association, 262,* 3452–3454.

Stoelting, R. K. (1983). Allergic reactions during anesthesia. *Anesthesia & Analgesia, 62,* 341–356.

Ulmas, J., & O'Neill, T. P. (1981). Heparin removal in an autotransfusor device. *Transfusion, 21,* 70–73.

Verstraaete, M. (1985). Clinical application of inhibitors of fibrinolysis. *Drugs, 29,* 236–261.

Viets, J. L., & Yawn, D. H. (1991). Impact of whole blood usage in massive transfusion. *Nurse Anesthesia, 2,* 184–187.

Walker, R. H. (1982). What is a clinically significant antibody? In H. F. Polesky & R. H. Walker (Eds.), *Safety and transfusion practices.* (p. 79). College of American Pathologists.

Wallace, E. L., Sturgenor, D. M., Hao, H. S., An, J., Chapman, R. H., & Churchill, W. H. (1993). Collection and transfusion of blood and blood components in the United States, 1989. *Transfusion, 33,* 139–144.

Wang, J. S., Lin, C. Y., Hung, W. T., & Karp, R. B. (1992). Monitoring of heparin-induced anticoagulation with kaolin-activated clotting time in cardiac surgical patients treated with aprotinin. *Anesthesiology, 77,* 1080–1084.

Wang, J. S., Lin, C. Y., Hung, W. T., Thisted, R. A., & Karp, R. B. (1992). In vitro effects of aprotinin on activated clotting time measured with different activators. *Journal of Thoracic & Cardiovascular Surgery, 104,* 1135–1140.

Watson, A. J., & Keough, J. A. (1983). Effect of 1-deamino-8-D-arginine vasopressin on the prolonged bleeding time in chronic renal failure. *Nephron, 32,* 49–52.

Williams, W. J., Beutler, E., Erslev, A. J., & Lichtman, M. A. (Eds.). (1983). *Hematology* (3rd ed.). New York: McGraw-Hill.

Woodman, R. C., & Harker, L. A. (1990). Bleeding complications associated with cardiopulmonary bypass. *Blood, 76,* 1680–1697.

Yawn, D. H. (1989). Autologous blood salvage during elective surgery. *Transfusion Science, 10,* 107–116.

Yawn, D. H. (1991). Characteristics of salvaged blood. In H. F. Taswell & A. A. Pineda (Eds.), *Autologous transfusion and hemotherapy* (pp. 87–122). Oxford: Blackwell Scientific.

Techniques of General Anesthesia and Conscious Sedation

Dolores A. Maxey

Conscious analgesia and general anesthetic techniques are discussed as a continuum. The interrelation between techniques and the standard guidelines from different professional societies also are discussed. It is the purpose of this chapter both to examine some of the standard techniques and to give the reader some alternative perspectives on conscious analgesia, sedation, and general anesthesia.

▶ SELECTION OF ANESTHETIC TECHNIQUES

Optimal anesthesia techniques, whether conscious sedation or general anesthesia, depend on many factors of equal consideration to the anesthetist. The primary goal of each technique is to obtain the best anesthetic outcome while minimizing any possibility of physiologic and pharmacologic problems. A comprehensive preoperative evaluation is vital to the success of the anesthetic technique.

Other indications for specific anesthetic techniques depend on some of the following: patient status, type of surgical procedure; expected duration of the procedure; location where the anesthesia is to be administered, surgeon's skills; anesthetist's skills and technique comfort; and patient's understanding of proposed anesthetic plan.

The patient's understanding of the proposed anesthetic technique may be based on experience with anesthesia, the surgeon's recommendations, the patient's expectations and knowledge, and known standards. One such example is a patient who had spinal anesthesia 10 years before and has had a backache ever since. This patient is likely to refuse spinal anesthesia now. Any past anesthetic problem probably will be remembered. Also, a patient who was aware during a prolonged surgical procedure under general anesthesia may be reticent to undergo general anesthesia again.

Knowledge of this type can help the clinician select the proper anesthetic technique. It also is important to keep in mind that the proposed technique may require modifications. When using conscious analgesia, a continuous assessment of the patient may require a decision to convert to general anesthesia at any time. The anesthetist must be prepared to make such a change. Patient safety and airway management always are the number-one priorities.

▶ MONITORED ANESTHESIA CARE

More and more surgical procedures are scheduled in an outpatient setting and Monitored Anesthesia Care (MAC) is required. Often hospitals and ambulatory care centers have no precise guidelines for practitioners regarding definitions, clinical indications, and technique for MAC with conscious sedation; however, anesthetists and surgeons should be aware of the acceptable criteria for MAC.

In every sense of the word, monitored anesthesia care means that a qualified medical professional, primarily an anesthesiologist or certified registered nurse anesthetist (CRNA), is providing careful observation of the patient. This may include the administration of specific sedatives, analgesics, and other therapies in collaboration with the surgeon or diagnostician. From the outset, the appropriate technique to meet the needs of the patient is discussed between surgeon and anesthesia provider. Both the AANA and the ASA have specific, well-defined guidelines for MAC. Both of these societies have proposed that only one person be responsible for the monitoring and administration of any sedatives, analgesics, or other therapies necessary to complete the procedure. The surgeon or diagnostician is not able to administer drug therapies and complete the proposed procedure simultaneously. For this reason, MAC has been established. On behalf of the welfare and safety of the patient, the anesthesia provider is autonomous in the administration of anesthetic agents or sedatives.

In many cases MAC is requested for minor procedures both in the operating room and in other settings. The most dangerous scenario may occur when an inexperienced anesthetist or individuals who have no anesthesia training are providing intravenous sedation as these procedures may quickly progress to deep sedation and even to general anesthesia. The leading causes of death are respiratory obstruction, hypoxemia, and cardiac instability. Untoward effects occur even in the most controlled situations and represent some of the major issues concerning provision of sedation and analgesia.

Sedation and analgesia have become much more in demand in both the pediatric and adult population as health care becomes more cost-effective and "efficient." More and more diagnostic procedures are performed outside the operating suite or in office settings. Many of these patients require sedation and/or analgesia for their comprehensive care. Frequently, anesthesia services are required where monitoring capabilities are limited. Emergent situations may arise in the diagnostic imaging area, endoscopy suite, cardiology laboratory, and even in the emergency room. Individual hospital policies regarding personnel and type of conscious analgesia vary according to the procedure and practitioner. It is very important for the anesthetist to understand the policies in their institution and to know what other professional societies use as guidelines regarding conscious sedation/analgesia.

▶ CONSCIOUS SEDATION/ANALGESIA

Sedation and analgesia occur on a continuum. Conscious sedation can quickly progress to require general anesthesia at the most unexpected time (Fig. 28-1). The definition of conscious sedation is a medically controlled state of consciousness in which protective reflexes are maintained (Guidelines of the American Association of Nurse Anesthetists [AANA, 1996] and the American Society of Anesthesiologists [ASA, 1996]). The patient retains the ability to maintain the airway and can respond appropriately to physical stimulation or verbal command such as "open your eyes" or "squeeze my hand."

Deep sedation is a medically controlled state of depressed consciousness in which the patient may or may not be able to maintain protective airway reflexes (ASA, 1995; Guidelines of the AANA, 1996; see Appendix 28-A). The patient may not be able to maintain a patent airway without support and cannot respond appropriately to verbal commands. It is this deeply sedated patient who will shift very quickly to a state of unconsciousness. Any medication, even in the appropriate dose, can cause deep sedation, hypoventilation, and hypoxemia by virtue of the individual pharmacokinetic variability of the drug. Understanding the guidelines set forth by the AANA will help determine practice parameters for CRNAs. However, these parameters may not be understood by registered nurses (RNs) performing conscious analgesia for patients in areas external to the operating suite, such as the endoscopy suite. The *Comprehensive Accreditation Manual for Hospitals* (JCAHO, 1995) states the following about anesthesia care:

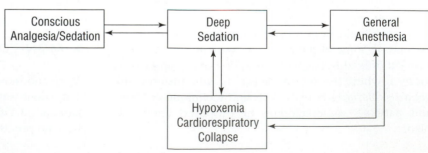

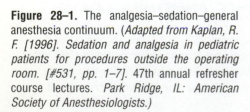

Figure 28-1. The analgesia–sedation–general anesthesia continuum. (*Adapted from Kaplan, R. F. [1996]. Sedation and analgesia in pediatric patients for procedures outside the operating room. [#531, pp. 1–7]. 47th annual refresher course lectures. Park Ridge, IL: American Society of Anesthesiologists.*)

The standards in this section apply when patients, in any surveyed setting, receive for any purpose, by any route, 1) general, spinal, or other major regional anesthesia; or 2) sedation (with or without analgesia) for which there is a reasonable expectation that, in the manner used, the sedation or analgesia will result in the loss of protective reflexes for a significant percentage of a group of patients. In addition, it is mandated that the patient has the right to know who is responsible for their care.

Many institutions do not have any formal competency programs for nonanesthesia providers administering conscious analgesia. Patients undergoing conscious analgesia must receive a comparable level of preoperative, intraoperative, and postoperative care as the patient undergoing a general anesthetic. This may be very difficult to accomplish when the individual providing the sedation is not a CRNA or anesthesiologist and the anesthetist must be called in an emergency to the cardiology laboratory for a deeper level of sedation or even a "stat" endotracheal intubation and resuscitation. All providers of this technique must remember that conscious sedation, conscious analgesia, deep sedation, and general anesthesia constitute a continuum (Fig. 28–1).

Goals of Conscious Sedation

The overall benefits of administering sedatives and analgesics are to minimize patient anxiety and discomfort while decreasing autonomic responses to painful stimuli. Sedation allows diagnostic procedures to be tolerated more comfortably for a longer time. Potent narcotics provide analgesia and are utilized when local anesthetics are administered by the surgeon.

A fine line divides the continuum of sedation between comfort and excessive or deep sedation (Table 28–1). Excessive sedation or analgesia can cause cardiac or respiratory depression and arrest and must be rapidly recognized and appropriately managed to avoid hypoxia, brain damage, cardiac collapse, and death. Patients have individual responses to both sedative agents and combinations of sedative/analgesic agents. One of the main questions is which agent to administer first. However, different studies from Smith (1996), Stoltzfus (1995), and Short and Chui (1991) clearly indicate that agents should be given individually and titrated slowly while waiting for the expected response. Once the response has been fully assessed, different agents can be introduced. An example is the use of intravenous benzodiazepines, such as midazolam, and narcotics, such as fentanyl. Used together, these very different drugs can produce deep sedation and loss of protective reflexes due to the synergistic or additive effects.

TABLE 28–1. Differences between Conscious Sedation and Deep Sedation Techniques

Conscious Sedation	Deep (Unconscious Sedation)
Mood altered	Patient unconscious
Patient cooperative/responsive to verbal stimuli or light touch	Patient unable to cooperate
Airway reflexes intact	Airway reflexes obtunded
Vital signs stable	Vital signs altered
Local anesthesia provides analgesia	Pain eliminated centrally
Commonly utilized outside OR	Utilized mainly in OR suite
Amnesia may be present	Amnesia always present
Short recovery room stay	Occasional prolonged recovery room stay or overnight admission required
Low risk of complications	Higher risk of complications
Postoperative complications uncommon	Postoperative complications reported in 25% to 75% of cases
Uncooperative or mentally handicapped patient cannot always be managed	Useful in managing difficult or mentally handicapped patients

Source: Stevens, M. H. & White, P. F. (1994). Monitored anesthesia care. In R. D. Miller (Ed.), Anesthesia (4th ed., p. 1470). Reprinted with permission.

Preoperative Assessment for Conscious Sedation/Analgesic Techniques

Whether the procedure is being performed in the operative suite, endoscopy suite, radiology suite, or cardiac catheterization laboratory, a complete preoperative assessment must be done when an anesthesia provider is involved. The practitioner must focus on cardiac and respiratory status, as well as any airway potential problems, because respiratory depression from sedatives can cause airway obstruction. As with any type of preoperative examination, the status of the airway must be fully documented for physical abnormalities as well as social habits, such as smoking. Factors which should signal the practitioner to use caution in the administration of sedation include, but are not limited to, previous problems with anesthesia or sedation (must be investigated fully); snoring, sleep apnea, dysphagia; obvious facial deformities (eg, trisomy 21); advanced rheumatoid arthritis; morbid obesity involving neck and facial areas; short neck, limited neck mobility; decreased hyoid-mental distance (less than 3 cm in adults); cervical spine disease or trauma; tracheal deviation; small mouth opening (less than 3 cm in adults); protruding incisors/micrognathia/macroglossia; nonvisible uvula. Preparation for a general endotracheal intubation must be considered for each patient regardless of technique to be utilized. Planning general anesthesia from the onset of conscious sedation can avoid a disastrous outcome in the end. Again, conscious sedation can quickly turn to respiratory arrest that necessitates quick airway intervention.

NPO Standards

Preprocedural fasting for elective conscious analgesic/sedative states is different for the adult and the pediatric patient. Factors that delay gastric emptying include intestinal obstruction, which may be the reason why the patient is having an endoscopy; pain, anxiety, trauma, pregnancy, diabetes, or other autonomic abnormalities. Sedatives and analgesic agents themselves can cause delayed gastric emptying. Preparation for elective procedures in an outpatient facility may include the use of H_2-blocking agents such as cimetidine, 300 mg, administered orally up to 1 hour prior to the procedure for adults. Pediatric patients should be offered clear liquids until 2 to 3 hours before sedation to minimize the risk of dehydration. Chapter 15 details perianesthetic considerations for the pediatric patient.

Monitoring for Conscious Sedation

Monitoring for conscious analgesia/sedation involves close observation and questioning to determine the depth of sedation. By definition conscious sedation means that protective reflexes remain intact. Deeply sedated patients may not respond to verbal commands such as "open your eyes" and are approaching the general anesthesia state. Pulmonary ventilation is used as the earliest indicator for air exchange and hypoventilation and subsequent hypoxemia may occur when depression is significant. Simple monitoring such as a precordial stethoscope placed at the left chest over the second intercostal space aids in the continuous assessment of ventilation. Continuous auscultation and visual assessment are sometimes not possible when the patient's airway is not physically accessible to the practitioner, such as during an MRI scanning of the head and neck. In this case, an apnea monitor, end-tidal CO_2 detector, or nasal thermistor may be indicated when providing supplemental oxygen. Preparation for this type of monitoring depends on knowledge of the surgeon's plan for the procedure as well as the anatomy involved.

Pulse oximeter readings are another continuous monitoring device for the patient undergoing conscious analgesia/sedation techniques. The audio "beep" correlates with the oxygen saturation as well as pulse rate. The pulse oximeter has made a tremendous impact on our ability to assess accurately response to the sedation level. During procedures in which the patient's airway is not visible to the anesthetist, hypoxemia can be assessed through the audio mode of the oximeter, which can detect early warning signs of hypoxemia. Supplemental oxygen given to the patient can, however, mask the onset of apnea because of the delay in the oximeter audio

tones. This emphasizes the need for independent ventilation monitoring of each patient.

Many health care societies, including the ASA and the AANA, continue to examine monitoring standards for conscious sedation/analgesia. Guidelines have been developed for practitioners within the anesthesia community and outside the field of anesthesia as well (Appendix 28–A). Within the operating room setting, patients who qualify for MAC anesthesia can certainly expect full monitoring techniques, including continuous ECG, pulse oximetry, ventilation assessment, temperature, interval blood pressure readings every 5 minutes, and chest auscultation. End-tidal CO_2 monitoring also is used for sedation procedures where supplemental oxygen is administered by nasal cannula or mask. However, outside the operating room suite there may be different established guidelines for monitoring the patient receiving conscious sedation. Whether the patient is in the operating suite or in the MRI scanner, full monitoring is mandatory when an anesthesia provider is involved.

It often is difficult for the practitioner performing the procedure to be fully cognizant of the patient's status during sedation. Undetected hypoxemia is the "final common pathway" through which hypoventilation, airway obstruction, and apnea lead to severe adverse outcomes, such as cerebral hypoxia, cardiac arrest, and death. All professional societies involved with the use of sedation and analgesic techniques agree that one individual must have the sole responsibility for monitoring the patient under sedation.

Drug Selection for Conscious Sedation/Analgesia

The goals for administering drugs that provide conscious sedation are sedation, anxiolysis, and amnesia, with or without analgesia. The most commonly utilized intravenous agents are the benzodiazepines, narcotics, and more recently hypnotics such as propofol. These drugs are fully discussed in Chapter 19, but specific considerations for use in conscious analgesia and anesthesia are described here.

Benzodiazepines

Until 1986 diazepam was the agent of choice because it offered the best amnestic property. Midazolam has since replaced diazepam for conscious sedation primarily because of its shorter duration of action, rapid metabolism, and water solubility. At physiologic pH, midazolam is highly lipid soluble, which allows rapid plasma-to-brain distribution. Clinical signs of sedative effects of midazolam can occur within 30 to 90 seconds. The elimination half-life of midazolam is 1 to 4 hours, which, with careful individual titration, can allow patients to be discharged from the surgical area in a more efficient manner. Certainly, one of the goals for clinical sedation is to achieve maximum effects for the limited time necessary to perform the procedure. The idea of micro dosing potent amnesia/analgesia and achieving adequate and controlled effects has brought about newer narcotics and hypnotic agents. The coadministration of narcotics with benzodiazepines can cause respiratory depression and hypoxemia. It is recommended that narcotic dosing for remifentanil be decreased by 50% when given with a benzodiazepine (Bailey, Pace, Ashburn, Moll, East, et al., 1990). Careful titration of drugs and observation of the patient's response are paramount.

Benzodiazepines reduce respiratory tidal volume. Early studies by Bailey et al. (1990) reported 86 deaths following the use of midazolam. Eighty-three of these reported cases occurred outside the operating room in clinical situations where patients were typically unattended by anesthesia personnel. It was reported that 78% of the deaths were associated with difficulties in ventilation and oxygenation. Midazolam in a dose of 0.1 mg/kg can cause as much as a 60% decrease in hypoxic ventilatory drive. The same researchers reported that midazolam also blunts the normal cardiovascular response to hypoxemia. Dosing by titration for sedation has become commonplace when utilizing midazolam. Additional sedatives can be given, however, too much can mandate ventilatory support or general anesthesia.

Midazolam

Midazolam is a water-soluble benzodiazepine that is supplied in either 1- or 5-mg/mL preparations. Because midazolam is water soluble, it has an extremely low incidence of venous irritation and therefore is well accepted by patients for both intramuscular and intravenous administration because of the lack of pain on injection. It is a rapid-acting agent, with onset of effect between 30 and 90 seconds when given intravenously and 60 to 90 minutes intramuscularly (Tanaka, 1992).

The pharmacokinetics of midazolam make it an excellent choice for outpatients because the alpha half-life is short and the elimination half-life is approximately 2 hours. It can be given intramuscularly at doses in the range 0.07 to 0.1 mg/kg, 1 hour prior to surgery, and additional doses of the drug can be titrated intravenously in the preoperative holding area to achieve a somnolent and calm, but arousable, patient. When titrating midazolam intravenously, it is recommended to start with 0.5 to 1 mg IV, followed every 2 to 5 minutes with additional doses up to 0.03 to 0.1 mg/kg until the desired level of sedation is achieved. The optimal level of sedation is reached when the patient appears calm and relaxed, yet is still cooperative. The clinical state of conscious sedation has then been achieved.

Midazolam has become increasingly popular to preoperatively medicate pediatric patients. Intramuscular injections for pediatric patients are restricted to only the most necessary cases, to reduce the traumatic and painful experience of an injection. The benefit of midazolam is its oral administration. Midazolam is diluted to a dose of 0.5 to 0.7 mg/kg (taken from the intravenous dose vial as this is the only preparation of midazolam presently available in the United States) in 3 to 10 mL of clear liquid solution such as apple or grape juice. To mask the slightly bitter taste, a sugar substitute may be added to the preparation. Because the child has been NPO (nothing by mouth) for several hours prior to arriving in the preoperative holding area, he or she generally welcomes "a little something to drink." The presence of the child's parents in the preoperative holding area and the perception of receiving a drink may lessen the patient's anxiety. Routinely, 10 to 20 minutes are required to achieve sedation by oral administration. It is recommended that an anesthesia practitioner be present who can quickly and properly manage a sedated child. The duration of action of midazolam when given orally is approximately 50 to 60 minutes. This is very useful in the radiology diagnostic suite because a cooperative sedated child may allow an intravenous line to be started.

Table 28–2 describes uses of benzodiazepines such as midazolam for sedation as well as induction of general anesthesia. The doses of midazolam for sedation and induction are on a continuum: 0.1 mg/kg is the upper limit for sedation; however, it is the mid-range dose for induction of general anesthesia. Careful titration and close observation of effectiveness are paramount when using midazolam as a sedative agent.

Narcotic Analgesics

Analgesics are administered to relieve pain prior to the induction of general anesthesia. They are most useful in patients already experiencing discomfort from a preexisting condition. Narcotics or opioids are the most frequently used analgesics, primarily because they offer superior pain relief. Narcotic premedications can be used to establish a baseline level of narcosis prior to induction, and they decrease the sympathetic response to endotracheal intubation and induction. Opioids decrease the minimum alveolar concentration of the inhalational agent when utilizing a balanced technique. Therefore, less inhalational agent is required to produce sufficient anesthesia to blunt the physiologic effect of surgical stimulation. Preoperative administration of intramuscular narcotics may provide pain relief postoperatively in relatively short surgical cases and may reduce postoperative narcotic analgesic requirements. The side effects, including drowsiness, mood alteration, and occasionally euphoria, are very helpful in conscious analgesia. Narcotics do not have hypnotic or amnestic properties and should

TABLE 28–2. Uses of Benzodiazepines

Agent	Use	Route	Dose
Diazepam	Premedication	Oral	0-2–0.5 mg/kg (max. dose 15 mg)
	Sedation	IV	0.04–0.2 mg/kg
	Induction	IV	0.3–0.6 mg/kg
Midazolam	Premedication	IM	0.07–0.15 mg/kg
	Sedation	IV	0.01–0.1 mg/kg
	Induction	IV	0.1–0.4 mg/kg
Lorazepam (not for children)	Premedication	Oral	0.05 mg/kg
		IM	0.03–0.05 mg/kg
	Sedation	IV	0.03–0.04 mg/kg

not be employed as the sole anesthetic agent. Individual titration and careful assessment of clinical effects must be noted.

All narcotics have side effects that are dose dependent. Respiratory depression due to direct central mechanisms is the most severe and life-threatening side effect as it causes hypoxemia. The newer opioids do not, with the exception of meperidine, cause direct myocardial depression and therefore can be used in anesthetic doses with remarkable cardiac stability. Histamine release is associated with morphine and meperidine. Nausea and vomiting are common side effects of narcotic administration. Narcotics also may induce spasm of the sphincter of Oddi, which may result in biliary colic; therefore they should be used with caution for patients prior to a cholecystectomy or a procedure exploring the biliary tract. Narcotics should be used judiciously (and possibly not at all) in a patient with increased intracranial pressure because hypoventilation-induced hypercarbia can enhance cerebral blood flow and elevate intracranial pressure (Tanaka, 1992).

It is important to premedicate patients who have a narcotic addiction with an appropriately long-acting narcotic, such as methadone, to prevent the sudden onset of withdrawal syndrome during the perioperative period. It is appropriate to use narcotics when indicated in these patients, realizing, however, that their tolerance to usual doses of narcotics may be overwhelmingly high. In addition, the anesthetist must ascertain from direct questioning the extent of the addiction, the type of narcotic, the last known use of that drug, and the quantity ingested or injected. If the administration of the substance was recent, the patient may require less than the usual amount of narcotic, inhalational anesthesia, or both. Individual assessment of anesthetic requirement will dictate the technique, dose requirements, and ultimately the outcome of the patient.

Conscious analgesia affords the patient pain relief while spontaneous respiration is maintained. The tidal volume remains constant while the respiratory rate is decreased. Incremental bolus doses of the drug to the respiratory rate desired are commonly employed during this technique. Caution must be taken when narcotics such as fentanyl and remifentanil are added to benzodiazepines or hypnotics. Concurrent administration will decrease doses of hypnotics as much as 75% after remifentanil administration (Glaxo Wellcome, 1996).

Narcotics of all types have been used successfully in both conscious sedation/analgesia and general anesthesia (Table 28–3). Fentanyl, alfentanil, sufentanil, and remifentanil have been effective in providing supplemental analgesia for local infiltration and regional blocks for short, closed-injury, realignment procedures. Each drug has specific uses and precautions in the operating room. Outside the operating room, meperidine and morphine frequently are utilized for endoscopy procedures. The practitioner's choice of narcotic plays a role in analgesia/sedation techniques.

Morphine and meperidine are the most commonly used preoperative narcotic agents, but hydromorphone also may be used for intramuscular premedication. Fentanyl and its sister agents, alfentanil, sufentanil, and remifentantil are not recommended for intramuscular injection as the pharmacokinetics of these agents preclude its effectiveness when given by this route. The magnitude of the clinical effects of these specific agents depends on the rapidity with which they cross the

TABLE 28–3. Uses and Doses of Common Opioids

Agent	Use	Route	Dose*
Morphine	Premedication	IM	0.05–0.2 mg/kg
	Intraoperatiave anesthesia	IV	0.1–1 mg/kg
	Postoperative analgesia	IM	0.05–0.2 mg/kg
	Premedication	IV	0.03–0.15 mg/kg
Meperidine	Intraoperative anesthesia	IM	0.5–1 mg/kg
		IV	2.5–5 mg/kg
	Postoperatiave analgesia	IM	0.5–1 mg/kg
	Intraoperative anesthesia	IV	0.2–0.5 mg/kg
Fentanyl	Postoperative analgesia	IV	2–150 µg/kg
	Intraoperative anesthesia	IV	0.5–1.5 µg/kg
Sufentanil	Intraoperative anesthesia	IV	0.25–30 µg/kg
Alfentanil	Loading dose	IV	8–100 µg/kg
	Maintenance infusion	IV	0.5–3 µg/kg/min
Remifentanil	Load	IV	0.5–1 µg/kg
	Infusion	IV	0.25–2 µg/kg/min

Note: The wide range of opioid doses reflects a large therapeutic index and depends on which other anesthetics are simultaneously administered. The relative potencies of fentanyl, sufentanil, and alfentanil are estimated to be 1 : 9 : 1/7.

Source: Mikhail, M. S., & Morgan, G. E. (1996). Clinical anesthesiology (2nd ed.). Norwalk, CT: Appleton & Lange. Reprinted with permission.

blood–brain barrier; therefore, they usually are given by intravenous bolus or infusion.

Morphine. Morphine is widely used in all patient populations. It is normally given in a dose of 0.1 mg/kg intramuscularly approximately 1 hour prior to surgery as a preoperative agent. In the immediate preoperative period, it can be titrated intravenously in 1- to 2-mg increments for a total dose of 0.1 to 0.25 mg/kg or until the desired effect is achieved. Intravenously, the onset of action of morphine is about 3 to 5 minutes, and the peak effect occurs at about 10 minutes. The duration of action of morphine is 4 to 5 hours, eliminating its wide use in the outpatient facility. Understanding how to match the proper drug with the proper environment is important when selecting the correct technique. Because of its ability to release histamine and its sympatholytic properties, morphine may act as a peripheral vasodilator. Care should be exercised when administering morphine to patients who are hypovolemic or exhibit a condition where the risk of hypotension is critical.

Meperidine. Meperidine is largely used as an intramuscular premedication agent at doses of 1 mg/kg. The onset of action of meperidine is faster than that of morphine, and the duration of effect is approximately 2 to 3 hours when used in analgesic doses. It is effective for pain relief and has a narrow therapeutic index. In the doses recommended for premedication and pain relief, the risk of tachycardia is relatively low. Normeperidine abiotransformation product is pharmacologically active.

Fentanyl and Its Analogs. Fentanyl is one of the most commonly used short-acting narcotics. It is commonly administered intravenously in the preoperative/preinduction period. Dosages of fentanyl depend on the desired sympatholytic effect, age, and overall physiological condition of the patient. Generally, doses of 1 to 2 μg/kg prior to anesthesia induction contribute to the blunting of the sympathetic response to intubation. Doses up to 5 to 7 μg/kg will not only blunt the response to intubation but will also decrease the dosage of other induction agents (eg, thiopental). The onset of action of fentanyl is 1 to 2 minutes, and it has a duration of action of 10 to 30 minutes. The elimination half-life is 2 to 4 hours. Because of its rapid onset of action, it is imperative that the anesthetist have resuscitation equipment and drugs readily available. The fentanyl analog alfentanil often is used for conscious sedation because of its rapid onset of action, but sufentanil is reserved for general anesthesia because of its longer action.

Remifentanil. Remifentanil hydrochloride is the newest narcotic agent employed for conscious analgesia. It is a mu-opioid agonist with rapid onset and distribution. The terminal elimination of 10 to 20 minutes makes it very useful for outpatient procedures in which the patient must be "street ready" within a few hours. Remifentanil is metabolized by nonspecific blood and tissue esterases, which allow its use in patients with renal and hepatic dysfunction.

Hypnotics

Perhaps the hypnotic agent most frequently administered for the greatest variety of techniques is propofol. It is a popular induction drug for general anesthesia for both inpatient and outpatient procedures. Propofol often is given by continuous infusion in combination with midazolam in the ICU setting. Propofol's use has spread outside the operating suite and ICU to areas where diagnostic procedures are conducted using conscious analgesia. Propofol's high clearance and rapid recovery when discontinuing the infusion allow for frequent assessment of neurological status. Propofol compares favorably to the inhalation agent sevoflurane for ambulatory surgery. Propofol's short onset and duration make it a valuable agent in this environment. Table 28–4 provides the doses for propofol and other intravenous agents for a variety of situations.

Total Intravenous Anesthesia or Analgesia for Conscious Sedation

Continuous infusion of narcotic agents and hypnotic agents is another method of providing intravenous sedation/analgesia. Another name for this technique is TIVA, or Total Intravenous Anesthesia or Analgesia. Some of the advantages of continuous infusion drugs include their water solubility, rapid onset of action, short duration of clinical effects, high clearance rate, minimal accumulation, absence of active metabolites, high therapeutic index, minimal side effects, and cost-effectiveness.

Comparison studies for different combinations of benzodiazepines, narcotics, and hypnotics search for the

TABLE 28–4. Uses and Doses of Ketamine, Etomidate, Propofol, and Droperidol

Agent	Use	Route	Dose
Ketamine	Induction	IV	3–5 mg/kg
		IM	3-5 mg/kg
Etomidate	Induction	IV	0.2–0.5 mg/kg
Propofol	Induction	IV	1.2–2.5 mg/kg
	Maintenance infusion	IV	50–200 μg/kg/min
	Sedation infusion	IV	25–100 μg/kg/min
Droperidol	Premedication	IM	0.04–0.07 mg/kg
	Sedation	IV	0.02–0.07 mg/kg
	Antiemetic	IV	0.05 mg/kg[a]

[a] Maximum adult dose without prolonging emergence is 1.25–2.5 mg.

ideal superior anesthetic technique. The controversy continues between balanced technique using inhalational agents and TIVA. Hemodynamic responses, emergence time, analgesic effects, and postoperative sequelae such as nausea and vomiting are some common indicators evaluated for a specific agent or technique. The site of the procedure also determines the use and dose of all agents.

Table 28-5 illustrates the clinical application of TIVA in conscious sedation for the adult. The combination of benzodiazepines, narcotics, and hypnotics such as propofol are commonly used in this technique. Other hypnotic agents, such as methohexital and ketamine, are used for TIVA. Achieving sedation and analgesia while maintaining adequate ventilation and cardiac stability is truly the "art of anesthesia."

▶ GENERAL ANESTHESIA TECHNIQUE

Each method of delivering general anesthesia whether by inhalation induction or intravenous induction relies

---

TABLE 28–5. Total Intravenous Anesthetic (TIVA) Technique (Conscious Sedation)

I. Premedication
  A. Anxiolytics/amnestics: midazolam 0.5–2.0 mg IV
  B. Antiemetics, optional (depends on patient's history of nausea/vomiting)
    1. Droperidol 0.625–1.25 mg IV (administer prior to narcotic) or
    2. Ondansetron 4 mg IV, either prior to induction of anesthesia or effective in treating nausea/vomiting in PACU or
    3. Metoclopramide 10 mg IV
II. Maintenance
  A. Hypnotics
    1. Propofol
      a. Infusion 50–75 μg/kg/min (may administer small bolus prior to infusion)
      b. Once desired level of sedation is achieved, adjust rate to maintain
  B. Analgesics
    1. Alfentanil
      a. Bolus: 5 μg/kg x 1 (do not exceed 5-μg/kg bolus in a spontaneously breathing patient, to prevent chest wall rigidity)
      b. Infusion: start at 1 μg/kg/min
      c. Range 0.25–2.0 μg/kg/min or
    2. Fentanyl
      a. Bolus: initially 1 to 2 μg/kg in divided doses (50 μg per bolus)
      b. Maintenance: 25 to 50 μg bolus prn or
    3. Remifentanil
      a. Bolus 0.1 μg/kg/min
      b. Infusion 0.25 μg/kg/min

Note: Titrate against respiratory rate. Monitor respirations with end-tidal CO_2 via nasal cannula while administering O_2.

---

on preoperative preparation both psychologically and, when appropriate, pharmacologically. Stress in itself produces the catecholamine outflow that causes multiple cardiovascular and endocrine responses undesirable for a general anesthetic induction.

Preoperative sedation with midazolam provides a more predictable anesthetic induction. In addition, narcotics such as fentanyl act by decreasing the central sympathetic outflow and increasing the parasympathetic outflow at the level of the medullary neurons (Tanaka, 1992). A patient who is adequately premedicated will have a much smoother induction to general anesthesia than one who is in pain, anxious, and nervous. If the patient is a healthy ASA Class 1 or 2 patient with sweaty palms and is tearful while in the preoperative holding area, it is appropriate to give an anxiolytic such as midazolam. If the same patient is having tremendous pain, narcotics should be given if not contraindicated. The importance of preparation and individualization of anesthesia technique cannot be stressed too much, and the CRNA must be responsive to changing techniques to meet the patient's needs.

Psychologic preparation goes hand in hand with pharmacologic preparation. Both cultural differences and personal beliefs must be addressed prior to general anesthesia. This is a much more difficult task, especially for practitioners of different cultures. Often there is a language barrier. It has been demonstrated that a simple and gentle touch or hand holding during a MAC anesthetic significantly lowers sympathetic responses to surgical stimulation. This may be very evident to the anesthetist during an intraocular procedure in which the face is covered by surgical drapes and the patient has had minimal sedation for the peribulbar block. Therapeutic touch adds to the sedative stress relief while allowing communication, comfort, and anxiety relief.

Levels of General Anesthesia

Willenkin and Polk (1994) described the levels of general anesthesia with the corresponding hemodynamic and physiologic responses as illustrated in Table 28-6. New intravenous agents given at induction doses allow passage from Level 1 to Level 3 to occur quickly. This avoids the excitement stage of anesthesia. However, in examining the levels of induced depression, two areas resemble deep sedation by our previous definition. Level 1 appears to be similar to deep intravenous sedation, where the patient responds to painful stimuli. Level 3, or the level of minimal anesthesia, resembles deep sedation when an intravenous muscle relaxant is not employed.

TABLE 28–6. Levels of Anesthesia-Induced Depression

Level	Manifestation
Level 1: Loss of consciousness (resembles deep sedation)	Passage from a fully awake state to unresponsiveness to verbal commands No loss of responsiveness to painful stimuli
Level 2: Depression-excitation	Irregular ventilation, breathholding, larygospasm, airway secretions Arrhythmias Hyperesthesia
Level 3: Minimal anesthesia (resembles deep sedation)	Regular respiratory rate and rhythm, respiratory response to stimulation Normal sinus rhythm, usually with mild hypotension Cardiovascular response to stimulation
Level 4: Light anesthesia	Respiratory depression, but response to maximal stimulation Hypotension with no stimulation Minimal cardiovascular response to major stimulation
Level 5: Deep anesthesia	Respiratory depression progressing to apnea Hypotension even with stimulation Arrhythmias No response to stimulation

Source: Willenkin, R. L. & Polk, S. L. (1994). Management of general anesthesia. In R. D. Miller (Ed.), Anesthesia (4th ed., p. 1049). Reprinted with permission.

Techniques of Induction and Maintenance of General Anesthesia

General anesthesia has four properties: (1) amnesia; (2) analgesia; (3) hypnosis; and (4) muscle relaxation. During conscious sedation or even deep sedation, these four properties are not completely achieved. General anesthesia generally is used to provide optimal conditions for laryngeal tracheal intubation where indicated, an adequate surgical depth of anesthesia, maintenance of hemodynamic stability throughout, hypnosis, elimination of the patient's recall of events, and muscle relaxation where indicated. This state is achieved with a variety of agents, intravenous or inhalational.

Induction of General Anesthesia

Very rarely is there only one best way to administer anesthesia, whether by intravenous or inhalation technique. The four phases for general anesthesia technique are (1) induction of anesthesia; (2) maintenance of anesthesia; (3) emergence from anesthesia; and (4) transfer of the patient from the operating room.

The primary goal of the general anesthesia induction phase is to produce unconsciousness and to move quickly to Level 3 of anesthesia while maintaining cardiovascular stability. Regardless of which technique is used, cardiovascular stability must be maintained. A secondary goal for general anesthesia is to provide an adequate airway to maintain ventilation for respiratory stability. This includes prevention of regurgitation of gastric contents, laryngospasm, excessive secretions, and any airway trauma. Step-by-step planning that begins with the preoperative assessment and consistent application of general anesthesia principles will ensure a positive outcome.

Intravenous Induction of General Anesthesia. Intravenous induction of general anesthesia is the most commonly employed general anesthesia technique. It is used in both the adult and pediatric population. It generally is accomplished by administering a rapid-acting barbiturate, such as thiopental, or other intravenous anesthetics, such as propofol. This technique may include laryngoscopy and the insertion of an endotracheal tube, or it can be used to induce anesthesia maintained with a conventional or laryngeal mask. Initially the patient is placed supine with the head in the "sniffing" or head up position to facilitate airway management and prepare for laryngoscopy if indicated. Appropriate monitoring parameters are applied to provide baseline cardiovascular and respiratory information. This includes placement of a precordial stethoscope at the sternal notch or left second intercostal space for auscultating ventilation.

Whenever it is not contraindicated, preoxygenation to denitrogenate the lungs is accomplished by placing a secure clear facemask on the patient's face and administering a 6 to 10 L/min flow of 100% oxygen for 2 to 5 minutes. Another method of preoxygenation is to ask the patient to take four slow "vital capacity" breaths. Patency of the intravenous line must be ensured before intravenous medications are administered. Willenkin and Polk (1994) suggest administering a 50-mg bolus of thiopental when this drug is used for induction of anesthesia to assess consciousness, hemodynamic response, and evaluation of allergic potential. Intravenous induction of anesthesia to produce unconsciousness can be accomplished with thiopental 2 to 5 mg/kg, propofol 1 to 2 mg/kg, or methohexital 1 to 2 mg/kg (Table 28–7). Doses may need to be adjusted depending on the degree of sedation from the premedicant. Once unconsciousness has been established from loss of lid reflex, establish a patent airway and begin ventilation. This may include inserting an oral pharyngeal airway or a laryngeal mask airway (LMA).

The anesthetist should then introduce an inhalational anesthetic agent when using a balanced technique of intravenous agent and volatile agents. Nitrous oxide is used

TABLE 28–7. Total Intravenous Anesthetic (TIVA) Technique (General Anesthesia for Outpatient Procedures)

I. Premedication
   A. Anxiolytics/amnestics
      1. Midazolam 0.5–3 mg IV,
   B. Antiemetics optional (depends on patient history of nausea/vomiting)
      1. Droperidol (Inapsine) 0.625–1.25 mg IV (administer prior to narcotic) or
      2. Ondansetron 4 mg IV, either prior to induction of anesthesia or effective in treating nausea/vomiting in PACU or
      3. Metoclopramide 10 mg IV
II. Induction
   A. Analgesics
      1. Alfentanil bolus
         a. 5 μg/kg ($\times$ 1 to 3 prior to propofol, number of boluses depends on patient's response)
         b. 20–25 μg/kg after administration of propofol and muscle relaxant and just prior to intubation or
      2. Fentanyl bolus: 2 to 3 μg/kg (at least 3–5 min prior to intubation)
   B. Hypnotics
      1. Propofol bolus: 1.5 to 2.5 mg/kg (decrease dose and rate of administration in patients with limited cardiac reserve)
   C. Muscle relaxants
      1. Nondepolarizing for intubation and maintenance whenever appropriate
         a. Atracurium intubation: 0.4–0.5 mg/kg or
         b. Mivacurium intubation: 0.25 mg/kg in divided doses (0.15 mg/kg followed by 0.1 mg/kg 30 s later)
         c. Rocuronium intubation: 0.6–0.8 mg/kg
         d. Vecuronium intubation: 0.8–1 mg/kg
III. Maintenance
   A. Analgesics
      1. Alfentanil infusion: start at 1 μg/kg/min; adjust PRN; stop infusion 5 min before end of procedure or
      2. Fentanyl
         a. Infusion: start at 1–2 μg/kg/hr; adjust PRN or
         b. Bolus: 0.5–1 μg/kg every 30 min; stop infusion or last bolus 30 min before end of procedure
         Total dose not to exceed 5 μg/kg
      3. Sufentanil
         a. Infusion: 0.1–0.2 μg/kg/hr; adjust PRN or
         b. Bolus: 0.05–0.1 μg/kg every 30 min; stop infusion or last bolus 15 min before end of procedure
         Total dose not to exceed 40 μg
      4. Remifentanil 0.25–0.1 μg/kg/min; stop infusion 5 min before end of procedure; be prepared for additional analgesics in postanesthesia recovery
   B. Hypnotic
      1. Propofol infusion:
         a. With O_2 and air: start at 150–200 μg/kg/min; range 100–200 μg/kg/min or
         b. With O_2 and N_2O: start at 100–150 μg/kg/min; titrate to clinical response, hemodynamic response
   C. Nondepolarizing muscle relaxants
      1. Start infusion after return of a single twitch on the train-of-four
      2. Adjust rate to maintain at least one twitch at all times
         a. Atracurium infusion: start at 10 μg/kg/min or
         b. Mivacurium infusion: start at 10 μg/kg/min or
         c. Rocuronium infusion: start at 10 μg/kg/min or
         d. Vecuronium infusion: start at 1 μg/kg/min

as a "carrier" agent for volatile agents, employing the second-gas effect for rapid uptake into the alveolus. Increase the volatile agent concentration by ½ minimum alveolar concentration (MAC) every three to four breaths to deepen anesthesia level and prevent severe sympathetic response to stimulation of surgical incision or laryngoscopy. Significant cardiovascular changes may occur while the anesthesia level deepens. Therefore, measuring blood pressure every 1 to 2 minutes may be necessary.

Evaluating baseline neuromuscular function with the "train-of-four" response measured by a peripheral nerve stimulator is indicated prior to the administration of any neuromuscular blocking agent. This measurement should be taken only after induction of general anesthesia and after sufficient depth of anesthesia has been established. An adequate dose of a neuromuscular blocking agent such as succinlycholine or rocuronium is indicated to facilitate endotracheal intubation. Loss of train-of-four response and other physical signs, such as jaw relaxation, indicate readiness for intubation. Intravenous narcotics or lidocaine 1 mg/kg may be given to attenuate sympathetic stimulation while performing laryngoscopy and endotracheal intubation. Endotracheal intubation generally is indicated for intracavitary surgical procedures, including abdominal, thoracic, and cranial cavities. Other indicators include position changes away from supine or when the airway is not directly visualized by the CRNA.

Once endotracheal intubation is accomplished, proper placement of the endotracheal tube is verified by observing peak inspiratory pressure, $ETCO_2$, and auscultation of bilateral breath sounds in the upper and lower lung fields after inflating the endotracheal cuff. Auscultation over the stomach will show whether the esophagus has been intubated. Once the endotracheal tube is secured with adhesive tape or another device, the concentration of the inhalation anesthetic agents is modified. Using an esophageal stethoscope with a thermistor continually to auscultate heart and breath sounds and to provide core temperature monitoring is recommended. During any period of minimal stimulation, cardiovascular depression can occur and may require the use of a vasopressor. Decreasing the inhaled concentration of volatile agents should be considered before administering any vasoactive drug. Continuous monitoring of hemodynamic status while administering maintenance anesthetic levels is necessary to provide safe and adequate anesthesia for the surgical procedure.

Technique of Balanced Anesthesia

The term *balanced anesthesia* describes the combination of intravenous or inhalation anesthetic agents that produces the four components necessary for general anesthesia. The term was first described by Lundy in 1926 and is still used as a technique for providing anesthesia. The variety of drugs produces amnesia, analgesia, hypnosis, and muscle relaxation while maintaining physiologic homeostasis throughout the surgical procedure. To date, no single agent provides all of these properties for general anesthesia. Knowledge of agents used singly, as well as in combination, will help in the selection of appropriate techniques for the best outcome.

Hypnosis can be achieved by a variety of agents including thiopental, propofol, and midazolam. Short and Chui (1991) studied more than 200 patients using midazolam and propofol in combination for inducing hypnosis of anesthesia. In this study, midazolam reduced the median effective dose of propofol by 52% and produced significantly better hypnosis than when each agent was used singly. In the same study, the best hypnosis was achieved with the combination of midazolam and alfentanil (46%) versus propofol/alfentanil (20%). Balanced anesthesia also

can be achieved by TIVA. As described with conscious sedation, the combination of agents administered on a continuous intravenous infusion basis can provide the same properties of amnesia, analgesia, hypnosis, and muscle relaxation while maintaining physiologic homeostasis. A combination of drugs such as propofol, midazolam, ketamine, and vecuronium offers the properties for general anesthesia. In a study by Dunnihoo, Wuest, Meyer, & Robinson (1994) the combination of propofol, ketamine, and vecuronium was used to maintain hemodynamic stability as well as provide rapid wakeup.

Currently, midazolam is the drug of choice for providing both retrograde and antegrade amnesia. Unlike diazepam, midazolam has been used in a variety of settings for conscious sedation as well as in the intensive care unit for long-term ventilation. Its dose can be easily titrated for amnesic effects in 0.5- to 1-mg boluses. Premedication enables the anesthetist to see individual pharmacodynamic results from therapy before the surgical procedure. Opioids may be administered by bolus or continuous infusion. The advantages of continuous opioid infusion include hemodynamic stability, decreased drug side effects, suppression of cortisol and vasopressin response to cardiopulmonary bypass, reduced total dose of opioids, a shorter recovery period, and a reduced need for opioid antagonists. Balancing analgesia and amnesia is truly the "art of anesthesia" in many aspects of current anesthesia practice.

Total Intravenous Anesthesia for General Anesthesia

Total intravenous anesthesia has four phases: (1) patient preparation or premedication; (2) induction; (3) maintenance; and (4) emergence. Premedication generally includes benzodiazepine administration to decrease the risk of awareness and smooth the induction process. In addition, patients undergoing TIVA should have an intravenous fluid preload of approximately 400 to 600 mL. Fluid administration can be adjusted to meet individual needs, but it will help maintain hemodynamic stability during the anesthetic process. Prior to commencing with TIVA, infusion lines should be purged using the purge mode of the pump to assess proper operation of the pump and the syringe. An antiemetic should be considered in patients with a history of postoperative nausea and vomiting. Monitors appropriate to patient management should be applied prior to induction.

Induction begins with administration of a small dose of narcotic (¼ the anticipated dose). Lidocaine 20 to 40 mg may be administered IV prior to the administration of propofol (especially if the IV is placed in a hand vein) to decrease any pain felt during injection. The patient should be apprised of the possibility of pain resulting from propofol injection prior to administration of the drug. The propofol induction dose is given in 2- to 3-mL increments to reduce the incidence of hypotension, especially in elderly patients. The infusion rates should be reduced by 25% to 50% for elderly patients or those who have been heavily premedicated prior to induction. Hypotension during induction can be minimized by administering narcotics and hypnotics slowly (30 to 90 seconds). Propofol infusion should be initiated as soon as possible after induction to maintain hypnosis or an additional 20- to 30-mg bolus should be administered prior to intubation, particularly when using a nondepolarizing muscle relaxant to facilitate intubation.

To maintain anesthesia the infusion is continued in accordance with individual patient needs. During the infusion recheck for adequate flow of carrier fluid: TIVA can become NIVA (no intravenous anesthesia) and the patient may awaken rapidly in the middle of the surgical procedure should the carrier fluid not flow properly. If the patient's blood pressure alone increases, administer a 20- to 40-mg bolus of propofol. Repeat the bolus and increase the infusion by 25 μg/kg/min if hypertension continues. Propofol administration as previously described and a small dose of narcotic can be given to treat an increase in blood pressure and pulse rate. The maximum potential of the drugs used in TIVA is achieved by titrating to effect. The dose should be adjusted for each drug as indicated. There is not one dose suited to all patients. The goal of this technique is to administer the smallest dose possible to achieve the desired effect.

The propofol infusion is discontinued 2 minutes before the end of the surgery if administering 100% oxygen or approximately 5 to 10 minutes before if using nitrous oxide. Nitrous oxide administration should be discontinued after reversal of muscle relaxant. Be prepared to give a 10- to 30-mg propofol bolus as needed once the infusion has been discontinued. Discontinue all narcotics, except remifentanil 15 to 30 minutes prior to the end of surgery. Nonsteroidal antiinflammatory agents such as ketorolac should be considered to treat postoperative pain prior to emergence. If possible, have the surgeon infiltrate local anesthetic into the surgical site to reduce postoperative pain. Table 28–7 describes TIVA used for general anesthesia in an adult undergoing an outpatient surgical procedure.

The use of continuous infusion devices for drug delivery in conscious sedation/analgesia and general anesthetic techniques may offer some advantages over the intermittent bolus technique. Cardiorespiratory stability and speed of recovery are two very significant considerations when employing the technique of continuous infusion. Current issues regarding the use of TIVA and sedation techniques in a target-controlled method are being tested and reviewed for clinical use. Concerns about the use of TIVA in conscious analgesia and general anesthesia involve some of the following:

(1) time involved in setting up multiple infusion devices for IV anesthetic drugs; (2) lack of convenient delivery systems; (3) unfamiliarity with pharmacokinetic concepts and widespread interpatient kinetic variability; (4) difficulty in monitoring depth of anesthesia during anesthesia; and (5) cost-effectiveness in setup and delivery.

Rapid-Sequence Induction

The rapid-sequence induction (RSI) technique is indicated for the patient with a full stomach. Full stomach has been defined as any solids within 6 hours and liquids within 4 hours of surgery. Patients with a history of hiatal hernia or esophageal reflux and parturients, as well as diabetics with a gastroparesis, are all considered candidates for rapid-sequence induction. Obvious abdominal trauma or mechanical restrictions for an empty stomach can be treated as a full stomach. One example is the patient with a small-bowel obstruction where passage is blocked and backflow occurs. The goal for rapid-sequence induction is to avoid further gastric distention during induction to prevent vomiting and aspiration of stomach contents. The technique for rapid-sequence induction is described in detail in Chapter 25. Although there are modifications, the basic principles of airway protection and prevention of aspiration remain paramount. Utmost care and preparation must be taken to ensure successful anesthesia for patients at high risk for pulmonary aspiration.

Inhalation by Mask

Face Mask

Newer inhalation agents such as the sweet-smelling sevoflurane have given the clinician alternatives for inhalation induction in the hospital and outpatient settings. Inhalation anesthesia can be induced using a traditional face mask. The low pungency of both N_2O and sevoflurane allows frightened children and adults to easily breathe in the agent and be maintained with a face mask, which assists ventilation. In addition, the clear face mask may be used to maintain anesthesia following an intravenous induction. It also is indicated in other patients in whom intravenous induction is not possible. The face mask selected should be disposable and clear, be properly sized for the patient, and have a secure seal around both nose and mouth. A clear face mask will alert the anesthetist to early signs of regurgitation of stomach contents. Maintenance of anesthesia via face mask may be ideal for short cases or those for which endotracheal intubation is not indicated. During maintenance of mask anesthesia, the anesthetist must be very aware of airway changes and quickly assess the need for possible endotracheal intubation. Understanding the respiratory rhythm and pattern of the patient under mask anesthesia is very valuable in determining the depth of anesthesia.

Critical to this technique is placement of the precordial stethescope for auscultation of ventilation. Assisting ventilation during mask anesthesia allows for rapid deepening of the anesthetic level as well as rapid emergence. Mask ventilation may be the only method to control a patient's airway, and the CRNA's skill with mask ventilation may be a lifesaving technique.

Laryngeal Mask Airway

The purpose of the LMA is to maintain the anesthetized patient's airway more efficiently and successfully than by conventional face mask ventilation. It has since become very useful in many situations for general anesthesia with a semi-closed or Bain circuit as well as for the patient with the potential for a difficult endotracheal intubation. It has not replaced endotracheal intubation, but it has become an integral part of the anesthetist's armamentarium. The procedure for inserting the LMA is described in Chapter 25.

The indications for LMA for delivering anesthesia or maintaining the airway have expanded. Benumof (1996) suggests that the LMA be utilized when ventilation and/or endotracheal intubation are difficult. Indeed this may be a lifesaving measure when the airway is unobtainable and may eliminate the need for an invasive cricothyrotomy. Baskett (1994) reports a 100% success rate for RNs who have been trained to insert an LMA. While this is an emergency use of the LMA, more practical indications in administering anesthesia include: surgical procedures where there is no need for mechanical ventilation (ie, extremity procedures); patients with a very irritable airway history where coughing could trigger a disaster; combined regional/general anesthetic technique; and professional singers. There are many indications for the LMA in anesthetic practice, especially in the ambulatory setting. Using the LMA reduces the risk of a postoperative sore throat, which often occurs following endotracheal intubation. Noncavitary procedures, such as hand or ankle procedures in which the patient may refuse a regional anesthetic block may be successfully done with the LMA.

Patients with a full stomach or suspected full stomach by definition are not candidates for the LMA. Severely traumatized victims by virtue of their injuries should not have their airways managed with LMAs. Patients with a history of hiatal hernia are also excluded from the use of the LMA. Any obvious pathology to the airway, such as subglottic stenosis or other periglottic conditions preclude successful use of an LMA. Indeed, airway preparation, as well as cautious evaluation, is paramount in any patient with a questionable airway. Any procedure in which the airway may not be in full view may be a relative contraindication for the use of the LMA. Such situations occur with certain surgical positioning. Patients placed in the prone position for pro-

cedures such as a laminectomy are not best managed with the LMA. The key concept is to choose an airway technique that will best manage the airway while not producing any undue risk of hypoxemia, aspiration, or airway compromise to the patient. Knowledge of the procedure, anatomy, patient history with complete assessment as well as the skill of the surgeon become vital factors when determining which airway technique to employ for the successful administration of general anesthesia.

Inhalation Induction

Volatile anesthetic agents can be used for the inhalation induction of general anesthesia in a number of clinical situations, such as for small children under 5 years of age who refuse an intravenous line. Short procedures such as myringotomy tube placement in a 3-year-old can be successfully done by inhalation induction as well as mask ventilation. Severely debilitated or uncooperative adult patients may be more easily managed with a mask induction. Patients who have difficulties with a complete airway assessment (ie, cannot open their mouth widely or have temporomandibular joint problems) may be evaluated fully after an inhalation induction. Historically, halothane was the volatile agent of choice for inhalation induction. One main reason for its use was the sweet smell and low irritability it produces in the upper respiratory tract.

Newer volatile agents such as desflurane and sevoflurane have made the inhalation induction technique easier on both patient and practitioner. Sevoflurane has a lower blood-to-gas partition coefficient than halothane, indicating rapid uptake and elimination. Inhaling sevoflurane at 1 MAC for 3 to 5 vital capacity breaths may produce enough anesthetic depth to permit the insertion of an intravenous infusion.

Spontaneous ventilation is the key concept to a smooth inhalation induction. Hand ventilation should not be forced. This can invoke coughing and laryngospasm and increased oral secretions from airway irritation. Eger (1994) suggests inhalation agents be described by a "pungency index" (Table 28–8). This may be an indicator of how volatile agents influence the upper respiratory tract.

Complete monitoring is ideal for inhalation induction; however, it may not be practical in an uncooperative child or adult. At a minimum, pulse oximetry provides the noninvasive information of oxygen saturation levels and pulse rate. Ideally the patient should have continuous ECG monitoring, pulse oximetry, and baseline blood pressure status. A precordial stethescope is recommended for auscultation of ventilation. A clear, well-fitting mask should be used to provide the best visualization of air exchange. The patient should be placed in a sniffing position or in a sitting position to maximize lung expansion and alveolar

TABLE 28–8. Pungency Index

Volatile Agent	Pungency Index
N$_2$O	0
Sevoflurane	0.5
Halothane	0.5
Enflurance	2.0
Isoflurane	2.5
Desflurane	3.0

Adapted from Eger, E. I. II. (1994). New inhaled anesthetics. Anesthesiology, 80, 906–922.

ventilation and comfort. A high flow of nitrous oxide-oxygen, 7 LPM/3 LPM, respectively, for three to four breaths allows for rapid denitrogenation and maximal analgesic effects. For halothane induction, traditionally concentrations have been introduced slowly moving from 0.5% to 3%. However, sevoflurane can be started at a higher concentration for rapid uptake into alveoli in order to produce unconsciousness and establish Level 3 general anesthesia quickly.

▶ CASE STUDY

The CRNA is summoned emergently to the endoscopy suite to assess a patient undergoing an upper gastrointestinal endoscopy. The patient is a 68-year-old female who is cyanotic and has shallow respirations. The only monitoring device on the patient is a pulse oximeter, which is reading 90%. A 20-gauge intravenous heparin lock is in place on the left hand. The registered nurse reports the patient has had meperidine 50 mg and midazolam 2 mg and has stopped breathing. The endoscopist is upset because he cannot finish the procedure.

1. What is your initial assessment and clinical diagnosis?

   In this chapter, conscious sedation and deep sedation are well differentiated. This patient has undetected hypoxemia under a state of deep sedation and must have assisted ventilation. A saturation of 90% may indicate a rapid change from conscious analgesia and deep sedation. This patient must be further assessed for any hemodynamic effects of the insult.

2. In managing this event, what should be done?

   Establish the level of consciousness; administer 100% oxygen by mask-assisted ventilation with an ambu bag if an anesthesia machine is not available; place ECG leads, a blood pressure cuff, and a precordial chest piece on the patient and monitor all vital signs. Monitoring procedures are the same whether in the operating room or outside the surgical area. The patient has a blood pressure of 90/50 and the ECG shows sinus bradycardia with a rate of 56 bpm.

3. Before administering any type of medication to this patient, what should the nurse anesthetist do?

   Obtaining pertinent information from the nurse and physician is vital to the successful treatment of this problem. In many cases the elderly patient is on a variety of medications, such as digoxin, which may cause the slowed heart rate. The patient also may be allergic to certain medications and knowing this will be very helpful in diagnosing and treating the incident. Endotracheal intubation may be indicated if apnea or airway obstruction has occurred. The patient shows no response to the prior treatment. Her respirations are shallow. However, the saturation monitor is registering 94%. The CRNA decides to intubate the patient.

4. What would be the technique of choice?

   This situation requires urgent endotracheal intubation utilizing the Sellick maneuver to help prevent aspiration of gastric contents. Upper gastrointestinal endoscopy further increases the risk of aspiration because the mechanical endoscope is inserted into the esophagus and stomach. In addition, the CRNA should be thinking ahead about any drug antagonism that should be administered to this patient once the airway is secured. If for some reason, intubation cannot be accomplished, the use of the LMA may be indicated. Barbiturate administration should probably be avoided as these drugs may compound the respiratory depression, resulting in increased apnea and possibly more cardiovascular depression.

▶ SUMMARY

Techniques for conscious sedation/analgesia and general anesthesia vary greatly according to the patient's needs and the environment. Clinical research for combinations of different agents, whether inhalational or intravenous, are ongoing. It is important for the anesthetist to provide continuous observation and assessment of the effects of both individual agents and synergistic effects. Recognizing and interpreting individual responses from anesthetic agents allow the CRNA to alter the anesthetic plan accordingly. Intravenous sedation or analgesia may progress to general anesthesia very quickly, therefore, vigilence is paramount. A full understanding of the whole environment, surgical needs, patient needs, and practitioner comfort level determines which technique is appropriate. A continuous process of assessment and evaluation of the applied practice will provide the best outcomes for each anesthetic administered.

► KEY CONCEPTS

- Conscious sedation is defined as a medically controlled state of consciousness in which protective reflexes are maintained.
- Deep sedation is a medically controlled state of depressed consciousness in which the patient may or may not be able to maintain protective airway reflexes.
- The four properties of general anesthesia are hypnosis, analgesia, amnesia, and muscle relaxation.
- Total intravenous anesthesia (TIVA) can be utilized

for deep sedation techniques as well as general anesthetic techniques.
- Undetected hypoxemia is characterized by hypoventilation, apnea, or airway obstruction.
- Balanced anesthesia is the combination of intravenous and inhalation agents to achieve general anesthesia.
- A rapid-sequence induction technique for general anesthesia is used for patients with a full stomach or a suspected full stomach.

► STUDY QUESTIONS

1. What is the continuum from sedation to anesthesia?

2. In selecting an anesthetic technique for a specific patient, when would you use TIVA?

3. In establishing individual hospital protocols for administering conscious sedation, should anesthesia providers set the standards for care?

4. If the risk of aspiration is common for all patients undergoing general anesthesia, should all patients be treated with a rapid-sequence induction technique?

5. What anesthetic techniques can be used for general anesthesia, and how are they accomplished?

KEY REFERENCES

Committee on Drugs, Section on Anesthesiology. (1985). Guidelines for the elective use of conscious sedation, deep sedation, and general anesthesia in pediatric patients. *Pediatrics, 76,* 317–321.

Booth, M. (1996). Clinical aspects of nurse anesthesia practice: Sedation and monitored anesthesia care. *Nursing Clinics of North America, 3,* 667–682.

Smith, I. (1996). Monitored anesthesia care: How much sedation? How much analgesia? *Journal of Clinical Anesthesia, 8,* 765–805.

REFERENCES

American Society of Anesthesiologists (ASA). (1995). ASA standards, guidelines and statements. Park Ridge, IL: ASA.

Bailey, P. L., Pace, N. L., Ashburn, M. A., Moll, J. W., East, K. A., & Stanley, T. H. (1990). Frequent hypoxemia and apnea after sedation with midazolam and fentanyl. *Anesthesiology, 73,* 826–830.

Baskett, P. J. (1994). The laryngeal mask in resuscitation. *Resuscitation, 28,* 93–95.

Benumof, J. L. (1996). Laryngeal mask airway and the ASA difficult airway algorithm. *Anesthesiology, 84*(3), 686–699.

Booth, M. (1996). Clinical aspects of nurse anesthesia practice. Sedation and monitored anesthesia care. *Nursing Clinics of North America, 3,* 667–682.

Dunnihoo, M., Wuest, A., Meyer, M., & Robinson, M. (1994). The effects of TIVA using propofol, ketamine, and vecuronium on cardiovascular response and wake up time. *AANA Journal, 62,* 261–266.

Eger, E. I. II. (1994). New inhaled anesthetics. *Anesthesiology, 80,* 906–922.

Epstein, B. S. (1996). Analgesia-sedation, how, when, and where? The role of the anesthesiologist. *47th annual refresher course lectures,* (#153, pp. 1–5). Park Ridge, IL: American Society of Anesthesiologists.

Fallacaro, M. D. (1993). A biting commentary on monitored anesthesia care with conscious sedation. *AANA Journal, 61,* 229–232.

Griner, R. L. (1996). Update for nurse anesthetists-the laryngeal mask airway: Attributes and inadequacies. *AANA Journal, 64,* 485–496.

Joint Commission on Accreditation of Healthcare Organizations (JCAHO). (1995). 1995 Comprehensive Accreditation Manual for Hospitals. Oakbrook Terrace, IL: JCAHO.

Kaplan, R. F. (1996). Sedation and analgesia in pediatric patients for procedures outside the operating room. (#531, pp. 1–7). *47th annual refresher course lectures.* Park Ridge, IL: American Society of Anesthesiologists.

Mikhail, M. S., & Morgan, G. E. (1996). *Clinical anesthesiology* (2nd ed.). Norwalk, CT: Appleton & Lange.

Glaxo Wellcome. (1996). Remifentanil. *Product monograph.* Research Triangle Park, NC: Author.

Reves, J. G. (1996). Intravenous anesthetics, how much should I administer and how? *47th annual refresher course lectures.* (#432, pp. 1–7). Park Ridge, IL: American Society of Anesthesiologists.

Short, T. G., & Chui, P. T. (1991). Propofol and midazolam act synergistically in combination. *British Journal of Anaesthesia, 67,* 539–545.

Smith, I. (1996). Monitored anesthesia care: How much sedation? How much analgesia? *Journal of Clinical Anesthesia, 8,* 765–805.

Stoltzfus, D. P. (1995). Advantages and disadvantages of combining sedative agents. *Critical Care Clinics, 11,* 903–911.

Tanaka, D. (1992). Pharmacology of intravenous anesthetics and adjuncts. In W. R. Waugaman, S. D. Foster, & B. M. Rigor (Eds.), *Principles and practice of nurse anesthesia* (2nd ed., pp. 437–460, chapter 26). Norwalk, CT: Appleton & Lange.

Twersky, R. S. (1995). *The ambulatory anesthesia handbook.* St. Louis: Mosby-Yearbook.

White, P. (1995). Sevoflurane for outpatient anesthesia: A comparison with propofol. *Anesthesia & Analgesia, 81,* 823–828.

Willenkin, R. L., & Polk, S. L. (1994). Management of general anesthesia. In R. D. Miller (Ed.), *Anesthesia* (4th ed., p. 1049). New York: Churchill Livingstone.

► APPENDIX 28–A

AANA GUIDELINES FOR NONANESTHESIA PRACTITIONERS ADMINISTERING CONSCIOUS SEDATION (June 1996)

A. Qualifications

1. The registered nurse is allowed by state law and institutional policy to administer conscious sedation.

2. The health care facility shall have in place an educational/credentialing mechanism that includes a process for evaluating and documenting the individual's competency relating to the management of patients receiving conscious sedation. Evaluation and documentation occur on a periodic basis.

3. The registered nurse managing and monitoring the care of patients receiving conscious sedation is able to:

   a. Demonstrate the acquired knowledge of anatomy, physiology, pharmacology, cardiac arrhythmia recognition, and complications related to conscious sedation and medications.

   b. Assess the total patient care requirements before and during the administration of conscious sedation, including the recovery phase.

   c. Understand the principles of oxygen delivery, transport and uptake, respiratory physiology, as well as understand and use oxygen-delivery devices.

   d. Recognize potential complications of conscious sedation for each type of agent being administered.

   e. Possess the competency to assess, diagnose, and intervene in the event of complications and institute appropriate interventions in compliance with orders or institutional protocols.

   f. Demonstrate competency, through ACLS or PCLS, in airway management and resuscitation appropriate to the age of the patient.

4. The registered nurse administering conscious sedation understands the legal ramifications of providing this care and maintains appropriate liability insurance.

B. Management and Monitoring

Registered nurses who are not qualified anesthesia providers may be authorized to manage and monitor conscious sedation during therapeutic, diagnostic, or surgical procedures if the following criteria are met. These criteria should be interpreted in a manner consistent with the remainder of this document.

1. Guidelines for patient monitoring, drug administration, and protocols for dealing with potential complications or emergency situations, developed in accordance with accepted standards of anesthesia practice, are available.

2. A qualified anesthesia provider or attending physician selects and orders the agents to achieve conscious sedation.

3. Registered nurses who are not qualified anesthesia providers should *not* administer agents classified as anesthetics, including but not limited to ketamine, propofol, etomidate, sodium thiopental, methohexital, nitrous oxide, and muscle relaxants.

4. The registered nurse managing and monitoring the patient receiving conscious sedation shall have no other responsibilities during the procedure.

5. Venous access shall be maintained for all patients having conscious sedation.

6. Supplemental oxygen shall be available for any patient receiving conscious sedation, and where appropriate in the postprocedure period.

7. Documentation and monitoring of physiologic measurements, including but not limited to blood pressure, respiratory rate, oxygen saturation, cardiac rate and rhythm, and level of consciousness should be recorded at least every 5 minutes.

8. An emergency cart must be immediately accessible to every location where conscious sedation is administered. This cart must include emergency resuscitative drugs, airway and ventilatory adjunct equipment, defibrillator, and a source for administration of 100% oxygen. A positive pressure breathing device, oxygen, suction and appropriate airways must be placed in each room where conscious sedation is administered.

9. Back-up personnel who are experts in airway management, emergency intubations, and advanced cardiopulmonary resuscitation must be available.

10. A qualified professional capable of managing complications that might arise is present in the facility and remains in the facility until the patient is stable.

11. A qualified professional authorized under institutional guidelines to discharge the patient remains in the facility to discharge the patient in accordance with established criteria of the facility.

Regional Anesthesia Techniques

Francis R. Gerbasi

Regional anesthesia offers the patient a safe and effective alternative to general anesthesia for certain types of surgical and diagnostic procedures. It provides a relatively pain-free state without necessitating a loss of consciousness. Analgesia and motor blockade result from the interruption of nerve impulses before they reach and after they leave the spinal cord. This is accomplished by the administration of a local anesthetic solution at a specific site along the pathway of a nerve. Local anesthetic solutions act by inhibiting nerve cell ion transfer and by stopping the propagation of nerve impulses. Various types of regional anesthetics can be used and are designated according to the specific site of blockade (eg, field blocks, specific nerve or plexus blocks, and ganglionic blocks).

This chapter discusses four major regional anesthetic techniques: (1) spinal; (2) epidural; (3) brachial plexus (axillary approach); and (4) intravenous regional anesthesia. The primary intent is to emphasize the administration process. The anesthetist sincerely interested in neural blockade must have a thorough understanding of pertinent anatomy, physiology, and pharmacology related to the local anesthetic agents. *It is recommended that additional references be consulted and that supervised clinical experience be acquired before performing any of the regional anesthetics discussed.*

▶ PREOPERATIVE ASSESSMENT

The patient must be evaluated to determine whether a specific regional anesthetic technique is suitable. This assessment should encompass four primary areas:

1. Patients should always willingly give permission for a regional anesthetic to be performed. If a block is attempted without authorized permission from the patient or guardian, the anesthetist may be liable for assault and battery charges.
2. Initially the patient's anatomic and pathophysiologic status should be evaluated. Specific anatomic landmarks must be identified for all regional anesthetics. Conditions such as obesity and severe arthritis may hamper the identification of these landmarks and the administration of a specific block. A thorough history and physical examination should be completed, including allergies, drug therapy, and evaluation of any pathophysiologic condition. Conditions such as infections, hypovolemia, neurologic disease, and coagulopathies may contraindicate a regional anesthetic.
3. A positive rapport should be established and the patient's psychologic status evaluated. One should explain the regional anesthetic being considered, its benefits and risks, and obtain consent to its use. Usually, increased patient understanding will promote acceptance and facilitate successful anesthetic management. Psychologically the patient must have a positive mental attitude to be cooperative during a regional anesthetic. Conditions such as hysteria and disorientation make administration and management of a regional anesthetic difficult. Often,

when there is a language barrier between the patient and provider, administration of blocks is difficult.

4. Finally, the proper anesthetic management is determined. This decision should be based on the findings of the aforementioned evaluation, the specific instructions and contraindications for a given block, the operative procedure, and the needs of the surgeon. No regional anesthetic can be guaranteed effective, and one should always be prepared to administer a general anesthetic.

Preoperative preparation should include nothing by mouth (NPO) for a minimum of 6 to 8 hours before surgery and the possible use of a narcotic and/or sedative as premedication. Although various opinions exist regarding the use of specific premedicants, a sedative (eg, midazolam) and narcotic (eg, meperidine, fentanyl) may be given to healthy patients to relieve anxiety and to facilitate anesthetic management. Anticholinergics are not commonly used because of their antisialagogue effect; however, they may be indicated for intraoperative treatment of bradycardia. Premedicants should be used with caution in the elderly or poor-risk patient.

▶ SPINAL ANESTHESIA

A spinal anesthetic, or subarachnoid block, consists of the injection of a local anesthetic solution into the subarachnoid space, with resultant blockade of the spinal nerve roots. August Bier is credited with the first planned spinal anesthetic in 1898, but it was not until 1921, when Gaston Labat published an article discussing methods to decrease the dangers of spinal anesthesia, that it became a relatively popular technique (Lund, 1983). Spinal anesthesia continues to be safe with the use of small-gauge needles, new local anesthetics, and intrathecal adjuvants such as opioids (Horlocker et al., 1997).

Advantages and Disadvantages

In selecting a subarachnoid block, as in the process of determining any anesthetic management, the anesthetist must consider the patient's emotional makeup and physical status and the needs of the surgeon. Usually, spinal anesthesia is administered for surgical procedures performed on the lower abdomen, inguinal region, or lower extremities. It may, however, be used in certain situations for upper abdominal procedures. The degree of muscle relaxation and contraction of bowel obtained with spinal anesthesia is unrivaled by any other anesthetic technique.

A subarachnoid block also presents certain disadvantages. The anesthetist must remember that the duration of anesthesia is limited and that there is a statistical chance of failure associated with administration. The possibility of hypotension, resulting from sympathetic blockade, may present concerns, particularly in the patient who has preoperative cardiovascular disorders. Also, the patient's airway and respiratory systems are not under the direct control of the anesthetist as with general anesthesia.

Anatomy

A basic knowledge of the vertebral column, spinal cord, and surrounding structures is of the utmost importance to the anesthetist administering a spinal anesthetic (Hahn, McQuillan, & Sheplock, 1996). The following discussion highlights the main areas that directly relate to spinal anesthetic administration.

The vertebral column comprises four curves, the thoracic and sacral being concave anteriorly and the cervical and lumbar being convex anteriorly (Fig. 29–1). Prior to the administration of a spinal anesthetic, the lumbar curve often is modified by having the patient arch his or her back posteriorly. This modification facilitates spinal needle placement by opening the interspinous spaces. Kyphosis, scoliosis, and lordosis can represent variations in the natural curvature of the spine and make the administration of a spinal anesthetic difficult.

The vertebral column is bound together by the ligamentum flavum and the supraspinous, interspinous, and longitudinal ligaments (Fig. 29–2). The vertebral canal runs vertically in the vertebral column and is bounded anteriorly by bodies of the vertebrae and the intervertebral discs. The vertebral canal is bounded posteriorly by the arch bearing the spinous process and the interspinous ligaments. The vertebral canal contains the spinal cord, spinal nerve roots, cerebrospinal fluid, and membranes that enclose the spinal cord. The spinal cord is protected by the vertebral column and three tissue membranes. These membranes are the dura mater, arachnoid mater, and pia mater. Although some anatomic variations are seen, the spinal cord usually extends down the spinal canal to the lower border of L-1 (Fig. 29–3; see Brown, 1994; MacIntosh, 1957; Reimann & Anson, 1944). To prevent possible spinal cord damage, a spinal needle, therefore, should not be inserted above the second lumbar vertebrae.

The initial placement of the spinal needle is determined by the specific relationship between the fourth lumbar vertebra and the top of the iliac crests. Based on the fact that these two structures lie at corresponding levels, each vertebra's location and respective interspaces can be determined. The anesthetist should select an interspace below L-2. The most commonly used interspace is that between the third and fourth lumbar vertebrae.

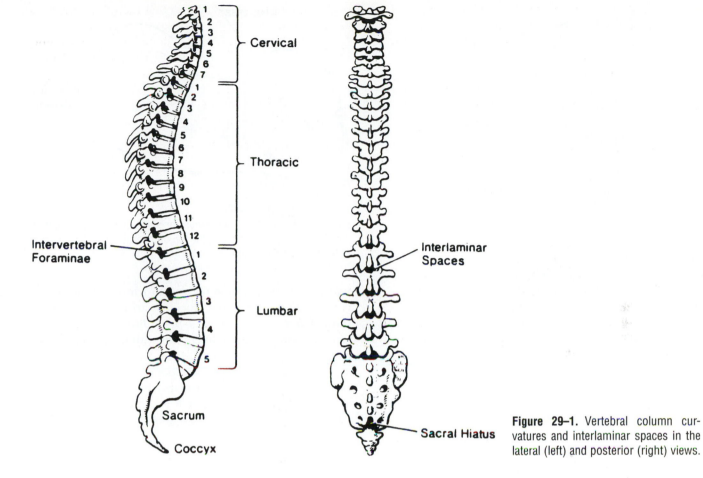

Cervical

Thoracic

Intervertebral
Foraminae

Lumbar

Sacrum

Coccyx

Interlaminar
Spaces

Sacral Hiatus

Figure 29–1. Vertebral column curvatures and interlaminar spaces in the lateral (left) and posterior (right) views.

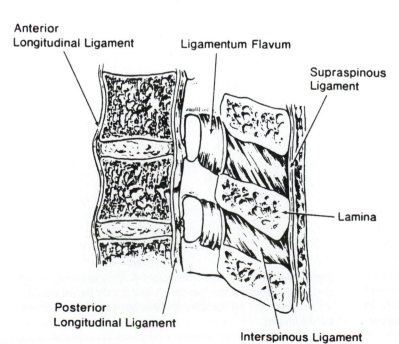

Anterior
Longitudinal Ligament

Ligamentum Flavum

Supraspinous
Ligament

Lamina

Posterior
Longitudinal Ligament

Interspinous Ligament

Figure 29–2. Cross-section of the vertebral column, showing ligaments.

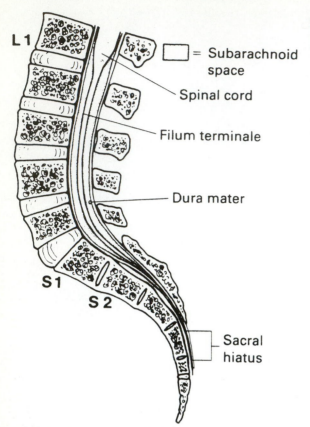

Figure 29–3. Cross-section of the lumbosacral vertebrae, showing spinal cord ending at lower border of L-1 with subarachnoid space continuing to S-2. *(From Miller, R. D. [1990]. Anesthesia [3rd ed]. New York: Churchill Livingstone. Reprinted with permission.)*

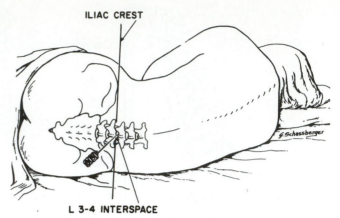

Figure 29–4. Anatomic orientation for spinal needle placement at the L3–4 interspace. Note that the top of the iliac crest corresponds to the fourth lumbar vertebra.

which then extends and divides into anterior and posterior divisions supplying specific areas of the body, termed *dermatomes* (Fig. 29–5; see Brown, 1994).

Sympathetic nerve fibers run with the spinal nerves and supply various organs. Figure 29–6 indicates the sympathetic innervation corresponding to specific levels of the vertebral column. Primarily because of the small size of the sympathetic fiber, it is thought that the sympathetic impulses are blocked above the corresponding

To place a spinal needle in the subarachnoid space, the correct intervertebral space must be identified and the needle inserted at an appropriate angle. Each of the spinal vertebrae has a spinous process extending posteriorly. The direction in which these spinous processes extend determines to a large extent the angle at which the spinal needle must be inserted. The spinous process of the last four lumbar vertebrae extends in a more horizontal plane than the other spinous processes. The spinal needle must be introduced parallel to this angle to reach the subarachnoid space (Fig. 29–4).

If a midline approach is used, the spinal needle pierces various ligaments while being introduced into the subarachnoid space. These ligaments, in order of their penetration, are the supraspinous ligament, interspinous ligament, and ligamentum flavum. If a paramedian or lateral approach is used, only the ligamentum flavum is pierced. Spinal anesthesia results primarily from blockade of the spinal nerve roots. These spinal nerves originate from the spinal cord as the anterior and posterior roots (Greene, 1981). The nerve roots unite in the intervertebral foramen to form the spinal nerve,

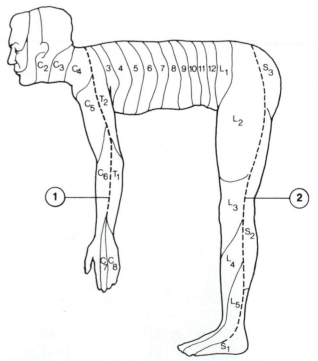

Figure 29–5. Dermatomes of the body indicating an orderly cranial-to-caudad sequence. The numbers 1 and 2 indicate the axial line around which the dermatomes of the upper and lower extremities are distributed.

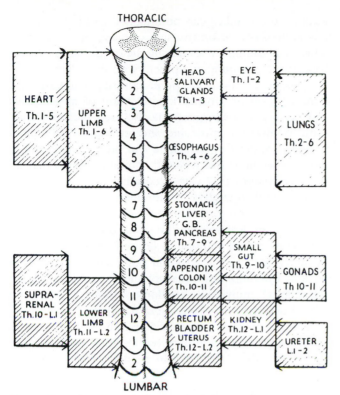

Figure 29–6. Spinal levels of sympathetic innervation.

TABLE 29–1. Indications for and Contraindications to Spinal (Subarachnoid) Anesthesia

Indications
    Procedures involving lower abdomen and extremities
    Obstetric procedures
    Patient preference
Contraindications
    Absolute
        Anticoagulant therapy or coagulation abnormalities
        Systemic or localized infection
        Allergy to anesthetic drug
        Increased intracranial pressure
        Presence of acute neurologic disease
        Patient refusal
    Relative
        Chronic neurologic disorders
        Backache
        Headache
        Psychologic disorders

sensory block; however, recent investigators have suggested that sympathetic block has less extent and intensity than sensory analgesia (Bengtasson, Lofstrom, & Malmquist, 1985). Motor blockade usually occurs approximately two spinal levels below the sensory level (Freund et al., 1967). A decrease in blood pressure often is the result of sympathetic blockade and may indicate a relatively high block if it occurs rapidly after spinal administration.

Indications and Contraindications

The indications for and contraindications to a spinal anesthetic are listed in Table 29–1. Contraindications can be viewed on an absolute or relative basis. A spinal anesthetic should not be administered in the presence of an absolute contraindication. If a relative contraindication is present, one must weigh the advantages and disadvantages of the technique to arrive at the appropriate anesthetic management decision.

Generally, spinal anesthesia is indicated for lower abdominal procedures, such as transurethral prostatectomy and inguinal herniorrhaphy. It is particularly useful in a patient whose condition may be aggravated by a general anesthetic or in the patient who fears losing consciousness. Spinal anesthesia has been used in obstetrics for vaginal deliveries or cesarean sections, although epidural anesthesia has gained preference.

Procedure

The following procedure describes the administration of a spinal anesthetic using a 25-gauge noncutting spinal needle and introducer. Compared with larger-bore cutting needles, the 25-gauge noncutting needle offers the advantage of a decreased incidence of postdural puncture headache (Greene, 1979; Halpern & Preston, 1994). However, larger-gauge noncutting needles (eg, 22-gauge Whitacre) may provide more stability in a difficult spinal and still have a relatively low incidence of spinal headache.

The importance of adequate preparation prior to administration of a spinal anesthetic cannot be overstressed. Table 29-2 indicates some important points about preparation and actual administration of the block. As with any anesthetic technique, this procedure should not be performed without the immediate availability of proper resuscitation equipment and medications. The anesthetist must remember that this is a sterile procedure; consequently, sterile technique must be used. Also, in preparation, the healthy patient should receive a preload of fluid (0.5 to 1 L) and have blood pressure, pulse, and respirations measured and recorded.

One of the most important aspects in preparing to administer a spinal anesthetic is patient positioning. Proper positioning of the patient ensures good anatomic orientation and maximum opening of the interspinous spaces. An assistant should be available at all times to help position and support the patient during the administration of a spinal anesthetic. Opening of the interspinous spaces can best be accomplished in the lateral position by having the patient "curl up" as much as pos-

TABLE 29–2. Important Steps in the Administration of a Spinal (Subarachnoid) Anesthetic

I. Preparation
  A. Prepare equipment.
    1. Arrange resuscitation equipment and medication so that they are immediately available.
    2. Obtain sterile gloves and prep solution.
    3. Verify spinal anesthesia tray sterility and prepare it for easy use.
  B. Prepare patient.
    1. Explain procedure.
    2. Check vital signs.
    3. Position appropriately sitting or lateral.
      a. Back at edge of table
      b. Proper body alignment with support
      c. Knees and head flexed
      d. Patient relaxed
II. Performance
  A. Identify landmarks.
  B. Raise skin wheal at site.
  C. Insert spinal needle.
    1. Insert 21-gauge introducer to ligamentum flavum.
    2. Introduce 25-gauge spinal needle, bevel parallel to dura fibers.
    3. Advance needle gently.
    4. Frequently check for cerebrospinal fluid.
    5. Identify subarachnoid space.
    6. Rotate needle 90 to 180 degrees.
  D. Inject medication.
    1. Attach needle-stabilized syringe.
    2. Aspirate cerebrospinal fluid, inject medication.
    3. Aspirate postinjection.
  E. Remove needle and syringe assembly.
  F. Reposition patient.

sible and flex his or her back posteriorly. Anatomic orientation is best accomplished by having the patient assume a sitting position. This may be particularly useful in the obese patient. Using a marking pen to indicate anatomic landmarks also can help maintain good anatomic orientation.

There are many variations in skin preparation. Which one to choose is an individual decision by the provider according to institutional policy or accepted practice standards of aseptic technique. Informing the patient that a disinfectant solution is going to be applied and that the needle is about to be inserted is particularly important to prevent movement and provides the patient with a more pleasant experience. Several sponges are used to remove the disinfectant solution and the area is draped to maintain sterility.

Presently, a number of spinal trays are commercially available and provide all the necessary syringes, needles, and medications to administer a subarachnoid block. The spinal tray may be prepared between application and removal of the disinfectant solution or prior to application of the solution. It should be prepared so that the med-

ications and needles can be obtained easily. The spinal tray is then placed on the side of provider dominance, which will facilitate maintaining the needle site with one hand while obtaining equipment with the other.

The medications are prepared using standard techniques to ensure proper identification of medications and sterility. Various agents may be used, including lidocaine, bupivacaine, procaine, and tetracaine. Table 29–3 provides dosages of tetracaine and bupivacaine in relation to specific spinal levels. It should be noted that individual dosages may vary according to patient characteristics and operative requirements. The effect of gravity in relation to patient positioning is a very important factor in determining the spinal level achieved. If a hyperbaric spinal solution is desired, tetracaine should be mixed with 10% dextrose in water solution. This may be done by combining equal volumes, on a millimeter basis, although individual variations of this ratio often are seen. Since the late 1980s there has been an explosive growth in the use of intrathecal opioids (Raj, 1992). Morphine and fentanyl administered intrathecally block the spinal reflexes related to pain stimuli (Abboud, Dror, & Mosaad, 1988).

Using the top of the iliac crest as a reference, the fourth lumbar vertebra (L-4) is identified and the appropriate interspace determined. One should not go above the second lumbar vertebra. The step-by-step technique is reviewed in Table 29–2. An introducer is used to facilitate placement of the small-gauge spinal needle and to prevent its contact with the skin. If a cutting spinal needle is used, the needle is inserted through the introducer with the bevel parallel to the fibers of the dura, which run cephalad to caudad. This decreases the number of transected dura fibers. When initially introduced, the spinal needle should be held securely; then two hands should be used gently to guide the needle inward. The anesthetist must maintain a firm understanding of the anatomic orientation during insertion. It is on this basis that he or she directs the needle into the subarachnoid space (Fig. 29–4).

The needle is advanced until a give or "pop" is elicited. The stylet is removed and a return of cere-

TABLE 29–3. Dosage of 1% Tetracaine and 0.75% Bupivacaine (in 8.5% Dextrose) Necessary to Achieve an Approximate T-10 Anesthetic Level in Relation to Patient's Height

Height (in)	Tetracaine Dosage (mg)[a]	Bupivacaine Dosage (mg)
60	10	8-10
66	12	10-12
72	14	14-16

[a] Tetracaine dosages assume mixture with an equal volume, on a milliliter basis, of 10% dextrose water. Please refer to text for factors that influence analgesic level achieved.

brospinal fluid indicates entry into the subarachnoid space. The normal "pop" felt on entering the subarachnoid space is less pronounced when the smaller-gauge needles (eg, 25- or 26-gauge) are used and the return of cerebrospinal fluid will be relatively slow.

Occasionally, blood is obtained on stylet removal. Usually, this clears after a few drops. If clearing does not occur, the needle may be repositioned until clear cerebrospinal fluid is obtained. *At no time should the agent be injected in the presence of a blood tap or abnormally appearing cerebrospinal fluid.*

Rotating the needle 90 to 180 degrees after obtaining cerebrospinal fluid will help ensure appropriate placement. Then, while the needle is firmly supported, the syringe is attached. One should support the needle with the hand, using the patient's back to assist in stabilizing the spinal needle. This is a very crucial point in the technique. The importance of maintaining needle placement cannot be overstressed. Even a very slight movement may reposition the needle outside the subarachnoid space. Cerebrospinal fluid is then aspirated to confirm needle placement and the local anesthetic is injected. After injection, cerebrospinal fluid is again aspirated as an indication of efficacy and the needle/syringe assembly removed. The patient should then be repositioned according to the level of analgesia desired.

Occasionally, a nerve fiber is touched by the spinal needle, causing a temporary paresthesia that dissipates rapidly. *The medication may be injected in this situation, but at no time should the local anesthetic agent be injected in the presence of persistent paresthesia.*

Management

Generally, a spinal anesthetic is administered to obtain a desired level of anesthesia. Specific factors that influence the level obtained are (1) the specific gravity of the agent employed; (2) the volume injected; (3) the speed of injection; and (4) the patient's position immediately after administration. Of these factors, patient positioning should be instituted immediately after injection. If a hyperbaric solution is used, the effect of gravity will move the medication to the lowest point of the vertebral column. If a unilateral block is desired, the patient should remain on the side to be anesthetized for approximately 5 minutes after administration. If the patient is supine, the table may be placed in a Trendelenburg position to increase the height of the block.

After the patient is repositioned, the vital signs should be assessed and recorded every minute for the first 20 minutes, then monitored every 5 minutes. Oxygen should be administered on a routine basis, and significant hypotension should be treated with appropriate fluids and a vasopressor (eg, ephedrine). The Trendelenburg position does not appear to be a reliable measure to prevent

or treat hypotension (Miyabe & Sato, 1997). The patient's respirations must be closely monitored. Although an approximate fixing time of 20 minutes is expected with tetracaine, this may vary and the spinal level can rise, causing respiratory embarrassment. The level of anesthesia can be assessed, after administration, by using a large-gauge needle and touching the skin lightly to determine patient sensitivity (pinprick method). Characteristically, onset of the block proceeds in the following order: sympathetic blockade, superficial pain and temperature, motor, proprioception, and, finally, loss of sensation to touch and deep pressure. Therefore, a patient may feel the touch and pressure associated with disinfectant solution application but be insensitive to pain. Effective communication is essential at this time to alleviate anxiety and assess the patient's status. Symptoms of a high spinal, such as numbness in the hands or difficulty in breathing can be detected and the appropriate treatment initiated.

Duration of action will vary and depends on the dosage of agent employed, level of anesthesia, type of local anesthetic used, and the patient's age. If epinephrine or phenylephrine has been added, a clinically significant prolongation of regression of analgesia and anesthesia with tetracaine is seen (Armstrong, Littlewood, & Chambers, 1983). Recovery is due primarily to diffusion and vascular absorption of the local anesthetic agent from the subarachnoid space (Greene, 1983; Reimann & Anson, 1944). Characteristically, nerve function recovers in reverse order of onset.

► EPIDURAL ANESTHESIA

The injection of a local anesthetic agent into the posterior lumbar epidural space that surrounds the dural sac in the vertebral canal is termed epidural anesthesia or epidural block. In 1885 Corning produced the first epidural block, and since that time various administration techniques have been developed. The following describes the loss of resistance technique and indicates specific points of importance in its administration.

Advantages and Disadvantages

Epidural anesthesia offers distinct advantages over a subarachnoid block. An epidural block has a slower onset of sympathetic blockade, which allows for compensatory vasoconstriction to occur. This may decrease the incidence of hypotension after administration. A larger number of agents are available for an epidural block then for a subarachnoid block, which allows the anesthetic to be tailored to the specific needs of the procedure. A distinct advantage is the absence of postlumbar puncture headache as long as the dura has not been penetrated. A disadvantage of the technique is its relative difficulty.

The technique requires careful administration and the importance of proper training and supervised experience cannot be overemphasized.

Anatomy

An understanding of anatomy also is important in the administration of an epidural block. The epidural space, which extends from the foramen magnum to the sacral hiatus, lies between the periosteal and investing layers of the dura. It is approximately 6 mm at its widest point and is bordered posteriorly by the ligamentum flavum (Ching, 1963). It contains the spinal nerve roots, blood vessels, and fatty areolar tissue.

The anterior and posterior spinal nerve roots pass through the epidural space, surrounded by a dural cuff, and then unite and exit through the intervertebral foramen. These nerves are characteristically less movable in the epidural space and, therefore, are vulnerable to needle trauma. It is postulated that an epidural anesthetic blocks the spinal nerves by a variety of pathways, including diffusion of the local anesthetic through arachnoid villi. The arachnoid villi are located in the dural cuff, which surrounds the nerve roots.

Another important feature of the epidural space is the demonstrable negative pressure that is encountered on initial entry. This is believed to be caused by the transmission of negative thoracic pressure through the intervertebral foramina. The negative pressure may be used to locate and verify the epidural space and can promote the cephalad spread of a local anesthetic agent. An exception is noted in advanced pregnancy where a positive epidural pressure is present (Aboulish, 1977; Moya & Smith, 1962).

Indications and Contraindications

Epidural anesthesia may be used for many types of operative and diagnostic procedures. Its popularity has increased in obstetrics because of its ability to provide a relatively pain-free labor and analgesia for either cesarean or vaginal delivery. Contraindications are similar to those associated with a subarachnoid block and are listed in Table 29–4.

Procedure

Initially, the procedure should be discussed with the patient and his or her consent obtained. Prior to administration, an intravenous cannula must be inserted and the appropriate fluid therapy initiated. Vital signs should be measured and recorded and standard resuscitation equipment should be immediately available to treat possible complications.

A standard commercial epidural tray generally contains all the necessary equipment to administer the

TABLE 29–4. Indications for and Contraindications to Epidural Anesthesia

Indications
  Postoperative pain relief
  Lower-abdominal operative procedures
  Normal- and high-risk obstetric procedures
Contraindications
  Absolute
    Anticoagulant therapy
    Hypovolemia
    Systemic or localized infection near needle puncture site
    Increased intracranial pressure
    Patient refusal
  Relative
    Inexperience with the technique
    Active disease of central nervous system
    Previous laminectomy

block, with the possible exception of the local anesthetic agent and the disinfectant solution. A wide range of local anesthetic agents of various concentrations may be used. The proper selection depends on the characteristics of the block required. Some specific local anesthetic agents are indicated in Table 29–5, along with their respective dosages and approximate durations of action. Currently, the use of narcotics (e.g., fentanyl) in combination with a local anesthetic agent is gaining popularity. Fentanyl 50 to 100 µg can be mixed with bupivacaine 0.125% to 0.25% to provide better analgesia without increasing the volume or concentration of the local anesthetic.

The patient is positioned and disinfectant solution applied using a technique similar to that described for subarachnoid block administration (Table 29–6). The appropriate interspace is identified according to the desired area being blocked. A skin wheal of local anesthetic is raised, and then a secondary skin puncture is made with a 15-gauge needle. This helps prevent the epidural needle from removing a piece of epidermis, which could lead to cyst formation.

TABLE 29–5. Local Anesthetic Agents: Concentrations and Approximate Durations of Epidural Anesthesia

Agents	Concentration (%)	mg/Segment[a]	Duration (min)
2-Chloroprocaine	3.0	45	60
Lidocaine	2.0	31	46
Mepivacaine	2.0	31	60
Bupivacaine	0.5	7	170

[a] These dosages should be decreased in elderly patients.

TABLE 29–6. Important Steps in the Administration of an Epidural Block: Loss of Resistance Technique

I. Preparation
   A. Prepare equipment.
      1. Arrange resuscitation equipment and medication so that they are immediately available.
      2. Obtain sterile gloves and disinfectant solution.
      3. Verify epidural tray sterility and prepare it for easy use.
   B. Prepare patient.
      1. Explain procedure.
      2. Position appropriately.
II. Performance
   A. Identify landmark and select site.
   B. Apply disinfectant solution.
   C. Raise skin wheal at site.
   D. Pierce skin with 15-gauge needle.
   E. Insert epidural needle.
      1. Introduce epidural needle.
      2. Attach lubricated 5-mL glass syringe to needle and check resistance.
      3. Advance slowly, checking for resistance.
      4. Identify epidural space and check for cerebrospinal fluid or blood.
   F. Inject medication.
      1. Aspirate, introduce test dose, and monitor for symptoms of spinal or toxic reaction
      2. If negative, administer remaining dosage in incremental doses.
   G. Insert catheter.
      1. After test dose, insert catheter 3 cm beyond needle tip.
      2. Remove needle.
      3. Tape catheter securely and attach syringe assembly.
   H. Reposition patient.

Using a midline approach, the anesthetist inserts an epidural needle in a median plane. The stylet must be firmly held in place during insertion to prevent the possible tearing of the epidermis. On entry into the interspinous ligament, which is identified by increased resistance, the stylet is removed. A well-lubricated air- or normal saline–filled 5-mL glass syringe is then attached and the feeling of resistance noted in the plunger (Saberski, Kondamuri, & Osinubi, 1997). The needle is advanced a few millimeters at a time and the plunger retested. If no change in resistance is noted after continued advancement, the needle may be withdrawn and redirected. Penetration into the epidural space is identified when a distinct "pop" through the ligamentum flavum is noted, associated with a loss of resistance to injection. At this point, if no paresthesia is present, the syringe is disconnected and viewed for cerebrospinal fluid or blood. If negative, a test dose of 2 to 3 mL is slowly administered and the patient is observed for signs of spinal anesthesia (eg, numbness of the extremities; Reisner, Hockman, & Plumer, 1980); an additional 3 to 5 mL is then administered to test for intravascular injection (eg, metallic taste, dizziness). If no adverse symptoms are

noted, a loading dose is administered in incremental injections, and the needle removed. This is termed *the single administration technique.*

If cerebrospinal fluid is noted after removal of the stylet, one may elect to administer a spinal anesthetic at that time or use an adjacent space. Sixty milliliters of norm saline should then be administered in the epidural space at termination of the technique. If blood is present, the needle should be repositioned to ensure against intravascular injection.

Continuous epidural analgesia is obtained by inserting a catheter through the epidural needle into the epidural space after administration of a test dose to verify needle position. Once the catheter has passed the tip of the needle, it is advanced approximately 3 cm. The needle is removed over the catheter and the catheter taped securely. *At no time must the catheter be removed from the needle after insertion because of the possibility of catheter shearing.* Prior to local anesthetic injection, catheter position should be verified by administering a test dose to ensure that the catheter does not communicate with a blood vessel or cerebrospinal fluid. Repeat dosages of the local anesthetic agent may then be administered to maintain continuous analgesia. The repeat dosages should consist of a test dose, with aspiration before and after injection, followed by repeated fractional doses to obtain the refill dose (Covino & Marx, 1980).

Problems may be encountered in association with catheter placement, such as difficulty in advancement and unilateral analgesia. These may be corrected by various catheter and needle maneuvers, but *at no time should the catheter be removed from the needle.*

Management

After administration the patient should be repositioned according to the procedure to be performed. The parturient may be positioned on her left side, thus providing left lateral displacement during labor. If a lower extremity or abdominal procedure is to be performed, the patient can be placed in a supine position. As with a spinal anesthetic, the patient's vital signs should be measured every minute for the first 20 minutes, and then monitored every 5 minutes.

An appropriate level of analgesia can be expected in approximately 20 minutes, although time varies according to the agent employed. Generally, the shorter-acting local anesthetic agents (eg, 2-chloroprocaine) have a faster onset than the longer-duration anesthetics (eg, bupivacaine). The level of analgesia can be determined by using the pinprick technique that was previously discussed in relation to spinal anesthesia assessment. After repositioning and initial assessment, the anesthetist must monitor the patient for possible complications, such as hypotension, respiratory insufficiency, and toxic reactions, throughout the procedure.

The epidural catheter is removed when analgesia is no longer required. At this time the catheter should be inspected to ensure complete removal, and the findings should be documented in the patient's record. Epidural catheters may remain in place for continuous postoperative pain relief. An infusion pump is used to maintain a continuous infusion of the local anesthetic. Nurses caring for these patients must be able to detect and treat possible complications, such as respiratory depression.

The combination of spinal and epidural (combined spinal-epidural anesthesia) was used in the 1930s. However since the 1980s it has gained popularity. The technique offers the advantages of rapid onset of analgesia, titration of a desired sensory level, variation of the intensity of block, and control of the duration and delivery of postoperative analgesia. Several techniques have been used; however, none offers significant advantages over the needle-through-needle technique using a long fine-gauge pencil-point spinal needle through a conventional epidural needle (Urmey, 1997).

▶ BRACHIAL PLEXUS ANESTHESIA

Axillary Approach

The technique of blocking nerve impulses to and from the arm by injecting a local anesthetic solution into the group of nerves, or plexus, or innervating the extremity is termed *brachial plexus anesthesia.* Blocking the brachial plexus can be performed in a variety of ways, such as using the subclavian, interscalene, or axillary techniques. These methods depend on the approach used to reach the plexus and the extent to which the extremity is blocked (Lanz, Theiss, & Janicovic, 1983). Blockade of the brachial plexus by the axillary approach is discussed in this section, with an emphasis on aspects of administration.

Advantages and Disadvantages

Brachial plexus anesthesia by the axillary approach has distinct advantages and disadvantages over the subclavian and interscalene techniques and general anesthesia. The axillary approach has the advantage of being less disturbing to general body physiology than general anesthesia, which may be of special importance in the poor-risk patient. Postoperative nausea and vomiting are less, and other complications of general anesthesia are avoided. Compared with the subclavian and interscalene techniques of blocking the brachial plexus, the axillary approach eliminates the risk of pneumothorax and thus is considered a safer technique. It

also is impossible to block the phrenic, vagus, and recurrent laryngeal nerves or the stellate ganglia with the axillary approach.

As with any anesthetic technique, the axillary approach has disadvantages. It has a prolonged onset time and produces less muscle paralysis than other approaches. Analgesia may be spotty and may be inadequate for surgery beyond the hand into the forearm. Complete anesthesia of the entire upper extremity is not possible, because the injection is made where the nerve fibers begin to leave the axillary sheath.

Anatomy

An understanding of the distribution and anatomic location of the various nerve fibers supplying the arm is useful in administering an axillary block (Table 29–7). On the basis of this knowledge, the anesthetist can relate paresthesias elicited during needle insertion to the needle's anatomic orientation. This can help to ensure adequate analgesia to a particular area of the extremity.

The brachial plexus is an arrangement of nerve fibers that send both sensory and motor nerve impulses to the arm. The nerve fibers originate from the fifth cervical vertebra (C5) through the first thoracic vertebra (T1) (Reese, 1977). The nerves leave their respective vertebral foramina, and the nerve roots form three groups, the upper, middle, and lower trunks (Fig. 29–7). An extension of the prevertebral fascia surrounds the nerves as a multicompartmented sheath (Thompson & Rorie, 1983).

The upper trunk is formed by the fifth and sixth cervical nerves. As the upper trunk progresses, it gives rise to the suprascapular and subclavicular nerves. The upper trunk then forms the lateral cord, which has two primary branches. One branch forms the musculocutaneous nerve, and a second branch assists in forming the median nerve. The lower trunk is formed by the eighth cervical and first thoracic nerves. The lower trunk progresses into the medial cord, which has two primary branches. One branch assists in forming the median nerve; a second branch forms the ulnar nerve. The middle trunk is formed by the seventh cervical nerve. The middle trunk, along with a branch from the upper and lower trunks, forms the posterior cord. The posterior cord branches into the suprascapular, axillary, and radial

TABLE 29–7. Major Nerves in the Arm and Their Distribution

Nerve	Area Supplied
Musculocutaneous	Brachial muscle
Medial	Lateral arm and thumb
Ulnar	Medial arm
Radial	Posterior arm and hand

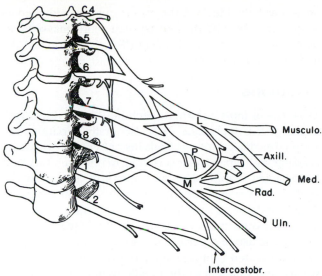

Figure 29–7. The nerve fibers composing the brachial plexus. The lateral, medial, and posterior cords give rise to the musculocutaneous axillary, median, radial, and ulnar nerves.

nerves. The intercostal brachial nerve, originating from the second thoracic vertebra (T-2), is important because it innervates the proximal inner arm.

Indications and Contraindications

An axillary block of the brachial plexus is indicated for surgical procedures involving the arm and hand. It can be used to differentiate central and peripheral pain. The technique is useful for surgical procedures on patients with a full stomach, patients who fear losing consciousness, and patients with complicating conditions.

An axillary block is contraindicated in patients with active infections of the extremity resulting from lymphadenopathy, and in patients with coagulation disorders, and in patients whose injury would prevent them from abducting the arm. The presence of a nerve injury also may be a contraindication because of legal implications. Difficulty should be anticipated in the markedly obese patient, whose axillary artery may be difficult to palpate.

Procedure

Proper preparation is very important. Table 29–8 offers a step-by-step approach for administration of an axillary block. One should have all the necessary equipment available for resuscitation before proceeding with the block. If the block is performed in the holding area, resuscitation equipment should be readily available. *At no time should this anesthetic technique be performed without equipment on hand to treat complications.*

TABLE 29–8. Important Steps in the Administration of a Brachial Plexus Block via the Axillary Approach

I. Preparation
  A. Prepare equipment.
    1. Arrange resuscitation equipment and medication so that they are immediately available.
    2. Obtain sterile gloves and disinfectant solution.
    3. Obtain two 20-mL syringes, stopcock, extension, and B-beveled needle.
  B. Prepare patient.
    1. Explain procedure.
    2. Position patient supine, with arm abducted 90 degrees and dorsum of hand by head.
    3. Note anatomic landmarks.
    4. Apply disinfectant solution.
II. Performance
  A. Identify landmarks and select site.
  B. Raise skin wheal at site.
  C. Insert needle.
    1. Insert and advance 22-gauge B-beveled needle.
    2. Aspirate continuously while inserting needle.
    3. Allow needle to enter sheath until "pop" is felt.
    4. Redirect needle until paresthesia is elicited.
  D. Inject medication.
    1. Withdraw needle slightly and apply digital pressure distal to injection site.
    2. Inject medication and monitor symptoms of toxicity.
    3. Leave medication in extension tubing for T-2 block.
  E. Withdraw needle to subcutaneous tissue.
  F. Institute blockade of intercostal brachialis (T-2).
    1. Advance needle upward in axilla and inject medication.
    2. Advance needle downward in axilla and inject medication.
  G. Remove needle and abduct arm with gentle massage of axilla.

The specific local anesthetic agent used may vary, and there is no one ideal agent. In deciding which agent to use, one must consider the duration of action needed and the degree of block required. The agent's potency, duration of action, toxic dosage, and effective concentration and the presence of allergies also must be considered. Table 29–9 lists commonly used agents, including their concentration and approximate duration of action.

TABLE 29–9. Various Anesthetic Agents Used for Brachial Plexus Blocks by the Axillary Approach, Their Concentrations, and Approximate Durations of Action

Agent	Concentration (%)	Duration
Bupivacaine	0.5 or 0.25	Long (4-6 h)
Lidocaine	1	Intermediate (2 h)
Mepivacaine	1	Intermediate (2 h)
2-Chloroprocaine	1, 2, 3	Short (1 h)

Use of a sufficient volume (40 to 50 mL) will help ensure adequate spreading of the agent, but the recommended maximum dose should not be exceeded. The use of epinephrine prolongs the action of shorter-acting agents, but is of little benefit to agents of longer duration. The local anesthetic agent is drawn up into two 20-mL syringes in an appropriate dosage, which are then labeled. The extension tubing and syringes are attached to a stopcock and any air is removed. The extension tubing is used to facilitate needle placement and injection.

Before proceeding with the block, the patient's full cooperation must be obtained. The importance of this cannot be overstated. If the patient is aware of what is to occur, success is more likely. Prior to administering the block, an intravenous catheter should be inserted and appropriate fluid therapy initiated. The appropriate monitoring equipment, such as cardioscope, blood pressure cuff, and precordial stethoscope, should be used.

After the appropriate monitoring equipment has been secured and checked, the patient's arm is abducted 90 degrees and the hand placed under the heart or the head. The artery is then identified by palpation and appropriate landmarks noted. Axillary hair may be removed at this time. Using sterile technique, the area is prepared with a disinfectant solution. The disinfectant solution is removed with a sterile sponge and the axillary artery is palpated. It is useful at this point to have an assistant manage the syringe and stopcock assembly. The artery is retracted downward by the underfinger and the needle is introduced above the artery just under the greater pectoralis muscle. A skin wheal of local anesthetic is then raised and the needle is advanced toward the axillary sheath. An assistant must keep aspirating during needle insertion to detect if a blood vessel has been entered.

When the axillary sheath is entered, a distinct "pop" is felt. The needle should then be advanced until a paresthesia is elicited in an area close to the surgical site. The needle is withdrawn slightly, digital pressure is applied distal to the needle site, and the local anesthetic solution is injected slowly. The patient must be carefully monitored for any symptoms of a toxic reaction during injection. The needle is removed to the subcutaneous tissue of the axilla, and the remaining solution is injected caudad to and cephalad from the insertion site to block the intercostal brachialis nerve (T-2) supplying the upper axilla. This helps eliminate tourniquet pain.

If during insertion the axillary artery is penetrated, as revealed by aspiration, the needle may be advanced dorsally, through the artery, and one half of the anesthetic agent injected. The needle is then removed until it is located ventral to the artery and the remaining half of the anesthetic agent is injected. A T-2 block is performed as previously described. After the intercostal brachial nerve has been blocked, the arm should be adducted as soon as possible and the axillary area gently massaged to help spread the anesthetic agent (Winnie, Radonjic, Akkineni, & Durrani, 1979).

Variations

As is true of most anesthetic techniques, individual variations of this technique exist. Generally, variations are adopted as the anesthetist finds his or her success rate increasing with a particular variation. In one such variation a tourniquet is applied to the upper arm, just below the axilla. This prevents the local anesthetic from spreading distally and encourages its upward movement, although digital pressure may be just as effective (Winnie et al., 1979). The use of a peripheral nerve stimulator also has been advocated (Montgomery, 1973). It is set at a low voltage and attached to the needle to help detect the location of specific nerves and provide a better perception of needle positioning. This variation can cause discomfort to the patient during testing (Smith, 1976).

After administering the block, the anesthetist must constantly assess the patient's status. Onset time varies depending on the local anesthetic agent employed, but enough time must be allowed for onset to occur. Informing the surgeon of the time necessary for onset may prevent undue stress. The first sign of onset is characterized by a loss of proprioception in the arm as evidenced by an inability of the patient to touch his or her nose. Then, motor blockade usually develops, followed by sensory blockade, depending on the agent used (Winnie et al., 1977).

Management

Adequate sedation during the procedure will help ensure effective patient management and make the operation a pleasant experience. Midazolam and fentanyl are useful agents in increasing patient comfort and allaying anxiety. As with any anesthetic technique, the anesthetist must be aware of the possible complications and their treatment. Although this technique is considered to be a very safe means of blocking the brachial plexus, still some possible complications must be considered.

A hematoma as a result of axillary artery puncture is always possible because the axillary artery lies in the axillary sheath with the plexus. Clinically, it usually has little significance, and vigorous massage of the injection site will help prevent its formation. In addition, intravenous or interarterial injection must be avoided because of the toxic reactions and arterial damage that may result. Aspirating while advancing and positioning the needle helps avoid this complication.

A spotty block always is a possibility and is due to incomplete blockade of all nerve fibers within the plexus. If this occurs, additional sedation and patient reassurance may be adequate to complete the operative procedure. If not, additional local infiltration or a specific nerve block may be administered to ensure that adequate anesthesia is present.

Whatever the route of administration, the local anesthetic eventually enters the bloodstream, and the possibility of a toxic reaction always exists. Prevention, of course, should be the primary goal. Toxic reactions can be prevented by limiting the dosage of local anesthetic and closely monitoring the patient. Premonitory signs, such as anxiety, muscle twitching, headache, drowsiness, and slurring of speech, may indicate an impending toxic reaction. Should a reaction occur, 100% oxygen should be administered with assisted ventilation. Diazepam may help by decreasing limbic system excitability and precluding focal seizure generation. In addition, sodium thiopental may be used as an anticonvulsant. The aim in treating a toxic reaction is to prevent cerebral hypoxia.

▶ INTRAVENOUS REGIONAL ANESTHESIA

Injecting a local anesthetic agent into a tourniquet-occluded arm is termed *intravenous regional anesthesia*. It is one of the oldest forms of peripheral nerve blockade and often is used today because of its simplicity and relative safety.

Advantages and Disadvantages

Intravenous regional anesthesia offers distinct advantages. It is relatively easy to perform as long as a step-by-step process is followed. In addition, the onset of anesthesia after injection is rapid (5 to 10 minutes), and the recovery time is short after tourniquet deflation. A major disadvantage of the technique is the limited amount of time the tourniquet can remain inflated without causing tissue damage to the extremity. Generally, the tourniquet should not remain inflated longer than 2 hours. After 2 hours it must be deflated, which causes a loss of anesthesia (Bruner, 1951; Kessler, 1966).

Anatomy

The technique of administering an intravenous regional anesthetic does not require specific anatomic landmarks, as is true of spinal or brachial plexus anesthesia. It is important to note that postinjection the local anesthetic is distributed throughout the extremity and is thought to work at three principal sites: (1) the peripheral nerve endings; (2) the neuromuscular junction; and (3) the nerve trunk (Reese, 1981). The primary site of action is controversial but appears to be on the small peripheral nerve branches (Holmes, 1980; Urban & McKain, 1982).

TABLE 29–10. Indications and Contraindications to Intravenous Regional Anesthesia

Indications
    Suturing of lacerations
    Reduction and manipulations of fractures
    Amputations
    Minor external operations (eg, ganglion removal)
Contraindications
    Severe peripheral vascular disease
    Infections of the extremity
    Patient refusal

Indications and Contraindications

Indications and contraindications to intravenous regional anesthesia are listed in Table 29–10. This technique is very useful for soft-tissue operations of the arm or hand (eg, ganglion removal). The block provides a bloodless field and anesthesia with relatively rapid onset and recovery. If the surgery is expected to last more than 2 hours, this technique is not advised. After 2 hours, the tourniquet must be deflated to prevent tissue damage. It is possible to reinflate the tourniquet and reinject, but, in actual practice, this is hard to accomplish.

Procedure

Administering an effective intravenous regional anesthetic requires specific attention to details. Table 29–11 emphasizes some of the important aspects. Various local anesthetic agents have been used, but only lidocaine hydrochloride is presently approved by the U.S. Food and Drug Administration (Fisher, 1980; personal communication). It is effective at low concentrations (0.5%) and relatively safe in large volumes. A dosage of 3 mg/kg lean body weight of a 0.5% solution is recommended.

Before proceeding with the block, the anesthetist must check all equipment for proper operation. This is true with any anesthetic technique, but it is particularly important with an intravenous regional anesthetic. Many unsuccessful blocks can be attributed to a leaky cuff or failure of the pressure system supplying the tourniquet. Before administering the block, the anesthetist must pressurize the tourniquet system to ensure that no leaks are present and identify that the connections are correct between the double-cuffed tourniquet and the selection switch.

The patient is placed in a supine position, and cottonwool (Webril) and a double-cuffed tourniquet are applied to the proximal aspect of the extremity. The cottonwool should be applied wrinkle-free and in an

TABLE 29–11. Important Steps in the Administration of an Intravenous Regional Block

I. Preparation
  A. Prepare equiprnent.
    1. Arrange resuscitation equipment and medications.
    2. Obtain double tourniquet with switch valve and inflationary device.
    3. Obtain Esmarch bandage and roller gauze.
    4. Obtain IV catheter (20 gauge), extension tubing, and 50-mL syringe.
  B. Prepare patient.
    1. Perform standard IV insertion.
    2. Explain procedure.
    3. Position patient supine.
    4. Apply cottonwool (Webril) to upper arm.
    5. Apply double tourniquet.
II. Procedure
  A. Insert IV catheter and connect to syringe assembly
  B. Elevate extremity and wrap tightly with Esmarch bandage
  C. Inflate proximal cuff.
  D. Remove Esmarch bandage and examine extremity for blanching.
  E. Inject local anesthetic agent and monitor for toxic symptoms.
  F. Remove IV catheter (optional).
  G. Inflate distal cuff and deflate proximal cuff to treat tourniquet pain.

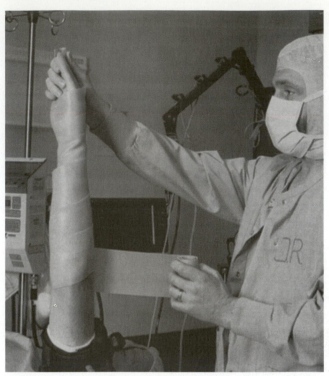

Figure 29–8. Application of double-tourniquet cuff to an extremity wrapped with an Esmarch bandage.

adequate amount to prevent skin damage from tourniquet pressure. The double-cuffed tourniquet should then be applied snugly to ensure that cuff pressure is applied to as large a surface area as possible on tourniquet inflation.

An intravenous catheter is inserted into a good-size vein using an appropriate aseptic technique. Individual opinion on the best site for the catheter placement varies, but, generally, the closer the catheter site is to the operation field, the better the anesthesia will be in that specific area (Dunbar & Mazzee, 1967). Leaving the catheter in place can facilitate reinjection of the local anesthetic, but it makes placement near the operative site difficult.

One of the most important points in administering an intravenous regional block is to ensure complete exsanguination of the extremity. Early elevation of the limb and tightly wrapping the extremity distally to proximally with an Esmarch bandage should facilitate adequate exsanguination (Fig. 29–8). The Esmarch bandage should be wrapped tightly up to the tourniquet and the proximal cuff inflated 100 to 150 mm Hg above the patient's systolic pressure. A maximum pressure of 300 mm Hg for the upper extremity should not be exceeded (Thorn-Alquist, 1971). After the Esmarch bandage has been removed, the extremity should have a pale, blanched appearance and no pulses. If this is not the case, it is advisable to rewrap the extremity to obtain better results. The presence of blood in the extremity will significantly decrease the action of the local anesthetic agent.

After the extremity has been exsanguinated adequately, the anesthetist slowly injects the local anesthetic agent while monitoring for signs of adverse reactions. After injection, the intravenous catheter may be removed and the disinfectant solution applied in preparation for the surgical procedure. The onset of anesthesia should occur within 5 to 10 minutes of injection.

Management

The management of an intravenous block is similar in many respects to the management of other regional anesthetic techniques. Adequate sedation and effective communication alleviate patient anxiety and help ensure a pleasant experience. Tourniquet pain may occur after prolonged tourniquet occlusion (Cole, 1952). It often can be eliminated by inflating the distal tourniquet and deflating the proximal one, a maneuver that must be performed with caution. If at any time both cuffs become deflated, the block is terminated. If this occurs, the anesthetist must monitor for signs of a toxic reaction caused by the bolus effect of local anesthetic agent entering the bloodstream.

A local anesthetic toxic reaction may occur any time but is more likely immediately after tourniquet release. The occurrence of a toxic reaction can be directly related to the duration of ischemia and the dosage and volume of medication administered. To help prevent toxic reactions, the recommended local anesthetic dosage should not be exceeded, a reliable tourniquet should be used, and tourniquet release should be delayed 20 to 30 minutes after injection (Bier, 1908; Morrison, 1931).

To terminate the block, the anesthetist should use an inflation–deflation technique, especially if the time from injection is less than 45 minutes. The cycled deflation technique consists of deflating the tourniquet for 5 seconds and then reinflating it for 2 to 3 minutes (Merrifield & Carter, 1965). This procedure is repeated two to three times. This decreases the local anesthetic bolus effect associated with tourniquet release.

► CASE STUDY

A 35-year-old healthy female is having a cesarean section for failure of her labor to progress. The preanesthesia assessment reveals the patient has had a normal pregnancy. Her height is 5 feet, 6 inches, and vital signs and lab tests are within normal ranges. Following a review of the preanesthetic assessment and discussion with the patient, a spinal anesthetic is selected for the surgery.

The patient is transported to the operating room, and vital signs are reassessed by the anesthetist prior to positioning for the spinal administration. An intravenous fluid bolus of 500 to 1000 mL is given and the patient is placed in a lateral position.

1. What is the procedure for administering a spinal anesthetic to this patient, including drug doses and other considerations?

   The back is cleansed, prepared, and draped. The patient can be placed in either a sitting or a lateral position. A 25-gauge noncutting spinal needle is inserted into the subarachnoid space at the L4 level. After obtaining clear, free-flowing cerebrospinal fluid, 1.6 mL of 0.75% bupivacaine is injected. The patient is then quickly repositioned supine with left uterine displacement, vital signs checked, and nasal oxygen administered.

2. When should the level of the block be assessed, and what level would be appropriate for the cesarean section?

   Prior to the start of surgery the level of anesthesia is determined to be at the T4 dermatome. At this time the patient's blood pressure decreases to 90/60 mm Hg.

3. How should hypotension be managed in this patient?

   The anesthetist administers ephedrine 10 mg IV and increases the rate of intravenous fluid infusion. This action increases the blood pressure, and a healthy baby is delivered without complications.

4. What postanesthetic monitoring and care is appropriate?

   Following surgery the patient is taken to the postanesthesia care unit and monitored. One hour after admission the patient's vital signs have remained stable and motor function has returned to the lower extremities. The patient is then discharged from the unit. On the postoperative assessment the following day, no complications were noted.

► SUMMARY

Regional anesthesia is a technique appropriate for many types of surgery and provides patients with a safe and effective alternative to general anesthesia. The nurse anesthetist must have a comprehensive knowledge of anatomy, physiology, and pharmacology as well as the technical skills to execute the various regional techniques. Utilization of regional anesthesia in the clinical practice setting requires effective communication skills with the patient to gain cooperation and provide essential information to the patient and family.

► KEY CONCEPTS

- Prior to regional anesthesia a patient's preoperative assessment should include (1) obtaining informed consent; (2) performing a thorough history and physical examination; (3) establishing rapport; and (4) determining the best anesthetic care plan.
- Spinal anesthesia is indicated for lower abdomen, inguinal, and lower extremity surgery. The possibility of hypotension is a concern particularly in patients with cardiovascular disease.
- Vigilance in monitoring the patient during a regional anesthetic is required. Monitoring should include the cardiovascular and respiratory systems. Early detection of changes and appropriate interventions are essential for safe patient care.
- A spinal should not be administered above the second lumbar vertebra because of the increased potential for causing damage to the spinal cord.
- In administering a spinal anesthetic positioning is very important. Positioning should maximize

opening of the interspinous spaces and good anatomic orientation.

- During the administration of a spinal anesthetic the local anesthetic should not be injected in the presence of a bloody tap, abnormal cerebrospinal fluid, or a persistent paresthesia.
- Epidural analgesia may be administered as a single injection or continuous technique. If an epidural catheter is used, the catheter should not be removed from the needle after being inserted because of possible catheter shearing.
- An axillary brachial plexus block is indicated for operations involving the arm or hand. The anesthetist should not perform any regional anesthetic technique without equipment or drugs available to treat complications.

- The possibility of a toxic reaction exists anytime the local anesthetic enters the bloodstream (epidural, axillary block, or intravenous regional). The anesthetist must focus on prevention and close monitoring for signs, and, should a reaction occur, appropriate treatment to prevent cerebral hypoxia.
- Prior to proceeding with an intravenous regional block it is very important that the anesthetist check all equipment for proper operation. A leaky tourniquet cuff or failure of the pressure system will result in loss of the block.
- A cycled deflation technique should be used when terminating an intravenous regional block to prevent a toxic reaction from a bolus of the local anesthetic suddenly being released into the bloodstream.

▶ STUDY QUESTIONS

1. What preoperative considerations determine the suitability of regional anesthesia for a patient?

2. Where does the spinal cord end in the adult and what are the landmarks for selecting the site for a lumbar spinal or epidural anesthetic?

3. What is the importance of patient positioning prior to performing a regional anesthetic?

4. What equipment should be immediately available when performing a Bier block?

5. What is the minimum volume of local anesthetic agent that should be used for a brachial plexus block?

6. How should epidural catheters ideally be placed and threaded?

KEY REFERENCES

Cousins, M. J., & Bredenbaugh, P. O. (1982). *Neural blockade* (2nd ed.). Philadelphia: Lippincott.

Hahn, M. B., McQuillan, P. M., & Sheplock, G. J. (1996). *Regional anesthesia.* St. Louis, MO: Mosby Yearbook.

Raj, P. P. (1992). *Practical management of pain* (2nd ed.). St. Louis, MO: Mosby-Yearbook.

Urmey, W. F. (1997). *Techniques in regional anesthesia and pain management.* Philadelphia: Saunders.

REFERENCES

Abboud, T. K., Dror, A., Mosaad, P., Zhu, J., Mantilla, M., Swart, F., Gangolly, J., *et al.* (1988). Mini-dose intrathecal morphine for the relief of post-cesarean section pain: Safety, efficacy and ventilatory responses to carbon dioxide. *Anesthesia & Analgesia, 67,* 137–143.

Aboulish, E. (1977). *Pain control in obstetrics.* Philadelphia:. Lippincott.

Armstrong, I. A., Littlewood, D. G., & Chambers, W. A. (1983). Spinal anesthesia with tetracaine—The effect of added vasoconstrictors. *Anesthesia & Analgesia, 62,* 793–795.

Bengtasson, M., Lofstrom, J. B., & Malmquist, L. A. (1985). Skin conductance responses during spinal analgesia. *Acta Anesthesiologica Scandinavica, 27,* 67–71.

Bier, A. (1908). Concerning a new method of local anesthesia of the extremities. *Arch. f. Klin. Chir. 86,* 1007–1016. [English translation by Hellijas, C. S. (1967). *Survey of Anesthesiology, classic file, 11,* 294–300.]

Brown, D. L. (1994). In R. D. Miller (Ed.), *Anesthesia* (4th ed., pp. 1505–1533). New York: Churchill Livingstone.

Bruner, J. M. (1951). Safety factors in the use of the pneumatic tourniquet for the hemostasis in surgery of the hand. *Journal of Bone & Joint Surgery, 3A,* 221–224.

Ching, D. (1963). Epidural space: Anatomical and clinical aspects. *Anesthesia & Analgesia, 42,* 398–407.

Cole, F. (1952). Tourniquet pain. *Anesthesia & Analgesia, 31,* 63064.

Cousins, M. J., & Bridenbaugh, P. O. (1982). *Neural blockade* (2nd ed.). Philadelphia: Lippincott.

Covino, B. G., & Marx, G. F. (1980). Prolonged sensory/motor deficit following inadvertent spinal anesthesia. *Anesthesia & Analgesia, 62,* 55–58.

Dunbar, R. W., & Mazzee, R. I. (1967). Intravenous regional anesthesia—Experience with 779 cases. *Anesthesia & Analgesia, 46,* 806–813.

Freund, F. G., Bonica, J. J., et al. (1967). Ventilatory reserve and level of motor block during high spinal and epidural anesthesia. *Anesthesiology, 28,* 834.

Greene, N. M. (1979). Present concepts of spinal anesthesia. *Refresher Courses Anesthesiology, 7,* 131.

Greene, N. M. (1981). *Physiology of spinal anesthesia* (3rd ed.). Baltimore: Williams & Wilkins.

Greene, N. M. (1983). Uptake and elimination of local anesthetics during spinal anesthesia. *Anesthesia & Analgesia, 62,* 1013–1024.

Hahn, M. B., McQuillan, P. M., & Sheplock, G. J. (1996). *Regional anesthesia.* St. Louis, MO: Mosby-Yearbook.

Halpern, S., & Preston, R. (1994). Postdural puncture headache and spinal needle design: Metaanalyses. *Anesthesiology, 81,* 1376–1383.

Holmes, C. M. (1980). *Intravenous regional neural blockade in clinical anesthesia and pain* (pp. 343–354). Philadelphia: Lippincott.

Horlocker, T. T., McGregor, D. G., Matsushige, D. K., Schroeder, D. R., Besse, J. A., & the Perioperative Outcomes Group. (1997). A retrospective review of 4767 consecutive spinal anesthetics: Central nervous systems complications. *Anesthesia & Analgesia, 84,* 578–584.

Kessler, F. (1996). The brachial tourniquet and local analgesia in surgery of the upper limb. *Journal of Trauma,* 43–47.

Lanz, E., Theiss, D., & Janicovic, D. (1983). The extent of blockade following various techniques of brachial plexus block. *Anesthesia & Analgesia, 62,* 55–58.

Lund, P. C. (1983). Reflections upon the historical aspects of spinal anesthesia. *Regional Anesthesia, 8.*

MacIntosh, R. (1957). *Lumbar puncture and spinal analgesia.* Edinburgh: Livingstone.

Merrifield, A. J., & Carter, S. J. (1965). Intravenous regional anesthesia—lidocaine blood levels. *Anaesthesia, 20,* 287–293.

Miyabe, M., & Sato, S. (1997). The effect of head-down tilt position on arterial blood pressure after spinal anesthesia for cesarean delivery. *Regional Anesthesia, 22*(3), 239–242.

Montgomery, S. T. (1973). The use of the nerve stimulator with standard unsheathed needles in nerve blockade. *Anesthesia & Analgesia, 52,* 827–831.

Morrison, J. T. (1931). Intravenous local anesthesia. *British Journal of Surgery, 18,* 642–647.

Moya, F., & Smith, B. (1962). Spinal anesthesia for cesarean section: Clinical and biochemical studies of the effects on maternal physiology. *Journal of the American Medical Association, 179,* 608.

Raj, P. P. (1992). *Practical management of pain* (2nd ed.). St. Louis, MO: Mosby-Yearbook.

Reese, C. (1977). Conduction anesthesia of the upper extremity—A literature and technique review. *AANA Journal,* 269.

Reese, C. (1981). Intravenous regional conduction anesthesia—A technique and literature review, Part I. *AANA Journal,* 357–373.

Reimann, A. F., & Anson, B. J. (1944). The spinal cord and meninges. *Anatomical Record, 88,* 127.

Reisner, L. S., Hockman, B. N., & Plumer, M. H. (1980). Persistent neurologic deficit and adhesive arachnoiditis following intrathecal 2-chloroprocaine injection. *Anesthesia & Analgesia, 59,* 452–454.

Saberski, L. R., Kondamuri, S., & Osinubi, O. (1997). Identification of the epidural space: Is loss of resistance to air a safe technique? *Regional Anesthesia, 22*(1), 3–15.

Smith, B. L. (1976). Efficacy of a nerve stimulator in regional analgesia: Experience in a resident training programme. *Anaesthesia, 31,* 778–782.

Thompson, G., & Rorie, D. (1983). Functional anatomy of the brachial plexus sheaths. *Anesthesiology, 59,* 117–122.

Thorn-Alquist, A. M. (1971). Intravenous regional anesthesia—A seven year survey. *Acta Anaesthiologica Scandinavica, 15,* 23–32.

Urban, B., McKain, C. (1982). Onset and progression of the intravenous regional anesthesia with dilute lidocaine. *Anesthesia & Analgesia, 61,* 834–838.

Urmey, W. F. (1997). *Techniques in regional anesthesia and pain management.* Philadelphia: Saunders.

Winnie, A., Radonjic, R., Akkineni, S. R., & Durrani, Z. (1979). Factors influencing distribution of local anesthetic injected into the brachial plexus sheath. *Anesthesia & Analgesia, 58,* 225–233.

Winnie, A. P., Tay, C. H., Patel, K. P., Ramamurthy, S., & Durrani, Z. (1977). Pharmacokinetics of local anesthetics during plexus blocks. *Anesthesia & Analgesia, 56,* 852–862.

30 CHAPTER

Postoperative Management and Critical Care

Cecil B. Drain

▶ THE ROLE OF THE CRNA IN THE PACU AND ACUTE CARE SETTING

Anesthesia nursing care of the surgical patient begins in the preoperative phase, moves into the intraoperative phase, and ends after the postoperative phase. During each phase, it is of the utmost importance that appropriate, informed anesthesia nursing care be used to facilitate positive outcomes for the surgical patient. The primary purpose of the postanesthesia care unit (PACU) is the critical evaluation and stabilization of postoperative patients. The emphasis must be on anticipating and preventing complications resulting from anesthesia or the operative procedure. Anesthesia care in the acute care setting of the postanesthesia care unit (PACU) has far-reaching implications as to whether the patient will survive even the best administered anesthetic. The role of the nurse anesthetist in the PACU is collaborative. The nurse anesthetist's expertise can enhance the quality of nursing care administered in the PACU.

Nurse anesthetists can have an expanded role in the PACU setting. More specifically, in the managed care environment the role of the CRNA in various clinical settings will change. In the PACU setting, the CRNA may take on the role of physician extender. This will be particularly true in the small hospital setting.

Perianesthesia nurses (PANs) are professional nurses who are well versed in postanesthesia and critical care nursing. As described by Goldiner (1997), the Phase I postanesthesia care unit is an acute care unit to which the patient arrives directly from the operating room. The

staffing ratio depends on the acuity of the postanesthesia patient. For example, the ratio can be one nurse for every two patients, when one patient is unconscious, but stable, has no artificial airway, and is older than age 9 and/or when the other patient is conscious, stable, and free of complications; or with two conscious, stable patients that are free from complications. A staffing ratio of 1 to 1 is required at the time of admission until critical elements are met. Other patients who require 1-to-1 nursing care are those on mechanical life support and/or artificial airway and unconscious patients younger than age 9. Two postanesthesia nurses to one patient are required when the patient is critically ill and/or unstable.

Goldiner (1997) describes the Phase II unit as the ambulatory surgery setting from which the patient is discharged to home. In this unit, the staffing ratio can be one nurse to three patients when the patients are older than age 5 and are within a half-hour of the procedure and discharge or when patients are younger than age 5, who have their family present and are within a half-hour of discharge. A staffing ratio of one nurse to two patients is required for patients younger than age 5 without family and support staff present at initial admission. A 1-to-1 ratio is necessary for patients who become unstable and are awaiting transfer to a critical care unit.

The nurse anesthetist can collaborate with the PAN on many administrative matters and provide expert input into the clinical process in the PACU. This chapter discusses the basic care of the patient emerging from anesthesia, including assessment of the postanesthesia patient, the various treatment modalities, review of the common postanesthesia problems, and a sample case study.

► ASSESSMENT OF THE POSTANESTHESIA PATIENT

It is imperative that a knowledgeable, skillful postanesthesia nurse and nurse anesthetist fully assess the condition of each patient—not only at admission and at discharge but also at frequent intervals throughout the postanesthesia period. Assessment must be a continuous and complete process, leading to sound nursing judgments and the implementation of therapeutic care. Assessment includes gathering information from direct observation of the patient (the primary source), from the physician and other health care personnel, and from the medical record and the care plan (McGaffigan & Christoph, 1994).

The nurse anesthetist has a professional obligation to present and assess all pertinent data about the patient, including the patient's history, clinical status, and psychosocial state. The necessary data may be gathered by chart review, personal preoperative visit, intraoperative events, and consultation with other health care members who are providing care to the patient. The collection of such information should be a coordinated effort with all involved members of the health care team. Nursing diagnoses are established based on analysis of data collected during the assessment phase, and then an appropriate plan of care is generated.

Subjective Data Collection

Postanesthesia care of the patient recovering from anesthesia is a critical part of the total anesthetic experience. It is imperative that the perianesthesia nurse and the nurse anesthetist collaborate during the admission phase to facilitate a positive surgical and anesthetic experience for the surgical patient. Subjective data to be collected during this phase include a report of the patient's history and intraoperative anesthesia care of the patient.

Upon arrival at the PACU, a rapid assessment of the life-sustaining cardiorespiratory system is of initial concern. First, ensure that the airway is patent and that respirations are free and easy. Next, determine and record the patient's blood pressure, pulse, rate of respiration, and oxygen saturation level. Finally, inspect all dressings and drains for gross bleeding. These baseline observations, made immediately on admission, should be recorded in the admission note.

The Postanesthesia Report

Ideally, the surgeon and the nurse anesthetist should accompany the patient to the PACU, where the nurse anesthetist should give the following information to the PAN (Campbell & Johnston, 1991; Frost & Andrews, 1983).

1. Patient's name, sex, age, hospital number, height and weight, and native language, including communication handicaps, if any
2. Surgical procedure, including the name(s) of the surgeon(s), complications, and surgical and anesthesia times
3. Anesthetic technique and all agents used for the procedure, including preoperative medication and reversal agents
4. Intraoperative course, including vital signs, estimated blood loss, urine output, fluid therapy, and monitoring techniques (eg, laboratory and radiologic studies) used during the procedure
5. Previous medical history, including American Society of Anesthesiologists (ASA) physical status, baseline vital signs, medications, mental status, drug addiction history, allergies, and any other disease processes that would have an impact on the postanesthesia care.

Postoperative management should be elaborated on, and the areas of concentration should include oxygen therapy, breathing exercises, airway care, pain management, diagnostic tests, and, if indicated, mechanical ventilation. The anesthetist and PAN should mutually determine the postanesthesia recovery score.

Objective Data Collection

Postanesthesia Recovery Score

At the completion of the postanesthesia report, the PAN and the nurse anesthetist should conduct an assessment of the patient to determine the postanesthesia recovery score (PARS). This score aids both the PAN and the anesthetist in a collaborative effort to determine the focus of postanesthesia care and potential postoperative problems and to develop discharge criteria for the patient (Drain, 1994).

The PARS should be initiated when the patient is admitted to the PACU. Jointly, the nurse anesthetist and the PAN who will be providing direct nursing care to the patient conduct the PARS assessment. The nursing assessment using the PARS system should be repeated every 15 minutes by the same PAN to verify the patient's improvement or deterioration. The five primary areas of assessment in the PARS are activity, respiration, circulation, consciousness, and color. A PACU patient can receive 0, 1, or 2 points in each area of assessment (2 being the best score). A total score of 10 indicates that the patient is in the best possible condition, scores of 8 or 9 are considered safe, and a score of 7 or less is considered unsafe (Fig. 30–1). More specifically, the PARS system consists of the following criteria.

```
┌─────────────────────────────────────────────────────────────────────────────────────────┐
│ Name _____    Age ____   Sex ____   Date _____  │
│ Arrival Time to PACU _____    Discharge Time from PACU _____  │
│ Type of Surgery _____    Surgeon _____   │
│ _____    Analgesics Administered in PACU     │
│ Anesthetic Agents & Drugs _____    Agent   Dosage  Route   Time Given   │
│                                                      _____   _____  _____   _____   │
│ _____    _____   _____  _____   _____   │
│ Preoperative History _____    _____   _____  _____   _____   │
│ _____    _____   _____  _____   _____   │
│ Preoperative Vital Signs                                                                  │
│ BP ____ / ____      P ____     R ____                 PAR Score at Admission _____   │
│ Temp _____     O₂ Saturation _____ %              PAR Score at Discharge _____   │
└─────────────────────────────────────────────────────────────────────────────────────────┘
```

Figure 30–1. Chart for detailing the postanesthesia recovery score (PARS).

Activity. Muscular activity is assessed by observing the patient's ability to move his or her limbs either spontaneously or on command. If the patient is able to move all four extremities, a score of 2 is given; if only two extremities can be moved, the score is 1; and if none of the extremities can be moved, a score of 0 is given. This evaluation is of particular importance when assessing patients who have received subarachnoid, epidural, brachial plexus, or Bier blocks.

Respiration. If the patient can deep-breathe or perform the sustained maximal inspiration maneuver, can freely cough, and has normal respiratory rate and depth, a score of 2 is given. If the respiratory effort is labored or limited or if dyspnea is present, a score of 1 is given. If no spontaneous respiratory activity is evident and the condition necessitates ventilator or assisted respiration, the patient receives a score of 0.

Circulation. Because circulation is probably the most difficult to evaluate by a simple sign, blood pressure evaluated by comparing the reading derived in the PACU with the baseline preanesthetic systolic blood pressure value is used. When the systolic arterial blood pressure is within plus or minus 20% of the preanesthetic baseline level, the patient receives a score of 2. If the systolic blood pressure is within plus or minus 21% to 50% of the same control level, a score of 1 is given. When the PACU systolic arterial blood pressure is plus or minus 51% or more from the baseline reading, a score of 0 is given.

Consciousness. If the PACU patient is fully alert, as evidenced by the ability to answer questions, a score of 2 is given. If the patient is aroused only when called by name, a score of 1 is given. A score of 0 is given when the patient does not respond to auditory stimulation. For this particular assessment parameter, painful stimulation should not be used because even decerebrated patients may react to the stimulus. In addition, in such patients, it is difficult to develop a consistent, reliable, practical method of assessment.

Color. Patients who have an obviously normal or pink skin color are given a score of 2. If normal pigmentation of the skin prevents an accurate evaluation, the color of the oral mucosa should be assessed. If there is any alteration from the normal pink appearance that is not obvious cyanosis, the patient receives a score of 1; this includes pale, dusky, or blotchy discolorations, as well as jaundice. When frank cyanosis is present, a score of 0 is given.

Once these initial observations are made, it is essential systematically to assess the patient's total condition. This assessment may be made from head to toe or by systems, whichever the individual nurse prefers—the observations are essentially identical. The systems approach for assessment in the PACU, will be presented in detail. It should be noted that each system of the body has an integral function, and therefore all observations are interrelated.

Assessment of Respiratory Function

Because the postanesthesia patient has experienced some interference with his or her respiratory system, maintaining adequate gas exchange is a crucial aspect of care in the PACU. Any change in respiratory function must be detected early so that appropriate measures can be taken to ensure adequate oxygenation and ventilation. The most significant respiratory problems encountered in the immediate postoperative period include hypoventilation, airway obstruction, aspiration, and atelectasis.

Respiratory assessment is coupled with the related responses of the cardiovascular and neurologic systems to provide for total evaluation of the adequacy of gas exchange and ventilatory efficiency. Respiratory function is evaluated by clinical assessment. In addition, pulse oximetry is used to assess arterial oxygenation, and capnography is used to evaluate the adequacy of ventilation. Arterial blood gas measurements also may be a part of the respiratory assessment. The clinical assessment of the respiratory system should include inspection, palpation, percussion, and listening and auscultation (McGaffigan & Christoph, 1994).

Inspection

The resting respiratory rate of a normal adult is approximately 16 to 20 breaths/minute. Infants and children have a higher respiratory rate and a lower tidal volume than adults. Respirations should be quiet and easy, with a regular rate and rhythm. The chest should move freely as a unit, and expansion should be equal bilaterally. Alterations in symmetry may be due to many factors, including pain that may cause splinting at the incision site, consolidation, and pneumothorax. Note the character of the respirations; intercostal retractions, bulging, nasal flaring, or use of the accessory respiratory muscles are signs of respiratory distress. The depth of respiration is as important as the rate. Shallow respiration is the cardinal sign of continuing depression from anesthesia or preoperative medications, but it may be caused by many other factors, including incisional pain, obesity, tight binders, and dressings that restrict movements of the thoracic cage or abdomen. Shallow respirations and use of the neck and diaphragmatic muscles also may indicate recurarization from the use of skeletal muscle relaxants, such as atracurium, pancuronium, and vercuronium. The presence of chest movements alone, however, does not provide evidence that adequate gas exchange is occurring.

Airway obstruction may be present when the normal duration of inspiration versus exhalation is altered. Restlessness, confusion or anxiety, and apprehension are the earliest signs of hypoxemia and carbon dioxide (CO_2) retention, and they should receive immediate attention to determine their cause. The patient's color also should be regularly evaluated. Although this assessment is difficult, it provides important information about the respiratory function. However, it is crucial to remember that cyanosis is a late sign of severe tissue hypoxia; when it appears, immediate and vigorous efforts must be instituted to determine and correct the cause of hypoxia. The noninvasive monitors that are increasingly used in the PACU provide an effective means of continuously and objectively assessing gas exchange; pulse oximeters monitor hemoglobin oxygen saturation, and capnographs evaluate the adequacy of ventilation.

Note the presence of an artificial airway; airways are used primarily to maintain a patent air passage so that respiratory exchange is not hampered. Four types of airways commonly used are (1) the balloon-cuffed endotracheal tube (extends from the mouth through the glottis to a point above the bifurcation of the trachea); (2) the balloon-cuffed nasotracheal tube (extends from the nose

to the trachea); (3) the oropharyngeal airway (extends from the mouth to the pharynx and prevents the tongue from falling back and obstructing the trachea); and (4) the nasopharyngeal airway (extends from the nose to the pharynx). The airway must be kept clear of secretions for adequate gas exchange to occur, and it may need to be suctioned if gurgling develops. The airway should not be removed until the laryngeal and pharyngeal reflexes return; these reflexes enable the patient to control the tongue, to cough, and to swallow. If the patient "reacts on the airway" (makes attempts to eject it), gagging may occur that progresses to retching and vomiting. The airway should be removed as soon as clinically possible in this instance to avoid aspiration. An endotracheal tube can be removed as soon as the patient is adequately reversed and able to maintain the airway without it and when the danger of aspiration is over.

Palpation

Palpation and inspection of the chest may be carried out simultaneously to validate observations such as symmetry of expansion. In addition, crepitation may be heard or fremitus may be felt. The temperature, the level of moisture and general turgor of the skin, and the presence of any edema should be noted.

Percussion

The normal sound over the lungs is resonance. Dullness heard where there should normally be resonance indicates consolidation or filling of the alveolar or pleural spaces by fluid.

Listening and Auscultation

First, listen to the patient's respirations unaided. Normal respiration should be quiet; noisy breathing indicates a problem. Extraneous sounds always indicate some kind of obstruction; however, quiet breathing does not always indicate the absence of problems. An accumulation of mucus or other secretions evidenced by gurgling in any of the respiratory passages may cause airway obstruction and should be removed immediately. Purposeful coughing with good expiratory airflow is the most effective way of clearing secretions. If the patient is not yet reactive enough to do this alone, the secretions must be suctioned out orally and nasally. Nasotracheal suctioning may be useful to clear secretions and to stimulate cough, but the catheter is ineffective for reaching secretions distal to the carina. Obstruction also may occur from poor oropharyngeal muscle tone, resulting from the muscle-relaxant effect of general anesthesia plus the rolling back of the tongue. To relieve this obstruction, provide anterior pressure support on the angle of the jaw to open the air passages.

Crowing may indicate laryngospasm—a sudden, violent contraction of the vocal cords that may result in complete or partial closure of the trachea. If spasms continue, the airway must be maintained by inserting an endotracheal tube. Total blockage of the airway caused by laryngospasm produces no sound because of the absence of moving air. Equipment and medications for emergency tracheostomy should be readily available in the PACU.

Wheezing may indicate bronchospasm caused by a reflex reaction to an irritating mechanism. Bronchospasm occurs most often in patients with preexisting pulmonary disease such as severe emphysema, reactive airway disease, pulmonary fibrosis, and radiation pneumonitis. Laryngeal edema following endotracheal intubation is not uncommon and can contribute significantly to airway obstruction. Acute changes in the patient's skin condition, cardiovascular status, and bronchospasm after regional anesthesia must alert the nurse to a possible allergic reaction, but this event is rare.

With a stethoscope, listen to the patient's chest for the quality and intensity of breath sounds; any abnormalities should be located and identified. The total absence of breath sounds on one side may signal the presence of pneumothorax, obstruction, fluid, or blood within the pleural space. Auscultation of breath sounds in the PACU often is difficult, because the patient frequently cannot sit up or respond to commands to breathe deeply with the mouth open. Positioning the patient on alternating sides during the stir-up regimen provides an opportunity to examine the posterior lung field.

Pulse Oximetry

A pulse oximeter noninvasively measures the arterial oxygen saturation (SaO_2) in the blood (referred to as SpO_2 when measured by pulse oximetry). Therefore, it is a valuable adjunct to the clinical assessment of oxygenation. Many clinical indicators, such as the patient's color and the characteristics of the respirations, are subjective, and the physical signs of cyanosis are not evident until hypoxia is severe. Pulse oximetry monitoring is objective and continuous, and it provides an early warning of developing hypoxemia, allowing intervention before signs of hypoxia appear. Consequently, pulse oximetry has been widely adopted in the PACU as a tool for both safety monitoring and patient management. This assessment tool should be used on every patient in the PACU (New, 1985).

A pulse oximeter consists of a microprocessor-based monitor and a sensor. In addition to SpO_2, most oximeters display the pulse rate and have an adjustable alarm system that sounds when values register outside a designated range. A variety of sensors is available, each intended for application to specific sites and for use on patients of various sizes. The sensor is applied to a site with a good arterial supply. The most common application site is a finger or toe (hand or foot in

neonates); other sites include the nose, the forehead, or the temple.

Pulse oximetry is used in the PACU setting for safety monitoring and as a patient management tool. As a safety monitor, a pulse oximeter detects hypoxemia caused by unanticipated events such as severe atelectasis, bronchospasm, airway displacement, disconnections or kinks in the breathing circuit, and cardiac arrest. As a patient management tool, it is valuable in titrating oxygen therapy, weaning a patient from mechanical ventilation, and evaluating response to medications or other interventions intended to improve oxygenation.

Interpretation of SpO₂ Measurements. In the PACU, a hypothermic patient may have a left-shifted oxygen-dissociation curve. In such a patient, a given SpO_2 as measured by pulse oximetry may correspond to a lower-than-normal PaO_2. Although oxygen saturation may be adequate, hemoglobin will have a greater affinity for oxygen and be less willing to release oxygen to meet tissue needs. Warming the patient to a normothermic range facilitates oxygen unloading from the hemoglobin molecule and helps maintain adequate tissue oxygenation.

As with any technology, important clinical issues must be considered to use pulse oximetry appropriately. Shifts in the oxyhemoglobin dissociation curve that are caused by abnormal values of pH, temperature, PCO_2, and 2,3-diphosphoglycerate must be considered. It also is important to consider the patient's hemoglobin level because a pulse oximeter cannot detect a depletion in the total amount of hemoglobin. When using pulse oximetry on a postoperative patient with a low hemoglobin level, a high SpO_2 value may not be reflective of adequate oxygenation. The amount of hemoglobin, although well saturated with oxygen, may be inadequate to meet tissue needs because there are fewer carriers available to transport oxygen.

Adequate oxygenation is a factor of not only adequate oxygen saturation and hemoglobin values but also adequate oxygen delivery (which necessitates appropriate cardiac output) and the ability of the tissues to utilize oxygen effectively. When oxygen demand exceeds oxygen supply, tissue hypoxia results. Pulse oximetry readings, therefore, should be assessed in conjunction with all other indices of oxygenation.

Dysfunctional hemoglobins, variants of the hemoglobin molecule that are unable to transport oxygen, present a similar problem. Despite the high SpO_2 level, there may be insufficient hemoglobin available to carry oxygen. Carboxyhemoglobin is hemoglobin that is bound with carbon monoxide and therefore unavailable for carrying oxygen. Its effect must be considered in patients with burns or carbon monoxide poisoning and those who smoke. In methemoglobinemia, the iron molecule on the hemoglobin is oxidized from the ferrous to the ferric state. This form of iron is unable to transport oxygen. Methemoglobinemia, although rare, may occur in patients receiving nitrate-based and other drugs, as well as those exposed to a variety of toxins. When dysfunctional hemoglobins are suspected, assessment of oxygenation by pulse oximetry must be supplemented with arterial blood gas saturations measured by a laboratory co-oximeter to determine whether dyshemoglobins are present and oxygenation is adequate.

Perfusion at the sensor application site must be sufficient for the pulse oximeter to detect pulsatile flow. This is an important consideration for some PACU patients, such as those treated with vasoconstrictors, those who are markedly hypothermic, and those who have significantly reduced cardiac output. When applying the sensor, select a well-perfused site. If in doubt, check the pulse and adjacent capillary refill. If the monitor is unable to track the pulse, first evaluate the patient for adverse physiologic changes. Next, ensure that blood flow is not being restricted, such as by a flexed extremity, a blood pressure cuff, an arterial line, any restraints, or a sensor that is applied too tightly. Local perfusion to the sensor site can be improved by covering the site with a warm towel or by using a convective warming device such as the Bair Hugger. Certain sensors, such as a nasal sensor, are designed for application to areas where perfusion is preserved even when peripheral perfusion is relatively poor. Finally, some pulse oximeters use an electrocardiogram (ECG) signal to help identify the pulse, thus enhancing the instrument's ability to detect a weak pulse.

Patient movement seen in the PACU can produce false signals that interfere with the pulse oximeter's ability to identify the true pulse, leading to unreliable SpO_2 and pulse rate readings. When movement presents a problem, check whether the sensor is properly and securely applied; a sensor that is loosely attached or incorrectly positioned can magnify the effect of motion. If the problem persists, consider moving the sensor to a less active site. Pulse oximeters that use the ECG signal to identify pulse also can have an enhanced ability to distinguish between the true pulse and artifacts produced by motion. The result is more reliable than SpO_2 readings.

Normally, venous blood is nonpulsatile and is not detected by a pulse oximeter. In the presence of venous pulsations, the SpO_2 value provided by the pulse oximeter may be a composite of both arterial and venous saturations. Venous pulsations may occur in patients with severe right-sided heart failure or other pathophysiologic states that create venous congestion and in patients receiving high levels of positive end-expiratory pressure. They also may occur when the sensor is placed distal to a blood pressure cuff or occlusive dressing and when additional tape is wrapped tightly around the sensor. When venous pulsations are present, the PACU nurse should

take care in interpreting the SpO_2 readings and, if possible, attempt to eliminate their cause.

Because pulse oximeters are optical measuring devices, additional factors can influence the reliability of SpO_2 readings. To ensure good light reception, the sensor's light sources and detector must always be positioned according to the manufacturer's specifications. In the presence of bright lights, such as infrared warming devices, fluorescent lights, direct sunlight, and surgical lights, the sensor must be covered with an opaque material, or else incorrect SpO_2 readings may result. Also, agents that significantly change the optical-absorbing properties of blood, such as recently administered intravascular dyes, can interfere with reliable SpO_2 measurements. The use of pulse oximetry with certain nail polishes, especially those that are blue, green, and reddish-brown in color, may result in inaccurate readings. If nail polish in these shades cannot be removed, the sensor should be applied to an alternate unpolished site.

Capnography

Monitoring CO_2 in respiratory gases provides an early warning of physiologic and mechanical events that interfere with normal ventilation. Capnography, which measures CO_2 at the patient's airway, is increasingly used in the PACU (Skoog, 1989). It allows continuous assessment of the adequacy of alveolar ventilation, the function of the cardiopulmonary system, ventilator function, and the integrity of the airway and the breathing circuit. Consequently, it enables the early detection of many potentially catastrophic events, including the onset of malignant hyperthermia, esophageal intubation, hypoventilation, partial or complete airway obstruction, breathing circuit leaks or disconnects, a large pulmonary embolus, and cardiac arrest.

To measure exhaled CO_2, the most common type of capnograph passes infrared light at a wavelength that is absorbed by CO_2 through a sample of the patient's respiratory gas. The amount of light that is absorbed by the patient's gas is reflective of the amount of CO_2 in the sample (Sanders, 1989).

Capnographs differ in the manner in which they obtain respiratory gas samples for analysis. Sidestream (or diverting) capnographs transport the sample through a narrow-gauge tubing to a measuring chamber. Mainstream (or nondiverting) capnographs position a flow-through measurement chamber directly on the patient's airway. Special adapters are available to allow sidestream capnographs to be used on nonintubated patients. The sample adapter should be placed as close to the patient's endotracheal tube or airway as possible.

In addition to the diagnostic usefulness of changes in the capnograph, capnography has specific applications that are particularly valuable in the PACU. Of primary importance is its ability to provide early warning of hypoventilation, which in the PACU may be secondary to anesthesia, sedation, analgesia, or pain. A falling $ETCO_2$ may indicate pulmonary hypoperfusion due to blood loss or hypotension. During rewarming, $ETCO_2$ values are likely to increase as metabolic activity increases. Capnography can signal when shivering is producing an unacceptable increase in oxygen consumption and metabolic rate. During ventilator weaning, capnography is valuable in assessing the adequacy of ventilation.

End-Tidal versus Arterial CO_2. Under normal conditions, when ventilation and perfusion are well matched, $ETCO_2$ closely approximates arterial CO_2 ($Paco_2$). The difference between the $Paco_2$ and the $ETCO_2$ levels is referred to as the alveolar–arterial CO_2 difference (a − $ADCO_2$). Usually the $ETCO_2$ values are as much as 5 mm Hg lower than $Paco_2$ levels. When the two measurements differ significantly, there is usually an anomaly in the patient's physiology, the breathing circuit, or the capnograph. Significant divergence between $ETCO_2$ and $Paco_2$ measurements often is attributable to increased alveolar dead space: CO_2-free gas from non-perfused alveoli mixes with gas from perfused regions, decreasing the $ETCO_2$ measurement. Clinical conditions that cause increased dead space, such as pulmonary hypoperfusion, cardiac arrest, and pulmonary embolus, can increase the a − $ADCO_2$. Changes in the a − $ADCO_2$ can be used to assess the efficacy of the treatment: as the patient's dead space improves, the $PAO_2 − PaO_2$ narrows. Alternatively, a significant $PAO_2 − PaO_2$ can indicate incomplete alveolar emptying (such as with reactive airway disease), a leak in the gas-sampling system that allows loss of respiratory gas, and contamination of respiratory gas with fresh gas.

Assessment of Cardiovascular Function and Perfusion

The three basic components of the circulatory system that must be evaluated are (1) the heart as a pump; (2) the blood; and (3) the arteriovenous system. The maintenance of good tissue perfusion depends on a satisfactory cardiac output. Therefore, most assessment is aimed at evaluating cardiac output.

Clinical Assessment

Observe the overall condition of the patient, especially skin color and turgor. Peripheral cyanosis, edema, dilatation of the neck veins, shortness of breath, and many other findings may be indicative of cardiovascular problems. In addition to checking all operative sites for blood loss, note the amount of blood lost during surgery and the patient's most recent hemoglobin level.

Blood Pressure Monitoring

Arterial blood pressure must be assessed in the preoperative physical assessment, on admission to and discharge from the PACU, and at frequent, regular intervals during the PACU stay. As Henneman and Henneman (1989) state, arterial blood pressure is currently measured either noninvasively (indirectly) or invasively (directly). Noninvasive methods include manual cuff measurement with either an aneroid or mercury sphygmomanometer and automatic measurements with an electronic blood pressure monitor. Invasive measurement may be accomplished via a transduced arterial line.

To assess their significance, blood pressure readings in the postoperative period must be compared with preoperative baseline measurements. A low postoperative blood pressure may be the result of a number of factors, including the effects of muscle relaxants, spinal anesthesia, preoperative medication, changes in the patient's position, blood loss, poor lung ventilation, and peripheral pooling of blood. The administration of oxygen to help eliminate anesthetic gases and to assist the patient in awakening causes an increase in blood pressure. Deep breathing, leg exercises, verbal stimulation, and conversation can be instituted to raise the blood pressure. A low fluid volume may be augmented by increasing the rate of intravenous fluids, which helps maintain the arterial pressure. Any method designed to raise the pressure must be instituted with consideration for the patient's overall condition.

An increase in blood pressure postoperatively is not uncommon because of the effects of anesthesia, respiratory insufficiency, or decreased respiratory rate and depth causing CO_2 retention. The surgical procedure, with its accompanying discomfort, also causes increased blood pressure. Emergence delirium, with its excitement, struggling, and pain, also may be a causative factor in a transient increase in blood pressure. Obviously, it is important to determine the cause before treatment is instituted. In patients with uncontrolled hypertension, continuous intravenous antihypertensive medications may be required. However, it is extremely important to diagnose the cause of the hypertension so that effective therapy may be employed rapidly.

Pulse Pressure Monitoring

Pulse pressure is an important determinant in the evaluation of perfusion. Because of the pulsatile nature of the heart, blood enters the arteries intermittently, causing pressure increases and decreases. The difference between the systolic and diastolic pressures equals the pulse pressure. The pulse pressure is affected by two major factors: the stroke volume output of the heart and the compliance (total distensibility) of the arterial tree. The pulse pressure is determined approximately by the ratio of stroke output to compliance. Therefore, any condition that affects either of these factors also affects the pulse pressure.

To evaluate the patient's cardiovascular status accurately, all signs and symptoms must be evaluated individually as well as within the body system as a whole. For example, cool extremities, decreased urine output, and narrowed pulse pressure may be indicative of decreased cardiac output, even when blood pressure is normal.

Pulses

The rate and character of all pulses should be assessed bilaterally. Examine the pulses simultaneously to determine their equality, and note the time of arrival in the PACU. Peripheral arterial occlusion is not uncommon; if it is suspected, a Doppler instrument can be of great value in detecting the presence or absence of blood flow. Occlusion is an emergency and must be reported to the surgeon at once. Irregularities in pulse are most frequently caused by premature beats, generally premature ventricular contractions (PVCs) or premature atrial contractions (PACs). These irregular rhythms should be thoroughly investigated before therapy is initiated.

Electrocardiographic Monitoring

The CRNA should have a basic understanding of cardiac monitoring and should be able to interpret the basic cardiac rhythms and dysrhythmias and correlate them with expected cardiac output and its effects on the patient's condition. Moreover, ECG monitoring should be available for each patient in a Phase I PACU and should be readily available for patients in Phase II units. Arrhythmias of any type may occur at any time and in any patient during the postoperative period. Any type of cardiac arrhythmia may be seen in the PACU. The causes of specific arrhythmias must be carefully differentiated before any treatment is instituted. All abnormal rhythms should be documented with a rhythm strip and recorded in the patient's progress record. Any questionable rhythms should be documented by a complete 12-lead ECG.

Electrical monitoring of the patient's heart is only one assessment parameter and must be interpreted in conjunction with other salient parameters before therapy is initiated. Cardiac monitors generally depict only a single lead. They do not detect all rhythm disturbances and alterations, and a 12-lead ECG is essential to define a conduction problem accurately.

In regard to lead placement in the PACU, the site on the chest is based on a triangular arrangement of positive, negative, and ground electrodes. Avoid placing electrodes directly over the diaphragm, areas of auscultation, heavy bones, or large muscles. Allow adequate space for application of defibrillator paddles in the event that defibrillation should become necessary. The modified lead II is the most commonly used because it is the most ver-

satile; it is useful in assessing P-waves, PR intervals, and atrial arrhythmias. The modified chest lead I is useful for assessing bundle branch block and differentiating between ventricular arrhythmias and aberrations. This lead is useful when the patient is known to have preexisting cardiac disease.

Hemodynamic Monitoring

Although more prominent in cardiac surgery, additional hemodynamic monitoring is commonly used with higher-acuity patients not cared for in many PACUs (McGaffigan & Christoph, 1994). Hemodynamic monitoring can be accomplished via the following invasive lines: a flow-directed pulmonary artery catheter, a central venous pressure catheter, a left-atrial or right-atrial catheter, a pulmonary artery thermistor catheter, or a peripheral arterial catheter (A-line).

Right-Atrial Pressure. The normal right-atrial pressure ranges from 0 to 7 mmHg. Pressures exceeding that level can be the result of fluid overload, right-ventricular failure, tricuspid valve abnormalities, pulmonary hypertension, constrictive pericarditis, or cardiac tamponade. Values in the lower range are usually indicative of hypovolemia.

Pulmonary Artery Pressure. Pulmonary artery systolic pressures normally range from 15 to 25 mmHg, whereas a normal pulmonary artery diastolic pressure is 8 to 15 mmHg. Hypovolemia contributes to low pressure readings. Increased volume loads that can develop with an atrial or ventricular septal defect or left-ventricular failure can create elevations in pressure. In addition, obstructions to forward flow that can be caused by mitral stenosis or pulmonary hypertension can lead to an elevation in pulmonary artery pressures.

Pulmonary Capillary Wedge Pressure. Normal pulmonary capillary wedge pressure (PCWP) recordings are between 6 and 15 mmHg. Values in this range can be caused by an increased volume load, as is seen in left-ventricular failure, or created by an obstruction to forward flow. Such obstructions may be caused by mitral stenosis or regurgitation or by a pulmonary embolism. Lower values may be a result of hypovolemia or indicative of an obstruction to left-ventricular filling, which could occur with a pulmonary embolism, pulmonary stenosis, or right-ventricular failure.

Left-Atrial Pressure. Normal left-atrial pressures range from 4 to 12 mmHg. As is seen with the PCWP, elevations in left-atrial pressure are associated with volume overloads or obstructions to forward flow, the latter of which may consist of left-ventricular failure states, mitral or aortic valve dysfunctions, or constrictive pericarditis.

Lower recordings generally are a consequence of hypovolemia from inadequate volume or related to an obstruction to forward flow. Such an obstruction may be a pulmonary embolism or pulmonic valve stenosis, or it may result from right-ventricular failure.

Mean Arterial Pressure. Normal mean arterial pressures generally range between 80 and 120 mmHg. In a postoperative cardiac surgical patient, pressures lower than 60 mmHg are generally avoided, because coronary artery filling may be limited or impeded when parameters reach this level and may contribute to an ischemic or infarction state. Conversely, pressures higher than 120 mmHg are avoided, because they place too much stress on newly created suture lines that could readily rupture under sustained pressures.

Cardiac Output and Cardiac Index. Cardiac output is the amount of blood ejected by the ventricle in 1 minute. Normal cardiac output is 5 to 6 L/min and the normal cardiac index (CI) ranges from 2.5 to 3.5 L/min/m^2. Because the cardiac index takes body size into consideration, it is a better indicator of the patient's perfusion status.

Systemic Vascular Resistance. Systemic vascular resistance (SVR) is the resistance the left ventricle must work against to eject its volume of blood. Normal SVR is 900 to 1300 dyne/s/cm^5. An elevated SVR can create enough resistance to left-ventricular ejection that cardiac output and cardiac index will decrease, which will lead to a state of hypoperfusion or shock. Infusion of vasodilators and afterload-reducing agents can counteract this elevation.

Pulmonary Vascular Resistance. Pulmonary vascular resistance (PVR) is the resistance the right ventricle must work against to eject blood into the pulmonary bed. Normal PVR is 80 to 240 dyne/s/cm^5. An elevated PVR can create enough resistance to right-ventricular ejection for right-sided failure or infarction to develop. Infusion of vasodilators or pulmonary artery dilators, such as aminophylline, can counteract these elevations.

Assessment of Central Nervous System Function

All anesthetics affect the central nervous system (CNS). At present, even though we do not know exactly how narcosis occurs, anesthetics are general, nonselective depressants. The complexity of the CNS, coupled with our incomplete knowledge of how it functions, makes it a most difficult system to evaluate. Assessment of the CNS in the PACU generally involves only gross evaluation of behavior, level of consciousness, intellectual performance, and emotional status.

Assessment of Thermal Balance

The measurement of the patient's body temperature in the PACU is particularly important. At minimum, the preoperative assessment, initial postoperative physical assessment, and discharge evaluation of the patient in Phases I and II PACUs should include documentation of temperature. Normal body temperature may vary from 35.9°C to 38°C. In the normal healthy adult, body temperature remains fairly constant, owing to the balance between heat production and heat loss. According to Shinozaki, Deane, and Perkins (1988), alterations in body temperature occur frequently in the postoperative patient.

Premedications, anesthesia, and the stress of surgery all interact in a complex fashion to disrupt normal thermoregulation. Both hypothermia (temperature below 36°C) and hyperthermia (temperature above 39°C) are associated with physiologic alterations that may interfere with recovery. Patients at the age extremes, and those who are extremely debilitated, are at even greater risk for the development of temperature abnormalities postoperatively.

The accuracy of axillary, rectal, or oral measurement is frequently debated. Core temperature (approximate value of temperature of blood perfusing the major metabolically active organs) is estimated only by oral and rectal temperature readings. Invasive techniques that use the thermistor on a pulmonary artery catheter, the tympanic membrane, or the bladder as a site for monitoring temperature are more accurate. Unless required during surgery or because of a specific problem, these temperature-monitoring modalities are seldom used in the PACU.

Shell (skin) temperature may be measured at the axilla or forehead with conventional thermometers or liquid crystal temperature strips. Shell temperature does not accurately reflect core temperature, although it may at least indicate gross trends.

Infrared tympanic membrane thermometry is increasingly used in the PACU. It is noninvasive and nontraumatic and may be used with patients of all sizes. When placed over the outer third of the auditory canal, the sensor on this otoscope-like thermometer gathers emitted infrared energy from the ear and translates this energy into a temperature reading within seconds. The infrared tympanic thermometer has been found to accurately track core temperature as measured by the thermistor tip of a pulmonary artery catheter (Shinozaki et al., 1988).

Management of the hypothermic patient is directed toward restoring normothermia and avoiding shivering.

Warm blankets may be placed over the patient as specific hospital protocol allows. Convective warming devices, such as the Bair Hugger, provide a safe and effective means of gradually rewarming the patient (Kruse, 1983).

Assessment of Fluid and Electrolyte Balance

Evaluation of a patient's fluid and electrolyte status involves total body assessment. Imbalances readily occur in the postoperative patient owing to a number of factors, including the restriction of food and fluids preoperatively, fluid loss during surgery, and stress. The normal body response to the stress of surgery is renal retention of water and sodium. In addition, patients often have abnormal avenues of fluid loss postoperatively.

Each patient must be evaluated to determine his or her baseline requirements and the fluid needed to replace abnormal losses. The normal adult deprived of oral intake requires 2000 to 2200 mL of water per day to make up for urinary output and insensible loss.

Most patients admitted to the PACU from the operating room will be receiving intravenous fluids. The anesthetist must have an open intravenous line for the administration of necessary medications and replacement fluids intraoperatively, and an open line is needed postoperatively to supply necessary fluids, electrolytes, and medications. Because all efforts to substitute for normal oral intake of electrolytes and adequate volumes of fluid are, at best, temporary and inadequate, the first objective is to return the patient to adequate oral intake as soon as possible.

Oral fluids should be prohibited after anesthesia until the laryngeal and pharyngeal reflexes are fully regained, as evidenced by the patient's ability to gag and swallow effectively. If the patient is permitted oral intake, it is best to start with small amounts of ice chips, because these are less likely to cause nausea and vomiting. Some PACUs use isotonic ice chips that are made from a balanced electrolyte solution, such as Lytren®. If ice chips are well tolerated, the patient can progressively increase oral intake to include water and other clear liquids. Kool-Aid® and fruit-flavored popsicles are well tolerated and accepted by both children and adults. In addition, carbonated beverages may be soothing to a patient who feels slightly nauseated.

Fluid Output

Normal output in the average adult results from obligatory urinary output and insensible avenues of loss, including evaporation of water from the skin and exhalation during respiration. The amount of urine necessary for the normal renal system to excrete the waste products of a day's metabolism is approximately 600 mL. Op-

timally, 30 mL/h or more of urine should be obtained from a catheterized adult to ensure proper hydration and kidney function. Urinary output should be closely monitored in the recovery phase; measurement of urinary output and urine specific gravity yields important clues to the overall status of the patient and may alert the nurse to overhydration or dehydration, or the development of shock.

A lower-than-normal urinary output can be expected in the postoperative patient as a result of the body's normal reaction to stress; however, an unduly small volume of urine (less than 500 mL in 24 hours) may indicate the presence of renal insufficiency.

▶ TREATMENT MODALITIES IN THE PACU

Nurse anesthetists use both respiratory therapy and mechanical ventilation in the perioperative setting. This section discusses treatment modalities utilized in the PACU and includes oxygen therapy and mechanical ventilation, along with the modified stir-up regime.

Respiratory Therapy

Oxygen Therapy

There are two types of oxygen therapy systems: high flow and low flow (McPherson, 1990; Shapiro & Cane, 1990). When determining which system is better suited for the patient, the comfort of the patient, humidification, and desired oxygen concentration should be considered.

A low-flow system for the administration of oxygen exists when air entrainment varies to provide the patient's inspiratory flow requirement. A low-flow system for the administration of oxygen supplies less than the total inspired volume of gas needed by the patient. The additional volume of gas required to meet the patient's inspiratory demand is supplied by room air entrained during active inspiration.

The actual concentration of inspired oxygen provided by a low-flow system depends on four factors. First, a reservoir for the accumulation of oxygen that will increase the inspired oxygen concentration must be available. The larger the reservoir, the greater the resultant increase in inspired oxygen concentration. The nasopharynx and oropharynx act as an anatomic reservoir, with a volume of approximately 50 mL. The oxygen therapy device itself also can serve as a reservoir of varying volume; for example, the area under a face mask or the reservoir bag, which is a part of many oxygen systems, serves as a reservoir. Second, the oxygen flow rate provided also varies with the inspired oxygen concentration. In general, the greater the flow rate of oxygen into the system, the higher the inspired concentration. This effect is limited by the volume of the available oxygen reservoir. Once this reservoir is filled, the excess flow escapes into the atmosphere. Third, the patient's ventilation pattern affects the inspired oxygen concentration. A more rapid respiratory rate and a greater-than-normal tidal volume reduce the inspired concentration. The degree to which this occurs varies with the degree of change in the patient's ventilatory pattern. Fourth, the oxygen therapy device must fit properly to achieve the desired result.

The nasal cannula and catheter are classified as low-flow devices that deliver low to midrange oxygen concentrations. The nasal cannula is comfortable for the patient, but it is easy to dislodge from its desired position. Mouth breathing or any obstruction to the flow of oxygen through the nasal route will reduce the concentration of inspired oxygen (F_{IO_2}). The nasal catheter is not as comfortable for the patient, but does offer greater stability. Both the cannula and the catheter, when used at excessive flow rates of oxygen, can cause considerable discomfort, such as drying of secretions, nasal bleeding, and gastric distension. The flow rate recommended by Oakes (1988) for the cannula and the catheter is 1 to 6 L/min. Actual inspired oxygen concentrations range from approximately 24 to 44% (Table 30–1).

Oxygen masks offer slightly higher oxygen concentrations than nasal devices. With the addition of a reservoir bag, masks of various types can deliver very high concentrations of inspired oxygen. To deliver the highest concentration possible, the mask must fit tightly, which may be uncomfortable for the patient. The oronasal face mask may be hazardous for patients at risk of regurgitation and aspiration. Oxygen masks should be operated at flow rates from 5 to 8 L/min. The inspired oxygen concentration ranges from approximately 40% to 60% (Oakes, 1988). A concentration greater than 60% is difficult to achieve because of the limited reservoir available.

Oxygen masks with an added reservoir bag can deliver very high inspired oxygen concentrations. These devices must be operated at flow rates high enough to prevent the reservoir bag from being emptied during inspiration. If this occurs, the patient will supplement the inspired volume with room air and dilute the oxygen concentration. Masks with a reservoir bag should be operated at a minimum flow rate of 6 L/min, with a maximum flow rate of about 10 L/min. The concentration of inspired oxygen will range from approximately 60% to approximately 80%, depending on the patient's ventilation pattern.

Tracheostomy masks and T-tubes are similar in their oxygen-delivery capabilities to those of other masks; however, because the upper airway is bypassed in the tracheotomized or intubated patient, the nasopharynx and oropharynx cannot be used as an oxygen reservoir. The loss of this reservoir causes a slight decrease in the inspired oxygen concentration. Loss of the anatomic reservoir can be compensated for, if necessary, by using an oxygen therapy device with a larger reservoir.

The simple, clear plastic face tent is a low-flow oxygen therapy device. It is well tolerated by the patient recovering from anesthesia and supplies extra humidity to the patient. The recommended flow rate for the face tent is 4 to 8 L/min through a bubble-through humidifier. The actual inspired oxygen concentration ranges from approximately 30% to 55% (Shapiro & Cane, 1990).

A high-flow system for the administration of oxygen is one in which the flow rate and reservoir capacity are adequate to provide the total inspired volume to the patient (McPherson, 1990; Shapiro & Cane, 1990). Consequently, the F_{IO_2} is premixed and predictable. An air entrainment principle is used to create this very high flow of gas. This type of system is capable of delivering both low and high concentrations of oxygen. The most common example of a high-flow system is the Venturi-type mask, which uses a Venturi device to produce a specific oxygen concentration. A relatively low flow of 100% oxygen is delivered

TABLE 30–1. Oxygen-Delivery Systems (F_{IO_2} Assumed on Eupnea)

Delivery System	Liter (L/m) Flow	F_{IO_2}	Comments
Low-flow delivery systems			
Nasal cannula	1–6	24–44	F_{IO_2} increases at 4% per L/m increase; comfortable
Nasal catheter	1–6	24–44	Same as nasal cannula
Simple mask	5–8	40–60	F_{IO_2} increases at 5% per L/m increase; less comfortable
Partial rebreathing mask	6–10	55–70	High F_{IO_2} delivered; same as simple mask; flow should be sufficient to keep reservoir bag from deflating on inspiration
Nonrebreathing mask	6–10	70–100	High F_{IO_2} delivered; same as partial rebreathing mask
High-flow delivery systems			
Venturi mask	Variable	24–50	Exact F_{IO_2} delivered to patient; device of choice for patient with hypoxic drive
Nebulizer with face tent, aerosol mask, or T-piece	6–12	30–100	Used to deliver oxygen and/or aerosol in high concentration; controls temperature of gas

through the Venturi device, creating a high velocity as it escapes. As a result of this high velocity, room air is entrained to mix with the 100% oxygen. This mixing, which is designed to occur at a specific ratio, produces a high flow with a relatively specific and consistent oxygen concentration. Depending on the manufacturer, various concentrations are available ranging from a low of 24% to a high of 50%. Because of the high flow created with this type of system, changes in the patient's ventilatory pattern do not greatly affect the inspired oxygen concentration. To achieve the desired oxygen concentration, the manufacturer's guidelines pertaining to oxygen flow rate to achieve a desired FIO_2 should be adhered to.

When a patient's drive to breathe is due mainly to hypoxic or secondary drive, oxygen therapy should not be omitted merely because of the fact that the patient will become apneic as a result of cessation of the hypoxic drive from high oxygen concentrations (Drain, 1994). The patient who is breathing on the hypoxic drive should receive oxygen at a precise FIO_2. In this case, a high-flow oxygen delivery system using the Venturi principle should be used. The minimal oxygen concentration for the patient can be dialed in on the Venturi mask. The patient can be monitored by oxygen saturations or arterial blood gases. For patients whose control of ventilation is through the secondary drive, the PaO_2 should be in the range of 60 to 70 torr, and the oxygen saturation should be greater than 96%.

Humidity Therapy

Humidity therapy, which is basically the addition of moisture to therapeutic gases, is a major therapeutic intervention used in the practice of anesthesia nursing. Humidification is indicated to enhance bronchial hygiene and when continuous gas therapy is being administered (McPherson, 1990). The intended outcomes of humidity therapy are hydration of inspired secretions, maintenance of the mucus blanket, and reduction of airway inflammation. Humidity therapy can be classified into two major categories based on purpose: (1) to supply enough water vapor to the inspired gas to enhance the patient's comfort; and (2) to heat the gas to prevent a reduction in the patient's body temperature by providing a more normal body humidity. The efficiency of humidification devices is increased by enhancing the time of contact between gas and water by increasing the surface area involved in the water–gas interface or heating the water (Shapiro & Cane, 1990).

Humidification devices are basically of two major types: simple humidifiers and heated humidifiers (McPherson, 1990). On the one hand, simple humidifiers are nonheating devices. Examples of simple humidifiers are given in Table 30–2. Heated humidifiers, on the other hand, enhance the efficiency of humidification by focusing on the heating properties of humidification. More specifically, bubble diffusion humidifiers or cascade humidifiers are used to replace the heat and moisture nor-

TABLE 30–2. Aerosol and Humidity Therapy Delivery Systems

Delivery System	Use	Comments
Aerosol Nebulizers		
Small-reservoir nebulizer: sidestream, mainstream, mininebulizer	Used to deliver aerosolized medications to a patient intermittently; usually 2 to 5 mL of solution, 1- to 40-μm particle size	Only precautions are those for the medications; use air for patients on hypoxic drive
Large-reservoir jet nebulizer	Used for continuous oxygen and/or aerosol therapy; 1- to 40-μm particle size, $\frac{1}{2}$- to 1-mL/min output	Condensation collects in tubing; correct solution level must be maintained
Ultrasonic nebulizer	Used to mobilize thick secretions in lower airways; 90% of the particles are 1–5 μm; usually used only intermittently, but can be used for continuous therapy, output is about 1–6 mL/min	Provides 100% humidity; may precipitate bronchospasm; may cause overhydration
Humidifiers		
Bubble diffuser	Used with all low-flow devices and Venturi masks	Provides only 20% to 40% of body humidity; may be heated to deliver 100% humidity; should not be used for patients with endotracheal tube or tracheostomy
Passover humidifier	Used for either low- or high-flow devices and ventilators	Effective humidity only when heated
Cascade humidifier	Mainstream humidifier for ventilators, for patients with endotracheal tube or tracheostomy	100% humidity at body temperature; correct H_2O level is required

Source: Oakes, D. (1998). Clinical practitioners pocket guide to respiratory care (p. 102). Old Town, ME: Health Educator Publications. Reprinted with permission.

mally supplied to the upper airways. In these humidifiers the gas is broken up into small bubbles that pass through heated water, which allows a greater production of small bubbles at higher flow rates than do cold-bubble humidifiers. Heated humidifiers are preferred for patients receiving mechanical ventilation in the intra- or postoperative period.

Aerosol Therapy. Devices that deliver water vapor along with very fine particles of liquid suspended in a gas are termed *aerosol therapy devices* (McPherson, 1990). These devices are used in patients in which secretions need to be effectively diluted and mucus production enhanced. Aerosol particles are usually spherical and range from 0.2 to 0.7 mm in diameter. The penetration and the deposition of an aerosol particle depend on the size of the particle, the patient's breathing pattern, and gravity. Particles larger than 30 mm are deposited in the upper airways; 5- to 30-mm particles penetrate the larger airways; and particles smaller than 5 mm enter the small airways (McPherson, 1990). A slow ventilatory frequency with large tidal volumes will enhance aerosol penetration.

The two most common types of nebulizers are the jet nebulizer and the ultrasonic nebulizer. Jet nebulizers can produce particles between 0.5 and 30 mm; ultrasonic nebulizers produce particles of about 5 mm. Intermittent therapy is advised because of the possibility of fluid overload and acute respiratory distress from airway obstruction, as the dried secretions can swell with water over time. Consequently, patients receiving aerosol therapy should never be left unattended (Harper, 1981).

Mechanical Ventilation

The use of mechanical ventilatory support and the subsequent weaning of the patient from this support have evolved to include numerous methods of ventilation. The various methods used clinically are briefly described in this section.

Modes of Mechanical Ventilation

Spontaneous Ventilation. In certain circumstances when the muscles of ventilation are not capable of supporting the total ventilatory needs of the patient, ventilator assistance is necessary. As it is commonly believed that spontaneous breathing is physiologically more effective in the distribution of ventilation than is positive-pressure ventilation, the patient should be permitted to breathe spontaneously to the clinical extent possible. When the patient has enough muscular power to ventilate adequately but an oxygenation problem exists, a ventilator may not be necessary. Various techniques asso-

ciated with spontaneous ventilation are available to improve oxygenation without using a ventilator. Each technique uses positive end-expiratory pressure (PEEP) to improve the oxygenation level of the patient (Nunn, 1984). It is therefore logical to begin the description of the various techniques with a discussion of PEEP.

Positive end-expiratory pressure is the application of a pressure greater than atmospheric pressure to the airway at the end of exhalation. This positive pressure is usually created by using some mechanical device that ends the exhalation phase of ventilation early. A certain volume of gas is maintained in the lung over and above the normal volume to achieve the desired airway pressure level. Basically, PEEP therapy improves oxygenation by expanding the gas-exchanging areas of the lung. Therefore, the clinical goal of PEEP is to raise the functional residual capacity (FRC). By successfully increasing the FRC, oxygenation can be improved without increasing the inspired oxygen concentration, and often the oxygen concentration can be reduced to nontoxic levels while maintaining an adequate PaO_2 and oxygen saturation level.

The therapeutic range of PEEP varies depending on the respiratory pathophysiology being treated. In most clinical situations, the therapeutic range of PEEP is 5 to 30 cm H_2O. The level of PEEP should be increased or decreased in increments of 2.5 to 5 cm H_2O. An appropriate level of PEEP is achieved when there is adequate arterial oxygenation and cardiac output with an inspired concentration of oxygen of 40% or less. Physiologic PEEP is equal to about 5 cm H_2O PEEP and is considered to be the same as the resistance normally offered by the intact respiratory system during expiration. Best PEEP is the level at which the patient has the best lung compliance (Barash, Cullen, & Stoelting, 1997). Optimal PEEP is the level at which optimal lung function is obtained. It is the level of PEEP that provides a maximum decrease in V_D/V_T and a maximum increase in PvO_2.

Expiratory positive airway pressure (EPAP) is the application of PEEP to the spontaneously breathing patient. Expiratory airway pressures are maintained above atmospheric pressure, whereas inspiratory pressures occur at subatmospheric levels created during normal inspiration. EPAP is indicated in patients who are capable of performing all the work of breathing but require PEEP therapy.

Continuous positive airway pressure (CPAP) is the application of PEEP to the spontaneously breathing patient (EPAP) and the maintenance of inspiratory pressure at a level greater than atmospheric pressure. Continuous positive airway pressure is clinically more effective when PEEP therapy is indicated (Kirby, Smith, & Desautels, 1985). However, as a result of the CPAP, cardiovascular function may be reduced, and, therefore, EPAP may be more beneficial for the administration of PEEP.

Assisted Ventilation. Assisted ventilation augments the patient's spontaneous breathing efforts. The patient, by initiating a spontaneous inspiration, creates a subatmospheric pressure that is sensed by the ventilator, triggering the inspiratory phase of ventilation. Once the ventilator initiates gas flow in response to the patient's breathing efforts, it takes control of inspiration, overriding the patient's efforts. The assisted mode of ventilation is commonly referred to as intermittent positive-pressure ventilation (IPPV) or positive-pressure ventilation (PPV). This mode of ventilation is used for both long-term ventilatory support and intermittent therapy. When it is used with a volume/time-cycled ventilator, the patient has control over respiratory rate only. During intermittent therapy, a pressure-cycled ventilator is usually used. In this situation, the patient not only controls the respiratory rate but can also influence the delivered tidal volume and inspiratory flow of the assist mode of ventilation, but this has little physiologic advantage over the control mode of ventilation. It does, however, alleviate the need for pharmacologic assistance in controlling the patient's ventilation.

Intermittent Mandatory Ventilation. As with assisted ventilation, intermittent mandatory ventilation (IMV) is a method of augmenting the patient's spontaneous ventilation. Intermittent mandatory ventilation differs from assisted ventilation in that the patient's spontaneous breath does not trigger the ventilator into the inspiratory phase. The patient breathes spontaneously from a flow of gas from the ventilator circuit. Intermittently, the ventilator provides a mandatory volume of gas at a predetermined rate. The IMV rate is determined by the patient's ability to assume a portion of the work of breathing. The patient's ventilatory pattern and delivery of the mandatory inspiration are independent of one an-

other. In an attempt to synchronize the mandatory breath from the ventilator with the patient's ventilatory pattern, various techniques have been developed. Synchronized intermittent mandatory ventilation (SIMV), intermittent assisted ventilation (IAV), and intermittent demand ventilation (IDV) are all systems designed to provide the mandatory breath in response to a spontaneous inspiration at predetermined intervals. This is nothing more than assisted ventilation during the mandatory cycle. The use of IMV, SIMV, IAV, and IDV as methods of weaning has increased significantly in recent years. The patient may assume more of the work of breathing while reducing the mandatory ventilation rate. An advantage to using one of these systems during weaning is that the patient is weaned while remaining attached to the ventilator. The patient thus can be better monitored and receives the same oxygen concentrations and humidification during both spontaneous and mandatory ventilation as during the weaning process.

Controlled Ventilation. Use of intermittent, positive-pressure ventilation has decreased significantly in recent years, primarily because of the use of intermittent mandatory ventilation for short- and long-term ventilatory support. The use of controlled ventilation (CV) is, however, still advocated in certain circumstances, such as in patients with central nervous system disorders, anesthetized patients, and critically ill patients whose condition has not been stabilized. The respiratory rate, tidal volume, and inspiratory/expiratory flow rates may all be manipulated during controlled ventilation to obtain the desired physiologic effects. Total control of the patient's ventilatory pattern is the only advantage of IPPV over other modes of ventilation. See Table 30–3 for the initial setup of a ventilator for controlled ventilation.

TABLE 30–3. Recommended Ventilator Setup Parameters

Parameter	Setting Range	Discussion
Minute ventilation ($\dot{V}_E$)	5–10 L/min	$\dot{V}_E$ determines alveolar ventilation ($\dot{V}_A$) as $V_E = 1/Paco_2$, which is usually controlled by V_T and f
Tidal volume (V_T)	10–15 mL/kg	Large V_T is preferred to improve $\dot{V}_A/\dot{Q}_C$, prevent atelectasis, and account for dead space lost to tubing
Peak pressure	<40 cm H_2O	Keep as low as possible to prevent pneumothorax and yet deliver desired V_T
Rate (f)	12–18 breaths/min	Combined with V_T to give desired V_E ($Paco_2$). Keep rate (f) low for large V_T
F_{IO_2}	≤40%	Adjust in 5%–10% increments to keep the PaO_2 between 60 and 100 torr
Sigh	6–12/hr $1^1/_2$–2 × V_T	Prevent miliary atelectasis, not critical if high V_T values are used
Flow rate (V_I)	25–60 L/min	Used to provide desired inspiratory pattern
PEEP/CPAP	5–10 cm H_2O	Indicated when PaO_2 <50 torr on 50% oxygen
Inspiratory time (T_I)	0.5–1.0 s	Normal physiologic time
I : E ratio	1:2 to 1:3	Longer time for obstructive lung disease
Sensitivity	−1–2 cm H_2O	Allows triggering of ventilator in assist mode
Pressure limit	10 cm H_2O above peak pressure	Prevents excess pressure from reaching lungs, warning for increased airway resistance or decreased compliance

Inverse Inspiratory-to-Expiratory Ratio Ventilation. In the early 1970s it was determined that infants were successfully ventilated using a technique that had an inspiratory phase longer than the expiratory phase, with a pressure hold. This technique has been used on adults in which the inspiratory-to-expiratory (I : E) ratio reaches 4 : 1 and is combined with low levels of PEEP or CPAP (Shapiro & Cane, 1990).

Pressure Support Ventilation. In pressure support ventilation (PSV) a gas is applied at a preset level above PEEP. When the patient's spontaneous inspiration is sensed, a demand valve is opened and the ventilator delivers a pressurized breath. Once a particular pressure is reached or flow is decreased, inspiration is ended and exhalation occurs.

Pressure support ventilation is particularly useful for patients requiring weaning from mechanical ventilation who have increased airway resistance. Consequently, PSV offers adjustable breath-to-breath ventilatory assistance and helps reduce the work of breathing.

High-frequency Ventilation. High-frequency ventilation (HFV) is a method of ventilation that uses rates higher than 60 per minute or greater than four times the standard positive pressure ventilation rate. Although the exact mechanism of action is not clearly defined, it has been established that in HFV, carbon dioxide exchange can and does occur even when the tidal volume is less than the patient's dead space.

High-frequency ventilation uses a commercially available ventilator called a high-frequency jet ventilator (HFJV) that delivers a pulse of gas from a high-pressure source between 5 and 50 psi. The pulse of gas is delivered through a small-bore cannula at rates up to 150 per minute. Advantages to the HFJV are few; however, it may have a place in one-lung ventilation, in patients with bronchopleural fistulas, and in anesthetic cases where minimal movement in the surgical field is desirable, as in computerized lithotripsy.

Indications for Mechanical Ventilation

Mechanical ventilation is instituted to correct one of three pathophysiologic processes: acute hypoventilation or apnea, high V_A/Q_C, or low V_A/Q_C. Acute hypoventilation may be caused by inadequate skeletal muscle relaxant reversal, prolonged emergence from anesthesia, or overdosage of narcotic agonist. The arterial blood gases of a patient with acute hypoventilation will demonstrate a decreased PaO_2 and an increased $Paco_2$ along with a reduced pH. Apnea, however, can result from multiple causes. When acute hypoxemia caused by acute hypoventilation or apnea is present, a volume-limited ventilator should be used. In this case, the intervention is intended to restore the patient's normal alveolar ventilation. The initial setup should be in accordance with the parameters described in Table 30–3. Twenty to thirty minutes after the institution of the mechanical ventilation, arterial blood gases should be drawn and evaluated, and the ventilator setting changed accordingly.

High V_A/Q_C (dead space) occurs when alveolar ventilation exceeds alveolar perfusion. A patient with an acute elevation of the FRC, as occurs during acute respiratory insufficiency caused by chronic obstructive pulmonary disease (COPD), is one example of a high V_A/Q_C. Another example is a pulmonary embolism. The arterial blood gases of a patient with a high V_A/Q_C will demonstrate acute hypoxemia and minimal hypercarbia. Another helpful test is to determine the amount of dead-space breathing by using the Bohr equation, commonly referred to as the V_D/V_T:

$$V_D/V_T = \frac{Paco_2 - PECO_2}{PECO_2}$$

Here, $PECO_2$ is mixed expired partial pressure of CO_2 and $Paco_2$ is partial pressure of arterial CO_2. If the VD/VT is greater than 0.6, mechanical ventilation should be instituted. The same basic considerations in setting up the ventilator (Table 30–3) should be used for the patient with high VA/QC, as for the patient with acute hypoventilation.

Low V_A/Q_C (shunt) is a pathophysiologic process that can occur intraoperatively and postoperatively. Severe atelectasis is a common cause of low V_A/Q_C. Arterial blood gases in the patient with low V_A/Q_C usually demonstrate hypoxemia, hypercarbia, and a low pH. Another helpful test to determine the amount of shunt is the Q_s/Q_t. The shunt equation can be used to determine the exact amount of right-to-left shunt; however, if the Fio_2 and the PaO_2 are known, the isoshunt line graph can be used to determine the approximate percentage of shunted blood (Fig. 30–2). If a patient has a shunt (Q_s/Q_t) that is greater than 15%, mechanical ventilation should be considered.

Usually FRC is low in patients with low V_A/Q_C because the patient often has low lung compliance and high lung recoil. Consequently, hyperinflation or PEEP may be required to return the FRC to normal levels. By returning the FRC to normal levels, the V_T will be elevated out of the closing capacity (CC) range, and ultimately alveolar ventilation will improve because there will be better matching of ventilation to perfusion in the lungs.

In patients who have undergone major operations and do not have underlying lung disease, mechanical ventilation may be required until the effects of anesthesia and surgery have dissipated. The patient initially should be provided with 100 mL/kg/min total ventilation. An IMV rate of 8 to 10 is usually acceptable, and a PEEP of 5 cm H_2O may be added to the ventilator circuit. The use of IMV has decreased the period of mechanical ventilatory support slightly and has probably made weaning safer.

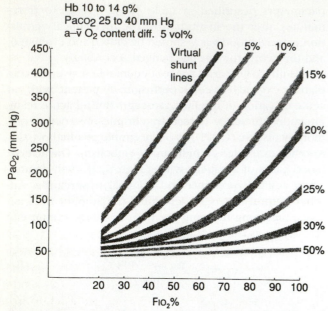

Hb 10 to 14 g%
Paco₂ 25 to 40 mm Hg
a–v̄ O₂ content diff. 5 vol%

Figure 30–2. Isoshunt chart indicating the relationship between partial pressure of arterial O_2 (PaO_2) and inspired O_2 concentration (FIO_2) for a range of shunt fractions (0%–50%). *(From Benatar, S. R., Hewlett, A. M., & Nunn, J. F. [1973]. The use of shunt lines for control of oxygen therapy. British Journal of Anaesthesia, 45, 713.)*

Weaning from Mechanical Ventilation

While the patient receives mechanical ventilatory support, cardiovascular stability is of utmost importance. This is particularly true when the patient is being weaned from mechanical ventilation. Special attention should be given to fluids and electrolyte balance. The patient should be afebrile and in a good nutritional state before the weaning process is instituted (Table 30-4).

The patient's respiratory status must be assessed before the weaning process can be started. The assessment parameters are usually grouped into three major categories: ventilation, oxygenation, and mechanics (Table 30-5) (Traver, Mitchell & Flodquist-Priestley, 1992).

Assessment of ventilation centers around the arterial blood gas analysis. The $Paco_2$ should be within normal limits (35 to 45 torr). The V_D/V_T should be less than 0.6. If PEEP was used, it should be less than 5 cm H_2O at the

TABLE 30–4. Physiologic Parameters to be Corrected before Weaning from Mechanical Ventilation

Cardiovascular stability
Improvement in underlying disease
Absence of fever/shivering
Absence of acid–base abnormalities
Absence of electrolyte abnormalities
Adequate nutrition

TABLE 30–5. Physiologic Criteria for Weaning a Patient off Mechanical Ventilation

Ventilation
$\quad$ $Paco_2$ = 35–45 torr (CO_2 retains about 55 torr)
$\quad$ V_D/V_T <0.6
$\quad$ $\dot{V}_E$ < 10 L/min
Mechanics
$\quad$ VC > 10–15 mL/kg
$\quad$ MIF = −20 cm H_2O
$\quad$ MVV = 2 V_E
Oxygenation
$\quad$ PaO_2 > 70 torr (PEEP< 5 cm H_2O and FIO_2 < 0.4)
$\quad$ P(A-a)O_2 at FIO_2 = 1 between 300 and 350 torr
$\quad$ $\dot{Q}_S/\dot{Q}_T$ at FIO_2 = 1.0 at < 10%–20%

beginning of the weaning process. Finally, if the minute ventilation (VE) is less than 10 L/min, the weaning process should be allowed to proceed.

As with ventilation, oxygenation is assessed by obtaining arterial blood gases. Before weaning is attempted, the PaO_2 should be greater than 70 torr with a FIO_2 less than 0.4 and less than 5 cm H_2O PEEP. The PaO_2 appears to be the best assessment parameter to evaluate adequacy for weaning from mechanical ventilation. The alveolar-arterial oxygen difference or gradient P(A − a)O_2 and the shunt equation (Q_s/Q_t) adds little additional information over the use of PaO_2 alone.

The best tests for assessing mechanical function are vital capacity (VC) and maximal inspiratory force (MIF). Assessment of VC reflects respiratory system compliance and mechanical muscle strength. The VC should be 10 to 15 mL/kg, and the MIF should be more negative than 20 cm H_2O. Maximum voluntary ventilation (MVV) can be used as an assessment criterion; however, the VC and MIF are usually adequate to make a decision on weaning from mechanical ventilation.

When the patient fulfills the criteria of the three categories of assessment, the actual process of weaning can begin. It is important to restate that the patient must possess good cardiovascular stability, including adequate nutrition and blood volume. The patient should not receive any drugs that would sedate or depress the respiratory drive. During the weaning process, constant psychologic and physiologic monitoring of the patient is mandatory. Vital signs, arterial blood gases, and mechanics should be recorded on a flowsheet. Once the patient is allowed to breathe spontaneously without the aid of mechanical ventilation, vital signs are recorded every 5 to 10 minutes for about half an hour and then every 30 minutes after that. Arterial blood gases are checked 15 minutes after spontaneous breathing off the ventilator has begun and thereafter on an hourly basis. Mechanical ventilation is resumed if any of the following signs appear: arrhythmia, hypertension or hypotension (change of 15 torr from baseline), tachycardia (>120 beats per minute), pallor, cyanosis, agitation, increasing Pa_{CO_2} greater than 1 torr/min, pH less than 7.25, or PaO_2 less than 70 torr (Drain, 1994).

Most patients who are receiving short-term mechanical ventilation can be weaned in several hours. Mechanical ventilation can be discontinued in two ways: (1) periodic removal from the ventilator using the Briggs T-piece; or (2) use of IMV. If the first method is used, the Briggs T-piece ensures that the patient will be adequately oxygenated. The patient who has received long-term ventilator care may tolerate only short periods (<30 minutes) every 2 to 4 hours of the T-piece weaning process. As tolerated, these patients should spend less time receiving mechanical ventilation and more time using the T-piece. If it is anticipated that the weaning process will be lengthy, the discontinuance from mechanical ventilation should be commenced in the morning when the patient can physiologically tolerate the weaning process.

Intermittent mandatory ventilation is an acceptable method of weaning a patient from mechanical ventilation and offers many advantages. It increases safety, decreases weaning time, preserves respiratory muscle strength and coordination by allowing ongoing spontaneous breathing efforts, and improves psychologic adjustments to weaning. This method focuses on reducing the number of breaths per minute and allowing the patient to increase control over ventilation. Finally, the patient breathes spontaneously without the aid of mechanical ventilation. The weaning process with IMV is the same as with the T-piece regarding time off the ventilator.

Some patients develop intolerance to the IMV method. The intolerance may be caused by increased resistance in the IMV circuit (as compared with the T-piece circuit), malfunctions in ventilator setup, or overoxygenation during the weaning period. Patients who are difficult to wean via IMV may respond well to the T-piece method.

The Modified Stir-Up Regime

Pulmonary complications are the single leading cause of morbidity and mortality in the postoperative period. An incidence of 4.5% to 76% (average of 11%) for pulmonary complications after abdominal operations has been reported. Most research has shown that the incidence of postoperative complications is highest after upper abdominal and thoracic surgery (Drain, 1994).

Atelectasis, or collapse of the alveoli, is a common postoperative pulmonary complication. Atelectasis accounts for more than 90% of postoperative pulmonary complications. Normally, adults breathe regularly and rhythmically and spontaneously perform a maximal inspiration or sigh every 5 to 10 minutes. During anesthesia and in the immediate postoperative period, sighless respirations occur. With this absence of the spontaneous

deep breaths with an inspiratory hold, lung compliance decreases, resulting in lower alveolar volume. As these lung volumes decrease in the immediate postoperative period, transpulmonary pressure decreases. Without periodic lung hyperinflations with inspiratory holds (sigh), the surfactant may not be allowed to form an appropriate layer about the terminal bronchioles and alveoli. Ultimately, the surfactant becomes bunched. Inappropriate surfactant function increases surface tension within the alveoli, which causes a higher lung recoil, or a stiff lung. One of the lung volumes reduced in the postoperative period is the functional residual capacity (FRC). When the FRC decreases into the closing capacity (CC) range, the airways leading to dependent lung zones may be effectively closed throughout the respiratory cycle. Ultimately, atelectasis, hypoxemia, and pneumonia can result (Nunn, 1984).

To reverse the events that lead to the reduction of the FRC, the patient should be encouraged to perform a sustained maximal inspiration (SMI) maneuver. In this respiratory maneuver, the patient is encouraged to take a deep inspiration and, at the peak of inspiration, to hold the inspired air for 3 seconds, then to exhale the air. The volume excursion and inspiratory hold attained by the use of an incentive spirometer are similar to those obtained with the SMI maneuver. This maneuver will increase the patient's lung volumes and, consequently, will reinflate the collapsed alveoli. The SMI is believed to increase alveolar inflation time and volume, increase lung compliance, and allow the surfactant to layer out, thus promoting an increase in lung volume, specifically the FRC. The end result should be a decrease in the amount of atelectasis and hypoxemia.

Anesthesia, surgery, immobility, and the absence of an adequate cough maneuver are some factors that cause the patient to retain secretions. Research indicates that the forced expiratory volume in 1 second (FEV_1) is reduced in the immediate postoperative period. It is important for the postanesthesia nurse to initiate the cough maneuver when the patient arrives in the PACU. The cascade cough is the most effective cough maneuver that can be used because the patient has a low FEV_1 in the immediate postoperative period.

To perform the cascade cough maneuver, the patient should be taught to take a slow deep inspiration, which will increase the lung volume and open the airways via a tethering effect, allowing air to pass beyond the secretions. At the peak of inspiration, the patient is encouraged to perform multiple "mini" coughs at succeeding lower lung volumes. With each "mini" cough during exhalation, the length of the airways undergoing dynamic compression increases, thus enhancing the effectiveness of secretion clearance. Patients with pulmonary pathology that includes a history of retained secretions benefit from chest percussion and postural drainage to enhance the movement of secretions to larger airways, where they can be removed by the cascade cough maneuver (Traver et al., 1992).

The original regimen of turn-cough-deep breathe has been significantly modified. Clinical research demonstrates that the SMI maneuver and cascade cough are more effective in reducing the incidence of postoperative complications. Repositioning of the patient every 15 minutes during the immediate postoperative period aids in better matching of ventilation to perfusion (V_A/Q_C), and secretion clearance continues to be an important part of this regimen. Hence, the *modified stir-up regimen,* consisting of turn–cascade cough–SMI, should be used on every patient recovering from anesthesia in the PACU.

► COMMON PROBLEMS IN THE PACU

Hypoxemia

Hypoxemia, which is deficient oxygenation of the blood, is a relatively common event that occurs in the PACU. Some possible causes of postoperative hypoxemia are a low inspired oxygen concentration, ventilation-perfusion mismatching (V_A/Q_C), hypoventilation, increased oxygen consumption, decreased cardiac output, or shunt (Levitzky, 1991).

The clinical signs of hypoxemia include hypertension, hypotension, tachycardia, bradycardia, cardiac arrhythmias, restlessness, diaphoresis, dyspnea, and tachypnea. Cyanosis, which is defined as 5 g of reduced hemoglobin, is not a reliable sign of hypoxemia; however, an oxygen saturation below 90% is an excellent quantitative symptom of hypoxemia. Central nervous system symptoms of hypoxemia should be evaluated in the context of other causes such as pain, full bladder, and disorientation and restlessness caused by postoperative excitement and somnolence.

Therapy for the hypoxemic patient begins with a positive assessment of hypoxemia. Objective assessment using arterial blood gases with a PaO_2 of less than 60 torr or an oxygen saturation via a pulse oximeter of less than 90% indicates the presence of hypoxemia. Because anesthesia, surgery, and narcotics depress respiratory mechanics and response to carbon dioxide, room air is insufficient for all patients recovering from general anesthesia. The same holds true for regional anesthesia in which any type of sedation was used. Along with this, high spinal or epidural anesthetics produce a reduced ventilatory effort with resultant hypoxemia. Another justification for an increased inspired oxygen concentration is that many patients in the PACU may shiver, have a fever, or be in disoriented or restless states. Consequently, the initial intervention to relieve hypoxemia is an increased F_{IO_2}. Also, the patient may require inter-

ventions that are designed specifically to combat the particular cause of the hypoxemia. Patients suffering from ventilation–perfusion mismatching, hypoventilation, and shunt will respond to a vigorous modified stir-up regimen along with chest physiotherapy. Patients who demonstrate possible increased oxygen consumption by shivering should be warmed to near-normal body core temperature. Patients demonstrating emergence excitement from general anesthesia will have an increased oxygen consumption. This phenomenon occurs frequently after scopolamine premedication. Intravenous physostigmine 1 to 3 mg usually reverses the scopolamine-induced delirium and ultimately reverses the hypoxemia.

Hypercapnia

Elevated carbon dioxide tensions can and do occur in the immediate postoperative period. Many factors contribute to the development of hypercapnia, including a depressed central response to carbon dioxide, inadequate muscular forces to move air, oversedation, or an increase in metabolic rate (Levitzky, 1991).

The pathophysiology leading to hypercapnia centers on ventilation-perfusion mismatch and a blunting of the carbon dioxide response in the respiratory center of the brain (Murray & Nadel, 1994). This is particularly important in the PACU when patients experience emergence excitement, shivering, or hyperthermia, all of which increase the metabolic rate and ultimately carbon dioxide production. Because of the residual effects of anesthesia, the central response to carbon dioxide is blunted; consequently, carbon dioxide cannot be adequately removed, leading to carbon dioxide retention or hypercapnia.

Assessment of hypercarbia may be difficult because of possible depression of other physiologic systems. The only definitive determinant of hypercarbia is direct blood gas analysis; however, objective signs of hypercarbia include low tidal volume and rapid respiratory rate, tachycardia, hypertension, and sternal retractions. Many hypercapnic patients subjectively demonstrate restlessness, confusion, lassitude, and somnolence. Preventive interventions for patients with hypercarbia include aggressive use of the modified stir-up regimen. If the patient continues to demonstrate objective and subjective signs of hypercarbia, reversal of the effects of anesthesia should be considered. If the residual anesthesia is due to narcotic depression, naloxone (Narcan®), an opiate receptor antagonist, should be used. Because of the unpredictable duration of action of naloxone, careful titration to effect and close monitoring are mandated. Also, titration to effect can be used should further administration of naloxone be required. It must be remembered that naloxone does not reverse the respiratory depressant effects of barbiturates and tranquilizers. If the patient does not respond to the dose of naloxone, mechanical support of ventilation may be required.

Nalbuphine (Nubain®), which is chemically related to both naloxone and the potent narcotic agonist oxymorphone, has been studied in the PACU for its agonist-antagonist properties. Clinically, it has been demonstrated that 5 mg of nalbuphine administered intravenously to a patient who has narcotic respiratory depression will reverse much of the respiratory depression, yet the patient will remain analgesic (Stoelting, 1991).

If the residual effects of anesthesia are due to inadequate skeletal muscle relaxant reversal, the patient should be evaluated for inadequate neuromuscular function. Tests to determine if neuromuscular function is depressed are the head lift, hand grip strength, vital capacity of 10 to 15 mL/kg, and inspiratory force of at least −20 to −25 cm H$_2$O. The best method of determining neuromuscular function is with the peripheral nerve stimulator, especially in patients with altered central nervous system function. If the assessment determines that a competitive neuromuscular blockade exists, an anticholinesterase such as neostigmine (0.07 mg/kg) and an anticholinergic such as glycopyrrolate (0.015 mg/kg) should be administered intravenously (Stoelting, 1991). Improvement in neuromuscular function should be observed within 2 to 5 minutes of injection of the reversal drug.

Airway Obstruction

Obstruction of the upper airway, which is considered to be an extrathoracic obstruction, may be caused by obstruction of the pharynx by the relaxed soft tissue or by partial or complete laryngospasm. An extrathoracic airway obstruction can be reliably assessed. As the patient inspires, stridor can be auscultated over the partially obstructed area. Inspiratory stridor occurs because the airway pressure is more negative than atmospheric pressure during inspiration. During expiration, less stridor is heard because the airway pressure is greater than atmospheric pressure. Certainly, if complete obstruction occurs, auscultation will reveal an absence of breath sounds and sternal retractions will be observed.

As the patient is emerging from anesthesia in the PACU, the tongue may be relaxed and can occlude the pharynx, especially when the head is flexed while the patient is supine. Intervention for this type of airway obstruction begins with hyperextension of the head. If the obstruction continues, the angle of the jaw should be lifted to move the tongue off the posterior pharynx. If more interventions are required, especially in the obtunded patient, an oral or nasal airway can be inserted; however, if the airway obstruction is due to masseter spasm and the jaws are clenched tightly, a nasal airway or

nasotracheal tube placed into the nasopharynx should relieve the obstructed airway.

Laryngospasm, or adduction of the vocal cords, is commonly caused by secretions or manipulation of the vocal cords. Laryngospasm can be partial or complete (Drain, 1994). Partial laryngospasm is due to a partial adduction of the vocal cords. On assessment of the patient having a partial laryngospasm, inspiratory stridor over the larynx will be heard. Physiologically, this occurs because the obstruction is extrathoracic. The recommended intervention for a partial laryngospasm is the administration of 100% oxygen under positive pressure using a bag-valve-mask system. High inflation pressures should be avoided, and the rate of ventilation should be timed to the patient's own rate. As the obstruction improves, careful oral suctioning should be performed to prevent further laryngospasm.

Complete laryngospasm is characterized by complete adduction of the vocal cords, resulting in an absence of ventilation to the point of hypoxemia. On auscultation, no breath sounds are heard and the patient exhibits the characteristic rocking motion in the lower abdominal area. At this point, a small dose of a rapid-acting depolarizing skeletal muscle relaxant (eg, succinylcholine 0.5 to 1 mg/kg) should be administered intravenously. Within 30 to 45 seconds postinjection, the vocal cords will begin to abduct. The patient should be ventilated gently via a bag-valve-mask system using 100% oxygen. Once the succinylcholine is administered, the anesthetist should be prepared to perform an endotracheal intubation if the patient cannot be ventilated adequately or if regurgitation and aspiration of stomach contents are imminent. Finally, cricoid pressure should be applied before and during intubation if the risk of aspiration is high.

In postintubation patients, especially in the pediatric age group, laryngeal edema and trauma may occur. These are significant obstructions of the extrathoracic airways because the narrowest portion of the larynx in the pediatric age group is the cricoid ring (Miller, 1994). If untreated, this pathophysiologic process can progress to complete obstruction of the airway. This obstruction is extrathoracic, and inspiratory stridor is heard audibly or by auscultation. To differentiate between partial laryngospasm and laryngeal edema, 100% oxygen is administered via a bag-valve-mask system. The obstruction will progressively worsen if laryngeal edema is present; whereas, if the patient is experiencing a partial laryngeal spasm, the stridor will be reduced and ventilatory function will improve. The assessment to differentiate between laryngeal spasm and edema should be carried out rapidly. Once laryngeal edema is determined as the cause of the airway obstruction, the patient should be placed in an upright position and administered humidified oxygen along with some nebulized racemic epinephrine. Dexamethasone should be administered intravenously to enhance the actions of the racemic epinephrine and to reduce the inflammation of the larynx (Miller, 1994).

In a younger patient, laryngeal edema can progress rapidly to complete obstruction. Hence, equipment for both an oral intubation and emergency laryngotomy should be available. Oral tracheal intubation should be attempted first. If this is unsuccessful, a cricothyroidotomy should be performed by incising the cricothyroid membrane and inserting a tracheostomy tube or endotracheal tube into the airway (Miller, 1994).

Hypotension

One of the more common problems in the immediate postoperative period is hypotension, which requires immediate corrective action. If the hypotension is allowed to progress, severe damage can occur to the brain, the heart, and the kidneys. Because of the high metabolic activity in these organs, any sustained abnormal decrease in the perfusion pressure can result in ischemia or infarction.

In the PACU, many situations can lead to hypotension. Hypotension can be caused by decreased cardiac output or decreased peripheral resistance. The decreased cardiac output can be a result of hypovolemia. Hypovolemia can result from excess fluid loss or inadequate fluid replacement. If the patient is being mechanically ventilated, positive airway pressure, especially PEEP, can cause hypotension. This positive pressure will, if in excess, inhibit the preload and reduce the cardiac output. Many anesthetic drugs, including halothane, isoflurane, enflurane, desflurane, sevoflurane, fentanyl, morphine, and meperidine, can cause myocardial depression to varying degrees, resulting in a reduced cardiac output. Finally, patients who have cardiac dysfunction, such as valvular disease, ischemia, and infarction, may have a reduced cardiac output.

Decreased peripheral resistance can result from several causes. Anaphylaxis and sepsis reduce peripheral resistance. The anesthetic drugs noted as causes of decreased cardiac output also decrease peripheral resistance.

Assessment for hypotension should begin with reaffirmation of the measurement. A blood pressure cuff improperly placed or of the wrong size will result in errors in blood pressure measurement. More specifically, blood pressure cuffs that are too large yield falsely low readings. It must be remembered that the cuff width should equal approximately two thirds of the arm circumference (Drain, 1994; Henneman & Henneman, 1989; Lake, 1990). Also, if arterial transducer measurement is being used, calibration of the monitor should be validated by a cuff or Doppler blood pressure measurement on the same arm in which the radial artery was cannulated. Improper calibration, dampening caused by air bubbles,

and catheter obstruction also lead to inappropriately low blood pressure readings. Rapid bedside clinical assessment should include level of consciousness to detect brain ischemia resulting from reduced cardiac output. If urine output is less than 0.5 mL/kg/hr, hypovolemia or inadequate cardiac output is the most likely cause of the hypotension.

Once the assessment reveals the existence of hypotension, assessment of the possible cause(s) of the hypotension should be implemented. The assessment should focus on checking for continued blood loss, adequate blood replacement intraoperatively or postoperatively, myocardial ischemia or infarction through ECG confirmation, pneumothorax, cardiac tamponade, and evidence of sepsis or adverse drug effects.

Interventions to return the patient to the normotensive state may include administration of oxygen, fluid infusion, reversal of the depressant effects of the anesthetics, and treatment of arrhythmias or bradycardia. The first intervention should be the administration of oxygen to ensure tissue oxygenation. If the patient is hypovolemic, depending on the degree of loss, blood or blood products or crystalloid solutions should be administered promptly. The type of fluid chosen may not be as crucial as adequate replacement in a timely manner with any fluid. An intravenous bolus of crystalloid solution of 300 to 500 mL should be considered as the first-line intervention for hypotension (Miller, 1994). Naloxone should be administered if it is determined that a narcotic is the cause of the hypotension. Vasopressors, especially those with positive inotropic action, can be used occasionally to raise the blood pressure and prevent coronary hypoperfusion. If the etiology of the hypotension is decreased peripheral resistance, vasopressors that are agonists on the alpha$_1$-receptors should be administered.

Many patients arrive in the PACU with excess vagal tone, which results in bradycardia and hypotension. This is especially true of patients with distended bladders or those in severe pain. Anticholinergic drugs, such as atropine (0.2 to 0.4 mg) and glycopyrrolate (0.1 to 0.2 mg) given intravenously will reverse the increased vagal effects. Finally, if the hypotension is due to excess positive airway pressure, a reduction in PEEP is required along with administration of fluids.

Hypertension

One of the more common sequelae in the immediate postoperative period is hypertension. The elevated blood pressure in the PACU usually is due to pain, hypercapnia, hypoxemia, or excessive fluids administered intraoperatively. About 50% of the patients who demonstrate hypertension in the PACU have a history of hypertension preoperatively. Consequently, the report to the postanesthesia nurse should include information on the patient's hypertension if it exists.

Assessment of the patient who is experiencing hypertension in the PACU should include hypothermia, pain, respiratory, and volume status. All patients with hypertension in the PACU should be aggressively treated with the modified stir-up regimen. If pain is present, appropriate medications should be administered. If hypothermia is present, it should be appropriately treated as discussed later in this chapter. If the systolic or diastolic pressure is 20% to 30% above the preoperative resting values or the patient complains of headache, ocular changes, or angina along with ST segment depression, antihypertensive treatment should commence.

Most patients can be treated with short-acting antihypertensive drugs. Beta-blocking drugs such as propranolol, labetalol, and esmolol are effective in treating hypertension in the PACU. Propranolol is effective in treating hypertension in patients who were on beta-blockers preoperatively. This drug is administered intravenously in 0.5- to 1-mg increments until a reduction in blood pressure is demonstrated. Labetalol can be titrated to effect using an initial dose of 0.25 mg/kg and increasing the dose to 0.5 mg/kg up to 1 mg/kg every 10 to 15 minutes via the intravenous route (Stoelting, 1991). Esmolol, an ultrashort-acting beta-blocker, can be used to treat both hypertension and tachycardia. Because of its short half-life of 9 minutes, it is usually given in a loading dose of 500 mg/kg and then followed by a continuous infusion at rates of 25 to 300 mg/kg/min (Stoelting, 1991). Other drugs that can be used to treat postoperative hypertension include hydralazine, nitroprusside, nifedipine, clonidine, and trimethaphan.

Postoperative Hypothermia

Hypothermia usually occurs during anesthesia and surgery. Consequently, hypothermia is a common syndrome in the immediate postoperative period. Hypothermia exists when a patient's core temperature is below her or his set point or when it is less than 36°C. The thermal set point is defined in the anterior hypothalamus and normally is 37.1°C (Flacke, & Flacke, 1983). Heat generation occurs by increasing the metabolic rate and shivering. Heat dissipation takes place by increasing blood flow to the skin, which is ultimately lost to the environment by radiation, conduction, and convection. Sweating and evaporation enhance heat loss. Finally, of particular importance to anesthesia and postoperative care, heat is lost via evaporation of water from the respiratory tract.

During the intraoperative anesthesia phase, many factors contribute to the development of hypothermia. The state of unconsciousness results in immobility and removal of the behavioral protection against the cold.

The thermal regulating center in the anterior hypothalamus is depressed along with all the autoregulatory mechanisms. There is an autonomic and accompanying motor blockade that impairs heat-generating mechanisms. Cooling also occurs when the patient inspires unheated, dry anesthetic gases. In addition, the operating room is cold (18°C to 21°C) and the patient's skin is wet in many exposed areas.

On arrival in the PACU, a patient usually is hypothermic. Studies indicate that 60% of the patients have temperatures less than 36°C, and 13% have temperatures less than 35°C. If hypothermia is allowed to progress, the patient can experience delayed awakening and inadequate peripheral blood flow leading to thrombosis and hypoxemia.

Treatment of hypothermia in the PACU first requires assessment of the degree of temperature loss. If the temperature is between 36°C and 37°C, the patient can simply be covered with warmed blankets and heat lamps can be used to keep the patient adequately warm. If the patient's temperature is less than 36°C, rapid rewarming is required to decrease the possible complications of hypothermia and decrease the postanesthesia recovery time. Rewarming prevents the thermoregulatory responses to cold such as shivering that increase the patient's discomfort and metabolic activity. It is suggested that a skin surface warming device such as the Bair Hugger be placed on the patient. In patients with a normal metabolic rate, a setting of low or medium increases the mean body temperature at about 1°C per hour. A high setting increases the mean body temperature about 1.5°C per hour (Flacke & Flacke, 1983). Other methods of rewarming are thermal mattresses, fluid and blood warming, and environmental warming.

Postoperative Nausea and Vomiting

Among the most difficult and dangerous problems that occur in the PACU are postoperative nausea and vomiting (PONV). Although the incidence of this syndrome occurring in the PACU is about 20% to 30% (range 2% to 70%), it is considered a grave concern because of the problems of airway management. In addition, studies indicate that the incidence of nausea and vomiting is higher in women than in men. Other factors that excite this reflex are a history of motion sickness; surgical procedures involving the eye, ear, and mouth; and certain narcotics such as morphine. Anesthetic agents that have been studied in this area and are associated with a significant incidence of nausea and vomiting are nitrous oxide, isoflurane, and etomidate (Barash et al., 1997).

The emetic center is located in the medulla of the brain. It is activated by afferent impulses from the pharynx, stomach, or other portions of the gastrointestinal tract to the chemoreceptor trigger zone (CTZ) in the medulla (Guyton, 1996). Certainly, anesthetic gases, blood, and mucus can initiate this reflex. Also, the emetic center can be excited by impulses received from other portions of the brain. For example, anesthetic agents and narcotics sensitize the vestibular apparatus, the center of balance. Consequently, one of the principal causes of nausea and vomiting is movement of the patient during transfer or even during repositioning. Other activators of this reflex are increased intracranial pressure, dehydration, and electrolyte imbalance. The hormones that affect the emetic center do this by first stimulating the CTZ. The major hormones are dopamine (D_2), central muscarinic receptors, histamine (H_1), and serotonin ($5\text{-}HT_3$). A patient experiencing nausea should be encouraged to cough and perform the SMI maneuver. Oxygen in a high concentration should be administered. A patient who begins to vomit actively should assume a head-down and lateral position. Oral suctioning should be instituted if the patient is not able to control the airway completely. Rapid assessment of the patient's respiratory status should be made during and after the vomiting episode. This is done by auscultation of the chest bilaterally, listening for adventitious sounds. The pulse oximeter should be used to ensure that oxygen saturation does not fall below 90%. If the patient is experiencing a low oxygen saturation and adventitious sounds, aspiration should be suspected and the appropriate therapy instituted.

Pharmacologic methods of reducing the incidence of nausea and vomiting include the use of metoclopramide preoperatively in the dose range 5 to 20 mg given orally, intramuscularly, or intravenously. Metoclopramide enhances the action of acetylcholine (ACh) at the muscarinic synapses and in the central nervous system to antagonize dopamine (Stoelting, 1991). This latter action is responsible for its antiemetic effect. Another drug that has a profound antiemetic effect is droperidol (Inapsine). This drug can be given preoperatively to patients who are anticipated to experience a high incidence of nausea and vomiting. The preoperative dose of this drug is 0.01 to 0.02 mg/kg IM or IV (Stoelting, 1991). Postoperatively, droperidol can be administered to treat the syndrome once it has commenced. Titration of this drug can begin with a dose of 0.02 mg/kg IV. It should be remembered that droperidol can cause oversedation, circulatory depression, and activation of the extrapyramidal system.

The serotonin ($5\text{-}HT_3$) antagonist ondansetron (Zofran) was first introduced as an antiemetic for chemotherapy and radiotherapy and now is becoming popular as the antiemetic of choice for PONV. Ondansetron can be used as a prophylactic at a dose of 4 or 8 mg intraoperatively or as an antiemetic in the postoperative period at a dose of 1, 4, or 8 mg. Excellent for PONV, this drug has a length of action of about 24 hours. This drug is effective in the treatment of PONV and is not associated with significant side effects, such as oversedation (Roberson & McLeskey, 1996).

Postoperative Pain

Acute pain is an unpleasant sensation and emotional experience usually caused by damage to tissue or by noxious stimuli (Altsberger & Shrewsbury, 1988). Pain receptors, called nociceptors, are located mainly in the skin, blood vessels, subcutaneous tissue, fascia, periosteum, and viscera, and are stimulated by noxious stimuli. Nociceptors act as transducers and convert the painful stimulus into impulses that are transmitted along peripheral fibers to the central nervous system. The degree of nociceptor input from the periphery to the central nervous system is influenced by temperature, sympathetic function, vasculature, and the chemical environment.

In the immediate postoperative period, even as the effects of anesthesia disappear, tissue injury continues, and liberation of pain-producing substances continues. These greatly reduce the high threshold of the nociceptors, leading to the production of pain. Moreover, stimulation of the cut ends of nerves further contributes to pain perception. For example, patients who have had thoracic surgery experience pain from the summation of sensory input from three sites of tissue injury: the skin, the deep somatic structures, and the involved viscera.

On reaching the central nervous system, the pain stimulus activates highly complex interactions among neural systems, psychologic factors, and cultural factors. These interactions of the sensory, motivational, and cognitive processes affect the motor system and initiate psychodynamic mechanisms that are translated physiologically into the affective responses characteristic of acute pain.

By activating the sympathoadrenal system, pain accelerates the cardiovascular system as observed by the parameters of pulse and blood pressure. If the patient has a significant degree of cardiovascular dysfunction, the pain should be lessened with appropriate intervention. It has been suggested that pain, especially at upper abdominal and thoracic surgical sites, will decrease or in fact eliminate the normal sighing (yawn) mechanism (Guyton, 1996). The absence of an appropriate sigh leads to reduced lung volumes and, ultimately, to the atelectasis/pneumonia sequela. Again, appropriate pain relief in these patients may reduce the incidence of atelectasis and pneumonia postoperatively.

Assessment of postoperative pain includes both behavioral and physiologic clues (Altsberger & Shrewsbury, 1988). Pain usually elicits an increased response by the sympathetic nervous system, which in turn produces a large amount of catecholamines, causes tachycardia, increases cardiac output, increases peripheral resistance, and ultimately increases blood pressure. Other assessment parameters of excessive sympathoadrenal activity resulting from acute pain include respiratory changes, excessive perspiration, changes in skin color, nausea, and vomiting. Other objective and subjective findings include generalized or local muscle tension or rigidity, writhing, unusual postures, knees drawn up to abdomen, restlessness, rubbing, and scratching. Finally, pain may affect the behavioral affect of the patient, so that the patient in acute pain may be irritable, depressed, or withdrawn or have behavioral reverses, such as hostility in an ordinarily quiet person.

Once the assessment has been made and it has been determined that the patient is indeed experiencing acute postoperative pain, certain interventions are suggested. If the patient has received an inhalational anesthetic, such as isoflurane, enflurane, or halothane, and demonstrates signs and symptoms of acute pain, postoperative pain relief by the use of narcotic agonists should be instituted early in the postanesthetic period. Similarly, patients receiving a nitrous oxide–narcotic technique should be medicated early in the immediate postoperative period if the intraoperative narcotics were of short duration of action. If narcotics such as sufentanil, meperidine, and morphine were used intraoperatively, the PACU patient should be administered narcotic agonists. Respiratory depression resulting from the synergistic actions of the intraoperative and postoperative narcotic agonists should be avoided. Finally, if the PACU patient was administered droperidol intraoperatively or preoperatively, great caution should be used because narcotic agonists as well as barbiturates are significantly potentiated by this butyrophenone tranquilizer. Therefore, the usual dosage of narcotic agonists should be reduced by one third to one half during the first 8 to 10 hours postoperatively. A complete discussion of pain management can be found in Chapter 31.

▶ CASE STUDY

A 30-year-old patient with mild asthma presented for surgery to relieve the symptoms of an obstructed bile duct. During the preoperative period, a very careful history was elicited as part of the preanesthetic assessment. The patient was using oral zafirlukast (Accolate), a leukotriene-3 blocker, triamcinoline (Azmacort), and a salmeterol (Serevent) inhaler four times a day. The patient also used a metaproterenol (Alupent) inhaler as needed for acute wheezing attacks. Because the patient states a positive history of asthma, it is important to determine the severity of the disease and exercise tolerance.

A history and physical was performed preoperatively to determine the patient's severity of wheezing. He stated that he had an expiratory wheeze only on exertion and that his FEV_1/FVC ratio was 68%, demonstrating mild reactive airways disease. He could walk up two flights of stairs and experience only mild shortness of breath. The patient was evaluated and treated by a medical internist to facilitate good pulmonary outcome before the hospitalization occurred. The patient had not been on steroids over the last year.

1. What anesthesia technique should be selected?

   A general endotracheal anesthetic technique was sellected. A regional technique was ruled out because the level (>T4) of the block would preclude the patient's use of his accessory muscles.

   Because of the pathophysiology of reactive airway disease, it was imperative that all reflex arcs that produce bronchospasm be suppressed with profound anesthesia. Propofol appears to have some bronchodilating effects and will block airway reflexes better than thiopental. Hence, propofol was administered for induction along with IV lidocaine. Nonhistamine-producing muscle relaxants, such as vecuronium, were used along with an inhalational anesthetic, isoflurane. However, it should be stated that, although all volatile anesthetic agents are good bronchodilators, halothane as a gas induction agent is well tolerated because it does not possess a noxious odor and is the best bronchodilator at low MACs (<0.5%). Nitrous oxide was used to assist in getting the volatile agent into the patient via the second-gas effect (Drain and Robinson, 1996).

   Narcotic agents such as remifentanil were given in the low dose range in an effort to reduce the MAC of isoflurane. Because remifentanil has a short half-life of 3 to 6 minutes, it is ideal for the patient. Moreover, because it is metabolized by cholinesterases, it will not cause any bronchospasm or blunt the ventilatory response to carbon dioxide in the immediate postanesthesia period.

   Much debate still exists about extubating the patient deep or awake (Drain, 1996). Both techniques have their advantages and disadvantages, but because the patient was considered a mild asthmatic, he was extubated when he was totally awake. Prior to extubation, he was given IV lidocaine to blunt any response to the procedure. The patient tolerated the extubation well and was transported to the PACU. Oxygen via mask was administered to the patient throughout the transport period.

2. Describe the assessment process for the postanesthesic period.

   Patient assessment using the PARS scoring system was performed by the CRNA and the post anesthesia nurse immediately upon arrival. The patient scored 8 (1 for activity and 1 for consciousness) on arrival and 10 after the first 15 minutes of arrival. The patient was constantly monitored via a continuous cardiac monitor and a blood pressure monitor. Oxygen saturation and pulse via pulse oximetry and body temperature also were monitored. Along with this, the patient's level of consciousness was monitored. All vital signs were documented, at the minimum, every 15 minutes. Following the assessment process, a short form was used to document the appropriate patient data. On the patient's arrival in the PACU, nursing interventions were focused on the modified stir-up regimen and on monitoring the patient's physiologic parameters.

In the immediate PACU phase, 30% oxygen was administered via a high-flow mask and the modified stir-up regimen was initiated along with the use of prolonged expiration with physiologic PEEP. His vital signs were within normal limits, including his core body temperature. However, warming blankets were used for the first 30 minutes of his recovery.

Many studies indicate that lung volume, particularly in patients who have had upper abdominal or thoracic surgery, remained lower 5 to 7 days postoperatively. Hence, the patient was educated to continue performing the SMI maneuver with the use of an incentive spirometer long into the postoperative phase. Cascade cough and early ambulation also were emphasized to facilitate secretion clearance and better ventilation-perfusion matching.

Because many cardiovascular parameters of blood pressure, pulse, and electrical activities of the heart are affected by anesthesia and surgery, constant surveillance of the cardiovascular system was performed in the PACU. Monitoring equipment for this ASA Class II patient included continuous ECG, pulse oximetry, blood pressure measurement by cuff, and chest auscultation. If there is any difficulty in hearing the Korotkoff or heart sounds, a Doppler or ultrasound indirect blood pressure device could be used. In this patient, urinary output was monitored to provide an index of renal perfusion, hydration, and overall adequacy of cardiac perfusion.

The postanesthesia blood pressure and pulse readings were compared to the baseline readings taken preoperatively to determine their significance. Possible interventions for any signs of hypotension included the administration of oxygen and the institution of the previously described modified stir-up regimen to help eliminate the anesthetic gases and thus accelerate the emergence process. If indicated, the rate of intravenous fluid therapy could be increased and the legs elevated. If the hypotension is still not resolved, direct and indirect vasoactive agents may be administered (Lake, 1990). In the case of this patient, no apparent hypotension was noted throughout his PACU stay.

3. If the patient experiences bradycardia, how should it be treated?

Mild bradycardia was treated by the vigorous use of the modified stir-up regimen and oxygen. It was determined that the bradycardia was due to anticholinesterase drugs, and therefore glycopyrrolate was titrated intravenously to raise the heart rate to an acceptable level. It should be noted that glycopyrrolate is the preferred drug in the awake PACU patient because it does not cross the blood-brain barrier (Stoelting, 1991).

4. Because this patient had been on sympathomimetics, would the development of tachycardia need to be aggressively monitored in the PACU?

Tachycardia is a very important postoperative sign and should be aggressively evaluated and resolved in all patients. In general, the patient with previously normal cardiac function can tolerate tachycardia up to 160 beats per minute without deleterious sequelae. The first intervention for tachycardia is oxygen administration. If an underlying problem, such as hypo-volemia, shock, fever, hypoxemia, or excess anticholinergic drug, is not present, the tachycardia is usually due to anxiety or pain. At that point, a narcotic agonist is indicated. Should the tachycardia persist, a (beta$_2$-agonist should be considered (Stoelting, 1991).

5. How should the patient be evaluated for discharge from the PACU?

The use of the PARS system to score patients who are recovering from anesthesia is helpful in setting up discharge criteria from the PACU. On arrival in the PACU, the patient's PARS was 8. After about 45 minutes and allowing for metabolism and excretion of the anesthetic agents, the PARS remained 10, at which point the patient was discharged from the PACU. Many factors determine readiness for discharge; however, the major areas to assess prior to discharge are the patient's general condition; cardiorespiratory function specifically including maintenance of a patent airway and a normal electrocardiogram; renal function (>30 mL/h); pain relief; and laboratory data. Also, discharging a patient who has been medicated with a narcotic agonist in the PACU should be delayed for 30 minutes postadministration of the drug so that the effects of the drug can be fully evaluated. Because this patient received ketorolac about 15 minutes prior to arriving in the PACU, 45 minutes after arriving in the PACU this patient had a PARS of 10 and was fully awake, responsive, and pain free.

Discharging patients from the PACU can be the responsibility of the patient's principal physician, the physician director of the PACU, the CRNA, or an anesthesiologist. The nurse anesthetist who administered the anesthesia intraoperatively was consulted during the discharge phase to enhance the decision-making process, and the decision was made to discharge the patient.

A follow-up postoperative visit was made by the anesthetist. The focus of the postoperative assessment was on the patient's cardiorespiratory status. Again, patients who are ASA Class III or higher or who have upper abdominal or cardiothoracic surgery should be visited until postoperative day 7 or the day of discharge to ensure adequate return of cardiopulmonary function.

► SUMMARY

The primary purpose of the postanesthesia care unit (PACU) is the critical evaluation and stabilization of postoperative patients, with emphasis on anticipation and prevention of complications resulting from anesthesia or the operative procedure. It is imperative that a postanesthesia nurse and the nurse anesthetist fully assess the condition of each patient, not only at admission and discharge but also at frequent intervals throughout the postanesthesia period. Assessment must be a continuous and complete process leading to sound nursing judgments and the implementation of therapeutic care. Nurse anesthetists will continue to expand their professional role in the PACU setting and throughout the managed care environment. The role of the CRNA in various clinical settings already is changing to that of physician extender. This will be of even greater significance in some settings, such as small hospitals, where the need for advanced practice nurses will continue to increase in response to demands of patients for quality accessible health care. Nurse anesthetists must fully appreciate their role throughout the entire perianesthetic period, including postanesthesia and critical care.

► KEY CONCEPTS

- The primary purpose of the postanesthesia care unit (PACU) is the critical evaluation and stabilization of postoperative patients, with emphasis on anticipation and prevention of complications resulting from anesthesia or the operative procedure.
- The nurse anesthetists have an expanded role in the PACU setting and in the managed care environment. The role of the CRNA in various clinical settings is changing to that of physician extender. This is particularly true in small hospitals.
- The Phase I Postanesthesia Care Unit is an acute care unit where the patient arrives directly from the operating room and the Phase II Postanesthesia Care Unit is the ambulatory unit where the patient is discharged to home from the unit.
- It is imperative that a postanesthesia nurse and nurse anesthetist fully assess the condition of each patient—not only at admission and at discharge but also at frequent intervals throughout the postanesthesia period. Assessment must be a continuous and complete process, leading to sound nursing judgments and the implementation of therapeutic care.
- The anesthetist and PAN should mutually determine the postanesthesia recovery score.
- Pulse oximetry monitoring is objective and continuous, and it provides an early warning of developing hypoxemia, allowing intervention before signs of hypoxia appear.
- Monitoring CO_2 in respiratory gases provides an early warning of physiologic and mechanical events that interfere with normal ventilation. Capnography, which measures CO_2 at the patient's airway, is increasingly used in the PACU. Under normal conditions, when ventilation and perfusion are well matched, $ETCO_2$ closely approximates arterial CO_2 ($Paco_2$).
- ECG monitoring should be available for each patient in a Phase I PACU and should be readily available for patients in Phase II units. Arrhythmias of any type may occur at any time in any patient during the postoperative period. Any type of cardiac arrhythmia may be seen in the PACU. The causes of specific arrhythmias must be carefully differentiated before any treatment is instituted.
- Measuring of the patient's body temperature in the PACU is particularly important. At minimum, the preoperative assessment, initial postoperative physical assessment, and discharge evaluation of the patient in Phases I and II PACUs should include documentation of temperature.
- Optimally, 30 mL/hr or more of urine should be obtained from a catheterized adult to ensure proper hydration and kidney function. Urinary output should be closely monitored in the recovery phase; measurement of urinary output and urine specific gravity yields important clues to the overall status of the patient and may alert the nurse to overhydration, dehydration, or the development of shock.
- The clinical goal of PEEP is to raise the functional residual capacity (FRC).
- Mechanical ventilation is instituted to correct one of three pathophysiologic processes: acute hypoventilation or apnea, high V_A/Q_C, and low V_A/Q_C.

- Intermittent mandatory ventilation (IMV) is a good method of weaning a patient from mechanical ventilation and offers many advantages. It increases safety, decreases weaning time, preserves respiratory muscle strength and coordination by allowing ongoing spontaneous breathing efforts, and improves psychologic adjustments to weaning.
- Pulmonary complications are the single leading cause of morbidity and mortality in the postoperative period. An incidence of 4.5% to 76% (average of 11%) of pulmonary complications after abdominal operations has been reported. Most research has shown that the incidence of postoperative complications is highest after upper abdominal and thoracic surgery.
- The modified stir-up regimen, consisting of turn-cascade cough-SMI, should be used on every patient recovering from anesthesia in the PACU.

▶ STUDY QUESTIONS

1. What subjective data should be communicated to the perianesthesia nurse when the patient is admitted to the PACU, and what information should be specifically included in the postanesthesia report?

2. What is the postanesthesia recovery score, and how is it assessed?

3. How is respiratory function assessed in the postanesthesia period, and what common problems may be seen?

4. How are cardiovascular function and perfusion assessed in the postanesthesia period, and what problems may be encountered during this period?

5. How are central nervous system and fluid balance assessed in the postanesthesia period?

6. What are the treatment modalities that may be instituted in the PACU?

7. What are the indications for mechanical ventilation in the postanesthesia period?

8. How are postoperative nausea, vomiting, and pain managed in the postanesthetic period?

KEY REFERENCES

Altsberger, D., & Shrewsbury, P. (1988). Postoperative pain management: The PACU nurse's challenge. *Journal of Post Anesthesia Nursing, 3*(6), 399–403.

Campbell, A., and Johnston, C. A. (1991). OR-PACU reports: What they should tell you about your postoperative patient. *Nursing 91, 21*(10), 49–51.

Drain, C. (1994), *The post anesthesia care unit: A critical care approach to post anesthesia nursing* (3rd ed.). Philadelphia: Saunders.

Goldiner, P. (1997): Are all post anesthesia care units created equal? *Audio-Digest Anesthesiology, 39*(7), 1–4.

Oakes D. (1988). *Clinical practitioners pocket guide to respiratory care.* Old Town, ME: Health Educator Publications.

REFERENCES

Altsberger, D., & Shrewsbury, P. (1988). Postoperative pain management: The PACU nurse's challenge. *Journal of Post Anesthesia Nursing, 3*(6), 399–403.

Campbell, A., & Johnston, C. A. (1991). OR-PACU reports: What they should tell you about your postoperative patient. *Nursing 91, 21*(10), 49–51.

Drain, C. (1994). *The post anesthesia care unit: A critical care approach to post anesthesia nursing* (3rd ed.). Philadelphia: Saunders

Drain, C. (1996). Anesthesia care of the patient with reactive airways disease. *CRNA: The Clinical Forum for Nurse Anesthetists, 7*(4), 207–212.

Drain, C., & Robinson, S. (1996). The pharmacology of respiratory disorders related to anesthesia. *CRNA: The Clinical Forum for Nurse Anesthetists, 7*(4), 193–199.

Flacke, J., & Flacke, W. (1983). Inadvertent hypothermia: Frequent, insidious, and often serious. *Seminars in Anesthesia, 2*(3), 183–196.

Frost, E., & Andrews, I. (1983). Recovery room care. *International Anesthesiology Clinics, 21*(1), 21–28.

Goldiner, P. (1997). Are all postanesthesia care units created equal? *Audio-Digest Anesthesiology, 39*(7), 1–4.

Guyton, A. (1996). *Textbook of medical physiology* (9th ed., pp. 311–342). Philadelphia: Saunders.

Harper, R. (1981). *A guide to respiratory care.* Philadelphia: Lippincott.

Henneman, E. A., & Henneman, P. L. (1989). Intricacies of blood pressure measurement: Reexamining the rituals. *Heart Lung, 18*(3), 263–273.

Kirby, R., Smith, R., & Desautels, D. (1985). *Mechanical ventilation.* New York: Churchill Livingstone.

Kruse, D. H. (1983). Postoperative hypothermia. *Focus on Critical Care, 10*(2), 48–50.

Lake C. (1990). *Clinical monitoring.* Philadelphia: Saunders.

Levitzky, M. (1991). *Pulmonary physiology* (3rd ed., pp. 281–342). New York, McGraw-Hill.

McGaffigan, P., & Christoph, S. (1994). Assessment and monitoring of the post anesthesia patient. In C. Drain (Eds.), *The post anesthesia care unit: A critical care approach to post anesthesia nursing* (3rd ed., pp. 12–50). Philadelphia: Saunders.

McPherson, S. (1990). *Respiratory therapy equipment* (4th ed.). St. Louis, MO: Mosby.

Mecca, R. S. (1997). In Barash, P. G., Cullen, B. F., & Stoelting, R. K. (Eds.), *Clinical anesthesia* (3rd ed., pp. 1279–1303). Philadelphia: Lippincott-Raven.

Miller, R. D. (1994). *Anesthesia* (4th ed.). New York: Churchill Livingstone.

Murray, J., & Nadel, J. (1994). *Textbook of respiratory medicine* (2nd ed.). Philadelphia: Saunders.

New, W. (1985). Pulse oximetry. *Journal of Clinical Monitoring, 1*(2), 126–129.

Nunn, J. (1984). Positive end-expiratory pressure. *International Anesthesiology Clinics, 22*(4), 149.

Oakes, D. (1988). *Clinical practitioners pocket guide to respiratory care.* Old Town, ME: Health Educator Publications.

Roberson, C., & McLeskey, C. (1996). Ondansetron: In a class (5-HT$_3$) of its own. *Seminars in Anesthesia, 15*(1), 41–46.

Sanders, A. (1989). End-tidal carbon dioxide monitoring during cardiopulmonary resuscitation: A prognostic indicator for survival. *Journal of the American Medical Association, 262*(10), 1347–1351.

Shapiro, B., & Cane, R. (1990). Respiratory care. In R. Miller (Ed.), *Anesthesia* (3rd ed., pp. 2169–2210). New York: Churchill Livingstone.

Shinozaki, T., Deane, R., & Perkins, F. M. (1988). Infrared tympanic thermometer: Evaluation of a new clinical thermometer. *Critical Care Medicine, 16*(2), 148–150.

Skoog, R. E. (1989). Capnography in the post anesthesia care unit. *Journal of Post Anesthesia Nursing, 4*(3), 147–155.

Stoelting, R. (1991). *Pharmacology and physiology in anesthetic practice* (2nd ed., pp. 719–751). Philadelphia: Lippincott.

Traver, G., Mitchell, J., & Flodquist-Priestley, G. (1992): *Respiratory care: A clinical approach* (pp. 165–185). Gaithersburg, MD: Aspen.

Pain Management

Margaret Faut-Callahan and Louis Heindel

The phenomenon of pain has been studied for hundreds of years, yet today it remains a major health issue. Bonica (1980) was one of the first to report in the anesthesia literature the importance of unmanaged pain. It was estimated that over 50 million Americans are disabled annually because of a pain problem. Hospitalized patients report significant levels of pain associated with various diagnoses, including postsurgical, oncologic, and medical entities (Cohen, 1980; Donovan, Dillon, & McGuire, 1987; Marks & Sachar, 1973; Mather & Mackie, 1981; Sriwantanakul, Weiss, & Alloza, 1983). Pain management remains a problem. The Agency for Health Care Policy and Research (AHCPR) focused its efforts on the unrelieved pain associated with operative and medical procedures and trauma, oncologic pain (1994), and pediatric pain (1992). No single group seems to be immune from the occurrence of pain.

Nurse anesthetists must familiarize themselves with the latest information and issues in pain management. For the surgical patient, it often is the nurse anesthetist who initiates the pain management plan of care. Furthermore, nurse anesthetists are being called upon to assist with the care of chronic pain patients. Proper assessment, application of current theories in pain management, development and evaluation of the care plan, and additional intervention are all within the realms of current nurse anesthesia practice.

The nurse anesthetist often is in the best position to assess the preoperative and intraoperative patient response to pain and the stress of surgery. On the basis of this assessment, the postoperative pain management plan is developed, incorporating all strategies in the management of pain, including pharmacologic and nonpharmacologic interventions. Developing a patient-centered approach for the management of pain provides the best mechanism for rapid resolution of patient discomfort. Pain management is not limited to patients with acute pain. Patients often present for surgery with chronic, unrelated pain conditions that also must be evaluated. Furthermore, nurse anesthetists are often found in pain centers providing needed pain assessment and management services.

▶ CONCEPTUAL MODEL

Recognizing the interaction between the patient, the care providers, and the delivery system is essential in developing an adequate pain management plan. One model identifies the interaction between nociception, pain experience, and pain behaviors (Loeser & Egan, 1989). A modification of that model is depicted in Figure 31–1 (Donovan, Slack, & Faut, 1989), and highlights the need to evaluate the systems response to the patient in pain. Success or failure in this area significantly impacts the patient. The modification to Loeser's early work focuses on the concept of system response. Health care providers must respond to the patients' assessment of pain; without appropriate and timely intervention, one could argue that the provider has not met his or her commitment to the patient.

Edwards (1990) identified many issues related to the failure of providers to administer or of patients to obtain adequate postoperative analgesia. He categorized the issues relative to the responsibility of health care professionals, patients and families, and system and administrators (Table 31–1). It is clear that the opportunity for inappropriate pain management is an obvious and complex issue.

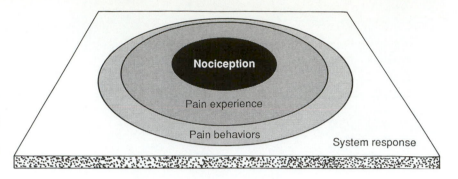

Figure 31–1. Model for pain management. *(Adapted from Loeser, J., & Egan, D. [1989]. Managing the chronic pain patient.* Theory and practice at the University of Washington Multidisciplinary Pain Clinic *[p. 6]. New York: Raven Press.)*

▶ THEORETICAL FRAMEWORK

It is important to understand historical and theoretical developments in pain management. Primitive man believed that pain was a reflection of evil spirits of objects intruding the body. The Egyptians thought that pain was caused by the dead wishing evil on the living while Hebraic societies believed that pain was a consequence of sin (Lundeberg, 1995).

The Greeks wrote about sensations extensively. Plato thought that the heart was at the center of all feelings while Aristotle believed it to be the "quale of the soul" (Lundeberg, 1995). It was not until early discoveries leading to the measurement of nerve conduction in the 1900s that the phenomena of pain, nerve conduction, and response of the brain, were linked.

▶ PAIN THEORIES

The evolution of pain theories has largely spanned the later part of the twentieth century, although references to pain have been made since the beginning of time. Although many theories have been posited, five major theories have been developed. Descartes and others believed that the brain was the center of all motor activities and sensation. However, it was not until 1858 that the specificity theory was presented by Schiff (Bonica, 1990). Schiff suggested that pain and touch were specific and independent. In his work, Schiff demonstrated that cutting into gray matter eliminated pain but had no affect on touch; conversely, cutting into white matter affected touch but not pain. Further work isolated areas dealing with warmth and cold (Fig. 31-2A).

TABLE 31–1. Barriers to Appropriate Postoperative Pain Management

	Deficit in Knowledge/Skill	Resultant Attitude	Inappropriate Resultant Behavior
Health care professionals	Anatomy, physiology, psychology of postop pain	"The pain well"	Therapy as needed; too little, too infrequently
	Pharmacology of opioid drugs	Fear of physiologic fallout	
	Understanding how to assess pain and response to therapy	"It doesn't make any difference"	
	Knowledge of spectrum of existing drugs	Conventional approaches	Wrong drug; wrong route of administration
	Understanding existing modern pain therapy technology, including advantages/disadvantages of patient-controlled analgesia, etc.	Patients cannot determine own needs or self-medicate safely	Therapy determined by patient's ability to convince staff of sincerity: the adversarial stance
Patients and families	Knowledge of availability of modern pain control	Expect pain around a procedure; should not burden staff	Grin and bear it
	Understanding of "signals" and language to make the system respond to pain control needs	Staff are cruel, uncaring; do not understand—the enemy	Cajole, argue, demand: the adversarial approach
System and administrator	Knowledge of role of pain control in marketing services	Pain management team/equipment too expensive	Stonewall requests for personnel/equipment
	Knowledge of potential for reduction of surgical complications/length of stay versus expense of providing service	Service is "unnecessary"	Stonewall requests for payment

From Edwards, W. T. (1990). U.S. Cancer Pain Relief Committee. New York: Elsevier.

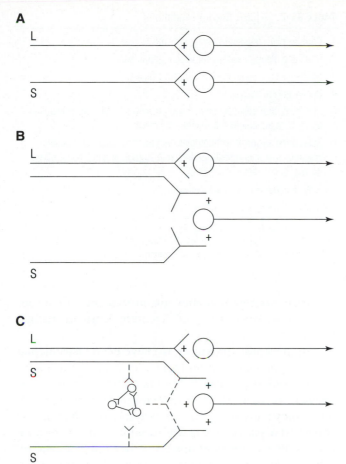

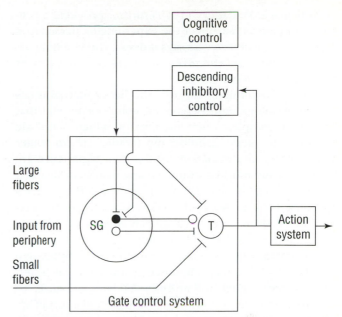

Figure 31–3. Gate control theory. *(From Melzack, R., & Wall, P. [1983]. The challenge of pain. New York: Basic Books.)*

Figure 31–2. Illustration of pain transmission theories. *(From Bonica, J. [1990]. History of pain concepts and therapies. In J. Bonica [Ed.]. The Management of Pain [1st ed., pp. 2–17]. Philadelphia: Lea & Febiger.)*

In 1874 Erbin posited the intensive theory of pain. This theory was based on previous work of Aristotle, Darwin, and others. This theory suggests that every stimulus can cause pain if the intensity is high enough. Pain is the summation of stimuli at the level of the dorsal horn and occurs if a critical level is exceeded (Fig. 31-2B).

In the mid-twentieth century, Livingston proposed the central summation theory. In his work Livingston suggested that intense stimulation of internuncial neuron pools in the central nervous system, specifically the spinal cord, activates the sympathetic nervous system and somatic motor systems. Stimulation of these systems causes vasoconstriction, increased work of the heart and skeletal muscle spasm, establishing a positive feedback loop (Fig. 31-2C).

The pattern theory of pain perception postulated that the brain recognized patterns of pain. This was based on the premise that it was the intensity of the stimulus and central summation that caused the signal to be perceived as pain.

Today, the most commonly discussed theory of pain is one that was posited by Melzack and Wall in 1965. The gate control theory of pain has been modified several times and has resulted in a 1983 adaptation (Fig. 31-3). This theory presents a holistic approach to understanding pain and acknowledges the sociocultural and psychologic issues that influence the perception of pain intensity and quality. The entire nervous system is involved in modulating both physiologic and psychologic responses of the body to painful stimuli. Peripheral nerves conduct excitatory signals to the spinal cord and upward to the thalamus and cortex. The major emphasis of this theory is that pain is modifiable. Melzack and Wall (1983) hypothesize that a gate mechanism in the substantia gelatanosia opens and closes in response to stimuli. They suggested that the gate opens in response to small-fiber (A delta and C) stimulation and closes in response to large fiber (A beta) stimulation. This theory has generated much discussion and controversy, and although is not universally accepted, it has been a significant contribution in the area of pain management.

▶ DEFINITIONS OF PAIN

Reluctance to explore beyond the boundaries of some early theories may have contributed to the limited understanding of the phenomenon of pain. In 1979, however, the International Association for the Study of Pain developed a definition of pain that has provided new direction. Accordingly, pain was defined as an unpleasant sensory and emotional experience associated with actual or potential tissue damage, or described in terms of such damage. McCaffery (1979) further provided a definition of pain as "whatever the experiencing person says it is, existing whenever he says it does." These definitions remind us that the caregiver should believe the patient and then intervene.

These definitions support the belief that pain has both physiologic and behavioral components and that pain is a complex phenomenon for which simplistic strategies for understanding and treating are no longer appropriate. All dimensions of the pain experience are important and must be evaluated and managed. Simply, if all providers understand the importance of the patient's response to pain and work to develop systems to assess and meet these needs adequately, then few patients should have complaints about pain.

Unfortunately, the issue is much more complex. System failures have been identified in areas such as health provider knowledge and attitude deficits, inadequate assessment/intervention strategies, and unavailability of appropriate analgesics and/or qualified providers to administer the best pain management regimen (Marks & Sachar, 1973; Cohen, 1980; Grossman & Sheidler, 1985; Lander, 1990; Portenoy & Kranner, 1985; Porter & Jick, 1980; Watt-Watson, 1987; Weis, Sriwatanakul, Alloza, Weintraub, & Lasagna, 1983; Weissman & Dahl, 1990). Furthermore, Faut et al. (1989), Donovan et al. (1989) and Paice, Mahon, and Faut-Callahan (1995) demonstrated system failures in both surgical and nonsurgical patients. Even in a system that recognized the need for advanced pain managment strategies, these researchers found repeated examples of suboptimal pain management.

When one reviews the practices of physicians, one finds that they undermedicate by at least 50% (Angell, 1982; Beaver, 1980; Marks & Sachar, 1973). When working with as needed (PRN) orders, nurses undermedicate by 50% (Rankin, 1984). It is no wonder that as high as 75%

TABLE 31–2. AHCPR Recommendations

1. Promise patients attentive analgesic care.
2. Chart and display assessment of pain and relief.
3. Define pain and relief levels to trigger a review.
4. Survey patient satisfaction.
5. Analgesic drug treatment should comply with several basic principles: use of both nonopioid and opioid analgesics.
6. Specialized analgesic technologies, including systemic or intraspinal continuous or intermittent opioid administration or patient controlled dosing, local anesthetic infusion.
7. Offer nonpharmacologic interventions.
8. Monitor the efficacy of pain treatment.

From Agency for Health Care Policy Research. (1992). Acute pain management: Operative or medical procedures and trauma. Clinical practice guidelines (pp. 75–76). AHCPR Publication 92-0032. Rockville, MD: Author.

of patients report that they are in moderate to severe pain (Coyle, 1985; Dewi, 1972; Shimm, Laque, & Malbie, 1979).

As anesthesia providers, we have been instrumental in solving much of the problem with pain management. However, there is still much work to be done. So much needs to be done that the federal government, through the Agency for Health Care Policy and Research (AHCPR) convened a panel specifically to address issues of concern in the management of patient in acute pain. The result has been the publication of standards (1992) to guide practice. As anesthesia providers we must be aware of the guidelines and implement them as appropriate in our practice.

The AHCPR guidelines specifically caution us to provide complete care to patients in pain. Eight recommendations were made and are found in Table 31–2. Many of the AHCPR recommendations rely heavily on a system-

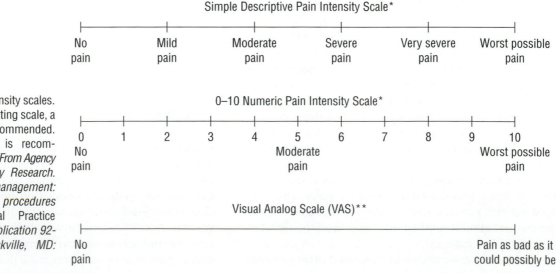

Figure 31–4. Pain intensity scales. *If used as a graphic rating scale, a 10-cm baseline is recommended. **A 10-cm baseline is recommended for VAS scales. *(From Agency for Health Care Policy Research. [1992]. Acute pain management: Operative or medical procedures and trauma. Clinical Practice Guidelines. AHCPR Publication 92-0032 [p. 116]. Rockville, MD: Author.)*

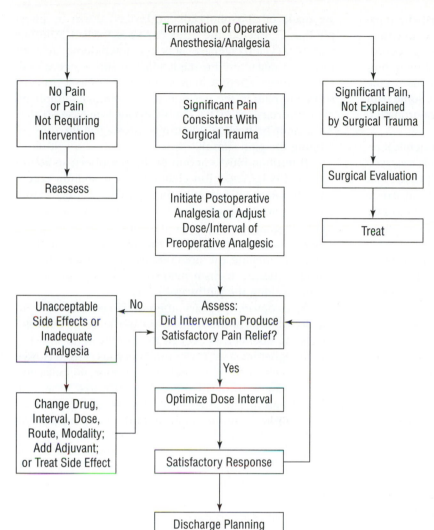

Figure 31–5. Pain treatment flowchart, post-operative phase. *(From Agency for Health Care Policy and Research [1992]. Acute pain management: Operative or medical procedures and trauma.* Clinical Practice Guidelines. AHCPR Publication 92-0032 [p. 10]. Rockville, MD: Author.)

atic plan to assess and reassess a patient's pain. The best way to accomplish this is to develop a system in which a consistent evaluation mechanism is employed. The use of a standardized assessment form provides the most effective overall way of managing a patient's pain. The proper use of such an assessment instrument is the clearest way to communicate among all health care providers caring for the patient in pain. Several suggested assessment instruments are presented in Figure 31–4 and will be discussed in greater detail later in this chapter. The AHCPR guidelines also suggest clear adherence to a pain treatment flowchart to assist providers in managing a patient's acute pain. This flowchart is depicted in Figure 31–5.

To treat pain adequately, one must constantly review the physiology of pain, the pharmacology of our agents, and the efficacy of adjuvant interventions. We must be aware and respect the behavioral principles that form the foundation of our work in the area of pain management. The use of established guidelines is effec-

tive in the management of these complex patient care situations.

▶ PHYSIOLOGY OF PAIN

It is necessary briefly to review the physiology of pain. Pain can be initiated by various types of stimuli. Chemical, thermal, and mechanical stimuli can initiate a pain message. The painful stimuli results from some form of trauma. The traumatized tissue then releases substances that stimulate the afferent nerve fibers or nociceptors. Several different types of afferent nerve fibers have been identified. They are classified as Type A, Type B, and Type C fibers. Painful stimuli will likely affect more than one type of afferent nerve fiber. This difference in affect is what causes, in part, the many characteristics of the transmission of a pain stimulus.

Pain is broadly characterized as nociceptive or neuropathic. Briefly, nociceptive pain is best illustrated by inflammatory disease processes such as arthritis. These patients do not have constant pain and only experience pain when the joints are actively or passively moved. Neuropathic pain is quite different. It is a dysfunction of the nervous system that allows for spontaneous excitation leading to severe pain (Lundeberg, 1995). Some pain syndromes exhibit both nociceptive and neuropathic pain components.

Once a pain reaction occurs, a series of chemical reactions are initiated (Fig. 31-6). Potassium is released from the interior of the cell. This causes the plasma that leaks into the traumatized tissue to produce a substance called bradykinin. Both potassium and bradykinin irritate the tissues and nerve fibers further. The tissue injury causes platelets to mount a response and thus release a substance called serotonin. In addition, the mast cells, which are responsible for fighting infection, release histamine. This reaction results in the development of an inflammatory response. Nerve fibers release chemicals called neurotransmitters. The best understood of these is Substance P. It potentiates and spreads the pain message through a series of electrochemical actions. An age-old remedy, capsaisin, works here by causing sensory neurons to release Substance P. Substance P is then depleted, decreasing the pain signal.

When an injury occurs, the cell membranes, which are made of phospholipids are broken down by phospholipase. Arachidonic acids (AA) are formed. Another enzyme, cyclooxygenase acts on arachidonic acid to form prostaglandin. Prostaglandin sensitizes nerve endings (primary afferent neurons) and serves as a primary source of pain in the periphery. Nonsteroidal antiinflammatory drugs (NSAIDs) inhibit cyclooxygenase so that AA cannot be broken down into prostaglandin, thus inhibiting the pain stimuli.

If nothing blocks action in the periphery, an action potential is initiated. Ion channels open, sodium enters the cell, and potassium exits the cell. This produces ionic changes that allows pain stimuli to pass along the neuron from the periphery to the spinal cord. Some drugs block sodium channels and stabilize the membrane. Membrane stabilizers include the anticonvulsants and anesthetics. Through this mechanism, pain stimuli are not allowed to continue along the pathway.

Nociceptors (primary afferent fibers) terminate in the dorsal horn of the spinal cord. In the spinal cord the ascending fibers cross over to the contralateral side and rise to higher levels in the central nervous system (CNS). These levels in the CNS include the pons, medulla, and hypothalamus. Messages must be transmitted from neuron to neuron. The afferent fiber message cannot jump from neuron to another neuron, so the neurons must re-

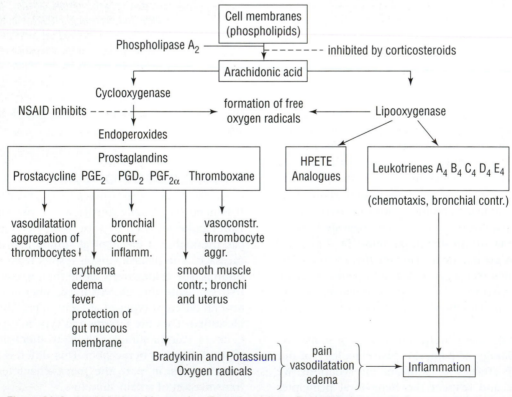

Figure 31–6. Arachidonic acid cascade. *(From Lundeberg, T. [1995]. Pain physiology and principles of treatment.* Scandinavian Journal of Rehabilitative Medicine *[Suppl. 32], 13–42.)*

lease neurotransmitters at the synaptic cleft. The best understood is once again Substance P. Substance P binds to the receptor on a spinothalamic tract (STT) neuron, the ascending fibers. When enough binding takes place, another action potential is initiated within the STT. This perpetuates the pain stimuli/message. The message continues until it is either blocked or terminates in the thalamus.

The synaptic cleft is a central part of the pain pathway. It is here where many opioids bind to block painful stimuli. Opioid receptors have been classified as mu-$_1$, mu-$_2$, delta, kappa, sigma, and epsilon. Opioid receptors have been further characterized by their actions (Table 31-3). Endorphins and enkephalins are naturally produced by the body and bind with the opioid receptors and are natural modulators; an endogenous system. This action inhibits the transmission of the pain stimuli.

Opioid receptors also are found higher in the central nervous system, in the pons, medulla, cortex, and brain stem. When opioids bind with these receptors, it is more likely that adverse reactions, such as respiratory depression, nausea and vomiting, increased sedation and decreased consciousness, will be seen.

If the pain message has not been blocked by this point, it will travel and terminate in the thalamus, where it will be relayed to the somatosensory cortex and the association cortex in the parietal lobe. From this point the pain message is sent to the limbic system and other areas in the brain. It is at this point that the patient perceives pain. The goal of pain management should be to inhibit pain before the patient can perceive the pain. Based on this observation, it is clear why cognitive behavioral techniques are helpful in alleviating some types of pain.

In addition to transmitting painful stimuli in an ascending manner, a descending system also plays a part in the modulation of pain. The descending system originates in the pons and medulla, where many of the ascending neurons end. The message then gets sent down the descending pathway to the dorsal horn of the spinal cord where substances such as serotonin and norepinephrine are released from their vesicle into the synaptic cleft. These substances then bind with the receptors in the afferent fibers to prevent the release of neurotransmitters and results in the inhibition of the pain stimuli.

Serotonin and norepinephrine are recycled by the body. They are released by the receptors and are taken back up in the vesicles where they remain to be used again if the descending signals continue. Antidepressant therapy works here. Antidepressants inhibit the reuptake of serotonin and norepinephrine into the vesicles, which ultimately increases the buildup of these substances in the synaptic cleft. This is why antidepressant therapy is often useful in the total management of a patient's pain.

▶ BEHAVIORAL COMPONENTS OF PAIN MANAGEMENT AND EFFECTS OF UNRELIEVED PAIN

There is now convincing evidence that unrelieved pain may result not only in harmful physiologic responses, but also in harmful psychologic effect (Kehlet, 1989; Yaeger, Glass Neff, & Brinck-Johnsen, 1987). Shorter hospital stay, morbidity, and mortality and increased patient satisfaction have been reported with effective pain relief (Cullen et al., 1985; Modig & Paalzow, 1981).

Pain, especially severe pain, can cause a number of changes in an individual's behavior, including increased self-absorption, withdrawal from interpersonal contact, and increased sensitivity to external stimuli such as light and sound. Emotional processes are central to the experience and expression of pain. In fact, signs of emotional distress such as fear and anxiety are frequently the most recognizable evidence that a patient is experiencing pain. Although Craig and Prkachin (1982) identified anxiety, fear, and depression as the most common emotional concomitant of pain, other emotions, including anger, aggression, guilt, and subservience may be observed.

Unrelieved severe pain can lead to depression and a feeling of helplessness as patients experience a loss of control over their environment. If the source of pain persists and is perceived as uncontrollable, high levels of anxiety can be precipitated (Johnson, Magnani, Chan, & Ferrante, 1989). In a few cases, the inability to cope with pain may create an acute psychotic reaction (Peck, 1986).

Unrelieved acute pain is one of the important factors contributing to the development of delirium in the intensive care unit, which can be further exacerbated by related sleeplessness (Cousins & Phillips, 1986). A vicious circle of pain, anxiety, fear, helplessness, and sleep

TABLE 31-3. Opioid Receptors

Mu$_1$	Supraspinal analgesia, miosis, hypothermia, prolactin release, catalepsy
Mu$_2$	Respiratory depression, physical dependence, sedation, bradycardia, decreased GI motility, euphoria
Delta	Analgesia, alterations in affective behavior
Kappa	Spinal analgesia, respiratory depression, miosis, sedation
Sigma	Psychomotor stimulation, hallucinations, mydriasis, tachycardia, tachypnea
Epsilon	Dysphoria, analgesia

Adapted from Noren, R. (1994). Opiate pharmacology. In R. Hamill & J. Rowlingson, (Eds.), Handbook of critical care pain management (p. 122). New York: McGraw-Hill.

deprivation occurs if pain persists unrelieved for several days.

In both the clinical setting and the laboratory, individual differences in responsiveness to noxious stimuli are documented. Clinical observations by Beecher (1956) of wounded soldiers constituted the first clear description of individual differences in pain response to injury. Beecher reported that 65% of soldiers who were severely wounded in battle felt little or no pain. This phenomenon was attributed to the positive meaning of the pain experience: being wounded meant the soldier would be sent home. Civilian surgical teams have reported similar findings of decreased pain response after surgery on patients in developing countries because the opportunity to have corrective surgery is viewed by the patients in a very positive sense. In a study of patients in an emergency unit, 30% did not feel pain at the time of injury, and some did not experience pain for several hours after the injury; Melzack, Wall, and Ty (1982) concluded that the link between injury and pain is highly variable and depends on the circumstances surrounding the injury.

Researchers have known for years that much of the variance in pain response is due to psychologic factors (Averill, 1973). Anxiety has been shown to be fostered by the anticipation of an unpleasant experience (Hodges & Spielberger, 1966). Uncertainty enhances anxiety. Pain that escalates because of anxiety is likely to be reduced when information is given that reduces the uncertainty regarding questions of concern. A number of studies have demonstrated that measures that reduce anxiety have an important bearing on the acute pain experienced by patients and the need for analgesia (Chapman & Cox, 1977; Fortin & Kirovac, 1976).

Another important area of study has been the interaction between coping style and the control the patient has over the situation. Patients who anticipate that they will have some control over stressful stimuli experience less anxiety (Andrew, 1970; Ball & Vogler, 1977; Mandler & Watson, 1966). Some of the effectiveness of patient-controlled anesthesia (PCA) is attributed to the sense of control that is fostered when the patient knows that he or she can administer analgesia on demand (Johnson, Magnani, Chan, & Ferrante, 1989).

Fear of the unknown and of death probably are the most intense emotions a person can experience. Circumstances associated with acute postoperative pain and trauma are most likely to aggravate such fears. Fear of the unknown produced by hospitalization and the possibility of disability, loss of life, loss of freedom, and separation from one's family are all very real stressors for patients. Furthermore, the anxiety experienced by family members often is transferred directly to the patient and serves to reinforce fear and anxiety. In a detailed analysis of the variance in pain response, Peck (1986) identified a

number of psychologic factors that can affect the individual's response to pain, including fear and anxiety, meaning of pain, observable learning, perceived control of events, coping style, cultural differences, and attention/distraction.

Some studies of pain relief suggest that the initial experience with pain management may be an important determinant of future relief (Craig, 1986; Graffam & Johnson, 1987). The patient's expectations may be conditional with the first experience. Therefore, if pain relief is inadequate, a negative expectation could adversely affect later pain control efforts. This has important implications for clinicians to provide adequate analgesia as quickly as possible to convey the expectation that pain control measures will continue to be effective.

▶ FACTORS THAT INFLUENCE THE EFFICACY OF PAIN MANAGEMENT

Clinicians' attitudes, institutional priorities, and factors associated with the patient can influence clinical decisions about pain management. A number of variables affect the clinician's decision to order or administer analgesia to patients. Studies of pain management have identified that no specific group of health care providers consistently accepts responsibility for pain relief (Faut et al., 1989; Sofaer, 1985). This has serious implications for patients because adequate analgesia must be ordered and administered to patients in a timely fashion.

One variable that influences clinicians' medication practices is the ability to assess accurately the level of pain intensity and intervene effectively to manage the patient's pain. If pain is assessed inadequately or too infrequently, relief may be inadequate. To manage pain effectively, one must understand what the experience of pain is like for the patient and accurately assess the intensity of pain. Specific issues related to measurement and assessment of pain are discussed later in this chapter.

In a study of 255 adult and pediatric patients, the clinician's stated goal for complete pain relief was not significantly related to the amount of analgesic administered or to the level of pain relief reported by the patients (Donovan et al., 1989). This lack of relationship between clinician attitudes and actual clinical practice requires further study to determine why it exists.

The clinician's perception of the severity of a patient's illness has also been reported to affect the selection of analgesic regimen. Higher pain levels are attributed to patients with objective signs of pathophysiologic disruption (Burgess, 1981). Yet, pain experts widely accept that physical pathology alone is not necessarily related to the amount of pain reported by an individual (Melzack et al., 1982). This finding has implications for the patient with chronic pain, who may or may not exhibit obvious pathophysiologic alterations. The pain management of the chronic pain patient may be a different type and quality from that provided to the acute pain patient.

In 1973 Marks and Sachar suggested that inadequate administration of analgesia occured because health care professionals have incorrect pharmacologic information about various analgesics and an excessive and unrealistic concern about addiction. In 1980 Cohen stated that undermedication may be the result of caregivers' lack of the basic knowledge necessary to manage pain effectively. She also found clinicians to be overly concerned with the possibility of addiction in their patients. They often lacked knowledge of the physiologic action of analgesics. A review of both medical and nursing curricula and textbooks reveals that very little formal instruction is provided about pain management. Even less information is provided about pharmacologic principles and use of analgesics. This inadequate knowledge base has probably contributed to misconceptions about pain and to ineffective use of pharmacologic and nonpharmacologic interventions for pain relief.

The use of narcotics to control pain often is associated with concerns about addiction and respiratory depression (Jaffee, 1985). The tendency on the part of clinicians to select nontherapeutic doses of narcotic analgesics is most likely influenced by overestimating the incidence of narcotic addiction (Cohen, 1980; Jaffee, 1985; Marks & Sachar, 1973). In a study by Porter and Jick (1980) only 4 of 11 882 patients became addicted during hospitalization.

The fear of side effects such as respiratory depression also is unwarranted unless a toxic dose of the narcotic is administered. In one study, clinicians erroneously attributed analgesia rather than uncontrolled pain to be the cause of respiratory changes on the day after surgery (Cohen, 1980). In another study of 134 surgical patients, patients receiving effective epidural analgesia in the early postoperative phase demonstrated significantly better postoperative recovery in relation to respiratory and ambulatory parameters than patients reporting inadequate pain relief (Slack & Faut-Callahan, 1990). Effective analgesia may be an important "overlooked" factor in the overall efforts of the health care system to decrease the length of patients' hospitalization.

Interestingly, clinicians continue to administer medications such as demerol to patients without apparent concern, even though there is a potential for serious side effects. Pellegrine, Paice, and Faut-Callahan (1996) found that 79% of the patients were being treated outside of the AHCPR acute pain management guidelines. Nine percent of patients receiving meperidine also were on medications that were contraindicated with this narcotic. Further, 12% were in moderate to severe renal failure.

Forty percent of the patients received concurrent analgesics to alleviate pain, and all reported lower pain scores and higher satisfaction scores. Clearly, an individual's pharmacologic knowledge and attitudes about narcotics can contribute to ineffective pain management.

Further complicating pain management decisions is the patient's belief about pain and analgesia. For example, if the patient believes that pain builds character, this may influence pain behavior (Weis et al., 1983). Patients do not always report pain accurately. Patients may minimize the intensity of pain to avoid receiving medications, either out of fear of injections or out of concern about anticipated side effects. One study reported that 17% of patients were believed to have minimized their pain (Lander, 1990).

Many patients who experience moderate to severe pain wait to ask for pain relief until the pain becomes unbearable. In a study of 259 patients, over two thirds of the patients would wait until they were in severe pain before requesting analgesia or not ask at all, expecting the clinician to know that they were experiencing pain. Furthermore, 75% of the patients expected that when analgesics were requested, they would be administered immediately (Owen, McMillan, & Rogowski, 1990). This lag time between patient request and clinician response contributes significantly to ineffective pain management.

Some patients fail to verbalize pain needs because of the attitude expressed verbally or nonverbally by their health care providers. The patient already is feeling dependent and threatened by the strange hospital environment and may be hesitant to ask for pain relief. In some cases patients are inconsistent in verbal reports of pain. A patient may complain of unrelieved pain to the nurse, but when questioned by a physician, the patient will deny having any pain. Such contradictions in patient communication can contribute to inadequate pain relief. Patients also may be concerned about potential side effects associated with analgesics. Side effects such as drowsiness, nausea, itching, and constipation often are identified as the reasons patients refuse or limit the use of narcotic analgesics.

Clinical decision making should be based not only on the behavior exhibited by the patient but also on the pathophysiologic disruption. The clinician should consider what alterations have occurred in the patient's anatomic and physiologic integrity, such as tissue anoxia, incisional repair, and fractures, that require pain control.

Patient traits also can influence clinical decisions about pain management. Individuals learn to express pain in ways particular to their cultural group (Zborowski, 1952). Therefore, the ethnic background of the patient may influence pain assessment and management. Other studies have demonstrated that the practitioner's beliefs about ethnic differences influence analgesic administration practices (Von Baeyer, Johnson, & McMillan, 1984).

Studies of health care providers' perceptions of pain in hypothetical cases demonstrated that greater pain was inferred for Jewish American and Hispanic American patients than for African American, Asian American, Mediterranean American, and European American patients (Davitz & Davitz, 1981). Greater pain also was inferred for low-socioeconomic-status patients than moderate- or high-socioeconomic-status patients.

Although studies of the effect of gender on decision making related to pain management have been contradictory, the age of the patient does influence pain management practices. In general, younger children and geriatric patients are prescribed and administered fewer analgesics because of the fear of side effects and myths about the patient's ability to feel pain and the misinterpretation of patient behavior (Faherty & Grier, 1984; Hargreaves, 1987).

What information do clinicians use to evaluate whether the patient is in pain or not? In a classic observational study of decision making related to pain, Hammond (1966) observed 165 cues exhibited by patients and 17 responses to the cues by the health care providers. Clinicians must attend to a wide variation in cues and possible responses when deciding (1) if a patient is in pain; (2) how much pain; (3) whether to provide analgesia; (4) how much to medicate; and (5) what other adjuvant interventions can enhance or potentiate the overall effect of the analgesic regimen.

Clinicians usually are the individuals implicated in poor pain management, but the patient also shares some responsibility. The patient is not a passive recipient of care and should be encouraged to participate in pain control measures. The clinician, however, must consider the patient's individual coping style and ability to use various pain relief measures.

Another factor that influences the efficacy of pain management is the expectation of the health care setting. Consideration of the impact of the health care organization has not been the focus of pain management research; however, the setting within which pain is managed can be a factor. For example, in the intensive care unit the primary focus is the management of the complex physiologic and technologic needs of the patient. Patient needs that are not life-threatening, such as the need for analgesia, often are not a priority. In emergency units, pain is useful for formulating the diagnosis, so analgesia may not be provided.

Other institutional factors that influence pain management include the ability of the organization to recruit and retain permanent staff. Inadequate and inconsistent care providers can further decrease accountability for providing pain relief. The changing health care reimbursement practice that restricts hospital admission of patients until the morning of major surgery is another variable that may influence the efficacy of pain manage-ment. The implication of this practice is that little or no opportunity is provided for the patient to learn various methods of pain control. In a study, Knorrel and Faut-Callahan (1997) found a significant lack of correct information about pain in an ambulatory surgery patient population. They found that the introduction of a simple preoperative teaching video used the morning of surgery signficantly increased patient knowledge, understanding of pain management principles, better use of analgesics, and greater patient satisfaction. The trend toward increased outpatient surgery places increasing importance on the patient's ability to understand and effectively use both pharmacologic and nonpharmacologic pain intervention techniques. As health care reimbursement and quality-of-care reviews become more focused on the outcomes experienced by patients, effective pain relief will gain increasing importance in relation to the overall recovery of the patient.

▶ PAIN ASSESSMENT

Pain is a multidimensional phenomenon in which intensity, quality, meaning, and impact must be considered as part of the assessment. Pain and its management cannot be separated from the individual who experiences the pain. Reporting of pain requires an interaction between caregiver and patient and depends to some extent on the relationship between the staff and patient.

If patients could always tell clinicians that they hurt and clinicians could accept the patient's report as fact, the assessment and management of pain would be significantly less complex; however, as discussed, a number of variables influence the efficacy of pain management. In the clinical setting, accurate assessment and reliable pain measurement are essential for monitoring fluctuations in the patient's pain levels and for evaluating the efficacy of pain relief therapies.

Just as methods of managing pain may vary, similarly, methods for pain assessment also may be different depending on whether the pain is acute or chronic. In the case of chronic pain, measures of behavioral functioning, coping style, and emotional state are important in the overall assessment of the patient's pain. The McGill Pain Questionnaire has greatly facilitated the assessment of the qualities of the pain experienced (Melzack, 1975). It provides intensity-graded scales of word descriptors that assess the sensory, affective, and evaluative aspects of the pain experience. The instrument has content and construct validity and is sensitive to the effects of different therapies of pain. The McGill Pain instrument is frequently used to measure clinical pain and patient response to treatment trials. The limitation of this instrument is that it is complex and time consuming and may not be appropriate for all acute settings.

To assist the clinician in identifying appropriate pain control strategies with the patient, a pain history should be obtained that considers the (1) previous experience(s) with pain and the impact of the current pain event; (2) patient knowledge and understanding of opioid and other sedative drugs; (3) history of drug usage or abuse, if any; (4) previous side effects that may have been experienced with certain drugs; and (5) the patient's coping style with stressful situations or pain (eg, does the patient want information and active involvement in pain control, or does the patient become more anxious and prefer a pain control approach that does not require active participation, such as is necessary with patient-controlled analgesia?).

Pain Rating Scales

Although the multidimensional nature of pain has been widely accepted, the most common approach to pain estimation continues to be unidimensional, in the form of self-report scales on which the patient is asked to rate one dimension of his or her pain, most often its intensity (Syrjala & Chapman, 1984). Such unidimensional rating scales fall into three main categories: the visual analog scale (VAS), the graphic rating scale (GRS), and the numerical rating scale (NRS).

Visual Analog Scale

The visual analog scale (VAS) consists of a 10-cm line with endpoint descriptors beyond the stops at either end (Fig. 31–4). The VAS is useful for patients with limited language skills because the choice points are not labeled. The VAS also has been shown to be sensitive to medication effects over time and to behavioral indicators of pain (Abu-Saad & Holzemer, 1981).

Graphic Rating Scale

A graphic rating scale is a straight-line continuum with four to seven verbal descriptors placed in ascending order of severity at equal intervals along the line (Fig. 31–4). This scale usually is intended for assessing the intensity of pain, so descriptors such as "none," "mild," "moderate," "severe," and "unbearable" are used.

Numerical Rating Scale

The numerical rating scale consists of a straight-line continuum numbered 0 to 10 or 0 to 100 (Fig. 31–4). Anchor points at the two ends are usually "no pain" and "worst pain." The numerical rating scale is a self-report scale that permits more definable choices than the graphic rating scale and increases the sensitivity of the instrument.

Pain Assessment in Children

Assessment of pain in children will vary depending on the child's ability to communicate verbally. For the pre-verbal child or for the child who is reluctant to admit pain, assessment of pain requires observations of physiologic signs and nonverbal behavior. The clinician must assess the pain associated with the procedures and pathologic processes and be especially alert to changes in the child's responses. Children, like adults, may deny pain or refuse analgesia.

Reliable and valid tools are available for assessing pain in children. Graphic rating scales often are used to assess pain in children with cartoon facial scale being one of the most frequently used rating scales (McGrath, de Veber & Hearn, 1985). However, children are sometimes able to communicate more effectively through their drawings than they are able to do verbally. Pain drawings usually convey much more information about the child's perception of pain than other pain assessment methods.

Limitations of Pain Assessment Tools

For research purposes, the self-report rating scales provide no basis for assigning numerical values to categories and using parametric statistics in analyzing the data. Studies have found that the word and numerical categories do not represent successive identical steps in pain intensity. Attachment of a numerical value to each word category descriptor means that the numerical scores are ordinal or rank-ordered scores so that nonparametric statistics are the appropriate level of analysis (Heft & Parker, 1984). The self-report scale scores obtained, however, often are treated as interval or ratio-level scaling in the absence of evidence that respondents have interpreted the self-report numbers as equal increments (Syrjala & Chapman, 1984). All of the self-report scales are notable for clarity and simplicity. The scales are versatile, can be adapted to different cognitive levels, and are practical in a variety of clinical settings.

A limitation of the unidimensional approach to pain measurement is that the patient's pain rating is likely to be influenced by the patient's affective state and all of the other components that contribute to the pain event. The oversimplification of the pain experience that occurs when one mark on a line represents the patient's pain has been criticized (Gracely, 1980). Because the self-report scales cannot assess the diverse qualities of the pain experience, a comprehensive pain history is most useful for determining effective pain control strategies for the individual patient.

To ensure accurate pain measurement, the clinician should review the pain measurement tool with the patient and indicate how frequently the patient will be asked to report pain intensity. The patient should understand the relationship between the pain rating score and pain control measures. It is essential that both the patient and the staff using the pain measurement tool be fully familiar with the scale.

In summary, there are numerous methods of assessing pain, but generally the quantification of pain should be systematic and simple and obtained at appropriate intervals. Some have suggested that it should be incorporated as the fifth vital sign. There should be consistency in interpretation and communication of pain ratings. Accurate assessment enables the clinician to have a clearer understanding of the patient's pain experience and a means of evaluating the effectiveness of pain relief measures and the patient's response.

▶ MANAGEMENT OF PAIN

The management of pain is a complex phenomenon that must be carefully planned. Pain management is best accomplished through a collaborative effort between physicians, nurses, and other health providers. Acute pain must be viewed as a multidimensional phenomenon and must be approached with that in mind. Complete assessment of all components of the patient's pain must be done and an intervention planned that will treat all aspects of the pain. This may mean a multiple drug regimen coupled with cognitive behavioral techniques. The World Health Organization (WHO) promotes the use of a "laddered" approach to pain management. This approach is depicted in Figure 31–7. Although this approach was developed for use with cancer patients, it also provides reference points for the management of all types of pain and is used with other patients as well.

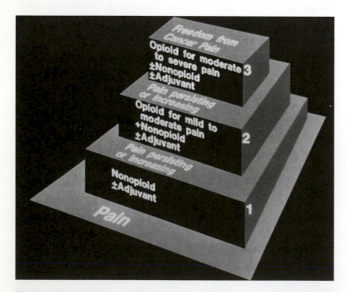

Figure 31-7. Analgesic Ladder. *(From World Health Organization [WHO]. [1990]. Cancer Pain Relief and Palliative Care [p. 9]. Geneva, WHO. Reprinted with permission.)*

Pharmacology

The pharmacologic management of pain is a complex phenomenon and must be managed with such an appreciation. Because the pain experience is not unidimensional, various strategies must be employed adequately to alleviate the patient's pain. To better understand the vast array of interventions, it is necessary to review the types of drugs available to treat a patient in pain.

The choice of appropriate analgesics should be based on the type of pain the patient is experiencing and the site of action of the drug. Once the necessary types of drugs are identified, they should be added to the treatment plan as indicated.

Analgesics are most commonly divided into three groups: opioids, nonopioids, and the adjuvants. As anesthesia providers, we are most familiar with the opioid analgesics. Opioids are used to treat moderate to severe pain and work at the level of the spinal cord by binding to receptors on the afferent neurons. It is here that they block the release of neurotransmitters that inhibits the transmission of the pain stimuli to the ascending fibers.

Opioid analgesics are commonly used to relieve pain. Opioids frequently used are listed in Table 31–4. Morphine was first purified by Serturner in 1806. Since that time, morphine and morphinelike drugs have become the foundation of analgesic therapy. Morphine works in the central nervous system to block painful stimuli. Morphine influences mu opiate receptors located in the brainstem modulating nuclei and the dorsal horn of the spinal cord. Specifically, it activates pain-modulating neurons that inhibit transmission from the primary nociceptor to the dorsal horn. Morphine also has a direct action at the spinal cord. It is known that opiate receptors and endogenous opioids are present at these sites. Morphine, then, works similarly to the endogenous opiates. Evidence of the specificity seen with opioid analgesia is the fact that no other analgesic works with such direct and limited effect as do the opioids. Opioids have very little effect on other central nervous system function.

Other morphinelike drugs work in a similar manner. They produce analgesia through the same central nervous system mechanism. All have different degrees of potency, but in equianalgesic dosages, if tolerated by the patient, a similar level of analgesia is achieved. Morphine and morphinelike substances also produce similar side effects. These include mood changes, nausea and vomiting, sedation, mental clouding, respiratory depression, cough suppression, and pupillary constriction. In addition to these central effects, peripheral effects include decreased gastrointestinal motility, increased biliary duct pressure, pruritus, histamine release, and urinary retention.

Prolonged use of morphine and morphinelike substances has been linked to undesirable drug or disease

TABLE 31–4. Dosing Data for Opioid Analgesics

Drug	Usual Adult Dose	Usual Pediatric Dose[a]	Comments
Oral NSAIDs			
Acetaminophen	650–975 mg q 4 h	10–15 mg/kg q 4 h	Acetaminophen lacks the peripheral antiinflammatory activity of other NSAIDs
Aspirin	650–975 mg q 4 h	10–15 mg/kg q 4 h[b]	The standard against which other NSAIDs are compared. Inhibits platelet aggregation; may cause postoperative bleeding
Choline magnesium trisalicylate (Trilisate)	1000–1500 mg bid	25 mg/kg bid	May have minimal antiplatelet activity; also available as oral liquid
Diflunisal (Dolobid)	1000 mg initial dose followed by 500 mg q 12 h		
Etodolac (Lodine)	200–400 mg q 6–8 h		
Fenoprofen calcium (Nalfon)	200 mg q 4–6 h		
Ibuprofen (Motrin, others)	400 mg q 4–6 h	10 mg/kg q 6–8 h	Available as several brand names and as generic; also available as oral suspension
Ketoprofen (Orudis)	25–75 mg q 6–8 h		
Magnesium salicylate	650 mg q 4 h		Many brands and generic forms available
Meclofenamate sodium (Meclomen)	50 mg q 4–6 h		
Mefenamic acid (Ponstel)	250 mg q 6 h		
Naproxen (Naprosyn)	500 mg initial dose followed by 250 mg q 6–8 h	5 mg/kg q 12 h	Also available as oral liquid
Naproxen sodium (Anaprox)	550 mg initial dose followed by 275 mg q 6–8 h		
Salsalate (Disalcid, others)	500 mg q 4 h		May have minimal antiplatelet activity
Sodium salicylate	325–650 mg q 3–4 h		Available in generic form from several distributors
Parenteral NSAID			
Ketorolac	30 or 60 mg IM initial dose followed by 15 or 30 mg q 6 h. Oral dose following IM dosage: 10 mg q 6–8 h		Intramuscular dose not to exceed 5 days

Note: Only the above NSAIDs have FDA approval for use as simple analgesics, but clinical experience has been gained with other drugs as well.
[a] Drug recommendations are limited to NSAIDs where pediatric dosing experience is available.
[b] Contraindicated in presence of fever or other evidence of viral illness.
From *Agency for Health Care Policy Research. (1992). Acute pain management: Operative or medical procedure and trauma. Clinical practice guidelines. Publication 92-0032 (pp. 16–17). Rockville, MD: Author.*

interaction. Liver and renal failure have been linked to narcotic use. Caution must be exercised when dealing with patients with these types of conditions or on these drugs.

When managing pain problems, the most efficacious approach to pain management includes the use of opioids employing a frontload approach, that is, rapid development of a serum analgesic level. One such scheme for determining appropriate dosages of analgesics is presented in Table 31–4.

Opioids can be used alone or in combination with other drugs. The most commonly used opioid for pain is morphine. It also is used as the standard when measuring the efficacy of other agents. Unfortunately, the adverse reactions seen with opioids, although usually transient,

often keep the health provider from applying the most appropriate drug to a specific patient situation. Adverse effects often seen with opioids are sedation, constipation, respiratory depression, nausea and vomiting, pruritus, and urinary retention. Tolerance develops within 24 to 48 hours with the subsequent elimination of most side effects. Because of this phenomenon, treating these side effects for a short time might be warranted to best manage a patient's pain.

The side effect most often affecting treatment is respiratory depression. This is caused by the binding of the opioid in the pons and medulla. Although this is a significant side effect, it often is assessed inappropriately. A slowing of a rapid respiratory rate may be in part attributed to the patient's becoming more comfortable. Discontinuance of an opioid in a patient who is in real need should be done with proper assessment of the patient's condition and with caution.

Opioids are categorized as agonists, antagonists, and mixed agonist-antagonists. Morphine, hydromorphone, and codeine are agonists and bind to the mu-receptors. Antagonists, such as naloxone and naltrexon are mu-, kappa-, delta-, and sigma-receptor antagonists and prevent opioids from binding. Mixed agonist-antagonists such as Stadol and Talwin bind at the agonist kappa-receptor and as antagonists at the mu-receptor. They should not be used in patients receiving agonists.

Meperidine has been heavily prescribed for years. It is interesting to note that with the development of much better opioids, with fewer side effects, meperidine is still used inappropriately (Pellegrine et al., 1995). Meperidine has significant side effects due to the metabolite normeperidine. Normeperidine causes increased central nervous system toxicity, which is especially problematic in the elderly population and in patients with renal dysfunction. Intramuscular injection of meperidine is very painful with unpredictable absorption, and the oral route provides poor bioavailability. Health providers must step beyond tradition and develop improved treatment strategies.

Another concern that limits the appropriate use of opioids is that of addiction. A surprising number of health providers believe patients can become addicted if given an opioid. This has no substantive basis and is most likely a "myth" that often is propagated. The nonopioid analgesics can be employed to provide adequate analgesia for a patient. Aspirin, acetaminophen, and other nonsteroidal antiinflammatory drugs (NSAIDs) are the most commonly used analgesics. Aspirin has been used since the turn of the century and is quite effective in managing mild to moderate pain. Taylor and Curran (1985) reported that 60% of all Americans used aspirin to relieve mild pain.

Aspirin and the nonsteroidal antiinflammatory agents (Table 31–5) do not work in the central nervous system like the morphinelike substances. Instead, these drugs work in the periphery, decreasing the inflammatory response to tissue damage that accompanies the onset of pain. They act to inhibit cyclooxygenase, which catabolizes arachidonic acid into prostaglandins. Prostaglandins induce inflammation and activate peripheral nociceptors. Thus, any drugs that interfere with this mechanism should also be effective in treating peripheral pain and pain associated with inflammation. Side effects of these drugs include decreased platelet aggregation and prolonged bleeding time, as well as gastric irritation. The most common of these agents are the nonsteroidal antiinflammatory drugs (NSAIDs). They are the largest group of nonopioid analgesics available and should be used to treat mild to moderate pain, either alone or in combination with opioids or other adjuvants. They work in the periphery at the site of injury. The mechanism of action is straightforward. When injury occurs, the injured cell membrane releases phospholipids that are converted into prostaglandin, which in turn sensitizes the nerve to pain. The NSAIDs block the release of enzymes that allow the conversion of phospholipids to prostaglandin. They are not prostaglandin antagonists. In cases of injury, one must wait for all previously released inflammatory mediators to be inactivated. The analgesic effect of the NSAIDs is rapid (10 to 60 minutes), the anti-inflammatory effect may take days.

The concept of preemptive analgesia is an important one. Preemptive analgesia theoretically blocks the pain pathways prior to the injury or surgical intervention (Dahl & Kehlet, 1993; Kehlet & Dahl, 1993a, 1993b; Woolf & Chong, 1993). The use of preemptive analgesia is currently under investigation and the advantages are promising. The NSAIDs seem to offer the most benefit in this area (Fletcher, Zetlaoui, Monin, Bombart & Samii, 1995; Mather, 1992; Sutters, Levine, Dibble, Savedra, & Miaskowski, 1995) and have been used in both adults and children. The NSAIDs most commonly used in the United States are found in Table 31–5 and demonstrate the large number of agents available to health providers in their search to treat a patient's pain adequately.

When looking at the benefits of the NSAIDs, one must clearly evaluate the potential side effects. The most common side effects are gastrointestinal (GI) ulcers and prolonged bleeding time. Both of these conditions occur due to the inhibition of prostaglandin. One must remember that the inhibition of this mechanism occurs not only in the periphery, which decreases the sensitization of the nerves to pain, but also in the stomach. Prostaglandins work in the stomach to produce a protective layer. Because NSAIDs inhibit prostaglandin activity, they can cause GI problems. Although some of these drugs are marketed in forms said to be gentle to the GI system, it is important to note that GI effects occur despite the route of administration because of the prostaglandin effects in the stomach.

Prostaglandin analogs have been administered in an attempt to reverse the deleterious effects of prostaglandin inhibition. Misoprostol (Cytotec®) has been effective. However, the cost associated with this therapy and concerns about polypharmacy have limited its use.

Gastrointestinal irritation is dose dependent, which supports the idea that short, deliberate courses of NSAIDs may be effective in decreasing the dose of opioids, especially in situations where respiratory function is most critical (eg, weaning from mechanical ventilation).

Increased bleeding times is a concern with the administration of NSAIDs because of the inhibition of cycloxygenase, which is necessary for clotting. Aspirin

TABLE 31–5. Dosing Data for NSAIDs

Drug	Approximate Equianalgesic Oral Dose	Approximate Equianalgesic Parenteral Dose	Recommended Starting Dose (adults more than 50 kg body weight)		Recommended Starting Dose (children and adults less than 50 kg body weight)[a]	
			Oral	Parenteral	Oral	Parenteral
Opioid agonist						
Morphine[b]	30 mg q 3–4 h (around-the-clock dosing) 60 mg q 3–4 h (single dose or intermittent dosing)	10 mg q 3–4 h	30 mg q 3–4 h	10 mg q 3–4 h	0.3 mg/kg q 3–4 h	0.1 mg/kg q 3–4 h
Codeine[c]	130 mg q 3–4 h	75 mg q 3–4 h	60 mg q 3–4 h	60 mg q 2 h (intramuscular subcutaneous)	1 mg/kg q 3–4 h[d]	Not recommended
Hydromorphone[b] (Dilaudid)	7.5 mg q 3–4 h	1.5 mg q 3–4 h	6 mg q 3–4 h	1.5 mg q 3–4 h	0.06 mg/kg q 3–4 h	0.015 mg/kg q 3–4 h
Hydrocodone (in Lorcet, Lortab, Vicodin, others)	30 mg q 3–4 h	Not available	10 mg q 3–4 h	Not available	0.2 mg/kg q 3–4 h[d]	Not available
Levorphanol (Levo-Dromoran)	4 mg q 6–8 h	2 mg q 6–8 h	4 mg q 6–8 h	2 mg q 6–8 h	0.04 mg/kg q 6–8 h	0.02 mg/kg q 6–8 h
Meperidine (Demerol)	300 mg q 2–3 h	100 mg q 3 h	Not recommended	100 mg q 3 h	Not recommended	0.75 mg/kg q 2–3 h
Methadone (Dolophine, others)	20 mg q 6–8 h	10 mg q 6–8 h	20 mg q 6–8 h	10 mg q 6–8 h	0.2 mg/kg q 6–8 h	0.1 mg/kg q 6–8 h
Oxycodone (Roxicodone, also in Percocet, Percodan, Tylox, others)	30 mg q 3–4 h	Not available	10 mg q 3–4 h	Not available	0.2 mg/kg q 3–4 h[d]	Not available
Oxymorphone[b] (Numorphan)	Not available	1 mg q 3–4 h	Not available	1 mg q 3–4 h	Not recommended	Not recommended
Opioid agonist-antagonist and partial agonist						
Buprenorphine (Buprenex)	Not available	0.3–0.4 mg q 6–8 h	Not available	0.4 mg q 6–8 h	Not available	0.004 mg/kg q 6–8 h
Butorphanol (Stadol)	Not available	2 mg q 3–4 h	Not available	2 mg q 3–4 h	Not available	Not recommended
Nalbuphine (Nubain)	Not available	10 mg q 3–4 h	Not available	10 mg q 3–4 h	Not available	0.1 mg/kg q 3–4 h
Pentazocine (Talwin, others)	150 mg q 3–4 h	60 mg q 3–4 h	50 mg q 4–6 h	Not recommended	Not recommended	Not recommended

Note: Published tables vary in the suggested doses that are equianalgesic to morphine. Clinical response is the criterion that must be applied for each patient; titration to clinical response is necessary. Because there is not complete cross tolerance among these drugs, it is usually necessary to use a lower than equianalgesic dose when changing drugs and to retitrate to response.

Caution: Recommended doses do not apply to patients with renal or hepatic insufficiency or other conditions affecting drug metabolism and kinetics.

[a] **Caution:** Doses listed for patients with body weight less than 50 kg cannot be used as initial starting doses in babies less than 6 months of age. *Consult the Clinical Practice Guideline for Acute Pain Management: Operative or Medical Procedures and Trauma* section on management of pain in neonates for recommendations.

[b] For morphine, hydromorphone, and oxymorphone, rectal administration is an alternate route for patients unable to take oral medications, but equianalgesic doses may differ from oral and parenteral doses because of pharmacokinetic differences.

[c] **Caution:** Codeine doses above 65 mg often are not appropriate because of diminishing incremental analgesia with increasing doses but continually increasing constipation and other side effects.

[d] **Caution:** Doses of aspirin and acetaminophen in combination opioid/NSAID preparations must also be adjusted to the patient's body weight.

From Agency for Health Care Policy Research. (1992). Acute pain management: Operative or medical procedure and trauma. Clinical practice guidelines. Publication 92-0032 (pp. 18–19). Rockville, MD: Author.

permanently blocks the cyclooxygenase in platelets. The length of effect is approximately 7 to 10 days and relates to the life of the platelet. Other NSAIDs work to inhibit platelet cyclooxygenase with an effect of much shorter duration, generally 6 to 24 hours. Ketorolac works in still another way to increase bleeding time. It does not alter platelet count, prothrombin time, or partial thromboplastin time.

Other side effects of the NSAIDs, although rare, include central nervous system (CNS) toxicity and renal dysfunction. In general NSAIDs should be used with caution in patients with renal insufficiency as prostaglandins promote renal vasodilatation. When this is inhibited, renal blood flow can be impaired.

Finally, acetaminophen often is listed as an NSAID. It does not possess any antiinflammatory effect and does not inhibit prostaglandin synthesis. It does possess good analgesic properties and should be used in patients with mild to moderate pain. However, concern over the total dose (4000 mg/day) of acetaminophen exists. Despite its relative safety, patients and health providers must be cautioned not to exceed these daily doses (Table 31–6).

A number of other drugs are used to treat patients in pain and are termed *adjuvants*. Adjuvants are classified as antidepressants, anticonvulsants, corticosteroids, muscle relaxants, and local anesthetics. These drugs do not typically possess analgesic properties but assist in interrupting the pain pathways in the transmission of stimuli.

The tricyclic antidepressants often are prescribed to treat neuropathic pain. This pain is characterized as tingling, burning, or electric sensations. Tricyclic antidepressants block the reuptake of serotonin and norepinephrine at the neuronal membrane that potentiates their activity. The most commonly used tricyclic antidepressants are Amitriptyline, Desipramine, Doxepin, and Nortriptyline. Side effects include anticholinergic effects (dry mouth), CNS effects (sedation, fatigue), and cardiovascular effects (orthostatic hypotension, arrhythmias, tachycardia).

Anticonvulsants also are used to treat neuropathic pain. The mechanism of action of these drugs is to block the ion channels along the nerve fiber, thus blocking the generation of action potentials. Commonly used anticonvulsants are Carbamazepine and Phenytoin.

Corticosteroids are used as adjuvants in pain therapy in situations where the mechanism of action directly affects the disease process. Often used to treat rheumatoid arthritis, connective tissue disorders, and tumors sensitive to steroids, they must be selected carefully and not used indiscriminately. Steroids inhibit cell-mediated immune responses and stabilize the lysosomal membranes. When appropriately applied, they can be helpful in managing complex pain syndromes.

Steroids often are seen in the treatment of adrenal insufficiency, cerebral edema, spinal cord injury, and respiratory problems such as asthma and postintubation stridor. Although not pain syndromes, therapeutic regimens often are concurrent and synergistic. Steroids often are used to treat cancer pain to alleviate the effect of tumor compression and swelling. However, the actual rationale for their administration must be clear and health providers should not confuse the use of steroids and analgesics. Steroid use is not without complication. Cushing-like syndromes may occur as well as gastrointestinal erosion and bleeding. Care must be used when administering these drugs.

As with the steroids, muscle relaxants often are used as adjuvants to treat pain, but should never be used as sole analgesics. When used as pain adjuvants, muscle relaxants are administered to decrease muscle tension and thus decrease the associated pain. They do not have analgesic or sedative effects. Patients treated with muscle relaxation for other reasons (ventilatory assistance) should never be paralyzed without other sedative and analgesic agents being administered.

A unique substance currently being used for the management of local pain is capsaicin (Zostrix HP®). Capsaicin stimulates the release of Substance P from the sensory neuron. Patients report transient local burning and skin redness. Eventually, there is a total depletion of Substance P with a concomitant reduction in pain.

Routes of Administration

We are all familiar with the traditional routes of analgesic administration. Although the intramuscular route often is used to administer analgesics, it is the least reliable way to give a medication. Transdermal routes offer an interesting advantage in chronic pain states, but offer nothing in acute states because it takes an average of 17 hours to see a response. Transnasal preparations have been studied, and butorphenol is available in this form. The sublingual and buccal routes are used with some medications, although analgesics are not marketed in this manner.

TABLE 31–6. Acetaminophen Dose in Commonly Used Drugs

Drug	Dosage (mg)
Arthritis formulas	325
Cold formulas	325–1000
Sinus medications	500
Tylenol #3	300
Vicodin ES	750
Percocet Caps	500
Darvocet-N	325

Patient-Controlled Analgesia

A valuable addition in the area of pain management has been the development of patient-controlled analgesia (PCA) devices. First introduced in the United States in the early 1980s, PCA has found wide acceptance from both patients and health care providers. This technique has been associated with better pain control, lower dosages of narcotic, and fewer narcotic-associated side effects (Graves et al., 1983).

Patients control the amount and timing of drug administration as their need indicates within preset limits. Most PCA devices use digital electronics to regulate the dose of narcotic delivered via an intravenous route. A lockout mechanism prevents overadministration of the narcotic.

Patient-controlled anesthesia decreases the long delays that often occur when the nurse must administer the narcotic. In addition, the use of the intravenous route facilitates the uptake and distribution of the drug. Pharmacokinetics theory suggests that a loading dose promotes the maintenance of a steady plasma level. The initial loading dose typically is administered by the nurse, as this may vary considerably from patient to patient. Graves et al. (1983) reported fewer postoperative complications when PCA was used. This was presumed to be the result of the decreased level of sedation with this type of drug regimen.

Continuous administration has been shown to decrease the overall dosage of opioids because it affords the patient control and the ability to titrate their medication to their actual need. Opioids and their suggested PCA, intravenous, and subcutaneous dosages are included in Table 31–7.

Regional Analgesia

The goal of postoperative pain control techniques is to provide maximum subjective comfort for the patient by blunting the surgically induced nociceptive impulses. For many years, anesthesia providers have used a variety of techniques to achieve optimal pain relief for patients. The combined use of opioid and nonopioid drugs has long been considered one method to improve pain relief. Today, central neural axial techniques and peripheral nerve blocks for both intraoperative and postoperative pain control also are widely used in anesthesia. Kehlet and Dahl (1993b) described use of these techniques as "multimodal or balanced" analgesia to achieve improved pain control and patient satisfaction. Improved analgesia facilitates patient mobilization and leads to earlier hospital discharge. An additional benefit may come from instituting analgesic measures early, before the surgical incision (Dahl & Kehlet, 1993). Preemptive analgesia theorizes that, by blocking the central neural axial impulses before they happen (ie, preincision), a noxious stimulus has less negative effects and overall analgesia is improved. The development of central sensitization induced by surgical incision may be prevented by preemptive techniques (Katz et al., 1992). Regional anesthesia techniques, specifically peripheral nerve blocks, are ideal preemptive analgesic strategies because they can be performed well in advance of the surgical procedure and combined with general anesthesia.

Peripheral Nerve Blocks

For many years, peripheral nerve blocks (PNB) have been administered to achieve excellent surgical anesthesia and recently have been used in combination with general anesthesia to provide improved postoperative analgesia for various extremity procedures. A nationwide shift to outpatient surgery or same-day surgery has resulted in the need for early discharge of patients undergoing major knee reconstructive procedures. The use of PNB has been shown to reduce or eliminate the amount of postoperative parenteral narcotics needed to achieve adequate analgesia, thereby reducing overall side effects and shortening hospital stays (Brown, Weiss, Greenberg, Flatow, & Bigliani, 1993; DeAndres, Bellver, Barrera, Febre, & Bolinches, 1993; Dorman, Conroy, Duc, Haynes, & Friedman, 1994; Edkin, Spindler, & Flanagan, 1995; Kinnard, Truchon, St. Pierre, & Montreuil, 1994; Lang, Yip, Chang, & Gerard, 1993; McQuay, Carroll, & Moore, 1988). Two safe and effective PNB techniques for postoperative analgesia in patients having extremity procedures are sciatic-femoral nerve block and brachial plexus blockade.

Femoral and Sciatic Nerve Block. For lower-extremity procedures, such as knee arthroplasty and reconstruction surgery, a femoral-sciatic nerve block is very effective in reducing postoperative pain. The advantage of performing a single-leg peripheral nerve

TABLE 31–7. Suggested Intravenous and Subcutaneous Patient-Controlled Anesthesia Doses

Drug	Dose (μg/kg)	Basal (μg/kg)	Lockout, (min)
Morphine[a]	10–30	10–30	8–10
Hydromorphone[a]	1.5–4	1.5–4	5–8[b]
Meperidine	100–300	100–300	8–10
Fentanyl	0.1–0.3	0.1–0.3	5–8
Sufentanil[a]	0.01–0.03	0.01–0.03	5–8[b]

[a] Due to the high potency of these drugs and the small volume needed, they are best choices for subcutaneous PCA (high-potency morphine: up to 100 mg/mL).
[b] Doses recommended apply to healthy, narcotic-naive patients.
From Rowlingson, & Hamill (1994). Techniques of narcotic and local anesthetic administration. In R. Hamill, & J. Rowlingson, Handbook of critical care pain management (p. 213). New York: McGraw-Hill, Inc.

block over central neural axis blockade (ie., epidural) are greatly reduced sympathectomy, no bladder tone changes, earlier ambulation using the nonblocked leg, and prolonged analgesia with single injection. The femoral nerve originates at L 2-4 and supplies sensory innervation to the entire anterior surface of the upper thigh and knee. It can be blocked with local anesthetic at the level of the inguinal ligament, just lateral to the femoral artery (Cousins & Bridenbaugh, 1988). A peripheral nerve stimulator (PNS) may be used to help locate the femoral nerve, indicated by a twitch of the quadriceps muscle. Following localization of the nerve, 20 mL of 0.25% to 0.5% of bupivacaine is deposited. This may provide 12 to 24 hours of postoperative analgesia (De-Andres et al., 1993; Edkin et al., 1995; Lang et al., 1993).

The sciatic nerve originates at L 4-5 and S 1-3 and is a large nerve supplying sensory innervation to the posterior aspect of the knee and entire foot. For most major knee joint procedures the sciatic nerve should be blocked in addition to the femoral nerve to provide optimal postoperative analgesia. For this technique, the patient is placed in the lateral position with the surgical leg up and flexed at the knee, the classic Labat approach. A line is drawn between the head of the greater trochanter and posterior superior iliac spine. A second line drawn downward approximately 3 to 4 cm from the midpoint of the first line indicates the point of injection. Using a 22-gauge spinal needle connected to a peripheral nerve stimulator (PNS), slowly advance the needle looking for muscle twitch to the calf or foot indicating localization of the sciatic nerve. Deposit approximately 20 mL of 0.25% to 0.5% bupivacaine. For short knee arthroscopy procedures that do not require a thigh tourniquet, this block combination may provide adequate anesthesia by itself. However, for procedures that require lengthy tourniquet times or last several hours, general anesthesia may be used to augment the nerve block.

Brachial Plexus Block: Interscalene Approach. In the late 1800s Dr. Crile described a technique to render the arm and shoulder insensitive to pain by blocking the brachial plexus (Cousins & Bridenbaugh, 1988). Today, several different approaches or techniques have been described to block the brachial plexus (Teltzlaff, Yoon, & Brems, 1994). The interscalene approach is widely accepted and performed for anesthesia and analgesia in surgical procedures involving the upper arm and shoulder. Interscalene approach to the brachial plexus is a highly effective nerve block that can produce excellent muscle relaxation, lower blood loss, and reduce postoperative opioid requirements in patients undergoing shoulder surgery. Patients have less immediate postoperative pain, sleep better the first postoperative night, and experience higher satisfaction with interscalene block than without the block. Used in combination with gen-

eral anesthesia or as the sole anesthetic, interscalene blocks facilitate early discharge and rapid mobilization of ambulatory patients undergoing shoulder surgical procedures (Brown et al., 1993; Dorman et al., 1994; Kinnard et al., 1994).

The brachial plexus (C 5-8 and T1) supplies most of the sensory innervation to the shoulder. The interscalene approach is performed by palpating the groove between the anterior and middle scalenus muscles at the level of C 5-6. The landmark to determine this level is the cricoid cartilage. The point of needle insertion is usually just posterior to the external jugular vein. Using a PNS, a 22-gauge needle is inserted perpendicular to the skin with a slight angle caudad. The depth of needle insertion to reach the plexus is approximately 2 to 4 cm. A shoulder or biceps twitch will indicate location of C 5-6. Injecting between 30 and 40 mL of 0.25% to 0.5% bupivacaine will produce a block that provides 12 to 24 hours of analgesia. General anesthesia in combination with the nerve block often is indicated because of the difficult patient position required for shoulder surgery or patient and surgeon preferences.

Peripheral nerve blocks provide excellent immediate postoperative pain management for most extremity procedures. The success of the blockade often is closely related to the time allowed to perform the block. These techniques can be safely performed well in advance of induction in the PACU or preanesthesia areas, avoiding a delay in the operating room schedule. Mild sedation should be used to help decrease the patient's anxiety and facilitate a successful block. Painless wakeups and early mobility using peripheral nerve blocks decrease hospital stay time and improve patient satisfaction.

Spinal and Epidural Analgesia

The use of epidural analgesia to control postoperative pain, especially in the critically ill, is growing in popularity. The first spinal anesthetics were reported in 1899, and the first epidural anesthetics were reported in 1901. Cleland (1949) first demonstrated the effectiveness of epidural analgesia in early postoperative ambulation in patients undergoing extensive abdominal surgery. In 1956 Dawkins reported the use of continuous epidural analgesia with local anesthetics for postoperative pain. In the 1980s several studies demonstrated the use of epidural narcotics as a means of managing postoperative pain, with decreased total dosage of narcotics and fewer central depressant effects (Lang, Theiss, Reiss, & Sommer, 1982; Soliman & Safwat, 1985) and provided the rationale using regional analgesia in both acute and chronic pain management.

Epidural analgesia occurs when a drug crosses the epidural space into the cerebrospinal fluid and diffuses into the dorsal horn of the spinal cord. The drug then binds with the opioid receptors in the dorsal horn,

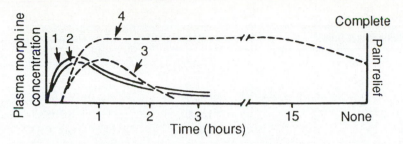

Figure 31–8. Plasma concentration of epidural drugs.

preventing the release of substance P, an excitatory transmitter, thus preventing the transmission of painful stimuli.

A second mechanism of action occurs when drugs are administered into the epidural space. Uptake of drugs by the epidural vasculature increases the plasma concentration, which is similar to the normal uptake and distribution of drugs given systemically (Fig. 31-8). Another pharmacologic action that must be recognized in the administration of epidural analgesia is the lipid solubility of the drugs administered. Fentanyl, meperidine, and sufentanil are highly lipid soluble, resulting in rapid absorption and rapid onset of drug action.

The duration of drug action also is affected by the lipid solubility of the drug. The greater the lipid solubility, the more likely the drug is to be absorbed by the epidural fat, limiting the degree to which the drug spreads within the epidural space and resulting in decreased duration of action. The opposite is true for drugs with low lipid solubility.

These drugs are not absorbed, which results in a higher concentration in the cerebrospinal fluid, with the possibility of cephalad spread. The degree to which the drug is absorbed by the epidural vasculature and diffuses into the cerebrospinal fluid determines the duration of drug effect.

Local anesthetics are used in a variety of ways to manage pain: local infiltration, topical application, and major nerve blocks. The local anesthetics commonly used and specific characteristics are found in Table 31-8. Local anesthetic effects are both dose and concentration dependent. The site of action is at the nerve ending, and the degree of blockade is determined by the concentration of the drug at the site.

Narcotics used for epidural analgesia are depicted in Table 31-9. Dosage, onset, and duration of drug action are shown. Wang, Nauss, and Thomas (1979) were the first to report success with the use of preservative-free morphine. Nautly, Datta, and Ostheimer (1985) used fentanyl to control postcesarean pain via the epidural route. In addition to narcotics and local anesthetics used alone, combination protocols have been studied to determine the best drug regimen. A comparison of narcotic and local anesthetic action is found in Table 31-10.

TABLE 31–8. Clinical Characteristics and Dosages of Local Anesthetics

	Procaine (Novocaine)	2-Chloroprocaine (Nesacaine)	Lidocaine (Xylocaine)	Mepivacaine (Carbocaine)	Prilocaine (Citanest)	Tetracaine (Pontocaine)	Bupivacaine (Marcaine)	Etidocaine (Duranest)
Latency (speed of onset)	Moderate	Fast	Fast	Moderate	Moderate	Very slow	Fast	Very fast
Penetration (diffusibility)	Moderate	Marked	Marked	Moderate	Moderate	Poor	Moderate	Moderate
Duration	Short	Very short	Moderate	Moderate	Moderate	Long	Long	Long
Optimal concentration (%)								
Infiltration	0.5	0.5	0.25	0.25	0.25	0.05	0.05	0.1
Spinal nerve and plexus block	1.5–2	1.0–2	0.5–1.0	0.5–1.0	0.5–1.0	0.1–0.25	0.25–0.5	0.5–1.0
Maximum amount (mg/kg)	12	15	6	6	6	2	2	2

From Wall, P. D., & Melzack, R. (1989). Textbook of pain (p. 726). New York: Churchill Livingstone. Reprinted with permission.

TABLE 31–9. Narcotics Used in the Epidural Space

Drug	Bolus Dose (mg)	Detectable Onset (min)[a]	Complete Pain Relief[a]	Duration (h)[a]
Morphine	5	23.5 ± 6	37 ± 6	$18.1 + 8$
Methadone	5	12.5 ± 2	17 ± 3	7.2 ± 4.6
Fentanyl	0.1	4–10	20	2.6–4
Meperidine	30–100	5–10	12–30	6.6 ± 3.3
Diamorphine	6	5	15	12.4 ± 6.5

[a] Values are means ± standard deviations or ranges.
From Cousins, M. J., & Mather, L. E. (1984). Intrathecal and epidural administration of opioids. Anesthesiology, 61, *276*. *Adapted with permission.*

Controversy over the optimal drugs to use via the epidural route waged through the early 1980s. Graham, King, and McCaughey (1980) showed that, although both epidural morphine and bupivicaine were effective, epidural morphine provided greater duration of analgesia with fewer side effects. One year later, Modig and Paalzow (1981) reported that epidural analgesia with bupivicaine produced a more profound analgesia than epidural morphine with concomitant motor blockade; however, epidural analgesia with morphine was not associated with motor or sympathetic blockade or loss of sensation. Finally, Torda and Pybus (1982) found that epidural bupivicaine produced greater intensity of analgesia but for a shorter duration than epidural morphine. As conflicting as these initial reports were, the search for best use of the epidural route was under way.

Because of the problems associated with the use of local anesthetics in the epidural space for continued pain management and the discovery of opiate receptors in the substantia gelatinosa, the use of narcotics via the epidural route has increased in popularity to manage pain after most types of surgery. Furthermore, epidural analgesia provides effective postoperative pain relief with few side effects, such as sedation and respiratory depression. In addition, analgesia is attained with lower total dosages than with other conventional forms of drug administration, including intravenous, intramuscular, and PCA (Wermaling, Foster, & Rapp, 1987).

Nonpharmacologic Interventions

Nonpharmacologic mechanisms to control pain have been viewed with both enthusiasm and indifference and should be used as adjuncts in the management of pain, rather than the sole approach. Lundeberg (1995) suggests that up to 60% of all patients with acute pain will benefit from the use of mechanisms to enhance the individuals own neurobiologic control mechanisms. Nonpharmacologic interventions are categorized as cognitive-behavioral strategies and physical agents. Cognitive-

TABLE 31–10. Effects of Local Epidural Anesthetics and Narcotics

	Local Anesthetics	Narcotics
Quality of blockade		
Sympathetic blockade	Yes, dose dependent	None
Locomotion blockade	Slight to complete, dose dependent	None
Sensory blockade	All modalities, dose dependent	Mainly pain
Vascular uptake	Dose dependent and reduced by adrenalin 1 : 200 000	
Possible to limit segmental blockade	Yes	Yes, but may spread rostrally
Tachyphylaxis	Yes	Yes
Duration of action	Short	Short or very prolonged, depending on agent
Side effects		
Central respiratory depression	No	Yes, dose dependent
Peripheral respiratory depression	Yes, if respiratory muscles are involved	No
Urinary retention	Yes, relatively short	Yes, may be very prolonged
Pruritus	No	Yes
Nausea and vomiting	No	Yes

From Wall, P. D., & Melzack, R. (1988). Textbook of pain *(p. 746)*. New York: Churchill Livingstone. *Reprinted with permission.*

behavioral strategies include education/instruction, relaxation, imagery, music/distraction, and biofeedback.

Relaxation and Guided Imagery

Relaxation is the most widely studied of these strategies. These interventions are often not complex, but yield effective results. Relaxation techniques have been used in the labor and delivery area for decades. Increased use in acute pain situations is recommended. According to McCaffery and Beebe (1989), imagery can be used as a distraction from pain or as a method to induce relaxation. Imagery techniques are intended to supplement standard analgesic therapy, not replace the need for pharmacologic support. Imagery can include simple conversations, standardized messages, individualized imagery techniques (Faut & Paice, 1990). The use of these techniques increases the patient's confidence and self-esteem as they feel they can to some degree control their pain experience. However, a considerable time commitment is necessary to learn these strategies successfully. Daake and Gueldner (1989) used imagery coupled with preprocedural information and found a significant ($P < .05$) difference in the total amount of analgesics administered and in the patients' pain intensity ratings.

Biofeedback

Principles of biofeedback also have been used successfully in postoperative populations (Madden, Singer, Peck, & Nayman, 1978; Moon and Gibbs, 1984). Biofeedback is based on principles of tension reduction in voluntary muscles. However, biofeedback requires significant involvement by a professional with specialized training and equipment. Essential to the use of biofeedback is the ability to provide measurable physiologic parameters for the patient to use as a benchmark. Such measurements have included skin temperature, pulse rate, blood pressure, muscle activity, and electroencephalographic activity. Biofeedback has been used most commonly to treat headache and stress-related syndromes.

Transcutaneous Electrical Nerve Stimulation

The use of transcutaneous electrical nerve stimulation (TENS) and acupuncture, although once thought to be significant advances in pain management, require a trained individual to implement in a pain practice. The first one, TENS, which is the use of electrical current delivered to the skin via electrodes, has been used in postsurgical patients. It is often used with orthopedic patients. The electrodes are placed along, but not on, the incision. The mechanism of action is thought to be the local release of endogenous substances as well as blockage of fast A fibers. The TENS literature presents a conflicting view of the effectiveness of this strategy (AHCPR,

1992; Benedetti et al., 1997; Carroll et al., 1996; Carroll et al., 1997). There appears to be a placebo effect in some patients.

Acupuncture and Acupressure

The use of acupuncture also is controversial. Acupressure is based on the same principles. Although it is often cited in the lay press, the analgesic efficacy has limited scientific support. Traditional acupuncture incorporates the Asian belief in disturbances in chi(qi), which means vital energy. Needles are placed in areas thought to be highly concentrated with chi(qi) to release the blockade of chi(qi) flow and restore harmony. Many ideas about the mechanism of action of acupuncture have been suggested, including an endogenous effect, stimulation of medium-size afferent fibers in muscles, and the concept that large-fiber stimulation may block small-fiber input (Hamill & Rowlingson, 1994).

Hypnosis

Hypnosis is one of the oldest methods used to decrease pain. It requires the cooperation of the patient and confidence in the therapist. Orne and Dinges (1989) claim that it is the manipulation of the patient's attention away from the pain. Hypnosis has been reported to alleviate many types of acute and chronic pain. Nonpharmacologic techniques in the management of pain should be considered as an adjunct to traditional therapy and when other pain management regimens do not completely control the patient's pain.

Other Adjuncts

Use of physical agents to alleviate pain and to supplement the use of analgesics is quite common in some surgical specialty areas. Applications of cold and heat are common, as are massage, exercise, and immobilization. The use of these types of adjuncts is becoming common, although research is limited in most areas.

Pediatric Pain

The management of pediatric pain is a specialty unto itself, and, although it is not the focus of this chapter, a few points must be raised. Kierney (1995) suggests that infants' and toddlers' response to pain often is ignored, most likely because of lack of knowledge and fear of complications in managing pediatric patients' pain. Infants from the age of 6 months consistently avoid painful stimuli. Children as young as 3 years can reliably use pain assessment strategies and effectively communicate their pain through the use of drawings. The important issue is that children do have pain, and it must not be ignored. The NSAIDs can be used safely in children. The pediatric dosages of NSAIDs are found in Table 31–11.

TABLE 31–11. Pediatric Dosages of NSAIDs

Drug	Single Dose (mg/kg)	Number of Daily Doses	Maximum Dose (mg/kg/day)
Acetaminophen	10–15	4–6	60
Aspirin	10–15	4–6	60
Diclofenac	1.0–2.0	3–4	?
Ibuprofen	10	3–4	40
Indomethacin	1	3	3
Ketoprofen	2.5	2	5
Naproxen	7	2	15
Piroxicam	0.4	1	?
Ketorolac (experimental)	0.5?	2–4	?

From Maunuksela, E. (1993). Nonsteroidal anti-inflammatory drugs in pediatric pain management. In N. Schechter, C. Berde, & M. Yaster, (Eds.), Pain in infants, children and adolescents (p. 140). Baltimore: Williams & Wilkins.

The use of opioids in children also has been viewed with caution. However, opioids have been successfully used in children (Table 31-12). Appropriate monitoring is necessary in this population. The use of PCA in children has been successfully implemented, provided appropriate precautions are in place. The most important precaution beyond care dosing, is that parents and visitors must not be allowed to administer the drug to the child. This type of intervention defeats the principles that underlie PCA use in children. A suggested routine for the use of PCA is presented in Table 31-13.

▶ QUALITY ASSURANCE IN PAIN MANAGEMENT

Pain is easier to prevent than it is to manage once it has become established. Therefore, beginning at the time of the initial encounter with the patient, the nurse anesthetist should encourage the patient to participate in pain control. The anesthetist should explain to the patient that pain can adversely affect the recovery process or an existing condition. The aim of pain management is to prevent significant pain from the onset. The patient must understand that dosages of analgesia may need to be increased or adjunctive therapies, such as relaxation and TENS, may be needed to provide effective pain management.

Documenting the efficacy of pain control measures is essential for quality pain control. A study of 100 surgical patients indicates that documentation of pain is incomplete and infrequent (Faut et al., 1989). Documentation is important for effective communication between the patient and health care providers and among health care providers. Without accurate and complete documentation, health care professionals cannot follow a consistent and appropriate plan of care to provide pain control. Documentation also is important for evaluating the effectiveness of pain control strategies. Without evaluation, the nurse anesthetist may continue to use ineffective methods or insufficient analgesia for pain management. Furthermore, inconsistent and inadequate documentation of pain assessment or effectiveness of interventions could potentially be viewed as a deviation from acceptable clinical practice.

Individuals who are responsible for patient care in health care organizations should evaluate their own process of pain management. Established standards of care and an organized process by which pain is acknowledged, assessed, effectively managed, and reassessed are essential. A pain care program that is sporadic and depends on patients' or families' demands for analgesia "as needed" is likely to result in intervals of inadequate pain relief and foster the patient's anxiety, loss of control, and fatigue.

TABLE 31–12. Opioids in Children

Drug	Oral Dose	Intramuscular Dose	Intravenous Dose	Subcutaneous Dose
Codeine	0.5–1 mg/kg			
Fentanyl			0.5–2 μg/kg q 1–2 h	
Morphine	0.2–0.4 mg/kg q 4 h	0.1–0.15 mg/kg q 3–4 h	0.08–0.1 mg/kg q 2 h	0.1–0.15 mg/kg q 3–4 h
Meperidine		0.8–1.3 mg/kg q 3–4 h	0.8–1 mg/kg q 2 h	0.8–1.3 mg/kg q 3–4 h

TABLE 31–13. Suggested Patient-Controlled Anesthesia Prescription for Acute Pediatric Pain

1. Syringe order:
   Add 1 mg/kg morphine to 60-mL syringe (maximum 60 mg) or add 0.5 mg/kg to a 30-mL syringe
   Note: equivalent meperidine, hydromorphone, or fentanyl dose may be used instead of morphine.

2. PCA settings:
   Bolus dose: 0.016 mg/kg (1 mL)
   Lockout interval: 5 min
   Background infusion: 0.016 mg/kg (0.016 mg/kg [1 mL/h])
   Concentration: 0.016 mg/kg/mL
   Note: this regime simplifies programming as the same number is used for all settings.
   Bolus dose volume remains constant irrespective of patient's weight.

3. Optional settings (varies with equipment):
   Loading dose: 0.05–0.1 mg/kg (most brands)
             1-h limit: 0.16 mg/kg (10 mL) (Pharmacia, Bard)
             4-h limit: 0.5 mg/kg (30 mL) (Abbott)
   Dose duration: Stat (Graseby)

4. Standing orders:
   a. Discontinue previous narcotic orders
   b. Nurse in close proximity to nursing station
   c. Ensure one-way valve is correctly positioned in IV line
   d. Observations:
          Respiratory rate and color q 1 h
          Syringe check q 1 h
          Pulse rate and BP q 2 h
          Pain, sedation, and vomiting scores q 2 h
   e. Problems:
          Page pain service or physician
          If respirations <10/min, or if oversedated:
              (1) Stop PCA
              (2) Administer oxygen
              (3) Call pain service
          If apneic:
              (1) Resuscitate
              (2) Call for help
              (3) Give naloxone 0.01 mg/kg IV
              (4) Stop PCA

From Gaukroger, P. (1993). Patient-controlled analgesia in children. In N. Schechter, C. Berde, & M. Yaster (Eds.), Pain in infants, children and adolescents (p. 206). Baltimore: Williams & Wilkins.

► CASE STUDY

A 20-year-old female with a negative medical history was diagnosed with a right thyroid mass and taken to surgery for a partial thyroidectomy. The surgical procedure was uneventful. She had received a balanced anesthetic with midazolam, fentanyl, and low-dose isoflurane. From the time she was admitted to the postsurgical unit she has reported that she was in the most pain she had ever been in her life. She rated her pain as a 10 on a scale of 0 to 10. It is now 2 hours postoperatively. She had received 2 extra-strength acetaminophen for pain 45 minutes earlier and was told by the nurse that the surgeon had only ordered plain acetominophen and aspirin.

1. What is wrong with this pain management plan?

   Any benefits from intraoperative analgesia have dissipated. The patient reports severe pain and "plain" acetominophen is inappropriate for this type of pain. The surgeon clearly underestimated the level of pain associated with this surgical procedure. Aspirin in a postoperative neck should be avoided because of bleeding problems and concern about airway maintenance.

   When questioned further, the nurse said that the surgeon never orders anything stronger for pain because he is concerned about respiratory depression. However, the patient insisted that she call the physician, and he then ordered Darvon. He states that he is concerned about postoperative respiratory depression related to the anesthesia.

2. Critique this plan.

   There is significant first pass hepatic metabolism of Darvon resulting in a weak analgesic effect, compared to 600 mg of aspirin. This is not an appropriate analgesic for severe postsurgical pain. More important, there is a significant knowledge deficit among the health care providers. Nurse anesthetists must work in health care systems to change attitudes and increase the knowledge level of those working with postoperative patients. This is where collaboration is critically important.

3. What analgesics or other medications should be ordered for this patient?

   An oral narcotic analgesic would be a good choice. Concern about postoperative respiratory depression due to residual operative medications should be evaluated. Respiratory depression due to airway edema and the potential for postoperative bleeding also should be assessed. These issues should not interfere with the development of an appropriate pain management plan. Furthermore, once postoperative bleeding is not a concern, the addition of a NSAID may be warranted to reduce inflammation.

► SUMMARY

Since the 1960s researchers have commented about poor pain management in health care institutions (Cohen, 1980; Faut, Paice, & Mahon, 1989; Marks & Sachar, 1973; Paice et al., 1995; Weis et al., 1983). Yet despite new technologies such as epidural analgesics, patient-controlled analgesia, and new medications, patients remain in pain. Attention should be given to how physicians and nurses make critical decisions about selecting methods of pain control and the amounts of analgesic medications ordered and administered. Much of the research on pain has focused on health care providers' beliefs and values about medicating patients in pain, but few research studies have investigated medication decisions of either physicians and nurses, as key players in the treatment of patients' pain. The development of a clinical decision-making model would be useful for identifying effective strategies for decreasing faulty judgments about pain management. Unfortunately, the recognition of ineffective practices in pain management has not led educators to improve the knowledge and clinical pain management skills of practitioners. Both clinicians and patients must be educated about the various options for pain control and the need for systematic assessment of interventions. Patients must understand the importance of effective pain control in the overall recovery process.

Effective pain management should begin with a comprehensive plan. The nurse anesthetist must be in the position, both by education and by conviction, to be an integral part of the planning, implementation, and evaluation process. This requires additional knowledge, skill, and patience, all of which are essential components of the nurse anesthetist role.

▶ KEY CONCEPTS

- Pain is a complex, multidimensional phenomenon encompassing both physiologic and psychologic components.
- The patient's assessment of his or her own pain should guide the practitioner in the development of a pain management plan. Providers must not impose their own biases about a patient's condition when developing the plan of care.
- Patients often require multimodal therapies for effective control of pain. This may include several different medications and routes of administration. This also may include nonpharmacologic interventions.
- Accurate documentation of the patient's pain is an essential component in the overall management. Documentation becomes the essential blueprint for all providers as they attempt to manage the patient's pain.

▶ STUDY QUESTIONS

1. What are the key components of the definition of pain?

2. What are the steps required to develop a pain management plan?

3. What are the pain control options and when is each indicated?

KEY REFERENCES

Bonica, J. (1990). History of pain concepts and therapies. In *The management of pain* (pp. 2–17). Philadelphia: Lea & Febiger.

Hamill, R., & Rowlingson, J. (1994). *Handbook of critical care pain management.* New York: McGraw-Hill.

Kehlet, H., & Dahl, J. (1993). The value of "multimodal" or "balanced analgesia" in postoperative pain treatment. *Anesthesia & Analgesia, 77,* 1048–1056.

Loeser, J., & Egan, D. (1989). Managing the chronic pain patient: Theory and practice at the University of Washington Multidisciplinary Pain Center. New York: Raven.

Lundeberg, T. (1995). Pain physiology and principles of treatment. *Scandinavian Journal of Rehabilitative Medicine, 32* (Suppl.), 13–42.

Wall, P., & Melzack, R. (1989). *Textbook of pain.* New York: Churchill Livingstone.

REFERENCES

Abu-Saad, H., & Holzemer, W. L. (1981). Measuring self-assessment of pain. *Issues in Comprehensive Pediatric Nursing, 5,* 337–349.

Agency for Health Care Policy Research. (1992). *Acute pain management: Operative or medical procedures and trauma. Clinical practice guidelines.* Publication 92-0032. Rockville, MD: Author.

Andrew, J. (1970). Recovery from surgery with and without preparation instruction for three coping styles. *Journal of Personality and Social Psychology, 15,* 233.

Angell, M. (1982). The quality of mercy. *New England Journal of Medicine, 306*(2), 98–99.

Averill, J. (1973). Personal control over aversive stimuli and its relationship to stress. *Psychological Bulletin, 80,* 286–303.

Ball, T., & Vogler, R. (1971). Uncertain pain and the pain of uncertainty. *Perceptual and Motor Skills, 3,* 1195–1203.

Beaver, W. (1980). Management of cancer pain with parenteral medication. *Journal of the American Medical Association, 244,* 2653–2657.

Beecher, H. (1956). Relationship of significance of wound to the pain experienced. *Journal of the American Medical Association, 161,* 1613–1617.

Benedetti, F., Amanzio, M., Casadio, C., Cavallo, A., Cianci, R., & Giobbe, R. (1997). Control of postoperative pain by transcutaneous electrical nerve stimulation after thoracic operations. *Annals of Thoracic Surgery, 63,* 773–776

Bonica, J. (1980). Pain research and therapy: Past and current status and future needs. In L. K. Y. Ng & J. Bonica (Eds.), *Pain, discomfort and humanitarian care* (pp. 1–46). Amsterdam: Elsevier.

Bonica, J. (1990). History of pain concepts and therapies. In *The management of pain* (pp. 2–17). Philadelphia: Lea & Febiger.

Brown, A. R., Weiss, R., Greenberg, G. G., Flatow, E. L., & Bigliani, L. U. (1993). Interscalene block for shoulder arthroscopy: Comparison with general anesthesia. *Arthroscopy: The Journal of Arthroscopic and Related Surgery, 9*(3), 296–300.

Burgess, A. (1981). Children's drawings as indication of sexual trauma. *Perspectives in Psychiatry, 19,* 50–58.

Carroll, D., Tramer, M., McQuay, H., & Moore, A. (1996), Randomization is important in studies with pain outcomes: Systematic review of transcutaneous electrical nerve stimulation in acute postoperative pain. *British Journal of Anaesthesia, 77,* 798–803.

Carroll, D., Tramer, M., McQuay, H., & Moore, A. (1997). Transcutaneous electrical nerve stimulation in labour pain: A systematic review. *British Journal of Obstetrics and Gynaecology, 104,* 169–175.

Chapman, C., & Cox, G. (1977). Anxiety, pain and depression surrounding elective surgery: A multivariate comparison of abdominal surgery patients with kidney donors and recipients. *Journal of Psychosomatic Research, 21,* 7–15.

Cleland, J. (1949). Continuous peridural analgesia in surgery and early ambulation. *Northwest Medicine, 48,* 26–32.

Cohen, F. (1980). Postsurgical pain relief: Patients' status and nurses' medication choices. *Pain, 9,* 265–274.

Cousins, M. J., & Bridenbaugh, P. O. (1988). Neural blockade. In *Clinical anesthesia and management of pain* (2nd ed., pp. 387–441). Philadelphia: Lippincott.

Cousins, M. J., & Phillips, G. D. (1986). *Acute pain management* (pp. 61–78). New York: Churchill Livingstone.

Coyle, N. (1985). Symptom management—pain: An overview of current concepts. *Cancer Nursing, I (Suppl.),* 44–49.

Craig, K. (1986). Social modeling influences: Pain in context. In R. A. Sternbach (Ed.), *The psychology of pain* (2nd ed., pp. 73–109). New York: Raven Press.

Craig, K., & Prkachin, K. (1982). Non-verbal measures of pain. In R. Melzack (Ed.), *Pain measurement and assessment* (pp. 173–179). New York: Raven.

Cullen, M., Staren, E., El-Ganzouri, A., Logas, W., Ivankovich, A., & Economou, S. (1985). Continuous epidural infusions for analgesia after major abdominal operations: A randomized, prospective, double-blind study. *Surgery, 98,* 718–728.

Daake, D., & Gueldner, S. (1989). Imagery instruction and the control of postsurgical pain. *Applied Nursing Research, 2*(3), 114–120.

Dahl, J., & Kehlet, H. (1993). The value of preemptive analgesia in the treatment of post-operative pain. *British Journal of Anaesthesia, 70,* 434–439.

Davitz, J., & Davitz, L. (1981). *Inferences of patient's pain and psychological distress: Studies of nursing behaviors.* New York: Springer.

Dawkins, C. J. M. (1956). Relief of postoperative pain by continuous epidural drip. *Proceedings of the Fourth Congress, of the Scandinavia Society of Anesthesiologists* (p. 77), Helsinki.

DeAndres, J., Bellver, J., Barrera, L., Febre, E., & Bolinches, R. (1993). A comparative study of analgesia after knee surgery with intraarticular bupivacaine, intraarticular morphine, and lumbar plexus block. *Anesthesia & Analgesia, 77,* 727–730.

Dewi, R. (1972). The distress of dying. *British Journal of Medicine, 3,* 105–107.

Donovan, M., Dillon, P., & McGuire, L. (1987). Incidence and characteristics of pain in a sample of medical-surgical inpatients. *Pain, 30,* 69–78.

Donovan, M., Slack, J., & Faut, M. (1989). Factors associated with inadequate management of pain. *Proceedings of the Eighth Annual Scientific Meeting of the American Pain Society.* Phoenix, AZ.

Dorman, B. H., Conroy, J. M., Duc, T. A., Haynes, G. R., & Friedman, R. J. (1994). Postoperative analgesia after major shoulder surgery with interscalene brachial plexus blockade. *Southern Medicine Journal, 87*(4), 502–505.

Edkin, B. S., Spindler, K. P., & Flanagan, J. F. K. (1995). Femoral nerve block as an alternative to parenteral narcotics for pain control after anterior cruciate ligament reconstruction. *Arthroscopy: The Journal of Arthroscopic and Related Surgery, 11*(4), 404–409.

Edwards, W. T. (1990). Optimizing opioid treatment of postoperative pain. *Journal of pain and symptom, 5,* S24–S27.

Faherty, B., & Grier, M. (1984). Analgesic medication for elderly people postsurgery. *Nursing Research, 33,* 369–372.

Faut, M., & Paice, J. (1990). Postoperative pain control for the parturient. *Journal of Perinatal and Neonatal Nursing, 4,* 27–40.

Faut, M., Paice, J., & Mahon, S. (1989). Factors associated with the adequacy of pain control in hospitalized surgical patients. *Proceedings of the 13th Annual Midwest Nursing Research Society* (p. 214), Cincinnati, OH.

Fletcher, D., Setlaoui, P., Monin, S., Bombart, M., & Samii, K. (1995). Influence of timing on the analgesic effect of intravenous ketorolac after orthopedic surgery. *Pain, 61,* 291–297.

Fortin, F., & Kirovac, S. (1976). A randomized controlled trial of preoperative patient education. *Educational Journal of Nursing Studies, 13,* 11.

Gaukroger, P. (1993). Patient-controlled analgesia in children. In N. Schecter, C. Berde, & M. Yaster, (Eds.), *Pain in infants, children and adolescents* (p. 206). Baltimore: Williams & Wilkins.

Gracely, R. H. (1980). Pain measurement in man. In J. J. Bonica (Ed.), *Pain, discomfort and humanitarian care* (p. 111). Amsterdam: Elsevier.

Graffam, C., & Johnson, A. (1987). A comparison of two relaxation strategies for the relief of pain and its distress. *Journal of Pain Symptom Management, 2,* 229.

Graham, J. L., King, R., & McCaughey, W. (1980). Postoperative pain relief using epidural morphine. *Anaesthesia, 35,* 158–160.

Graves, D. A., Foster, T. S., Batenhorst, R. S., et al. (1983). Patient controlled analgesia. *Annals of Internal Medicine, 99,* 360–366.

Grossman, S., & Scheidler, V. (1985). Skills of medical students and house officers in prescribing narcotic medications. *Journal of Medical Education, 60,* 552–557.

Hamill, R., & Rowlingson, J. (1994). *Handbook of critical care pain management.* New York: McGraw-Hill.

Hammond, K. R. (1966). Clinical inference in nursing: Analyzing cognitive tasks representative of nursing problems. *Nursing Research, 15,* 134–138.

Hargreaves, S. A. (1987). *Implementing TENS to control postoperative pain.* Master's Thesis, Edmonton, University of Alberta, Alberta.

Heft, M. W., & Parker, S. R. (1984). An experimental basis for revising the graphic rating scale for pain. *Pain, 19,* 153–161.

Hodges, W., & Spielberger, C. (1966). The effects of threat of shock on heart rate for subjects who differ in manifest anxiety and fear of shock. *Psychophysiology, 2,* 287.

Jaffee, J. (1985). Drug addiction and drug abuse. In L. Goodman, A. Gilman, T. Ral, & F. Murad (Eds.), *Pharmacologic basis of therapeutics* (pp. 535–584). New York: Macmillan.

Johnson, L., Magnani, B., Chan, V., & Ferrante, M. (1989). Modifiers of patient-controlled analgesia efficacy: Locus of control. *Pain, 39,* 17–22.

Katz, J., Kavanagh, B. P., Sandler, A. N., Niernberg, H., Boylan, J. F., Friedlander, M., & Shaw, B. F. (1992). Preemptive analgesia. *Anesthesiology, 77,* 439–446.

Kehlet, H. (1989). Surgical stress: The role of pain and analgesia. *British Journal of Anaesthesia, 63,* 189.

Kehlet, H., & Dahl, J. (1993a). Preemptive analgesia: A misnomer and a misinterpreted technique. *American Pain Society Journal, 2,* 122–124.

Kehlet, H., & Dahl, J. (1993b). The value of "multimodal" or "balanced analgesia" in postoperative pain treatment. *Anesthesia & Analgesia, 77,* 1048–1056.

Kierney, K. (1995). Pain management in children. Rush Presbyterian St. Luke's Medical Center, Chicago, Illinois.

Kinnard, P., Truchon, R., St. Pierre, A., & Montreuil, J. (1994). Interscalene block for pain relief after shoulder surgery. *Clinics in Orthopaedics and Related Research, 304,* 22–24.

Knorrel, D., & Faut-Callahan, M. (1997). The effect of a video-based structured preoperative teaching program on patient's use of patient-controlled analgesia to manage postoperative pain. Unpublished manuscript. Chicago: Rush University.

Lander, J. (1990). Clinical judgements in pain management. *Pain, 42,* 15–22.

Lang, E., Theiss, D., Reiss, W., & Sommer, V. (1982). Epidural morphine for postoperative analgesia: A double-blind study. *Anesthesia & Analgesia, 61,* 236–240.

Lang, S. A., Yip, R. W., Chang, P. C., & Gerard, M. A. (1993). The femoral 3 in 1 block revisited. *Journal of Clinical Anesthesia, 5,* 292–296.

Loeser, J., & Egan, D. (1989). Managing the chronic pain patient: Theory and practice at the University of Washington Multidisciplinary Pain Center. New York: Raven.

Lundeberg, T. (1995). Pain physiology and principles of treatment. *Scandinavian Journal of Rehabilitation Medicine, 32* (Suppl.), 13–42.

Madden, C., Singer, G., Peck, C., & Nayman, J. (1978). The effect of EMG biofeedback on postoperative pain following abdominal surgery. *Anaesthesia and Intensive Care, 6,* 333–336.

Mandler, G., & Watson, D. (1966). Anxiety and the interruption of behavior. In C. Speillberger (Ed.), *Anxiety and behavior.* New York: Academic Press.

Marks, R., & Sachar, E. (1973). Undertreatment of medical patients with narcotic analgesics. *Annals of Internal Medicine, 78,* 173–181.

Mather, L. (1992). Do the pharmacodynamics of the nonsteroidal antiinflammatory drugs suggest a role in the management of postoperative pain? *Drugs, 44*(Suppl. 5), 1–5.

Mather, R., & Mackie, J. (1981). The incidence of post operative pain in children. *Pain, 15,* 271–282.

Maunuksela, E. (1993). Nonsteroidal anti-inflammatory drugs in pediatric pain management. In N. Schecter, C. Berde, & M. Yaster (Eds.), *Pain in infants, children and adolescents.* Baltimore: Williams & Wilkins.

McCaffery, M. (1979). *Nursing management of the patient in pain* (p. 11). Philadelphia: Lippincott.

McCaffery, M., & Beebe, A. (1989). *Pain: Clinical manual for nursing practice.* St. Louis, MO: Mosby.

McGrath, P. A., de Veber, L. L., & Hearn, M. T. (1985). Multidimensional pain assessment in children. In H. L. Fields, R. Dubner, & F. Cervro (Eds.), *Advances in pain research and therapy* (pp. 387–393). New York: Raven.

McQuay, H. J., Carroll, D., & Moore, R. A. (1988). Postoperative orthopaedic pain—The effect of opiate premedication and local anaesthetic blocks. *Pain, 33,* 291–295.

Melzack, R. (1975). The McGill pain questionnaire: Major properties and scoring methods. *Pain, 1,* 275–299.

Melzack, R., & Wall, P. (1965). Pain mechanisms: A new theory. *Science, 150,* 971–979.

Melzack, R., Wall, P., & Ty, T. (1982). Acute pain in the emergency clinic: Latency of onset and descriptor patterns. *Pain, 14,* 33.

Melzack, R., & Wall, P. (1983). *The challenge of pain.* New York: Basic Books.

Mersky, H. (1986). Classification of chronic pain: Description of chronic pain syndromes and definitions of pain terms. *Pain, 3*(Suppl.), S217.

Modig, J., & Paalzow, L. (1981). A comparison of epidural morphine and epidural bupivicaine for postoperative pain relief. *Acta Anaesthesiologica Scandinavica, 25,* 437–441.

Moon, M., & Gibbs, J. (1984). The control of postoperative pain by EMG biofeedback in patients undergoing hysterectomy. *New Zealand Medicine Journal, 97,* 643–646.

Nautly, J., Datta, S., & Ostheimer, G. (1985). Epidural fentanyl for post cesarean delivery pain management. *Anesthesiology, 63,* 694–698.

Noren, R. (1994). Opiate pharmacology. In R. Hamill, & J. Rowlingson (Eds.), *Handbook of critical care pain management.* New York: McGraw-Hill.

Orne, M. T., & Dinges, D. F. (1989). Hypnosis. In P. D. Wall & R. Melzak (Eds.), *Textbook of pain* (pp. 1021–1031). Edinburgh: Churchill Livingstone.

Owen, H., McMillan, V., & Rogowski, D. (1990). Pain management and patient expectations. *Pain, 41,* 303–307.

Paice, J., Mahon, S., & Faut-Callahan, M. (1995). Pain control in hospitalized postsurgical patients. *Medical Surgical Nursing, 4*(5) 367–372.

Peck, C. (1986). Psychological factors in acute pain management. In M. Cousins & G. Phillips (Eds.), *Acute pain management* (pp. 61–78). Edinburgh: Churchill Livingstone.

Pellegrine, J., Paice, J., & Faut-Callahan, M. (1996). Meperidine utilization and compliance with AHCPR guidelines at a tertiary care hospital. *Proceedings of the 63rd AANA Annual Meeting* (p. 58), Philadelphia.

Portenoy, R., & Kranner, R. (1985). Patterns of analgesic prescription and consumption in a university-affiliated community hospital. *Archives of Internal Medicine, 145,* 439–441.

Porter, J., & Jick, H. (1980). Addiction rare in patients treated with narcotics. *New England Journal of Medicine, 302*(2) 123.

Rankin, M. (1984). Nurses' perception of cancer patient's pain. *Cancer Nurse, 7,* 149–155.

Rowlingson, J. (1993). Pain relief before pain starts? *American Pain Society Journal, 2,* 125–127.

Rowlingson, J., & Hamill, R. (1994). Techniques of narcotic and local anesthetic administration. In R. Hamill, & J. Rowlingson. *Handbook of critical care pain management* (pp. 207–228). New York: McGraw-Hill.

Schecter, N., Berde, C., & Yaster, M. (1993). *Pain in infants, children and adolescents.* Baltimore: Williams & Wilkins.

Shimm, D., Lague, G., & Malbie, A. (1979). Medical management of chronic cancer pain. *Journal of the American Medical Association, 241,* 2408–2412.

Slack, J., & Faut-Callahan, M. (1990). Efficacy of epidural analgesia for pain management of critically ill patients and the implications of nursing care. *AACN Clinical Issues in Critical Care Nursing, 2*(4), 729–740.

Soliman, I. E., & Safwat, A. M. (1985). Successful management of an elderly patient with multiple trauma. *Journal of Trauma, 25*(8), 806–807.

Sriwantanakul, K., Weiss, O., & Alloza, J. (1983). Analysis of narcotic usage in the treatment of postoperative pain. *Journal of the American Medical Association, 250,* 926–929.

Sofaer, B. (1985). Pain management through nursing education. In L. Coop (Ed.), *Recent advances in nursing: Perspectives on pain.* London: Churchill Livingstone.

Sutters, K., Levine, J., Dibble, S., Savedra, M., & Miaskowski, C. (1995). *Pain, 61,* 145–153.

Syrjala, K. L., & Chapman, C. R. (1984). Measurement of clinical pain: A review and integration of research findings. In C. Benedetti, C. R. Chapman, & G. Moricca (Eds.), *Advances in pain research and therapy* (pp. 71–101). New York: Livingstone Press.

Taylor, H., & Curran, N. H. (1985). *The Nuprin pain report.* New York: Louis Harris and Associates.

Teltzlaff, J. E., Yoon, H. J., & Brems, J. (1994). Interscalene brachial plexus block for shoulder surgery. *Regional Anesthesia, 19*(5), 339–343.

Torda, T. A., & Pybus, D. A. (1982). Comparison of four narcotic analgesics for extradural analgesia. *British Journal of Anaesthesia, 54,* 291.

Von Baeyer, C., Johnson, M., & McMillan, M. (1984). Consequences of nonverbal experience of pain: Patient distress and observer concern. *Social Science and Medicine, 19,* 1319–1324.

Wall, P., & Melzack, R. (1989). *Textbook of pain.* New York: Churchill Livingstone.

Wang, J. K., Nauss, L. A., & Thomas, J. E. (1979). Pain relief by intrathecally applied morphine in man. *Anesthesiology, 50,* 149–151.

Watt-Watson, J. (1987). Nurses' knowledge of pain issues: A survey. *Journal of Pain Symptom Management, 2,* 207–211.

Weis, O., Sriwatanakul, K., Alloza, J., Weintraub, M., & Lasagna, L. (1983). Attitudes of patients, housestaff and nurses toward postoperative analgesic care. *Anesthesia & Analgesia, 62,* 70–74.

Weissman, D., & Dahl, J. (1990). Attitudes about cancer pain: A survey of Wisconsin's first year medical students. *Journal of Pain Symptom Management, 5,* 345–349.

Wermaling, D. P., Foster, T. S., & Rapp, R. P. (1987). Evaluation of a disposable, nonelectric patient controlled analgesia device for postoperative pain. *Clinical Pharmacology, 6,* 307–314.

Woolf, C., & Chong, M. (1993). Preemptive analgesia — Treating postoperative pain by preventing the establishment of central sensitization. *Anesthesia & Analgesia, 77,* 362–379.

Yaeger, M., Glass, D., Neff, R., & Brinck-Johnsen, T. (1987). Epidural anesthesia and analgesia in high risk surgical patients. *Anesthesiology, 66,* 729–736.

Zborowski, M. (1952). Cultural components in responses to pain. *Journal of Social Issues, 8,* 16–30.

32

Case Planning and Management by Patient Classification

Donna Jean Funke

The text has provided the reader with information necessary to assess and manage anesthesia for patients undergoing surgical or diagnostic procedures. This chapter will help the reader use this information and skills acquired and apply them to case analysis of a variety of anesthetic situtations commonly encountered in clinical practice.

▶ CASE 1 Transurethral Resection of the Prostate

Age: 69   **DX:** BPH
Sex: male   **Proposed Operation:** TURP
Problems: multiple bladder infections with diagnosed stone and bladder obstruction
smoker; 1 ppd for 50 y

PAST HISTORY
Allergies: Clindamycin—rash
Tobacco: 1 ppd for 50 y
Cardiovascular: negative HTN, CHF, or MI
Respiratory: negative asthma or TB
GI: negative hepatitis, cirrhosis, or PUD

Medications: acetaminophen with codeine, haloperidol
Drug Use: negative

GU: multiple bladder infections with DX stones and bladder obstruction. Pain and burning with urination

Bleeding Disorder: none
Previous Operations and Anesthetics: T and A as a child, no complications

LABORATORY
Hgb: 11.3   **Hct:** 40.2   **BUN:** 16   **CR:** 0.9
CXR: cardiac enlargement noted
ECG: sinus tach. with occ. PVCs

EXAMINATION
BP: 148/84   **P:** 101   **R:** 24   **T:** 37.0   **WT:** 73 kg   **HT:** 183 cm
Heart: S1–S2, no S3 or S4
Lungs: scattered rhonchi; morning productive cough
Airway: *Mouth opening:* 3 FB   *Neck:* full range of motion   *Submental space:* >6.5 cm
Uvula and pillars seen: Class I   *Teeth:* upper dentures, lower teeth intact

1. What is a TURP?

A TURP is transurethral resection of the prostate. It involves the application of a high-frequency current to a wire loop and the removal of fragments of obstructive tissue under direct endoscopic vision. Hemostasis is effected by sealing vessels with the coagulating current. Continuous irrigation with fluids is required to improve visibility through the cystoscope, distend the prostatic urethra, and maintain the operative field free of blood and dissected tissue. This procedure involves the elderly population. Therefore, assess for coexisting diseases. These patients have a relatively high prevalence of both pulmonary and cardiovascular disorders.

2. What are the anesthesia options for this case?

When discussing anesthetic techniques the patient indicates that the anesthesia provider should "pick whatever is best." Both a general or regional anesthetic would be appropriate. However, the technique of choice is either a spinal or epidural anesthesia with a T9 sensory level. Regional anesthesia decreases surgical blood loss and reduces the incidence of postoperative thrombosis. In addition, an awake patient is capable of providing early warning of complications. This patient also has a potential irritable airway because of his smoking history and would benefit from less manipulation in this area. If a general anesthetic is given, the anesthesia provider could place a laryngeal mask airway (LMA) or perform it under a mask technique, unless otherwise contraindicated.

3. Why is it difficult to estimate blood loss in this case?

Once a T9 level is obtained following regional anesthesia, the patient is placed into the lithotomy position and surgical procedure begins. You are monitoring the estimated blood loss (EBL) and are a bit perplexed with estimating an accurate number. It is difficult to assess EBL because the irrigating fluid dilutes the blood. Perkins and Miller (1969) state that the average loss is 4 mL/min of resection time. A type and screen laboratory assessment is adequate for most patients. Decreases in hematocrit may simply reflect hemodilution from absorption of irrigation fluid.

4. Approximately 1 hour into the case the patient begins to get mentally confused and complains of nausea. What may be the cause?

You make a differential diagnosis of *hypervolumic hyponatremia*. Desmond (1970) reports that the absorption of large volumes of nonelectrolyte irrigating solutions (glycine 1.5% or a mixture of sorbitol 2.7% and mannitol 0.54%) results in increased intravascular volume and dilutional hyponatremia, with early symptoms like the ones the patient exhibited. Other signs include visual disturbances, headache, restlessness, cyanosis, dyspnea, arrhythmias, hypotension, or seizures. Because the patient received regional rather than a general anesthetic, these symptoms were assessed in a timely manner. Hypertension and reflex bradycardia may have been the only clues in an asleep patient.

5. Why does intravascular absorption of irrigating fluids occur, and what are the main causes?

The open venous sinuses of the prostatic bed result in absorption of irrigating fluid. What are the primary determinants of the fluid absorption? Height (pressure) of the irrigation container, the number and size of the venous sinuses opened, and the duration of the resection. A study by Hagstrom, Dennise, and Rowlands (1955) revealed that approximately 10 to 30 mL of fluid are absorbed per minute of resection time, hence the recommendation to limit resection time to 45 to 60 minutes.

6. What is the treatment for this patient, if any?

Treatment of *TURP syndrome* depends on early recognition and should be based on severity of symptoms. The absorbed water needs to be eliminated and hypoperfusion and hypoxia avoided (Emmet, Gilbough & McLean, 1969). Endotracheal intubation may be necessary to prevent aspiration until the patient's mental status normalizes. Hyperventilation provides cerebral protection. Assess serum sodium levels. Henderson and Middleton (1980) state that, if the sodium level is lower or equal to 120 mEq/L, you should limit fluids and administer furosemide. Symptomatic hyponatremia resulting in seizures or coma should be treated with hypertonic (3%–5%) saline, not to be given at a rate faster than 100 mL/h. Seizure activity can be terminated with small doses of a benzodiazepine (midazolam or diazepam) or a barbiturate (thiopental). A proactive stance to this potential situation involves calculating the patient's serum osmolality in the preoperative area: 2 (Na) + glucose/18 + BUN/2.8. At 1 hour resection time, redraw select laboratory studies (electrolytes and serum osmolality). Calculate the difference between new and control serum osmolalities. If it is larger than 40, start 3% normal saline at 100/mL/h. If it is lower than 40, give lasix IV.

7. What other potential complications could happen to this patient?

Other potential complications that could have happened to this patient include: bladder perforation, glycine toxicity, coagulopathy, and/or hypothermia.

1. *Bladder perforation* may result when the resectoscope goes through the bladder wall or from

overdistention of the bladder with irrigation fluid. Awake patients may complain of retropubic or lower abdominal pain or referred pain from the diaphragm to the precordial region or shoulder, diaphoresis, and/or nausea. Initially, hypertension and tachycardia may be seen followed by hypotension, especially with bradycardia (vagally mediated). Suspect perforation of the prostatic capsule if irrigation fluid fails to return. If this occurs, prepare for an open surgical procedure.

2. *Glycine toxicity* may occur because a metabolite of glycine is ammonia. Glycine absorption can produce central nervous system (CNS) symptoms such as mild depression, confusion, and transient blindness, to a coma. Avoid this complication by limiting the duration of the resection as well as the height of the irrigation fluid.

3. *Coagulopathy,* specifically disseminated intravascular coagulation (DIC), is thought to result from the release of thromboplastins from the prostate into the circulation during surgery. The diagnosis of coagulopathy may be suspected from diffuse uncontrollable bleeding, but must be confirmed by laboratory tests. The treatment may require heparin in addition to replacement of clotting factors and platelets.

4. *Hypothermia* may occur because large volumes of irrigating fluids can be a major source of heat loss. Warming solutions should prevent hypothermia.■

▶ CASE 2   Excision of Hemorrhoids or Hemorrhoidectomy

Age: 60   **DX:** large external hemorrhoids
Sex: male   **Proposed Operation:** excision of hemorrhoids and rigid sigmoidoscopy
Problems: history of bleeding hemorrhoids for 2–3 mo
                     history of MI in 1980, was treated in the ICU. Currently asymptomatic for chest pain, shortness of
                        breath, or dyspnea on exertion. The patient is able to walk one block without any complaints
                     history of HTN for 1 y; currently controlled by diet
                     history of bilateral carotid endarterectomy
                     history of chronic nasal congestion, possibly due to sinusitis (never formally worked up)

PAST HISTORY
Allergies: NKDA   **Medications:** vitamins, baby aspirin each AM
Tobacco: 10 cigarettes a day for 40 y   **Drug Use:** none
Cardiovascular: positive HTN   **CAD:** MI 1980
Respiratory: chronic nasal congestion
GI: negative   **Endocrine:** negative
Neuro: negative
Bleeding Disorder: currently, bright red blood noted in stools and on toilet paper
Previous Operations and Anesthetics: T&A as a child; right carotid endarterectomy 2 y ago; left carotid
                                         endarterectomy 1 y ago;
                                         all under general anesth. without c/o

LABORATORY
Hgb: 9.7   **Hct:** 30
CXR: NSAD
ECG: minimal voltage for LVH, inferior infarct, age undetermined

EXAMINATION
BP: 136/70   **P:** 76   **R:** 20   **T:** 35.8   **WT:** 72 kg   **HT:** 183 cm
Heart: S1–S2, no murmurs
Lungs: BBS, CTA
Airway: *Mouth opening:* 3 FB   *Neck:* full range of motion   *Submental space:* 3 FB
           Uvula and pillars seen: Class II   *Teeth:* intact

1. How long is this case expected to last?

Excision of hemorrhoids is a relatively noninvasive, brief procedure. Hemorrhoids are masses of vascular tissue found in the anal canal. Internal hemorrhoids are found above the pectinate line, arising from the superior hemorrhoidal venous plexus, and are covered with mucosa. External hemorrhoids are found below the pectinate line, arising from the inferior hemorrhoidal venous plexus, and are covered by anoderm and perianal skin.

2. What are the anesthesia options for this case, and will the surgical position affect the decision?

Hemorrhoidectomy and perirectal abscess are approached in prone or lithotomy position. General anesthesia by mask is possible when the patient is placed in the lithotomy position. However, intubation is necessary for prone cases. If general anesthesia is selected, either a short-acting muscle relaxant or deep planes of anesthesia are necessary so that the anal sphincter is relaxed. Hypobaric spinals work in the flexed prone (jackknife) or knee-chest position. Hyperbaric spinals can be administered for the lithotomy or prone position. If you choose to administer a hyperbaric spinal for a prone case, administer the agent with the patients in the sitting position, allow them to remain there for 5 to 10 minutes, placing the "local" anesthetic to the sacral region. Solicit assistance to reposition the patient for the surgical procedure once the regional technique is complete.

3. A spinal anesthetic is selected, hypobaric technique, with the use of tetracaine. What level of anesthesia is necessary for surgery? After positioning the patient and injecting the medication, the surgeon comes into the room and startles the patient with a question, which causes him to move his position significantly, specifically, his hips and head. Does this pose an anesthetic concern?

Analgesia to S2–5 level is required. After verification of lumbar puncture, the tetracaine solution is injected and can be expected to move in a nondependent manner away from the head, resulting in anesthesia from the level of injection and caudally to block the sacral dermatones. A solution of tetracaine mixed in preservative free water will have a specific gravity slightly less than that of cerebrospinal fluid and when injected will move away from the dependent area. Because your patient moved both his head and hips, he has completely altered what was dependent and nondependent. This is of great concern as movement will affect the final migration of the local anesthetic to the extent that the agent is unbound at the time the postural changes occurred.

4. After repositioning the patient, the breath sounds have diminished and he has become nauseated. What parameter regarding patient status can be assessed?

As the level of sensory anesthesia ascends, the degree of physiologic insult increases. With high thoracic or cervical levels, profound bradycardia (T1-T4 cardiac accelerator fibers), severe hypotension, and respiratory insufficiency (C3-5 diaphragm and C6-8 phrenic innervation) will occur. Therefore, the other parameters that can be obtained include heart rate as seen on the ECG monitor, and the blood pressure that can be "stat" cycled on the noninvasive blood pressure monitor.

5. What is the treatment for this patient?

If profound hypotension persists, hypoperfusion of the medullary respiratory center will lead to apnea. This is the most common presentation of *high spinal* anesthesia. The diagnosis should be made as quickly as possible and can be made in combination with treatment. Treatment consists of initially supporting the airway and circulation. Supplemental oxygen is mandatory. The patient should be given oxygen, preferably by mask attached to the anesthesia circuit. Assess tidal volume and negative inspiratory function. Ask the patient to take a deep breath, and observe intercostal muscle function and movement of the reservoir bag. Inability to perform this is indicative of a high spinal. This means the patient needs to be placed in the supine position and intubated. Decreases in heart rate and blood pressure are expected. Administration of intravenous fluid and use of vasopressors are required to stabilize the blood pressure. Elderly patients with cardiac and cerebrovascular disease may be at risk if the blood pressure is allowed to decline to low levels during spinal anesthesia. It is best not to allow the mean blood pressure to decline more than 20% in these individuals. The profound bradycardia is treated with an anticholinergic agent to counteract the unopposed action of vagal parasympathetic tone on the heart after complete block of the sympathetic cardiac accelerators. This may be refractory to the anticholinergic drug. If necessary, begin the ACLS protocol. If respiratory and hemodynamic control can be achieved after high or total spinal anesthesia, surgery may proceed. It is advisable to keep the patient sedated with a small dose of potent inhalation agent once intubation of the trachea has been accomplished. It is important that the event be discussed with the patient in your postoperative rounds.■

► CASE 3   D&C/Incomplete Abortion

Age: 17   **DX:** pregnancy
Sex: female   **Proposed Operation:** D&C/incomplete abortion
Problems: G_2P_0 **s/p TAB** $\times$ **1:** currently + HCG
                     smoker 1 ppd $\times$ $1\frac{1}{2}$ y, none in last 2 mo
                     extremely anxious; crying

PAST HISTORY
Allergies: NKDA   **Medications:** none
Tobacco: +1 ppd $\times$ $1\frac{1}{2}$ y; none in last 2 mo   **Drugs Use:** none
Cardiovascular: negative
Respiratory: negative
GI: negative   **Endocrine:** negative
Neuro: negative
Bleeding Disorder: none known
Previous Operations and Anesthetics: T&A, GA without complications;
                                         TAB x 1 GA without complications

LABORATORY
Hgb: 12.7   **Hct:** 37.3
CXR: N/A
ECG: N/A

EXAMINATION
BP: 126/78   **P:** 78   **R:** 22   **T:** 37.2   **WT:** 70 kg   **HT:** 173 cm
Heart: RRR NL. S1 S2
Lungs: CTA
Airway: *Mouth opening:* wide   *Neck:* full range of motion   *Submental space:* 3 FB
            Uvula and pillars seen: Class I   *Teeth:* intact

---

1.   What is a D&C?

A dilation and curettage is the expansion of the cervix and scraping of the uterine endometrium. It is performed for diagnostic or therapeutic purposes, such as the removal of retained products of conception.

2.   What preoperative medications might be administered?

One goal with preoperative medication is to minimize the risk of aspiration pneumonitis by decreasing gastric volume and acidity. Outpatients have an increase in gastric volume; pregnancy causes a decrease in gastric emptying, an increase in gastric volume, and incompetence in the physiologic sphincter mechanism. A mask anesthetic technique, if used, may cause insufflation of air into the stomach. All of these can potentially lead to problems. Metoclopramide (10–20 mg IV) increases lower-esophageal sphincter tone, speeds gastric emptying, and lowers gastric fluid volume. Ranitidine (50 mg IV), and

cimetidine (300 mg IV), are H_2-histamine receptor antagonists and inhibit gastric acid secretion. Antacids (30 mL PO) have an immediate H_2-receptor antagonist effect compared to ranitidine or cimetidine, but they increase intragastric volume. A nonparticulate antacid (sodium citrate or citrate acid), should be administered within 30 minutes of induction of anesthesia or the effectiveness is lost. The patient may also be lightly sedated with benzodiazepines and short-acting narcotics because her anxiety level is probably elevated as she is observed to be crying.

3.   What anesthetic options should be considered?

The anesthetic choices consist of local with sedation, regional blockade with analgesia to T6–T8, or a general anesthetic. The general anesthetic may be administered by mask, LMA, or an endotracheal tube if the patient has a full stomach, a poor airway, or is obese. This case could be performed as a monitored anesthesia care (MAC). The surgeons would administer a paracervical block with local anesthetic, usually chloroprocaine or lidocaine. The anesthesia provider would sedate the patient with small doses of benzodiazepines, narcotics, and/or propofol. The patient must always remain spontaneously breathing during a MAC procedure. Most likely oxygen through a nasal cannula or mask would be administered.

4. What IV drug should be available if bleeding is suspected?

If the surgeon suspects bleeding, you may be asked to administer oxytocin. This drug will increase uterine contraction and should decrease bleeding. Gilman, Rall, Nies, and Taylor (1990) suggest the dose be administered as 10 to 30 units diluted in 1000 mL of crystalloid. It appears that the request for oxytocin is secondary to weeks of gestational age and/or the age of the patient. Both of these can increase the chance of hemorrhage.

5. What altered vital sign might occur because of manipulation of the pelvic organs, and what pharmacologic intervention should be used?

A drop in heart rate may be witnessed during manipulation of the pelvic organs. Vasovagal reflexes also have been implicated in the production of arrhythmias. Atropine and glycopyrrolate have vagal-blocking effects and can be administered if necessary.

6. When performing the postoperative visit, the patient complains of diminished sensation over the superior aspect of the thigh and medial and anteriormedial aspect of the leg. What is the cause of this? What is the most frequently damaged nerve in the lower extremity?

The complaints of diminished sensation over the areas described may have resulted from excessive angulation of the thigh when the patient was placed in the lithotomy position. The anesthesia provider must consider that there may be femoral nerve injury. The saphenous nerve (which is a branch of the femoral nerve) can be compressed by the stirrups used to elevate the legs when padding is inadequate. This is not the most frequently damaged nerve in the lower extremity. The common peroneal nerve, which is a branch of the sciatic nerve, is injured more often. Injury of this nerve manifests as foot drop, loss of dorsal extension of the toes, and inability to evert the foot. Proper padding greatly reduces the likelihood of this complication by preventing compression of the nerve between the head of the fibula and the metal brace used in the lithotomy position. When positioning the patient in the lithotomy position, both legs should be elevated and flexed simultaneously to avoid stretching the peripheral nerves. The thigh should be flexed at no more than 90 degrees before rotating the stirrups laterally.

7. What other complication may be associated with a D&C?

Molar pregnancy should always be ruled out by the obstetric physician via ultrasound before performing a D&C. A molar pregnancy can lead to multiple complications. According to Changigian (1994), the patient may present with: vaginal bleeding after a delayed menses, absence of fetal heart rate, large beta HCG, and a large uterus for the gestational age. These women are at higher risk for hyperemesis, PIH, anemia, hyperthyroidism, and pulmonary edema. When evacuation of the uterus occurs, one must expect a large blood loss. Anesthesia for this condition is performed under a general with the application of cricoid pressure and rapid-sequence tracheal intubation. Administration of an antacid half an hour before induction of anesthesia will usually increase the pH of the gastric fluid. Large-bore IV access must be in place and blood within easy access. It is recommended that a thorough baseline pulmonary evaluation be performed. This may include pulse oximetry reading, chest x-ray, and/or arterial blood gas analysis. If the results are within normal range, proceed. If not, consider using an arterial line and/or pulmonary artery catheter during the surgical case to obtain additional discriminatory information through-out the procedure. ■

▶ CASE 4   Appendectomy

Age: 22   **DX:** acute appendicitis
Sex: female   **Proposed Operation:** appendectomy
Problems: right lower-quadrant pain for 1 day associated with vomiting

PAST HISTORY

Allergies: NKDA
Tobacco: few per day: 1–2
Cardiovascular: negative
Respiratory: negative
GI: + abdominal guarding, right lower-quadrant pain for 1 day
  associated with vomiting
Endocrine: negative
Bleeding Disorder: heavy menstrual cycles, "when they occur"
Menses: irregular cycles
Previous Operations and Anesthetics: D&C 2 y ago, local
with sedation, no c/o

Medications: acetaminophen
Drug Use: none

Neuro: negative

LABORATORY

Hgb: 16.1   **Hct:** 47   **WBC:** 16.8   **PLAT:** 154
CXR: N/A
ECG: N/A

EXAMINATION

BP: 96/50   **P:** 70   **R:** 18   **T:** 38.2   **WT:** 46.7 kg   **HT:** 155 cm
Heart: RRR
Lungs: BBS CTA
Airway: *Mouth opening:* 3 FB   *Neck:* full range of motion   *Submental space:* 3 FB
  Uvula and pillars seen: class 1   *Teeth:* caps on upper incisors

---

1. **What would you expect to find in the history/ physical and diagnostic tests when dealing with this appendicitis case? Is all the essential preoperative information available?**

When questioned in detail, this patient states that she has been sexually active and has not had a period for about 4 months. She believes that she is pregnant, even though she has received no prenatal care or confirmation of pregnancy through testing. Immediately order a blood pregnancy test since it is likely this patient is pregnant. Apart from trauma, Morgan and Mikhail (1996) reveal that the most common pregnant emergencies are abdominal, involving torsion or rupture of an ovarian cyst and acute appendicitis. Patients point to localized pain at "McBurney's point," which is midway between the iliac crest and umbilicus. The patient will complain of rebound tenderness, muscle rigidity, and abdominal guarding. Abdominal films if indicated may show the appearance of fecalith (formed, hard mass of feces) in the right lower quadrant or a localized ileus. X-rays would be contraindicated in the pregnant patient. The white blood cell (WBC) count will be elevated with a shift to the left (75% neutrophils). When a patient presents with an acute appendicitis, the long narrow tube of the appendix is obstructed. Hypoxia of the organ develops, the mucosa ulcerates, and bacteria invade the wall.

2. **What are the three major objectives for managing of anesthesia in parturients undergoing nonobstetric surgery?**

Shnider and Levinson (1993) indicate that the three major objectives for managing anesthesia in parturients undergoing nonobstetric surgery are (1) avoidance of teratogenic drugs; (2) avoidance of intrauterine fetal hypoxia and acidosis; and (3) prevention of premature labor.

1. *Avoidance of teratogenic drugs.* In humans, the critical period of organogenesis is between 15 and 56 days of gestation. Three stages of susceptibility are generally recognized. In the first 2 weeks of intrauterine life, teratogens have either a lethal or no effect on the embryo. During the third to eighth week, drug exposure can produce major development abnormalities. From the eighth week onward, organogenesis is complete and organ growth takes place. Teratogen exposure during this last period usually results in only minor morphologic abnormalities but can produce significant physiologic abnormalities and growth retardation. To reduce fetal hazard, it appears preferable to choose drugs with a long history of safety in pregnant clients such as: thiopental, morphine, meperidine, muscle relaxants, and low concentrations of nitrous oxide and anesthetic gases. Ketamine may be preferable to thiopental as an induction agent if severe hypovolemia is suspected. The use of benzodiazepines has been linked to congenital anomalies.

2. *Avoidance of intrauterine fetal hypoxia.* This can be avoided with prevention of maternal hypoten-

sion, hypovolemia, severe anemia, hypoxemia, and excessive changes in the $PaCO_2$. All of these conditions can compromise the transfer of oxygen and of other nutrients across the uteroplacental circulation and promote intrauterine aphyxia.

3. *Prevention of premature labor.* Premature labor may be treated with beta$_2$-agonists (ritodrine or terbutaline). These drugs relax uterine smooth muscle, resulting in inhibition of uterine contractions and increased uteroplacental blood flow. However, be aware of the side effects, which include: hypokalemia, cardiac dysrhythmias, and fetal tachycardia and hypoglycemia.

3. What would be the most ideal anesthetic technique in this patient?

The most ideal anesthetic for this patient is regional anesthesia (analgesia to T6–T8). Regional anesthesia decreases the risks of pulmonary aspiration and failed intubation, which are the major causes of maternal morbidity and mortality, and minimizes drug exposure to the fetus. The higher incidence of failed intubations in pregnant patients may be due to airway edema, a full dentition, or large breasts that can interfere with insertion of the laryngoscope in patients with short necks. A clear plan should be formulated if intubation will be implemented. It is important to remember that the health of the mother takes priority over that of the fetus. Administration of a nonparticulate antacid half an hour before induction of anesthesia will usually increase the pH of the gastric fluid. Beginning in the second trimester, mothers should not be transported or placed in supine position on the operating table without left uterine displacement. This maneuver minimizes the risk of aortocaval compression. Displacement of the uterus to the left can be accomplished manually or by elevating the right hip 10 to 15 cm with a blanket or foam rubber wedge. Hypotension related to spinal or epidural anesthesia should be prevented by rapid IV infusion of crystalloid (500–1000 mL lactated Ringer's) solution before induction. If hypotension develops, a predominantly beta-adrenergic vasopressor such as ephederine should be administered. Ephedrine is a useful sympathomimetic to raise blood pressure in parturients because uterine blood flow is maintained in the presence of this vasopressor. If regional anesthesia cannot be performed and general anesthesia is selected, it must be preceded with denitrogenation. Regardless of the time interval since ingestion of food, the parturient must be treated as having a full stomach. The risk of aspiration should be minimized by applying cricoid pressure and performing a rapid-sequence induction technique with tracheal intubation. Inhaled concentrations of oxygen should be at least 50%.

4. What special monitors are indicated perioperatively?

In addition to the standard monitors, Shnider and Levinson (1993) state that fetal heart rate with a Doppler should be utilized from the 16th week of pregnancy, although you should ensure that the placement of the transducer does not encroach on the surgical field. Intraoperative monitoring of fetal heart rate is helpful in providing early warning signs of fetal distress from impaired uteroplacental perfusion. If the uterus has grown to reach the umbilicus or above, monitoring of uterine activity will allow early treatment to abort preterm labor. The presence of a member of the obstetrical team may be warranted to assess fetal/uterine monitoring while the case is in progress.∎

► CASE 5   Tonsillectomy

Age: 40   **DX:** sleep apnea
Sex: male   **Proposed Operation:** tonsillectomy
Problems: obese
                    difficult airway
                    hiatal hernia

PAST HISTORY
Allergies: shellfish-rash

Tobacco: few per day × 20 y, stopped 2 y ago
Cardiovascular: negative chest pain; positive SOB with exertion; difficult to climb one flight of stairs
Respiratory: negative asthma or TB, C-PAP worn at night
GI: positive hiatal hernia
Bleeding Disorder: none
Previous Operations and Anesthetics: broken wrist repaired at age 22, GA, c/o post-op n/v

Medications: cimetidine, olprezolam, ibuprofen
Drug Use: none

Endocrine: denies, but Accucheck = 178
Neuro: negative CVA or seizures

LABORATORY
Hgb: 14.1   **Hct:** 42.0   **Accucheck:** 178   **SpO₂:** room air, 97%
CXR: decreased lung volumes
ECG: left ventricular hypertrophy

EXAMINATION
BP: 160/88   **P:** 98   **R:** 26   **T:** 36.3   **WT:** 131 kg   **HT:** 178 cm
Heart: positive murmur III/VI
Lungs: diminished throughout
Airway: *Mouth opening:* 2 FB   *Neck:* short, thick neck with a large tongue
          Submental space: 2 FB,   and soft tissue noted in the oropharynx
          Uvula and pillars seen: II   *Teeth:* left lower-right molar chipped

---

1. What are some indications for an adenotonsillectomy?

Some indications for a tonsillectomy and adenoidectomy include recurrent infection, hearing loss, airway obstruction, distorted speech, and obstructive sleep apnea. This patient's indication for surgery is obstructive sleep apnea. During rapid-eye-movement sleep, the pharyngeal muscles relax, along with other muscles of the body. In patients with obstructive sleep apnea, Hall (1986) states that this relaxation produces airway obstruction that can lead to episodes of hypoxia, eventually resulting in pulmonary hypertension, cor pulmonale, and congestive heart failure.

2. What medications might be administered in the preoperative area?

In all patients scheduled for an adenotonsillectomy, one must consider whether or not airway obstruction is a significant factor. If it is a factor, sedative-hypnotics should be avoided for preoperative sedation. Because it is an intraoral procedure, and a potential difficult intubation, an antisialagogue would be appropriate. An antiemetic may provide prophylaxis for postoperative nausea and vomiting, particularly if the patient has a significant history.

3. Are there any concerns regarding this patient's airway, and will this have an impact on induction?

When the assessment of the patient's airway indicates that tracheal intubation may be difficult, as in this case, an awake intubation maintaining spontaneous breathing should be performed. Characteristics that help to identify that this is a difficult airway include an obese individual with a short, thick neck, relatively large tongue, and redundant soft tissue in the oropharynx. The anesthesia provider should be prepared for a difficult tracheal intubation. Essential equipment includes a stylet, an assortment of laryngoscopes, and a fiberoptic laryngoscope.

Equipment should also be available for performing a cricothyrotomy and ventilating through it if necessary.

4. Once the airway has been secured, where should the endotracheal tube be located?

Once the airway has been secured and taped, the surgeon inserts a mouth gag into the patient's oral cavity. This requires that the (RAE) endotracheal tube be located in the midline. The endotracheal tube usually is held in place by being pressed between the tongue blade of the mouth gag and the tongue.

5. After the surgeon has placed the mouth gag, there is a decrease in breath sounds on the left side. Why, and what should be done?

The tongue blade has a groove so that it will accept an endotracheal tube. The endotracheal tube can be moved or kinked while the surgeon is placing the mouth gag. Thus, it is essential to check breath sounds after gag placement. The tube can be taped in place, or a piece of tape can be placed on the tube to serve as a visual marker indicating whether or not the surgeon has inserted or withdrawn the tube during the mouth gag placement. Because there are diminished breath sounds on the left side, the endotracheal tube has most likely been repositioned into the right mainstem bronchus during mouth gag placement. It is important slowly to move the tube out of the area until bilateral breath sounds are again auscultated equally. Another cause of decreased breath sounds could be a pneumothorax. The anesthesia provider must differentially diagnose all problems to make an accurate assessment.

6. Describe the maintenance of anesthesia for this type of case?

Maintenance of anesthesia for these short surgical procedures is acceptably achieved with oxygen, nitrous oxide, low doses of a volatile agent, and alfentanil. Sometimes, a succinylcholine drip or a short-acting nondepolarizing muscle relaxant may be introduced. The tonsillar area may also be sprayed with 4% lidocaine or the surgeon may choose to inject a local anesthetic with epinephrine. The advantage of this inhalational method is a rapid, comfortable awakening in a patient whose protective airway reflexes are intact. Thus, the use of long-acting IV drugs is probably unwise. Tonsillectomies also can be performed under local anesthesia in a spontaneously breathing patient. Intraoperative arrhythmias may result from light anesthesia or hypoventilation. Continuous ECG, pulse oximetry, and precordial stethoscope monitoring is essential. An IV line must be in place and functioning in case there is sudden bradycardia or excessive bleeding.

7.   What is the expected blood loss?

Blood loss during tonsillectomy averages 4 mL/kg, according to Joseph (1998), but usually is underestimated because of an undetermined amount of blood draining directly from the operative site into the stomach. A graduated suction should be used by the surgical team, and blood loss replaced with crystalloid or blood transfusion, if necessary. A small orogastric tube may be placed to empty the stomach at the end of the procedure. This may reduce the likelihood of nausea and emesis because blood in the stomach is a potent stimulus for nausea. Be cautious when performing this action because stimulating the surgical site may cause bleeding.

8.   Are there special considerations during emergence from anesthesia?

Before awakening the patient, inspect the mouth for active bleeding, blood clots, and debris. Carefully suction the nasopharynx and oral cavity to prevent dislodging of clots and slow oozing of blood, which can result in a laryngospasm after extubation of the trachea. After breathing 100% oxygen, the patient should be extubated awake, when protective airway reflexes are intact. A study by Gefke, Andersen, and Friese (1983) showed that "bucking" on the endotracheal tube may be reduced with the administration of lidocaine (1.0–1.5 mg/kg).

9.   What is the best position to transport the patient to the postoperative area?

Patients are transported to the recovery room in the lateral head-down position, known as the "tonsil position," and are kept in this position until they are fully awake. This will help prevent aspiration of blood from either the nasopharynx or the tonsillar bed. It prevents also blood and secretions from dripping into the posterior pharynx, which could cause a laryngospasm. Once in the recovery room, the patient should be given humidified oxygen by mask and observed for a dry pharynx before discharge. In patients with sleep apnea, the use of steroids to help reduce tissue edema may be considered.

10.   What is the most common postoperative complication and its treatment?

The most frequent complication associated with adenotonsillectomy is postoperative bleeding, with resultant hypovolemia and airway obstruction. Expectorant of bright red blood, persistent swallowing, tachycardia, pallor, orthostatic hypotension, and restlessness all suggest an ongoing blood loss. The extent of blood loss often is underestimated until the patient vomits a large amount of swallowed blood. Crysdale and Russel (1986) state thate there are two likely periods for postoperative bleeding. The first period is 4 to 6 hours postoperatively. The second period is from 5 to 10 days postoperatively. A large IV catheter must be inserted so that the patient may be rehydrated prior to surgery to achieve hemostasis. Surgery may be indicated if the bleeding cannot be controlled through electrocautery, silver nitrate, or topical vasoconstrictors. Coagulation laboratory studies should be reassessed and blood available for transfusion. An "awake look" intubation of the trachea is preferred, but may not be possible. An assistant during the induction process and patent suction is essential to ensure an optimal view for intubation. A rapid-sequence induction with cricoid pressure and preoxygenation is indicated if an awake technique cannot be performed because the patient has a full stomach (blood). An alternative induction drug to thiopental may be needed because the patient's intravascular status may not be stable. An acceptable alternative is ketamine or etomidate. The stomach can be emptied by means of an orogastric tube after placing the endotracheal tube. The criteria for extubation of the trachea after surgery for hemostasis are the same as for the original procedure.■

▶ CASE 6   Laparoscopic Cholecystectomy

Age: 38   **DX:** gallstone pancreatitis
Sex: female   **Proposed Operation:** laparoscopic vs. open cholecystectomy
Problems: history of epigastric pain prior to admission associated with nausea and vomiting
                     ultrasound reveals multiple gallstones
                     moderate obesity

PAST HISTORY
Allergies: NKDA

Tobacco: none
Cardiovascular: negative HTN, CHF, or MI
Respiratory: negative asthma, COPD, TB, or URI
GI: history of epigastric pain associated with n/v, last
   episode, 24 h ago
Endocrine: negative thyroid or hepatitis
Bleeding Disorder: unaware of any
Previous Operations and Anesthetics: C-section for second child 15 y ago, regional anesthesia without c/o

Medications: calcium carbonate and
   acetaminophen
Drug Use: none

Neuro: negative seizures, CVA, or musculoskeletal

LABORATORY
Hgb: 14.5   **Hct:** 41.5   **Amylase:** 61   **Alk. phos.:** 255   **AST:** 89   **ALT:** 230   **TB:** 1.0
HCG: negative
CXR: n/a
ECG: n/a

EXAMINATION
BP: 132/86   **P:** 98   **R:** 24   **T:** 36.0   **WT:** 90 kg   **HT:** 160 cm
Heart: S1–S2 without deficit
Lungs: BBS, but diminished
Airway: *Mouth opening:* 3 FB   *Neck:* full range of motion   *Submental space:* >6.5 cm
          Uvula and pillars seen: class II   *Teeth:* intact

1. **What anesthetic choices are available for a patient undergoing laparoscopy? Would this patient benefit from one choice compared to the other?**

The anesthetic choices for a laparoscopy consist of a regional or a general technique. Epidural and spinal anesthesia are generally not tolerated well because of the increased ventilatory load associated with pneumoperitoneum and the nausea/vomiting complaints leading to an increased risk for pulmonary aspiration. Most anesthesia providers feel uncomfortable ventilating a patient undergoing a laparascopy with a mask because of potential problems with hypoventilation and aspiration. Risk factors that would favor intubation include abdominal pressures exceeding 20 mmHg, a Trendelenburg position of greater than 10 degrees, pelvic adhesions, or preexisting respiratory and/or cardiac dysfunction. The obese patient presented here would benefit from a general anesthetic with intubation (rapid-sequence induction with cricoid pressure) to lessen the likelihood of hypoxia, hypercapnia, and aspiration. It might be suggested that the patient have prophylactic antacid with ranitidine and metoclopramide to neutralize acid present in the stomach, encourage gastric emptying, and prevent reflux of gastric contents.

2. **Are there any concerns when the surgeon inserts a trocar into the abdomen?**

To prepare for a laparoscopy, the surgeon inserts a trocar into the abdominal cavity and distends it with a gas, usu-ally carbon dioxide or nitrous oxide. Introduction of the trocar may cause hemorrhage if a major abdominal vessel is lacerated or peritonitis if a viscus is perforated. Some anesthesia providers remove the patient from the mechanical ventilator and hand-ventilate during trocar insertion. This prevents the patient from exhaling at the same moment that the trocar device would be inserted. There has been documentation of bowel injury and bowel gas explosions from the use of electrocoagulation during the procedure.

3. **What considerations must be in the anesthesia plan when the CO_2 insufflation begins?**

Anesthesia for a patient undergoing laparoscopy with CO_2 insufflation involves several important considerations. Rising intraabdominal pressure by gas insufflation may result in cardiovascular depression, reflux of gas contents, cardiac arrhythmias, and hypoxia, or hypercarbia.

   1. *Cardiovascular depression.* Researchers (Pillalamarri et al., 1983) concluded that increases in intraabdominal pressures, especially greater than 30 mmHg, cause decreases in central venous pressure (CVP), systolic pressure, pulse pressure, and cardiac output. This suggests the impairment of venous return (decrease right-heart filling) as the primary cause of the changes. High peripheral resistance and elevated peak respiratory pressure also might contribute to circulatory depression. Gas insufflation at pressures of

20 to 25 cm H_2O produces increases in CVP and cardiac output secondary to central redistribution of blood volume. The clinical revelance is that elevation of intraperitoneal pressure above 20 mmHg may be potentially dangerous. If it occurs, the release of intraabdominal pressures by the surgeon would result in a rapid return of cardiovascular stability.

2. *Increased reflux* risk secondary to insufflation. An elevation in abdominal pressure may increase the risk of aspiration by raising gastric pressure and altering the function of the gastroesophageal junction. The incidence of this can be reduced by inserting an oral or nasal gastric tube once the patient has been intubated. The gastric tube can be withdrawn upon completion of the surgical procedure.

3. *Bradyarrhythmias.* Vasovagal reflexes have been implicated in the production of bradyarrhythmias. This may be related to CO_2 insufflation, manipulation of the pelvic organs, or the rise in CVP. Atropine and glycopyrrolate have vagal-blocking effects. Increased arrhythmias have been noted in patients who have maintained spontaneous ventilation once carbon dioxide insufflation was implemented. The occurrence of arrhythmias is greatly reduced by control of ventilation.

4. *Hypoxia.* Atelectasis and a decreased functional residual capacity may lead to hypoxia.

5. *Hypercarbia.* Hypercarbia results from decrease pulmonary compliance, decreased FRC, and absorption of the CO_2 used for pneumoperitoneum. Impairment by mechanical factors such as abdominal distention and the Trendelenburg position, as well as the administration of premedicants or anesthetic drugs, also will have an influence on the respiration and ventilatory status. Adequate removal of CO_2 can be ensured by increasing ventilation to one and one-half times the normal ventilation required.

4. Describe the anesthetic technique you would select?

The preferred anesthetic technique involves administering a balanced N_2O (debatable)–O_2–narcotic–muscle re-laxant. The use of a low-concentration inhalation agent also may be indicated. Intraoperative monitoring should include electrocardiography, blood pressure measurement, precordial stethoscope, end-tidal CO_2, temperature, and peripheral nerve stimulation. Intraabdominal pressure is monitored to observe any marked increases during insufflation.

5. What drugs have been associated with sphincter spasms during a cholecystectomy?

Opioids (morphine, meperidine, fentanyl) can produce spasm of the choledochoduodenal sphincter, which elevates common bile duct pressures. This spasm could impair passage of contrast media into the duodenum, erroneously suggesting the need for a sphincteroplasty or the presence of common bile duct stones. However, opioids have been used without adverse effects, revealing that not all patients respond to opioids with spasm. If medical treatment becomes necessary, atropine, nitroglycerine, glucagon, and narcan have been used successfully.

6. What laboratory tests are important to assess prior to anesthetizing the patient for a cholecystectomy?

In patients scheduled for a cholecystectomy, liver function tests are usually normal, but elevated serum bilirubin or alkaline phosphate concentrations suggest the presence of choledocholithiasis (common bile duct stone) or chronic cholangitis.

7. What differential diagnoses must be considered when a patient becomes hypoxic, difficult to ventilate, or hypotensive during a laparoscopic cholecystectomy?

If the patient becomes hypoxic, difficult to ventilate, or hypotensive, a pneumothorax or pneumomediastinum must be considered. The gas may pass retroperitoneally through congenital foraminae, through defects in the diaphragm, or weak points of the aortic or esophageal hiatus. Gas embolism also may occur.

8. Your patient begins to complain of shoulder pain in the postoperative care unit. Why?

Shoulder pain may be caused by referred absorption of CO_2 used for the pneumoperitoneum. ∎

▶ CASE 7   Inguinal Hernia Repair

Age: 45   **DX:** right inguinal hernia (RIH), possible incarceration
Sex: male   **Proposed Operation:** repair of RIH, possible mesh, possible bowel resection
Problems: C/O severe pain in right inguinal area × 2 days, surgeons unable to reduce the hernia
                   smoker × 10 y

PAST HISTORY
Allergies: NKDA
Tobacco: 1/2 ppd for 10 y
Cardiovascular: N/A
Respiratory: C/O early morning cough
GI: negative hepatitis, cirrhosis, hiatal hernia, or PUD

Medications: acetaminophen, last taken 2 days ago
Drug Use: a few beers on the weekend

Endocrine: negative
Neuro: negative seizure or CVA

Bleeding Disorder: none
Previous Operations and Anesthetics: T&A as a child without incident

LABORATORY
Hgb: 12   **Hct:** 48
CXR: WNL
ECG: unchanged from 2 y ago

EXAMINATION
BP: 104/52   **P:** 51   **R:** 20   **T:** 36.4   **WT:** 79 kg   **HT:** 180 cm
Heart: S1–S2 without deficit
Lungs: scattered rhonchi cleared with coughing
Airway: *Mouth opening:* 3 FB   *Neck:* full range of motion   *Submental space:* >6.5 cm
                    Uvula and pillars seen: Class II   *Teeth:* poor dentition; upper incisors rotted,
                                                                                                                                                    mult. missing teeth

1.   What events occur when a patient is scheduled for outpatient surgery?

The surgeon is responsible for scheduling outpatient surgery, obtaining a medical history, performing a physical examination, initiating the laboratory studies, and providing instructions to the patient. The surgeon may be asked to describe and explain the anesthetic management to the patient, but it is the anesthesia provider's responsibility to consult with the client on the day of surgery. After the patient arrives for outpatient surgery, compliance with preoperative instructions is verified. It is especially important to confirm that fasting has been maintained. All questions regarding anesthesia must be answered and a preanesthetic worksheet completed. Elicit any change in medical condition that may have developed since the outpatient surgery was scheduled.

2.   The patient tells you that he is interested in being told all the anesthesia options for an inguinal hernia repair. What are they?

Inguinal herniorrhaphies can be done under local, regional (spinal or epidural), or general anesthesia. Closure of large fascial defects is facilitated by muscle relaxation, which is best provided by regional anesthesia.

3.   Since the patient has decided to have a local anesthetic performed, he wants to know if it is necessary "to have one of those tubes" put in his arms?

Regardless of the technique of anesthesia selected, an intravenous catheter should probably be inserted into the peripheral vein before the institution of anesthesia, unless the surgery is very short and only superficial tissues are involved. The catheter is necessary to allow administration of fluids to offset dehydration associated with preoperative fasting. Additionally, IV access makes the administration of drugs to produce anesthesia or treat adverse intraoperative events possible. Local infiltration with lidocaine at the IV site might decrease any discomfort during IV insertion.

4.   What area is the local anesthetic administered?

Ilioinguinal and iliohypogastric blocks are performed for local anesthesia for inguinal or genital surgery, such as an inguinal herniorrhaphy or orchiopexy. Anesthesia of these nerves alone is not sufficient for hernia repair and subcutaneous infiltration also is necessary. Infiltration of anesthetic is performed along the skin crease of the groin through an imaginary line extending to the umbilicus. Further anesthesia of the spermatic cord is required. This usually is performed with local anesthesia injections given by the surgeon in the area of the cord and internal ring.

5.   Are there any complications that could arise from this local administration?

Complications from the local anesthetic administration are extremely rare. Hematoma formation and unwanted motor blockade of the femoral nerve are possible. The patient must be monitored for signs and symptoms of a hypersensitivity reaction to the local anesthetic. Local hypersensitivity reactions may present as local erythema, urticaria, edema, or dermatitis. Systemic hypersensitivity is rare and presents as generalized erythema, urticaria, edema, bronchoconstriction, or hypotension. Treatment is symptomatic and supportive. Hypotension should be managed with the administration of fluids and vasopressors. Cutaneous reactions may respond to an antihistamine (diphenhydramine). A severe reaction may require the administration of a systemic steroid (methylprednisolone). Bronchoconstriction is treated with the administration of epinephrine 0.3 mg SC. An astute anesthesia provider would also be monitoring for the potential intravascular injection.

6. What are the most common local anesthetic drugs used for an inguinal hernia, and what is the dosage?

The most common anesthetic drugs for a local procedure without inhalation agents are 1% lidocaine or 0.25% bupivacaine. This patient weighs 175 lb, or 79.5 kg. The maximum dose of lidocaine is 7 mg/kg and 3 mg/kg for bupivicaine, with epinephrine. The maximum dose of lidocaine is 556.5 mg/kg, or 55.65 mL. The maximum dose of bupivacaine is 238.5 mg/kg, or 95.4 mL.

7. Do you think that the patient will be able to have the surgical procedure performed under local anesthesia with sedation?

The injection of local anesthetics often is associated with severe discomfort. The use of an intravenous sedative and analgesic drug during local anesthetic injections will allow the patient to remain comfortable throughout the procedure. This is known as a conscious sedation or conscious analgesia technique.

8. If this patient has the procedure under a general anesthetic, what is a concern with emergence?

If general anesthesia is administered, then either a mask technique or a deep extubation should be performed to decrease the possibility of coughing on emergence, which can strain the hernia repair. However, the risks of laryngospasm and aspiration are increased by deep extubation. Patients who require awake intubations or rapid-sequence inductions are not candidates for a deep extubation.■

▶ CASE 8   Reattachment of Right Index Finger

Age: 36
Sex: male
Problems:

DX: hand trauma
Proposed Operation: reattachment of right index finger tip
right hand caught in assembly press 2 h ago; tip of index finger removed
smoker, 1 ppd for 20 y
alcohol, cocaine, and marijuana use
full stomach: consumed a few beers with his sandwich about 2½ h ago

PAST HISTORY
Allergies: NKDA
Tobacco: positive smoker 1 ppd for 20 y

Medications: aluminum hydroxide
Drug Use: cocaine: last used 3 days ago; alcohol: last used 2½ h ago; marijuana: last used in the AM yesterday

Cardiovascular: c/o "fluttering" after cocaine usage
Respiratory: positive TB dx. 5 y ago, noncompliant with treatment
GI: positive ulcer, negative hepatitis
Endocrine: negative diabetes or thyroid

Neuro: positive seizure ×1 when using LSD 15 y ago, affect: slow to answer questions

Bleeding Disorder: none
Previous Operations and Anesthetics: open reduction internal fixation mandible 8 y ago without complications

LABORATORY
Hgb: 11.0   **Hct:** 33.2
CXR: not taken
ECG: ? septal infarct, age undetermined

EXAMINATION

BP: 130/72   **P:** 102   **R:** 18   **T:** 37.4   **WT:** 72 kg   **HT:** 185 cm

Heart: regular, irregular

Lungs: "harsh" throughout

Airway: *Mouth opening:* 2½ FB   *Neck:* full range of motion   *Submental space:* >6.5 cm

Uvula and pillars seen: Class II   *Teeth:* Poor dentation with multiple teeth missing

---

1. What anesthetic options are possible for an upper-extremity procedure such as this one?

Upper-extremity procedures can be done under IV regional (Bier block), brachial plexus, peripheral nerve blocks, and general anesthesia.

2. What are the potential risks of these options?

Intravenous regional blocks are quick in onset and recovery, but their duration is limited by the time the tourniquet can be tolerated. The supraclavicular approach to the brachial plexus block has the risk of phrenic nerve block and pneumothorax. The interscalene block may cause recurrent laryngeal nerve block, phrenic nerve block, or Horner's syndrome, and the axillary approach can result in a hematoma, nerve injury, or intravascular injection. Regional anesthesia usually has the advantage of less postoperative drowsiness and nausea than seen with general anesthesia, but often requires a longer induction period. Frequently, regional anesthesia is supplemented with IV sedation. The patient stated that he ate lunch only 1 hour before and is, therefore, considered to have a full stomach. If a general anesthetic is performed, he will be at risk for pulmonary aspiration. After discussing all of these options with the patient, because the surgeon claims to be able to finish the procedure in 1 hour, the patient has decided to have a Bier block performed.

3. Are there any contraindications to performing a Bier block?

Relative contraindications to a Bier block include bifascicular and trifascicular block on the ECG, history of syncope, distal infection of the extremity, and seizure disorders.

4. What anesthetic drugs are used in the administration of a Bier block?

Local anesthetics used for intravenous regional blocks on the upper extremity are 40 to 50 mL 0.5% lidocaine or prilocaine without epinephrine. Bupivacaine is avoided because of systemic toxic effects, especially on the cardiac system if the drug enters the circulation. Chloroprocaine is not used for intravenous regional blocks because of its association with thrombophlebitis.

5. The patient complains of discomfort 45 minutes into surgery. What can be done?

A double tourniquet technique can be used to eliminate tourniquet pain. The proximal tourniquet is initially inflated, and when the patient experiences pain, the more distal (second) tourniquet over anesthetized skin is inflated and the proximal cuff deflated. In long operations, tourniquet pain usually is the limiting factor for success. The duration of anesthesia depends on the time the tourniquet is inflated, not on the local anesthetic selected. If a heparin lock was placed on the IV catheter, reinjection may be considered after 90 minutes.

6. What is the minimum time that a tourniquet should be inflated when performing a Bier block?

With very short procedures, Purdman (1997) states that the tourniquet must remain inflated for a total of 20 to 30 minutes to avoid a rapid intravenous bolus of local anesthetic. Deflation with immediate reinflation repeated several times provides a safety margin to prevent excessive plasma concentrations of local anesthetics from developing. Limiting extremity movement after the release of the tourniquet also is useful to minimize anesthetic blood levels. Signs and symptoms that a local anesthetic has flooded the circulation include arrhythmias (usually bradycardia), restlessness, tachypnea, dizziness, nausea, and in extreme cases centrally triggered convulsions and apnea.

7. What is the treatment of central nervous system toxicity?

Treatment of central nervous system toxicity begins with airway management. The convulsing patient should be hyperventilated with a mask at 100% oxygen. In the presence of a full stomach, as in this case, endotracheal intubation with rapid-sequence induction and cricoid pressure should be performed. Hypotension is treated by the administration of fluids, peripheral vasoconstrictive drugs, and the placement of the patient into the Trendelenburg position. Cardiac arrhythmias are difficult to treat, but subside over time if the patient can be hemodynamically maintained.

8. **An hour and fifteen minutes into the case the patient remains comfortable, but the surgeon states that the procedure is going to take at least another hour. What are you going to do?**

When administering a Bier Block and the surgical case is prolonged, as in this one, the anesthesia provider more than likely will need to convert the case into a general anesthetic. Supplementation of the Bier block with IV sedation will not suffice for another hour or more. It is not advisable to risk sedating a patient who is undergoing emergency surgery too deeply without airway protection. A general anesthesia by mask is ruled out because of the patient's full stomach. It will be necessary to intubate the patient following a rapid sequence induction (RSI) with cricoid pressure (CP) to prevent aspiration. The anesthesia provider must be prepared for this change of anesthetic plan by having all the necessary equipment within reach. This patient also might have been a candidate for prophylactic antacid preoperatively with ranitidine and metoclopramide. This would have neutralized the acid present in the stomach, encouraged gastric emptying, and prevented reflux of gas contents. Because of the patient's history of noncompliance with TB treatment, precautions must be taken to prevent contamination of the anesthesia equipment by placing filters on the ventilatory circuit.

9. **What specific findings given by this patient will have an impact on your anesthetic management?**

There are specific principles to be aware of when providing anesthesia to a patient who indulges in alcohol and illicit drugs. The management of anesthesia in the sober alcoholic patient may be accompanied by functional tolerance to anesthetics where more anesthesia is needed to produce loss of consciousness than in other patients. Dispositional tolerance to anesthetics also may occur where hepatic metabolism to drugs is enhanced. Isoflurane may be associated with the optimal maintenance of hepatic blood flow and hepatocyte oxygenation. Injected anesthetics (narcotics and benzodiazepines) are useful, but a cumulative effect is possible. Alcohol-induced cardiomyopathy also is a consideration. In contrast to the chronic, but sober, alcoholic, the acutely intoxicated patient requires less anesthetic, as there is an additive depressant effect between alcohol and anesthetics. If the patient was truthful during his anesthesia evaluation period, he will not be considered acutely intoxicated with alcohol or cocaine. Cocaine prevents the reuptake of norepinephrine to the postganglionic sympathetic nerve endings. Increased levels of norepinephrine cause an increase in blood pressure, heart rate, and temperature. Cocaine-induced patients are vulnerable to myocardial ischemia and cardiac dysrhythmias because of an increase in circulating catecholamines. Cocaine produces a sympathetic nervous system stimulation of the cardiovascular system. This may present as hypertension, pulmonary edema, and coronary artery constriction. Esmolol or labetalol is useful in blunting the effects of the sympathetic nervous system stimulation. Diazepam may be effective in terminating cocaine-induced seizures. Appropriate medications should be ordered in the postoperative period to prevent this patient from experiencing withdrawal symptoms.■

► CASE 9 Open Reduction Internal Fixation (ORIF) Mandible

Age: 23 **DX:** open mandible fracture and laceration
Sex: male **Proposed Operation:** ORIF mandible with internal fixation
Problems: patient involved in a fight 24 h ago, c/o painful trismus but facial swelling and nasal/oral bleeding
    have subsided
  potential difficult airway

PAST HISTORY
Allergies: NKDA **Medications:** acetaminophen (elixir), meperidine, penicillin
Tobacco: none **Drug Use:** few beers a day (2)
Cardiovascular: negative
Respiratory: negative
GI: negative
Endocrine: negative
Neuro: negative
Bleeding Disorder: none, but sickle cell trait
Previous Operations and Anesthetics: none, but multiple dental visits without problems

LABORATORY
Hgb: 13.5   **Hct:** 41.5
CXR: N/A
ECG: sinus bradycardia on ER monitor

EXAMINATION
BP: 108–130/60–72   **P:** 60–64   **R:** 20   **T:** afebrile   **WT:** 65 kg   **HT:** 179 cm
Heart: S1–S2
Lungs: BBS CTA
Airway: *Mouth opening:* 1–1½ FB   *Neck:* full range of motion   *Submental space:* >6.5 cm
Uvula and pillars seen: Class III   *Teeth:* upper incisors broken and/or chipped, malalignment noted

---

1. What type of intubation is necessary for this case?

The anesthesia provider must be aware that mandibular fractures may be associated with loose teeth, blood, displaced fragments, malocclusion, limitation of mandibular movements, sublingual hematoma, or swelling at the fracture site. All of these could complicate securing the airway. Elective surgery on this particular case scenerio has a patient presenting with painful trismus, but facial swelling and nasal/oral bleeding have subsided. This patient is scheduled for an interdental fixation, so a nasal tracheal intubation is indicated. It is important that a thorough airway assessment be performed. It is not uncommon to have patients complain of jaw pain and be unwilling or unable to open their mouths. Temporary pain must be differentiated from anatomical compromise. One important diagnostic test to assist with airway assessment is to evaluate and discuss x-ray findings with the surgeon. This will provide information to the anesthesia provider on the location of the fracture, whether there is any joint relocation, and how long ago the injury occurred. If the time to surgery is greater than 72 hours, fixation of the trismus begins, adding difficulty to the intubation. Some anesthesia providers administer a narcotic intravenously and have the patient perform a mouth opening in the preoperative area to evaluate the difference pre- and post-narcotic administration. When this technique is performed, the patient is able easily to open his mouth three fingerbreadths. Following airway assessment, an asleep induction is performed. It also would be wise to have the fiberoptic bronchoscope available in the room should the equipment be necessary. If this patient presented with a compromised airway, safe anesthetic options would include awake direct laryngoscopy after topical block, awake fiberoptic evaluation of the airway, or tracheostomy under local anesthesia.

2. What preoperative medications should be considered?

Patients undergoing internal fixation should be given an antiemetic, especially if there is any history of nausea and vomiting. To decrease airway secretions, an anticholinergic such as glycopyrrolate should be administered. Preoperative assessment includes evaluation and preparation of the nares. Once patency is confirmed, the larger of the two nares usually is the location for placing the nasotracheal tube. However, both nares should be prepared. For nasal endotracheal tube placement, application of swabs soaked in either 4% cocaine or 4 mL 4% lidocaine mixed with 5 mg phenylephrine will provide both topical anesthesia and vasoconstriction of the mucosa. The areas blocked with the topical anesthetic solution should include branches of the ethmoidal nerve; the sphenopalatine ganglion and branches of the maxillary division of the trigeminal nerve; and topical anesthesia for passage of the endotracheal tube through the nasopharynx. Some anesthesia providers introduce a lubricated nasal airway (trumpet) once the local anesthetic has been administered and given adequate time to take effect. A RAE (preformed) or armored endotracheal tube should be used for this procedure.

3. Are there any special anesthesia equipment needs?

Magill forceps may be necessaray to guide the tip of the endotracheal tube through the vocal cords once visualization is accomplished. It is not uncommon for the patient to be moved away from the anesthesia provider once induction is completed. A long anesthesia circuit ensures that minimal pulling or tugging will occur on the RAE or armored endotracheal tube. You may want to disconnect the endotracheal tube from the circuit when moving the patient and OR table. Remember to reconnect after relocating the table. Ensure that the breathing circuit is "snug" at all connection sites. Reassess lung sounds and the $ETCO_2$ waveform. Some surgeons may suggest suturing the tube in place to prevent accidental movement or dislodging. It is appropriate to discuss what direction the table will be relocated to prevent tangling of the ECG, pulse oximeter, precordial, temperature, and ETCO₂ monitors.

4. What is an important technique to implement during emergence in a patient undergoing ORIF with fixation of the mandible?

Patients recovering from mandibular fixation should demonstrate cognitive and physical ability to clear the airway before the trachea is extubated. An awake extubation is preferred. Residual neuromuscular paralysis reduces the patient's ability to cough. The risk of aspiration is possible and the incidence of postoperative nausea and emesis is significant. The anesthesia provider must completely suction the nares and pharynx and extubate the trachea at end-inspiration or with positive airway pressure to avoid aspiration of material trapped below the vocal cords but above the endotracheal cuff.

5. What must be available in the PACU for the patient's airway safety?

Mandibular fixation makes expulsion of vomitus, blood, or secretions from the mouth almost impossible. Equipment for immediate release of fixation should be at hand throughout the postoperative period. A pair of wire cutters must be within immediate access. The best position for the patient may be on the side with his head slightly elevated during the recovery phase.

6. During the postoperative visit, the patient complains of a sensation of a foreign body and tearing in his eyes. What might be the cause of this, and what is the treatment?

A corneal abrasion must be suspected when a patient complains of the sensation of a foreign body, tearing, photophobia, and pain. It is desirable to obtain an ophthalmology consultation. The treatment usually consists of patching the injured eye and applying a prophylactic antibiotic ointment such as erythromycin. According to McGoldrick (1997), healing normally occurs within 24 to

48 hours. A variety of circumstances could result in corneal abrasions. The anesthesia provider must evaluate what might have been the cause to prevent this from occuring in future patients undergoing this procedure. During the intubation, the sleeve of the scrub suit may have caused the trauma, or perhaps it was the anesthetic mask, surgical drapes, or spillage of solutions used to clean the surgical site. Taping the eyelids closed and applying petroleum-based ointments (artificial tears) into the conjunctival sac may provide protection against eye injury. Disadvantages of ointments include allergy, flammability (making this a contraindication during laser surgery), and complaints of blurred vision upon emergence.

7. What are important considerations when working with a patient who has sickle cell disease?

Management of anesthesia is not likely to be altered by sickle cell trait. Sickle cell trait is the heterozygous manifestation of sickle cell disease. Sickle cell disease presents with an inherited defect in hemoglobin structure, hemoglobin S. Forrester (1986) states that hemoglobin S differs from normal adult hemoglobin A by the substitution of amino acid valine for glutamic acid at the sixth position of the beta chain in the hemoglobin molecule, creating two new reactive sites. Desaturated Hb S is 50 times less soluble than deoxygenated Hb A. The oxyhemoglobin dissociation curve is shifted to the right, facilitating oxygen unloading at the tissue level. Chronic sickling produces permanently distorted cells that are subject to elimination, accounting for the chronic mild to moderate hemolytic anemia. The lifelong hemolytic anemia leads to physiologic adaptation by expansion of plasma volume and increased cardiac output. Splenic enlargement, jaundice, bone marrow cavity enlargement, and reticulosis are common sequelae. Factors that tend to exacerbate the sickling of red cells include hypoxia, infection, reduction in temperature, acidosis, and dehydration. All of these must be avoided during the administration of anesthesia.■

▶ CASE 10   Vaginal Hysterectomy

Age: 59   **DX:** high-grade cervical dysplasia
Sex: female   **Proposed Operation:** total vaginal hysterectomy with BSO
Problems: rheumatoid arthritis
                   moderate obesity
                   difficult airway
                   depression

PAST HISTORY

Allergies: NKDA

Tobacco: negative
Cardiovascular: negative HTN or MI, but dyspnea with exertion
Respiratory: positive chronic cough
GI: positive anorexia
Endocrine: negative thyroid or diabetes

Bleeding Disorder: none

Medications: aspirin, corticosteroid, gold salt, and fluoxetine hydrochloride
Drug Use: one glass of wine with dinner

Neuro: positive rheumatoid arthritis for 20 y, positive depression for 10 y

Previous Operations and Anesthetics: cervical bx. 3 mo ago, local with sedation; foot surgery for joint replacement, 2 y ago GA; T&A as a child; no anesthetic complications

LABORATORY

Hgb: 10.0   **Hct:** 30.2   **Accucheck:** 125
CXR: pulmonary fibrosis
Pulm FXN Tests: within acceptable range
ECG: left vent. hypertrophy
ECHO: possible rheumatoid nodules on myocardium, aortic regurgitation

EXAMINATION

BP: 128/74   **P:** 88   **R:** 20   **T:** 36.7   **WT:** 78 kg   **HT:** 168 cm
Heart: + murmur
Lungs: BBS but diminished
Airway: *Mouth opening:* 2 FB   *Neck:* limited cervical spine   *Submental space:* 3 FB
                Uvula and pillars seen: Class II   movement   *Teeth:* upper and lower dentures
                Other: + hoarseness in voice

---

1. What medications is the patient currently taking that will impact anesthesia?

The patient is on three medications to help with her rheumatoid arthritis: aspirin, a corticosteroid, and gold salt. Aspirin produces drug-induced platelet dysfunction. This reflects irreversible interference with platelet release of adenosine diphosphate (ADP) and subsequent platelet aggregation. The patient should be withdrawn from the medication at least 7 days prior to surgery to prevent bleeding problems during the procedure. Preoperative assessment of bleeding time the morning of surgery will reveal platelet function. This patient manifests suppression of the pituitary adrenal axis because of the medical treatment with a corticosteroid. This suppression includes patients who have been treated for at least 1 month during the past 6 to 12 months. The patient has been receiving corticosteroids for 20 years. One approach to anesthesia management is to administer a supplemental dose of a corticosteroid, cortisol 25 mg IV at induction and 100 mg IV over the next 24 hours. Remember that corticosteroid therapy has multiple side effects that may impact the patient. According to Klinenberg (1992), these include: increased risk of infection, osteoporosis, gastrointestinal bleeding, hypertension, and hyperglycemia. Gold salts have been known to cause skin rashes and painful mouth ulcers. It is important that a thorough oral exam be performed since this patient will have an oral endotracheal tube placed. Other potential manifestations of gold salts include bone marrow suppression, renal damage, and rarely a nephrotic syndrome.

2. What indications identify this patient as having a difficult airway?

Indications identifying this patient as a difficult airway include the patient's history of rheumatoid arthritis with limited neck movement and the ability to open her mouth only minimally. A thorough evaluation of the cervical spine and temporomandibular and cricoarytenoid joint function is essential. Cervical spine involvement may include atlantoaxial subluxation and flexion deformities. Arnett (1992) states that atlantoaxial subluxation may result in odontoid displacement causing impingement on the cervical spine, medulla, or vertebral arteries. Symptoms would include headache, neck pain, and numbness or tingling in the arms or legs with neck motion. Patients should be evaluated preoperatively for these symptoms during flexion, extension, and rotation of the head. The head and neck must be manipulated carefully during positioning and intubation. Acute subluxation can occur with neck flexion, resulting in paralysis or sudden death. Flexion deformities of the cervical spine may result in airway obstruction with the induction of anesthesia, and intubation may be difficult because of the inability to extend the neck. Prior to surgery, cervical spine radiographs and flexion-extension films should be obtained to assess the degree of cervical spine involvement. Involvement of the cricoarytenoid joints may result in narrowing of the glottic opening. A smaller-size endotracheal tube may be required. Symptoms such as fullness or tightness in the throat, hoarseness or stridor, dysphagia, pain when swallowing, and dyspnea may indicate the presence of cricoarytenoid arthritis.

3. What preoperative medications should be administered?

As soon as the decision is made to proceed with fiberoptic endoscopy, an antisialagogue, either atropine or glycopyrrolate should be administered. This will prevent failure of intubation because of excessive oral secretions. Antisialagogues produce dry airway mucosa, which prevents dilution of the local anesthetic and formation of a barrier between mucosa and the local anesthetic agent by saliva. In this patient obesity and drug taking could affect the stomach mucosa. Therefore, the administration of prophylactic antacid and ranitidine or metoclopramide must be considered to neutralize acid present in the stomach, encourage gastric emptying, and prevent reflux of gastric contents.

4. What methods may be implemented to prepare a patient for a fiberoptic intubation?

To gain maximal patient cooperation, preoperative preparation must include a careful explanation of the procedure. Intravenous sedation should be titrated so that no obtundation or airway obstruction occurs. It is essential that this patient maintain adequate spontaneous respiration. Depending on the patient's response, a sedative, opioid, or a combination may be used. However, the patient may now be more susceptible to aspiration of gastric contents if regurgitation or vomiting occurs. Topical anesthesia of the oropharynx is provided by spraying 5 mL of 4% lidocaine with an atomizer or 10% aerosolized lidocaine to the base of the tongue and the lateral pharyngeal walls. Translaryngeal injection with 3 mL of 4% lidocaine and superiorlaryngeal injection with 3 mL of 1% lidocaine can be administered. Another approach for effective spraying of local anesthetic is to inject local anesthetic through the fiberscope channel using a "spray-as-you-go" technique. The goal is to prevent poor topical anesthesia, which represents a major cause of failure with fiberoptic intubation in the awake patient. Instrumentation of the airway in the presence of poor topical anesthesia causes

gagging, coughing, vomiting, and increases in blood pressure and heart rate, forcing abandonment of the technique.

5. What concerns should the anesthesia provider be aware of when positioning a patient with rheumatoid arthritis?

Positioning patients who have rheumatoid arthritis must be performed very carefully. Some practitioners suggest positioning the patients while they are awake. Care must be taken not to flex the neck excessively. Joints should not be moved beyond their normal range of motion. Excessive motion may result in nerve injury, joint dislocation or stretch, or muscle trauma. Preoperative assessment of joint motion will aid in intraoperative positioning. Technical concerns include flexion deformities of the wrist making arterial line placement challenging, and central venous lines may be difficult to insert because of fusion and flexion of the neck.

6. The surgeons decide that they must perform an abdominal incision after the case has been in progress for 2 hours. What implications might this have on the anesthetic plan?

The anesthetic implications of the surgeons converting from a vaginal to an abdominal hysterectomy might include:

1. When was the last time the patient received a narcotic? Are there any clues through the vital signs that the patient is experiencing pain with the abdominal incision? Consider the administration of additional narcotic medications. Narcotics must be titrated to treat pain from the procedure while preserving the ventilatory drive. Too little narcotic will result in discomfort, and excessive narcotic will decrease the respiratory drive. Hypoventilation will prolong emergence. Ideally, at the end of the surgical case, the patient will not complain of pain, the respiratory rate will be greater than 12 breaths per minute, $Paco_2$ will be less than 50, and the patient will respond appropriately to questions.

2. What is the patient's temperature at this time, and are there enough warming modalities? Evaporation from mucosa surfaces of the peritoneum during a laparotomy is a dramatic source of heat loss and is increased by the use of cold liquids for irrigation. However, some warming modalities already have been initiated with this patient, and the fact that the procedure has progressed longer than originally planned will not be cause for alarm. Review the methods to pre-

vent inadvertent hypothermia, which include: control of ambient room temperature, insulating the patient, warming fluids, heating humidified anesthetic gases, using a heating mattress, and implementing a forced-air exchange blanket.

3. Has the anesthetic caused any potential difficulty for the surgical team? Gaseous bowel distention may be caused from nitrous oxide, which prevents the surgical team to access abdominal contents easily. Nitrous oxide also has been implicated in causing a surgical challenge for abdominal closure. Perhaps, an oxygen–air versus oxygen–nitrous oxide combination would be a more appropriate selection for anesthesia maintenance.

4. Has fluid replacement been maintained with crystalloids and colloids? Do not forget to replace NPO fluids and insensible looses based on patient size and surgical procedure. Every 1 mL of blood loss must be replaced with 3 mL of crystalloids.

7. As the doctors begin their wound closure, they complain about the patient's "being tight." When the patient's neuromuscular response is assessed with the peripheral nerve stimulator, there are no twitches noted. An appropriate dose of muscle relaxant was administered recently. What does this mean, and what produced the lack of neuromuscular response assessed by the peripheral nerve stimulator?

When the surgeons complain that a patient is "tight," they are inferring that the musculature is difficult to manipulate. In this particular case, it has to do with the ability to ease peritoneal closure. It is important to remain calm when this discussion occurs. Do not get defensive, even though it may seem as if they are complaining about the anesthetic technique. Have a systematic approach to identifying the potential cause. Assess the nerve stimulation response first. Do not be fooled into thinking that the peripheral nerve stimulator is free of mechanical error. Are the batteries in the monitor functioning? Are all the connections intact? This includes connections to the patient's skin surface. What type of muscle relaxant is being used? Review the expected duration of the drug chosen. If the drug action appears to be lasting longer than expected, how is the drug eliminated? Perhaps the patient has a disease process that would alter the elimination. If a nitrous oxide–oxygen technique was selected for maintenance, it may be prudent to discontinue the nitrous oxide. Abdominal closure is a difficult phase because the peritoneal cavity may be overcrowded from edema and intestines inflated with nitrous oxide. Do not complicate the issue by con-

tinuing to use nitrous oxide. Consider decreasing the volume of the stomach by oral or nasal gastric suctioning. This might allow room for intestinal manipulation that eases abdominal closure. After reviewing all of these concepts, it would be an appropriate time to communicate openly to the surgical team. It may be advisable to preface the discussion with, "I am aware of the need to provide adequate relaxation at this time, however, this conflicts with the goal of having a patient ready for extubation shortly after the closure is completed. I have systemically reviewed potential reasons and cannot find how else to assist." Do not administer more muscle relaxant if the surgical team requests. It would be inappropriate. If mandated to do so by the surgeon, consult with the supervising CRNA or anesthesiologist and document carefully. Some individuals have been known to fill a syringe with saline and administer that through the peripheral IV so that the surgeons visualize some type of anesthesia action being taken. However, this is unethical and not recommended.

8. The surgeons decided to allow the third-year medical student to assist with abdominal closure. The time for the incisional closure has increased greatly. In fact, additional muscle relaxant must be administered. As soon as the drug is given the attending surgeon decided to complete the suturing because he has another case to follow. What should the anesthesia provider do?

When emergence is initiated, it is important to assess the status of neuromuscular blockade. If there is not at least one twitch on the train-of-four peripheral nerve stimulator, the blockade is too intense to be antagonized. If an anticholinesterase is administered, the muscle relaxant will probably outlast the reversal. The patient then will likely have complications in the recovery room. The most appropriate action is to call the PACU and ask for a ventilator. The patient should be taken to the postoperative area with the endotracheal tube in place. When the muscle relaxant wears off and reversal can be safely administered (at least one twitch on a train-of-four), extubation can occur. It may be necessary to administer small doses of a benzodiazepine while the endotracheal tube remains in place. Cucchiara, Miller, Reves, Roizen, et al. (1994) suggest that the anesthesia provider ask the following questions regarding reversal of nondepolarizing muscle relaxants:

1. Has enough time been allowed for the anticholinesterase to anatagonize the block, that is, at least 15 to 30 minutes?

2. Is the neuromuscular blockade too intense to be antagonized?

3. Has an adequate dose of antagonist been given?

4. Has the concentration of anesthetic vapor been reduced as much as possible?

5. Has the half-life of the relaxant been taken into consideration, especially if a long-acting drug has been given?

6. What is the acid–base and electrolyte status?

7. What is the temperature?

8. Is the patient receiving any drugs that may make antagonism difficult?

9. Has excretion (clearance) of the relaxant been reduced by a possibly unrecognized process?■

▶ CASE 11   Cataract Extraction

Age: 70   **DX:** cataract OD
Sex: male   **Proposed Operation:** cataract extraction with intraocular lens implant
Problems: HTN for 15 y, controlled with meds
                     NIDDM for 6 y, controlled with oral meds
                     smoker, 1 ppd for 15 y

PAST HISTORY

Allergies: sulfa, rash

Tobacco: positive 1 ppd × 15 y
Cardiovascular: positive HTN, negative CHF or MI
Respiratory: negative asthma, TB, or URI
GI: negative peptic ulcer or hiatal hernia

Bleeding Disorder: none
Previous Operations and Anesthetics: Right-eye surgery in El Salvador, local without complication

Medications: glyburide 5 mg each AM, benezepril 5 mg each day
Drug Use: occasional beer on the weekend

Endocrine: positive diabetes × 6 y
Neuro: negative CVA or seizures

LABORATORY

Hgb: 15   **Hct:** 43   **Glucose:** 117   **BUN:** 21   **CR:** 1.2
CXR: normal
ECG: right vent., hypertrophy, mult. PVCs and PACs

EXAMINATION

BP: 156/80   **P:** 86   **R:** 20   **T:** 36   **WT:** 67.8 kg   **HT:** 156 cm
Heart: S1–S2 with an irregular rate
Lungs: few rhonchi noted in right lower lobe
Airway: *Mouth opening:* adeq.   *Neck:* full range of motion   *Submental space:* >6.5 cm
            Uvula and pillars seen: Class II   *Teeth:* upper and lower dentures
NPO: advised, except for antihypertensive

---

1. **What are the types of anesthesia used for cataract surgery?**

The requirements for ophthalmic surgery include akinesia, analgesia, minimal bleeding, and no patient movement (coughing or retching). Usually, the anesthesia provider is positioned remote from the patient's airway, which will require astute monitoring. Most ophthalmic procedures may be performed in adults under either local or general anesthesia. The choice of technique reflects a balanced judgment of patient safety, cooperation, and surgical difficulty. When local anesthesia is chosen, the ophthalmologist will most likely administer the local or regional blockade. Although in some locales, the anesthesia provider administers the regional block. The anesthesia provider is present throughout the procedure to monitor the patient's vital signs, provide sedation, treat potential complications of local anesthesia, and induce general anesthesia if necessary. This is referred to as *monitored anesthesia care.* If the patient is cooperative and able to communicate, and the surgeon has no objection, local anesthesia should provide satisfactory conditions for most individuals. Patients who speak a foreign language, are deaf, have an involuntary tremor, have a history of anxiety or claustrophobia, are experiencing a cough, and/or are unable to lie flat, are poor candidates for local anesthesia. When general anesthesia is selected for cataract surgery, it is essential to maintain an adequate depth. Sudden movement or attempts to cough when the globe is open can result in extrusion of ocular contents and cause permanent damage. In addition, skeletal muscle paralysis or a "deep" anesthesia often is included to minimize the chance of unexpected movement. Modest hyperventilation of the lungs to produce hypocarbia and a 10-degree head-up tilt to promote venous drainage will help reduce intraocular pressure during surgery.

2.   Because a cataract procedure frequently is performed under regional anesthesia, what regional block techniques are performed?

Regional anesthesia for eye surgery may consist of retrobulbar block, facial nerve block, or peribulbar block. Retrobulbar block is a means of achieving akinesis of the globe. It involves injecting local anesthesia behind the eye into the muscle cone. The facial nerve block prevents squinting of the eyelids during surgery and allows placement of the lid speculum. Peribulbar block achieves akinesis of the globe and provides a large volume of injection so that it diffuses into the eyelids, making a lid block superfluous.

3.   What is the usual choice of local anesthetic?

The choice of local anesthetic varies, but lidocaine and bupivacaine are most common. Hyaluronidase, a hydrolyzer of connective tissue polysaccharides, is commonly added to enhance the retrobulbar spread of the local anesthetic.

4.   During the retrobulbar blockade, bradycardia and cardiac dysrhythmias occur. Is this expected or cause for alarm?

Oculocardiac reflex (OCR) manifests as bradycardia and occasionally as cardiac asystole. This response is elicited by pain, pressure on the globe, and by traction on the extraocular muscles, especially the medial rectus. The afferent pathway of the OCR involves the ciliary branch of the ophthalmic division of the trigeminal nerve. The efferent impulse arises in the brainstem and is carried by the vagus nerve. When it occurs, the OCR should be promptly treated by cessation of the stimulus. Occasionally atropine administration IV and local infiltration of lidocaine near the extrinsic eye muscles may be necessary.

5.   What other complications may occur from the administration of regional anesthesia?

Complications of retrobulbar injection of local anesthetics may be local or systemic and may result in blindness or even death. The most common complication is retrobulbar hemorrhage secondary to puncture of vessels within the retrobulbar space. Other complications include globe perforation, optic nerve atrophy, extrusion of intraocular contents, direct intravascular injection presenting as frank convulsions, and respiratory arrest. Forceful injection of local anesthetic causes retrograde flow toward the brain and may cause a gradual onset of unconsciousness and apnea. A facial nerve block may cause subcutaneous hemorrhage.

6.   What effect may the preoperative ophthalmic eye solutions have on the patient?

Ophthalmic eye solutions are used in the preoperative period to produce vasoconstriction and pupillary dilation or constriction. The solutions are absorbed from the lacrimal duct and may cause systemic effects, including tachycardia, bradycardia, hypertension, arrhythmias, angina, bronchoconstriction, or headaches. Occluding the nasolacrimal duct by pressing on the inner canthus of the eye for a few minutes after each instillation greatly decreases systemic absorption.

7.   How should sedation be administered?

The goal with sedation is to have a calm, cooperative, spontaneously breathing patient during the local administration by the ophthalmologist. Less-than-adequate sedation may cause tachycardia and hypertension, producing deleterious effects in patients with coronary artery disease. Deep sedation increases the risk of apnea and unintentional patient movement during the procedure. The particular drug chosen is less important than dosage. Many advocate the administration of methohexital or propofol IV immediately before ocular regional anesthesia, provided that no contraindication exists. These drugs should produce a brief state of relaxation and amnesia. Steps to reduce the likelihood of postoperative nausea and vomiting should be included in the anesthesia plan. An antiemetic avoidance of opioids in the preoperative/intraoperative period may decrease the incidence of nausea and vomiting.

8.   After the patient has been sedated, rocking movements on the chest and abdomen are observed. What may be the cause?

Airway obstruction may be revealed by snoring sounds, by failure of the reservoir bag to empty and fill with the respiratory cycle, and by "rocking" movements of the chest and abdomen. Rocking is seen when the chest retracts rather than expands as the diaphragm descends with inspiration. The anesthesia provider must initiate basic airway management techniques immediately. Perhaps the patient's jaw has relaxed and the tongue fallen backward, obstructing the glottis. Lifting the jaw forward and upward by exerting pressure behind the mandible and hyperextending the neck to carry the tongue forward and upward should solve the problem. Perhaps a nasopharyngeal or oropharyngeal airway will relieve the obstruction. Turning the head to a lateral position also has proved to be a good technique. If these do not resolve the problem, the case must progress to a general anesthetic because of the danger of oversedation and its untoward effect. The majority of cataract patients include the geriatric population and the risks of respiratory depression, airway obstruction, hypotension, and prolonged recovery time exist. Patients under conscious sedation must be capable of responding rationally to commands and be able to maintain airway patency. Avoid using the combination of local anesthesia with heavy sedation in the form of high doses of opioids, benzodiazepines, or hypnotics. Careful monitoring of drug administration and patient response should have prevented this airway obstruction. Monitoring includes ECG, blood pressure, precordial stethoscope, pulse oximeter, and observations of ventilations. Unfortunately, the anesthesia provider must distance him- or herself and the usual anesthetic apparatus from the surgical field when providing care for a patient undergoing cataract surgery. Eventually, the patient will be draped distanced from the anesthesia provider, making the airway inaccessible. Adequate ventilation near the face is essential for all patients to avoid carbon dioxide accumulation. Some individuals build a "tent" to provide air circulation. Supplemental oxygen via nasal cannula or face mask also is recommended. Remember that undue restlessness may be a sign of hypoxia or oversedation in the elderly.

9. What are the goals with this patient's glucose management?

Management of anesthesia for the diabetic patient undergoing elective surgery is intended to mimic normal metabolism. This includes avoiding hypoglycemia and preventing excessive hyperglycemia, ketoacidosis, and electrolyte disturbances. Because an oral hypoglycemic agent is being taken by the patient, it may be continued until the evening before surgery, but not on the day of surgery. Preadmission to the hospital is probably indicated only for the patient with poorly controlled IDDM. It is important that a blood glucose level be obtained the day of surgery. The anesthesia provider may choose to monitor this value every hour in the operating room. Values below 100 mg/dL and over 250 mg/dL are typically treated with additional glucose or exogenous insulin, respectively.

10. The postoperative nurse reports that the patient has had an increased blood pressure since arriving in the unit and asks how it should be treated?

Hypertension during the early postoperative period is not an unexpected response in the patient with preoperative hypertension. The development of postoperative hypertension warrants assessment of potential causes: pain, fluid overload, or inappropriate lapses of medication (the patient should not discontinue their antihypertensive medication dosage prior to surgery). Treatment should be implemented: opioids, hydralazine, nitroprusside, labetalol. The goal is to decrease the risks of myocardial ischemia, cardiac dysrhythmias, congestive heart failure, stroke, and bleeding.

11. What medication could have been administered in the preoperative area that treats hypertension and promotes sedation?

Clonidine is a centrally acting alpha$_2$-agonist that acts as an antihypertensive drug. Administered orally as a preoperative medication, the drug attenuates autonomic nervous system reflex responses, such as increases in blood pressure and heart rate associated with intraoperative stimulation. Anesthetic requirements also are reduced in patients treated with clonidine.■

▶ CASE 12   Septorhinoplasty

Age: 60   **DX:** trauma to the septum
Sex: female   **Proposed Operation:** septorhinoplasty
Problems: recent passenger in a car accident 1 wk ago, head hit dashboard during incident
                    anemic; Jehovah's Witness and refusing blood products

PAST HISTORY
Allergies: NKDA   **Medications:** multivitamins, iron
Tobacco: negative   **Drug Use:** none
Cardiovascular: negative

Respiratory: Difficult to take deep breaths since incident
GI: negative
Endocrine: negative
Neuro: no LOC with accident
Blood Products: refusing
Previous Operations and Anesthetics: appendectomy, GA; laparoscopy, ovarian cyst, GA; breast mass excision, MAC; no anesthetic complications

LABORATORY
Hgb: 9.4   **Hct:** 28.0   **SPO$_2$:** 99% room air   **BUN:** 8   **CR:** 0.6
CXR: normal, no broken ribs noted
ECG: sinus tachycardia

EXAMINATION
BP: 102/60   **P:** 103   **R:** 22   **T:** 37.6   **WT:** 55 kg   **HT:** 165 cm
Heart: RRR
Lungs: CTA but diminished, patient c/o pain with breathing, currently taking small, shallow breaths
Airway: *Mouth opening:* 3 FB   *Neck:* full range of motion   *Submental space:* >6.5 cm
              Uvula and pillars seen: Class II   *Teeth:* upper-right incisor broken, oral mucosa with noted tears and poor oral hygiene

---

1. How may the anesthesia for nasal surgery be performed?

Nasal surgery may be performed under either local anesthesia or general anesthesia. If general anesthesia is implemented, amnesia and toleration of the (RAE) endotracheal tube should be ensured. The painful stimuli of surgery are attenuated by administering local anesthesia, which is usually given under all anesthesia options. The surgeon will inject lidocaine with epinephrine and place cocaine nasal packs for vasoconstrictive effect.

2. An increase in the heart rate and blood pressure after the surgeon has prepared the nares is observed. What may be the cause?

Cocaine, the local anesthetic used by the surgeon to prepare the nares, has sympathomimetic effects by blocking the synaptic reuptake of norepinephrine. The effects of cocaine and epinephrine together may cause tachycardia, and/or hypertension. If it becomes necessary, these reactions may be attenuated with a beta-blocker, propanolol or esmolol.

3. What are the philosophies of a Jehovah's Witness regarding transfusional therapies?

The philosophy of a Jehovah's Witness regarding transfusional therapies must be discussed completely before entering the operating room. It is an individualized decision that needs clarification. Mann (1992) states that generally accepted blood substitute products include: crystalloids (Ringer's lactate, normal saline, hypertonic saline); colloids (dextran, gelatin, hetastarch); perfluorochemicals; and erythropoietin. Generally not accepted are whole blood and its components: packed red blood cells, leukocytes, platelets, plasma, albumin, and autotransfusion of blood or blood components.

4. What are the most effective methods to manage the Jehovah's Witness who is anemic?

The most effective ways to manage the Jehovah's Witness who is anemic is to minimize blood loss by reducing iatrogenic loss (microchemistry analyzers, pediatric-size blood samples, analyze the necessity of tests); reduce hemorrhagic loss (hemodilution, red cell scavenging devices, hypotensive anesthesia, desmopressin, progesterone); maximize blood production (erythropoietin, intravenous iron dextran, nutritional support); maximize cardiac output (volume expansion, hemodilution); and decrease metabolic rate (hypothermia, sedation, and paralysis).

5. Because the patient is a Jehovah's Witness and refuses blood products, the surgeon requests that the anesthesia provider help decrease blood loss, even though he is expecting the amount to be small. What might be one of the first anesthesia techniques implemented?

To assist with minimizing surgical blood loss and increase wound visualization, controlled hypotension may be instituted. This is elective lowering of the patient's arterial blood pressure.

6.   How is controlled hypotension accomplished?

Methods to electively lower blood pressure include the administration of hypotensive drugs and/or proper patient positioning. In the presence of adequate anesthesia, as provided by volatile anesthetics, the addition of pharmacologic agents will effectively lower blood pressure. Nitroprusside is administered as a continuous intravenous infusion using a pump. The dose is slowly titrated to produce hypotension. Seldom is more than 3 to 5 μg/kg/min necessary. The effect of nitroprusside is easily reversed by slowing or discontinuing the drug infusion. Nitroprusside is converted to cyanide, and arterial pH should be monitored to detect metabolic acidosis related to cyanide toxicity. Alternative drugs include nitroglycerin, hydralazine, and trimethaphan. Vasodilators decrease BP by dose-related direct effects on vascular smooth muscle, independent of alpha- or beta-receptors. These drugs often evoke baroreceptor-mediated increases in heart rate. One can offset this reflex tachycardia by administering a beta-antagonist: propanolol or esmolol. Positioning involves elevation of the surgical site so that blood pressure at the wound is selectively reduced.

7.   Are there any complications with using a controlled hypotension technique?

Complications of controlled hypotension include cerebral thrombosis, hemiplegia, acute tubular necrosis, hepatic necrosis, myocardial infarction, and cardiac arrest. Miller (1994) states that healthy individuals tolerate mean arterial pressures as low as 50 to 60 mmHg. However, hypertensive patients have altered autoregulation of cerebral blood flow and should not have their mean arterial blood pressure lowered more than 50 mmHg below their normal pressure. Intraarterial blood pressure monitoring is strongly recommended.

8.   Are there any contraindications to controlled hypotension?

Contraindications of controlled hypotension include severe anemia, cerebrovascular disease, hypovolemia, atherosclerotic vascular disease, and renal or hepatic insufficiency.

9.   What actions might prevent gastric aspiration of blood and decrease postoperative vomiting?

Blood loss during nasal surgery may be difficult to estimate because blood drains into the pharynx or esophagus posteriorly. A pharyngeal pack helps prevent gastric aspiration of blood and decreases postoperative nausea and vomiting. The stomach may be emptied with an oral gastric tube if the surgeon declines using a throat pack. The administration of an antiemetic may reduce the incidence of vomiting.

10.   As emergence is initiated, the patient begins "bucking" and straining on the endotracheal tube. How can this be prevented?

"Bucking" and straining on the endotracheal tube may be reduced with the administration of lidocaine (1–1.5 mg/kg). The patient may be straining on the endotracheal tube because of discomfort from the stimulus. One may desire to remove that stimulus. However, before removing the endotracheal tube, inspect the nares and mouth for active bleeding, blood clots, and debris. Carefully suction the oral cavity and nasopharynx to prevent dislodging and slow oozing of blood and secretions, which can result in a laryngospasm after extubation of the trachea. After breathing 100% oxygen, the patient should be extubated awake when protective reflexes are intact. If following nasal surgery the nose is unstable and face mask application is difficult, humidified oxygen could be administered by a Venturi mask.

11.   During the postoperative visit, the patient complained of bilateral swelling of her neck. There was an associated pain aggravated by touch and movement. The patient stated that she could not feel her ears. There was no rash, hives, fever, or difficulty with breathing. Is this expected after sinus surgery?

The complaint of bilateral neck swelling, with associated pain aggravated by touch and movement of the neck, is not normal after sinus surgery. There is no reason why the patient should not feel her ears. These complaints need to be investigated further. A consultation by phone can be performed to the attending surgeon or an ENT specialist.

12.   What is acute parotitis, and what are the factors that may predispose to the development of this etiology?

Upon further investigation, it is determined that the patient has acute postoperative parotitis. The parotid gland is located anterior and inferior to the external ear, on the posterior surface of the masseter muscle. It is composed of a superficial and deep lobe. Each parotid gland drains into a Stensen's duct that crosses the masseter muscle, pierces the buccinator muscle, and empties into the vestibule opposite the second upper molar tooth. The inflammatory parotid gland disorders are categorized as suppurative or nonsuppurative. Suppurative disorders result from a bacterial infection of the gland. It is believed that oral microorganisms ascend in a retrograde manner up the Stensen's duct. Signs and symptoms involve facial pain accompanied by fever, headache, malaise, and leukocytosis. Edema may tend to the periorbital area and cheeks. Nonsuppurative disorders result from obstruction of the duct with mucous plugs and secretions. Recurrent obstruction can lead to chronic inflammation of the gland and permanent fibrous enlargement. Signs and symptoms include complaints of a dry mouth and pain that resolves spontaneously over several hours following oral rehydration. According to Rubin and Cozzi (1986), factors that may predispose to the development of acute postoperative parotitis include dehydration, malnutrition, vomiting; poor oral hygiene; the suppression of oral secretions by the restrictions of fluid or administration of diuretics; middle age or older; and being African American.

13.   What anesthesia factors play a role in transient postoperative swelling of the salivary glands?

Reilly (1970) found anesthesia factors that play a role in transient postoperative swelling of the salivary glands, including inhalation of unhumidified gases; use of medication with antisialagogue properties; use of depolarizing neuromuscular blocking drugs; use of succinylcholine; and straining and coughing on the endotracheal tube or the Valsalva maneuver.

14.   What is the treatment for parotitis?

Treatment for acute postoperative parotitis is symptomatic according to Orser (1990). This usually resolves spontaneously within several days. It may be difficult for the patient to swallow, so a bland diet of custards, nonfruit gelatin, and ice cream is recommended. It is highly suggested that the patient increase his oral and parenteral intake. Analgesics may be given for pain. If suppurative parotitis is suspected, then smears and cultures should be obtained from material milked from the Stensen's duct. Initiation of antimicrobial therapy with type-specific antibiotics is essential.■

► CASE 13   Thyroidectomy

Age: 35   **DX:** hyperthyroidism
Sex: female   **Proposed Operation:** thyroidectomy
Problems: hyperthyroid; under medical management × 2 mo
                   exercise- and anxiety-induced asthma

PAST HISTORY
Allergies: iodine dye, rash and SOB

Tobacco: none
Cardiovascular: negative HTN, CHE, or MI
Respiratory: positive asthma: exercise and anxiety induced, last episode 7 mo ago
GI: negative

Bleeding Disorder: none
Previous Operations and Anesthetics: D&C 5 y ago, ? anesth., but no c/o

Medications: albuterol PRN, propanolol, propylthiouracil, methimazole
Drug Use: none

Endocrine: negative
Neuro: generalized muscle weakness × 3 mo

LABORATORY
Hgb: 13   **Hct:** 40.1   **T3:** 70   **T4:** 5.2   **TSH:** 5.0   **HCG:** negative   **SPO$_2$:** 99% room air
CXR: hyperinflated lung
ECG: sinus rhythm

EXAMINATION
BP: 133/84   **P:** 72   **R:** 24   **T:** 37.0   **WT:** 49 kg   **HT:** 170 cm
Heart: S1–S2 without deficit
Lungs: BBS CTA
Airway: *Mouth opening:* 3 FB   *Neck:* full range of motion   *Submental space:* >6.5 cm
          Uvula and pillars seen: Class I   *Teeth:* intact

1. What is the anesthesia goal when working with thyroid surgical procedures?

All elective surgical thyroid procedures should be postponed until the patient is rendered euthyroid. Preoperative assessment includes evaluation of thryroid function tests, which should be within normal range. An evaluation of the cardiovascular system should reveal a resting heart rate of less than 90 beats/minutes. Antithyroid medications and beta-adrenergic antagonists are continued through the morning of surgery. Once the goal of a euthyroid state has been achieved, and provided vital organs have not been damaged, choice of anesthetics is influenced minimally by the history of endocrine pathology.

2. What might the medical management of this patient consist of?

Medical management for a hyperfunctioning thyroid consists of beta-blockers, iodide, methimazole, and propylthiouracil. Beta-blockade alleviates symptoms of excessive sympathetic nervous system activity, such as tachycardia and anxiety. Iodide inhibits the synthesis and release of thyroid hormones. The traditional antithyroid medications methimazole and propylthiouracil inhibit hormone synthesis and later inhibit peripheral conversion of T4 to T3. However, both will require several weeks to optimize a preoperative regimen. Medical management also must be performed with the asthma history. Dawson and Simon (1984) states that hyperthyroidism can increase the severity of asthma. Our patient has a history of exercise-induced asthma. This population has bronchoconstriction with activity. Symptoms are short-lived, self-limiting, and totally reversible. It is felt that the asthma may be related to transmucosal temperature gradients associated with inhaling cold, dry air. Preoperatively, the absence of wheezing during breathing and a total blood eosinophil count below 50 mm suggests that the patient is not experiencing an acute exacerbation of bronchial asthma. Bronchodilator drugs should be continued until the morning of surgery. Supplementation with cortisol may be indicated before surgery if adrenal cortex suppression from corticosteroids is used to treat the asthma, which is not the case with this patient. Evaluate the chest x-ray. A hyperinflated lung with downward displacement of the diaphragm may be seen because of increased lung volume and alveolar pressure during expiration. The ECG usually is normal, showing changes during an attack. Sinus tachycardia may be noted, as may right ventricular strain and right-axis deviation. If this patient had a severe history of asthma, Cherniack (1988) recommends pulmonary function tests be performed before and after bronchodilator treatment. This test assesses the degree of ventilatory impairment and the reversibility of any bronchospastic component. One would expect to see an increase in residual volume (RV), functional residual capacity (FRC), and total lung capacity (TLC) if the patient has a history of asthma because there is an increased volume of trapped gas beyond closed airways and a decreased ability of the lung to deflate secondary to long-standing airway obstruction. If the FEV_1 is less than 70 to 80, the patient should be treated with bronchodilators.

3. What specific airway evaluation needs to be performed?

It is important to perform a thorough airway evaluation. If the patient presents with a large goiter, there may be tracheal shift; a chest x-ray would help confirm or invalidate the diagnosis. It also is useful to evaluate baseline vocal cord function in the early preoperative period by assessing the patient's ability to say the letter *E*.

4. What are some concerns with preoperative medications and this patient?

Because this patient has a history of asthma, anticholinergics in the preoperative area must be administered with caution. These drugs can decrease airway resistance and increase the viscosity of secretions, which should be avoided. The drug also can cause an increase in heart rate, which is undesirable with hyperthyroidism. The administration of H_2-antagonists is debatable because antagonism of H_2-mediated bronchodilation could unmask histamine-mediated H_1-receptor bronchoconstriction.

5. What are your anesthesia plans for induction and management of the case?

Plans for induction should include adequate anesthesia depth before laryngoscopy and surgical stimulation. The goal is to avoid tachycardia, hypertension, and dysrhythmias. Induction of anesthesia can be accomplished with intravenous administration of thiopental. The chemical structure of thiopental is similar to that of antithyroid drugs, but it is unlikely that a significant antithyroid effect is produced by an induction dose of thiopental. Avoid stimulating the sympathetic nervous system, which may cause an exaggerated elevation in heart rate and blood pressure. Ketamine, pancuronium, and indirect-acting adrenergic agonist are examples of medications to avoid. In view of the increased oxygen consumption of hyperthyroid patients, it would seem appropriate to limit the inhaled concentration of nitrous oxide to 50%. If the patient has an elevation in body temperature, one may need to increase anesthetic requirements by 5% for every degree of body temperature that exceeds 37°C. Constant monitoring of body temperature is important, as are means of lowering the body temperature, should that become necessary. The patient's eyes should be well protected because the exophthalmos of Graves' disease increases the risk of corneal abrasions. Muscle relaxants must be administered carefully and responses monitored with a peripheral nerve stimulator as the patient may present with skeletal muscle weakness. When it is time to reverse the nondepolarizing muscle relaxant blockade, it might be better to combine glycopyrrolate rather than atropine with anticholinesterases to minimize potential excessive increases in heart rate.

6. After the intubation is performed, wheezing is noted with auscultation and high peak airway pressures. What might be happening?

After intubation, wheezing is noted upon auscultation and high peak airway pressures are observed. It is imperative that the anesthesia provider have a methodical system of determining the cause of the problem. Reauscultate the lung sounds. Is ventilation occuring only in the right lung? If so, slowly remove the endotracheal tube from the right mainstem bronchus. If bilateral wheezing is noted, consider other potential causes. Delay medical treatment until mechanical obstruction of the breathing circuit and the patient's airway are evaluated. This includes kinking, secretions, or overinflation of the cuff. Next, ask whether there is inadequate depth of anesthesia, as noted by active expiratory efforts or decreased functional residual capacity? It may be time to deepen the anesthesia with a volatile anesthetic. If a bronchospasm is occurring, keep in mind that it will respond to deepening of anesthesia, but not to skeletal muscle paralysis. Finally, begin medical treatment. Administer 100% oxygen until the problem is resolved. Consideration should be given administering a bronchodilator drug, beta$_2$-agonist, theophylline, and/or an anticholinergic. Albuterol may be delivered into the patient's airway by attaching the metered dose inhaler to the anesthesia delivery system. Sympathomimetics basically cause an increase in cyclic 3′-5′-adenosine monophosphate (cAMP), which produces bronchodilation. They inhibit the release of mediators, improve mucociliary transport, and inhibit vascular permeability. Terbutaline 0.25 mg may be administered SC. This dosage may be repeated once again in 15 to 30 minutes if necessary. A theophylline bolus (5 mg/kg over 15 minutes) followed by a continuous drip (0.5–1 mg/kg) may be instituted. The dosage should be calculated on lean body weight as theophylline does not distribute to body fat. The goal is to obtain a serum level of 10 to 20 μg/mL. Theophylline inhibits the enzyme phosphodiesterase, which then decreases the degradation of cAMP. Beware, you may notice an increase in arrhythmias. Some practitioners also would consider administering a corticosteroid, hydrocortisone 1 to 3 mg/kg and methyprenisolone 0.5 to 1 mg/kg. In addition to mem-

brane-stabilizing actions that may reduce the release of vasoactive substances (histamine) from mast cells, it has antiinflammatory effects. Cromolyn (2 mg) is a membrane stabilizer that prevents degranulation of mast cells and the subsequent release of vasoactive substances responsible for bronchoconstriction. This drug is effective only for prophylaxis and is of no value in managing acute exacerbations.

7. What is the most serious threat to the hyperthyroid patient in the postoperative period? Describe the signs and symptoms and expected onset.

The most serious threat to the hyperthyroid patient in the postoperative period is a thyroid storm. Bonner (1989) and Stoelting and Dierdorf (1993) state that this can occur intraoperatively, but it is most likely to manifest in the first 6 to 18 hours after surgery. Symptoms are due to the sudden and excessive release of thyroid gland hormones. The signs and symptoms are hyperpyrexia, tachycardia, altered consciousness, hypotension, dehydration, and shock. Some of these tend to mimic malignant hyperthermia. However, it is not associated with muscle rigidity, elevated creatine kinase, or a marked degree of lactic and respiratory acidosis, as are seen with malignant hyperthermia. Treatment of thyroid storm includes cooling, hydration with cold solutions (some of which contain glucose), and administration of drugs to treat specific manifestations of excessive thyroid gland hormone concentrations. According to Burman (1990), intravenous propanolol (0.5-mg increments until the heart rate is less than 100/min) is necessary to alleviate the peripheral effects of thyroid gland hormones on the cardiovascular system. Schwartz, Rosenbaum, and Graf (1997) state that propylthiouracil (250 mg every 6 hours by nasogastric tube or orally) and sodium iodide (1 g intravenously over 12 hours) are effective in acutely reducing the release of active hormones from the thyroid gland. Dobyns (1978) suggests cortisol (100–200 mg every 8 hours), as indicated to offset the increased endogenous use of corticosteroids that could result in acute primary adrenal insufficiency. Thyroid storm is considered a medical emergency, so call for assistance and treat aggressively.

8. What other postoperative complications exist specific to a thyroidectomy?

Other postoperative complications associated with a thyroidectomy are recurrent laryngeal nerve palsy, hematoma, hypoparathyroidism, and pneumothorax.

1. *Recurrent laryngeal nerve palsy.* Results in unilateral hoarseness or bilateral aphonia (inability to say *E*) and paralyzed vocal cords that can flap together during inspiration to produce airway

obstruction (stridor). Vocal cord functioning may be evaluated by laryngoscopy immediately after a deep extubation. Failure of cord movement requires reintubation and wound exploration.

2. *Hematoma.* Compression of the trachea leading to airway obstruction may reflect a hematoma at the operative site or tracheomalacia due to weakening of the tracheal rings by chronic pressure from a goiter. Immediate treatment includes opening the neck wound and evacuating the clot, as well as reassessing the need for reintubation.

3. *Hypoparathyroidism.* Hypoparathyroidism may occur because of inadvertent removal of the parathyroid glands. Stoelting and Dierdorf (1993) state that this can manifest as early as 1 to 3 hours after surgery, but most likely will not appear until 24 to 72 hours according to Graf and Rosenbaum (1992). Hypocalcemia signs will be revealed. Laryngeal muscles are sensitive to hypocalcemia, and inspiratory stridor leading to laryngospasm may be the first sign. Other manifestations include paresthesias; carpopedal spasm (Trousseau's sign) masseter spasm; (Chvostek's sign) and cardiac irritability (prolonged Q–T interval on the ECG).

4. *Pneumothorax.* A pneumothorax is a possibility with any neck exploration.

9. What medication should be avoided when treating postoperative pain in this patient?

For complaints of postoperative pain Stoelting and Dierdorf (1993) suggest avoiding administering aspirin and nonsteroidals. There is an increased sensitivity when asthmatics take these products. Aspirin blocks cyclooxygenase, but allows production of leukotrienes, which can cause bronchonconstriction.■

► CASE 14 Hip Repair

Age: 71   **DX:** fractured right hip
Sex: female   **Proposed Operation:** open reduction and internal fixation of subtrochanteric fracture of the femur
Problems: HTN × 15 y
                   PVD × 5 y
                   diabetic × 15 y
                   smoker

PAST HISTORY
Allergies: NKDA

Tobacco: positive smoker × 50 y,
  quit for 3 mo
Cardiovascular: positive HTN × 15 y,
  positive PVD × 5 y
Respiratory: positive chronic cough in AM
GI: negative PUD or hiatal hernia
Endocrine: positive diabetic × 15 y
Neuro: negative
Bleeding Disorder: none
Previous Operations and Anesthetics: hysterectomy 23 y ago; right-leg bypass 2 y ago; both procedures
  under GA without problems

Medications: baby aspirin, mefedipine, Micronase®, docusate
  sodium
Drug Use: none

LABORATORY
Hgb: 9.9   **Hct:** 30.4   **SPO₂:** 98%
CXR: unable to locate
ECG: NSR, LAH

EXAMINATION
BP: 150–180/80–90   **P:** 78   **R:** 24   **T:** 37.4   **WT:** 80 kg   **HT:** 163 cm
Heart: RRR
Lungs: bilateral crackles in bases, cleared with coughing
Airway: *Mouth opening:* 3 FB   *Neck:* decreased movement to the right   *Submental space:* >6.5 cm
          Uvula and pillars seen: Class II   *Teeth:* upper dentures, lower
                                                                                                    with mult. missing teeth

1. What are the anesthesia options for the surgical procedure?

Hip fractures are common in the elderly. Regional (spinal or epidural) to level T8 or a general anesthetic may be implemented. Blood loss and thromboembolism may occur less frequently with regional anesthesia because of peripheral vasodilation and maintenance of venous blood flow in the lower extremities. Local anesthetics also inhibit platelet aggregation and stabilize endothelial cells. Cardiovascular changes are usually are limited to a fall in arterial blood pressure as sympathetic blockade is obtained. This reduction in blood pressure can be minimized with prophylactic fluid loading if there is no contraindication, such as congestive heart failure (CHF). A vasopressor within easy access also might be suggested. If administering a general anesthetic, IV induction agents must be given slowly as the elderly population has a slow blood circulation time (decreased cardiac output). The onset of action will be delayed, so do not get impatient and administer large doses of drugs. There is a decrease in esophageal and intestinal motility that results in delayed gastric emptying. Elderly patients are, therefore, at increased risk for pulmonary aspiration. However, this does not mandate all elderly patients to receive a rapid sequence induction (RSI). A slow induction with firm cricoid pressure during mask ventilation to prevent cardiovascular compromise may be indicated. Initial hypotension may be replaced by hypertension and tachycardia during laryngoscopy and intubation. As with anesthetic drugs, the doses of muscle relaxants probably should be decreased because of the reduced skeletal muscle mass and altered renal clearance mechanisms that are likely to accompany aging.

2. How will the induction be performed since the patient has chosen to have a general anesthetic?

The position chosen to facilitate surgical access is not always easy to obtain. It is common to find a "fracture table" in the operating room versus the normal type seen. The patient will most likely present in pain preoperatively and be in traction. Therefore, anesthetizing this patient in bed before positioning her on the table will be necessary, as she has chosen to have a general anesthetic. This places an additional burden on the anesthesia provider to ensure safety for the unconscious and paralyzed patient during the bed-to-operating room (OR) table transfer. The goal is to provide optimal exposure without circulation or ventilation compromise. It is important that no pressure points be allowed throughout the procedure and at the end of the case when the patient is transferred on to the bed from the OR table prior to emergence.

3. What lead on the ECG monitor should be placed on the patient?

The ECG is the only practical way to monitor the balance between myocardial oxygen requirements and myocardial oxygen delivery in an unconscious patient. When this balance is altered, myocardial ischemia occurs as seen on the ECG by at least 1 mm downsloping of the ST segment from baseline. A precordial V5 lead is useful for detecting ST segment changes of the left ventricle in the elderly population.

4. What additional protection in the OR should be available during orthopedic procedures?

Additional protection from radiation should be available for the anesthesia provider who works in an orthopedic case as x-rays and fluoroscopy are frequently needed. The anesthesia provider should obtain a standard lead apron and be positioned as far away from the axial beam as possible and turn away during exposure time to minimize exposure to radiation.

5. Why are orthopedic procedures performed with laminar flow?

Laminar flow ventilation removes airborne particles with filters and increases air movement at the operative site. Infection can be disastrous for an orthopedic patient, and this is one of the prevention techniques. Laminar flow provides up to 500 air exchanges per hour as opposed to 12 to 15 exchanges in the ordinary OR. However, the increased air flow at the operative site promotes drying of the operative field and increases patient cooling. Other infection-control methods include meticulous skin preparation of the patient, multilayered draping, covering of the head and neck of personnel, and limiting traffic flow in and out of the OR.

6. Why is methylmethacrylate administered?

Methylmethacrylate is an acrylic bone cement used in hip replacement operations to provide a tight fit and fixation of the prosthesis. During the preparation of the substance, an odor may be noted in the room. It is nontoxic, but offensive. Hardening occurs in a few minutes and is accompanied by release of heat.

7. What are the anesthetic implications when methylmethacrylate cement is used?

The insertion of methylmethacrylate has been associated with sudden episodes of hypotension related to the vasodilating effects of the absorbed monomer. Hypotension effects may occur within 30 to 60 seconds after insertion of the cement, usually terminating spontaneously according to Purdman (1997). Plan ahead when the smell is first noted in the OR and problems can be avoided. Determine the level of volume in the patient's vasculature. If the vessels are constricted because of hypovolemia, sudden vasodilation will result in a decrease in arterial blood pressure. Perhaps it is necessary to administer a fluid bolus. Some practitioners remove the patient from nitrous oxide and decrease the amount of vasodilating inhalation agent prior to the application. It may be wise to have vasopressor drugs, neo-synephrine or ephedrine, availabe to treat potential hypotension.

8.   What are alternative strategies for managing of blood loss during surgery?

Orthopedic procedures may be quite bloody. Deliberate hypotension is a means of reducing surgical blood loss when the benefits outweigh the risks. Despite the efforts to reduce bleeding, it may become necessary to administer blood products. Meticulous attention to blood loss must be paid by monitoring sponges, suction bottle contents, and estimated blood loss (EBL) on the drapes. The aim of fluid therapy is to maintain adequate amounts of hemoglobin and normal circulating blood volume. Alternative strategies for blood loss management during surgery include autologous transfusions, blood salvage and reinfusion, hemodilution, donor-directed transfusions, and plasma volume expanders.

1. *Autologous transfusions.* These involve patients donating their own blood. Collection usually starts a few weeks prior to the operation and are ended 72 hours before surgery to permit restoration of plasma volume. This approach eliminates the chances of hemolytic reactions or transmission of viral disease.
2. *Blood salvage and reinfusion.* Blood salvage and reinfusion involves collecting shed blood intraoperatively together with an anticoagulant, usually heparin. The red blood cells (RBC) are concentrated and washed to remove debris and anticoagulant and then reinfused into the patient. The technique requires blood losses greater than 500 to 1000 mL to be effective.
3. *Hemodilution.* Blood is removed from the patient before the procedure, replaced with crystalloids or albumin solutions, and reinfused at the end of the operation. The concept is that, if the concentration of RBC is decreased, total red cell loss is reduced when large amounts of blood are shed.
4. *Donor-related transfusions.* Donor-related transfusions involve donated blood from ABO-compatible family or friends.
5. *Plasma volume expanders.* Plasma volume expanders includes dextran, hetastarch (20 mL/kg), albumin and crystalloids (3–4 mL for every 1 mL of EBL).

9.   It is necessary to administer packed red blood cells (PRBC) intraoperatively. What are some basic principles of transfusion?

Administering PRBC is facilitated by reconstituting them in isotonic saline or plasma. Stored blood should always be administered through micron filters. Use of hypotonic glucose solutions may cause hemolysis, hypertonic solutions will cause dehydration and crenation of red blood cells, and lactated Ringer's may cause clotting because of the calcium. One may choose to administer the blood product through a warmer to prevent hypothermia.

10.   If this were an emergency, how would the patient be crossmatched for transfusion? What type of blood products are acceptable?

If the patient were in an emergency situation and the need to transfuse arose prior to completion of a crossmatch, screen, or even blood typing, the patient should be given O Rh-negative blood. Packed red blood cells should be used instead of whole blood to minimize the transfer of antibodies. Once type O Rh-negative whole blood is used, further transfusions should be type O Rh-negative until anti-A and anti-B titers are determined in the patient's serum.

11.   What types of reactions may occur with the administration of blood products?

Complications of blood therapy must be considered when administering such treatment. Reactions are categorized as febrile (most common), allergic, and hemolytic. Febrile nonhemolytic reactions may be caused by an interaction between the recipient's antibodies and antigens present on the leukocytes and/or platelets of the donor. Treatment involves slowing the infusion and administering antipyretics. Allergic reactions may be revealed as increased temperatures, pruritus, and urticaria. Treatment begins with administration of antihistamines and slowing down the rate of infusion. Hemolytic reactions occur when the wrong blood type (ABO-incompatible) is administered. Naturally acquired antibodies can react against the foreign antigens, activate complement, and result in intravascular hemolysis. Signs include hypotension, lumbar pain, fever, chills, dyspnea, skin flushing, and free hemoglobin in the plasma or urine. Unfortunately, many of these clinical signs are masked by anesthesia. Intraoperatively, an increase in temperature with a change in vital signs and urine color may indicate a reaction. Treatment consists of immediately discontinuing the infusion and preventing renal failure by administering crystalloids, mannitol, and/or furosemide.

12. What happens to components in stored blood?

Once blood is collected, a preservative anticoagulant solution is added. CPD-A is the most common. It contains citrate, phosphate, dextrose, and adenine. Citrate is an anticoagulant by binding calcium. Phosphate is a buffer. Dextrose is a red cell energy source, and adenine is a precurser for adenosine triphosphate (ATP) synthesis. Over time, changes occur with stored blood. The pH falls. There is excess free potassium, which only increases with time. There is a decrease in 2,3-DPG levels that results in decreased tissue oxygen delivery. Citrate may metabolize to bicarbonate and contribute to metabolic alkalosis, whereas the binding of calcium by citrate could result in hypocalcemia. Eventually, one will find a decrease in ATP and an increase in lactate levels.

13. The patient requests that the anesthesia provider review possible infections spread through blood products. What are they?

Possible infections spread through blood products include, hepatitis; acquired immune deficiency syndrome; viral infections such as cytomegalovirus and Epstein-Barr virus; and parasites, including malaria, toxoplasmosis, and bacteria.

14. During the procedure, tachycardia, a decreased end-tidal carbon dioxide pressure, and arterial hypoxemia are noted. What may be the cause, and how should this problem be treated?

If the patient presents with tachycardia, a decreased end-tidal carbon dioxide pressure, and arterial hypox-

emia during an orthopedic procedure, you will want to rule out a fat embolus. Morgan and Mikhail (1996) report that a triad of dyspnea, petechiae, and mental confusion has been noted in some of these patients in the preoperative area. It should be suspected with individuals who have long-bone fractures. During portions of the surgical procedure, especially with reaming, physicians may mobilize marrow fat from the bone cavity, causing the aforementioned signs and symptoms. Fat droplets can embolize to pulmonary capillaries and mechanically obstruct blood flow. Lipases then degrade the neutral triglyceride emboli and release free fatty acids that are toxic to the lung. Treatment for fat emboli is supportive. The goal is to maintain adequate tissue perfusion to promote normal lipid metabolism and reduce the likelihood that a coagulopathy will develop. Immediately, place the patient on 100% oxygen, intubate (if not done already), and consider the addition of positive end-expiratory pressure. Start to hydrate the patient and begin ACLS protocol. It most likely will be necessary to abort the surgical procedure.■

SUMMARY

Case analysis is a challenge to the nurse anesthetist. Critical case analysis enables the nurse anesthetist to synthesize knowledge from a variety of resources and to apply them to clinical scenarios encountered in clinical practice. This chapter has focused on applying assessment and management skills in a variety of clinical situations to prepare the student for clinical practice or hone the skills of the experienced practitioner.

▶ KEY CONCEPTS

- Each case must be approached individually and require the anesthetist to synthesize information from a variety of resources to prepare the anesthetic plan.
- A thorough history must be conducted on all patients to elicit information critical to the anesthetic plan. This may include discussion with one or more family members.
- Objective and diagnostic data must be evaluated for each case before initiating the anesthetic.

- Critical thinking is essential to evaluate and solve problems that arise in the course of anesthetic management.
- The nurse anesthetist must be ready to treat complications as they arise by thoroughly preparing for each anesthetic and anticipating any problems that occur before initiating the anesthetic.

▶ STUDY QUESTIONS

1. As the anesthesia provider, how do you assimilate information from a patient's chart and history and physical exam to develop an anesthesia plan?

2. How many safe methods to administer anesthesia might there be for any given surgical case?

3. If challenged by another health care provider, how would you articulate why an anesthesia plan was chosen?

4. When preparing the anesthesia setup for a scheduled local with sedation case, how should you prepare to convert the anesthesia technique to a general anesthetic at any time?

5. If an adverse, unforeseen event were to occur in the operating room, what steps should be taken quickly to identify and implement proper treatment?

REFERENCES

Arnett, F. C. (1992). Rheumatoid arthritis. In J. B. Wyngaarden, L. H. Smith, & J. C. Bennett (Eds.), *Cecil textbook of medicine* (19th ed., pp. 1508–1515). Philadelphia: Saunders.

Bonner, S. (1989). The patient for thyroidectomy. *Middle Eastern Journal of Anesthesiology, 10,* 47–57.

Burman, K. D. (1990). Hyperthyroidism. In K. L. Becker, J. Bilezikian, & W. Bremner (Eds.), *Principles and practice of endocrinology and metabolism* (pp. 331–347). Philadelphia: Lippincott.

Changigian, R. (1994). Molar pregnancy. In D. Chestnut (Ed.), *Obstetric anesthesia principles and practice* (pp. 268–269). St Louis, MO: Mosby-Year Book.

Cherniack, R. M. (1988). Pulmonary function testing. In R. S. Mitchell , T. L. Pety, & M. Schwartz (Eds.), *Synopsis of clinical pulmonary diseases* (4th ed.). St. Louis, MO: Mosby-Year Book.

Crysdale, W. D., & Russel, D. (1986). Complications of tonsillectomy and adenoidectomy in 9409 children observed overnight. *Canadian Medical Association Journal,* 1139.

Dawson, A., & Simon, R. (1984). *The practical management of asthma* (pamphlet). FL: Grune & Stratton.

Desmond J. (1970). Serum osmolality and plasma electrolytes in patients who develop dilutional hyponatremia during transurethral resection. *Canadian Journal of Surgery, 13,* 116–121.

Dobyns, B. M., (1978). Prevention and management of hyperthyroid storm. *World Journal of Surgery, 2,* 293–306.

Emnet, J., Gilbough, J. H., & McLean, P. (1969). Fluid absorption during transurethral resection: Comparison of mortality and morbidity after irrigation with water and non-hemolytic solutions. *Journal of Urology, 101,* 884.

Forrester, K. (1986). Anesthetic implications in sickle cell anemia. *AANA Journal, 54,* 19–24.

Gefke, K., Andersen, L.W., & Friese, E. (1983). Lidocaine given intravenously as a suppressant of cough and laryngospasm after tonsillectomy. *Acta Anesthesiologica Scandinavica, 27,* 1211.

Gilman, G., Rall, T., Nies, A. & Taylor, P. (1990). *Goodman and Gilmans' The pharmacological basis of therapeutics* (9th ed., pp. 939–942). New York: Pergamon.

Hagstrom, R. S., Dennise, S. A., & Rowland, H. S. (1955). Studies on fluid absorption during transurethral prostatic resection. *Journal of Urology, 73,* 852.

Hall, J. B. (1986). The cardiopulmonary failure of sleep-disoriented breathing. *Journal of the American Medical Association, 255,* 930.

Henderson, D. J., & Middleton, R. G. (1980). Coma from hyponatremia following transurethral resection of the prostate. *Urology, 15,* 267.

Joseph, M. M. (1998). Anesthesia for ear, nose, and throat surgery. In D. E. Longnecker, J. H. Tinker, & G. E. Morgan, Jr. (Eds.), *Principles and practice of anesthesiology* (2nd ed., pp. 2208–2209). St. Louis, MO: Mosby-Year Book.

Klinenberg, J. R. (1992). Rheumatoid arthritis. In J. R. Hurst (Ed.), *Medicine for the practicing physician* (3rd ed., pp. 189–193). Boston: Butterworth-Heinemann.

Mann, M. C. (1992) Management of the severely anemic patient who refuses transfusion: Lessons learned during the care of a Jehovah's Witness. *Annals of Internal Medicine, 12,* 1042–1048.

McGoldrick, K. (1997). Anesthesia and the eye. In P. G. Barash, B. F. Cullen, & R. K. Stoelting (Eds.). (2nd ed., pp. 924–925). Philadelphia: Lippincott.

Miller, E. D., Jr. (1994). Deliberate hypotension. In R. D. Miller (Ed.), *Anesthesia* (4th ed., pp. 1481–1503). New York: Churchill Livingstone.

Miller R. D., Cucchiara, R., Miller, E., Reves, J., Roizen, M., & Savarese, J. (1994). *Anesthesia* (4th ed., p. 470). New York: Churchill Livingstone.

Morgan, G., & Mikhail, M. (1996). *Clinical anesthesiology* (2nd ed.). Norwalk, CT: Appleton & Lange.

Orser, B. (1990). Facial pain in the recovery room secondary to acute parotitis. *Anesthesiology, 72,* 1090–1091.

Perkins, J. B., & Miller, H. C. (1969). Blood loss during transurethral prostatectomy. *Journal of Urology, 101,* 93–97.

Pillalamarri, E. D., Bhangdia, P., Rudin, R. S., Chadry, R. M., Tudoon, P. R., & Abadir, A. R. (1983). Effects of CO_2 pneumoperitoneum during laparoscopy on A.B.G.'s, end-tidal CO_2, and cardiovascular dynamics. *Anesthesiology, 59,* 424.

Purdman, R. (1997). Anesthesia and orthopedics. In J. Nagelhout & K. Zaglaniczny (Eds.), *Nurse anesthesia* (pp. 1090–1121). Philadelphia: Saunders.

Reilly, M. (1970). Postanesthetic parotid swelling. *Anesthesia & Analgesia, 49*(4), 560–563.

Rothenberg, D. M. (1990). The approach to the Jehovah's Witness patient. *Anesthesiology Clinics of North America* (pamphlet), *8*(3).

Rubin, M. & Cozzi, G. (1986). Acute transient sialadenopathy associated with anesthesia. *Oral Surgery, 61,* 227–229.

Schwartz, J., Rosenbaum, S., & Graf, G. (1997). Anesthesia and the endocrine system. In P. G. Barash, & R. K. Stoelting (Eds.), *Clinical anesthesia* (pp. 1039–1058). Philadelphia: Lippincott.

Shnider, S. M., & Levinson, G. (1993). *Anesthesia for obstetrics* (3rd ed., pp. 259–280). Philadelphia: Williams & Wilkins.

Stoelting, R. K., & Dierdorf, S. F. (1993). *Handbook for anesthesia and co-existing disease* (pp. 225–227). New York: Churchill Livingstone.

West, J. B., Smith, L. H., & Bennett, J. C. (1990). *The essentials* (4th ed.). Baltimore: William & Wilkins.

Outcomes and Evaluation

Documentation of Anesthesia Care

Elizabeth Sodbinow

Documentation of anesthesia care began in 1894 when Cushing and Codman first recorded pulse and respirations during the administration of ether at the Massachusetts General Hospital. Since that time, the recording of anesthesia care has evolved into a complex written account of all aspects of anesthesia care (Mastropietro & Bruton-Maree, 1994). Today documentation of anesthesia care provides information about one of the most important events in a patient's clinical life. It chronicles information gathered about a patient in the course of a preanesthetic evaluation from which a specific anesthesia management plan is derived. It presents a record of the patient's responses to a surgical procedure and any actions and interventions taken to maintain a safe and comfortable anesthetic. Documentation also describes the postanesthetic status of the patient and any additional steps taken to maximize the patient's comfort. The culmination of all this information may be found on a single, dedicated, comprehensive form or on separate, specialized preanesthetic evaluation forms, intraanesthetic records, and postoperative progress notes. Together, records from these three phases of care are known as the anesthetic record. The way in which different institutions design and implement this record of care can vary, but the practice of completing a preanesthetic assessment, maintaining an intraoperative record, and conducting a postanesthetic review remains relatively standard.

According to Markarian (1991), the intraoperative or intraanesthetic record, the central and major component of the anesthetic record, must be prepared in such a way as to allow an accurate reconstruction of events during the administration of anesthesia. Entries should be clear, concise, legible, and accurate. It must offer proof of adequate care and document professional practices and decision making in accordance with accepted standards of care. The best and perhaps only way to verify that appropriate and accepted standards of care have been met is by reviewing written perioperative documentation of the anesthetic course.

Anesthesia records serve a variety of purposes. They communicate information about the continuum of patient care to all health care providers involved in the care of that patient. In this role, records relate important preoperative and intraoperative events that may be critical in developing a sound plan for postoperative management. Informative documentation also can help develop an appropriate anesthesia plan for future operations, particularly in patients who have a difficult or complex anesthetic course. In addition, statistics derived from anesthesia records can be used as a source of data for education and research.

Moreover, anesthesia records are important business records that can be used for billing purposes and inventory management. These records also can be an instrument of accountability in determining the extent to which an anesthesia provider complied with standards of care, clinical care guidelines, and peer-review standards. Last, the anesthesia record serves as a permanent record of care that is provided to a particular patient at a specific point in time (Gunn, 1992).

The technologies for patient monitoring and recordkeeping continue to develop. Automated systems in anesthesia exist, but their utilization is limited and their acceptability by the anesthesia community is varied. Future generations of these systems will be more advanced anesthesia information managers whose implications, capabilities, and potentials will be far-reaching for case planning, patient safety, and clinical decision making. The potential impact of these systems themselves on the evolution of the health professions remains to be seen.

▶ DOCUMENTING THE PHASES OF ANESTHESIA CARE

Documentation of anesthesia care can be said to fall into three major phases: (1) the preanesthetic period; (2) the intraanesthetic period; and (3) the postanesthetic period. These time intervals have traditionally been referred to as the preoperative, intraoperative, and postoperative periods. Information derived in the preanesthetic period help develop an appropriate anesthesia management plan for a specific patient about to undergo a specific procedure. In this phase, there is information exchange between patient and provider, as well as patient education and counseling. The intraanesthetic period includes that period when the patient arrives in the anesthetic setting and undergoes the actual administration of anesthesia and surgical procedure and ends when the patient is transferred to appropriate postanesthesia staff. In this phase adjustments and changes to the original anesthesia management plan can be made based on the responses of the patient to surgical interventions. During the postanesthetic period the patient is evaluated for any lingering effects of anesthesia and the care itself can be evaluated. Appropriate interventions still may be required and given by the anesthesia provider in this phase. These include antiemetic therapy, continued administration of fluid, or pain management techniques. Anesthesia care responsibilities end once the patient has fully recovered from the effects of the anesthetic or when the anesthetist no longer is directly responsible for the care of that patient.

The Preanesthetic Period

The preanesthetic period is the time before anesthesia is administered until induction of anesthesia; this is the time when patients are interviewed and evaluated by the anesthesia provider or their designee. Major goals of this evaluation period are to determine the patient's health status, prepare the patient for anesthesia and surgery, and institute measures to optimize the patient's postoperative outcome. Important aspects of the preanesthetic interview and evaluation process are summarized in Table 33–1.

TABLE 33–1. Important Aspects of the Preanesthetic Interview and Evaluation

Determine patient's medical, surgical, and anesthesia histories
    Review of organ systems
    Past surgeries and anesthetics
    Family anesthetic history
    Use of dental appliances, contact lenses, or other artificial devices
    Exercise level, tolerance, and frequency
    Allergies
Determine patient's demographic data
    Age
    Height
    Weight
Determine medication use
    Current medications
    Significant past medications
Determine social history impacting on anesthesia and surgery
    smoking
    alcohol use
    recreational drug use
Perform an appropriate physical examination
    Heart and lung auscultation
    Examination of circulation and extremities
    Airway examination and inspection
    Range of motion of head and neck
    Vital sign measurements
Review or order appropriate laboratory or diagnostic tests
Assignment of ASA classification
Discussion of anesthetic options and risk
Informed consent
Preanesthetic education, instructions, and counseling

The methods by which preanesthetic information is gathered can vary among institutions. These techniques also differ depending on the needs and requirements of the patient, institutional design, and technologies available. For example, in some outpatient surgery settings, healthy patients may not be interviewed until the day of surgery and specific instructions such as NPO status and laboratory or diagnostic workups may be ordered by the operating surgeon ahead of time. In these cases, the actual anesthesia interview may be short and concise and occur immediately prior to the anesthetic and surgery.

In other situations, where patients have significant medical compromise, such as heart or lung disease, patients may be instructed to consult with anesthesia personnel days or weeks before the actual surgery to determine what regimens can best optimize the patient for anesthesia and surgery. In some cases, these patients may be admitted days before surgery for additional testing, invasive line placement, or other presurgical preparations.

In other institutions, nonanesthesia personnel may be responsible for interviewing the patient and conducting limited physical examinations in preparation for a final interview by an anesthesia professional. With this process other health care providers can work on anesthesia-related tasks, such as obtaining histories, gathering data, or assisting patients with computer-generated questionnaires. These sessions may be followed by other counseling sessions about the process of anesthesia, surgery, or other presurgical activities. Information relevant to the development of a final anesthetic plan is then flagged for a final interview by an anesthesia professional. This method allows the anesthesia provider to concentrate on pertinent patient and anesthesia-related items. The mechanics of when, how, and who gathers preanesthetic information can vary significantly, but ultimately an anesthesia provider must discuss specific anesthesia plans and risks with the patient before the procedure. Under no circumstances should a nurse anesthetist attempt to conduct an anesthetic before a preanesthetic evaluation is complete, even when extreme, life-threatening emergencies may make waiting difficult.

Informed Consent

The preanesthetic period permits disclosure and discussion about events that will occur in the operating room, anesthetic options available, and the risks of anesthesia. By definition, informed consent means that the patient has agreed to undergo a procedure after receiving a clear description of the nature of the procedure and any potential side effects. Informed consent protects the caregiver from libelous acts and educates the patient about the events surrounding the procedure to be performed. Informed consent can be given by persons of legal age, legal guardians, or emancipated minors. Patients who may not understand the information being given because of a language barrier, presence of medications, alcohol ingestion, or other debilitated physical condition must have alternative arrangements made to obtain the consent. If this is not possible, informed consent should be delayed. Life-threatening circumstances are the only exception to these situations (Mastropietro & Bruton-Maree, 1994).

Usually, consents for surgical procedures are written contracts that state the name of the procedure and are signed by the patient, dated, and witnessed. The consent for anesthesia may be a separate form (Fig. 33-1) or may be incorporated as part of the surgical consent form. Regardless of the format, informed consent must involve effective and thorough communication so that the anesthesia provider has a strong sense that the patient has understood all the details given about anesthetic options and risks.

A health care provider other than the one who is to administer the anesthetic can obtain a patient's informed consent, provided that the information given is essentially the same as that given by the actual provider (Markarian, 1991). The discussion of risk does not have

to include every possible and potential complication. According to Markarian (1991), only "substantial risks" must be disclosed, and these include risks that are inherent in the instrumentation of the mouth, invasive line placement, or blood transfusion. Disclosure of risk should be accomplished as not to unduly alarm the patient and should be simultaneously balanced with information about measures to minimize harm. A statement about the rarity of such risks also should be included, if applicable.

Other Important Aspects of the Preanesthetic Evaluation

Written reference should be made by the interviewer about the preanesthetic interview, findings, plan, and informed consent on the patient's preanesthetic evaluation, progress note, or other designated form. Where a detailed discussion has taken place and the patient's condition and upcoming surgical procedure warrants a lengthy and necessary review, appropriate notations should be made to designate this extensive review.

Forms for documenting preanesthetic evaluations vary by institution or setting and can range from very cursory blocks requesting "any significant medical history" to an extensive check list for every organ system and type of question to be asked of patients. One format that is fairly standard is presented by the AANA (1996) in Figure 33-2. Whatever format is used, the information gathered by an anesthesia provider in the preanesthetic period must be consistent and give valuable information about a patient to allow specific anesthesia management plans to be developed.

The assignment of an ASA classification depicting a pathophysiologic baseline for all patients is a required standard in anesthesia practice and is usually assigned as a result of the preanesthetic review. The specific criteria by which various categories of patients and problems are assigned this classification are discussed in Chapter 9.

The discussion and documentation of appropriate anesthesia management options should be conducted so as not to "lock" the provider into a specific anesthetic technique in the event that circumstances change. This allows flexibility in cases where the interviewing provider is not the actual provider of the anesthetic itself. In either case, options that the patient specifically and/or adamantly objects to must be clearly identified in the written preanesthetic evaluation.

The preanesthetic period also is a time when appropriate instructions can be given to the patient. These include medications to be continued or taken, NPO instructions, and other important preparations. Documentation of patient instruction on the preanesthetic evaluation will alert the entire anesthesia team to particular

CONSENT FOR ANESTHESIA SERVICES

I, _____ , acknowledge that my doctor has explained to me that I will have an operation, diagnostic or treatment procedure. My doctor has explained the risks of the procedure, advised me of alternative treatments and told me about the expected outcome and what could happen if my condition remains untreated. I also understand that anesthesia services are needed so that my doctor can perform the operation or procedure.

It has been explained to me that **all** forms of anesthesia involve some **risks** and no guarantees or promises can be made concerning the results of my procedure or treatment. Although rare, unexpected *severe complications* with anesthesia can occur and include the remote possibility of *infection, bleeding, drug reactions, blood clots, loss of sensation, loss of limb function, paralysis, stroke, brain damage, heart attack or death*. I understand that these risks apply to all forms of anesthesia and that additional or specific risks have been identified below as they may apply to a specific type of anesthesia. I understand that the type(s) of anesthesia service checked below will be used for my procedure and that the anesthetic technique to be used is determined by many factors including my physical condition, the type of procedure my doctor is to do, his or her preference, as well as my own desire. It has been explained to me that sometimes an anesthesia technique which involves the use of local anesthetics, with or without sedation, may not succeed completely and therefore another technique may have to be used including general anesthesia.

☐ General Anesthesia	Expected Result	Total unconscious state, possible placement of a tube into the windpipe.
	Technique	Drug injected into the bloodstream, breathed into the lungs, or by other routes.
	Risks	Mouth or throat pain, hoarseness, injury to mouth or teeth, awareness under anesthesia, injury to blood vessels, aspiration, pneumonia.

☐ Spinal or Epidural Analgesia/ Anesthesia
  ☐ With sedation
  ☐ Without sedation
	Expected Result	Temporary decreased or loss of feeling and/or movement to lower part of the body.

	Technique	Drug injected through a needle/catheter placed either directly into the spinal canal or immediately outside the spinal canal.
	Risks	Headache, backache, buzzing in the ears, convulsions, infection, persistent weakness. numbness, residual pain, injury to blood vessels, "total spinal".

☐ Major / Minor Nerve Block
  ☐ With sedation
  ☐ Without sedation
	Expected Result	Temporary loss of feeling and/or movement of a specific limb or area.

	Technique	Drug injected near nerves providing loss of sensation to the area of the operation.
	Risks	Infection, convulsions. weakness, persistent numbness. residual pain, injury to blood vessels.

☐ Intravenous Regional Anesthesia
  ☐ With sedation
  ☐ Without sedation
	Expected Result	Temporary loss of feeling and/or movement of a limb.

	Technique	Drug injected into veins of arm or leg while using a tourniquet.
	Risks	Infection, convulsions, persistent numbness, residual pain, injury to blood vessels.
☐ Monitored Anesthesia Care (with sedation)	Expected Result	Reduced anxiety and pain, partial or total amnesia.
	Technique	Drug injected into the bloodstream, breathed into the lungs, or by other routes producing a semi-conscious state.
	Risks	An unconscious state, depressed breathing, injury to blood vessels.
☐ Monitored Anesthesia Care (without sedation)	Expected Result	Measurement of vital signs, availability of anesthesia provider for further intervention.
	Technique	None.
	Risks	Increased awareness, anxiety and/or discomfort.

I hereby consent to the anesthesia service checked above and authorize that it be administered by_____or his/her associates, all of whom are credentialed to provide anesthesia services at this health facility. I also consent to an alternative type of anesthesia, if necessary, as deemed appropriate by them. I expressly desire the following considerations be observed (or write "none"):

_____

BLOOD TRANSFUSIONS

The likelihood of needing a blood transfusion for this procedure is: ☐ highly unlikely, ☐ possible, ☐ probable.

I understand that there are potential risks from blood transfusions, though rare, and that some of these include transfusion reaction, hepatitis, and AIDS (Acquired Immune Deficiency Syndrome). *Initial in appropriate box:*

☐ I give consent to receive blood or blood products as determined by my anesthetist and doctor to be necessary for my well-being.
☐ I give consent to receive blood or blood products only as an emergency life-saving measure.
☐ I do not want to receive blood or blood products under any circumstance.

I certify and acknowledge that I have read this form or had it read to me, that I understand the risks, alternatives and expected results of the anesthesia service and that I had ample time to ask questions and to consider my decision.

PATIENT IDENTIFICATION

_____   _____
Patient's Signature   Date and Time

_____   _____
Substitute's Signature   Relationship to Patient

_____   Developed by the American Association
Witness   of Nurse Anesthetists - 1991

Figure 33–1. Sample informed consent. *(From the American Association of Nurse Anesthetists. [1996]. Professional Practice Manual for the Certified Registered Nurse Anesthetist. Park Ridge, IL: Author. Reprinted with permission.)*

PREANESTHESIA EVALUATION

Age	Sex M F	Height in / cm	Weight lb / kg

Proposed Procedure	Pre-Procedure Vital Signs B/P P R T

Previous Anesthesia / Operations	None ☐	Current Medications	None ☐

Family History of Anesthesia Complications	None ☐	Allergies	NKDA ☐

AIRWAY / TEETH / HEAD & NECK

History From:
☐ Patient   ☐ Significant Other
☐ Parent / Guardian   ☐ Chart
☐ Communication / Language Problems
☐ Poor Historian

SYSTEM	WNL	COMMENTS	DIAGNOSTIC STUDIES
RESPIRATORY	☐	Tobacco Use: ☐ Yes ☐ No _____ Packs / Day for _____ Years	EKG
Asthma Productive Cough Bronchitis Recent URI COPD SOB Dyspnea Tuberculosis Orthopnea Pneumonia			Chest X-ray
CARDIOVASCULAR	☐		
Abnormanl EKG Hypertension Angina MI ASHD Murmur CHF Pacemaker Dysrhythmia Rheumatic Fever Exercise Tolerance Valvular Disease			Pulmonary Studies
HEPATO / GASTROINTESTINAL	☐	Ethanol Use: ☐ Yes ☐ No Frequency _____ "Street Drug" Use: ☐ Yes ☐ No Frequency _____	Other
Bowel Obtruction Cirrhosis Hepatits / Jaundice Hiatal hernia / Reflux Nausea & Vomiting Ulcers			
NEURO / MUSCULOSKELETAL	☐		**LABORATORY STUDIES**
Arthritis Muscle Weakness Back Problems Neuromuscular Dis. CVA / Stroke / TIAs Paralysis DJD Paresthesia Headaches / ↑ ICP Syncope Loss of Consciousness Seizures			Hgb / Hct / CBC
RENAL / ENDOCRINE	☐		Electrolytes
Diabetes Renal Failure / Dialysis Thyroid Disease Urinary Retention Urinary Tract Infection Weight Loss / Gain			Urinalysis
OTHER			
Anemia Immunosuppressed Bleeding tendencies Pregnancy Cancer Sickle Cell Dis. / Trait Chemotherapy Recent Steroids Dehydration Tranfusion History Hemophilia			Other

Problem List / Diagnoses	PHYSICAL STATUS 1 2 3 4 5 E	**POSTANESTHESIA NOTE**
Planned Anesthesia / Special Monitors		
		Signed _____ Date _____ Time _____
Pre-Anesthesia Medications Ordered		PATIENT IDENTIFICATION
Evaluator Signature	Date Time	

Figure 33–2. Sample of a preanesthesia evaluation form. (*From the American Association of Nurse Anesthetists [1996]. Professional Practice Manual for the Certified Registered Nurse Anesthetist. Park Ridge, IL: Author. Reprinted with permission.*)

discussions and preparatory activities that have taken place.

The development of interpersonal rapport between the patient and provider is crucial during this period. This relationship becomes even more relevant when a patient is about to undergo an anesthetic. Many patients' fears, anxieties, and misconceptions about anesthesia can be openly addressed and alleviated at this time. Reassurances and teaching also can assist in clarifying a patient's postanesthetic expectations. Discussion can include antiemetic techniques, pain management options, and/or expectations about invasive lines or the presence of an endotracheal tube, if these are to be left in place at the end of an operation. A brief narrative in the patient's chart about these discussions also may help provide continuity of care among care team members.

In instances where the best anesthetic plan for the patient is monitored anesthesia care or a regional technique, anxiety and fear about anesthesia and surgery can become even more heightened. It is imperative that the anesthesia provider explain the benefits of these techniques and the availability of sedatives and other methods of support, including music via earphones. In all instances, it is important to reinforce the fact that an anesthesia provider is in attendance with the patient at all times. This verbalized reassurance allows some patients to feel more comfortable knowing that their anesthesia provider can administer medications or institute other measures for continued comfort. Brief documentation of any discussion about backup plans or supplemental activities are important in the event changes to the original anesthesia plan occur. Preanesthetic evaluations remain an important aspect of every patient's anesthesia care. As newer technologies in computerization and anesthesia information management systems emerge, methods for preanesthetic information gathering and documentation will necessarily change. Pressures in the future to streamline and maximize efficiencies in the operating suite may result in preanesthetic evaluations derived from national resource databases, clinical care guidelines, or best-practice models. Whatever the method or model, anesthesia providers must continue to do their best to acquire this important information as it will remain, perhaps, the single most important data source in managing a successful anesthetic.

Documentation of Intraanesthetic Care

Intraanesthetic care (Table 33-2) begins when the patient is brought to the operating area and ends when a final report has been given to postanesthesia care unit (PACU) personnel. The documentation of events in this phase usually is accomplished on the intraanesthetic record and includes induction, maintenance, and emergence from anesthesia.

TABLE 33-2. Summary of Documentation of Intra-anesthetic Care

Preinduction and induction
  Preanesthetic checks
    Patient identification, consents, and evaluations
    Machine, drug, and equipment checks
    Laboratory, radiologic, and diagnostic data
    NPO status
  Medications taken, fluids given
  Preanesthetic measures instituted
    Monitors used
    Baseline vital signs
    Invasive lines placed
    Preoxygenation techniques
    Warming devices used
  Patient's preanesthetic psychological state
  All aspects of laryngoscopy and intubation
  Auscultation of breath sounds
  Postintubation hemodynamic status
Maintenance of anesthesia
  Patient positioning
    Auscultation of breath sounds
    Eye care, safety of head and extremities,
    Placement of rolls, padding, and devices for maximizing safety and circulation
    All infusions, transfusions, outputs, and losses
  All anesthetic agents, gases, and drugs
  Degree of neuromuscular blockade
  All hemodynamic measurements, including temperature
  All ventilatory measurements and settings
  All interventions, therapies, and measures
  All additional directives and consultations
  All complications and unusual events
Emergence from anesthesia
  Termination of all anesthetics and gases
  Supplemental oxygenation
  Hemodynamic status at emergence
  Reversal drugs and their effects
  Evaluation of recovery from neuromuscular blockade
  Extubation parameters and maneuvers
  Totals for all infusions, outputs, and losses
  Summary of all medications administered
  Level of patient wake up and awareness
  Adequacy of ventilation
  Levels of sensory and motor blockade
  Safety and stability of patient at transfer
Reports of patient to PACU staff
  Patient demographics and health history
  Surgical procedure and tolerance of anesthetic
  Anesthetic techniques and medications given
  All intake and output
  Unusual events, reactions, or complications
  Vital sign trends throughout anesthetic
  Current hemodynamic status
  Any postanesthetic interventions to be carried out
  Any areas for close observation

The Intraanesthetic Record

The intraanesthetic record, commonly called the anesthesia record, usually is a multiple-copy document with no carbon required (NCR) paper. As a written record of anesthetic events, it is a surveyable and time-continuous monograph of the entire course of anesthesia administration. According to Mastropietro and Bruton-Maree (1994), documentation in this format stimulates continuous observation of the patient and allows the user to track the trends elicited by a patient's responses to specific anesthetic interventions. Documentation arranged in a logical and sequential manner also can facilitate review of pertinent data.

There are various parts to the anesthesia record (Fig. 33-3) that are intended as reminders about the care to be given and are easy to use. These major areas can be seen as preprinted blocks, the open central grid, and the narrative section. The preprinted blocks usually contain items that can be easily checked off. These generally pertain to patient demographics, patient and equipment safety checks, and personnel- and time-related factors. Actual forms will vary by institution, but the information to be documented is fairly standard.

The largest portion of the anesthesia record is the open, central grid that permits time-continuous tracking of the patient's vital signs, agents employed, position changes, and fluids given, to name a few. These and other informational items usually contained in the anesthesia record are outlined by an anesthetic record prototype from the Professional Practice Manual for the Certified Registered Nurse Anesthetist (1996).

A blank space on the record accommodates narrative entries that cannot be graphically noted or checked. Documentation of surgical events, patient responses, and anesthetic interventions that are written in the narrative should follow an appropriate, chronological sequence when charted. Observable trends, both on the grid and in the narrative section, can then be easily reviewed and subsequent intervention readily noted. Items that are missed in charting at the time they occur may be added to the record or in the progress note with a specific notation of time, date, and provider signature. It is unacceptable practice to make late entries onto the chart by "squeezing" them in between or among previously recorded information.

Induction of Anesthesia

On entry into the anesthetizing area, the anesthetist should document that all appropriate preanesthetic checks have been completed. One document listing recommendations for checking the anesthesia machine and its various components is presented in Fig. 33-4. Other checks that must be made and noted are verification of patient identity and the type or name of the contemplated surgical procedure, presence of all appropriate consents, presence of adequate preanesthetic evaluations, including laboratory, diagnostic, and radiologic data, time of last intake, medications taken or administered, and the

patient's preanesthetic psychological state. Patients who present in a confused, uncooperative, or unresponsive state may warrant additional remarks in the narrative section.

All preinduction and induction maneuvers must be documented to reflect an appropriate standard of care. These include the placement of monitors and establishing baseline vital signs; temperature monitoring in all pediatric and hyperpyrexic patients; placement of intravenous catheters and other invasive monitoring lines; the administration of fluids and drugs in preparation for induction; utilization of warming devices; and preoxygenating techniques.

When the anesthesia has been induced and the patient's airway secured, the intubation technique used and endotracheal tube verification procedures followed also must be documented. Specific notations in this area may be difficulty of mask ventilation; specific laryngoscopy maneuvers; visualization or nonvisualization of vocal cords; utilization of rapid-sequence methods; auscultation of bilateral breath sounds; and verification of end-tidal CO_2. A narrative description of the successful intubation procedure should be fully described in the narrative, including tube size, ease of laryngoscopy, and confirmation of ventilation by both direct auscultation and an end-tidal CO_2 waveform. If intubation is initially unsuccessful, alternative techniques and procedures employed should be described as this information will help providers of subsequent surgical procedures ensure a safe anesthestic course.

If regional techniques are used, documentation must include a narrative description of the procedure followed, equipment used, and medications administered. Pertinent items to document a regional anesthetic are listed in Table 33-3. Notations regarding the state of the patient's hydration, sedative medication employed, and assessment of the patient's physiologic status after a regional technique also must be made. In addition, notations of any complications or difficulties encountered and the interventions used to rectify problems should be clearly documented as this information will be helpful for postanesthetic care and to prepare for future anesthetics.

Documentation of patient positioning and actions taken to ensure there is no nerve or circulatory impairment during surgery is critical. Patients who undergo general anesthesia have no means of alerting their provider to potential positional compromise. Thus, the use of adequate padding to vulnerable sites, measures to minimize undue stretch or nerve injuries, adequate eye protection, appropriate adjustments of the head and extremities, and any additional rolls or pads to maximize ventilation should all be noted. In addition, patients that are placed in the prone, lithotomy, or lateral positions, or who have their arms tucked at their sides, should be

ANESTHESIA RECORD

						START	STOP
	Procedure				Anesthesia		
Date	OR No.	Page	of	Surgeon(s)	Procedure		

PRE-PROCEDURE	MONITORS AND EQUIPMENT	ANESTHETIC TECHNIQUE	AIRWAY MANAGEMENT	RECOVERY

PRE-PROCEDURE
- ☐ Identified: ☐ ID Band ☐ Questioning
- ☐ Chart Reviewed ☐ Permit Signed
- ☐ NPO Since _____
- **Pre-anesthetic State:** ☐ Calm
- ☐ Awake ☐ Asleep
- ☐ Apprehensive ☐ Confused
- ☐ Uncooperative ☐ Unresponsive

PATIENT SAFETY
- ☐ Anes. Machine # _____ Checked
- ☐ Safety Belt On ☐ Axillary Roll
- ☐ Armboard Restraints ☐ Arms Tucked
- ☐ Pressure points checked and padded
- **Eye Care:** ☐ Ointment ☐ Saline
- ☐ Taped ☐ Pads ☐ Goggles

MONITORS AND EQUIPMENT
- ☐ Steth: ☐ Precord ☐ Esoph ☐ Other
- ☐ Non-Invasive B/P: ☐ Left ☐ Right
- ☐ Continuous EKG ☐ V Lead EKG
- ☐ Pulse Oximeter ☐ Oxygen Sensor
- ☐ End Tidal CO_2 ☐ Gas Analyzer
- ☐ Temp. _____ ☐ Nerve Stimulator
- ☐ Warming Blanket ☐ EEG ☐ Doppler
- ☐ Airway Humidifier ☐ Fluid Warmer
- ☐ NG / OG Tube ☐ Foley Catheter
- ☐ Art.Line _____
- ☐ CVP _____
- ☐ PA Line _____
- ☐ IV(s) _____
- ☐ _____

ANESTHETIC TECHNIQUE
- **General:** ☐ Pre-Oxygenation ☐ L.T.A.
- ☐ Rapid Sequence ☐ Cricoid Pressure
- ☐ Intravenous ☐ Inhalation
- ☐ Intramuscular ☐ Rectal
- **Regional:** ☐ Spinal ☐ Epidural
- ☐ Axillary ☐ Bier Block ☐ Ankle Block
- ☐ _____ ☐ Position _____
- ☐ Prep _____ ☐ Local _____
- ☐ Needle _____
- ☐ Drug(s) _____
- ☐ Dose _____ ☐ Attempts x _____
- ☐ Site _____ ☐ Level _____
- ☐ Catheter _____ ☐ See Remarks
- **Other:** ☐ M.A.C. ☐ _____

AIRWAY MANAGEMENT
- **Intubation:** ☐ Oral Tube size _____
- ☐ Stylet used ☐ Nasal ☐ Regular
- ☐ Magill's ☐ Direct ☐ RAE
- ☐ Fiber optic ☐ Blind ☐ Armored
- ☐ Blade _____ ☐ Laser
- ☐ Secured at _____ cm ☐ Endobronch.
- ☐ Attempts x _____ ☐ $ET CO_2$ present
- ☐ Breath sounds _____
- ☐ Uncuffed, leaks at _____ cm H_2O
- ☐ Cuffed ☐ Min. occ. pres. ☐ Air ☐ NS
- **Airway:** ☐ Oral ☐ Nasal ☐ Difficult,
- **Circuit:** ☐ Circle ☐ NRB see Remarks
- ☐ Mask Case ☐ Nasal Cannula
- ☐ Via Tracheostomy ☐ Simple O_2 mask

RECOVERY

Location		Time
B/P		O_2 Sat.
P	R	T

- ☐ Awake ☐ Stable ☐ Nasal Oxygen
- ☐ Drowsy ☐ Unstable ☐ Mask Oxygen
- ☐ Somnolent ☐ Intubated ☐ T-piece Oxygen
- ☐ Unarousable ☐ Ventilator ☐ Oral/nasal airway

Recovery Notes

FLUID TOTALS

Crystalloid _____   EBL _____
Blood _____   Urine _____

REMARKS

FLUIDS / AGENTS

TIME:														
Oxygen (L/min)														TOTALS
☐ N_2O ☐ Air (L/min)														
(%)														

| Urine (ml) | | | | | | | | | | | | | |
| EBL (ml) | | | | | | | | | | | | | |

MONITORS

EKG													SYMBOLS
% O_2 Inspired													
O_2 Saturation													
End Tidal CO_2													
Temp.: ☐ °C ☐ °F													

✕ ANESTHESIA

⊙ OPERATION

VITAL SIGNS

Baseline Values	200												
	180												
	160												
	140												
B/P	120												
	100												
	80												
P	60												
	40												
R	20												

∨∧ B/P CUFF PRESSURE

⊥T ARTERIAL LINE PRESSURE

▲ MEAN ARTERIAL PRESSURE

• PULSE

○ SPONT. RESP

∅ ASSISTED RESP

⊠ CONTROLLED RESP

T TOURNIQUET

VENT

Tidal Volume													
Resp. Rate													
Peak Pressure													
PEEP													

| Symbols for Remarks | | | | | | | | | | | | | |
| Position | | | | | | | | | | | | | |

PATIENT IDENTIFICATION

Anesthesia Provider

CONTROLLED DRUGS

Drug	Issued	Used	Destroyed	Returned	Provider
					Witness

Figure 33–3. Sample of an intra-anesthetic record. *(From the American Association of Nurse Anesthetists [1996].* Professional Practice Manual for the Certified Registered Nurse Anesthetist. *Park Ridge, IL: Author. Reprinted with permission.)*

Anesthesia Apparatus Checkout Recommendations, 1993

This checkout, or a reasonable equivalent should be conducted before administration of anesthesia. These recommendations are only valid for an anesthesia system that conforms to current and relevant standards and includes an ascending bellows ventilator and at least the following monitors: capnograph, pulse odometer, oxygen analyzer, respiratory volume monitor (spirometer) and breathing system pressure monitor with high and low pressure alarms. This is a guideline which users are encouraged to modify to accommodate differences in equipment design and variations in local clinical practice. Such local modifications should have appropriate peer review. Users should refer to the operator's manual for the manufacturer's specific procedures and precautions, especially the manufacturer's low pressure leak test (step #5).

Emergency Ventilation Equipment

*1. Verify Backup Ventilation Equipment is Available & Functioning

High Pressure System

*2. Check Oxygen Cylinder Supply
   a. Open O_2 cylinder and verify at least half full (about 1000 psi).
   b. Close cylinder.

*3. Check Central Pipeline Supplies
   a. Check that hoses are connected and pipeline gauges read about 50 psi.

Low Pressure Systems

*4. Check Initial Status of Low Pressure System
   a. Close flow control valves and turn vaporizers off.
   b. Check fill level and tighten vaporizers' filler caps.

*5. Perform Leak Check of Machine Low Pressure System
   a. Verify that the machine master switch and flow control valves are OFF.
   b. Attach "Suction Bulb" to common (Fresh) gas outlet.
   c. Squeeze bulb repeatedly until fully collapsed.
   d. Verify bulb stays fully collapsed for at least 10 seconds.
   e. Open one vaporizer at a time and repeat 'c' and 'd' as above.
   f. Remove suction bulb, and reconnect fresh gas hose.

*6. Turn On Machine Master Switch and all other necessary electrical equipment.

*7. Test Flowmeters
   a. Adjust flow of all gases through their full range, checking for smooth operation of floats and undamaged flow tubes.
   b. Attempt to create a hypoxic O_2/N_2O mixture and verify correct changes in flow and/or alarm.

Scavenging System

*8. Adjust and Check Scavenging System
   a. Ensure proper connections between the scavenging system and both APL (pop-off) valve and ventilator relief valve.
   b. Adjust waste gas vacuum (if possible).
   c. Fury open APL valve and occlude Y-piece.
   d. With minimum O_2 flow, allow scavenger reservoir bag to collapse completely and verify that absorber pressure gauge reads about zero.
   e. With the O_2 flush activated allow the scavenger reservoir bag to distend fully, and then verify that absorber pressure gauge reads < 10 cm H_2O.

Breathing System

*9. Calibrate O_2 Monitor
   a. Ensure monitor reads 21% in room air.
   b. Verify low O_2 alarm is enabled and functioning.
   c. Reinstall sensor in circuit and flush breathing system with O_2.
   d. Verify that monitor now reads greater than 90%.

*If an anesthesia provider uses the same machine in successive cases, these steps need not be repeated or may be abbreviated after the initial checkout.

10. **Check Initial Status of Breathing System**
   a. Set selector switch to "Bag" mode.
   b. Check that breathing circuit is complete, undamaged and unobstructed.
   c. Verify that CO_2 absorbent is adequate.
   d. Install breathing circuit accessory equipment (e.g. humidifier, PEEP valve) to be used during the case.

11. **Perform Leak Check of the Breathing System**
   a. Set all gas flows to zero (or minimum).
   b. Close APL (pop-off) valve and occlude Y-piece.
   c. Pressurize breathing system to about 30 cm H_2O with O_2 flush.
   d. Ensure that pressure remains fixed for at least 10 seconds.
   e. Open APL (pop-off) valve and ensure that pressure decreases.

Manual and Automatic Ventilation Systems

12. **Test Ventilation Systems and Unidirectional Valves**
   a. Place a second breathing bag on Y-piece.
   b. Set appropriate ventilator parameters for next patient.
   c. Switch to automatic ventilation (Ventilator) mode.
   d. Fill bellows and breathing bag with O_2 flush and then turn ventilator ON.
   e. Set O_2 flow to minimum, other gas flows to zero.
   f. Verify that during inspiration bellows delivers appropriate tidal volume and that during expiration bellows fills completely.
   g. Set fresh gas flow to about 5 L/min.
   h. Verify that the ventilator bellows and simulated lungs fill and empty appropriately without sustained pressure at end expiration.
   i. Check for proper action of unidirectional valves.
   j. Exercise breathing circuit accessories to ensure proper function.
   k. Turn ventilator OFF and switch to manual ventilation (Bag/APL) mode.
   l. Ventilate manually and assure inflation and deflation of artificial lungs and appropriate feel of system resistance and compliance.
   m. Remove second breathing bag from Y-piece.

Monitors

13. **Check, Calibrate and/or Set Alarm Limits of all Monitors**

Capnometer	Pulse Oximeter
Oxygen Analyzer	Respiratory Volume Monitor (Spirometer)
Pressure Monitor with High and Low Airway Alarms	

Final Position

14. **Check Final Status of Machine**
   a. Vaporizers off.
   b. AFL valve open.
   c. Selector switch to "Bag".
   d. All flowmeters to zero.
   e. Patient suction level adequate.
   f. Breathing system ready to use.

Figure 33–4. Anesthesia apparatus checkout recommendations, 1993. Documentation that this checklist has been performed is required on every anesthetic case record. (*From Department of Health and Human Services, Food and Drug Administration, Rockville, MD.*)

TABLE 33–3. Specific Items to Be Charted When Performing a Regional Anesthetic Technique

Patient position
Hydration status
Sedatives given
Specific technique performed
Preparation of skin
Local anesthetic used, baricity, and amount
Additional medications used
Regional anesthetic kit and lot number
Number of attempts to accomplish technique
Site of insertion
Type and size of needle used
Character and flow of CSF, if present
Aspiration techniques and results
Any quadrant changes in CSF flow
Patient position after regional technique
Levels of sensory and motor blockade achieved and time achieved
Patient's physiologic and vital sign responses to procedure
Any difficulties encountered in accomplishing the regional technique

checked and appropriate notations made. All measures taken to verify patient safety after position changes should be charted in the patient's anesthetic record. This would include rechecking and documenting endotrachael tube position via direct ausculation.

Maintenance of Anesthesia

Maintenance of anesthesia is that period of time from the start to completion of the surgical procedure. In the case of a general anesthetic, the patient should be in a pain-free, relaxed, and unconscious state. Documentation should verify that the patient is physiologically stable, given any preexisting health condition or untoward effect of the surgical procedure. All activities at this time are directed toward optimizing the patient's postoperative outcomes (Mastropietro & Bruton-Maree, 1994).

Documentation of care during maintenance usually entails a time-continuous log of the patient's physiologic responses and all anesthetic interventions. All patient data, including fluid infusions, blood transfusions, fluid outputs and losses, hemodynamic and ventilatory measurements, monitoring measurements, neuromuscular blockade, and the administration of anesthetic agents, gases, and drugs are charted as well. Anesthetic gases should be noted in L/min, drugs in milligrams or micrograms, and volatile agents in percentages.

Notations regarding patient's responses, administration of nonroutine medications, any unusual physiologic occurrences, as well as consultations and complications must be accurately recorded. Any laboratory values, interventions, or other therapies must be noted and explained. Any surgical interventions that impact on the patient's condition, such as clamping and unclamping of vessels or tourniquet usage, must be charted. Directives given by physician consultants or surgeons should be documented with the physician's name, the order, and the time and date the order was carried out. Finally, if an anesthetist is relieved by another provider, their name and the time relief begins and ends should become part of the permanent record. According to Mastropietro and Bruton-Maree (1994), relief must never be accepted during induction, emergence, or when a patient is unstable.

Emergence from Anesthesia

Documentation about emergence from anesthesia should include the time that anesthetic gases were terminated; administration and liter flow of supplemental oxygen; reversal drugs administered, including assessment and evaluation of recovery from neuromuscular blockade; a description of how the patient met extubation criteria; totals for all infusions, fluid outputs, and losses; summary of all administered drugs; level of patient consciousness; concerns for patient safety relative to transport to postanesthesia care unit (PACU); and use of any monitors or supplemental oxygen during transport. Patients who have undergone regional anesthesia techniques also must meet safety and stability requirements as well as notation of sensory and motor blockade levels. Prior to transferring care, the anesthetist must ensure that the patient is hemodynamically stable and that ventilation is adequate.

Transfer to the Postanesthesia Care Unit

A verbal report to PACU staff should include chronologic presentation of surgical events prefaced by pertinent patient demographics and health history. The anesthetist also should provide the following data to the PACU nurse: surgical procedure and anesthesia technique employed; medications given; totals of intakes and outputs; any unusual events, reactions, or complications; vital sign trends; closing hemodynamic values; and any areas of close observation or caution warranted (Markarian, 1991). The chart should also note that a verbal report was given and that an appropriately credentialed provider accepted care of the patient. The CRNA's responsibilities regarding postanesthetic care are summarized in the AANA *Postanesthesia Care Standards* (1992). Despite various pressures for minimizing surgical turnover times and initiating subsequent anesthetics quickly, the burden remains on the anesthetist to make sure all aspects of the previous case, including records, are complete and that the patient is safe and stable in another's care.

Postanesthetic Evaluations

Evaluation of the patient after an anesthetic is a standard of care and has traditionally been intended to demonstrate continuity of care. This visit allows a patient to voice an evaluation of the anesthetic experience from his or her point of view. It also allows an opportunity for the anesthesia provider to determine whether there are any postanesthetic complications, discomfort, or questions from the patient. It is a time when difficulties encountered during anesthesia care, such as a difficult intubation or an untoward reaction to a medication or procedure, can be explained and discussed with the patient for future reference. Notations regarding the postanesthetic evaluation can be made in the patient's chart, either on a dedicated section of the anesthetic record or on the patient's progress note. Any findings, complaints, or measures taken should be documented clearly. If complications are noted, or additional follow-up evaluations or treatments are necessary, these should be written as well. Postanesthetic notations on patients that are discharged prior to a postoperative visit are managed either by an appropriate chart review or by specific institutionally designed mechanisms that address this component of care such as telephone interviews.

▶ DOCUMENTATION OF CARE OUTSIDE THE OPERATING ROOM

Notations of care given by an anesthesia provider outside of the operating room should follow the same principles for accuracy, completeness, legibility, and vigilance. Work performed by the nurse anesthetist in areas such as the delivery room, emergency room, or other patient care area must be noted on appropriate patient progress notes, consultation reports, anesthesia record, or other departmental form. Records regarding care given to obstetric patients for epidural pain management or during a cesarean-section delivery also must reflect identical standards given to the surgical patient. In addition, the time of a baby's birth, the sex of the baby, Apgar readings, time of placental delivery, and all drugs given to the mother, including the anesthetic technique employed, should be documented. Guidelines for the anesthetic care of the obstetric patient are outlined in the AANA *Guidelines for Obstetrical Anesthesia* (1991).

Anesthesia services may be required frequently in ancillary care areas for resuscitation, intubation, line placement, pain management services, cardioversion, or anesthesia consultation. These events should be noted on patient progress notes or specific departmental forms. The narrative must indicate the reasons for the request, interventions performed, patient status, and responses to anesthetic interventions, stability of the patient at the end of the consultation period, and who is assuming care for the patient when the anesthetist leaves.

▶ DOCUMENTATION OF SPECIAL CIRCUMSTANCES

Increasingly, the complexity of care given in today's clinical environment, the current emphasis on patients' rights, and a litigious climate have made documentation of care provided in special circumstances very important. Examples of these considerations are the presence of "do not resuscitate" orders and their impact for anesthesia care; the seriously ill Jehovah's Witness patient and the need for lifesaving transfusions; the mechanics of maintaining accuracy and continuity in charting during emergencies; the management of incident reports; and the use of personal notes about patients.

The AANA ethical guidelines on do not resuscitate (DNR) orders (1994) state that these orders acknowledge a patient's right to choose to die with dignity without prolonging his or her life by artificial means. Automatic suspension of DNR orders during a perioperative period fails to comply with a patient's right to make decisions about his or her own medical care and raises the potential for a charge of "battery" or a "wrongful life" suit. In clinical situations where a patient with a DNR order must undergo an anesthetic, there must be clear communication between all parties involved regarding the extent of lifesaving interventions in the event of adverse developments. Participants involved in this discussion include the patient, family, surgeon, primary physician, anesthesia providers, and others who are closely involved in the care of the patient. Specific discussion should clarify all possible scenarios in the perioperative period and exactly what DNR means in those circumstances. These responses should then be documented. Health care providers should have the option to withdraw from a case and find a replacement if they are uncomfortable with the extent of DNR orders (Lewis, 1996). Finally, anesthesia departments must have a clear policy statement on how to manage DNR orders on patients undergoing anesthesia and surgery. This considers and respects both the patient's rights to make end of life decisions and the moral, ethical, and professional rights of the anesthesia provider (AANA, 1994).

When a patient who is a Jehovah's Witness undergoes an anesthetic and surgery, there should be clear documentation of the extent to which the patient's wishes transfusion of blood or blood products under life-threatening conditions. Modell, Layon, and Modell (1994) state that in instances where the patient is a child, parents need to be extremely well informed about all perioperative possibilities and that transfusion therapy could occur in the event of a life-threatening hemorrhage.

The authors continue by stating that a court order for transfusion therapy for a child could be obtained if time allows. However, in the author's view, this kind of legal intervention is rarely required if there is good communication between all parties. These types of situations highlight the importance of having clear policy statements within anesthesiology departments about how to manage these special patient care circumstances. In all cases, the family's wishes should be noted on the patient's record and witnessed by another competent, licensed individual.

The acuity of patients presenting for anesthesia and surgery is ever increasing. Because of the severity of illness sometimes seen in hospitalized or emergency room patients, the possibilities for anesthetist involvement in life-threatening situations occurs more frequently. In these emergent cases, it can be difficult for the anesthesia provider to chart in a consistent and accurate fashion the multitude of interventions taking place. It is imperative when emergencies arise, and especially when these events become prolonged, that a person be assigned whose sole function is to document all activities and interventions that take place. The charting of time, vital signs taken, medications administered, and therapeutic measures initiated can help the anesthetist significantly in capturing data and events that are as nearly accurate as possible for the anesthesia record or progress note. All names of members involved in the emergency, patient responses, and disposition of the patient must be noted on the record as well.

Philipsen and McMullen (1993) state that unusual circumstances can happen to patients and these must be documented on patient records. However, if an incident report is written, the fact that this note has been written should not be referred to in patient charting. These authors further state that incident reports are designed and intended to improve quality within an institution rather than to communicate the needs of a patient. An incident report that is referred to in patient charting becomes part of the patient's permanent medical record and not just part of the institution's quality assurance program. This documentation then, becomes an official document and is admissible in courts, along with the patient's other records.

Milstead and Rodriguez-Fisher (1992) comment on personal notes that are kept by some clinicians about specific patients. They state that clinicians must remember that personally kept notes may be subject to subpoenas and used as evidence if litigation occurs. Personal notes should not read differently from what is already written in the patient's record.

▶ LEGAL ASPECTS OF CHARTING

The charting of anesthesia care follows all the rules and dictates that govern documentation in all other clinical areas. In addition, an anesthetic record should be prepared in such a manner that anyone at a later time can reconstruct exactly what occurred during the administration of the anesthetic. If any element is omitted or documented in a haphazard manner, then the events that took place become tainted and any later attempt at reconstruction becomes difficult or impossible (Markarian, 1991).

If legal questions arise concerning care, an anesthetic record is admissible in court as evidence demonstrating the kind, standard, or quality of care delivered. Although accurate and complete documentation does not prevent anesthetic complications or potential legal concerns, it can help minimize the discussion surrounding the appropriateness of anesthesia management or compliance with nationally accepted standards of care. In addition, thorough and complete records assist in the recall of events in the event of litigation. A summary of legal aspects of clinical documentation is listed in Table 33–4. Further legal ramifications are discussed in Chapter 3.

In addition, narrative charting should be clear, concise, factual, and objective. Comments should not be conclusory or give vague suggestion. Examples given by Philipsen and McMullen (1993) include stating "200 mL of emesis," rather than "moderate amount." Also, "crying on admission to the OR," rather than "appears depressed."

Mastropietro and Bruton-Maree (1994) cite additional aspects of anesthesia records that require special clarification. If pertinent information is not present on the anesthesia record, there must be statements to ex-

TABLE 33–4. Summary of Legal Aspects of Charting

Never alter or falsify a record

If errors are made in charting, draw one line through it, initial, and make the correction

Never use white-out or paste a sticker over an error

Document in clear, chronological order

If back charting is necessary, place a late note and designate this as a late entry

Do not leave gaps in the narrative section

Make statements that are objective and factual

Use proper spelling

Make entries legible

Use language and abbreviations that are accepted and accurate

Explain omissions in anesthesia record (ie, preanesthetic evaluations)

Denote where important data can be found if not directly on the record (ie, lab, x-ray)

State rationale for blood transfusions when administered

Chart unit donor numbers and time and amount of transfusions

Chart laboratory data determined during anesthetic administrations

Document reasons for administering nonroutine medications

Always sign your legal name and title

plain reasons for omission and where the information can be found. These include reports of pertinent X-rays, consultations, or laboratory data. Medications that are given without a clear rationale must also be explained. Examples include the use of intravenous lidocaine for suppressing laryngeal reflexes or labetalol for treating hypertension. If a medication is given or an action is taken as a result of a directive from a physician, then that physician's name must be included in the record.

Finally, documentation regarding the termination of anesthesia is just as important as preoperative activities. There should be clear notation about the termination of gases and agents, actions taken to reverse, awakening the patient, and remarks about the stability, safety, and transfer of care to postanesthesia personnel. Any postanesthetic actions taken after the patient is assigned to the PACU also should be documented to provide evidence of adequate evaluation of the perioperative course.

► COMPUTERIZATION OF ANESTHESIA CARE DOCUMENTATION

Systems that automate recordkeeping and use anesthesia information management databases will become important in the future. To put these topics into appropriate context, it is important to discuss automated recordkeeping in its current application within anesthesia and the scope of information management systems, including their potential effects on the anesthesia provider.

Much of the anesthesia community still uses manual anesthesia records. Some departments do employ full computerized documentation and fully integrated information systems in all phases of anesthesia care, but they are not standard. However, the acceptance of these new technologies in business and industry indicates that it is only a matter of time before the anesthesia profession becomes comprehensively involved in similar technologic developments.

Merritt (1995) states that some practitioners still prefer the written record in anesthesia care. The reasons given are that manual records are simple to use, easy to learn, easy to chart on, permit individual variation in writing style, take up little space in the anesthetic workspace, are low in maintenance, inexpensive, and user-friendly. However, the number of advocates promoting computerized recordkeeping is growing, and the rationale for maintaining the handwritten record in an information age is declining. Smith and Gravenstein (1993) summarize some of the common concerns surrounding the manual anesthesia record in Table 33-5.

Two common phenomena that occur easily with manual charting and contribute greatly to the artifactual nature of handwritten records are "batch recording" and "smoothing." Batch recording occurs when no recording

TABLE 33–5. Issues Concerning the Manual Anesthetic Record

Manual recordings may be unreadable or illegible

Information may be incompletely or inaccurately recorded

Manual recordings take 10% to 15% of total anesthesia time; the more monitors used in anesthesia care, the more time spent in charting

Batch recording easily occurs

Phenomenon of smoothing can occur

Use of abbreviations, symbols, and other notations may be inconsistent

Manual records can get soiled during anesthetics

Manual records can get lost or misplaced

is done during critical moments spent with the patient and subsequent recording occurs in catch-up fashion, after the fact, and in "batches." When this happens, it may be difficult to record everything that has happened accurately, especially if multiple events have occurred or several monitors are used. Still, monitors that record patients' vital signs and other hemodynamic data do help significantly in transferring information to the manual record. However, the integration of these data on to one dedicated intraanesthetic form is generally left to the provider.

Smoothing occurs when selective manual recording every 5 minutes removes the true variability of instant data recording. Smoothing tends to record high heart rates and high blood pressures at lower values while low heart rates and low blood pressures tend to be recorded at higher values. Values that tend toward normal reveal less smoothing with manual charting.

Merritt (1995) states that anesthesia records can become easily soiled during surgery. This is increasingly important in an era when vigilance about infection control is critical and universal precautions in the care of all patients is mandatory. Soiled manual records can be difficult to review, not only during medico-legal proceedings, but also when data tracking and utilization reviews of personnel, equipment, and pharmaceuticals is required.

Manual charts can get lost or misplaced, and this can create gaps in the evaluation and continuity of patient care, particularly in patients who have long-term chronic illnesses. These situations can result in loss of time and personnel and can increase the costs of care as well as create undue hardships for patients when procedures and tests must be repeated. In addition, unspecified costs are incurred when there is inability to decipher important information about patients in handwritten charts. Finally, the financial implications of information not applied or used to its fullest potential is not cost-effective. As the health care sector continues to feel the pressures to improve efficiency, increase quality, and streamline costs, the dilemma to resolve many of these concerns with new and evolving anesthesia information management systems will be greatly enhanced.

Two studies have confirmed the advantages of automated recordkeeping in anesthesia. In 1992, Edsall, Jones, and Smith found that computerized anesthesia information management systems used in a community hospital setting did not complicate the anesthesia working environment, but, rather, showed that recordkeeping took less time and produced higher-quality anesthesia records. Supporting these findings, Coleman, Moyer, Sanderson, Gilbert, and Sibert (1995) surveyed anesthesia personnel in a major university medical center 2 years after an anesthesia information management system was introduced. This survey found that 89% of respondents favored the automated system over a manual system of recordkeeping. This preference increased to 97% when the complexity of care increased, as in major trauma or emergency cases. Smith and Gravenstein (1993) have summarized the major advantages in using automated recordkeeping in Table 33–6.

The greatest concerns about the use of computerized recordkeeping in anesthesia appear to center around liability, cost, and confidentiality. The potential liability question is posed by the capturing and recording of artifact on permanent patient anesthesia records. Some practitioners feel that records showing artifactual data may be interpreted as poor-practice patterns by a medical or legal examiner. Merritt (1995) counters that much artifact is nonphysiological and with critical review, there should be little confusion to what artifact truly is. Furthermore he adds that the written record, our "gold standard," in anesthesia is almost entirely artifactual because of smoothing and batch recording.

Other concerns that have been raised about automated recordkeeping include the high costs of these technologies, the costs of training, teaching, and learning computerized recordkeeping systems, the addition of more items into an already tight anesthesia workspace, and the dilemma of what to do with data that are not used. Concerns relative to confidentiality involve who owns recorded data and who can access, retrieve, and utilize the data (Edsall et al., 1992). These and other questions will continue to be debated as various information management systems are developed and introduced commercially.

▶ FUTURE USES OF ANESTHESIA INFORMATION MANAGEMENT SYSTEMS

Merritt (1995) comments that the acquisition of raw data in manual recordkeeping reveals little about the patterns of care, the uses of drugs, supplies, and equipment, or ways in which cost outcomes can be maximized. He states that, as the practice of anesthesia is examined, many areas of care will be probed for insights into how overall care can be improved, money can be saved, and efficiencies can be optimized. Merritt further adds that the computerization of anesthesia recordkeeping can give the anesthesia community an opportunity to document the care it provides and analyze the processes of that care to improve patient outcomes.

In 1992 Edsall et al. stated that the greatest potential of anesthesia information management systems lies in its ability to generate useful reports that could answer almost any question asked by providers; questions related to equipment and drug utilization, anesthesia care outcomes, clinical benchmarks, and personnel utilization, just to name a few. They further stated that, until this stage is reached, the value of computerized anesthesia information systems will not be fully realized. Pettus (1995) concurred with these statements and added that anesthesia information management systems could greatly benefit a technology-intensive specialty such as anesthesia care.

Lagasse (1996) found that one of the greatest values of anesthesia information management systems was in its ability to generate data bases that could allow a true look at technology in anesthesia. He believed that monitoring technologies in anesthesia have been advancing at a rate that far exceeds our abilities to assess their effectiveness.

TABLE 33–6. Advantages of Computerized Anesthesia Records

Automatic recording of vital signs and other anesthetic variables maintains continuity in documentation even during emergencies

Records are more accurate, complete, and legible

There is more opportunity for data input

Preconfiguration of a computerized database allows documentation of more events and more rapid recording of those events

Computerized entry and access can be accomplished rapidly and easily

There is more real-time entry of data

Less time can be spent on recording, which increases time spent directly with patients

Pertinent anesthetic information can be placed and viewed on one centralized display

Anesthesia information can be stored and integrated with other clinical data

Integrated systems allow information to be retrieved from other areas for more rapid review

Voice feedback mechanisms on automated systems can provide regular reminders, alerts, or alarms

Computerized systems allow data retrieval for statistics development and inventory management

Medical legal credibility of records can be increased

Data can be easily accessed for future quality assurance or outcome management studies

Opportunities for compiling adequate and more valid data for education and research are enhanced

Furthermore, he added that using good information management and informative data bases could allow monitoring devices to undergo a serious and formal process of technologic assessment before being adopted into clinical practice. The ability to develop data bases and conduct large-scale studies from routine practice settings could lead to better methods of comparing outcome indicators on a much wider basis than before. Data from multiple institutions could then be combined into a national data base when uniform standards are developed. These national data bases, in turn, could allow departments to compare their outcomes to those of the rest of the country. These kinds of data could further lead to clinical benchmarking, best practices, and clinical care guidelines that could ultimately contribute to patient care improvements.

▶ CASE STUDY

A 3-year-old boy is admitted to the same-day surgery center for bilateral myringotomy with insertion of tubes. He has no significant medical history, has never been hospitalized before, and first presents for his preanesthetic evaluation prior to surgery scheduled for the same day.

1. What information should be documented during the preanesthetic evaluation?

   The patient has no significant medical history nor any previous surgeries or anesthetics, so the preanesthetic evaluation should reflect this negative history. Any family history of allergies or reactions to anesthetics should be documented. Any medications taken and loose teeth should be noted. The patient's demographic data (age, height, and weight) are recorded. The anesthetist should perform a physical exam appropriate for the procedure and document the heart and lung examination, airway assessment, including range of motion of neck and head and vital sign measurements. Any appropriate laboratory data should be reviewed and/or ordered. The ASA classification should be assigned, and the type of anesthetic and risks should be discussed with the parent and the child. An informed consent for anesthesia must be obtained from the parent. If a separate anesthesia consent form is not utilized, a note can be written in the progress notes and the parent can sign affirming that an informed consent has been given. During the preanesthetic assessment patient education, instructions and counseling should be conducted and documented.

   The inhalation anesthesia induction with halothane proceeds without incident and an oral airway is inserted for the brief case. Ventilation is maintained via a face mask, respirations are assisted, and the patient receives halothane 1%, nitrous oxide 60%, oxygen 40%. Shortly after the surgeon begins the procedure, the oxygen saturation drops to 85%. The surgeon stops operating and the oral airway is readjusted, improving the oxygen saturation to 99%. The surgery is resumed and completed within 10 minutes. The vital signs remained stable throughout the procedure. The anesthetic is discontinued. The child awakens, the airway is removed. He is placed on his side and taken to the PACU where his admission vital signs are BP: 100/65; pulse: 116; respirations: 22; and oxygen saturation: 100% (on facemask oxygen).

2. The anesthetist has documented all anesthetic agents, vital signs, monitoring equipment (including preanesthetic equipment check), anesthesia and surgery "times," oxygen saturation, end-tidal carbon dioxide monitoring, and heart rhythm as measured on the ECG. What additional information should be documented during the intraanesthetic period?

   The patient's preanesthetic psychological state and any premedication given should be documented. The type of induction performed and size of airway inserted should be described. The patient positioning, including the placement of rolls or padding, eye care, and ausculation of breath sounds are recorded. The inspired oxygen concentration (F_{IO_2}) delivered from the anesthesia machine should always be noted on a continuum throughout the graphic part of the anesthesia record. This records the percentage of oxygen being delivered to the patient. The respiratory volumes of the patient should be recorded in a timely sequence. The repositioning of the airway that resulted in improved oxygen saturation should be noted and the time this was done should be recorded. The emergence from anesthesia should be described and the patient's condition upon arrival in the PACU, including vital signs and level of consciousness, should be recorded.

3. During the intraanesthetic portion of the graphic record, the anesthetist wrote the name of a medication not given after realizing that it had been drawn up but never administered. How should the charting error be handled?

   The anesthetist should draw one line through the error, initial it, and write in the correct drug name if another drug was given. If no other medication was given, just correct the error as previously described.

4. The anesthetist's signature reads "WRW." Is this the correct way to sign an anesthesia record?

   No, the anesthetist should always sign his or her legal name and title.

► SUMMARY

Gunn (1992) states that the anesthesia provider's expertise in anesthesia care documentation lies in knowing how and when to document. Complete and accurate charting must always reflect actual patient care findings, events, and interventions that are appropriate, reasonable, and in time sequence. She further adds that anesthesia care must be defensible from the standpoint of quality and the provider must be willing to be held accountable for the care that is provided and documented. With the advent of information technology and anesthesia information management systems, documentation of care will continue to be a valuable source for improving the care that is provided to all patients now and in the future. Documentation of care that is given is the most important and essential component done for patients, next to the care itself.

► KEY CONCEPTS

- The anesthetic record must provide sufficient data to allow an accurate reconstruction of events during the administration of anesthesia.
- Anesthesia care documentation includes the preanesthetic assessment, the patient's vital signs and physiologic responses to the anesthetic, intraoperative treatments imposed, complications encountered, and events of the postanesthetic course.
- The mechanics of performing a preanesthetic evaluation varies among institutions. However, obtaining pertinent information about the patient's history, presenting complaint, and planned therapies allows the anesthetist to develop an optimal plan of anesthesia care.
- Documentation of care for the obstetric patient should not differ from the care given any surgical patient and should reflect the same level of vigilance and standard of practice.

- The legal aspects of recordkeeping for anesthesia care follows the same rules and dictates for legibility, accuracy, and completeness as charting in any other clinical area.
- The emergence of anesthesia information management systems creates possibilities for improving all aspects of anesthesia care including, direct patient care by setting uniform patient and provider outcomes, improving utilization and efficiencies of anesthesia care technologies, setting high clinical standards and benchmarks, developing databases that allow ease of access of patient information, developing optimal care strategies, and identifying new avenues of research.
- From a legal perspective, the only clear proof of the quality of care provided to the patient is the evidence contained on the anesthetic record and patient chart.

► STUDY QUESTIONS

1. List all the important pieces of information that must be gathered about a patient before developing an anesthesia management plan.

2. List the key phases of intraanesthetic care and the important items to be documented on the anesthesia record.

3. Review the care of the obstetric patient and how this does or does not differ from the care of a surgical patient.

4. List all the important and specific aspects of legally defensible charting on the anesthesia record.

5. Summarize five possibilities for anesthesia information management systems in optimizing anesthesia care and delivery in the future.

KEY REFERENCES

American Association of Nurse Anesthetists. (1996). *Professional Practice Manual for the Certified Registered Nurse Anesthetist.* Park Ridge, IL: Author.

American Association of Nurse Anesthetists. (1991). *Guidelines for obstetrical anesthesia and conduction analgesia for the certified registered nurse anesthetist.* Park Ridge, IL: Author.

American Association of Nurse Anesthetists. (1992). *Postanesthesia care standards for the certified registered nurse anesthetist.* Park Ridge, IL: Author.

Gunn, I. P (1992). Documentation of anesthesia care. In W. R. Waugaman, S. D. Foster, & B. M. Rigor (Eds.), *Principles and practice of nurse anesthesia* (2nd ed., pp. 27–37). Norwalk, CT: Appleton & Lange.

Markarian, C. J. (1991). The anesthesia record. In W. H. Dornette (Ed.), *Legal issues in anesthesia care* (pp. 93–109). Philadelphia: F. A. Davis.

Mastropietro, C. A., & Bruton-Maree, N. (1994). In S. D. Foster, & L. M. Jordan (Eds.), *Professional aspects of nurse anesthesia* (pp. 251–271). Philadelphia: F. A. Davis.

REFERENCES

American Association of Nurse Anesthetists. (1991). *Guidelines for obstetrical anesthesia and conduction analgesia for the certified registered nurse anesthetist.* Park Ridge, IL: Author.

American Association of Nurse Anesthetists. (1992). *Postanesthesia care standards for the certified registered nurse anesthetist.* Park Ridge, IL: Author.

American Association of Nurse Anesthetists. (1994). *Considerations for development of an anesthesia department policy on do-not-resuscitate orders* (No. 4.1). Park Ridge, IL: Author.

American Association of Nurse Anesthetists. (1996). *Professional Practice Manual for the Certified Registered Nurse Anesthetist.* Park Ridge, IL: Author.

Coleman, R. L., Moyer, G. A., Sanderson, I. C., Gilbert, W. C., & Sibert, K. S. (1995). Satisfaction after the installation of an automatic anesthesia record keeping system in an academic anesthesia department (STA Abstract). *Journal of Clinical Monitoring, 4*(11), 274.

Edsall, D. W., Jones, B. R., & Smith, N. T. (1992). The anesthesia database, the automated record, and the quality assurance process. In T. Vitez, (Ed.), *International anesthesiology clinics: Quality improvement systems* (pp. 71–92). Philadelphia: Saunders.

Gunn, I. P. (1992). Documentation of anesthesia care. In W. R. Waugaman, S. D. Foster, & B. M. Rigor (Eds.), *Principles and practice of nurse anesthesia* (2nd ed., pp. 27–37). Norwalk, CT: Appleton & Lange.

Lagasse, R. S. (1996). Monitoring and analysis of outcome studies. In J. S. Vender (Ed.), *International anesthesiology clinics—Clinical monitoring* (pp. 263–277).

Lewis, S. (1996). DNR means "Do Not Relax" to avoid liability. *Anesthesia Malpractice Prevention 1*(1), pp. 1–3.

Markarian, C. J. (1991). The anesthesia record. In W. H. Dornette (Ed.), *Legal issues in anesthesia care* (pp. 93–109). Philadelphia: F. A. Davis.

Mastropietro, C. A., & Bruton-Maree, N. (1994). In S. D. Foster, & L. M. Jordan (Eds.), *Professional aspects of nurse anesthesia* (pp. 251–271). Philadelphia: F. A. Davis.

Merritt, W. T. (1995). Automation and anesthesia information management. In C. D Blitt & R. L. Hines (Eds.), *Monitoring in anesthesia and critical care medicine* (pp. 617–642). New York: Churchill Livingstone.

Milstead, J. A. & Rodriguez-Fisher, L. (1992, August). Legally, defensible, effective charting. *Critical Care Nurse,* 103–105.

Modell, J. H., Layon, A. J., & Modell, C. S. (1994). Ethical and legal concepts. In R. D. Miller (Ed.), *Anesthesia* (4th ed., pp. 2579–2602). New York: Churchill Livingstone.

Pettus, D. C. (1995). An automated information management system can produce ROI and improve anesthesia practice (STA Abstract). *Journal of Clinical Monitoring, 4*(11), 267.

Philipsen, N., & McMullen, P. (1993). Charting basics 101. *Nursing Connections, 3*(6), 62–64.

Smith, N. T. & Gravenstein, J. S. (1993). Manual and automated anesthesia management systems. In L. J. Saidman, & N. T. Smith (Eds.), *Monitoring in anesthesia* (3rd ed., pp. 575–590). New York: John Wiley & Sons.

Anesthetic Complications

Lucille Y. Osaki

The adage "do no harm" is the consummate goal of any health professional who provides patient care. As anesthetists, we deliberately manipulate the physiologic equilibrium of every patient whenever anesthetics or pharmacologic agents are administered. Although the premise of anesthesia practice is to safely establish and maintain optimal conditions of unconsciousness, amnesia, analgesia, anesthesia, and muscle relaxation, anticipated, as well as unanticipated disruptions in physiologic states do occur. Fortunately, many of the accidental or provocational events that happen are transient and have negligible effects on patient outcome. Still, there are those less frequently reported incidents, some with life-threatening potential, which are attributable to the anesthetic itself or provider error. The goal of this chapter is to expose the anesthesia practitioner to common clinical problems attendant to the administration of anesthesia: pharmacologically induced, surgical or mechanical-type, and patient-related complications.

Certain concepts presented here are unquestionably rare in occurrence. Nonetheless, all anesthetists, including the novice, must be prepared to recognize any given problem that can arise at any point along the anesthesia continuum, perform a systematic differential diagnosis, and treat the situation as expeditiously and appropriately as possible. Of all the anesthesia cases encountered, 99% will be uncomplicated and routinely managed. It is the remaining 1% that will test one's preparedness for unexpected events, challenge the anesthetist's ability to correct the ensuing chain of events, and minimize patient morbidity and mortality.

▶ PATHOPHYSIOLOGIC RESPONSES TO ANESTHESIA

Unexpected complications may occur following delivery of a pharmacologic agent or a routine anesthetic procedure. The observed variability in patient reaction may be linked to individual differences in biochemical sensitivities and physiologic conditions. For instance, following traumatic extubation, the development of negative-pressure pulmonary edema (NPPE) in otherwise young healthy patients is not always a predictable or avoidable event. Nevertheless, through awareness of potential anesthetic complications such as NPPE and symptom recognition, appropriate treatment measures can be implemented to attenuate morbidity.

Pulmonary Aspiration

Active vomiting or passive gastroesophageal reflux (GER) results in oropharyngeal pooling of gastric contents that can lead to tracheal aspiration in the unprotected airway. Studies of adult patients undergoing elective and emergent surgical procedures suggest that the incidence of clinically significant pulmonary aspiration is 1 in 3 216 anesthetics with an overall mortality of 1 in 71 829 (Chadwick, Posner, Caplan, Ward, & Cheney, 1991; Warner, Warner, & Weber, 1993). Although the number of pulmonary aspiration is seemingly rare, the true incidence may be higher than figures published in the literature. According to Illing, Duncan, & Yip (1992), 48% of patients who presumably aspirate often are clinically asymptomatic.

Traditionally, patients considered to be at risk for pulmonary aspiration are those patients with gastroesophageal sphincter incompetence and/or increased gastric pressures (Table 34–1). Gastroesophageal valve function may be affected by abnormal anatomy and pharmacologic agents, such as metoclopramide, whereas increased gastric pressures can be magnified by conditions associated with a delayed emptying of stomach contents, pregnancy, intraoperative body positioning, and gastrointestinal obstruction. Currently, however, it is unclear whether regurgitation of gastric contents may be more likely to occur in nonelective conditions necessitating specialized anesthetic management, such as emergency cases, the critically ill, patients with difficult airways, or on predictive patient characteristics (Illing, Duncan, & Yi, 1992). Although GER tends to occur during induction and emergence, rapid-sequence induction, antiemetics, and antacids are utilized as conventional prophylaxis to guard against aspiration pneumonitis. Nevertheless, GER is still possible during the intraoperative period.

The severity of pulmonary injury depends on the volume and pH of the aspirate as well as the presence of bacteria-contaminated material. Generally, chemical pneumonitis is unlikely to occur if the aspirate is less than 25 mL and has a measured pH greater than 2.5. Recognition of this complication is based on the witnessed event. Subsequently, symptom development evolves rapidly, typically within 2 hours, and the earliest signs of aspiration are tachypnea, tachycardia, and hypoxemia (Gwirtz, 1996). Impaired oxygenation due to intrapulmonary shunting and altered diffusion gradients may be reflected in a lowered arterial hemoglobin oxygen saturation despite the use of supplemental oxygen. Coughing, wheezing, and rales may be present. Bronchospasm is possible and acute respiratory distress syndrome (ARDS) may occur in the more serious cases. Radiographic changes will be detectable on chest x-rays, the right side being more affected because of the angulation of the right mainstem bronchus, although abnormalities may not become apparent for several hours.

TABLE 34–1. Conditions That May Predispose to Pulmonary Aspiration

---

Gastrointestinal obstruction

Emergency surgery

Increasing ASA physical status

Difficult upper airway

Recent solid-food intake

Abdominal distension (obesity, pregnancy, ascites)

Depressed level of consciousness

Diabetes mellitus (?)

From Stoelting, R. K. (1995). NPO—Facts and fictions. IARS 1995 Review Course Lectures. Anesthesia & Analgesia, 80(Suppl.), 1. Reprinted with permission.

Treatment for clinically significant pulmonary pneumonitis includes vigorous measures for protecting and maintaining the airway. Immediate oropharyngeal suctioning should be performed and tracheal saline lavage considered, especially if particulate matter is observed. Fiberoptic bronchoscopy may be indicated when aspirated material is obstructing the airways. Because of the high mortality rate associated with severe pulmonary aspiration, the patient with stained cords should be promptly intubated, mechanically ventilated with positive end-expiratory pressure (PEEP), and provided appropriate cardiopulmonary support. Steroids are no longer routinely administered and antibiotics are generally withheld until positive culture results are obtained.

Laryngospasm

An important function of the larynx is to reflexively protect the airway by preventing secretions, foreign bodies, and noxious fumes from reaching the lung fields. However, an abnormal and potentially life-threatening laryngeal constriction, termed *laryngospasm,* may occur as a result of light planes of anesthesia, upper-airway surgeries, direct instrumentation, and/or bloody secretions around the vocal cords, and certain volatile gases known to sensitize the airways (Rex, 1970). Laryngospasm postendotracheal extubation produces a sustained closure of the glottis by forceful contraction of the laryngeal musculature and adduction of the vocal cords. This complex laryngeal reflex is especially common among the pediatric population from heightened airway reactivity due to upper-respiratory tract infections or light planes of anesthesia (Young & Skinner, 1995).

During laryngospasm, manual bag and mask ventilation of the patient's airway will be difficult because of upper-airway obstruction. A high-pitched crowing sound may sometimes be audible. Once identified, prompt treatment measures must be undertaken to prevent the development of further complications, such as NPPE and hypoxemia. Usually, laryngospasm can be relieved by delivering gentle positive-pressure mask ventilation with 100% oxygen. Alternatively, intravenous lidocaine (0.5–1 mg/kg) deepens the stage of anesthesia, and small doses of succinylcholine (20–30 mg) have been effective in sufficiently relaxing the laryngeal muscles to reestablish airway patency (Miller, Harkin, & Bailey, 1995).

Bronchospasm

Bronchospasm is a hyperresponsive reflex mechanism often associated with individuals who have reactive airway disease, such as asthma. These patients tend to have an exaggerated respiratory response to various stimuli that result in severe bronchoconstriction of the upper and peripheral airways.

The mechanism underlying airway hyperreactivity appears to be an imbalance in autonomic control of the airways. Although it is unclear which system plays the more dominant role, there is either a relative increase in parasympathetic tone or diminished sympathetic tone that results in airway constriction (Gal, 1996). The sympathetic system produces bronchodilation via stimulation of beta$_2$-receptors by circulating catecholamines. The neurally controlled parasympathetic system is intimately linked to one of several types of sensory receptors that line the mucosa of cartilaginous airways, trachea, and carina. Airway caliber of bronchial smooth muscle is affected by various sensory receptor stimulants. Triggering factors include inhalational and mechanical stimulants to the airway, light anesthesia, and allergenic responses (eg, histamine).

Preoperative identification of patients at risk for bronchospasm and efforts to optimize their pulmonary function are the most effective approaches in avoiding this complication. Patients who present with upper-respiratory infections are at increased risk for airway hyperreactivity. The traditional advice of having active smokers abstain during the preoperative period (48 to 72 hours) to improve postoperative outcome may actually result in increased mucous production (Pearce & Jones, 1984). Generally, the risk-to-benefit ratio for smoking cessation requires several weeks. Whenever possible, regional anesthesia should be considered the technique of choice to avoid airway instrumentation, especially in susceptible patients.

Intraoperative bronchospasm usually is accompanied by a sudden rise in peak inspiratory pressure and a drop in oxygen saturation. However, other conditions can mimic these complications and must be ruled out (Table 34–2). One should first ascertain that wheezing and oxygen desaturation are not the result of endotracheal tube (ETT) misplacement, such as carinal irritation by the ETT tip or endobronchial migration. Bronchospasm can be obviated by increasing the anesthetic depth and the concentration of the volatile agent. In treating hypoxemia, nitrous oxide should be discontinued and the oxygen concentration increased to 100%.

TABLE 34–2. Conditions Confused with Bronchospasm during General Anesthesia

Endobronchial intubation

Persistent coughing and straining

Mechanical obstruction of the endotracheal tube

Pulmonary edema

Tension pneumothorax

Pulmonary aspiration of gastric contents

Pulmonary embolism

From Gal, T. J. (1996). Bronchial hyperresponsiveness and the patient for anesthesia. IARS 1996 Review Course Lectures. Anesthesia & Analgesia, 82(Suppl.), 42. Reprinted with permission.

Because coughing and straining on the endotracheal tube can raise inspiratory pressures (PIP) substantially, complete muscle relaxation should be verified. Finally, selective beta$_2$-agonists (eg, albuterol), administered as metered aerosol puffs directly into the endotracheal tube and/or terbutaline 0.25 mg, subcutaneously often are effective for eliciting rapid bronchodilatation.

For known asthmatics, the first line of treatment is 0.1% epinephrine, 0.1 to 0.5 mg, subcutaneously. Extubating the patient at deep surgical planes of anesthesia is a controversial technique for avoiding bronchospasm; however, there is insufficient clinical support to substantiate any real risk-to-benefit ratio (Miller, Harkin, & Bailey, 1995).

Allergic Reactions

Although allergic reactions are differentiated as anaphylactic or Type I (immunologic or mediated by IgE) or anaphylactoid or Type II (chemically mediated), the constellation of symptoms produced by either mechanism is clinically indistinguishable (Goldberg, 1996). In Type I reactions, the allergen binds with IgE antibodies on the cell surface of mast cells and basophils. Subsequent degranulation of these cellular elements results in the release of vasoactive substances such as prostaglandins, leukotrienes, and histamine. In a cascading effect, many of these mediators stimulate other pathways, such as the complement system, which provokes an inflammatory process associated with increased patient morbidity and mortality. In contradistinction, anaphylactoid events are not associated with immunoglobins or sensitization to a prior offending agent. In Type II reactions, there is direct release of mediators, of which histamine is the most clinically significant and the probable basis for most allergic responses seen in anesthesia (Moss, 1995).

Allergic reactions are acute and potentially fatal occurrences involving multiple organ systems and can result in hypotension, urticaria, dysrhythmias, cutaneous flushing, airway swelling, and bronchospasm. The majority of factors associated with Type I and Type II reactions include many standard anesthetic and pharmacologic agents (Table 34–3). Furthermore, mild allergic symptoms can be provoked by the customary and inadvisable practice of rapid intravenous drug boluses.

In the event that an allergic reaction occurs, primary treatment is supportive (Table 34–4). Efforts should be made immediately to discontinue the offending allergen and sustain respiratory and hemodynamic stability. Because of their antiinflammatory activity, steroids may be helpful, although the onset of action will not be immediate. Bronchodilators are considered useful adjuncts only if bronchospasm develops.

TABLE 34–3. Substances with Allergenic Potential

> Thiopental
> Muscle relaxants
> Protamine
> Antibiotics (penicillin, vancomycin, cephalosporins)
> Methylmethacrylate
> Latex
> Narcotics
> PABA, methylparaben preservatives
> Dextran (high molecular weight)

Hypercarbia and Hypocarbia

The use of capnography during anesthesia has enabled anesthesia providers to monitor extremes of end-tidal carbon dioxide ($ETCO_2$) levels during anesthetic management. Neither hypercarbia nor hypocarbia are benign conditions: They can affect multiple organ systems in adverse ways. An arterial partial pressure of CO_2 ($Paco_2$) greater than 45 mmHg is considered hypercarbic, and hypocarbia is defined when $Paco_2$ is less than 35 mmHg. Generally, the $ETCO_2$ value is 5 to 6 mmHg less than the actual $Paco_2$ measured because of dead-space ventilation.

TABLE 34–4. Treatment of Anaphylactic Reactions Occurring During Anesthesia

Primary Measures
1. Stop administration of antigen
2. Maintain airway; administer 100% oxygen
3. Discontinue anesthesia
4. Institute rapid intravascular volume expansion: crystalloid 2–4 L to help maintain blood pressure
5. Epinephrine 3–8 μg/kg, intravenous bolus, with dose adjusted to degree of hypotension

Additional considerations for intravenous medication (depending on signs and symptoms)

1. Aminophylline 5–6 mg/kg over 20-min period (loading dose); then 0.5–0.9 mg/kg/h infusion (maintenance dose), with dosage reduced 50% in patients with cardiac or renal failure
2. Epinephrine 1–4 μg/min, norepinephrine 2–4 μg/min, or isoproterenol 0.5–1 μg/min, adjusted to degree of hypotension
3. Hydrocortisone 0.25–1 g, methylprednisolone 0.1–1 g, or dexamethasone 4–20 mg, all intravenously
4. Diphenhydramine 25–50 mg intravenously
5. Atropine 0.5–2 mg intravenously

From Goldberg, M. (1996). Treatment of anaphylactic reactions occurring during anesthesia. In N. Gravenstein & R. R. Kirby (Eds.), Complications in anesthesiology (2nd ed., p. 616). Philadelphia: Lippincott-Raven. Reprinted with permission.

There are myriad conditions responsible for producing hypercarbic states intraoperatively (Table 34–5). Hypermetabolic states, laparoscopic procedures, and intravenous sodium bicarbonate are the more frequent causes for observed increases in $ETCO_2$ over 45 mmHg. However, by accelerating minute ventilation, $ETCO_2$ levels can be easily adjusted to fall within physiologic parameters. Ophthalmologic procedures that involve monitored anesthesia care (MAC) often predispose the patient to rebreathing of CO_2 when surgical drapes create a closed-chamber effect. A reliable suction apparatus positioned under the drapes will usually prevent CO_2 buildup. Any persistent and/or rapid increase in $ETCO_2$ should alert the practitioner to the potential for malignant hyperthermia.

In the postoperative spontaneously breathing patient, ventilatory drive from CO_2 may be altered by residual sedative-hypnotics, nondepolarizing muscle relaxants and opioids (Rose, Cohen, Wigglesworth, DeBoer, & Math, 1994). Subsequently, higher levels of $Paco_2$ are required to overcome the apneic threshold. Typically, the observed patient response is somnolence with hypoventilation. The rising $Paco_2$ activates the sympathetic nervous system which produces tachycardia and vasoconstriction. Generally, as $Paco_2$ levels approach 90 mmHg, which may happen in patients with chronic obstructive pulmonary disease (COPD), a state of narcosis will ensue with eventual progression to cardiovascular collapse.

Hypocarbic states under anesthesia can result from incorrect parameter settings of minute ventilation during positive-pressure ventilation or settings deliberately altered for managing certain neurosurgical procedures. With increases in minute ventilation, cardiac output diminishes and hypotension will develop as venous return is compromised. In addition, with induced respiratory alkalosis, there is increased protein binding of ionized calcium, which may cause a negative inotropic effect on the myocardium from hypocalcemia. More important, a sustained $Paco_2$ of less than 20 mmHg can cause a critical reduction in cerebral and myocardial blood flow that may lead to ischemia. To maintain normocarbia, the cause for CO_2 imbalance needs to be identified and appropriately treated (Table 34–6).

TABLE 34–5. Factors Contributing to Hypercarbia during Anesthesia

Exhausted carbon dioxide granules
Hypermetabolic states, malignant hyperthermia, sepsis, seizure activity
Sodium bicarbonate administration
Peritoneal insufflation of CO_2 during laparoscopic procedures
Rebreathing of CO_2

TABLE 34–6. Considerations for Managing Hypercarbic States

> Perioperatively
> > Replace canister with fresh CO_2 granules
> > Adjust minute ventilation
> > Adequate ventilation system during MAC cases
> > Treat the underlying cause of hypermetabolism
>
> Postoperatively
> > Optimal pain management
> > Treat "shivering" with low-dose merepidine
> > Reverse residual nondepolarizing muscle relaxants
> > Cautious use of opiate antagonists

Unintentional Hypothermia

Unintentional hypothermia commonly results from exposure to a chilled operating room during anesthesia. The greatest amount of heat loss occurs during the first hour by virtue of skin exposure (radiation) and body contact (conduction) with cold equipment and an unheated surgical environment. General anesthetics and sedative-narcotics aggravate heat loss via vasodilation and impairment of the central thermoregulatory center. Other factors contributing to hypothermia include rapid infusion of cold intravenous solutions, application of surgical scrub preparations to the patient's operative field and the delivery of unhumidified gases to the respiratory tract. Core body temperatures are typically monitored with esophageal and tympanic membrane probes. Temperatures lower than 35°C are considered hypothermic.

The major effects of unintentional hypothermia during the intraoperative period include coagulation disorders involving platelet function, clotting factor enzyme function and fibrinolytic activity whereby the incidence of hemorrhage may be increased (Sessler, 1994). In addition, the blood solubility of volatile gases increases, necessitating a reduction in the minimum alveolar concentration (MAC) of the inhalational agent. Drug metabolism is effectively prolonged as a result of reduced blood flow to the kidneys and liver, so muscle relaxants and other intravenous adjuncts require judicious titration. The autonomic thermoregulatory response to hypothermia produces peripheral vasoconstriction that can be disastrous during plastic surgeries involving free flap muscle transfers.

Postoperatively, the time necessary to restore normothermia is typically prolonged. In addition, studies suggest that hypothermic conditions in the PACU predispose patients to an increased risk of myocardial infarction (Faraday, Rosenfeld, & Herfel, 1995; Frank et al., 1993). Although not always associated with hypothermia, postoperative shivering is a common occurrence

and results in a dramatic 600% increase in oxygen consumption.

The prevention of unintentional hypothermia begins before the patient is transferred to the operating room. Whenever possible, the operating table should be heated with a bed warmer (especially for pediatric and geriatric patients), and conscious efforts should be made to keep patients draped with warmed blankets. For lengthy surgical cases or operative procedures associated with large blood loss, fluid/blood warmers, forced-air heating devices (Bair hugger), humidification devices, and low-flow or closed-circuit anesthesia should be maintained throughout the intraoperative course. To treat postoperative shivering, small doses of intravenous meperidine (20 mg) are usually effective.

Negative-Pressure Pulmonary Edema

Following an acute episode of upper-airway obstruction, negative-pressure pulmonary edema (NPPE) may develop. Negative-pressure pulmonary edema is known to occur in any patient predisposed to developing laryngospasm, but has also been associated with healthy children and young adults with no significant medical history or cardiac disease. Case reports describe the most common triggering event as laryngospasm following endotracheal extubation (Harlow & Ford, 1993; Umbrain & Camu, 1993). As the patient attempts to forcefully inspire against a closed glottis, high negative intrapleural pressures are generated, accompanied by a sudden increase in peripheral venous return. This combination of events provokes a sudden increase in stroke volume to the right side of the heart that rapidly overwhelms pulmonary circulation, resulting in transudation of fluid across the pulmonary arteries and into the central alveoli (Severinghaus, 1996). The onset of this phenomenon occurs within minutes of the obstructive episode, but can be delayed for a few hours (Lang, Duncan, Shepherd, & Hung, 1990). Postoperatively, the typical clinical manifestations include an acute onset of respiratory distress and oxygen desaturation. Arterial blood gas analysis and chest x-ray are confirmatory tests (Cascade, Alexander, & Mackie, 1993).

Treatment is supportive. Diuresis, supplemental oxygen, and fluid restriction often will promptly resolve the short-lived pulmonary edema. Some patients may require reintubation with controlled ventilatory support until symptoms resolve. Measures for avoiding laryngospasm would be equally prudent to prevent triggering this complex phenomenon.

▶ HAZARDS OF ANESTHESIA

During the course of anesthesia, there may be times when problems arise as a direct result of surgical risks, the biochemical makeup of the patient, mechanical failures or accidents, or an omission in application of anesthesia monitoring devices (eg, peripheral nerve stimulator). Unquestionably, total vigilance in monitoring the physiological state of the patient and all activities encompassing the surgical field are cardinal behaviors expected of the anesthetist. Although advances in technology have improved patient safety through sophisticated monitoring equipment, their proper functioning and reliability can only be ensured by daily inspection and when alarms are properly engaged.

Air Embolism

Venous air embolism (VAE) is a complication associated with various surgical and invasive procedures whereby a communicating pressure gradient exists between the atmosphere and the venous circulation. The entrained air traverses the heart and accumulates in the lungs, eventually forming an "air lock" that causes mechanical obstruction to the right ventricular outflow tract (Durant, Lanf, & Oppenheimer, 1947). Acute cardiovascular collapse results depending on the amount and rate of air entry.

Neurosurgical procedures that require the head to be positioned above the heart are frequently associated with VAE, with a reported incidence of 25% (Albin, 1993). However, VAEs are also known to occur in orthopedic, trauma, and obstetrical-gynecological cases in the supine position (Williamson, Webb, & Russell, 1993). In addition, central venous line disconnections and rapid fluid and blood infusers have resulted in significant morbidity and mortality attributed to air embolism. Occasionally, air bubbles may enter the arterial circulation, referred as paradoxical air embolism, by way of a patent foramen ovale.

The earliest signs of VAE include a rise in ETN_2 and drop in $ETCO_2$. Subsequently, hemodynamic changes, including hypotension, tachycardia, ECG changes, dysrhythmias, and increases in central venous pressure (CVP) and pulmonary artery pressure (PAP), may rapidly ensue. In the spontaneously breathing patient, a remarkable gasping episode may precede the expression of symptoms. A change in heart sounds, characteristically described as a mill-wheel murmur, may be detected. However, this sign may not be a sensitive indicator (Albin, 1993). Cyanosis and cardiovascular collapse result in severe cases of VAE (Fig. 34–1).

The most sensitive monitoring device is transesophageal echocardiography (TEE) followed by precordial Doppler and capnography for early detection of VAE (Albin, 1993). Once VAE is identified, the surgeon should be alerted to flood the operative field immediately with saline or apply surgical packing. Nitrous oxide should be discontinued to prevent air bubble enlargement and oxy-

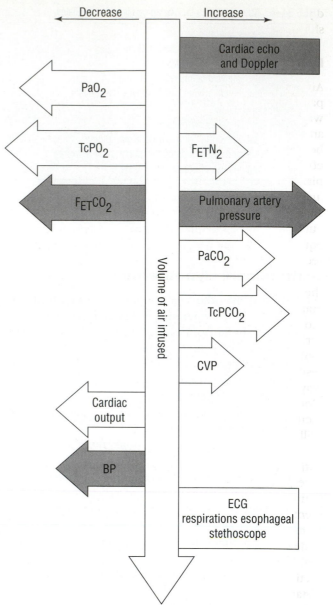

Figure 34–1. Changes in detection parameters for venous air embolism with increasing air volume. Data are from human and animal studies under a wide variety of circumstances. *(From Black, S., & Cucchiara, R. F. [1990]. Tumor surgery. In R. F. Cucchiara & J. D. Michenfelder [Eds.], Clinical neuroanesthesia [p. 296]. New York: Churchill Livingstone. Reprinted with permission from the Mayo Foundation.)*

gen concentration should be increased to 100%. When feasible, the anesthetist should reposition the patient in the supine and/or left lateral decubitus position to prevent further air entrainment and minimize the chance for right ventricular outlet obstruction. Intravenous fluids should be maximized and the patient hand-ventilated during hypotensive episodes. For hemodynamically unstable patients, attempts at aspirating air from an indwelling CVP or PA catheter and vasopressor therapy should be attempted.

Difficult Intubations

Airway management is the anesthesia provider's principal responsibility. Although anticipation of a difficult airway generally commences with the preoperative history and physical evaluation, not every airway problem will be positively identified. According to the American Society of Anesthesiologists (ASA) Closed Claim Project, respiratory events constituted the single largest class of injury (Cheney, Posner, & Caplan, 1991). The most common causes of respiratory morbidity and mortality were difficult tracheal intubation, esophageal intubation, and inadequate ventilation. Thirty percent of the deaths were directly attributable to anesthesia (Benumof, 1991).

Not surprisingly, recognition and management of the obvious difficult airway (eg, distorted anatomy) generally are not the basis for the majority of morbidity and mortality case reports. As Benumof (1996a) aptly describes, it is the subtle airway deviations that are overlooked during preoperative physical examinations and result in unexpected airway catastrophes. Successful airway management, therefore, necessitates not only meticulous evaluation, but also alternative plans. Proper equipment should be available and the practioner should be skilled in using these tools.

Every airway evaluation should include the Mallampati Classification (refer to Fig. 25-3) for determining ease of laryngoscopy (Mallampati, Gatt, Gugino, Desai, Waraksa, Freiberger, & Liu, 1985). Correct visual assessment of the uvula, tonsillar pillars, and soft palate is performed with the patient seated upright, the mouth open widely, and the tongue fully extended without phonating. Patient characteristics that should alert the anesthetist to intubating difficulties include a thyromental distance of less than 6 cm (predictive of an anteriorly positioned larynx), limited head and neck range of motion (inability to assume sniffing position), prognathism, short and thick neck, large breast size, a full beard, and presence of pathological states (Benumof, 1996). Once a determination, or even a suspicion, is made regarding potential difficulty intubating the patient's trachea, the ASA Difficult Airway Algorithm should be followed (Fig. 34-2).

Recently, with the introduction and proven efficacy of the laryngeal mask airway (LMA), the Difficult Airway Algorithm has been revised to include this device (Benumof, 1996a). If a patient with an unrecognized difficult airway is rendered unconscious and the anesthetist cannot ventilate or intubate, despite oral and/or nasal airway in situ, use of the LMA as an emergency airway is recommended over transtracheal jet ventilation (TTJV) because of its wider use among anesthesia providers and the reduced potential for trauma.

Other maneuvers during the course of intubation attempts that may assist the anesthetist are to ensure that the patient is properly positioned in the sniffing configuration. In addition, once laryngoscopy is undertaken and the larynx is not directly visualized, manipulation of the thyroid cartilage, described as optimal external laryngeal manipulation (OELM) by Benumof (1996a), and exchanging laryngoscope blade sizes or types may facilitate successful intubation.

Awareness under Anesthesia

Intraoperative awareness is a terrifying anesthetic complication patients may experience as a result of the anesthetic technique and type of surgery, as well as their preoperative emotional condition. Generally unrecognized by the anesthesia provider, the seemingly asymptomatic patient is able to describe or recall postoperatively vivid operating room conversations and specific body manipulations that occurred during the surgical procedure. Persistent nightmares with disturbing psychological sequelae have been reported, adding to discharge concerns (Blacher, 1984). The incidence of awareness under anesthesia, is estimated by Bogetz and Katz (1984) to be as high as 43%, although most researchers agree that the reported incidence is probably closer to 1% or 2%. Awareness tends to be associated with those procedures where lighter planes of anesthesia are necessitated because of the hemodynamic instability associated with trauma and shock patients (Bogetz & Katz, 1984), fetal protection during cesarean sections (Lyons & Macdonald, 1991), and nitrous-narcotic techniques used for cardiac patients (Blacher, 1975). The routine use of muscle relaxants also has contributed to the likelihood of awareness through a masking effect of light anesthesia (Dierdorf, 1996).

The difficulty in recognizing this phenomenon is that patients may not elicit any detectable symptoms, such as an increase in blood pressure and heart rate, diaphoresis and dilated pupils. Although not proven, administering amnestics and hypnotics to every patient may prevent intraoperative awareness. Discretion in operating room conversation is an advisable course to follow. In the event that a patient does experience intraoperative awareness, the anesthesia provider should encourage open discussion of the event.

Pharmacologically Prolonged Muscle Relaxation

The development of nondepolarizing muscle relaxants (NDMRs) has resulted in fewer side effects than the depolarizing agent succinylcholine and has provided the "quiet" field surgeons required to achieve success in many surgical procedures. However, not all operations necessitate the continuous use of muscle relaxants. In certain cases, muscle relaxants are contraindicated because of sur-

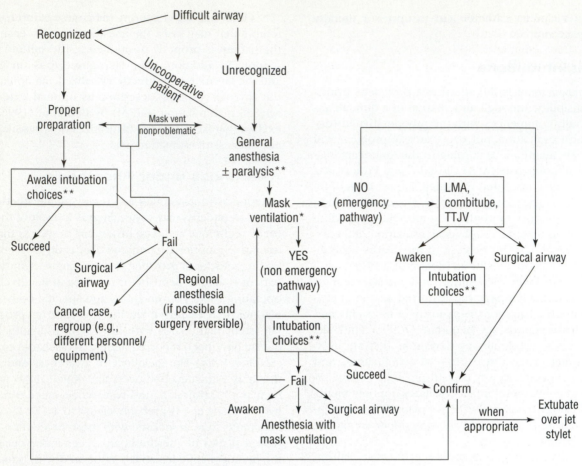

Figure 34–2. The ASA Difficult Airway Algorithm.

[a] Nonsurgical tracheal intubation choices consist of laryngoscopy with a rigid laryngoscope blade (many types), blind orotracheal or nasotracheal technique, fiberoptic/stylet technique, retrograde technique, illuminating stylet, rigid bronchoscope or percutaneous dilational tracheal entry.

*Always *consider* calling for help (eg, technical, medical, surgical) when difficulty with mask ventilation and/or tracheal intubation is encountered.

**Consider the need to preserve spontaneous ventilation.

(From Benumof, J. L. [1996b], Laryngeal mask airway and the ASA Difficult Airway Algorithm. Anesthesiology, 84, 687. Reprinted with permission.)

gical dissections in areas of nervous innervation whereby visible reactivity of the nerve branch assists the surgeon in preserving regional neurological function. One should be cautioned against the habit of overzealously administering muscle relaxants to patients undergoing general anesthesia to avoid embarrassment from sudden patient movement during surgery. However, skill is required in the judicious use of muscle relaxants because undesirable complications may arise from the indiscriminate administration of these adjuncts to anesthesia.

Apart from the many factors known to influence the pharmacodynamics of muscle relaxants (eg, drugs or disease states affecting neuromuscular junction activity), continued muscle paralysis may mask inadequate levels of anesthesia, resulting in intraoperative awareness, as discussed. Furthermore, excess administration of any

NDMR may result in a dose-dependent prolongation of muscle paralysis. Once the train-of-four monitoring response has been obliterated, a timely reversal of paralysis may not be predictable. Repeated administration of reversal agents will not only be ineffective in reestablishing muscle function, but also may place the patient at risk for a cholinergic crisis (Gwirtz, 1996). Because of the limited or ceiling effect of anticholinesterase agents, additional injections of neostigmine or edrophonium will be ineffective in reversing a prolonged neuromuscular blockade (Bartkowski, 1987).

Recurarization also may occur (Hershey, Wahrenbrock, & DeJong, 1965). This is a condition in which recurrence of neuromuscular blockade occurs following a seemingly successful reversal. Patients susceptible to this phenomenon include those with renal insufficiency, who are unable to eliminate NDMRs that depend on kidney function. Likewise, an inadequate dosage of reversal agent or a short-acting anticholinesterase used for treating a long-acting muscle relaxant may produce a similar outcome.

To avoid the pitfalls of prolonged neuromuscular blockade, the anesthetist should learn to utilize those agents only for surgical cases necessitating muscle relaxation. With the use of the peripheral nerve stimulator, maintenance of one twitch, as monitored during train-of-four stimulation, will generally ensure reversibility of paralysis. The practitioner should keep in mind that with return of the train-of-four twitch response, 70% of receptors may still be blocked.

Transurethral Resection of the Prostate Syndrome

Transurethral resection of the prostate (TURP) is a common surgical procedure typically seen among males over 60 years of age. Because of the anatomy of the prostate and the surgical manipulations involved in removing pathologic tissue, a constellation of symptoms regarded as the TURP syndrome may occur. During the procedure, copious amounts of irrigating fluid are employed to distend the bladder and flush the surgical field of blood and tissue debris. Because the prostate is supplied with large venous sinuses, a substantial volume of fluid is absorbed into the systemic circulation as a result of concomitant surgical exposure time and irrigation pressure. In addition to the TURP syndrome, inadvertent surgical complications of bacteremia, bladder perforation, hemorrhage, hypothermia, and coagulopathy also are possible.

The syndrome (Table 34–7) may develop perioperatively or postoperatively and often reflects signs and symptoms of intravascular fluid overload, dilutional hyponatremia (water intoxication), or occasionally, the toxicity from the irrigating fluid used (eg, glycine or Cytal®). Reports indicate that up to 3 L of irrigating fluid can be absorbed during a 2-hour procedure (Sunderrajan, Bauer, Vopat, Wanner-Barjenbruch, & Hayes, 1984). Although most patients appear clinically asymptomatic, signs of hyponatremia usually do not become evident until the serum sodium concentration falls below 120 mEq/L.

Depending on the patient's preoperative medical condition, water intoxication and subsequent cardiovascular collapse can develop rapidly. Although gastrointestinal complaints may herald hyponatremia, the predominant symptoms are reflective of central nervous system effects, such as confusion, lethargy, seizures, and eventual coma. Patients often initially exhibit bradycardia and systemic hypertension as a direct reflection of vascular fluid overload. Clearly, it is understandable why regional anesthesia is the preferred technique for early detection of TURP syndrome. Treatment of mild symptoms is aimed at eliminating the absorbed fluid through fluid restriction. Patients with severe symptomatology will require correction of the hyponatremia with normal or hypertonic saline, diuresis, and supportive care.

Intraoperative Hypotension

Patients who present with preoperative dehydration stemming from various conditions such as chronic hypertension, bowel obstruction, or surgical bowel preparation, will be predisposed to intraoperative hypotension. Under anesthesia, these patients may exhibit a sustained lowering of systolic blood pressures exceeding 30% of normal baseline values. The morbidity associated with hypotension is related to reduced perfusion of vital organs. Of critical importance, cerebral perfusion pressure becomes compromised as mean arterial pressure (MAP) falls below 50 mmHg. Hypotensive patients with a history of atherosclerotic disease may be at increased risk for developing ischemic changes on the electrocardiogram and possible myocardial injury.

In healthy patients inhalation agents produce a dose-dependent decrease in systemic vascular resistance (SVR), resulting in mild to moderate hypotension. Confounding the drop in blood pressure are intravenous adjuncts, which can contribute to further reductions in SVR and/or myocardial depression. However, in dehydrated patients, hemodynamic instability, as evidenced by persistent hypotension and reflex tachycardia, may

TABLE 34–7. Signs and Symptoms of TURP Syndrome

Symptoms
  Apprehension
  Disorientation
  Irritability
  Twitching
  Nausea
  Vomiting
  Shortness of breath
Signs
  Bradycardia
  Hypertension
  Anemia
  Jaundice
  Cyanosis
  Altered sensorium
  ECG changes
  Seizures

From Sunderrajan, S., Bauer, J. H., Vopat, R. L., Wanner-Barjenbruch, P., & Hayes, A. (1984). Posttransurethral prostatic resection hyponatremic syndrome: Case report and review of the literature. American Journal of Kidney Disease, 4(1), 83. Reprinted with permission.

occur suddenly when intravascular volume has not been judiciously maintained and surgical blood loss becomes significant.

Having ascertained that a hypotensive event is not a direct result of surgical compression of the vena cava, release of a tourniquet or arterial cross-clamp, or lowering of the legs from lithotomy position, hypotension should be primarily treated with crystalloid or colloid fluid replacements and a vasopressor, as needed. Additional maneuvers for attenuating decreases in blood pressure include reducing the concentration of the inhalation agent and substituting manual ventilation for positive-pressure machine ventilation.

Circuit Disconnect

Although more than a decade has elapsed since Cooper, Newboer, and Kitz (1984) analyzed preventable anesthesia-related errors that identified breathing circuit disconnects as one of the most frequently reported incidents, the principal source of morbidity and mortality in anesthetic mishaps continues to be associated with the airway and ventilation (Cullen, 1994). Despite the development of alarm systems and safety features that aid in respiratory monitoring, breathing system disconnections rank as the single most frequently occurring adverse incident (Vistica, Posner, Caplan, & Cheney, 1990). Anesthesia provider error has been described as a major contributing factor to this complication (Cooper et al., 1984). The most common human causes associated with circuit disconnects include failure to check the machine, disabling alarm systems, lack of vigilance, inadequate provider, experience and unfamiliarity with equipment (Allnutt, 1987).

Attending to breath sounds via the esophageal stethoscope, observing the rise and fall of the bellows, monitoring oxygen saturation and end-tidal CO_2, and listening for airway pressure and apnea alarms have not been foolproof measures in preventing ventilatory mishaps. To eliminate these preventable occurrences, established standards of practice need to be rigorously enforced (inspection of machines/equipment and ensuring functional alarm systems that cannot be permanently disabled). Anesthesia learners also need to be sensitized to those mishaps which are known to occur frequently (reinforcing disconnection sites with tape and familiarity with the different alarms to react reflexively to the problem at hand). Judicious supervision and relief personnel need to be available for providing breaks to alleviate fatigue and improve vigilance. Although circuit disconnections may be unavoidable, even for the most vigilant anesthetist, the source of the circuit violation must be immediately located and corrected to prevent an accidental break in the system from becoming a critical incident.

▶ POSTOPERATIVE DISTURBANCES

Although patient homeostasis may have been maintained successfully throughout the intraoperative period, the recovery phase of anesthesia delivery, likewise demands diligence in ensuring the return of normal physiologic function. In fact, this is a period when surgical and anesthetic effects that have been elicited perioperatively, become evident.

Nausea and Vomiting

Postoperative nausea and vomiting (PONV) is one of the most common, yet highly underreported, recovery room and discharge complaints, with a documented incidence of 39% to 73% (Cohen, Duncan, DeBoer, & Tweed, 1994). Although perceived as a minor complication, problems associated with its occurrence can result in significant sequelae. Persistent vomiting can lead to an unanticipated delay in the patient's hospital discharge, certainly a critical issue in today's cost-saving emphasis on outpatient surgeries. More important, disrupted suture lines and bleeding, requiring hemostasis, may result in a return trip to the operating room. In addition, pulmonary aspiration becomes a risk factor among those patients with depressed protective reflexes from residual anesthesia or analgesia.

Postoperative nausea and vomiting is complex and multifactorial phenomenon that is influenced by patient factors, the anesthetic technique, postoperative causes, and the type of operative procedure (Table 34-8). Younger patients with no previous health problems seem to have a greater incidence of PONV than the geriatric population. Females, especially premenopausal, are more likely to suffer from this complication than their male counterparts, suggesting a possible hormonal link to vomiting. Certain surgical procedures that involve peritoneal insufflation or middle-ear or ophthalmic manipulations and operations associated with swallowing of occult blood have a significant incidence of PONV. Finally, PONV may be triggered by severe pain and/or further provoked by postoperative analgesics.

A variety of anesthetic techniques and pharmacologic agents have been employed preoperatively and intraoperatively with varying degrees of success in blocking specific receptors interfacing with the brainstem's vomiting center or chemoreceptor trigger zone (Fig. 34-3). Regional techniques have no clear advantage over general anesthetic methods in minimizing PONV. Among drugs commonly used, narcotics and etomidate have been associated with a high incidence of PONV, whereas propofol and benzodiazepines appear to be less stimulating (Stoelting, 1996).

A number of drugs are available as prophylactic and "rescue" agents against PONV (Table 34-9). Because a

TABLE 34–8. Risk Factors for PONV

Patient factors
  Anxiety
  Gender (female)
  Age (younger)
  Known history of PONV or motion sickness
  Gastroparesis
  Obesity
Operative procedures
  ENT
  Gynecological
  Ophthalmic
  Plastic surgery
  Abdominal
Anesthesia factors
  Narcotics (morphine and synthetic opioids)
  Anesthetic agents (nitrous oxide, etomidate, inhalational agents, methohexital, balanced techniques)
  Gastric distension
  Longer duration and depth of anesthesia
Postoperative factors
  Pain
  Blood in stomach
  Early ambulation
  Hypotension
  Premature oral intake
  Opioid analgesics

Modified from Glaxo Pharmaceuticals. (1994). Risk factors for PONV. Brochure on Zofran, p. 3.

few of the antiemetics produce extrapyramidal side effects, it is recommended that these drugs be selectively used only in those patients at risk for or with a prior history of PONV (Miller & Jankovic, 1989). Although some anesthetists may espouse administering multireceptor antagonists for wide-coverage prophylaxis, there are no studies to support the efficacy of this practice. Ondansetron, the new serotonin receptor antagonist, has been effective in minimizing protracted emesis among oncology patients. Although this drug holds promise in treating surgical patients at risk for PONV, the precise role of this drug in anesthesia prophylaxis remains clouded by the cost-to-benefit ratio when compared with standard antiemetics (Tang, Watcha, & White, 1996).

Hypertension

A common hemodynamic disturbance seen in patients postoperatively is hypertension. Other than preexisting hypertension, contributing factors postoperatively often include urinary retention, postoperative shivering, surgical pain, and fluid overload. Sympathetic effects secondary to hypercarbia and hypoxemia are additional considerations to evaluate when assessing causes of sustained pressure elevation. Patients with preexisting hypertensive conditions tend to experience postoperative increases in blood pressure regardless of any identifiable cause. Uncontrolled hypertension can result in increased bleeding, disruption of vascular suture lines, arrhythmias, and myocardial ischemia.

Primary interventions are aimed at mitigating the offending stimuli, such as low-dose meperidine given intravenously to treat shivering or bladder catheterization. Antihypertensive agents (Table 34–10) generally are not administered until all other reasonable efforts to lower the blood pressure have failed and only if systolic pressures exceed baseline values by 20% or for sustained pressures higher than 160/90 mmHg. Those patients with limited cardiac reserve who are at risk for significant hemodynamic compromise may require aggressive pharmacologic therapy, such as intravenous nitroglycerin, and invasive monitoring to control their hypertension.

Hypoxemia

Aside from obvious anesthetic complications, such as significant pulmonary aspiration, other causes for postoperative hypoxemia should be considered, most commonly atelectasis. This condition, which occurs immediately postextubation can persist 7 to 10 days and is due to a reduction in both lung volume and chest compliance attributable to the general effects of perioperative anesthesia (Craig, 1981). As alveolar airways collapse in well-perfused areas of the lung, intrapulmonary shunting or ventilation-perfusion mismatch result. Additional risk factors of obesity, extremes of age (particularly, infants), smoking history, perioperative body positioning, and surgical procedures involving the upper abdomen and chest will reflect the severity of atelectasis and early postrecovery hypoxemia (Xue, Huang, Tong, Liu, Liao, An, Luo, & Deng, 1996).

Fortunately, deleterious pulmonary effects in most patients recovering from general anesthesia will have safely resolved after a few hours (Marshall & Wyche, 1972). Hypoventilation due to drug-induced central nervous system (CNS) depression is another consideration when evaluating hypoxemia in the recovery room. The CNS depressants most commonly implicated are volatile inhalants and narcotics (Gwirtz, 1996). Characteristically, volatile agents tend to produce fast, shallow breathing, whereas narcotics cause slow, deep patterns of breathing. Other possible causes of hypoventilation include pain, hypothermia, airway obstruction, and residual effects of nondepolarizing muscle relaxants.

Primary measures in minimizing postoperative hypoxemia include the use of supplemental oxygen when transporting patients to the recovery room. Airway ob-

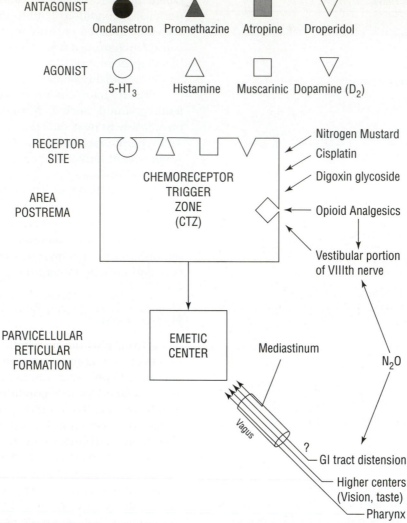

Figure 34–3. The chemoreceptor trigger zone and the emetic center with the agonist and antagonist sites of action of various anesthetic-related agents and stimuli. *(From Watcha, M. F., & White, P. F. [1992]. Postoperative nausea and vomiting: Its etiology, treatment, and prevention. Anesthesiology, 77, 164. Reprinted with permission.)*

struction from oral secretions or excessive analgesia or anesthetics requires suctioning and cautious administration of reversal agents.

► PHARMACOGENETIC COMPLICATIONS

Anesthesia and select pharmacologic agents are capable of initiating a cascade of physiologic disturbances secondary to an aberrant genetic expression. Although rare, the importance in identifying this subpopulation of patients preoperatively is imperative if a potential anesthetic disaster is to be avoided. With advance notifica-

tion, preventive preparations can be implemented to ensure safe anesthetic exposure and outcome.

► OTHER PROBLEMS TRIGGERED BY ANESTHESIA

Malignant Hyperthermia

All inhalation agents (except nitrous oxide) and succinylcholine are responsible for triggering the onset of a genetically inherited disorder known as malignant hyperthermia (MH). Although the etiology of MH is not entirely clear, it may involve the sarcoplasmic reticu-

TABLE 34–9. Antiemetics and Associated Receptor Affinity

Drug	Receptor
Droperidol	Dopamine (D_2)
Diphenhydramine	Histamine (H_1)
Metoclopramide	Dopamine (D_2)
Ondansetron	Serotonin (5-HT_3)
Prochlorperazine	Dopamine (D_2)
Scopolamine	Cholinergic (muscarinic)

TABLE 34–11. Clinical Findings of Malignant Hyperthermia

Increasing $ETCO_2$ (early sign)
Unexplained tachycardia
Dysrhythmias
Mottling of skin
Skeletal muscle rigidity
Acidosis
Cyanosis
Rising body temperature (late sign)
Hemodynamic instability
Rhabdomyolysis
Myoglobinuria

lum of skeletal muscle whereby a defect in some aspect of the calcium-release mechanism leads to toxic intracellular accumulation of this ion. Masseter spasm and neuroleptic malignant syndrome (NMS) are two of several coincidental disorders associated with MH. Over 2% of strabismus patients who develop severe masseter spasm under anesthesia are diagnosed to be MH susceptible (Carroll, 1987). However, NMS, although clinically indistinguishable from MH, is pharmacologically distinct and can occur without any genetic predisposition. With NMS, dopamine receptor antagonists are the definitive triggering agents and, contrary to MH, nondepolarizing muscle relaxants are effective adjuncts in alleviating skeletal muscle rigidity (Caroff, Mann, & Campbell, 1994).

There is significant variability in the clinical presentation of MH. A susceptible MH patient can be asymptomatic during previous anesthetics before a life-threatening crisis occurs. Children and young adults have the greatest predilection for developing MH, and the highest incidence is between the ages of 3 and 30 years (Carroll, 1987). The severity of the MH presentation depends on patient susceptibility and dose-dependent exposure time to the triggering agents (Allen, 1994). Although the speed of onset can be acute (eg, during induction), the full expression of MH also can be delayed for several hours, even into the recov-

ery phase of care (Larach, Rosenberg, Larach, & Broennle, 1987).

Episodes of MH are characterized by a syndrome of hypermetabolism, skeletal muscle rigidity, and hyperthermia (Table 34–11). Depending on the rapidity of symptom progression, any high level of suspicion for MH mandates prompt and vigorous intervention as outlined by the Malignant Hyperthermia Association of the United States (MHAUS) to prevent patient demise (see enclosed computer disk). The indispensable drug of choice used in successfully treating MH is dantrolene. This centrally acting muscle relaxant acts directly on skeletal muscle by inhibiting calcium release from the sarcoplasmic reticulum, thereby interfering with excitation-contraction coupling. Currently, there is little evidence to support routine prophylaxis of known MH-susceptible patients with dantrolene prior to anesthetic exposure (Allen, 1994). Recommendations for management of these patients include avoidance of triggering agents, especially volatile inhalants and succinylcholine, and evacuating volatile gas contaminants from the anesthesia machine by flushing the system with 10 L of oxygen for 5 minutes; changing accessible plastic and rubber components, such as the fresh gas outlet hose, removing vaporizers, and ensuring fresh CO_2 absorbent in the canister (Beebe & Sessler, 1988).

Acute Intermittent Porphyria

The so-called acute or hepatic porphyrias are a rare group of inherited metabolic disorders of the heme biosynthetic pathway that can be destabilized through the administration of certain anesthetic agents and drugs. Of the three types represented in this group (intermittent, variegate, and coproporphyria), intermittent porphyria is the most common and has a high prevalence among northern Europeans. The disease, characterized by episodes of life-threatening abdominal, neurologic, and mental symptoms, is due to enzymatic

TABLE 34–10. Antihypertensive Agents for Acute Episodes of Hypertension

Calcium-channel blockers
Nifedipine SL
Nicardipine
Beta-blockers
Labetolol
Vasodilators
Hydralazine
Sodium nitroprusside
Nitroglycerin

dysfunction in the heme synthetic pathway that results in overproduction and accumulation of heme precursors proximal to the metabolic block (Jensen et al., 1995). Disease presentation may be due to increased amino levulinic acid (ALA) synthetase activity, the enzyme responsible for catalyzing the rate-limiting step in heme synthesis. Other possibilities include toxic tissue buildup of porphyrins or decreased heme production that would affect hemoglobin synthesis and cytochrome systems.

Over two thirds of genetically susceptible acute in-termittent porphyria (AIP) individuals will remain asymptomatic throughout their lifetime. Of those who develop crisis, clinical manifestations of severe abdominal pain, paralysis, seizures, mental confusion, electrolyte imbalances, hypertension, and tachycardia may progress to hemodynamic instability and respiratory failure (Dover, Plenderleith, Moore, & McColl, 1994). Factors known to trigger acute attacks include infection, poor nutritional status, dehydration, emotional stress, pregnancy, and porphyrogenic drugs (Table 34-12). However, with advanced preparation, AIP patients can be safely

TABLE 34–12. Porphyria and Anesthetic Drugs

Group	Safe to Likely Safe	Unsafe to Likely Unsafe	Unclear
Intravenous drugs			
	Midazolam	Barbiturates	Diazepam
	Lorazepam	Etomidate	Ketamine
	Propofol	Chlordiazepoxide	
		Flunitrazepam	
		Nitrazepam	
Inhaled drugs			
	Nitrous oxide	Enflurane	Isoflurane
			Halothane[a]
Neuromuscular blockers			
	Succinylcholine		
Pancuronium			
	Vecuronium		Atracurium
	D-Tubocurarine		
Premedicants			
	Scopolamine		
	Atropine		
	Droperidol		
	Promethazine		
	Chloral hydrate		
	Diphenhydramine		
	Cimetidine		
Opioids			
	Morphine	Pentazosine	Sufentanil
	Fentanyl		
Anticholinesterases			
	Neostigmine		
Local anesthetics			
	Bupivicaine		Lidocaine
	Procaine		
Cardiovascular			
	Atenolol	α-methyldopa	
	Labetolol	Hydralazine	
	Guanethadine	Phenoxybenzamine	
	Reserpine		
	Phentolamine		
Other			
	Glucose loading	Oral contraceptive	
	Anticonvulsants	Griseofulvin	
		Endogenous steroids	

[a] Despite lack of definitive evidence of its safety, halothane still is recommended as the inhaled anesthetic of choice.

anesthetized through a number of anesthetic techniques by simply avoiding the use of precipitating agents.

In the event of an unexpected porphyric crisis, immediate efforts should be aimed at treating those factors that may be stimulating an increase in ALA synthetase activity: discontinuation of triggering agents, intravenous fluids increased to maintain adequate hydration, administration of a carbohydrate load (glucose 10–20 g/hr) and propranolol (Jensen, Fiddler, & Striepe, 1995). Although Hematin is an effective therapeutic agent and considered the standard drug for treating acute porphyric crisis, the significant side effects of coagulopathy and renal failure have discouraged its use. Depending on the variability in symptom development and duration, postoperative monitoring may be prolonged.

Exacerbation of Sickle Cell Trait

Sickle cell disease is a chronic condition predominately associated with African Americans. As a result of a hereditary defect in heme synthesis, Hgb S affected individuals are faced with repeated "sickle cell crisis" involving vascular-occlusive episodes that result in diffuse tissue infarction and multi-organ dysfunction. Conditions known to trigger a crisis include hypoxemia, dehydration, hypothermia, infection/fever, acidosis, and circulatory stasis.

TABLE 34–13. Complications of Sickle Cell Disorders

Painful (vasoocclusive) crisis
Cardiac irregularities
Hepatic crisis
Cholelithiasis
Aseptic necrosis of bone
Cerebral vascular occlusion
Hematuria
Priapism
Splenic infarction and sequestration
Postsplenectomy sepsis

From Sears, D. A. (1992). Hematologic diseases requiring critical care. In J. M. Civetta, R. W. Taylor, & R. R. Kirby (Eds.), Critical care (2nd ed., p. 1729). Philadelphia: Lippincott. Reprinted with permission.

Surgery and anesthesia have the propensity for disrupting a sickle cell patient's delicate physiologic balance.

Complications (Table 34–13) associated with sickle cell disease are a direct result of conformational changes in the erythrocytes that increase blood viscosity and sludging of red blood cells in the microcirculation. A vicious cycle (Figure 34–4) rapidly ensues as tissue hypoxia and acidosis develop, igniting conditions for further Hgb S sickling.

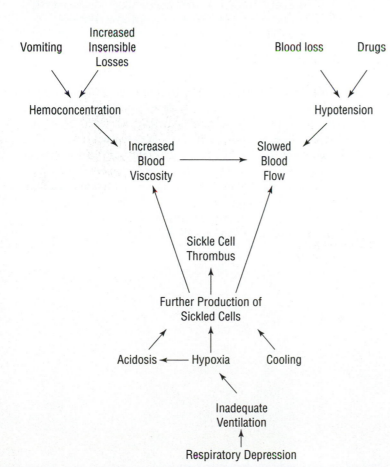

Figure 34–4. The vicious cycle of sickle cell disease and the interrelation of factors precipitating crisis in the patient undergoing anesthesia and surgery. *(From Platt, O. S. & Orkin, F. K. [1996]. Difficulties in sickle cell states. In N. Gravenstein & R. R. Kirby [Eds.], Complications in anesthesiology [2nd ed., p. 533]. Philadelphia: Lippincott-Raven. Reprinted with permission.)*

Anesthetic management is aimed at keeping the patient warm and hydrated, maintaining a urinary output at a minimum rate of 0.5 mL/kg/h, and maintaining an oxygen saturation of 100%, regardless of whether regional or general techniques are used. Although the use of limb tourniquets for orthopedic procedures and intravenous nerve blocks may theoretically predispose the sickle cell patient to crisis, tourniquet-induced ischemia is only a relative contraindication (Stein & Urbaniak, 1980).

▶ CASE STUDY

A 21-year-old, 80-kg male underwent a tonsillectomy under general inhalation anesthesia with isoflurane. No neuromuscular blockade was utilized after intubation facilitated by succinylcholine 100 mg. At the end of the case, all anesthetic agents are discontinued, the oropharynx is suctioned. The patient is spontaneously breathing a 550-mL tidal volume. Extubation is performed at the height of inspiration. Immediately following extubation, the anesthetist is unable to ventilate the patient with positive pressure and a high-pitched crowing sound is audible.

1. What treatment should be instituted?

   Gentle positive-pressure mask ventilation with 100% oxygen should be delivered. Alternatively, administer intravenous lidocaine (0.5–1 mg/kg), deepen anesthesia, or administer small doses of succinylcholine (20–30 mg) to relax the laryngeal muscles to reestablish airway patency.

2. What condition may develop following an acute episode of upper-airway obstruction such as in this case?

   The patient is at risk for developing negative-pressure pulmonary edema (NPPE). A common triggering event for NPPE in young healthy adults is laryngospasm following endotracheal extubation.

3. What is the physiological basis for the development of NPPE?

   As the patient attempts to inspire against a closed glottis forcefully, high negative intrapleural pressures are generated, accompanied by a sudden increase in peripheral venous return. This combination of events provokes a sudden increase in stroke volume to the right side of the heart that rapidly overwhelms the pulmonary circulation, resulting in transudation of fluid across the pulmonary arteries and into central alveoli of the lung.

4. When does this phenomenon typically develop, and what are the typical clinical manifestations observed postoperatively?

   This phenomenon can occur within minutes following the resolution of the laryngospasm, but it can be delayed for a few hours. Postoperatively, the typical clinical manifestations include an acute onset of respiratory distress and oxygen desaturation. Arterial blood gas analysis and chest radiographs can confirm the diagnosis.

5. How should NPPE be treated?

   Treatment is supportive. Diuresis, supplemental oxygen, and fluid restriction often will resolve the usually short period of pulmonary edema. Some patients may require reintubation with controlled ventilatory support until symptoms resolve.

▶ SUMMARY

Anesthesia can on occasion be complicated by a variety of critical incidents that stem from several sources, including iatrogenic, preexisting pathology, provider error, or equipment failure. Although advances in anesthetic agents and monitoring devices have substantially improved patient safety statistics since the mid-1980s, complications continue to occur. Detailed preoperative evaluations, provider vigilance, and awareness of potential anesthetic complications will further reduce morbidity and mortality in those rare cases of untoward anesthetic events.

► **KEY CONCEPTS**

- Aspiration pneumonitis is more likely to occur if the tracheal aspirant is greater than 25 mL and has an acid pH lower than 2.5.
- Laryngospasm may result in further complications, such as negative-pressure pulmonary edema and hypoxemia.
- One of the first measures in treating bronschospasm is to increase the depth of anesthesia.
- Although Type I and Type II allergic reactions may be clinically indistinguishable, Type II histamine-related reactions are the most commonly seen in anesthesia, whereas Type II antibody-complex reactions are capable of producing more deleterious effects.
- The greatest amount of body heat loss in the operating room occurs during the first hour.
- The earliest signs of venous air embolism are a rise in ETN_2 and a decrease in $ETCO_2$.
- Seventy percent of the neuromuscular junction

receptors may remain blocked despite return of train-of-four response and sustained tetany, as measured by the peripheral nerve stimulator.
- In TURP procedures, clinical symptoms of hyponatremia may not become evident until the serum sodium concentration falls below 120 mEq/L.
- Anesthetic mishaps associated with the airway and ventilation are the leading cause of morbidity and mortality.
- The most common postoperative complaint is nausea and vomiting.
- Atelectasis is the most common cause of postoperative hypoxemia.
- One of the earliest signs of malignant hyperthermia is a rising $ETCO_2$.
- Triggering factors for sickle cell crisis are hypoxemia, dehydration, infection, acidosis, hypothermia, and venous stasis.

► **STUDY QUESTIONS**

1. What is the mechanism most commonly responsible for hypoxia in recovery room patients?

2. Describe the hierarchy of treatment for a laryngospasm and any complications that can develop.

3. What is the earliest and most reliable sign of malignant hyperthermia during general anesthesia?

4. How can the incidence of postoperative nausea and vomiting be reduced in the surgical population?

5. What disease states can be exacerbated by anesthesia?

6. If a mill-wheel murmur is heard on precordial Doppler ultrasound, what observed parameter is consistent with venous air embolism?

KEY REFERENCES

Albin, M. S. (1993). Air embolism. In L. M. Caplan & S. M. Miller (Eds.), *Anesthesiology Clinics of North America: Embolism II, 11,* 1–24.

Benumof, J. L. (1996). Laryngeal mask airway and the ASA Difficult airway algorithm. *Anesthesiology, 84,* 686–699.

Caroff, S. N., Mann, S. C., & Campbell, E. C. (1994). Hyperthermia and neuroleptic malignant syndrome. In R. C. Levitt (Ed.), *Anesthesiology Clinics of North America: Temperature Regulation During Anesthesia, 12,* 491–512.

Cullen, B. F. (1994). Diagnosis and prevention of intraoperative mishaps. *Anesthesia & Analgesia, 80*(Suppl.), 8–11.

Dierdorf, S. F. (1996). Awareness during anesthesia. In S. F. Dierdorf (Ed.), *Anesthesiology Clinics of North America: Practical Solutions for Difficult Problems I, 14,* 369–384.

Gal, T. J. (1996). Bronchial hyperresponsiveness and the patient for anesthesia. *Anesthesia & Analgesia, 82*(Suppl.), 37–45.

Goldberg, M. (1996). The allegic response and anesthesia. In N. Gravenstein & R. R. Kirby (Eds.), *Complications in anesthesiology* (2nd ed., pp. 605–618). Philadelphia: Lippincott-Raven.

Gwirtz, K. H. (1996). Management of recovery room complications. In S. F. Dierdorf (Ed.), *Anesthesiology Clinics of North America: Practical Solutions for Difficult Problems, 14,* 307–339.

Illing, L., Duncan, P. G., & Yip, R. (1992). Gastroesophageal reflux during anaesthesia. *Canadian Journal of Anaesthesia, 39,* 466–470.

Jensen, N. F., Fiddler, D. S., & Striepe, V. (1995). Anesthetic considerations in porphyrias. *Anesthesia & Analgesia, 80,* 591–599.

Rex, M. A. E. (1970). A review of the structural and functional basis of laryngospasm and discussion of the nerve pathways involved in man and animals. *British Journal of Anaesthesia, 42,* 891–899.

Rose, D. K., Cohen, M. M., Wigglesworth, D. F., DeBoer, D. P., & Math, M. (1994). Critical respiratory events in the postanesthesia care unit. *Anesthesiology, 81,* 410–418.

Sessler, D. I. (1994). Consequences and treatment of perioperative hypothermia. In R. C. Levitt (Ed.), *Anesthesiology Clinics of North America: Temperature Regulation During Anesthesia, 12,* 425–456.

Severinghaus, J. W. (1996). Negative pressure pulmonary edema causes analyzed. *Anesthesia Patient Safety Foundation Newsletter, 11*(2), 23–24.

Stein, R. E., & Urbaniak, J. (1980). Use of the tourniquet during surgery in patients with sickle cell hemoglobinopathies. *Clinical Orthopaedics, and Related Research, 151,* 231–233.

Stoelting, R. K. (1995). NPO—facts and fiction. IARS 1995 Review Course Lectures. *Anesthesia & Analgesia, 81*(Suppl.) 4–8.

Sunderrajan, S., Bauer, J. H., Vopat, R. L., Wanner-Barjenbruch, P., & Hayes, A. (1984). Posttransurethral prostatic resection hyponatremic syndrome: Case report and review of the literature. *American Journal of Kidney Disease, 4,* 80–84.

REFERENCES

Allen, G. C. (1994). Malignant hyperthermia susceptibility. In R. C. Levitt (Ed.), *Anesthesiology Clinics of North America: Temperature Regulation During Anesthesia, 12,* 513–535.

Albin, M. S. (1993). Air embolism. In L. M. Caplan & S. M. Miller (Eds.), *Anesthesiology Clinics of North America: Embolism II, 11,* 1–24.

Allnutt, M. F. (1987). Human factors in accidents. *British Journal of Anesthesia, 59,* 856–864.

Bartkowski, R. B. (1987). Incomplete reversal of pancuronium neuromuscular blockade by neostigmine, pyridostigmine, and edrophonium. *Anesthesia & Analgesia, 66,* 594–598.

Beebe, J. J. & Sessler, D. I. (1988). Preparation of anesthesia machines for patients susceptible to malignant hyperthermia. *Anesthesiology, 69,* 395–400.

Benumof, J. L. (1991). Management of the difficult airway. *Anesthesiology, 75,* 1087–1110.

Benumof, J. L. (1996a, September). The ASA Difficult Airway Algorithm: New thoughts/considerations. In T. F. Sanchez (Chair), *The society for airway management.* Annual Scientific Meeting, Newport Beach, CA.

Benumof, J. L. (1996b). Laryngeal mask airway and the ASA Difficult Airway Algorithm. *Anesthesiology, 84,* 686–699.

Blacher, R. S. (1975). On awakening paralyzed during surgery. *Journal of the American Medical Association, 234,* 67–68.

Blacher, R. S. (1984). Awareness during surgery. *Anesthesiology, 61,* 1–2.

Bogetz, M. S. & Katz, J. A. (1984). Recall of surgery for major trauma. *Anesthesiology, 61,* 6–9.

Caroff, S. N., Mann, S. C. & Campbell, E. C. (1994). Hyperthermia and neuroleptic malignant syndrome. In R. C. Levitt (Ed.), *Anesthesiology Clinics of North America: Temperature Regulation During Anesthesia, 12,* 491–512.

Carroll, J. B. (1987). Increased incidence of masseter spasm in children with strabismus anesthetized with halothane and succinylcholine. *Anesthesiology, 67,* 559–561.

Cascade, P. N., Alexander, G. D. & Mackie, D. S. (1993). Negative-pressure pulmonary edema after endotracheal intubation. *Radiology, 186,* 671–675.

Chadwick, H. S., Posner, K., Caplan, R. A., Ward, R. J., & Cheney, F. W. (1991). A comparison of obstetric and nonobstetric anesthesia malpractice claims. *Anesthesiology, 74,* 242–249.

Cheney, F. W., Posner, K. L. & Caplan, R. A. (1991). Adverse respiratory events infrequently leading to malpractice suits: a closed claim analysis. *Anesthesiology, 75,* 932–939.

Cohen, M. M., Duncan, P. G., DeBoer, D. P. & Tweed, W. A. (1994). The postoperative interview: Assessing risk factors for nausea and vomiting. *Anesthesia & Analgesia, 78,* 7–16.

Cooper, J. B., Newboer, R. S. & Kitz, R. J. (1984). An analysis of major error and equipment failures in anesthesia management: Considerations for prevention and detection. *Anesthesiology, 60,* 34–42.

Craig, D. B. (1981). Postoperative recovery of pulmonary function. *Anesthesia & Analgesia, 60,* 46–52.

Cullen, B. F. (1994). Diagnosis and prevention of intraoperative mishaps. *Anesthesia & Analgesia, 80*(Suppl.), 8–11.

Dierdorf, S. F. (1996). Awareness during anesthesia. In S. F. Dierdorf (Ed.), *Anesthesiology Clinics of North America: Practical Solutions for Difficult Problems I, 14,* 369–384.

Dover, S. B., Plenderleith, L., Moore, M. R., & McColl, K. E. L. (1994). Safety of general anaesthesia and surgery in acute hepatic porphyria. *Gut, 35,* 1112–1115.

Durant, T. M., Long, J. & Oppenheimer, M. J. (1947). Pulmonary (venous) air embolism. *American Heart Journal, 33,* 269–281.

Faraday, N., Rosenfeld, B. A. & Herfel, B. M. (1995). Hypothermia increases intrinsic platelet reactivity in vitro. [Abstract.] *Anesthesia & Analgesia, 80,* 14.

Frank, S. M., Beattie, C., Christopherson, R., Norris, E. J., Perler, B. A., Williams, G. M. & Gottlieb, S. O. (1993). Unintentional hypothermia is associated with postoperative myocardial ischemia. *Anesthesiology, 78,* 468–476.

Gal, T. J. (1996). Bronchial hyperresponsiveness and the patient for anesthesia. IARS 1996 Review Course Lectures. *Anesthesia & Analgesia, 82*(35), 37–45.

Goldberg, M. (1996). The allergic response and anesthesia. In N. Gravenstein & R. R. Kirby (Eds.), *Complications in anesthesiology* (2nd ed., pp. 605–618). Philadelphia: Lippincott-Raven.

Gwirtz, K. H. (1996). Management of recovery room complications. In S. F. Dierdorf (Ed.), *Anesthesia Clinics of North America: Practical Solutions for Difficult Problems, 14,* 307–339.

Harlow, K. D. & Ford, E. G. (1993). Pulmonary edema following post-operative laryngospasm: A case report and review of the literature. *American Surgery, 59,* 443–447.

Hershey, W. N., Wahrenbrock, E. A., & DeJong, R. H. (1965). Residual curarization. *Anesthesiology, 26,* 834.

Illing, L., Duncan, P. G. & Yip, R. (1992). Gastroesophageal reflux during anaesthesia. *Canadian Journal of Anaesthesia, 39,* 466–470.

Jensen, N. F., Fiddler, D. S., & Striepe, V. (1995). Anesthetic considerations in porphyrias. *Anesthesia & Analgesia, 80,* 591–599.

Lang, S. A., Duncan, P. G., Shephard, D. A. E. & Hung, C. H. (1990). Pulmonary oedema associated with airway obstruction. *Canadian Journal of Anaesthesia, 37,* 210–218.

Larach, M. G., Rosenberg, H., Larach, D. R. & Broennle, A. M. (1987). Prediction of malignant hyperthermia susceptibility by clinical signs. *Anesthesiology, 66,* 547–550.

Lyons, G. & Macdonald, R. (1991). Awareness during caesarean section. *Anaesthesia, 46,* 62–64.

Mallampati, S. R., Gatt, S. P., Gugino, L. D., Desai, S. P., Waraksa, B., Freiberger, D., & Liu, P. L. (1985). A clinical sign to predict difficult tracheal intubation: A prospective study. *Canadian Anaesthesia Society Journal, 32,* 429–434.

Marshall, B. E., & Wyche, M. Q., Jr. (1972). Hypoxemia during and after anesthesia. *Anesthesiology, 37,* 178–201.

Miller, K. A., Harkin, C. P. & Bailey, P. L. (1995). Postoperative tracheal extubation. *Anesthesia & Analgesia, 80,* 149–172.

Miller, L. G. & Jankovic, J. (1989). Metoclopramide-induced movement disorders: Clinical findings with a review of the literature. *Archives of Internal Medicine, 149,* 2486–2492.

Moss, J. (1995). Muscle relaxants and histamine release. *Acta Anaesthesiologica Scandinavica, 39,* 7–12.

Pearce, A. C. G., & Jones, R. M. (1984). Smoking and anesthesia: Preoperative abstinence and postoperative morbidity. *Anesthesiology, 61,* 576–584.

Rex, M. A. E. (1970). A review of the structural and functional basis of laryngospasm and discussion of the nerve pathways involved in man and animals. *British Journal of Anaesthesia, 42,* 891–899.

Rose, D. K., Cohen, M. M., Wigglesworth, D. F., DeBoer, D. P. & Math, M. (1994). Critical respiratory events in the postanesthesia care unit. *Anesthesiology, 81,* 410–418.

Sessler, D. I. (1994). Consequences and treatment of perioperative hypothermia. In R. C. Levitt (Ed.), *Anesthesiology Clinics of North America: Temperature Regulation During Anesthesia, 12,* 425–456.

Severinghaus, J. W. (1996). Negative pressure pulmonary edema causes analyzed. *Anesthesia Patient Safety Foundation Newsletter, 11*(2), 23–24.

Stein, R. E. & Urbaniak, J. (1980). Use of the tourniquet during surgery in patients with sickle cell hemoglobinopathies. *Clinical Orthopaedics and Related Research, 151,* 231–233.

Stoelting, R. K. (1995). NPO—Facts and fiction. IARS 1995 Review Course Lectures. *Anesthesia & Analgesia, 80*(Suppl), 4–8.

Stoelting, R. K. (1996). Comparative pharmacology of intravenous anesthetics. *Anesthesia & Analgesia, 83,* 121–127.

Sunderrajan, S., Bauer, J. H., Vopat, R. L., Wanner-Barjenbruch, P., & Hayes, A. (1984). Posttransurethral prostatic resection hyponatremic syndrome: Case report and review of the literature. *American Journal of Kidney Disease, 4,* 80–84.

Tang, J., Watcha, M. F. & White, P. F. (1996). A comparison of costs and efficacy of ondansetron and droperidol as prophylactic antiemetic therapy for elective outpatient gynecologic procedures. *Anesthesia & Analgesia, 83,* 304–313.

Umbrain, V., & Camu, F. (1993). Acute pulmonary edema after laryngospasm. *Acta Anaesthesiologica Belgica, 44,* 149–153.

Vistica, M. F., Posner, K. L., Caplan, R. A. & Cheney, F. W. (1990). Role of equipment failure and misuse in anesthetic-related malpractice claims. [Abstract.] *Anesthesiology, 73,* 1007.

Warner, M. A., Warner, M. E., & Weber, J. B. (1993). Clinical significance of pulmonary aspiration during the perioperative period. *Anesthesiology, 78,* 56–62.

Watcha, M. F. & White, P. F. (1992). Postoperative nausea and vomiting: Its etiology, treatment, and prevention. *Anesthesiology, 77,* 162–184.

Williamson, J. A., Webb, R. K., & Russell, W. J. (1993). Air embolism—An analysis of 2000 incident reports. *Anaesthesia and Intensive Care, 21,* 638–641.

Xue, F. S., Huang, Y. G., Tong, S. Y., Liu, Q. N., Liao, X., An, G., Luo, L. K., & Deng, X. M. (1996). A comparative study of early postoperative hypoxemia in infants, children, and adults undergoing elective plastic surgery. *Anesthesia & Analgesia, 83,* 709–715.

Young, A. & Skinner, T. A. (1995). Laryngospasm following extubation in children. [Correspondence.] *Anaesthesia 50,* 827.

Anesthesia Outcomes and Evaluation

Denise Martin-Sheridan

► A FOCUS ON QUALITY ASSURANCE

Hospitals and health care providers are facing significant pressure to increase their level of efficiency by providing cost-effective anesthesia services and service-related effectiveness by improving the quality and appropriateness of anesthesia care. Concern over the cost and quality of health care has produced a variety of responses ranging from remedial programs to the creation of hospital committees and departments whose responsibility it is to monitor quality in performance and to identify strategies to ensure that the highest quality care is provided at the lowest possible cost.

Historically, formalized quality review in the United States is rooted in concepts employed in the business sector in problem solving and productivity development (Cummings & Huse, 1989). Since the late 1970s American companies have enhanced their ability to compete in the market by improving their overall quality of performance. In a 1991 report from the U.S. General Accounting Office, corporations that instituted quality improvement activities demonstrated improved market share and profitability, greater customer satisfaction and quality, lower costs, and better employee relations. In hospitals, steps to ensure quality began to emerge when the American College of Surgeons published the American College of Surgeons' Hospital Standardization Program in 1913, outlining requirements for the structure of professional staff, case reviews, medical record documentation, and support services (Lord & Kraus, 1994). Later, during the 1950s, the elements of the program served as the foundation for a hospital accreditation process developed by the newly formed Joint Commission on Accreditation of Hospitals, later renamed the Joint Commission on Accreditation of Healthcare Organizations (JCAHO, 1996).

The JCAHO requirements fostered the development of quality assurance programs and departments to monitor compliance to established quality standards. *Quality Assurance (QA)* may be viewed establishing a consensus of what standards constitute adequate, acceptable, and excellent care; finding out what level of care was being given and received; and taking some action to maintain or improve the care (Lang & Marek, 1995). In its early stages, retrospective review of patient records was employed to monitor variances in the QA process. For example, a QA reviewer would randomly sample anesthesia records to determine whether each was signed by the appropriate anesthesia provider or to record how many ICU admissions were anesthesia related. Although these examples are an oversimplification of the context of the actual review, they are meant to illustrate the emphasis on structure and process measures that could easily be compared to some established industry standard. Meeting established standards for patient care is important for health care institutions not only from a quality of care perspective, but also from a reimbursement perspective. According to the Social Security Amendments of 1965, Public Law 89-97, hospitals and health care facilities that seek Medicare reimbursement for services must satisfy certain predetermined conditions of participation; meeting JCAHO standards satisfies those conditions.

From Quality Assurance to Quality Improvement

While the QA movement made strides toward ensuring quality standards of care were met, the nature of its measurement and monitoring approach reflected the achievement of structural criteria (eg, existence of written anesthesia department policies) and process criteria (eg, that evidence anesthesia department policies were followed). However, measurement and monitoring data should be used to assess the quality of care and make improvements in practice.

To make changes in practice, objective feedback from quality assurance data is a potentially powerful means of enhancing performance. Specific objective feedback promotes goal-setting behavior that has consistently positive effects on behavior and performance (Kopelman, 1986). Striving to continuously improve performance, while promoting excellence, effectiveness, and efficiency, has become the emphasis of new programs in quality assurance.

Changing Forces in the Health Care Environment

In this era of increased competition, cost control, and marketing, the establishment of an organizationwide culture of service excellence and quality is being discussed (Kalafat & Siman, 1991). The processes of establishing priorities, strategic planning, policies and procedures, and staff attitudes need to permeate the organizational structure. Such approaches have been referred to as total *quality management (TQM)* and *continuous quality improvement (CQI)*.

Originally developed by Deming in the United States and subsequently implemented in Japanese manufacturing corporations, TQM is the integration of: (1) a customer-focused, continuous-improvement philosophy; (2) analytical skills; (3) people skills; and (4) a structure and organization within an internal and external culture affected by the leadership. It is a combination of philosophy, knowledge, and skills uniquely effective in accomplishing organizational change through improvement in quality, cost-effectiveness, and human relations (Gaucher & Coffey, 1993). The following is a summary of the TQM philosophy.

1. Customer-focused, continuous-improvement philosophy strives to meet or exceed customer-defined requirements while continuously improving the way those requirements are met. Increased emphasis is directed toward judging how successful service strategies are, based on the customer's definition of quality service (Kalafat & Siman, 1991). Continuous improvement calls on the employee to participate with management and administration in decision making about how to do their jobs better and increase productivity and task performance.

2. Using qualitative and quantitative tools to gather, analyze, interpret, and apply data is a fundamental premise of TQM. Specific objective information serves as an instrument to direct organization decisions based on analytical knowledge and skills.

3. In the TQM environment, work is accomplished in a multidisciplinary approach, where everyone within the organization is considered critical to successful achievement of goals. This participative management style requires a high degree of interpersonal and people-oriented skills, self-organization, and empowerment to facilitate individuals and groups to understand they have ownership of their jobs. This helps create a situation more conducive to effective quality assurance (LaPointe, 1996).

4. Leaders in the organization must be actively involved in TQM efforts and establish the structure required to make quality the highest priority. This means that employees must be able to participate in a wide range of activities. Although the concepts are the same, TQM should be tailored to the organization's internal and external environments, taking into account the particular needs and predispositions that are uniquely their own. Such things as client characteristics, work schedules, and financial resources are factors that must be taken into account.

Total Quality Management stresses the importance that a new paradigm, or model, must be adopted for organizations to be successful in the future. The paradigm is a shift in focus from managing to leading; control to coaching; quantity to quality; opinion to data; resistance to openness for change; people as commodities to people as resources; suspicion to trust; compliance to commitment; internal focus to customer focus; individual to team; and detection to prevention (Gaucher & Coffey, 1993).

A critical piece of any program that attempts to quantify and assess the quality of service provided to a client (eg, the quality of anesthesia services provided to the surgical patient) must include evidence of effectiveness. Demonstrating the link between a particular intervention (eg, service or care) and benefit (to the patient or client) is a measurement of outcome.

What Are Outcomes?

Outcomes are measures, or variables, that describe the result or effect of a particular intervention. When patients are considered, the result of an intervention may be the effect a method of treatment has on the patient. For the patient who undergoes anesthesia, an example of a desirable outcome could be a postoperative course during which time there was zero incidence of postoperative nausea and vomiting. Other examples of outcomes are variables such as the incidence of morbidity and mortality, complication rates, rating of satisfaction by the client (patient), and length of stay (Bidwell-Cerone, Krainovich-Miller, Haber, Penney, & Carter, 1995).

Outcomes also can be used to measure the extent to which a learner has met clinical education standards (Martin-Sheridan, Bruton-Maree & Horton, 1993). Clinical objectives (outcomes) are established by the faculty to assess whether graduate students in nurse anesthesia education programs have successfully assimilated requisite skills and knowledge. Requisite skills and knowledge might include such things as performing an induction sequence and articulating a rationale supporting the selection of a particular induction drug. Recent advances in technology, such as computer-based simulations in anesthesiology, are being used by many education programs to help assess outcome achievement in clinical practice.

The Role of the CRNA

The American Association of Nurse Anesthetists (AANA) and CRNAs have a long history of commitment to quality assurance endeavors. Examples include the AANA *Guidelines for the Practice of the Certified Registered Nurse Anesthetist,* first published in 1980. Now called the *Professional Practice Manual for the CRNA,* it describes the practice of the CRNA, delineates standards for nurse anesthesia practice, offers guidelines for CRNAs (AANA, 1996) and health care institutions regarding granting of clinical privileges, and provides a model position description for the CRNA (Table 35-1). In 1987 the JCAHO convened an Anesthesia Task Force charged with developing a list of clinical outcomes that could be used to evaluate performance data. Members of the Anesthesia Task Force included CRNAs who represented the nurse anesthesia community of interest (Zambricki, 1994). The AANA joined as a patron of the Anesthesia and Patient Safety Foundation (APSF). The APSF is a nonprofit foundation established in 1984 by the American Society of Anesthesiologists (ASA), whose stated mission it is "to assure no patient shall be harmed by the effects of anesthesia" (Siker, 1996). Other activities that focus on patient standards and quality patient care include continuing education offerings sponsored by the AANA. At the institutional level, CRNAs are responsible for developing, implementing, and participating in quality assurance and TQM programs. It is clear that CRNAs feel strongly that an essential component of practice is to define and maintain high-quality standards.

TABLE 35-1. Standards for Nurse Anesthesia Practice

Table of Contents

From the American Association of Nurse Anesthetists. (1996). Professional Practice Manual for the CRNA. *Park Ridge: IL: Author. Reprinted with permission.*

► CONCEPTS, PRINCIPLES, AND STRATEGIES OF OUTCOME EVALUATION

What Is Outcome Evaluation?

On March 11, 1847, a 21-year-old woman underwent surgery for removal of a tumor from her thigh. A diethyl ether anesthetic was administered to the patient, who

40 hours later was dead. According to officials who reviewed the case, later cited in *Medical Jurisprudence,* "The death of this person did result from the effects of the vapor of ether, and not from the tumor under which she was laboring." (as cited in Biddle, 1994). This case is an example of outcome evaluation in anesthesia.

Outcome evaluation, or analysis, entails observing and reviewing interventions (eg, surgical and anesthetic techniques in the case described) and results (eg, death) to determine whether there are any relationships between observed events. In basic terms, the purpose of outcome evaluation is to identify problems so that untoward events, such as death, can be avoided in the future. Outcome evaluation should provide a structured approach by which deviations from the norm or an established standard can be examined and alternatives developed to change the practice so as to promote quality improvement.

From a quality improvement perspective, standards may be viewed as expectations that should serve to drive the achievement of specified behaviors. In some situations, standards are used as yardsticks against which results can be measured. Standards often are established by a profession as a means of self-regulation to ensure quality in performance (Lang & Marek, 1995). In nurse anesthesia for example, the Council on Accreditation of Nurse Anesthesia Educational Programs (COA) uses the *Standards for Accreditation of Nurse Anesthesia Educational Programs* to "improve the quality of nurse anesthesia education and to provide a competent anesthetist for health care consumers and employers" (COA, 1997). Table 35-2 is Standard V: Evaluation, an example of the standards used by the COA to evaluate nurse anesthesia education programs.

Foundations of Quality Improvement

Quality as a concept in any environment will be perceived differently according to who has defined the term. For a systematic quality improvement program to succeed, quality must first be defined. In the health care environment, practitioners, consumers, payers, and society all have a stake in defining quality parameters. A model developed in 1988 by Boland (as cited in Lanning & O'Connor, 1990) that describes the different perspective of each stakeholder is represented in Figure 35–1.

The model includes (1) inputs, comprised of human resources and capital resources required to complete the work; and the patient population required to drive demand for service; (2) process or throughputs, which are the services provided; and (3) the outcomes or consequences of the services provided. Efficiency is described by achieving the specific result at the minimum human and capital resource cost. Appropriateness considers the fit between patient population and the continuum of ser-

TABLE 35-2. Standard V: Evaluation 1994 Standards for Accreditation of Nurse Anesthesia Educational Programs

A program of nurse anesthesia, in conjunction with its community of interest, must perform an ongoing assessment to determine its integrity and educational effectiveness. This process should assess not only the program's present status but determine its future goals for improvement and its methods for achieving them.

Specific criteria: Such a program is required to

E1. Provide for periodic review by external agencies.

E2. Evaluate the relevance of its mission statement, educational purposes and outcomes, curriculum plan, faculty and methods of instruction.

E3. Assess systematically its curriculum to determine if it accomplishes stated purposes, attains identified outcomes and uses the results of this evaluation to make appropriate adjustments to improve student achievement.

*E4. Employ a variety of indicators to evaluate student's clinical and cognitive skills as they progress through the program.

E5. Evaluate administrative policies and procedures to ensure that they are current and relevant and are used as a basis for making appropriate changes.

E6. Require students to periodically complete written evaluations of the faculty and program.

*E7. Require faculty members to complete formative and summative evaluations of each student's performance in the clinical and didactic area.

E8. Provide for periodic student and faculty self-evaluations.

E9. Provide for periodic faculty evaluations by superior(s).

E10. Conduct evaluation of all clinical and academic sites on a regular basis.

E11. Monitor and evaluate its indicators of success on a continual basis and correct deficiencies.

E12. Evaluate program length, tuition and fees relative to career opportunities and credentials earned.

E13. Utilize evaluative criteria to assess the adequacy of current and future resources to achieve the program's purposes and outcomes.

*E14. Resolve previously identified areas of partial compliance or noncompliance with the standards.

E15. Assess its responsibility as prescribed by law and devise plans for corrective action as necessary.

E16. Review default rates in the student loan programs under Title IV of the Act, based on the most recent data provided by the U.S. Secretary of Education.

* Noncompliance with one or more of these criteria is considered to be of critical concern in decisions regarding nurse anesthesia program accreditation.
From the American Association of Nurse Anesthetists. (1994). Standards for accreditation council on accreditation of nurse anesthesia educational programs. *Park Ridge, IL: Author.*

vices provided to meet the patient's needs and predispositions. Effectiveness assesses whether improved or maintained health status is achieved and whether perceptions of effectiveness held by the patient were satisfied.

In the model, structure is the variable measured by the stakeholder; process is the what and how valued by the stakeholder; and outcome is the specific indicator

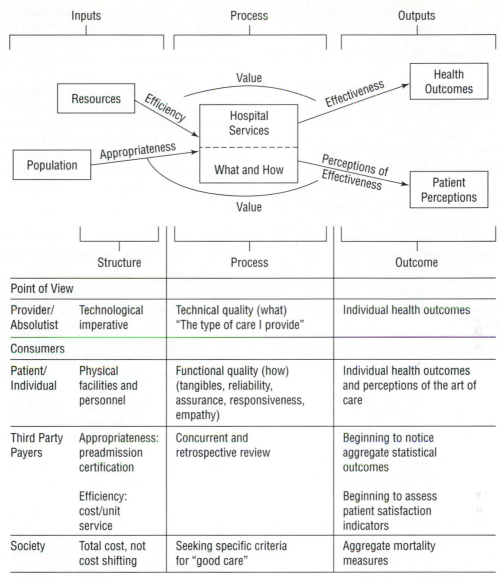

	Structure	Process	Outcome
Point of View			
Provider/ Absolutist	Technological imperative	Technical quality (what) "The type of care I provide"	Individual health outcomes
Consumers			
Patient/ Individual	Physical facilities and personnel	Functional quality (how) (tangibles, reliability, assurance, responsiveness, empathy)	Individual health outcomes and perceptions of the art of care
Third Party Payers	Appropriateness: preadmission certification	Concurrent and retrospective review	Beginning to notice aggregate statistical outcomes
	Efficiency: cost/unit service		Beginning to assess patient satisfaction indicators
Society	Total cost, not cost shifting	Seeking specific criteria for "good care"	Aggregate mortality measures

Figure 35–1. Definitions of quality health care. *(From Lanning, J. A., O'Connor, S. J. [1990]. The health care quality quagmire: Some sign posts. Hospital and Health Services Administration, 35[1], 42. Reprinted with permission. Adapted from Boland, P. [Ed.]. [1988]. The New Healthcare Market [p. 720]. Rockville, MD: Aspen.)*

(result) that defines quality for the stakeholder. For any quality improvement plan or process to succeed, it is critical to define and understand the perspective each stakeholder has about quality before problems can be identified and any improvements can be achieved. For example, from the perspective of the anesthesia provider, quality may mean that, because a CRNA has a high degree of technical competence and of scientific and nursing knowledge, he or she is able to provide anesthesia services with a low incidence of anesthesia-related patient morbidity and mortality. From the perspective of the patient, quality not only is good individual outcomes, but also includes perceptions of how anesthesia services were provided (was the service prompt, reliable, com-

passionate, and attentive to individual needs and predispositions) and quality-of-life issues (does the intervention provide any overall health benefit to the patient). From a payer's perspective, quality may consider the aggregate incidence of morbidity and mortality for an institution or group of providers, the cost of care, and the appropriateness of care. Although these examples are not all inclusive, they are points that should be considered when issues of quality in relation to health care services are discussed.

Most health care organizations have detailed quality improvement programs. Many have been developed to meet JCAHO requirements and to satisfy other state and national agency specifications. Lord and Krause (1995) outline major sections of a plan commonly utilized by organizations to assess and improve quality:

1. General description of the plan with goals and objectives
2. Outline and scope of activities to be assessed
3. Delineation of who is responsible for assessment activities
4. Methods for collecting data
5. Mechanisms for reporting and oversight
6. Process for assessment of effectiveness

Over the last several years, the changing complexion of health care has dictated that payers, providers, and employers join forces to identify strategies that achieve high levels of effectiveness while lowering costs. Doing better and more with less are driving forces in the environment.

Objective Assessment and Analysis of Outcomes

Understanding the link between effectiveness, outcome, and patient care is a matter of concern for those involved in analyzing outcomes. Analysis of outcome involves linking the type of care received by a variety of patients with a particular condition to positive and negative results (outcomes) in order to identify what works best for which patients (Guadagnoli & McNeil, 1994). An example of analysis of outcome might be to determine how effective a drug is on the incidence of postoperative nausea and vomiting (PONV) in a group of outpatients known to be at risk. Because PONV may prolong hospital stay and affect overall patient satisfaction, finding solutions to the problem may decrease costs and improve customer relations. Although this appears to be a relatively straightforward example, in practice several variables could call into question whether results from the analysis were based on objective measurements.

For example, if the risk of PONV was not similar across all patients, the homogeneity of the study population could be questioned. Nonpatient-related variables, such as the availability of nursing staff (human resources issues), may prolong hospital stay. The importance of identifying objective, measurable outcome criteria cannot be emphasized enough. If results of outcome analyses are not objective, decision making by consumers, payers, providers, and policymakers may be compromised (Martin-Sheridan, 1996).

Currently, research is being conducted to develop criteria for objective measurement of the "right" treatment, that is, application of defined diagnostic and treatment approaches, as well as responses to complications. These criteria provide a common language that may make it possible better to compare results from one hospital to another and from one provider to another. An example is the patient classification system APACHE (Acute Physiologic And Chronic Health Evaluation) that was developed better to identify risk of death in intensive care units (Knaus, Draper, & Zimmerman, 1985). Theoretically, classification systems of this type would make quantitative analysis of patient data possible to determine those organizations, or providers, that need to improve their performance, and furnish scorecards to consumers. It should be stressed again, while quantitative analysis of outcome is important, qualitative aspects, especially patient satisfaction and quality of life issues, also must be taken into account, when comparisons are made.

The Link between Outcome Evaluation and Improving Anesthesia Care

Understanding the link between outcome evaluation and patient care is a matter of concern for those involved in outcome analysis. An essential component of any program or process whose purpose is to ensure quality, evaluate outcome, and foster continuous quality improvement, must include feedback mechanisms to enhance performance, change behavior, and modify clinical practice patterns. Fundamentally, changes in practice should be driven by studies that systematically evaluate the effectiveness and efficiency of a patient intervention (Kaplan & Ries, 1996). In anesthesia, for example, the intervention may include such things as the application of end-tidal carbon dioxide ($ETCO_2$) monitoring to detect esophageal intubation.

Many poor outcomes during anesthesia are related to the effects of hypoventilation. Capnography, specifically $ETCO_2$ monitoring, is described in the literature as the best continuous monitor of ventilation and indicator of esophageal intubation (Wagner, 1992). Based on these studies, the AANA (1996) and ASA (Wagner, 1992) have published patient monitoring standards mandating that correct placement of an endotracheal tube be verified by auscultation, chest excursion, and $ETCO_2$ monitoring. The use of $ETCO_2$ monitoring is perceived to be so important that its use is a standard of care against which contemporary anesthesia practice is measured. Therefore, $ETCO_2$ monitoring is used to decrease the probability or risk of poor patient outcome during the perioperative period.

▶ RISK MANAGEMENT AND ANESTHESIA PRACTICE

What Is Risk Management?

Managing risk in organizations can be viewed as a systematic process designed to identify mishaps or failures that are likely to occur (probability) and to develop strategies to avoid poor outcomes to minimize financial losses. In the airline and nuclear power industries, for example, ongoing training, data gathering, standard operation procedures, and simulators to model critical events are used to prepare employees to manage adverse situations and avoid poor outcomes.

Managing risk is especially critical when the potential risk involves harm to a patient. Since the late 1970s there has been significant growth in the frequency and size of payments for medical malpractice claims as well as growth in the premiums paid for professional liability insurance. In health care the greatest risk of claims is associated with clinical care areas and patient care management (American Hospital Association, 1991). In anesthesia, the frequent cause of mishaps appears to be preventable human error (Cooper, Neubower, Long, & McPeek, 1978). The following section presents an overview of risk management as a process and the role it plays in promoting quality patient outcomes.

Components of a Risk Management Process

Fundamentally, risk management as a process may be viewed as a comprehensive plan that includes issues of health care, medical malpractice, risk of financial loss, and liability as parts of overall decision making. In this context, risk management goes beyond considering medical malpractice and liability and becomes an important part of strategies that emphasize quality and continuous improvement.

Taking Inventory

One of the first steps in a risk management process is to take inventory of the risk issues or factors in the organization or environment under consideration. In anesthesia practice, for example, before developing a risk management program, it would be essential to know what factors or issues generally place a patient who undergoes an anesthetic at risk. Acquiring this information may include such things as reviewing malpractice claims experience, such as closed-claims studies (Caplan, Posner, Ward, & Cheney, 1988), institutional claims reports, and reports of risk identified in the literature (Goldman & Caldera, 1979).

Accumulating Data

Once the risk factors in the environment in general have been identified, an assessment is made to determine the likelihood those factors could occur in a particular setting (eg, anesthesia department), and the impact it would have if they did occur. The impacts might include financial losses (payment of malpractice claims), loss of credibility with the public and consumers, and low staff morale. From this assessment risk priorities are developed for which solutions, or treatments, can be identified. Treatments will include ways to control risk and risk financing (insurance).

Education

Tailoring risk management to a particular organization or group requires members of the group to become shareholders in the process. It is important that all members actively participate to identify and modify situations that are inherently risky (Masta-Gornic & Youngberg, 1996). This means that information about the risks being faced must be shared with members of the organization. Ongoing teaching and staff education sessions can be used to increase involvement, active participation, and collaboration in the risk management process.

Evaluation and Improvement

The final step in the risk management process is to review and evaluate how well the objectives were met and to initiate strategies to revise and improve the plan. Measuring the degree of success or failure should be honest and difficulties encountered where objectives were not achieved should be identified. The evaluation should be especially sensitive to feedback from all participants to enhance the program's effectiveness in the future.

The creation of a risk management program can be expected to achieve several important objectives. The program should prevent financial losses and control insurance claims, produce positive employee health and safety data, and improve patient satisfaction. In addition, when the process is well conducted, it should foster a participative and collaborative work environment that may reap many subjective positive returns for the institution or department (DeMask & Welke, 1993).

▶ MANAGING RISK AND IMPROVING OUTCOME DURING ANESTHESIA

Anesthesia-related medical liability claims account for about 3% to 4% of total claims, although the indemnity paid exceeds 10%, which likely reflects the severity of injury experienced by the claimant. When reviews of anesthesia-related claims are summarized, certain factors (also called indicators or problems) recur (Brown, 1992). For example, human error has been found to be a significant factor contributing to anesthesia-related claims, especially complications involving inadequate ventilation, inadvertent extubation, ventilator disconnects, esophageal intubations, and equipment utilized during the perioperative period (Cooper et al., 1978).

In anesthesia, information about department-specific occurrences needs to be gathered to avoid risk and

TABLE 35–3. Joint Commission on Accreditation of Healthcare Organizations 10-Step Model of Quality Improvement

1. Assign responsibility for monitoring the evaluation activities.
2. Delineate the scope of care provided by the organization.
3. Identify the most important aspects of care provided by the organization.
4. Identify indicators (and appropriate clinical criteria) for monitoring the important aspects of the care.
5. Establish thresholds (levels, patterns, trends) for the indicators that trigger evaluation of care.
6. Monitor the important aspects of care by collecting and organizing the data for each indicator.
7. Evaluate care when thresholds are reached in order to identify opportunities to improve care or resolve problems.
8. Take actions to improve care or to correct identified problems.
9. Assess the effectiveness of actions and document the improvement in care.
10. Communicate the results of the monitoring and evaluation process to relevant individuals, departments, or services and to the organizationwide quality improvement program.

improve outcome and patient satisfaction. Before this can be accomplished, a plan (TQM) is essential. Often, the plan follows the JCAHO (1996) 10-step model of quality improvement (Table 35-3). Based on this model, responsibility in the anesthesia department to coordinate the plan is assigned, the scope of anesthesia services are defined, aspects of anesthesia care are identified, anesthesia indicators are developed (Table 35-4), trig-

TABLE 35–4. Examples of Anesthesia Indicators

Airway related
  Failed intubation
  Difficult intubation
  Traumatic intubation
  Esophageal intubation
Pulmonary related
  Diffuse rhonci
  Pulmonary edema
  Pulmonary aspiration
  Pneumothorax
Cardiovascular related
  Hypotension
  Hypertension
  Cardiac arrest
  Cardiac dysrhythmias
  Low PCWP
General
  PONV
  Failed regional technique
  Postoperative pain
  Recall after anesthesia

gers that set review in motion are established, data are collected and evaluated, remediation steps are taken if required, events are documented, and findings are communicated.

The following is an example of the components of a risk management guide for nurse anesthetists.

Anesthesia Management

Anesthesia management is comprised of three interrelated phases about which the anesthetist should have detailed information and a specific plan of action to avoid risk and ensure a satisfactory patient outcome. The phases are preanesthetic evaluation, intraoperative monitoring, and postoperative evaluation.

During preanesthetic evaluation, a determination is made concerning whether the patient can safely undergo anesthesia for the surgical procedure scheduled, what precautions should be taken, and what special considerations apply. The anesthetic technique is selected based on patient information and a plan of anesthetic patient care management is developed. During this phase, patient teaching takes place about the purpose, alternatives, and risks of anesthesia. It is an opportunity to establish patient–provider rapport and answer questions the patient may have about the process of anesthesia.

The second phase of anesthesia management is patient monitoring. Based on work by Cooper et al. (1978), vigilant monitoring of the patient and attention to the conduct of the anesthetic are critical elements of patient safety. The AANA endorsed the Harvard Standards for Monitoring Patients under Anesthesia (Table 35-5), which specify detailed mandatory standards for minimal patient monitoring under anesthesia. Required in the standards are blood pressure and heart rate monitoring, ECG, continuous monitoring of ventilation and circulation, breathing system disconnection monitoring, oxygen analyzer usage, and the ability to monitor temperature. In addition, the anesthetist must monitor patient position, fluids, response to pharmacologic agents, acid–base balance, and surgically induced problems.

The third phase of anesthesia management is postoperative evaluation, during which time the patient is assessed to identify any anesthesia-related problems. If problems are identified, actions should be taken to resolve them.

Anesthesia Equipment

A study by Cooper, Newbower, and Kitz (1984) that analyzed anesthesia critical incidents found a significant association between failure to perform a normal preuse check of anesthesia equipment and occurrences of critical incidents. Serious patient injury related to anesthesia equipment and malfunction or misuse can be avoided

TABLE 35–5. Harvard Standards for Monitoring Patients under Anesthesia

These standards apply for any administration of anesthesia involving department of anaesthesia personnel and are specifically referable to preplanned anesthetics administered in designated anesthetizing locations (specific exclusion; administration of epidural analgesia for labor or pain management). In emergency circumstances in any location, immediate life support measures of whatever appropriate nature come first with attention turning to the measures described in these standards as soon as possible and practical. These are minimal standards that may be exceeded at any time based on the judgment of the involved anesthesia personnel. These standards encourage high-quality patient care, but observing them cannot guarantee any specific patient outcome. These standards are subject to revision from time to time, as warranted by the evolution of technology and practice.

Anesthesiologist's or Nurse Anesthetist's Presence in Operating Room

For all anesthetics initiated by or involving a member of the department of anaesthesia, an attending or resident anesthesiologist or nurse anesthetist shall be present in the room throughout the conduct of all general anesthetics, regional anesthetics, and monitored intravenous anesthetics. An exception is made when there is a direct known hazard, e.g., radiation, to the anesthesiologist or nurse anesthetist, in which case some provision for monitoring the patient must be made.

Blood Pressure and Heart Rate

Every patient receiving general anesthesia, regional anesthesia, or managed intravenous anesthesia shall have arterial blood pressure and heart rate measured at least every five minutes, where not clinically impractical.

Electrocardiogram

Every patient shall have the electrocardiogram continuously displayed from the induction or institution of anesthesia until preparing to leave the anesthetizing location, where not clinically impractical.

Continuous Monitoring

During every administration of general anesthesia, the anesthetist shall employ methods of continuously monitoring the patient's ventilation and circulation. The methods shall include, for ventilation and circulation each, at least one of the following or the equivalent:

For Ventilation.—Palpation or observation of the reservoir breathing bag, auscultation of breath sounds, monitoring of respiratory gases such as end-tidal carbon dioxide, or monitoring of expiratory gas flow. Monitoring end-tidal carbon dioxide is an emerging standard and is strongly preferred.

For Circulation.—Palpation of a pulse, auscultation of heart sounds, monitoring of a tracing of intra-arterial pressure, pulse plethysmography/oximetry, or ultrasound peripheral pulse monitoring.

It is recognized that brief interruptions of the continuous monitoring may be unavoidable.

Breathing System Disconnection Monitoring

When ventilation is controlled by an automatic mechanical ventilator, there shall be in continuous use a device that is capable of detecting disconnection of any component of the breathing system. The device must give an audible signal when its alarm threshold is exceeded. (It is recognized that there are certain rare or unusual circumstances in which such a device may fail to detect a disconnection.)

Oxygen Analyzer

During every administration of general anesthesia using an anesthesia machine, the concentration of oxygen in the patient breathing system will be measured by a functioning oxygen analyzer with a low concentration limit alarm in use. This device must conform to the American National Standards Institute No. Z.79. 10 standard.

Ability to Measure Temperature

During every administration of general anesthesia, there shall be readily available a means to measure the patient's temperature.

Rationale.—A means of temperature measurement must be available as a potential aid in the diagnosis and treatment of suspected or actual intraoperative hypothermia and malignant hyperthermia. The measurement/monitoring of temperature during *every* general anesthetic is not specifically mandated because of the potential risks of such monitoring and because of the likelihood of other physical signs giving earlier indication of the development of malignant hyperthermia.

From the Department of Anaesthesia, Harvard Medical School. Adopted March 25, 1985; Revised July 3, 1985.

by establishing a policy for maintaining, use and daily checking of equipment.

Please refer to Figure 33–4 as an example of a preuse anesthesia equipment checklist developed by the FDA, with input from the ASA and AANA. It should be noted that to be effective the checklist must be used routinely to detect anesthesia equipment faults (Manley & Cuddeford, 1996).

Anesthesia Records and Documentation

A complete, accurate, and legible anesthesia record stands as documentation of patient care and may be used to evaluate the quality of anesthesia services rendered. The anesthesia record should include documentation about the perioperative period relevant to preoperative events, intraoperative management, and postoperative care. For an in-depth discussion of documentation of anesthesia care, the reader is referred to Chapter 33.

► UTILIZING OUTCOME MEASURES IN NURSE ANESTHESIA EDUCATION

The system of education in the United States is in a stage of transition comparable to that experienced in health care. There is a growing demand, and need, to do more with less and to make more efficient use of limited resources. Mechanisms developed to ensure that students receive the educational preparation required are critical. This is especially important in higher education, as there appears to be a direct link between the economic strength of a nation and the quality of its system of higher education (Lenn, 1995).

In nurse anesthesia education, the process of accreditation is used as a tool to assist programs develop critical self-assessment mechanisms and implement continuous quality improvement strategies. As in any other quality assurance or quality improvement process, assessment and improvement can be viewed as two ends of a continuum that undergird the process of accreditation and of evaluation of program effectiveness. Whereas accreditation processes have always been concerned with institutional and program effectiveness, the current emphasis on assessment recognizes the central importance of student learning and development and documents such learning and development in terms of outcomes related to instructional goals (Martin-Sheridan et al., 1993).

As Lanning and O'Connor (1990) described in Figure 35–1, one method of assessing quality in organizations is by examining inputs (what), throughputs (how), and outputs (outcomes/results). In nurse anesthesia education programs, inputs might include such things as financial resources, clinical resources, qualified clinical and didactic faculty, office space, and the prospective applicant pool. Examples of throughputs might include measures of how well graduate students achieve clinical skills, their success meeting didactic instructional goals, grade point average, and predicting how well they will perform in anesthesia practice after completing the program. Evaluating outputs might include verification from employers that program graduates are competent to practice, successful completion of the certification examination, and publication of a manuscript in a peer-reviewed journal.

Finally, as in any organization committed to improving the manner and method by which it conducts business, outcome assessment in nurse anesthesia education should be perceived as an opportunity to determine what needs to be retained, improved, or discarded. Ultimately the process should increase the overall effectiveness and efficiency of the nurse anesthesia education system.

▶ CASE STUDY

Outcome evaluation in anesthesia can take many forms. Morbidity and mortality review, chart audit, accreditation analysis and patient satisfaction surveys are examples of assessment strategies. The following case study discusses how members of an anesthesia department evaluated the effectiveness of a program allowing parents to be present while their children were being induced. It demonstrates a practical approach to quality assessment, based on qualitative and quantitative analysis, the results of which produced changes in clinical practice and promoted self-improvement.

The fact children experience fear and anxiety during the perioperative period was well known to members in the department. In our experience, one of the most difficult periods, especially for children over 2 years of age, appears to be when they are separated from their parents or significant person at the time of induction of anesthesia. We found that the impact of separation anxiety often led to a stormy induction, and others noted behavioral changes, such as bed wetting, temper tantrums, and attention disorder.

Traditionally, anesthesia providers have used pharmacologic agents to allay anxiety in children. However, we questioned the suitability of premedicating every pediatric outpatient, where an atraumatic route of administration and rapid and reliable onset and elimination are critical. Because the volume of pediatric outpatient surgery was on the rise and to improve the quality of services provided to pediatric patients and their families (improve discharge time and increase satisfaction), alternative strategies were investigated.

We found that allowing parents to be present during anesthesia induction was well documented in the literature and coincided with the emphasis on parental roles in pediatric health care in general. Many researchers reported that parental presence resulted in a significant decrease in the number of upset children during preinduction and induction periods and minimized the need for premedication.

A program was developed to allow parents to be present while their children were being induced. Protocols were written based on what was published in the literature, and on the input from those members of our department who were experienced at providing anesthesia care to pediatric patients.

After implementing the practice of allowing parents to be present during induction, we undertook two major reviews of the program (Jabour & Martin-Sheridan, 1996). This was accomplished through qualitative and quantitative assessment of factors that influenced parental anxiety and satisfaction. The results of the review demonstrated high overall satisfaction and low anxiety. However, results also identified a perception that preoperative patient teaching and the quality of information provided were not consistent.

Based on the results of our review, it was recommended that a more structured process of providing preoperative patient teaching and information be instituted. We have discussed two strategies to address this issue: (1) reviewing with anesthesia and PACU staff the purpose and process of the program allowing parents to be present at induction, emphasizing the importance of detailed preoperative patient teaching and information; and (2) developing a preoperative patient teaching and information booklet and video detailing the program.

▶ SUMMARY

As the health care environment evolves into the 21st century ongoing demands will be placed on anesthesia practitioners to increase the overall quality, effectiveness, and efficiency of the services they provide. To attain these goals organized and systematic planning, evaluating, and decision making at the institution, department, and individual practitioner level are necessary. Although new names may be assigned to the process in the future, outcome assessment and evaluation in anesthesia will be critical to longevity in the specialty.

▶ KEY CONCEPTS

- Irrespective of the terminology utilized (QA, TQM, CQI), quality assessment in health care should be an ongoing process designed to improve the quality, effectiveness, and efficiency of anesthesia services, as well as patient outcome.
- Risk management is a process designed to determine the likelihood of a poor outcome, estimate the probability a poor outcome will occur, and develop strategies to avoid the poor outcome in the future.
- Risk management is a process designed to decrease the probability an organization will suffer financial loss as a result of medical liability.
- Quality assessment and risk management programs assess inputs (what), throughputs (how), and results (outcomes).
- The AANA has been involved in quality assessment and risk management activities for many years and has established or endorsed policies to guide CRNA practice.
- Quality assessment and risk management activities were first developed to improve efficiency and effectiveness in service and manufacturing organizations. Experiences in the business sector later served as the foundation for similar initiatives in health care.
- The Joint Commission on Accreditation of Healthcare Organizations (JCAHO) establishes the minimum standards for quality in health care organizations required for accreditation.
- Accreditation by JCAHO is desirable because meeting JCAHO standards satisfies Medicare condition of participation for reimbursement.

STUDY QUESTIONS

1. Cooper et al., (1984) analyzed anesthesia critical incidents that lead to poor patient outcome. What are two factors associated with mishaps under anesthesia? Discuss the rationale for your answer.

2. Discuss three contemporary mechanisms established at the national level to ensure quality standards in health care. Describe how they impact nurse anesthesia practice.

3. What is outcome evaluation? What roles can CRNAs play in outcome evaluation?

4. Describe the process of risk management and outline three of its basic components.

5. Describe how outcome evaluation and risk management can lead to changes in nurse anesthesia practice.

KEY REFERENCES

American Association of Nurse Anesthetists. (1996). *Professional Practice Manual for the CRNA.* Park Ridge, IL: Author.

Cooper, J. B., Newbower, R. S., Long, C. D., McPeek, B. J. (1978). Preventable anesthesia mishaps: A study of human factors. *Anesthesiology, 49,* 399–406.

Joint Commission on Accreditation of Healthcare Organizations. (1996). *Accreditation manual for hospitals.* Oakbrook Terrace, IL: Author.

LaPointe, G. (1996). Management of an anesthesia department. In J. Nagelhout & K. Zaglaniczny (Eds.), *Nurse anesthesia* (pp. 28–43). Philadelphia: Saunders.

Lord, J. T. & Krause, G. P. (1995). Quality assessment and improvement in the 1990s. In S. D. Foster & L. M. Jordan (Eds.), *Professional aspects of nurse anesthesia practice* (pp. 291–305). Philadelphia: Davis.

REFERENCES

American Association of Nurse Anesthetists. (1996). *Professional Practice Manual for the CRNA.* Park Ridge, IL: Author.

American Hospital Association. (1991). *Risk management self assessment manual.* Washington, DC: Author.

Biddle, C. (1994). Outcome measures in anesthesiology: Are we going in the right direction? *AANA Journal, 62*(2), 117–124.

Bidwell-Cerone, S., Krainovich-Miller, B., Haber, J., Penney, N., & Carter, E. (1995, September). Nursing research and patient outcomes: Tools for managing the transformation of the health care delivery system. *The Journal of the New York State Nurses Association, 26*(3), 12–17.

Brown, D. L. (1992). Anesthesia risk: A historical perspective. In D. Brown (Ed.), *Risk and outcome in anesthesia* (pp. 1–35). Philadelphia: Lippincott.

Caplan, R. A., Posner, K., Ward, R. J., & Cheney, F. W. (1988). Peer reviewer agreement for major anesthetic mishaps. *Quality Review Bulletin, 14,* 363–368.

Cooper, J. B., Newbower, R. S., Long, C. D., & McPeek, B. J. (1978). Preventable anesthesia mishaps: A study of human factors. *Anesthesiology, 49,* 399–406.

Cooper, J. B., Newbower, R. S., & Kitz, R. J. (1984). An analysis of major errors and equipment failures in anesthesia management: Considerations for prevention and detection. *Anesthesiology, 60,* 34–42.

Council on Accreditation of Nurse Anesthesia Educational Programs. (1997). *Standards for accreditation.* Park Ridge, IL: Author.

Cummings, T. G., & Huse, E. F. (1989). *Organization development and change* (4th ed., p. 272). St. Paul, MN: West Publishing.

DeMask, D., & Welke, F. C. (1993). An anesthesia quality improvement program utilizing a computer database to effect change. *AANA Journal, 61*(1), 42–47.

Gaucher, E. J., & Coffey, R. J. (1993). *Total quality in healthcare: From theory to practice.* San Francisco: Jossey-Bass.

Goldman, L., & Caldera, D. L. (1979). Risks of general anesthesia and elective operation in the hypertensive patient. *Anesthesiology, 50,* 285–292.

Guadagnoli, E., & McNeil, B. (1994). Outcomes research: Hope for the future or the latest rage? *Inquiry, 31*(1): 14–24.

Jabour, J. L., & Martin-Sheridou, D. M. (1996). Examination of parental anxiety and satisfaction while attending anesthesia induction. *AANA Journal, 64*(4), 383.

Joint Commission on Accreditation of Healthcare Organizations. (1996). *Accreditation manual for hospitals.* Oakbrook Terrace, IL: Author.

Kalafat, J., & Siman, M. L. (1991). A systematic health care quality service program. *Hospital & Health Services Administration, 36*(4), 571–587.

Kaplan, R. M., & Ries, A. L. (1996). Outcomes of rehabilitation for patients with chronic obstructive pulmonary disease. *Cost and Quality, 2*(3), 39–49.

Knaus, W. E., Draper, D., & Zimmerman, J. (1985). APACHE: A severity of disease classification system. *Critical Care Medicine, 13*(10), 818–829.

Kopelman, R. E. (1986). Objective feedback. In E. A. Locke (Ed.), *Generalizing from laboratory to field settings.* Lexington, MA: DC Heath.

Lang, N. M., & Marek, K. D. (1995, March). Quality assurance: The foundation of professional care. *The Journal of the New York State Nurses Association, 26*(1), 48–50.

Lanning, J. A., & O'Connor, P. (1990). The health care quality quagmire: Some signposts. *Hospital and Health Services Administration, 35*(1), 39–54.

Lenn, M. P. (1995). Quality assurance in international education. *AANA Journal, 63*(1), 17–20.

LaPointe, G. (1996). Management of an anesthesia department. In J. Nagelhout & K. Zaglaniczny (Eds.), *Nurse anesthesia* (pp. 28–43). Philadelphia: Saunders.

Lord, J. T., & Krause, G. P. (1994). Quality assessment and improvement in the 1990s. In S. D. Foster & L. M. Jordan (Eds.), *Professional aspects of nurse anesthesia practice,* (pp. 291–305). Philadelphia: Davis.

Manley, R., & Cuddeford, J. D. (1996). An assessment of the effectiveness of the revised FDA checklist. *AANA Journal, 64*(3), 277–282.

Martin-Sheridan, D. M. (1996). Anesthesia providers, patient outcomes, and costs: A critique. *AANA Journal, 64*(6), 528–534.

Martin-Sheridan, D. M., Bruton-Maree, N., & Horton, B. J. (1993, June). Outcome assessment in education programs. *Nurse Anesthesia, 4*(2), 73–79.

Masta-Gornic, V., & Youngberg, B. J. (1996). Developing tools to identify and manage risks of managed care. In B. Youngberg (Ed.), *Managing risks of managed care* (pp. 33–48). Rockville, MD: Aspen.

Siker, E. S. (1996, Fall). Historical perspective of APSF shows safety advocacy. *Anesthesia Patient Safety Foundation Newsletter, 11*(3), 25–36.

U.S. General Accounting Office. (1991, May). *Management practices: U.S. Companies improve performance through quality efforts.* Report to the Honorable Donald Ritter, House of representatives, GAO/NSLAD-91-190 *Management Practices* (pp. 2–3). Washington, DC: National Security and International Affairs Division.

Wagner, D. L. (1992). Hemodynamic monitoring. In D. Brown (Ed.), *Risk and outcome in anesthesia,* (pp. 283–312). Philadelphia: Lippincott.

Zambricki, C. (1994). Joint commission on anesthesia clinical indicators: An update. *AANA Journal, 62*(3), 212–213.

Index

A

AANA. *See* American Association of Nurse Anesthetists (AANA)

Abdomen, closure of, 751–752

ABO blood group, 610–611, 610*t*

Abortion, incomplete, 735–736

Abruptio placentae, 328

Acebutolol, 488*t*

Acetaminophen
  and hepatic disease, 259*t*
  in postoperative pain management, 718, 718*t*

Acetazolamide, 237*t*
  cerebrospinal fluid and, 211
  renal insufficiency and, 246*t*

Acetylcholine (ACh), 207, 353
  extracellular calcium and, 435
  presynaptic effect of, 438
  structure of, 444*f*
  synthesis of, 435, 437*f*
  tetanic impulses and, 435
  venomous snake bite and, 435

Acetylcholinesterase (AChE), 207, 353, 434, 435
  mechanism of action of, 462, 464*f*

Acetylcholinesterase inhibitors. *See* Anticholinesterase agents

Acid-base balance, 347, 348–349
  kidneys in, 240, 349

Acidosis. *See also* Diabetic ketoacidosis (DKA)
  fetal heart rate and, 323
  metabolic, 186
    aortic surgery and, 156
  respiratory, 113, 186

Acinus, 264
  hepatic, 250–251, 251*f*
  pulmonary, 162

Acquired immunodeficiency syndrome (AIDS), 193. *See also* Human immunodeficiency viruses (HIV)
  occupational exposure to, 71
  transfusion transmission of, 626–627

Activated clotting time, 617

Activated partial thromboplastin time, 616, 616*t*

Acupressure, for postoperative pain management, 723

Acupuncture, for postoperative pain management, 723

Acute intermittent porphyria, 797–799, 798*t*

Adenosine monophosphate. *See* Cyclic adenosine monophosphate (cAMP)

Adenosine triphosphate (ATP), 350, 435

Adenyl cyclase, 355, 355*f*
  in asthma treatment, 191
  bronchial smooth muscle and, 163

Adiabatic compression, and gas cylinders, 88

Adjustable pressure-limiting (APL) valve, 105, 105*f*–106*f*, 107–108, 107*f*

Adrenal glands, 265, 267

α-Adrenergic blockers, 482–484
  for autonomic hyperreflexia, 222, 483
  for pheochromocytoma, 483–484

β-Adrenergic agonists, for asthma, 191, 193

β-Adrenergic blockers, 482, 483
  as antiarrhythmics, 488*t*, 491
  calcium channel blockers and, 483, 487
  cirrhotic patient and, 262
  diabetic patient and, 483
  digoxin and, 483
  hydralazine with, 486
  for idiopathic hypertrophic subaortic stenosis, 150
  intraoperative hypertension and, 249
  nifedipine and, 487
  for portal hypertension, 262
  renal insufficiency and, 246*t*
  for ventricular hypertrophy, 154
  verapamil and, 487

Adrenergic neurons, 207

Adrenergic receptors, 355*f*
  of airways, 163

Adrenocorticotropin (ACTH), 263, 264*t*
  etomidate and, 392

Page numbers followed by *t* and *f* indicate tables and figures, respectively.

Page numbers followed by *t* and *f* indicate tables and figures, respectively.

Page numbers followed by *t* and *f* indicate tables and figures, respectively.

C

Page numbers followed by *t* and *f* indicate tables and figures, respectively.

Page numbers followed by *t* and *f* indicate tables and figures, respectively.

Page numbers followed by *t* and *f* indicate tables and figures, respectively.

I

N

O

Page numbers followed by *t* and *f* indicate tables and figures, respectively.

Page numbers followed by t and f indicate tables and figures, respectively.

Page numbers followed by *t* and *f* indicate tables and figures, respectively.

Page numbers followed by *t* and *f* indicate tables and figures, respectively.